Illustrated Textbook of
Paediatrics

Illustrated Textbook of Paediatrics

FIFTH EDITION

Edited by

Tom Lissauer MB BChir FRCPH
Honorary Consultant Paediatrician, Imperial College Healthcare Trust, London, UK
Centre for International Child Health, Imperial College London, UK

Will Carroll BM BCh MD MRCPCH
Consultant in Paediatric Respiratory Medicine,
University Hospital of the North Midlands, Stoke-on-Trent, UK

Foreword by

Professor Sir Alan Craft
Emeritus Professor of Child Health, Newcastle University,
Past President Royal College of Paediatrics and Child Health

ELSEVIER

ELSEVIER

© 2018, Elsevier Limited. All rights reserved.

First edition 1997
Second edition 2001
Third edition 2007
Fourth Edition 2012

The right of Tom Lissauer and Will Carroll to be identified as author of this work has been asserted by them in accordance with the Copyright, Designs, and Patents Act 1988.

No part of this publication may be reproduced or transmitted in any form or by any means, electronic or mechanical, including photocopying, recording, or any information storage and retrieval system, without permission in writing from the publisher. Details on how to seek permission, further information about the Publisher's permissions policies and our arrangements with organizations such as the Copyright Clearance Centre and the Copyright Licensing Agency, can be found at our website: www.elsevier.com/permissions.

This book and the individual contributions contained in it are protected under copyright by the Publisher (other than as may be noted herein).

Notices
Knowledge and best practice in this field are constantly changing. As new research and experience broaden our understanding, changes in research methods, professional practices, or medical treatment may become necessary.

Practitioners and researchers must always rely on their own experience and knowledge in evaluating and using any information, methods, compounds, or experiments described herein. In using such information or methods they should be mindful of their own safety and the safety of others, including parties for whom they have a professional responsibility.

With respect to any drug or pharmaceutical products identified, readers are advised to check the most current information provided (i) on procedures featured or (ii) by the manufacturer of each product to be administered, to verify the recommended dose or formula, the method and duration of administration, and contraindications. It is the responsibility of practitioners, relying on their own experience and knowledge of their patients, to make diagnoses, to determine dosages and the best treatment for each individual patient, and to take all appropriate safety precautions.

To the fullest extent of the law, neither the Publisher nor the authors, contributors, or editors, assume any liability for any injury and/or damage to persons or property as a matter of products liability, negligence or otherwise, or from any use or operation of any methods, products, instructions, or ideas contained in the material herein.

ISBN: 978-0-7234-3871-7
978-0-7234-3872-4

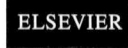
www.elsevierhealth.com

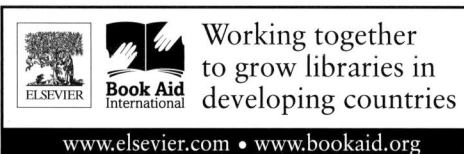

Printed in Europe
Last digit is the print number: 9 8 7 6 5 4 3 2 1

Content Strategist: *Pauline Graham*
Content Development Specialist: *Fiona Conn*
Project Manager: *Anne Collett*
Design: *Miles Hitchen*
Illustration Manager: *Amy Heyden*
Illustrator: *Graphic World US, Cactus*
Marketing Manager: *Deborah Watkins*

Contents

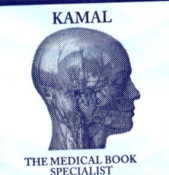

	Foreword	vi
	Preface	vii
	List of Contributors	viii
	Acknowledgements	xii
1.	The child in society	1
2.	History and examination	9
3.	Normal child development, hearing and vision	27
4.	Developmental problems and the child with special needs	44
5.	Care of the sick child and young person	64
6.	Paediatric emergencies	80
7.	Accidents and poisoning	97
8.	Child protection	109
9.	Genetics	121
10.	Perinatal medicine	142
11.	Neonatal medicine	166
12.	Growth and puberty	194
13.	Nutrition	211
14.	Gastroenterology	234
15.	Infection and immunity	256
16.	Allergy	288
17.	Respiratory disorders	294
18.	Cardiac disorders	320
19.	Kidney and urinary tract disorders	344
20.	Genital disorders	367
21.	Liver disorders	375
22.	Malignant disease	385
23.	Haematological disorders	401
24.	Child and adolescent mental health	424
25.	Dermatological disorders	442
26.	Diabetes and endocrinology	453
27.	Inborn errors of metabolism	472
28.	Musculoskeletal disorders	482
29.	Neurological disorders	500
30.	Adolescent medicine	525
31.	Global child health	535
	Appendix	544
	Index	560

Foreword

When the late Frank A. Oski wrote the foreword for the first edition of this book in 1997, he gave it generous praise and predicted that it would become a 'standard by which all other medical textbooks will be judged'. He was a great man and a wonderful writer, so his prediction was no doubt welcomed by the editors, Tom Lissauer and Graham Clayden, both well known for their contribution to undergraduate and postgraduate medical education and assessment.

I have a much easier task in writing the foreword for the fifth edition. The mere fact that there is a fifth edition is testimony in itself, but there is also the fact that this book has become the recommended paediatric textbook in countless medical schools throughout the world and has been translated into 12 languages. I have travelled the world over the last 20 years and wherever I have been in a paediatric department, the distinctive sunflower cover of *Lissauer's Illustrated Textbook of Paediatrics* has been there with me. Whether it is Hong Kong, Malaysia, Oman, or South Shields, it is there!

It is not surprising that it has won major awards for innovation and excellence at the British Medical Association and Royal Society of Medicine book awards. The book is well established and widely read for the simple reason that it is an excellent book. Medicine is now so complex and information so vast that students are no longer expected to know all there is to know about medicine. What they need are the core principles and guidance as to where to find out more. This book not only gives the core principles, but also provides a great deal more for the student who wishes to extend his or her knowledge. It is in a very accessible form and has a style and layout which facilitates learning. There are many diagrams, illustrations and case histories to bring the subject to life and to impart important messages. This new edition includes summaries to help revision and there is also a companion book for self-assessment.

This edition has a new editor, Will Carroll, who has succeeded Graham Clayden, and is also a paediatrician with great expertise in medical education and assessment. He has helped ensure that the book continues to provide the paediatric information medical students need. It has been thoroughly updated and has many new authors, each of whom is an expert in their field and who has been chosen because of their ability to impart the important principles in a non-specialist way. The book continues to focus on the key topics in the undergraduate curriculum, and in keeping with this aim there are new, expanded chapters on child protection and global child health.

There are now countless doctors throughout the world for whom this textbook has been their introduction to the fascinating and rewarding world of paediatrics.

For students, it is all they need to know and a bit more. For postgraduates, it provides the majority of information needed to get through postgraduate examinations. It stimulates and guides the reader into the world of clinical paediatrics, built on the sound foundation of the knowledge base provided by this book.

The editors are to be congratulated on the continuing success of this book.

I can only echo what Frank Oski said in his preface to the first edition: 'I wish I had written this book'!

Professor Sir Alan Craft
Emeritus Professor of Child Health,
Newcastle University
Past President Royal College of Paediatrics
and Child Health

Preface

Children are frequent users of healthcare. In the UK approximately one-third of all health consultations are about a child. Therefore, a good working knowledge of paediatrics is essential for all doctors and is a major part of the undergraduate medical syllabus. This textbook has been written to assist undergraduates in their studies. Our aim has been to provide the core information required by medical students for the 6 to 10 weeks assigned to paediatrics in the curriculum of most undergraduate medical schools. We are delighted that it has become so widely used, not only in the UK, but also in northern Europe, India, Pakistan, Australia, South Africa, and other countries. We are also pleased that nurses, therapists and other health professionals who care for children have found this book helpful. It will also be of assistance to doctors preparing for postgraduate examinations such as the Diploma of Child Health (DCH) and Membership of the Royal College of Paediatrics and Child Health (MRCPCH).

The huge amount of positive feedback we have received on the first four editions from medical students, postgraduate doctors and their teachers in the UK and abroad has spurred us on to produce this new edition. The book has been fully updated, many sections rewritten, new diagrams created and illustrations redone. There are new, separate chapters on child protection and global child health to accommodate their increasing importance in paediatric practice. There is also a companion book of self-assessment questions.

In order to make learning from this book easier, we have included many diagrams and flow charts and followed a lecture-note style with short sentences and lists of important features. Illustrations have been used to help in the recognition of important signs or clinical features. To make the topics more interesting and memorable, each chapter begins with some highlights, key learning points are identified, and case histories chosen to demonstrate particular aspects within their clinical context. Summary boxes of important facts have been included to help with revision.

We are fully aware of the short time allocated specifically to paediatrics in the curriculum of many medical schools, in spite of the rapid expansion in medical knowledge and therapies. We have therefore tried to focus on clinical presentation and principles rather than details of management, whilst providing sufficient background information to understand the care patients receive.

We would like to thank Graham Clayden, editor for the previous editions, for the fresh ideas and inspiration he brought to the book, and all our contributors, both to this and previous editions, without whom this book could not be produced. Thanks also to our families, in particular Ann Goldman, Rachel and David and Sam Lissauer, and Lisa Carroll, Daniel, Steven, Natasha, and Belinda for their ideas and assistance, and for their understanding of the time taken away from the family in the preparation of this book.

We welcome any comments about the book.

Tom Lissauer and Will Carroll

List of Contributors

Mark Anderson BM BS BSc BMedSci MRCPCH

Consultant Paediatrician, Great North Children's Hospital, Newcastle upon Tyne Hospitals NHS Foundation Trust, Newcastle upon Tyne, UK

7. Accidents and poisoning

Ian W. Booth BSc MSc MD FRCP FRCPCH DCH DRCOG

Professor Emeritus, Paediatrics and Child Health, University of Birmingham, UK

14. Gastroenterology

Robert Boyle BSc MB ChB MRCP PhD

Clinical Senior Lecturer in Paediatrics, Imperial College London and Honorary Consultant Paediatric Allergist, Imperial College Healthcare NHS Trust, London, UK

16. Allergy

Will Carroll BM BCh MD MRCPCH

Consultant in Paediatric Respiratory Medicine, University Hospital of the North Midlands, Stoke-on-Trent, UK

17. Respiratory disorders

Subarna Chakravorty PhD MRCPCH FRCPath

Consultant Paediatric Haematologist, King's College Hospital London, UK

23. Haematological disorders

Gabby Chow MBBChir MD MBA BSc BA DCH FRCPCH

Consultant Paediatric Neurologist, Nottingham Children's Hospital, Queens Medical Centre, Nottingham, UK

29. Neurological disorders

Angus J. Clarke BM BCh DM FRCP FRCPCH

Professor and Honorary Consultant in Clinical Genetics, Institute of Medical Genetics, University Hospital of Wales, Cardiff, UK

9. Genetics

Rory Conn MBBS BSc MRCPsych

Higher Trainee in Child and Adolescent Psychiatry, Tavistock and Portman NHS Foundation Trust, London, UK

24. Child and adolescent mental health

Max Davie MB BChir MA MRCPCH

Consultant Community Paediatrician, Evelina London Children's Hospital, Guy's and St Thomas' NHS Foundation Trust, London, UK

24. Child and adolescent mental health

Paul Dmitri BSc MBChB FRCPCH PhD

Honorary Professor of Child Health and Consultant in Paediatric Endocrinology, Sheffield Children's NHS Trust, Sheffield, UK

12. Growth and puberty
26. Diabetes and endocrinology

Rachel Dommett BMBS PhD BMedSci

Consultant Paediatrician in Haematology/Oncology, Bristol Royal Hospital for Children, Bristol, UK

22. Malignant disease

Saul Faust FRCPCH FHEA PhD

Professor of Paediatric Immunology & Infectious Diseases, University of Southampton and University Hospital Southampton NHS Foundation Trust, Southampton, UK

15. Infection and immunity

Helen E Foster MB BS MD FRCPCH FRCP DCH CertClinEd

Professor of Paediatric Rheumatology, Newcastle University and
Honorary Consultant in Paediatric Rheumatology, Great North Children's Hospital,
Newcastle Hospitals NHS Foundation Trust, Newcastle upon Tyne, UK

28. Musculoskeletal disorders

Andrea Goddard MB BS MSc FRCPCH

Consultant Paediatrician, Imperial College Healthcare NHS Trust and Honorary Senior Lecturer in Paediatrics, Imperial College London, UK

8. Child protection

Anu Goenka MB ChB BSc DFSRH DTM&H MRCGP MRCPCH

Clinical Research Fellow, Manchester Collaborative Centre for Inflammation Research, University of Manchester, Manchester, UK and
Honorary Specialist Registrar in Paediatric Immunology, Royal Manchester Children's Hospital, Manchester, UK

31. Global child health

Jane Hartley MB ChB MRCPCH MMedSc PhD

Consultant Paediatric Hepatologist, Birmingham Children's Hospital, Birmingham, UK

21. Liver disorders

David P. Inwald MB BChir PhD FRCPCH

Consultant Paediatrician and Honorary Senior Lecturer in Paediatric Intensive Care, Imperial College Healthcare NHS Trust, London, UK

6. Paediatric emergencies

Elisabeth Jameson MBBCh BSc MSc MRCPCH

Consultant in Paediatric Inborn Errors of Metabolism, Manchester Centre for Genomic Medicine, Central Manchester University Hospitals NHS Foundation Trust, St Marys Hospital, Manchester, UK

27. Inborn errors of metabolism

Sharmila Jandial MBChB MRCPCH MD

Consultant Paediatric Rheumatologist, Great North Children's Hospital, Newcastle upon Tyne, UK and
Honorary Clinical Senior Lecturer, Newcastle University, UK

28. Musculoskeletal disorders

Huw Jenkins MB BChir MA MD FRCP FRCPCH DL

Consultant Paediatric Gastroenterologist, Children's Hospital for Wales, Cardiff, UK

14. Gastroenterology

Deirdre Kelly MD FRCP FRCPI FRCPCH

Professor of Paediatric Hepatology, Birmingham Children's Hospital, Birmingham, UK

21. Liver disorders

Larissa Kerecuk MBBS BSc FRCPCH

Consultant Paediatric Nephrologist, Birmingham Children's Hospital, Birmingham, UK

19. Kidney and urinary tract disorders

Anthony Lander PhD FRCS (Paed) DCH

Consultant Paediatric Surgeon, Birmingham Children's Hospital, Birmingham, UK

14. Gastroenterology

Tom Lissauer MB BChir FRCPCH

Honorary Consultant Paediatrician, Imperial College Healthcare Trust, London, UK and
Centre for International Child Health, Imperial College London, UK

2. History and examination
5. Care of the sick child and young person
10. Perinatal medicine
11. Neonatal medicine
20. Genital disorders

Andrew Long MA MB FRCP FRCPCH FAcadMEd DCH

Vice President (Education), Royal College of Paediatrics and Child Health; Consultant Paediatrician, Great Ormond Street Hospital,
London, UK

5. Care of the sick child and young person

Chloe Macaulay BA MBBS MRCPCH MSc PGCertMedEd

Consultant Paediatrician, Evelina London Children's Hospital, London UK

2. History and examination

Janet McDonagh MB BS MD

Senior Lecturer in Paediatric and Adolescent Rheumatology, Centre for Musculoskeletal Research, University of Manchester, UK

30. Adolescent medicine

Dan Magnus BM BS BMedSci MSc MRCPCH

Paediatric Emergency Consultant, Bristol Royal Hospital for Children, Bristol, UK

31. Global child health

Daniel Morgenstern MB BChir PhD FRCPCH

Staff Physician – Solid Tumor Program, Assistant Professor, Department of Paediatrics, University of Toronto, Division of Haematology/Oncology, The Hospital for Sick Children, Toronto, Canada

22. Malignant disease

Rob Primhak MD FRCPCH

Consultant Paediatric Respiratory Physician (ret), Sheffield Children's Hospital, Sheffield, UK

17. Respiratory disorders

John Puntis BM DM FRCP FRCPCH

Consultant in Paediatric Gastroenterology and Nutrition, Leeds Teaching Hospitals NHS Trust, Leeds, UK

13. Nutrition

Irene A.G. Roberts MD FRCPath

Professor of Paediatric Haematology, Oxford University Department of Paediatrics, John Radcliffe Hospital, Oxford, UK

23. Haematological disorders

Damian Roland BMedSci MB BS MRCPCH PhD

Consultant and Honorary Senior Lecturer in Paediatric Emergency Medicine, University Hospitals of Leicester NHS Trust, Leicester, UK

5. Care of the sick child and young person

Don Sharkey BMedSci BM BS PhD FRCPCH

Associate Professor of Neonatal Medicine, University of Nottingham, Nottingham, UK

10. Perinatal medicine
11. Neonatal medicine

Diane P.L. Smyth MD FRCP FRCPCH

Honorary Consultant Paediatric Neurologist / Neurodisability, Imperial College Healthcare NHS Trust, London, UK

3. Normal child development, hearing and vision
4. Developmental problems and the child with special needs

Marc Tebruegge DTM&H MRCPCH MSc FHEA MD PhD

NIHR Clinical Lecturer in Paediatric Infectious Diseases & Immunology, Academic Unit of Clinical & Experimental Sciences, The University of Southampton, Southampton, UK

15. Infection and immunity

Tracy Tinklin BM FRCPCH

Consultant Paediatrician, Derbyshire Childrens Hospital, Derby, UK

12. Growth and puberty
26. Diabetes and endocrinology

Robert M. Tulloh BM BCh MA DM FRCP FRCPCH

Professor, Congenital Cardiology, University of Bristol, Bristol, UK and
Consultant Paediatric Cardiologist, Bristol Royal Hospital for Children, Bristol, UK

18. Cardiac disorders

Ian Tully MBBCh MRCPCH

Academic Clinical Fellow in Genomic Medicine, Cardiff University & University Hospital of Wales, Cardiff, UK

9. Genetics

Julian Verbov MD FRCP FRCPCH CBiol FSB FLS

Honorary Professor of Dermatology, University of Liverpool;
Consultant Paediatric Dermatologist, Royal Liverpool Children's Hospital, Liverpool, UK

25. Dermatological disorders

Premila Webster MBBS DA MSc MFPHM FFPH DLATHE DPhil

Director of Public Health Education & Training, Nuffield Department of Population Health, University of Oxford, Oxford, UK

1. The child in society

William P Whitehouse MB BS BSc FRCP FRCPCH

Clinical Associate Professor and Honorary Consultant Paediatric Neurologist, University of Nottingham and Nottingham Children's Hospital, Nottingham University Hospital's NHS Trust, Nottingham, UK

29. Neurological disorders

Lisa Whyte MBChB MSc

Consultant Paediatric Gastroenterologist, Birmingham Children's Hospital, Birmingham, UK

14. Gastroenterology

Bhanu Williams MB BS BMedSci MRCPCH DTMH BA MAcadMed

Consultant in Paediatric Infectious Diseases, London North West Healthcare NHS Trust, Harrow, UK

31. Global child health

Clare Wilson BA MBBChir MRCPCH

Academic Clinical Fellow, Institute of Child Health, University College London, UK

6. Paediatric emergencies

Neil Wimalasundera MBBS MRCPCH MSc

Consultant in Paediatric Neurodisability, The Wolfson Neurodisability Service, Great Ormond Street Hospital, London, UK

3. Normal child development, hearing and vision
4. Developmental problems and the child with special needs

Acknowledgements

The editors would like to acknowledge and offer grateful thanks for the input of all previous editions' contributors, without whom this new edition would not have been possible as we have widely reused their contributions.

The child in society Dr Rashmin Tamhne, Prof Mitch Blair, Dr Peter Sidebotham

History and examination Prof Dennis Gill, Dr Graham Clayden, Prof Tauny Southwood, Dr Siobhan Jaques, Dr Sanjay Patel, Dr Kathleen Sim

Normal child development, hearing, and vision Dr Angus Nicoll

Developmental problems and the child with special needs Dr Richard W Newton

Care of the sick child and young person Prof Raanan Gillon, Dr Graham Clayden, Prof Ruth Gilbert, Dr Maude Meates, Dr Vic Larcher

Paediatric emergencies Dr Nigel Curtis, Prof Nigel Klein, Dr Simon Nadel, Dr Rob Tasker, Dr Shruti Agrawal

Accidents and poisoning Prof Jo Sibert, Dr Barbara Phillips, Dr Ian Maconochie, Dr Rebecca C Salter

Child protection Prof Jo Sibert, Dr Barbara Phillips

Genetics Dr Elizabeth Thompson, Dr Helen Kingston

Perinatal medicine Dr Karen Simmer, Prof Michael Weindling, Prof Andrew Whitelaw, Prof Andrew R Wilkinson

Neonatal medicine Dr Karen Simmer, Prof Michael Weindling, Prof Andrew Whitelaw, Prof Andrew R Wilkinson

Growth and puberty Dr Tony Hulse, Dr Jerry K H Wales

Nutrition Prof Ian Booth, Dr Jonathan Bishop, Dr Stephen Hodges

Gastroenterology Dr Jonathan Bishop, Dr Stephen Hodges

Infection and immunity Prof Nigel Klein, Dr Nigel Curtis, Dr Hermione Lyall, Dr Andrew Prendergast, Dr Gareth Tudor-Williams

Allergy Dr Tom Blyth, Prof Gideon Lack

Respiratory disorders Dr Jon Couriel, Dr Iolo Doull, Dr Malcolm Brodlie, Dr Michael C McKean, Mr Gerard P S Siou

Cardiac disorders Prof Andrew Redington

Kidney and urinary tract disorders Prof George Haycock, Dr Lesley Rees

Genital disorders Mr Nicholas Madden, Mr Mark Stringer, Prof David Thomas, Mrs Aruna Abhyankar

Liver disorders Dr Ulrich Baumann, Dr Jonathan Bishop, Dr Stephen Hodges

Malignant disease Prof Michael Stevens, Dr Helen Jenkinson

Haematological disorders Dr Lynn Ball, Prof Paula Bolton-Maggs, Dr Michelle Cummins

Child and adolescent mental health Prof Peter Hill, Prof Elena Garralda, Dr Sharon E Taylor, Dr Cornelius Ani

Dermatological disorders Dr Gill Du Mont

Diabetes and endocrinology Dr Tony Hulse, Dr Jerry K H Wales

Metabolic disorders Dr Ed Wraith

Musculoskeletal disorders Dr John Sills, Prof Tauny Southwood

Neurological disorders Dr Richard W Newton, Dr Alison Giles

Adolescent medicine Dr Terry Segal, Prof Russell Viner

Global child health Prof Stephen J Allen, Dr Ike Lagunju, Raúl Pardíñaz-Solís

The child in society

The child's world	1	Major public child health initiatives	7
Well-being	5	Conclusion	8
Important public health issues for children and young people	5		

Regarding the society in which we live:
- in combination with our genes, it determines who we are
- it is responsible for the country's health outcomes – which is why the infant mortality in the UK is 3.8 per 1000 live births, but in Sweden is 2.7 whilst in Bangladesh it is 47 and in Malawi 77 per 1000 live births
- important public health issues for children and young people in the UK are reduction in mortality, health inequalities, variations in health outcomes, obesity, emotional and behaviour problems, teenage pregnancy, smoking and drug abuse, and improving child protection services
- many of the causes and determinants of childhood morbidity and mortality are preventable. Doctors can play a role by raising society's awareness of how this can be achieved and improving the health systems and healthcare services they provide.

Most medical encounters with children involve an individual child presenting to a doctor with a symptom, such as difficulty breathing or diarrhoea. After taking a history, examining the child and performing any necessary investigations, the doctor arrives at a diagnosis or differential diagnosis and makes a management plan. This disease-oriented approach, which is the focus of most of this book, plays an important part in ensuring the immediate and long-term well-being of the child. Of course, the doctor also needs to understand the nature of the child's illness within the wider context of their world, which is the primary focus of this chapter.

 In order to be a truly effective clinician, the doctor must be able to place the child's clinical problems within the context of the family and of the society in which they live.

Important goals for a society are that its children and young people are healthy, safe, enjoy life, make a positive contribution and achieve economic well-being (*Every Child Matters*, 2003 at: http://www.dcsf.gov.uk/everychildmatters). This chapter will focus on environmental factors that affect children in the UK and other high-income countries. Those in low and middle-income countries are considered in Chapter 31, Global Child Health.

The child's world

Children's health is profoundly influenced by their social, cultural and physical environment. This can be considered in terms of the child, the family and immediate social environment, the local social fabric and the national and international environment (Fig. 1.1). Our ability to intervene as clinicians needs to be seen within this context of complex interrelating influences on health.

The child

The child's world will be affected by gender, genes, physical health, temperament and development. The impact of the social environment varies markedly with age:
- Infant or toddler: life is mainly determined by the home environment
- Young child: in addition to home environment by school and friends
- Young person: physical and emotional changes of adolescence, but also aware of and influenced by events nationally and internationally, e.g. in music, sport, fashion or politics.

Immediate social environment

Family structure

Although the 'two biological parent family' remains the norm, there are many variations in family structure. In

The child in society

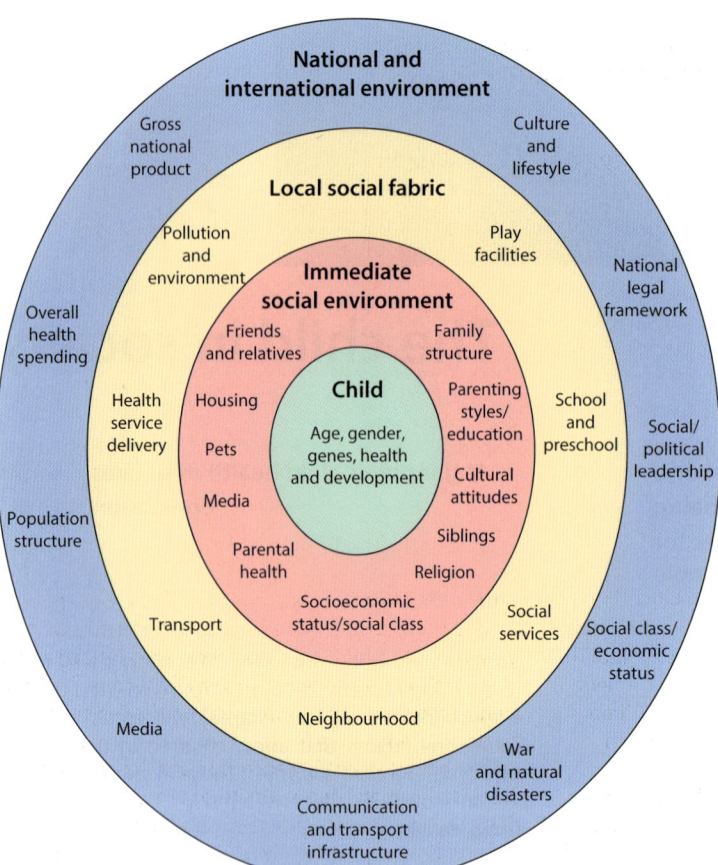

Figure 1.1 A child's world consists of overlapping, interconnected and expanding socioenvironmental layers, which influence children's health and development. (After Bronfenbrenner U. 1979. Contexts of child rearing – problems and prospects. *American Psychologist* 34:844–850.)

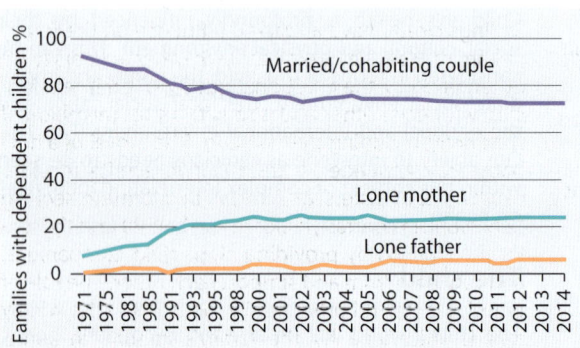

Figure 1.2 Changing structure of the family 1971–2014. (ONS, General Lifestyle Survey 2016).

the UK, the family structure has changed markedly over the last 30 years (Fig. 1.2).

Single-parent households – One in four children now live in a single-parent household (91% living with their mother). Disadvantages of single parenthood include a higher level of unemployment, poor housing and financial hardship (Table 1.1). These social adversities may affect parenting resources, e.g. vigilance about safety, adequacy of nutrition, take-up of preventive services such as immunization and regular screening, and ability to cope with an acutely sick child at home.

Reconstituted families – The increase in the number of parents who change partners and the

accompanying rise in reconstituted families (1 in 10 children live in a step-family) mean that children are having to cope with a range of new and complex parental and sibling relationships. This may result in emotional, behavioural and social difficulties.

Looked after children – The term 'looked after children' is generally used to mean those children who are looked after by the state. Approximately 3% of children under 16 years old in the UK live away from their family home. Children enter care for a range of reasons including physical, sexual or emotional abuse, neglect or family breakdown. There are currently over 92 000 children in care in the UK. They have significantly increased levels of health

Table 1.1 Comparison between parents who are single or couples (General Household Survey, Office for National Statistics, England 2008.)

	Lone-parent family	Couple family
Median weekly family income (£)	280	573
In lowest income quintile (%)	48	7
Living in social housing (%)	44	12
Parent with no educational qualification (%)	15	3
Child with school behaviour problems (%)	14	8

needs than children and young people from comparable socio-economic backgrounds who have not been "looked after". Past experiences, including a poor start in life, removal from family, placement location and transitions mean that these children are often at risk of having poor access to health services, both universal and specialist.

Asylum seekers – These are people who have come to the UK to apply for protection as refugees. They are often placed in temporary housing and moved repeatedly into areas unfamiliar to them. In addition to the uncertainty as to whether or not they will be allowed to stay in the country, they face additional problems as a result of communication difficulties, poverty, fragmentation of families and racism. Many have lost family members and are uncertain about the safety of friends and family. All of these can have a serious impact on both physical and mental health. Children have particular difficulties as the frequent moves can disrupt continuity of care. It also disrupts childhood friendships, education, and family support networks thereby having an inevitable impact on a child's well-being.

Parental employment – With many parents in employment, many young children are with child-minders or at preschool nurseries. Parents are receiving conflicting opinions on the long-term consequences of caring for their young children at home in contrast to nursery care. Also, increasing attention is being paid to the quality of day-care facilities in terms of supervision of the children and improving the opportunities they provide for social interaction and learning.

Parenting styles

Children rely on their parents to provide love and nurture, stimulation and security, as well as catering for their physical needs of food, clothing and shelter. Parenting that is warm and receptive to the child, while imposing reasonable and consistent boundaries, will promote the development of an autonomous and self-reliant adult. This constitutes 'good enough' parenting as described by the paediatrician and psychotherapist, Donald Winnicott, and can reassure parents that perfection is not necessary. However, some parents are excessively authoritarian or extremely permissive. Children's emotional development may also be damaged by parents who neglect or abuse their children. The child's temperament is also important, especially when there is a mismatch with parenting style, for example, a child with a very energetic temperament may be misperceived in a quiet family as having attention deficit hyperactivity disorder (ADHD).

Siblings and extended family

Siblings clearly have a marked influence on the family dynamics. How siblings affect each other appears to be determined by the emotional quality of their relationship with each other and also with other members of the family, including their parents. The arrival of a new baby may engender a feeling of insecurity in older brothers and sisters and result in attention-seeking behaviour. In contrast, children can benefit greatly from having siblings by providing close child companions, and can learn from and support each other. The role of grandparents and other family members varies widely and is influenced by the family's culture. In some, they are the main caregivers; in others, they provide valued practical and emotional support. However, in many families they now play only a peripheral role, exacerbated by geographical separation.

Cultural attitudes to child-rearing

The way in which children are brought up evolves within a community over generations, and is influenced by culture and religion, affecting both day-to-day issues to fundamental lifestyle choices. For example, in some societies children are given considerable self-autonomy, from deciding what food they want to eat to their education and even to participating in major decisions about their medical care. By contrast, in other societies, children are largely excluded from decision-making. Another example of marked differences between societies is the use of physical punishment to discipline children; in the UK it is not illegal for a parent to smack their child to administer "reasonable punishment" as long as it does not leave a mark or harm the child and is not administered with an instrument, whereas corporal punishment for children is illegal in 46 countries. The expected roles of males and females both as children and as adults differ widely between countries.

Peers

Peers exert a major influence on children. Peer relationships and activities provide a 'sense of group belonging' and have potentially long-term benefits for the child. Conversely, they may exert negative pressure through inappropriate role modelling. Relationships can also go wrong, e.g. persistent bullying, which may result in or contribute to psychosomatic symptoms, misery and even, in extreme cases, suicide.

Socioeconomic status

Poverty is the single greatest threat to the well-being of children, as it can affect every area of a child's development – social, educational and personal. Low socioeconomic status is often associated with multiple disadvantages, e.g. food of inadequate quantity or poor nutritional value, substandard housing or homelessness, lack of 'good enough' parenting, poor parental education and health, and poor access to healthcare and educational facilities. Families are usually considered to live in poverty when they "lack resources to obtain the type of diet, participate in the activities, and have the living conditions and amenities which are customary, or at least widely encouraged and approved, in the societies in which they belong' (P Townsend, Poverty in the United Kingdom, Allen Lane, 1979). The most widely used poverty measure in the UK is 'household income below 60 percent of median income' (Fig. 1.3). Data for 2013–2014 estimates that there are 3.5 million children living in poverty in the UK. The groups that are more at risk from poverty include lone parents, large families, families affected by disability, and black and minority ethnic groups.

In the UK, prevalence of the following are increased by poverty:
- low birthweight infants
- injuries
- hospital admissions
- asthma
- behavioural problems
- special educational needs
- child abuse.

Even a few years of poverty can have negative consequences for a child's development and is especially harmful from the ages of birth to five. Research indicates that being poor at both 9 months and 3 years is associated with increased likelihood of poor behavioural, learning and health outcomes at age 5 years (Magnuson, 2013). By the age of four, a development gap of more than a year and a half can be seen between the most disadvantaged and the most advantaged children (Sutton Trust, 2012). Babies whose development falls behind the norm during the first year of life are much more likely to fall even further behind in subsequent years rather than to catch up with those who have had a better start.

Local social fabric

Neighbourhood

Cohesive communities and amicable neighbourhoods are positive influences on children. Racial tension and other social adversities, such as gang violence and drugs, will adversely affect the emotional and social development of children, as well as their physical health. Parental concern about safety may create tensions in balancing their children's freedom with overprotection and restriction of their lifestyles. The physical environment itself, through pollution, safe areas for play and quality of housing and public facilities, will affect children's health.

Health service delivery

The variation in the quality of healthcare is an important component in preventing morbidity and mortality in children. Health services for children are increasingly provided within primary care. Some aspects of specialist paediatric care are also increasingly provided within the child's home, local community or local hospital through shared care arrangements and specialist community nursing and medical teams working within clinical networks. However, access to and the range of these services varies widely.

Schools

Schools provide a powerful influence on children's emotional and intellectual development and their subsequent lives. Differences in the quality of schools in different areas can accentuate inequalities already present in society. Schools provide enormous opportunities for influencing healthy behaviour through personal and social education and through the influence of peers and positive role models. They also provide opportunities for monitoring and promoting the health and well-being of vulnerable children.

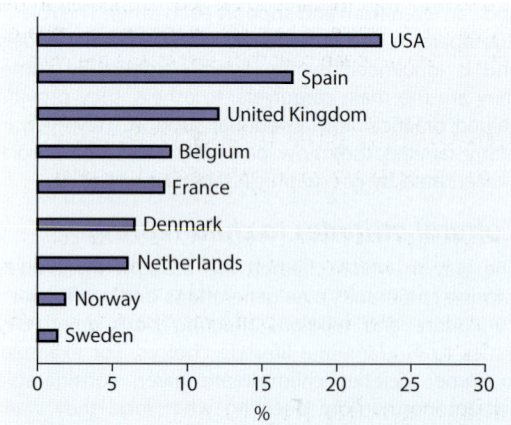

Figure 1.3 Percentage of children living in poverty. In this international comparison, the UNICEF definition of relative poverty is households with income below 50% of national median (Data from UNICEF report card, Innocenti Research Centre 2012).

Travel

The increasing ease of travel can broaden children's horizons and opportunities. Especially in rural areas, the ease and availability of transport allow greater access to medical care and other services. However, the increasing use of motor vehicles contributes to the large number of injuries sustained by children from road traffic accidents, mainly as pedestrians. It also decreases physical activity, as shown by the high proportion of children taken to school by car. Whereas 80% of children in the UK went to school by foot or bicycle in 1971, only 42% of children aged 5–16 years walked to school in 2013. This contributes to the rise in childhood obesity.

National and international environment

Economic wealth

In general, there is an inverse relationship between a country's gross national product and income distribution and the quality of its children's health. The lower the gross national income:

- the greater the proportion of the population who are children
- the higher the childhood mortality.

However, as described above, even in countries with a high gross national product, many children live in poverty.

In all countries, including those with high gross national product, difficult choices need to be made about the allocation of resources. Difficult decisions also have to be faced in deciding the affordability of very expensive procedures, such as heart or liver transplantation, neonatal intensive care for extremely premature infants and certain drugs, such as genetically engineered enzyme replacement therapy for Gaucher disease or cytokine modulators ('biologics') and other immunotherapies. The public are becoming more engaged in these debates.

Media and technology

The media has a powerful influence on children. It can be positive and educational. However, the impact of television and computers and mobile technology can be negative owing to reduced opportunities for social interaction and active learning, lack of physical exercise and exposure to violence, sex, and cultural stereotypes. The extent to which the aggressive tendencies of children may be exacerbated or encouraged by media exposure to violence is unclear.

The internet is enabling parents and children to become better informed about and gain support for their children's medical problems. This is especially beneficial for the many rare conditions encountered in paediatrics. A disadvantage is that it may result in the dissemination of information which is incorrect or biased, and may result in requests for inappropriate or untested investigations or treatment.

War and natural disasters

Children are especially vulnerable when there is war, civil unrest or natural disasters. Not only are they at greater risk from infectious diseases and malnutrition but also they may lose their caregivers and other members of their families and are likely to have been exposed to highly traumatic events. Their lives will have been uprooted, socially and culturally, especially if they are forced to flee from their homes and become refugees. Recently, the huge increase in the number of refugee children following war and ethnic violence in parts of the Middle East, South-East Asia and Africa, with families displaced internally or in other countries, often in refugee camps, is resulting in deterioration in even their basic health outcomes.

Well-being

The concept of well-being encompasses a number of different elements and includes emotional, psychological and social well-being. The well-being of children is key to the development of healthy behaviours and educational attainment and impacts on their childhood and life chances and on their families and communities. The Children's Society survey in 2014 found that 9% of children in the UK (aged 8–15 years) report low life satisfaction. Having low satisfaction increases with age, rising from just 4% of 8 year olds to 14% of 15 year olds. There is a gender gap, with girls tending to report lower well-being than boys. Having a low level of well-being appears to be related to sociodemographic factors such as household income and family structure. Children who have recently been bullied also report a lower level of well-being. One of the most important factors in promoting children's well-being appears to be the quality of family relationships and parental behaviours and in particular the availability of emotional support. Interventions which can result in improvement in childhood well-being include parenting support programmes, emotional health and well-being programmes in schools, access to green spaces and opportunities to be active. Children in the UK do much worse in terms of well-being compared with other European countries and across the world.

Important public health issues for children and young people

Important public health issues for the 11 million children and young people in the UK include reduction in mortality, health inequalities, child protection, obesity, emotional and behaviour problems, disability, smoking and drug abuse.

Child mortality (Fig. 1.4)

In 1900–1902, 146 out of every 1000 children born in England and Wales would die before their first birthday, by 1990–1992 the rate had fallen to 7 deaths per 1000 live births and to 3.8 per 1000 live births in 2013. This dramatic reduction in childhood mortality over the last

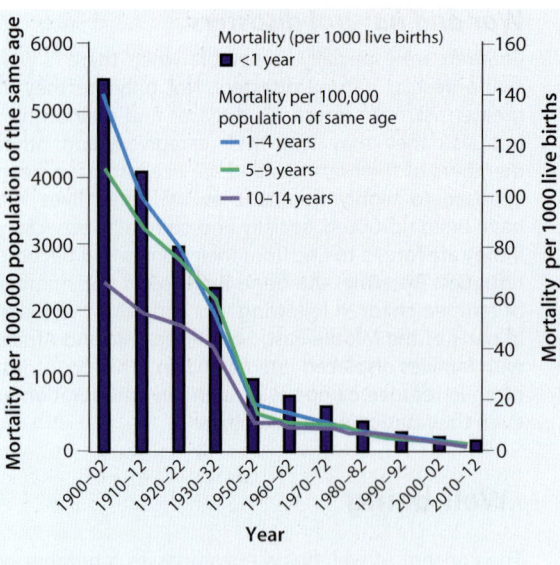

Figure 1.4 Marked reduction in childhood deaths between 1900 and 2012 in the UK. This is shown as deaths by age group per 100 000 population of the same age and infant mortality per 1000 live births.

century was primarily due to improvements in living conditions such as better sanitation and housing and access to food and clean water. There has also been a marked reduction in childhood deaths from infectious disease, augmented by the increased range and uptake of immunizations.

Currently over half of deaths in childhood in the UK occur during the first year of life. Prematurity and/or low birthweight contribute considerably to infant mortality. The wide variation in the proportion of babies born preterm between countries, almost 8% in the UK, 12% in the USA, but only 5.5% in Finland and 5.9% in Sweden is of uncertain origin, but is likely to be predominantly environmental. This wide variation in prematurity rate has a marked effect on infant mortality rate and outcomes. Infant mortality rates for very low birthweight babies (<1500 g) and low birthweight babies (<2500 g) are 164 and 32.4 deaths per 1000 live births respectively. This is much higher than the 1.3 deaths per 1000 live births among babies of normal birthweight (>2500 g).

Environmental factors that influence infant mortality include:

- maternal age – infant mortality rates are lowest for babies of mothers aged 25–29 years (3.4 per 1000 live births) and highest for mothers aged under 20 years (6.1 per 1000 live births)
- maternal country of birth – for babies of mothers born outside the UK, the infant mortality rate is 4.2 compared with 3.8 per 1000 live births for mothers born in the UK
- social class – in 2013, infant mortality rates were highest for those in routine and manual occupations, the long term unemployed and those who have never worked and lowest for those in higher managerial and professional occupations.

Amongst 1–9 year olds the main causes of death are injuries and poisoning, cancer, and congenital anomalies. Sociodemographic factors are important in mortality from injuries and poisoning and from congenital anomalies, though they are usually poorly understood. A good example of the role of sociodemographic factors in congenital anomalies is neural tube defects. Their prevalence varies markedly between different countries; maternal nutrition, particularly with folic acid, as well as genetic factors play a role. In addition, the birth prevalence of neural tube defects is affected by antenatal screening practices and attitudes towards termination of pregnancy if an affected fetus is identified.

Between the ages of 10 to 14 the most common causes of death in the UK are injuries and poisoning and cancer. Their mortality rate has declined over the last 50 years (see Fig. 30.2).

Comparison with other European countries

Although childhood mortality rates have declined over the past three decades, the UK continues to have a much higher child mortality rate compared with some other European countries. In 2013, the under 5 mortality rate for the UK was 4.9 deaths per 1000 live births, compared with 3.7 deaths per 1000 live births in France and 2.7 deaths per 1000 live births in Sweden. The reasons for this are complex, but it is in part due to the UK having higher rates of low birthweight and preterm rates when compared with some other European countries, both of which have a strong influence on infant mortality rates. In addition, the UK has one of the highest rates of child poverty compared with other comparable wealthy countries. Childhood mortality rates are higher in countries with a high proportion of deprived households. The Nordic countries have low levels of deprivation and also show some of the lowest child mortality rates. There is also evidence that the UK performs less well in the recognition and management of serious illness in primary and secondary care and in the community. In addition, outcome measures for chronic illnesses such as asthma, epilepsy and diabetes are poorer. More effective prevention and better medical care of these children could reduce mortality and morbidity.

Inequalities in child heath

What causes inequalities?

Inequalities in health refer to the marked differences in health outcomes within a given population. As there are so many factors that influence the health of a child the explanations about the causes of inequalities in health are complex. The World Health Organization uses the terms "equity" and "inequity to refer to "differences in health which are not only unnecessary and avoidable but, in addition, are considered unfair and unjust". A quarter of all deaths under the age of 1 year would potentially be avoided if all births had the same level of risk as those of women with the lowest level of deprivation.

Child protection and variation in outcomes

Child protection is the process of protecting individual children identified as either suffering, or likely to suffer, significant harm as a result of abuse or neglect. It involves measures and structures designed to prevent and respond to abuse and neglect. A substantial minority of children in high-income countries are maltreated by their caregivers. In 2013–2014 over 48 000 children in England were identified as needing protection from abuse, about 0.4% of the total child population (Child protection is considered in detail in Chapter 8, Child Protection.).

Obesity

The proportion of children in the UK who are overweight (BMI > 91st centile) is about 25% between 2–5 yrs, 30% between 6–10 years and 37% between 11–15 years. Doctors can help promote healthy eating through supporting breastfeeding in infancy, advising parents and young people on healthy lifestyles, monitoring growth parameters and the consequences of obesity, and through advocacy and support for local and national healthy lifestyle programmes. Further details are described in Chapter 13, Nutrition.

Emotional and behavioural difficulties

11% of boys and 8% of girls in the UK suffer from a defined emotional or behavioural problem. In addition, these problems are often unrecognized but have significant ongoing impact on children's overall well-being. Doctors can contribute to ameliorating them by being alert to and responding to the signs of mental health problems in childhood, and by promoting an equitable distribution of resources to child and adolescent mental health services.

Disability

Up to 5.4% have some form of disability and 7% have a long-standing illness that limits their activity. Doctors need to work closely with children and young people, families, local communities and other services to ensure that the needs of individual children are appropriately catered for. This may include outlining a child's health needs for a statement of special educational need, formulating an individual healthcare plan, and advocating for the resources to implement this. Doctors can also provide education and social services with data on the numbers and levels of need within their own population.

Smoking, alcohol, and drugs

A 2013 survey found that 8% of 15-year-olds smoke regularly; 6% had taken drugs in the past month, and 9% had drunk alcohol in the past week. Doctors have been instrumental in campaigning for legislation to protect young people from targeted advertising and to raise awareness of the dangers of smoking, alcohol, and drugs. There is evidence that prevalence of all three behaviours are decreasing.

Major public child health initiatives

A range of public health initiatives were introduced over the last decade to improve the health and well-being of children. Some are described below.

National Service Framework

This was a 10 year programme between 2004 and 2014 aimed at everyone who had contact with pregnant women, children or young people and was developed to ensure fair, high quality and integrated services, designed and delivered around the needs of children and their families, from pregnancy through to adulthood.

The Children's National Service Framework also led to the introduction of a Child Health Promotion Programme which was designed to promote the health and well-being of children from prebirth to adulthood.

Every Child Matters

In order to implement the Children's National Service Framework, Every Child Matters described the commitment to support all children to "Be Healthy, Stay Safe, Enjoy and Achieve, Make a positive contribution and Achieve economic well-being". Every Child Matters was underpinned by The Children Act 2004 which provided the legal basis for how agencies should deal with issues relating to children. The implementation of Every Child Matters meant a multi-agency approach ensuring that organizations shared information in order to help promote the health and well-being of children and young people. It included the role of a Children's Commissioner which gave children a voice in parliament.

The Healthy Child Programme and Family Nurse Partnership

The Healthy Child Programme was developed as part of an integrated approach to support children and their families. It is an early intervention and prevention public health programme which offers every family screening checks, immunizations, developmental reviews and guidance to support parenting and healthy choices. It is described in Chapter 3, Normal child development, hearing and vision.

Sure Start

Sure Start is a child health initiative which aims to "give children the best possible start in life". The emphasis is on improving childcare, early education, health and family support. The first Sure Start children's centres were focused on areas with higher levels of deprivation but with the intention that eventually there would be a children's centre in every community. Initiatives include early learning and childcare, support and advice on parenting, child and family health services such as antenatal and postnatal support, and breastfeeding support.

Conclusion

Children are vulnerable members of society. They rely on their parents and society to care for them and provide an environment where they can grow both physically and emotionally to reach their full potential. Their health is dependent on a nurturing environment and good health services.

Doctors can help children by the wider use of their knowledge about child health. This may be through advocacy about children's issues and by providing information to inform public debate.

Acknowledgements

We would like to acknowledge contributors to this chapter in previous editions, whose work we have drawn on: Dr Rashmin Tamhne (1st and 2nd Edition, Dr Tom Lissauer (2nd and 3rd Edition), Prof Mitch Blair (3rd Edition) and Dr Peter Sidebotham (4th Edition).

Further reading

Blair M, Stewart-Brown S, Waterston T, et al: *Child Public Health*, ed 2, Oxford, 2010, Oxford University Press.

Health and Social Care Information Centre: Smoking, drinking and drug use among young people in England in 2013. 2014

Magnuson K: Reducing the effects of poverty through early childhood interventions. Institute for Research on Poverty, 2013.

Royal College of Paediatrics and Child Health, National Children's Bureau, British Association for Child and Adolescent Public Health: Why Children Die: deaths in infants, children and young people in the UK. 2014.

The Sutton Trust: *Poorer Toddlers need Well Educated Nursery teachers*, London, 2012, Sutton Trust.

Wang H, Liddell CA, Coates MM, Mooney MD, Levitz CE, et al: Global, regional and national levels of neonatal, infant and under 5 mortality during 1990–2013: a systematic analysis for the global burden of disease study 2013. *Lancet* 384:957–979, 2014.

Websites (Accessed November 2016)

Well-being references

The Good Childhood Report 2015. The Children's Society and University of York. 2015

Available at http://www.childrenssociety.org.uk/sites/default/files/TheGoodChildhoodReport2015.pdf

Child health initiatives

Healthy Child Programme Public Health England 2015: Available at: https://www.gov.uk/government/publications/healthy-child-programme-pregnancy-and-the-first-5-years-of-life

Better health outcomes for children and young people: Available at: https://www.gov.uk/.../better_health_outcomes_children_young_people_pledge.pdf

Start4Life: Available at: http://www.nhs.uk/start4life.

From evidence into action: opportunities to protect and improve the nation's health: *Public Health England. October 2014.* Available at: https://www.gov.uk/government/uploads/system/uploads/attachment_data/file/366852/PHE_Priorities.pdf

History and examination

Taking a history	10	Communicating with children	24
An approach to examining children	12	Investigations during consultation	24
Obtaining the child's cooperation	13	Summary and management plan	24
Examination	13		

Features of history and examination in paediatric practice are:

- in contrast to adult medicine, the questions asked in the history and the way the examination is conducted need to be adjusted according to the child's age
- examination is opportunistic, e.g. listening to the chest and heart in an infant or young child when quiet, or may require distraction or play
- in order to achieve a successful and complete examination in young children, ingenuity is often required
- parents are acutely concerned and anxious about their children – they quickly recognize and appreciate doctors who demonstrate interest, empathy, and skill.

Despite advances in technology and the availability of ever more sophisticated investigations, history-taking and clinical examination continue to be the cornerstone of clinical practice. These skills are even more crucial in paediatrics, where most diagnoses are made on the basis of a good history, augmented by astute observation of the child and targeted examination.

When considering clinical history and examination of children, it is helpful to think about some of the common clinical presentations in which children are seen by doctors, and also the age of the child involved. All have an impact on the history taking and examination process.

Common clinical scenarios are:

- an acute illness, e.g. respiratory tract infection, a febrile child, appendicitis
- a chronic problem, e.g. faltering growth, constipation
- a newborn infant with a congenital malformation or abnormality, e.g. developmental dysplasia of the hip, Down syndrome
- suspected delay in development, e.g. delayed walking or speech
- behavioural problems, e.g. temper tantrums, hyperactivity, eating disorders.

The aims and objectives of all clinical encounters are to:

- establish the relevant facts of the history; this is usually the most fruitful source of diagnostic information – a parent's description of an event provides valuable information
- elicit all relevant clinical findings
- collate the findings from the history and examination
- formulate a working diagnosis or differential diagnosis
- assemble a problem list and management plan.

Key features in a paediatric history and examination are:

- the child's age – this is crucial in the history and examination (Fig. 2.1) as it determines:
  - the nature and presentation of illnesses, developmental or behavioural problems
  - the way in which the history-taking and examination are conducted
  - the way in which any subsequent management is organized
- the nature of the problem – assessment of the acutely ill child will need to be more focused and concise ("how unwell is this child at *this* particular moment?"), whereas a developmental assessment will require detailed evaluation
- observing the child – their appearance, behaviour, play, and gait. The continued observation of the child during the whole interview may provide important clues to diagnosis and management.

History and examination

Paediatrics is a specialty governed by age

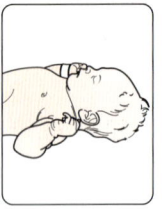
Infant
Neonate (<4 weeks)
Infant (<1 year)

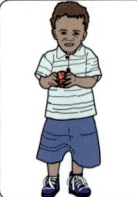
Toddler
Approx 1–2 years

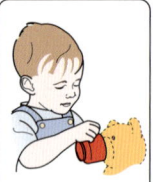
Preschool
Young child (2–5 years)

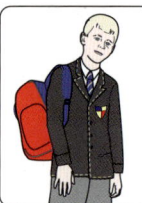
School-age
Older child

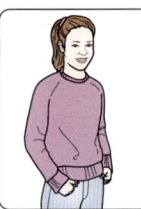
Teenager
Adolescent

Figure 2.1 The illnesses and problems children encounter are highly age-dependent. The child's age will determine the questions you ask on history-taking; how you conduct the examination; the diagnosis or differential diagnosis and your management plan.

 Paediatrics stretches from newborn infants to adolescents. Whenever you consider a paediatric problem, whether medical, developmental or behavioural, first consider "What is the child's age?"

To maximize the value of each consultation it is important to organize the environment so that it is welcoming and unthreatening. Have suitable toys or activities available. Avoid desks or beds between you and the family.

 Parents or carers know their children best – never ignore or dismiss what they say.

Taking a history

Introduction

- Make sure you have read any referral letter and/or hospital notes *before* the start of the consultation.
- When you greet the child, parents, and siblings, check that you know the child's first name and gender. Ask how the child prefers to be addressed.
- Introduce yourself.
- Determine the relationship of the adults to the child.
- Establish eye contact and rapport with the family, but keep a comfortable distance. Infants and some toddlers are most secure in parents' arms or laps. Young children may need some time to feel at ease.
- Observe how the child plays and interacts with any siblings present.
- Do not forget to address questions to the child, when appropriate.
- There will be occasions when the parents will not want the child present or when the child should be seen alone. This is usually to avoid embarrassing older children or teenagers or young adults to impart sensitive information. This must be handled tactfully, often by negotiating to talk separately to each in turn. Give an adolescent the opportunity to talk to you alone. This can be introduced as "It is my usual practice to …" See the adolescent after the parents so he/she knows that confidential information imparted to the doctor has not been disclosed.

Presenting symptoms

Full details are required of the presenting symptoms. Start with an open question. Let the parents and child recount the complaints in their own words and at their own pace. Note the parent's words about the presenting complaint: onset, duration, previous episodes, what relieves/aggravates them, time course of the problem, if getting worse and any associated symptoms. Has the child's or the family's lifestyle been affected? What has the family done about it? If describing a rash or an event such as a seizure, parents may have a photograph or video on their mobile phone. These can be very helpful, but you may need to ask for them!

Make sure you know:
- what prompted the referral
- what the parents think or fear is the matter. Have the parents been searching the internet or discussed it with others?

The scope and detail of further history taking are determined by the nature and severity of the presenting complaint and the child's age. While the comprehensive assessment listed here is sometimes required, usually a selective approach is more appropriate (Fig. 2.2). This is not an excuse for a short, slipshod history, but instead allows one to focus on the areas where a thorough, detailed history is required. For example, in a young child with delayed speech, a detailed birth

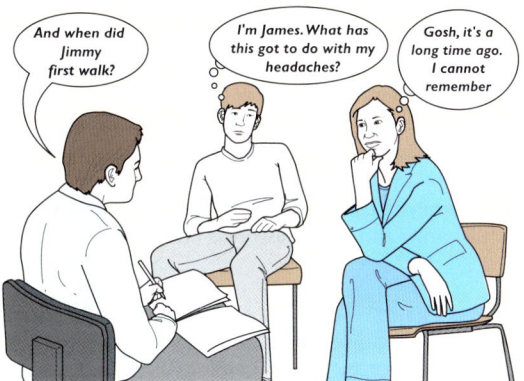

Figure 2.2 The history must be adapted to the child's age. The age when a child first walks is highly relevant when taking the history of a toddler or child with a developmental problem but irrelevant for a teenager in secondary school with headaches.

and neonatal history and details of developmental milestones should be established, but would not be appropriate for an adolescent with headaches (Fig. 2.2).

General enquiry and systems review

Check:

- general health – how active and lively? When were they last their normal self?
- normal growth – is the child following their weight and height centiles?
- feeding/drinking/appetite
- any recent change in behaviour or personality?

Selected, as appropriate:

- general rashes, fever (if measured)
- respiratory – cough, wheeze, breathing problems
- ear, nose, throat – earache, throat infections, snoring, noisy breathing (stridor)
- cardiovascular – cyanosis, exercise tolerance, faints
- gastrointestinal – vomiting, diarrhoea/constipation, abdominal pain
- genitourinary – dysuria, frequency, wetting, toilet-trained
- neurological – development, vision, hearing, seizures, headaches, abnormal or impaired movements, change in behaviour
- musculoskeletal – gait, limb pain or swelling, other functional abnormalities
- pubertal development.

Make sure that you and the parent or child mean the same thing when describing a problem. For example, parents may use the word 'wheeze' to describe any respiratory sound.

 Smartphones are particularly helpful in paediatric practice as parents will often have photographs showing what they are concerned about or taken videos, e.g. of abnormal movements of the limbs or eyes.

Past medical history

Often easiest to follow in chronological order:

- maternal obstetric problems including antenatal scans and screening bloods, delivery
- birthweight and gestation
- perinatal problems, whether admitted to special care baby unit, jaundice, etc.
- immunizations (ideally from the personal child health record)
- past illnesses, hospital admissions, and operations, accidents and injuries.

Medication

Check:

- past and present medications, both prescribed and "over the counter"
- known allergies.

Family history

Families share houses, genes, and diseases!

- Have any members of the family or friends had similar problems or any serious disorder?

Any neonatal/childhood deaths?

- Draw a family tree (see Ch. 9, Genetics). If there is a positive family history, extend family pedigree over several generations.
- Is there consanguinity?

Social history

Check:

- Relevant information about the family and their community – parental occupation, economic status, housing, relationships, parental smoking, marital stresses. "Who lives with you at home?" Adding this to the family tree is a convenient way to document it. (See Case history 2.1). Is the child "looked after" (i.e. under the care of social services)?
- Is the child happy at home? What are the child's preferred play or leisure activities? In an older child it may be appropriate to take a psychosocial history (see Table 30.2, use of HEADS acronym).
- Is the child happy at nursery/school?
- What has been the *impact* of this illness on the child and family?
- Are the family eligible to claim any benefits?
- Is there a social worker involved? This can often be tricky to ask. One approach is to simply ask "Do you have a health visitor? A social worker?" This should identify if families are known to social services, for example, if the child is subject to a Child Protection Plan.

This 'social snapshot' is crucial, since many childhood illnesses or conditions are caused by or affected by adult problems, for example:

- alcohol and drug abuse
- long-term unemployment/poverty
- poor, damp, cramped housing
- parental mental health disorders
- unstable partnership.

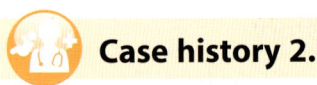
Case history 2.1

Drawing social arrangements on a family tree

Jade, a 3 year old girl, presents with faltering growth. She has two "full" siblings, but her mother has another two older children by a previous partner who gives her no financial support. Her current partner Simon, is out of work. Chris, his 17 year old son from a previous relationship is also living in the house. This can most easily be understood by drawing the family's social arrangements on the family tree (Fig. 2.3). These details could be missed if a full family and social history is not taken.

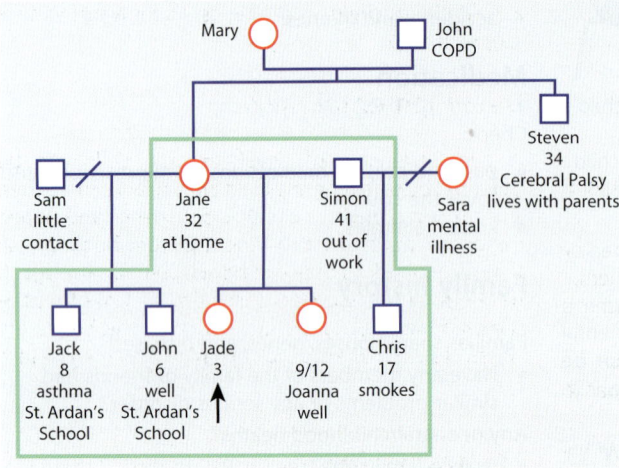

Figure 2.3 Drawing the family's social arrangements on the family tree can be helpful in understanding the child's social environment. The green box shows the members of the family living together in the family home.

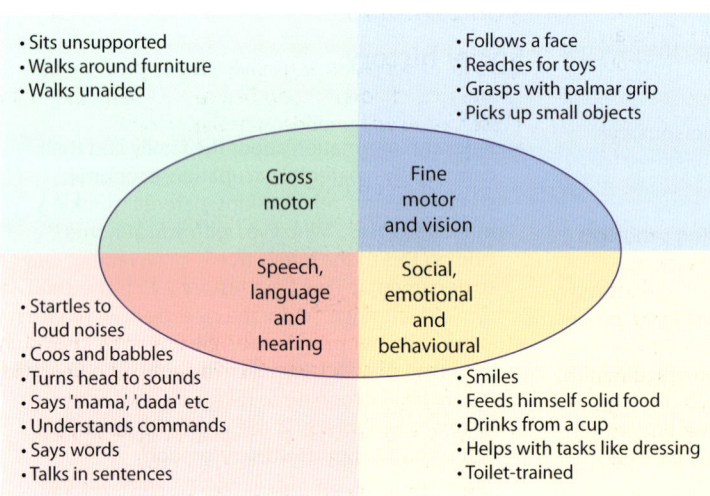

Figure 2.4 Some key developmental milestones in infants and young children. These are considered in detail in Chapter 3. Normal child development, hearing and vision.

Development

Check:
- parental concerns about development, vision, hearing
- key developmental milestones. It is helpful to consider the developmental history in domains (Fig. 2.4)
- previous child health surveillance developmental checks
- bladder and bowel control in young children
- child's temperament, behaviour
- sleeping problems
- concerns and progress at nursery/school.

Look through the personal child health record.

An approach to examining children

Adapting to the child's age

Adapt the examination to suit the child's age. While it may be difficult to examine some toddlers and young

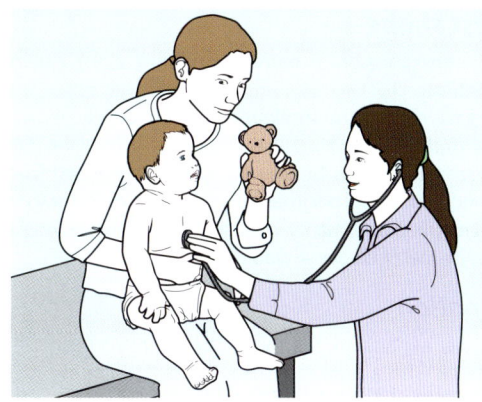

Figure 2.5 Distracting a toddler with a toy allows auscultation of the heart.

children fully, it is usually possible with resourcefulness and imagination on the doctor's part.

- Babies in the first few months are best examined on an examination couch with a parent next to them.
- A toddler is best initially examined on his mother's lap or occasionally over a parent's shoulder.
- Parents are reassuring for the child and helpful in facilitating the examination if guided as to what to do (Fig. 2.5).
- Preschool children may initially be examined while they are playing.
- Older children and teenagers are often concerned about privacy. Young people (males and females) should normally be examined in the presence of a parent or a nurse or suitable chaperone. Be aware of cultural sensitivities in different ethnic groups.

Obtaining the child's cooperation

- Make eye contact and smile. This will build trust: even very young children can judge your intentions from your facial expression and attitude. If the child still looks scared don't just press on but wait, allowing the parent to reassure them.
- Get on the child's level and try and engage in play or conversation. Try to make sure that your eye line is at the same height or lower than theirs if at all possible. It is intimidating to have an adult tower over you!
- Explain what you are about to do and what you want the child to do, in language he or she can understand. As the examination is essential, not optional, it is best not to ask for permission, as it may well be refused!
  - Be confident but gentle.
  - Short mock examinations, e.g. auscultating a teddy or a parent's hand, may allay a young child's fears.
- When first examining a young child, start at a non-threatening area, such as a hand or knee. In general, the more distant the site examined is from the face, the more likely a child is to cooperate.
- Leave unpleasant procedures such as ear and throat examinations until last.

Undressing children

Be sensitive to children's modesty. The area to be examined must be inspected fully but this is best done in stages, redressing the child when each stage has been completed. It is easiest, kindest and helpful to ask the child or parent to do the undressing.

Warm, clean hands

Hands must be washed before (and after) examining a child. Warm smile, warm hands, and a warm stethoscope all help.

Developmental skills

A good overview of developmental skills can be obtained by watching the child play. A few simple toys, such as some bricks, a car, doll, ball, pencil and paper, pegboard, miniature toys, and a picture book, are all that is required, as they can be adapted for any age. If developmental assessment (see Ch. 3) is the focus of the examination, it is advisable to assess this before the physical examination, as co-operation may then be lost.

Examination

Initial observations – watch before you examine

Careful observation is usually the key to success in examining children. Look before touching the child. Observation will provide information on:

- severity of illness
- growth and nutrition
- behaviour and social responsiveness
- level of hygiene and care.

Severity of illness

Is the child sick or well? If sick, how sick? For the acutely ill infant or child, perform the '60-second rapid assessment' (Fig. 6.2):

- airway and breathing – respiration rate and effort, presence of stridor or wheeze, cyanosis
- circulation – heart rate, pulse volume, peripheral temperature, capillary refill time
- disability – level of consciousness.

The care of the seriously ill child is described in Chapter 6. Paediatric emergencies

Measurements

Abnormal growth may be the first manifestation of illness in children, and faltering growth is a "red flag" sign. Always measure and plot growth on centile charts for:

- weight, noting previous measurements from personal child health record
- length (in infants, if indicated) or height in older children

- head circumference in infants and in older children if there is a neurological/developmental problem.

See Chapter 12. Growth and puberty for further details. Also, as appropriate:

- temperature
- blood pressure.

Approach to examination

Examination in younger children needs to be opportunistic; if a baby is quiet you may choose to auscultate the chest before undressing the infant, which may make the infant cry. There is no strict order and there is no 'right place to stand or sit' when examining an individual child, but by the end of the examination a thorough examination needs to have been performed. Some components of the examination, like abdominal examination are easier to do from the child's right hand side if you are using your right hand to palpate for organomegaly.

General appearance

The face, head, neck, and hands are examined. The general morphological appearance may suggest a chromosomal or dysmorphic syndrome. Is the head large or small? In infants, palpate the fontanelle and sutures. Look for any congenital abnormalities. Is the child dehydrated, jaundiced, or anaemic?

Respiratory system

Cyanosis

Is the child pink or blue (or are they on an oxygen saturation monitor)? Central cyanosis is best observed on the tongue.

Clubbing of the fingers and/or toes

Clubbing (Fig. 2.6a) is usually associated with chronic suppurative lung disease, e.g. cystic fibrosis, or cyanotic congenital heart disease. It is occasionally seen in inflammatory bowel disease or cirrhosis. It is obvious when severe but can be difficult to detect when mild; it starts with fluctuation (bogginess) of the nail bed.

Tachypnoea

Count the rate, or determine from a monitor. Rate of respiration is age-dependent (Table 2.1).

Dyspnoea

Laboured or increased work of breathing, from increased airway resistance. Increased work of breathing is judged by:

- nasal flaring
- expiratory grunting – to increase positive end-expiratory pressure
- use of accessory muscles, especially sternomastoids
- retraction (recession) of the chest wall, from use of suprasternal, intercostal, and subcostal muscles
- difficulty speaking (or feeding).

Chest shape

- Hyperexpansion or barrel shape (Fig. 2.6b), e.g. in asthma.
- *Pectus excavatum* (hollow chest) or *pectus carinatum* (pigeon chest).
- Harrison's sulcus (indrawing of the chest wall from long term diaphragmatic tug), e.g. from poorly controlled asthma.
- Asymmetry of chest wall movements.

Palpation

- Chest expansion: if it looks abnormal you can check with a tape measure, this is 3–5 cm in school-aged children. Check for symmetry.
- Trachea: checking that it is central is seldom helpful and is disliked by children. To be done selectively, e.g. if concerned about mediastinal shift in pneumothorax.
- Location of apex beat to detect mediastinal shift.

Percussion

- Needs to be done gently, comparing one side with the other, using middle fingers.
- In infants, only informative when clear cut signs.
- Localized dullness: collapse, consolidation, fluid.

Auscultation (ears and stethoscope)

- Note quality of breathing and symmetry of breath sounds and any added sounds.
- Cough – note its character.
- Hoarse voice – abnormality of the vocal cords.
- Stridor – harsh, low-pitched, mainly inspiratory sound from upper airways obstruction.
- Harsh breath sounds from the upper airways are readily transmitted to the upper chest in infants.
- Breath sounds – normal are vesicular; bronchial breathing is higher-pitched and the length of inspiration and expiration equal. Prolonged expiratory phase usually denotes gas trapping as in asthma.
- Wheeze – high-pitched, expiratory sound from distal airway obstruction (Table 2.2).
- Crackles – discontinuous 'moist' sounds from the opening of bronchioles (Table 2.2).
- Abnormal respiratory sounds may be inaudible in a child who is taking shallow, rapid breaths but may be detectable when the child takes big breaths.

Cardiovascular system

Cyanosis

Observe the tongue for central cyanosis.

Clubbing of fingers or toes

Check if present.

Pulse

Check:

- rate (Table 2.3)
- rhythm – sinus arrhythmia (variation of pulse rate with respiration) is normal

Respiratory system

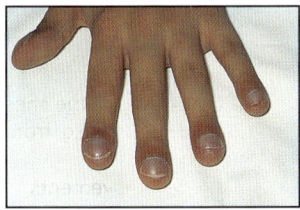

Figure 2.6a Clubbing of the fingers. There is increased curvature, loss of nail angle and fluctuation. This child had cystic fibrosis.

Table 2.1 Respiratory rate in children (breaths/min)

Age	Normal	Tachypnoea
Neonate	30–50	>60
Infants	25–40	>50
Young children	25–35	>40
Older children	20–25	>30

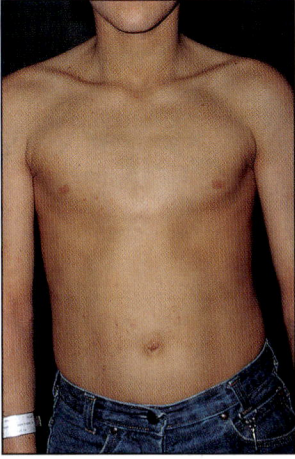

Figure 2.6b Hyperexpanded chest from chronic obstructive airways disease. This boy had severe asthma.

Table 2.2 Chest signs of some common chest disorders of children

	Chest movement	Percussion	Auscultation
Bronchiolitis	Laboured breathing Hyperinflated chest Chest recession	Hyper-resonant	Fine crackles in all zones Wheezes may/may not be present
Pneumonia	Reduced on affected side Rapid, shallow breaths	Dull	Bronchial breathing Crackles
Asthma	Reduced but hyperinflated Use of accessory muscles Chest wall retraction	Hyper-resonant	Wheeze
Croup	Stridor Chest wall retraction	Normal	Stridor from upper airways

 Infants with pneumonia – tachypnoea may be the only respiratory sign; may not have any abnormal signs on auscultation.

 Tachypnoea is the most sensitive marker of respiratory disease, but is less specific than chest recession.

 Sputum is rarely produced by children, as they swallow it. The main exception is suppurative lung disease, e.g. from cystic fibrosis.

- volume – small in circulatory insufficiency or aortic stenosis; increased in high-output states (stress, anaemia); collapsing in patent ductus arteriosus, aortic regurgitation.
- operative scars – mostly median sternotomy or left lateral thoracotomy.

Inspection

Look for:
- respiratory distress
- precordial bulge – caused by cardiac enlargement
- ventricular impulse – visible if thin, hyperdynamic circulation or left ventricular hypertrophy

Palpation

Identifies:
- apex at 4th to 5th intercostal space, mid-clavicular line, but not palpable in some normal infants, plump children, or dextrocardia
- a thrill, which is a palpable murmur
- heave from ventricular hypertrophy, e.g. at lower left sternal edge from right ventricular hypertrophy.

Cardiovascular system

Table 2.3 Normal resting pulse rate in children

Age	Beats/min
<1 year	110–160
2–5 years	95–150
5–12 years	80–120
>12 years	60–100

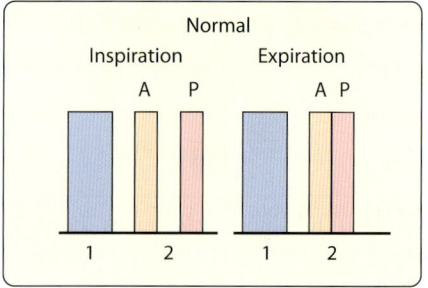

Figure 2.7 The splitting of the second heart sound is easily heard in children. (A is closing of Aortic valve, P is closing of Pulmonary valve).

 Features of heart failure in infants:
- Poor feeding/faltering growth
- Sweating
- Tachypnoea
- Tachycardia
- Gallop rhythm
- Cardiomegaly
- Hepatomegaly

 Features suggesting that a murmur is significant:
- Conducted all over the precordium
- Loud
- Thrill (equals grade 4–6 murmur)
- Any diastolic murmur
- Accompanied by other abnormal cardiac signs.

Percussion

Cardiac border percussion is rarely helpful in children. You may wish to percuss the upper border of the liver though (you are going to feel the lower border later).

Auscultation

Listen for heart sounds and murmurs.

Heart sounds

- Splitting of second sound is usually easily heard and is normal (Fig. 2.7).
- Fixed splitting of second heart sound in atrial septal defects.
- Third heart sound in mitral area is normal in young children.

Murmurs

- Timing – systolic/diastolic/continuous.
- Duration – mid-systolic (ejection)/pansystolic.
- Loudness – systolic murmurs graded:
  - 1–2: soft, difficult to hear
  - 3: easily audible, no thrill
  - 4–6: loud with thrill.
- Site of maximal intensity – mitral/pulmonary/aortic/tricuspid areas.
- Radiation:
  - to neck in aortic stenosis
  - to back in coarctation of the aorta or pulmonary stenosis.

Draw your findings (see Ch. 18. Cardiac disorders).

Hepatomegaly

An important sign of heart failure in infants. An infant's liver is normally palpable 1–2 cm below the costal margin.

Femoral pulses

Always palpate for femoral pulses in neonates. In coarctation of the aorta the femoral pulses are often difficult to palpate whilst upper limb pulses are easy to feel; in older children there is brachiofemoral delay.

Blood pressure (see later in chapter)

 Heart disease is more common in children with other congenital abnormalities or syndromes, e.g. Down or Turner syndrome.

Abdomen

Abdominal examination is performed in three major clinical settings:

- part of the routine clinical examination
- an 'acute abdomen' (see Ch. 14, Gastroenterology)
- recurrent abdominal pain/distension /constipation.

Associated signs

If not already done, examine:

- the eyes for signs of jaundice and anaemia
- the tongue for cyanosis
- the mouth for oral health and ulcers
- the fingers for clubbing.

Inspection

The abdomen is protuberant in normal toddlers and young children.

Occasionally, abdominal distension is caused by a grossly enlarged liver and/or spleen or kidney or mass.

Other abdominal signs are:

- dilated veins and spider naevi in liver disease
- abdominal striae

- operative scars (draw a diagram)
- peristalsis – from pyloric stenosis, intestinal obstruction.

Are the buttocks normally rounded, or wasted as in malabsorption, e.g. coeliac disease or malnutrition?

Palpation

The abdominal wall muscles must be relaxed for palpation.

- Kneel down so your face is level with the child's face. Use warm hands, explain, relax the child, and keep the parent close at hand. First ask if it hurts.
- Palpate in a systematic fashion – liver, spleen, kidneys, bladder, through the four abdominal quadrants. First, gently in each quadrant, then more deeply in each.
- Ask about tenderness. Watch the child's face for grimacing as you palpate. A young child may become more cooperative if you palpate first with their hand or by putting your hand on top of theirs.

Tenderness

- *Location* – localized in appendicitis, hepatitis, pyelonephritis; generalized in mesenteric adenitis, peritonitis.
- *Guarding* – often unimpressive on direct palpation in children. Pain on coughing, on moving about/walking/bumps during car journey suggests peritoneal irritation. Back bent on walking may be from psoas inflammation in appendicitis. By incorporating play into examination, more subtle guarding can be elicited. For example, a child will not be able to jump on the spot if they have localized guarding. You could ask them to blow out their tummy as big as they can, then suck it in as far as they can. This will elicit pain if they have peritoneal irritation.

Hepatomegaly

Normal size is shown in Fig. 2.8.

Abdomen

Table 2.4 Causes of hepatomegaly

Infection	Congenital, infectious mononucleosis, hepatitis, malaria, parasitic infection
Haematological	Sickle cell anaemia, thalassaemia
Liver disease	Chronic active hepatitis, portal hypertension, polycystic disease
Malignancy	Leukaemia, lymphoma, neuroblastoma, Wilms' tumour, hepatoblastoma
Metabolic	Glycogen and lipid storage disorders, mucopolysaccharidoses
Cardiovascular	Heart failure
Apparent	Chest hyperexpansion from bronchiolitis or asthma

On examining the abdomen:
- Inspect first, palpate later
- Superficial palpation first, deep palpation later
- Guarding may be subtle in children
- Silent abdomen – serious!
- Immobile abdomen – serious!

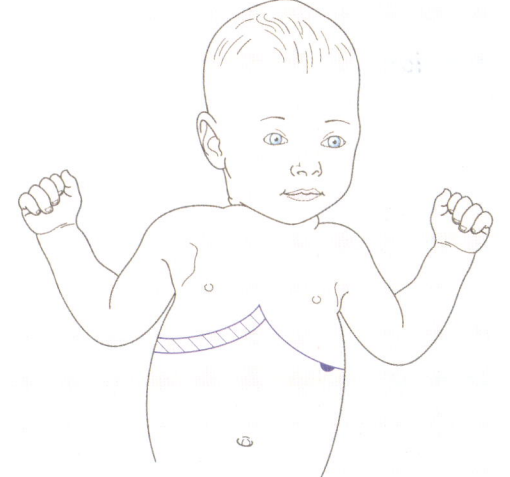

Figure 2.8 Normal findings. The liver edge is 1–2 cm below the costal margin in infants and young children. The spleen may be 1–2 cm below the costal margin in infants.

Table 2.5 Causes of splenomegaly

Infection	Viral, bacterial, protozoal (malaria, leishmaniasis), parasites, infective endocarditis
Haematological	Haemolytic anaemia
Malignancy	Leukaemia, lymphoma
Other	Portal hypertension, systemic juvenile idiopathic arthritis (Still's disease)

To identify hepatomegaly:

- Palpate from right iliac fossa.
- Locate edge with tips or side of finger.
- Edge may be soft or firm.
- Unable to get above it.
- Moves with respiration.
- Measure (in cm) extension below costal margin in mid-clavicular line.

Percuss downwards from the right lung to exclude downward displacement due to lung hyperinflation for example in bronchiolitis.

Liver tenderness is likely to be due to inflammation from hepatitis.

The causes of hepatomegaly are listed in Table 2.4.

Splenomegaly

To identify splenomegaly:

- Palpate from right iliac fossa.
- Edge is usually soft.
- Unable to get above it.
- Notch occasionally palpable if markedly enlarged.
- Moves on respiration (ask the child to take a deep breath).
- Measure size below costal margin (in cm) in mid-clavicular line.

If uncertain whether it is palpable:

- use bimanual approach to spleen
- turn child onto right side.

A palpable spleen is at least twice its normal size! Causes of splenomegaly are listed in Table 2.5.

 Lung hyperexpansion in bronchiolitis or asthma may displace the liver and spleen downwards, mimicking hepato/splenomegaly

Kidneys

These are not usually palpable beyond the neonatal period unless enlarged or the abdominal muscles are hypotonic.

On examination:

- palpate by balloting bimanually
- they move on respiration
- one can "get above them" (unlike the spleen or liver where you cannot palpate the upper border).

Tenderness implies inflammation.

Abnormal masses

- *Wilms' tumour* – renal mass, sometimes visible, does not cross midline.
- *Neuroblastoma* – irregular firm mass, may cross midline; the child is usually very unwell.
- *Faecal masses* – mobile, non-tender, indentable, often in left iliac fossa.
- *Intussusception* – acutely unwell, mass may be palpable, most often in right upper quadrant.

Percussion

- *Liver* – dullness delineates upper and lower border. Record span.
- *Spleen* – dullness delineates lower border.
- *Ascites* – shifting dullness. Percuss from most resonant spot to most dull spot.

Auscultation

Not very useful in 'routine' examination, but important in 'acute abdomen':

- increased bowel sounds – intestinal obstruction, acute diarrhoea
- reduced or absent bowel sounds – paralytic ileus, peritonitis.

Genital area

The genital area is examined routinely in infants and young children, but in older children and teenagers this is done only if relevant, e.g. vaginal discharge, is there an inguinal hernia or a perineal rash?

In *males*

- Is the penis of normal size? Is there hypospadias or chordee (head of the penis curves downward or upward, at the junction of the head and shaft of the penis)?
- Is the scrotum well developed?
- Are the testes palpable? With one hand over the inguinal region, palpate with the other hand. Record if the testis is descended, retractile, or impalpable.
- Is there any scrotal swelling (hydrocele or hernia)?

In *females*

- Do the external genitalia look normal?

Rectal examination

- Not performed routinely.
- Does the anus look normal?

Neurology/neurodevelopment

Brief neurological screen

A quick neurological and developmental overview should be performed in all children. When doing this:

- use common sense to avoid unnecessary examination
- adapt it to the child's age
- take into consideration the parent's account of developmental milestones.

Watch the child play, draw, or write. Does vision and hearing appear to be normal? Are the manipulative skills normal? Can he walk, run, climb, hop, skip, dance? Are the child's language skills and speech satisfactory? Are the social interactions appropriate?

In infants, assess primarily by observation:

- observe posture and movements of the limbs
- when picking the infant up, note their tone. The limbs and body may feel normal, floppy

(hypotonic), or stiff. Head control may be poor, with abnormal head lag on pulling to sitting.

Most children are neurologically normal and do not require formal neurological examination of reflexes, tone, etc.

More detailed neurological examination

If the child has a neurological problem, a detailed and systematic neurological examination is required.

Cranial nerves

Before about 4 years old you need some ingenuity to test for abnormal or asymmetric signs – make it a game; ask them to mimic you:

I	Smell – need not be tested in routine practice. Can be done by recognizing the smell of a hidden mint sweet, or hand towel splashed with hand-cleaning gel.
II	Visual acuity – determined according to age. Direct and consensual pupillary response tested to light and accommodation. Visual fields can be tested if the child is old enough to cooperate.
III, IV, VI	Full eye movement through horizontal and vertical planes. Is there a squint? You may need to hold the chin or head still. Nystagmus? – but avoid extreme lateral gaze, as it can induce nystagmus in normal children.
V	Clench teeth and waggle jaw from side to side against resistance.
VII	Close eyes tight, smile, and show teeth.
VIII	Hearing – whisper in each ear while supplying white noise with fingers outside the other ear. Ask the child what you have whispered. If in doubt, needs formal assessment in a suitable environment.
IX	Levator palati – saying 'aagh'. Look for deviation of uvula.
X	Recurrent laryngeal nerve – listen for hoarseness or stridor.
XI	Trapezius and sternomastoid power – shrug shoulders and turn head against resistance.
XII	Put out tongue and look for any atrophy or deviation.

Inspection of face

- Myopathic face – expressionless, often with ptosis and drooping of corners of the moth, is suggestive of neuromuscular disease, e.g. myotonic dystrophy.
- Ptosis. Unilateral ptosis suggestive of a third nerve palsy, bilateral ptosis, e.g. in myasthenia gravis.
- Tongue fasciculation – in spinal muscular atrophy.

Inspection of limbs

Muscle bulk

- Wasting – may be secondary to cerebral palsy, meningomyelocele, muscle disorder, or from previous poliomyelitis.
- Increased bulk of calf muscles – may indicate Duchenne muscular dystrophy, or myotonic conditions.
- Contractures or a 'windswept posture' suggests increased tone, or a child with hypotonia and restricted movements in utero.
- Fasiculation of muscles – lower motor neurone lesions.

Muscle tone
Tone in limbs

- The posture of the limbs may give a clue as to the underlying tone, e.g. scissoring of the legs, pronated forearms, fisting, extended legs – suggests increased tone (see Figs 4.3, 4.4 and 4.5). Sitting in a frog-like posture of the legs suggests hypotonia (see Fig. 9.2a), while abnormal posturing and extension suggests fluctuating tone (dystonia).
- Assess by taking the weight of the whole limb and then bending and extending it around the joints. Assess the resistance to passive movement as well as the range of movement.
- Increased tone (spasticity) in adductors and internal rotators of the hips, clonus at the ankles or increased tone on pronation of the forearms at rest – usually from pyramidal dysfunction. This is different from the lead-pipe rigidity seen in extra-pyramidal conditions, which, if accompanied by a tremor is called 'cog-wheel' rigidity.

Truncal tone

- In extra-pyramidal tract disorders, the trunk and head tend to arch backwards (extensor posturing).
- In muscle disease and some central brain disorders, the trunk may be hypotonic (Fig. 2.9a). The child feels floppy (hypotonic) to handle and cannot support the trunk in sitting.

Head lag

- This is best tested by pulling the child up by the arms from the supine position (Fig. 2.9b).

Power

Ask the child to hold his arms out straight with palms of hands upwards and close his eyes, and then observe for drift or tremor.

Power can be graded using the Medical Research Council (MRC) power scale:

5. normal
4. weak but active movements against gravity and resistance
3. able to move against gravity but not against resistance
2. unable to move against gravity
1. minimal movement/flicker
0. no movement.

Power is difficult to assess in babies. Eliciting a Moro reflex (see Table 3.1) can be used to see if there are symmetrical movements of all four limbs, as lack of movement suggests reduced power. Watch for anti-gravity movements and note motor function. Both provide information about power. From 6 months onwards, watch the pattern of mobility and gait. Watch the child standing up from lying and climbing stairs.

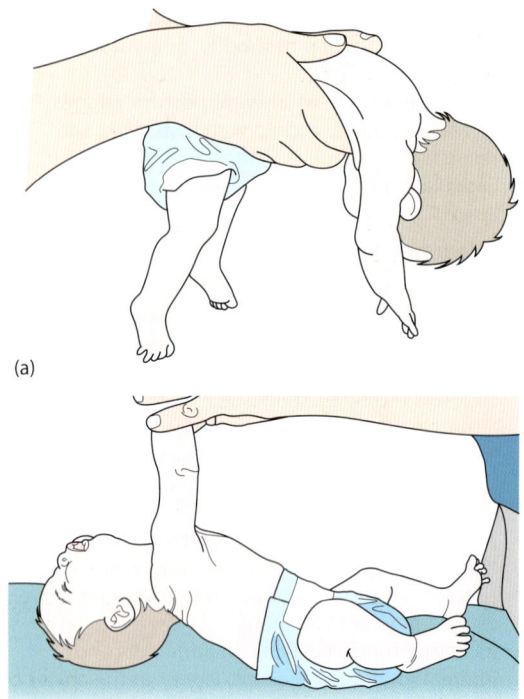

Figure 2.9 Hypotonic infant. (a) When held prone, the infant flops like a rag doll. (b) Marked head lag on traction of the arms.

From the age of about 4 years, power can be tested formally against gravity and resistance, first testing proximal muscle and then distal muscle power and comparing sides.

Coordination

Assess this by:

- finger–nose testing (use mother or teddy's nose to reach out and touch if necessary)
- asking the child to walk heel–toe, jump, and hop
- asking the child to build one brick upon another or using a peg-board, or do up and undo buttons, draw, copy patterns, and write.

Sensation

Ability to feel light touch can be used as a screening test. If loss of sensation is likely, e.g. meningomyelocele or spinal lesion (transverse myelitis, etc.), more detailed sensory testing with a wooden stick or neurotip is performed as in adults. In spinal and cauda equina lesions there may be a palpable bladder or absent perineal sensation.

Reflexes

Test with the child in a relaxed position and explain what you are about to do before approaching with a tendon hammer, or demonstrate on a parent or toy first. Brisk reflexes may reflect anxiety in the child or a pyramidal disorder. Absent reflexes may be due to a neuromuscular problem or a lesion within the spinal cord, but may also be due to inexpert examination technique. Children can reinforce reflexes by biting hard or squeezing their hands to make fists.

Plantar responses

They are unreliable under 1 year of age. Up-going plantar responses provide additional evidence of pyramidal dysfunction.

Patterns of movement

Assessment of walking and running can be incorporated into playing a game, for example: 'how fast can you run?' Children over 5 years of age can usually manage to walk heel-toe. Ask them to walk on a line on the floor 'as though they were walking on a tightrope'.

- In a hemiplegic gait the child holds one arm flexed whilst dragging the ipsilateral affected leg.
- A toe–heel pattern of walking (toe-walkers), although often idiopathic, may suggest pyramidal tract (corticospinal) dysfunction or pelvic girdle neuromuscular weakness. If you are unsure whether a gait is heel-toe or toe–heel, look at the pattern of shoe wear. Examining the wear of shoe soles can also show you if there is asymmetry.
- A broad-based gait may be due to an immature gait (normal in a toddler), secondary to a cerebellar disorder or a sign of lower limb weakness.
- Waddling gait may be due to proximal muscle weakness around the pelvic girdle.
- Difficulty walking on the heels may suggest foot drop e.g. in Hereditary Motor Sensory Neuropathy.
- Children may develop tight Achilles tendon due to weakness suggesting hemiplegia or myopathy.

Subtle asymmetries in gait may be revealed by Fogs' test – children are asked to walk on their toes, heels, the outside, and then the inside of their feet. Watch for the associated movements in the upper limbs. Observe them running. Look for asymmetry. Ask the child to stand up from lying down supine. Children up to 3 years of age will turn prone in order to stand because of poor pelvic muscle fixation; beyond this age, it suggests proximal neuromuscular weakness (e.g. Duchenne muscular dystrophy) or low tone, which could be due to a central (brain) cause. The need to turn prone to rise or, later, as weakness progresses, to push off the ground with straightened arms and then use hands to walk up the legs to stand is known as Gowers sign (see Fig. 29.6).

To complete the neurological examination examine the child's spine. Check the base of the spine for skin lesions such as birth marks and hair, which may be suggestive of spina bifida occulta, or a tethered cord.

Bones and joints

A rapid screen to identify disorders of the musculoskeletal is paediatric gait, arms, legs, spine (pGALS; Fig. 2.10). If an abnormality is found, a more detailed regional examination of the affected joint as well as the joint above and below should be performed (Fig. 2.11).

pGALS – musculoskeletal screening for school-aged children
(Differences from adult GALS highlighted in bold)

Screening questions
- Do you (or your child) have any pain or stiffness in your joints, muscles or your back?
- Do you (or your child) have any difficulty getting yourself dressed without any help?
- Do you (or your child) have any difficulty going up and down stairs?

POSTURE AND GAIT

Observe standing (from front, back and sides)

Observe walking **'Walk on your tip-toes, walk on your heels'**

ARMS

'Put your hands out straight in front of you'

'Turn your hands over and make a fist'

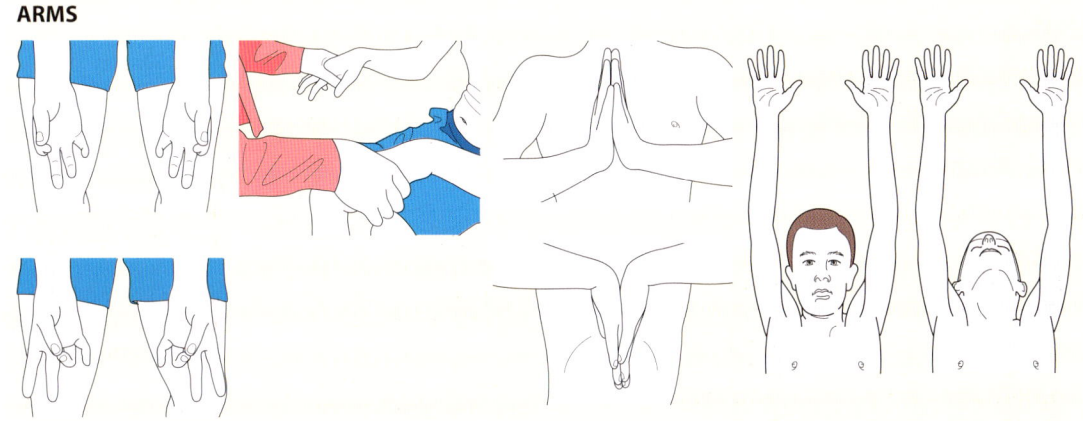

ARMS

'Pinch your index finger and thumb together'

'Touch the tips of your fingers with your thumb'

Squeeze the metacarpo-phalangeal joints for tenderness

'Put your hands together palm to palm'

'Put your hands back to back'

'Reach up and touch the sky'

'Look at the ceiling'

Figure 2.10 Paediatric gait, arms, legs, spine (pGALS) musculoskeletal screening for school-aged children (From Foster HE, Kay LJ, Friswell M, et al., Musculoskeletal screening examination (pGALS) for school-aged children based on the adult GALS screen. Arthritis Rheum 2006; 55:709–16 and see http://www.arthritisresearchuk.org/health-professionals-and-students/video-resources/pgals.aspx to view video of the examination).

Continued

pGALS – musculoskeletal screening for school-aged children—cont'd
(Differences from adult GALS highlighted in bold)

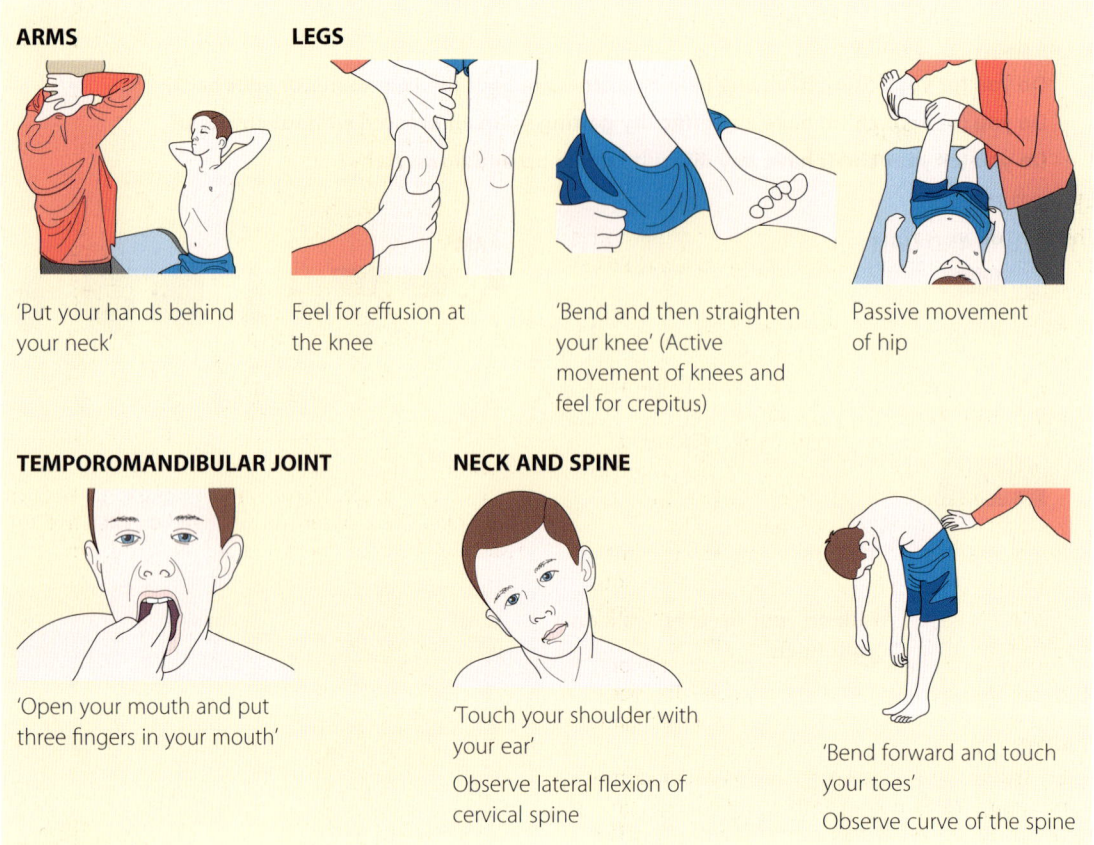

ARMS
'Put your hands behind your neck'

LEGS
Feel for effusion at the knee

'Bend and then straighten your knee' (Active movement of knees and feel for crepitus)

Passive movement of hip

TEMPOROMANDIBULAR JOINT
'Open your mouth and put three fingers in your mouth'

NECK AND SPINE
'Touch your shoulder with your ear'
Observe lateral flexion of cervical spine

'Bend forward and touch your toes'
Observe curve of the spine

Figure 2.10, cont'd

Regional musculoskeletal assessment

Look:
- For signs of discomfort
- Skin abnormalities – rashes, scars, bruising, colour, nail abnormalities
- Limb alignment, leg length, muscle bulk and evidence of asymmetry
- Bony deformity, soft tissue, joint swelling or muscle changes

Feel:
- Each joint, long bones and neighbouring soft tissues:
- Palpate along bones and joint line for tenderness
- Feel for warmth *(infection or inflammation)*
- Delineate bony or soft tissue swellings
- Check for joint effusion, most readily at the knee

Move:
- For each joint, ask the child to move the joint first (active movement).
  Observe for discomfort, symmetry and range of movement.
- Passively move the joint, noting range of any restriction of movement (compare sides but note bilateral changes)
- Lateral and rotational movements may be as important as flexion and extension.

Function:
- For lower limb joints – check gait
- For small joints such as hands – check grip

Figure 2.11 A regional musculoskeletal assessment. (From Foster HE and Brogan P: *Oxford Handbook of Paediatric Rheumatology,* Oxford, 2011, Oxford University Press with permission and http://www.arthritisresearchuk.org/shop/products/publications/information-for-medical-professionals/student-handbook/clinical-assessment-of-the-musculoskeletal-system.aspx).

Neck

Thyroid

- Inspect – swelling uncommon in childhood; occasionally at puberty.
- Palpate from behind and front for swelling, nodule, thrill.
- Auscultate if enlarged.
- Look for signs of hypo/hyperthyroidism.

Lymph nodes

Children often have easily palpable lymph nodes, particularly in the anterior cervical, inguinal and axillary regions.

- Bilateral anterior cervical lymph nodes, up to 2 cm in diameter, are often found in older healthy children or if experiencing or recovering from an upper respiratory tract infection.
- Bilateral axillary nodes up to 1 cm and inguinal nodes up to 1.5 cm in diameter are also found in older children. They may be encountered in younger children with eczema.
- Generalized lymphadenopathy may be present with viral infections, e.g. exanthems or infectious mononucleosis or systemic diseases, e.g. juvenile idiopathic arthritis or Kawasaki disease.
- Supraclavicular nodes of any size at any age or nodes that are firm, non-tender of variable size and matted together warrant further investigation, as they can be associated with malignancy.
- Erythema, warmth, tenderness and fluctuation of a node suggest lymphadenitis of infective origin.
- Nodes of variable size and consistency – is it TB?

Eyes

Examination

Inspect eyes, pupils, iris, and sclerae. Are eye movements full and symmetrical? Is nystagmus detectable? If so, may have ocular or cerebellar cause, or testing may be too lateral to the child. Are the pupils round (absence of posterior synechiae), equal, central, and reactive to light? Is there a squint? (See Figs 4.8 and 4.9.) Epicanthic folds are common in Asian ethnic groups.

Ophthalmoscopy

- In infants, the red reflex is best seen from a distance of 20–30 cm. Partial or complete absence of red reflex occurs in corneal clouding, cataract, and retinoblastoma.
- Fundoscopy requires experience and cooperation. In infants, mydriatics are needed and an ophthalmological opinion may be required.
- In older children with headaches, diabetes mellitus or hypertension, optic fundi should be examined. Mydriatics are not usually needed.

Ears and throat

Examination is usually left until last, as it can upset a previously cooperative child. Explain what you are going to do. Show the parent how to hold and gently

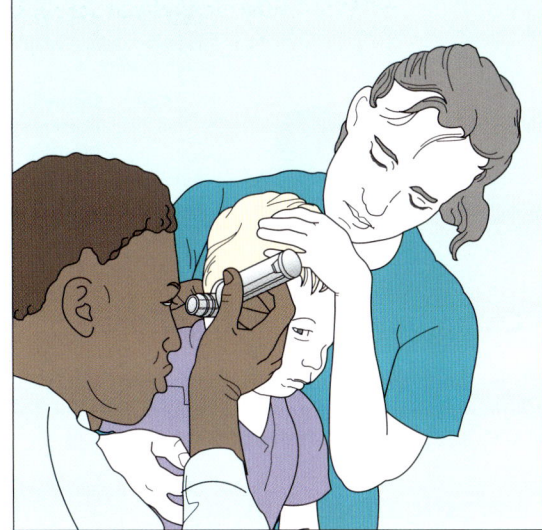

Figure 2.12 Holding a young child correctly is essential for successful examination of the ear with an auroscope. The mother has one hand on the child's head and the other hand holding the upper arm.

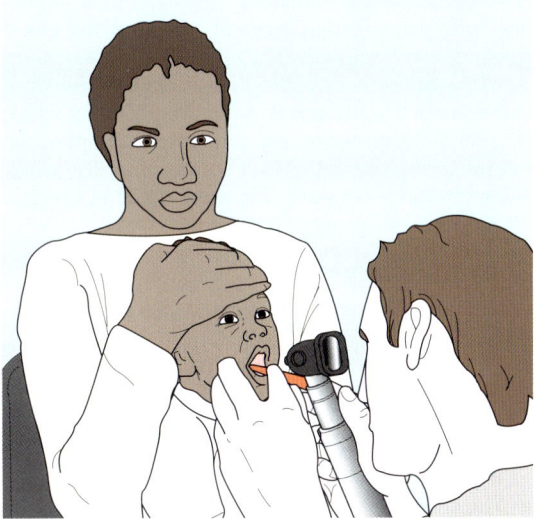

Figure 2.13 Holding a young child to examine the throat. The mother has one hand on the head and the other across the child's arms.

restrain a younger child to ensure success and avoid possible injury (Figs 2.12 and 2.13).

Ears

Examine ear canals and drums gently, trying not to hurt the child. Look for anatomical landmarks on the ear drum and for swelling, redness, perforation, dullness, fluid.

Throat

Rapidly observe the tonsils, uvula, pharynx, and posterior palate. Older children (5 years +) will open their mouths as wide as possible without a spatula. A spatula is required for young children. Look for redness, swelling, pus, or palatal petechiae. Also check the teeth for dental caries and other gross abnormalities.

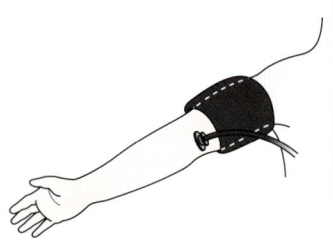

Cuff >2/3 upper arm. (Smaller cuffs give artificially high readings)

Age	Upper limit of normal systolic blood pressure
1–5 years	110 mmHg
6–10 years	120 mmHg

Figure 2.14 Measurement of blood pressure.

Communicating with children

Throughout the consultation, make sure that your communication with the child is appropriate for the child's age and stage of development (Table 2.6).

Investigations during consultation

Blood pressure

Blood pressure must be measured in acutely unwell children as part of assessing "Circulation". It should also form part of the assessment whenever the blood pressure may be abnormal for example when assessing a child with renal or cardiac disease, diabetes mellitus, is overweight or obese, receiving drug therapy which may cause hypertension, e.g. corticosteroids, and some neurological presentations or disorders, e.g. headaches. Hypertension is considered in more detail in Chapter 19. Kidney and urinary tract disorders.

Sphygmomanometer

When blood pressure is measured with a sphygmomanometer:
- Show the child that there is a balloon in the cuff and demonstrate how it is blown up.
- Use largest cuff which fits comfortably, covering at least two-thirds of the length of the upper arm (Fig. 2.14).
- The child must be relaxed and not crying.
- Systolic pressure is the easiest to determine in young children and clinically the most useful.
- Diastolic pressure is when the sounds disappear. May not be possible to discern in young children.

Measurement

Must be interpreted according to a centile chart for gender and height (see Appendix Fig. A.4). Blood pressure is increased by tall stature. Charts relating blood pressure to height are available and preferable; however, for convenience, charts relating blood pressure to age are often used. An abnormally high reading must be repeated, with the child relaxed, on at least three separate occasions; the lowest value is used.

Urinalysis

Urinalysis using a dipstick is required to identify protein, blood, and glucose ketones in the urine. The presence

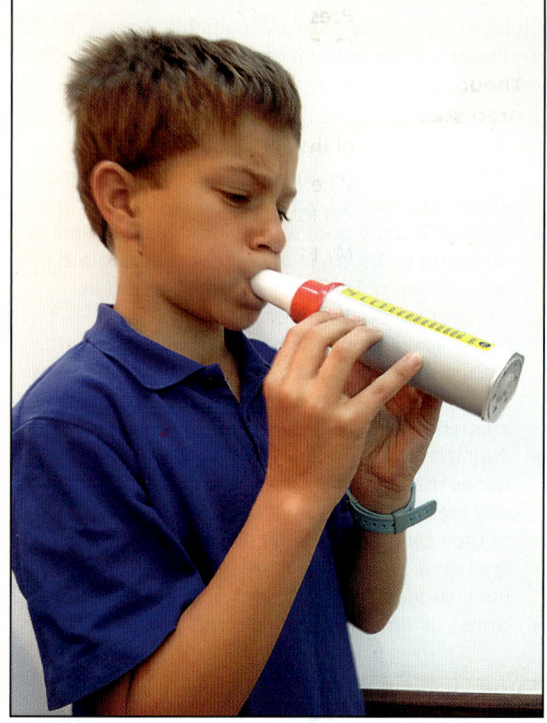

Figure 2.15 Measurement of peak flow rate with a peak flow meter.

of leucocytes and nitrites may assist with screening for a urine infection. In infants and young children, obtaining an uncontaminated sample for microscopy, culture, and sensitivity to identify a urinary tract infection can be problematic. This is considered in Chapter 19. Kidney and urinary tract disorders.

Peak flow or lung function tests

Measuring peak flow or obtaining spirometry is a part of the respiratory examination in school age children. It can be performed in most children from 5 years and is reliable in most 7 year olds. It is most often used to monitor control of asthma (Fig. 2.15 and Appendix 5).

Summary and management plan

By the end of the consultation, have you covered the 'ideas, concerns and expectations' (ICE) of the child and parents, not only for the consultation but also about their attitudes to illness in general. It provides a better

Table 2.6 The reasons for talking with children

Why talk to children when you can get the information from the parent? The reasons are:
- To establish rapport
- To obtain the child's own views about their problems
- To know how the child feels about their health and life
- To reduce anxiety and fear and to improve compliance with assessment and treatment
- To determine the presence of associated emotional or psychiatric problems

	Preschool child (2–5 years)	**School-age child (6–11 years)**	**Adolescent (12–18 years)**
Thought processes	I am asleep, so everyone is asleep (they are the centre of their world) When I fell, the floor hurt me (objects are alive) My toy elephant is crying because the other elephants won't play with him (involvement in pretend play)	I want to watch TV but George is on the Playstation – I'll ask Dad how much longer she's allowed (concrete problem solving) Will Amy still be my friend when I move schools (worries about the future) I know mum gets very upset when I wet the bed, but I can't help it (understands the feelings of others)	I can handle things without Mum's help (seeking autonomy and separation) Should our country be at war? (develops concern about social issues)
Effect on the way we talk to them	Use short, concrete questions within their immediate experience To avoid yes/no answers use a choice of options, e.g. when you go to nursery, what do you like to do – draw or dress up or something else? Use toys or puppets while interviewing, e.g. to represent different people in the child's life	Use familiar examples of experience of others to explore the child's feelings and behaviour, e.g. when a boy was bullying another boy at school, he came to see me so we could talk about how he controls his temper. Do you ever get angry and bully others? You can get at their hopes and dreams by asking them, 'If I was a magician and could give you three wishes, what would they be?'	Should be given an opportunity to be seen alone as they may have problems and difficulties not known to the parents and that the adolescent does not want to share with them Upsetting thoughts can be explored in some adolescents using metaphors

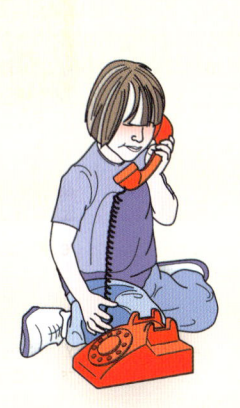

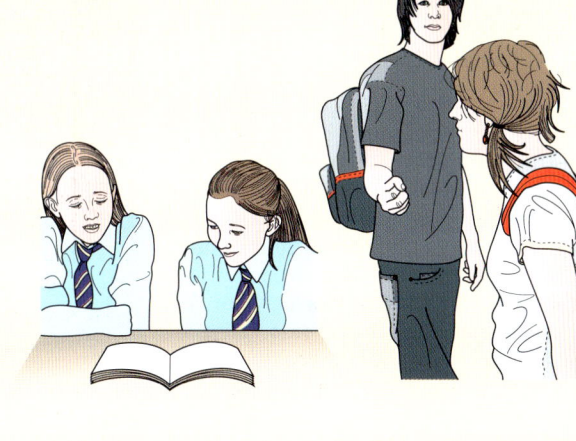

History and examination

understanding of where the family is coming from. If you go one step further and incorporate the information into your management plan, you are more likely to be in tune with the family's way of thinking. This might include:

- Ideas – 'What do you think is the matter?'
- Concerns – 'What particular worries or concerns did you have?'
- Expectation – 'And what are you hoping that we might be able to do for you?'

Finally:

- Summarize the key problems (in physical, emotional, social, and family terms, if relevant).
- List the diagnoses and if possible differential diagnoses. Draw up a management plan to address the problems, both short and long term. This could be reassurance, a period of observation, performing investigations or therapeutic intervention.
- Provide an explanation to the parents and to the child, if old enough. Consider providing further information, either written or on the internet.
- If relevant, discuss what to tell other members of the family.
- Consider which other professionals should be informed.
- Write a brief summary in the child's personal child health record.
- Ensure your notes are dated and signed.

Acknowledgements

We would like to acknowledge contributors to this chapter in previous editions, whose work we have drawn on: Tom Lissauer (1st, 2nd, 3rd, 4th Editions), Graham Clayden (1st Edition), Denis Gill (2nd Edition), Tauny Southwood (3rd Edition), Siobhan Jaques (4th Edition), Sanjay Patel (4th Edition), Kathleen Sim (4th Edition). We thank Laura Haynes and Noa Keren for reviewing the chapter.

Summary

In taking a history and performing a clinical examination:
- The child's age is a key feature – it will determine the nature of the problem, how the consultation is conducted, the likely diagnosis and its management.
- The interview environment should be welcoming – with suitable toys for young children.
- Most information is usually obtained from a focused history and observation, rather than detailed examination, although examination is also important.
- Check growth, including charts in personal child health record, and development.
- With young children – be confident but gentle, do not ask their permission to examine them or they may say 'no', and leave unpleasant procedures (ears and throat) until last.
- Involve children with the consultation, as appropriate to their age.

Always consider if there are child protection issues. Do you have any concerns that this child is not adequately cared for, or at risk? Any concerns must be reported to a senior member of the paediatric team.

Further reading

Brugha R, Mariais M, Abrahamson E: *Pocket Tutor Paediatric Clinical Examination*, London, 2013, JP Medical Ltd.

Gill D, O'Brien N: *Paediatric Clinical Examination Made Easy*, ed 5, Edinburgh, 2007, Churchill Livingstone.

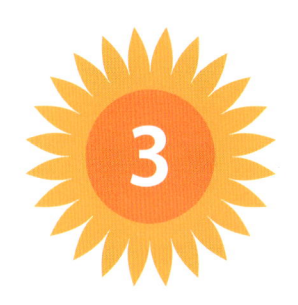

Normal child development, hearing and vision

Influence of heredity and environment	27	Analysing developmental progress	36
Fields of development	28	Developmental screening and assessment	37
Developmental milestones	28	Child health surveillance	38
Is development normal?	29	Hearing	39
Pattern of child development	30	Vision	42
Cognitive development	30		

Features of normal child development, hearing and vision are:

- children's acquisition of developmental abilities follow a similar pattern
- for developmental screening of young children, there are age limits by which time most children have achieved specific developmental milestones
- there is an integrated programme of screening tests, immunization, developmental reviews and health promotion for all children – the Healthy Child Programme
- all newborn infants have their hearing screened
- assessment of vision relies on parental observation; screening of visual acuity and squint occurs at school entry.

Children acquire functional skills throughout childhood. The term child development is used to describe the skills acquired by children between birth and about 5 years of age, during which there are rapid gains in mobility, speech and language, communication and independence. During school age, evidence of developmental progression is predominantly through cognitive development and abstract thinking, although there is also some further maturation of early developmental skills.

Normal development in the first few years of life is monitored:

- by parents, who are provided with guidance about normal development in their child's personal child health record and in the book *Birth to Five*, given to all parents in the UK
- at regular child health surveillance checks
- whenever a young child is seen by a healthcare professional. A brief opportunistic overview should always be made at those times.

The main objective of assessing a young child's development is to confirm normality of progress or the early detection of disordered development in order to:

- help children achieve their maximum potential
- provide treatment or therapy promptly (particularly important for impairment of hearing and vision)
- act as an entry point for the investigation, care and management of the child with special needs.

This chapter covers normal development. Delayed or disordered development and the child with special needs are considered in Chapter 4.

Influence of heredity and environment

A child's development represents the interaction of heredity and the environment on the developing brain. Heredity determines the potential of the child, while the environment influences the extent to which that potential is achieved. For optimal development, the environment has to meet the child's physical and psychological needs (Fig. 3.1). These vary with age and stage of development:

- infants are totally dependent on their parents for all physical needs, and also require a limited number of carers to meet their psychological needs

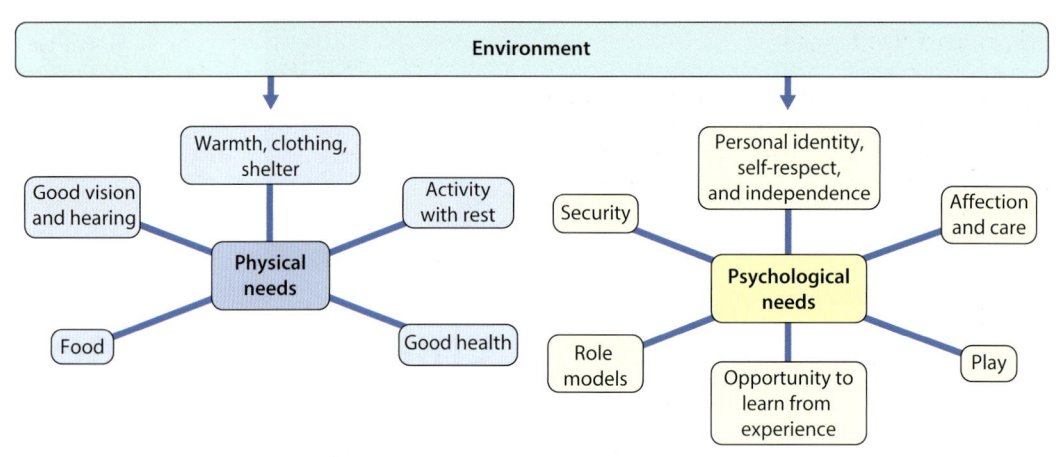

Figure 3.1 Development can be impaired if the environment fails to meet the child's physical or psychological needs.

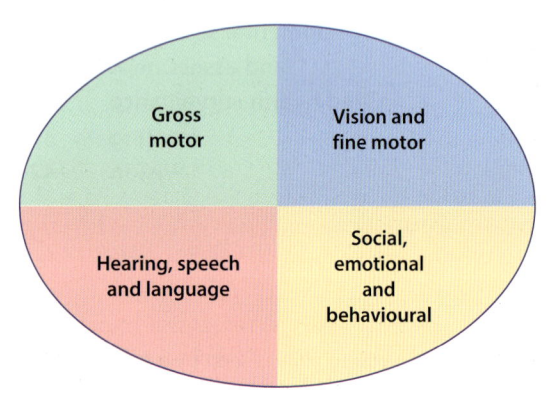

Figure 3.2 The four functional areas of child development and their core features.

- primary school age children can meet some of their physical needs and cope with many social relationships
- adolescents and young adults are able to meet most of their physical needs while experiencing increasingly complex emotional needs.

Fields of development

There are four fields of developmental skills to consider whenever a young child is seen (Fig. 3.2):

- gross motor
- vision and fine motor
- hearing, speech and language
- social, emotional and behavioural.

Gross motor skills are the most obvious initial area of developmental progress. As fine motor skills require good vision, these are grouped together. Similarly, normal speech and language development depend on reasonable hearing and so these are considered together. Social, emotional and behavioural skills are a spectrum of psychological development.

The acquisition of developmental abilities for each skill field follows a remarkably constant pattern between children, but may vary in rate. It is like a sequential story. Thus the normal pattern for acquisition of skills:

- is sequentially constant
- should always be considered longitudinally, relating each stage to what has gone before and what lies ahead
- varies in rate between children.

A deficiency in any one skill area can have an impact on other areas. For instance, a hearing impairment may affect a child's language, social and communication skills and behaviour. As a child grows, additional skills become important, such as attention and concentration and how an individual child manages to integrate their skills. Neglect or child abuse can affect a child at any age but may have a global detrimental effect in younger children.

Developmental milestones

Chronological age, physical growth and developmental skills usually evolve hand in hand. Just as there are normal ranges for changes in body size with age, so there are ranges over which new skills are acquired. Important developmental stages are called developmental milestones.

When considering developmental milestones:

- the *median age* is the age when half of a standard population of children achieve that level; it serves as a guide to when stages of development are likely to be reached but does not tell us if the child's skills are outside the normal range
- *limit ages* are the age by which the developmental milestones should have been achieved. Limit ages are usually two standard deviations (SDs) from the mean. They are more useful as a guide to whether a child's development is normal than the median ages. Failure to meet limit ages gives guidance for action regarding more detailed assessment, investigation or intervention.

Median and limit ages

The difference between median and limit ages is shown by considering the age range for the developmental milestone of walking unsupported. The percentage of children who take their first steps unsupported is:

- 25% by 11 months
- 50% by 12 months
- 75% by 13 months
- 90% by 15 months
- 97.5% by 18 months.

The median age is 12 months and is a guide to the common pattern to expect, although the age range is wide. The limit age is 18 months (2 SDs from the mean). Of those not achieving the limit age, many will be normal late walkers, but a proportion will have an underlying problem, such as cerebral palsy, a primary muscle disorder or global developmental delay. A few may be understimulated from social deprivation. Hence any child who is not walking by 18 months of age should be assessed and examined. Thus 18 months can be set as a 'limit age' for children not walking. Setting the limit age earlier may allow earlier identification of problems, but will also increase the number of children labelled as 'delayed' who are in fact normal.

Variation in the pattern of development

There is variation in the pattern of development between children. Taking motor development as an example, normal motor development is the progression from immobility to walking, but not all children do so in the same way. While most achieve mobility by crawling (83%), some bottom-shuffle and others become mobile with their abdomen on the floor, so-called commando crawling or creeping (Fig. 3.3). A very few just stand up and walk. The locomotor pattern (crawling, creeping, shuffling and just standing up) determines the age of sitting, standing and walking.

The limit age of 18 months for walking applies predominantly to children who have had crawling as their early mobility pattern. Children who bottom-shuffle or commando crawl tend to walk later than crawlers, so that within those not walking at 18 months of age there will be some children who demonstrate a locomotor variant pattern, with their developmental progress still being normal. For example, of children who become mobile by bottom-shuffling, 50% will walk independently by 18 months and 97.5% by 27 months of age, with even later ages for those who initially commando crawl. Some children who walk late have joint hypermobility.

Why motor development is most rapid in the first years of life

Motor development generally follows a cephalocaudal pattern (head to toe) in relation to maturation of the central nervous system and myelination. Myelin is required for nerves to function properly. The process of myelination in the brain begins in utero and most occurs in the first 2 years of life, allowing rapid motor development. Thereafter, it continues to develop at a slower rate; in some structures, such as the frontal lobes, myelination is only complete during adolescence.

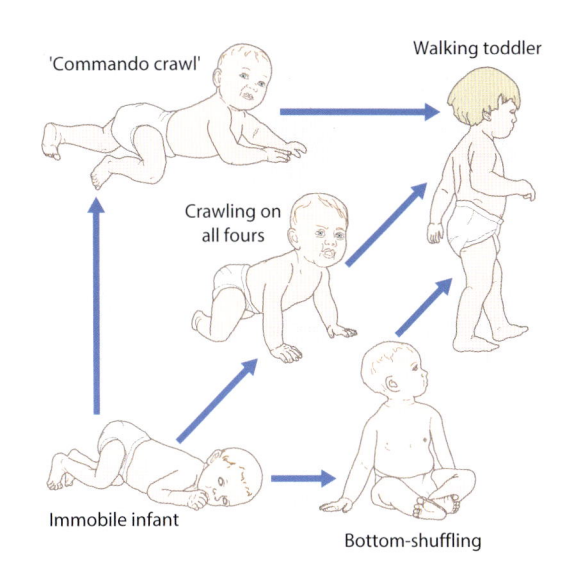

Figure 3.3 Early locomotor patterns. Most children crawl on all fours prior to walking, but some 'bottom-shuffle' and others 'commando crawl' (creep). Bottom-shuffling often runs in families. The late walking that often goes with this locomotor variant needs to be differentiated from an abnormality such as cerebral palsy.

Adjusting for prematurity

If a child has been born preterm, this should be allowed for when assessing developmental age by calculating it from the expected date of delivery. Thus the anticipated developmental skills of a 9-month-old baby (chronological age) born 3 months early at 28 weeks' gestation are more like those of a 6-month-old baby (corrected age). Correction is not required after about 2 years of age when the number of weeks early the child was born no longer represents a significant proportion of the child's life.

Is development normal?

When evaluating a child's developmental progress and considering whether it is normal or not:

- concentrate on each field of development (gross motor; vision and fine motor; hearing, speech and language; social, emotional and behavioural) separately
- consider the developmental pattern by thinking longitudinally and separately about each developmental field. Ask about the sequence of skills achieved as well as those skills likely to develop in the near future
- determine the level the child has reached for each skill field

- now relate the progress of each developmental field to the others. Is the child progressing at a similar rate through each skill field, or does one or more field of development lag behind the others?
- then relate the child's developmental achievements to age (chronological or corrected).

This will enable you to decide if the child's developmental progress is normal or delayed. Normal development implies steady progress in all four developmental fields with acquisition of skills occurring before limit ages are reached. If there is developmental delay, does it affect all four developmental fields (global delay), or one or more developmental field only (specific developmental delay)? As children grow older and acquire further skills, it becomes easier to make a more accurate assessment of their abilities and developmental status.

> **Summary**
>
> **Assessing child development**
> When assessing a young child's development:
> - consider the four fields of developmental skills: gross motor; vision and fine motor; hearing, speech and language; social, emotional and behavioural
> - the acquisition of developmental abilities follows a similar pattern between children, but may vary in rate and still be normal.
>
> Terms used are:
> - developmental milestones: the age of acquisition of important developmental skills
> - median age: the age when half the population acquire a skill; serves as a guide to normal pattern of development
> - limit age: the age when a skill should have been acquired; further assessment is indicated if not achieved.
>
> When evaluating a child's development, consider:
> - each skill field separately
> - the sequence of developmental progress
> - the stage the child has reached for each skill field
> - if progress is similar in each skill field
> - only at the end, the child's overall developmental profile and how that relates to the child's age.

Pattern of child development

This is shown pictorially for each field of development, including key developmental milestones and limit ages:

- gross motor development (Fig. 3.4 and Table 3.1)
- vision and fine motor (Fig. 3.5)
- hearing, speech and language (Fig. 3.6)
- social, emotional and behavioural (Fig. 3.7).

Table 3.1 The primitive reflexes evident at birth gradually disappear as postural reflexes essential for independent sitting and walking emerge

Primitive reflexes	Postural reflexes
Moro – sudden extension of the head causes symmetrical extension, then flexion of the arms	**Labyrinthine righting** – head moves in opposite direction to which the body is tilted
Grasp – flexion of fingers when an object is placed in the palm	**Postural support** – when held upright, legs take weight and baby may push up (bounce)
Rooting – head turns to the stimulus when touched near the mouth	**Lateral propping** – in sitting, the arm extends on the side to which the child falls as a saving mechanism
Stepping response – stepping movements when held vertically and dorsum of feet touch a surface	**Parachute** – when suspended face down, the baby's arms extend as though to save himself
Asymmetrical tonic neck reflex – lying supine, the infant adopts an outstretched arm to the side to which the head is turned	
Sucking reflex – child sucks when nipple/teat placed in their mouth (automatic feeding action)	

In order to screen a young child's development, it is only necessary to know a limited number of key developmental milestones and their limit ages.

Cognitive development

Cognition refers to higher mental function. This evolves with age. In infancy, thought processes are centred around immediate experiences. The thought processes at different ages are described in Table 2.6. Those of preschool children (which have been called preoperational thought by Piaget, who described children's intellectual development) tend to be that:

- they are the centre of the world
- inanimate objects are alive and have feelings and motives
- events have a magical element
- everything has a purpose. Toys and other objects are used in imaginative play as aids to thought to help make sense of experience and social relationships.

In middle-school children, the dominant mode of thought is practical and orderly, tied to immediate

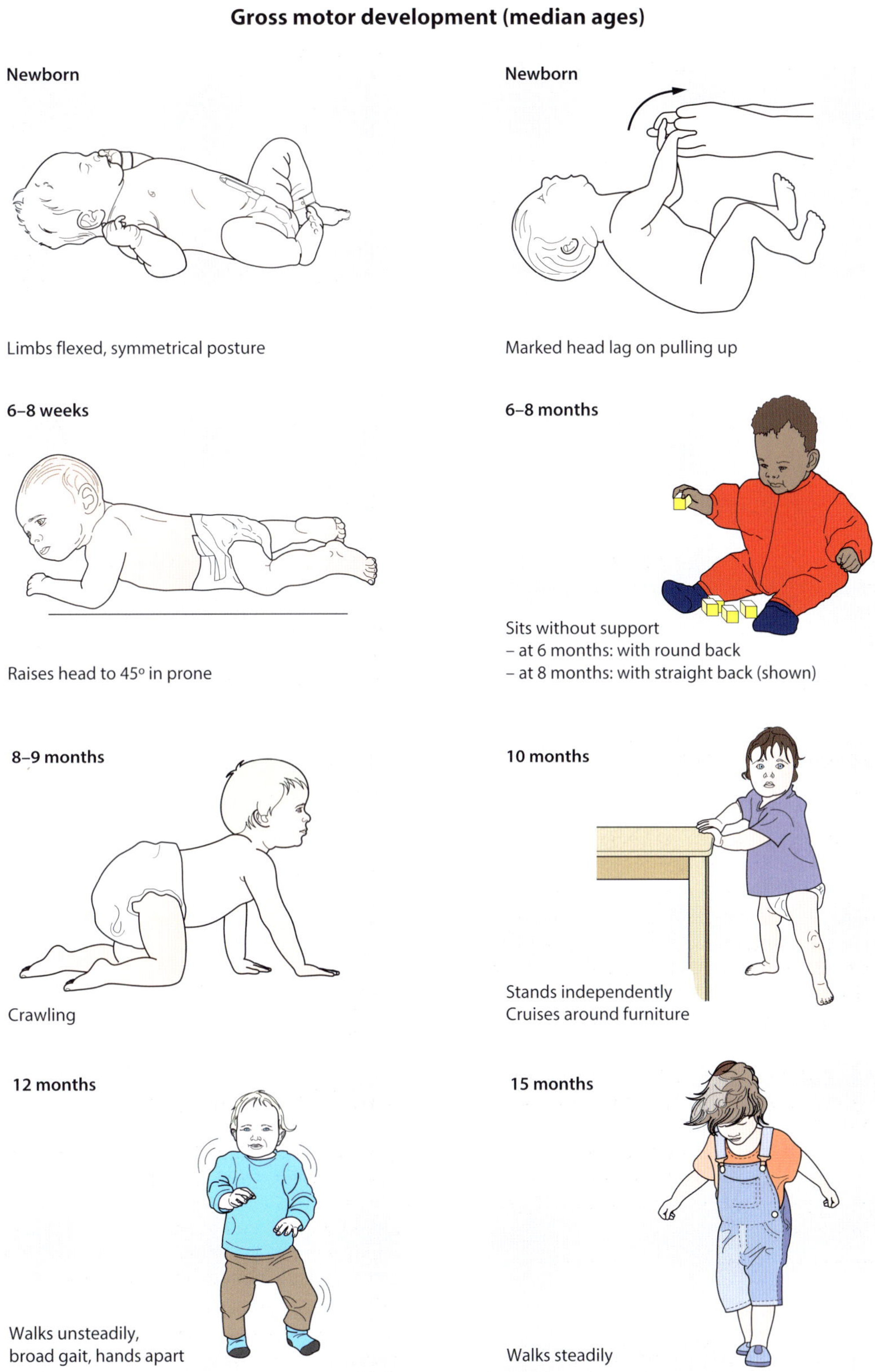

Gross motor development (median ages)

Newborn

Limbs flexed, symmetrical posture

Newborn

Marked head lag on pulling up

6–8 weeks

Raises head to 45° in prone

6–8 months

Sits without support
– at 6 months: with round back
– at 8 months: with straight back (shown)

8–9 months

Crawling

10 months

Stands independently
Cruises around furniture

12 months

Walks unsteadily, broad gait, hands apart

15 months

Walks steadily

Figure 3.4 Gross motor development (median ages).

Normal child development, hearing and vision

Vision and fine motor (median ages)

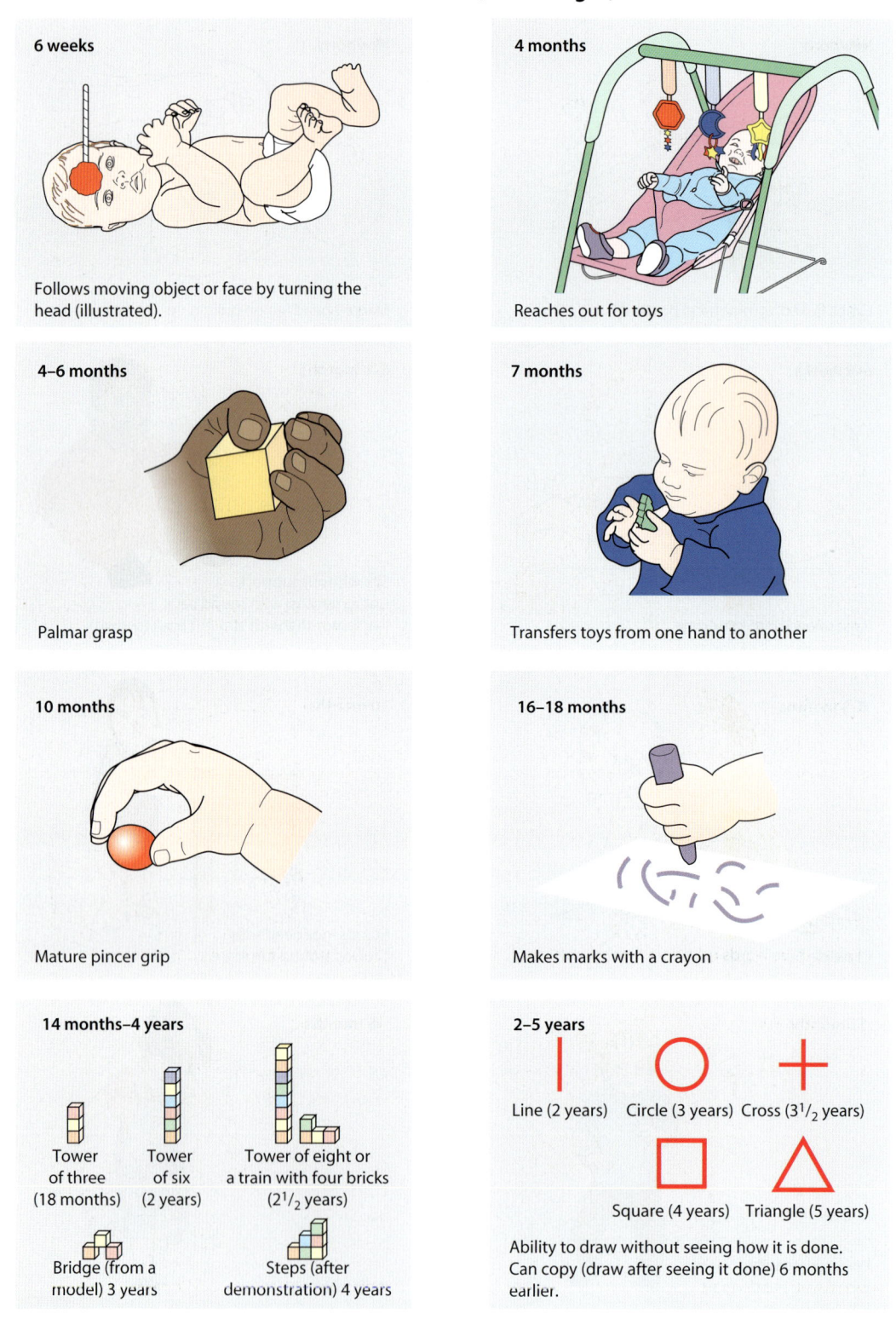

6 weeks
Follows moving object or face by turning the head (illustrated).

4 months
Reaches out for toys

4–6 months
Palmar grasp

7 months
Transfers toys from one hand to another

10 months
Mature pincer grip

16–18 months
Makes marks with a crayon

14 months–4 years
Tower of three (18 months)
Tower of six (2 years)
Tower of eight or a train with four bricks (2½ years)
Bridge (from a model) 3 years
Steps (after demonstration) 4 years

2–5 years
Line (2 years)   Circle (3 years)   Cross (3½ years)
Square (4 years)   Triangle (5 years)

Ability to draw without seeing how it is done. Can copy (draw after seeing it done) 6 months earlier.

Figure 3.5 Vision and fine motor skills (median ages).

Hearing, speech and language (median ages)

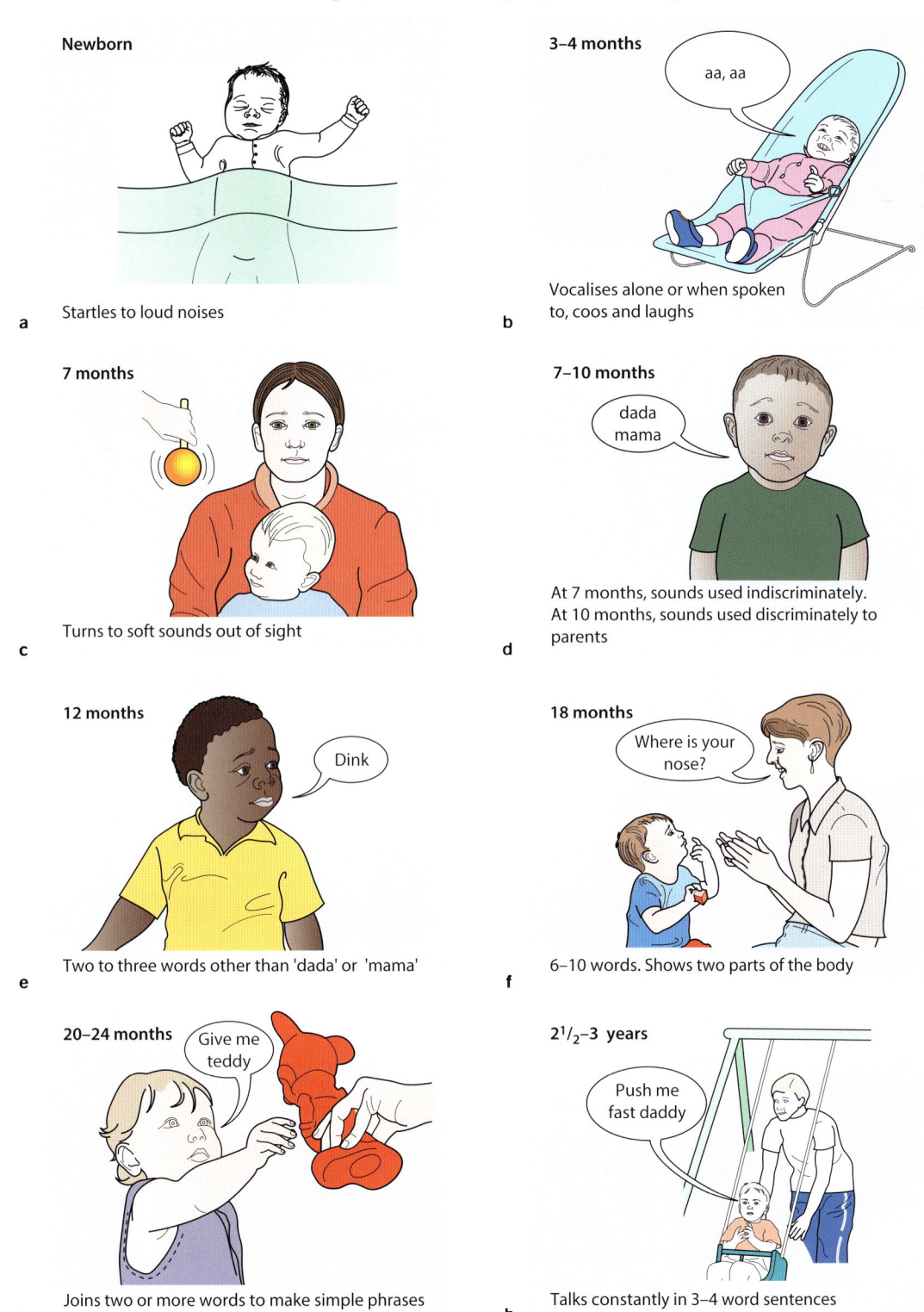

a Newborn — Startles to loud noises

b 3–4 months — "aa, aa" — Vocalises alone or when spoken to, coos and laughs

c 7 months — Turns to soft sounds out of sight

d 7–10 months — "dada mama" — At 7 months, sounds used indiscriminately. At 10 months, sounds used discriminately to parents

e 12 months — "Dink" — Two to three words other than 'dada' or 'mama'

f 18 months — "Where is your nose?" — 6–10 words. Shows two parts of the body

g 20–24 months — "Give me teddy" — Joins two or more words to make simple phrases

h 2½–3 years — "Push me fast daddy" — Talks constantly in 3–4 word sentences

Figure 3.6 Hearing, speech and language (median ages).

Social, emotional and behavioural development (median ages)

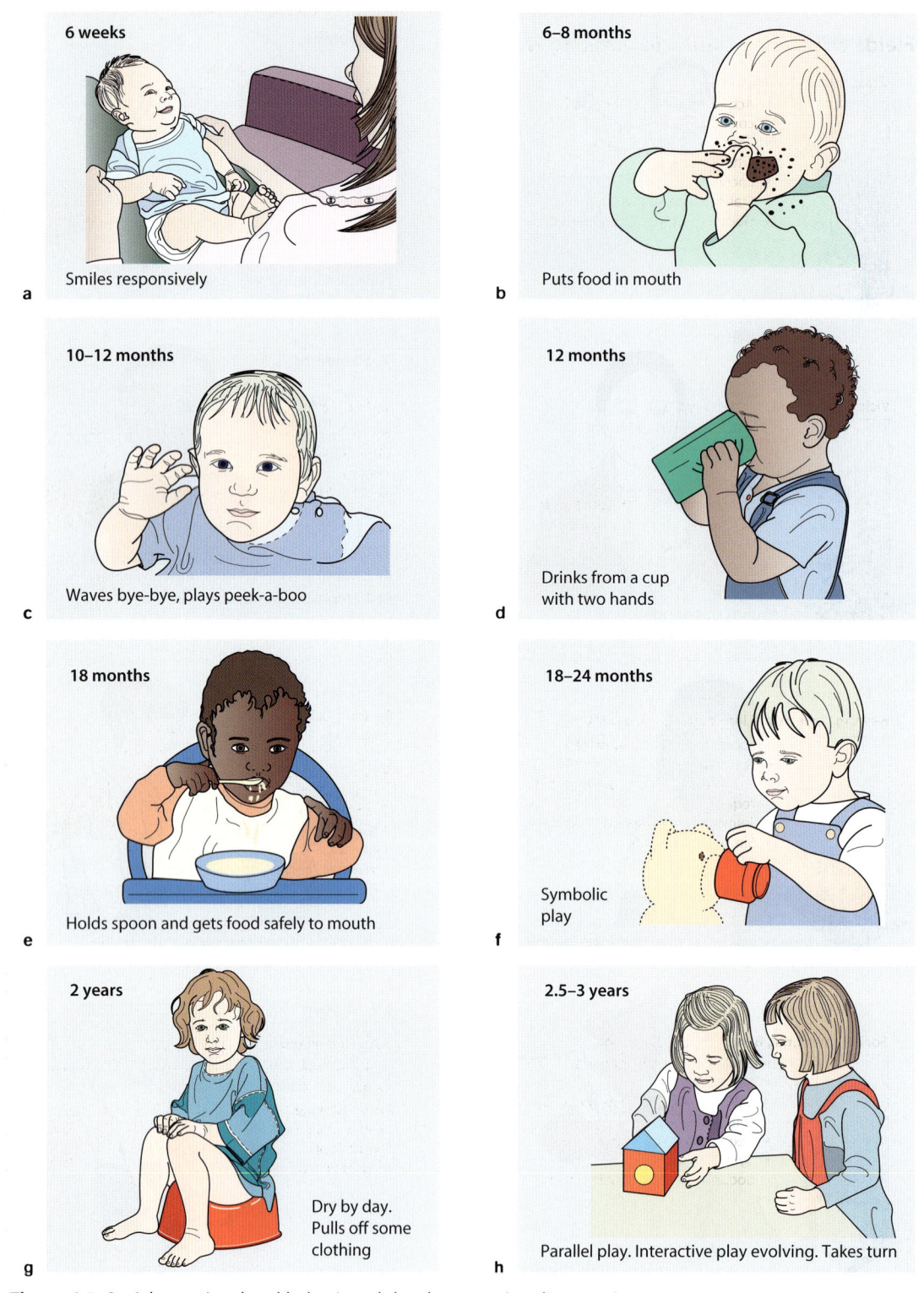

a 6 weeks — Smiles responsively

b 6–8 months — Puts food in mouth

c 10–12 months — Waves bye-bye, plays peek-a-boo

d 12 months — Drinks from a cup with two hands

e 18 months — Holds spoon and gets food safely to mouth

f 18–24 months — Symbolic play

g 2 years — Dry by day. Pulls off some clothing

h 2.5–3 years — Parallel play. Interactive play evolving. Takes turn

Figure 3.7 Social, emotional and behavioural development (median ages).

Summary

Fields of development with limit ages

Gross motor development
- Acquisition of tone and head control
- Primitive reflexes disappear
- Sitting
- Locomotor patterns
- Standing, walking, running
- Hopping, jumping, peddling

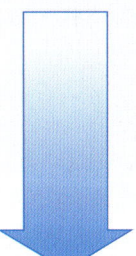

Gross motor	Limit ages
Head control	4 months
Sits unsupported	9 months
Stands with support	12 months
Walks independently	18 months

Vision and fine motor development
- Visual alertness, fixing and following
- Grasp reflex, hand regard
- Voluntary grasping, pincer, points
- Handles objects with both hands, transfers from hand to hand
- Writing, cutting, dressing

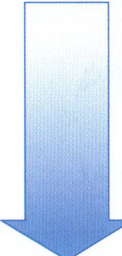

Vision and fine motor	Limit ages
Fixes and follows visually	3 months
Reaches for objects	6 months
Transfers	9 months
Pincer grip	12 months

Hearing, speech and language development
- Sound recognition, vocalisation
- Babbling
- Single words, understands simple requests
- Joining words, phrases
- Simple and complex conversation

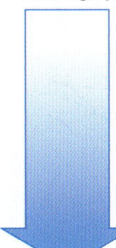

Hearing, speech and language	Limit ages
Polysyllabic babble	7 months
Consonant babble	10 months
Saying 6 words with meaning	18 months
Joins words	2 years
3-word sentences	2.5 years

Social, emotional, behaviour development
- Smiling, socially responsive
- Separation anxiety
- Self-help skills, feeding, dressing, toileting
- Peer group relationships
- Symbolic play
- Social/communication behaviour

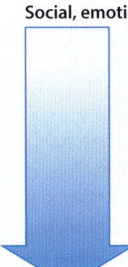

Social behaviour	Limit ages
Smiles	8 weeks
Fear of strangers	10 months
Feeds self/spoon	18 months
Symbolic play	2–2.5 years
Interactive play	3–3.5 years

Normal child development, hearing and vision

Summary

Developmental milestones by median age

Age	Gross motor	Vision and fine motor	Hearing, speech, and language	Social, emotional, and behavioural
Newborn	Flexed posture	Follows face or light by 2 weeks	Stills to voice Startles to loud noise	Smiles by 6 weeks
7 mo	Sits without support	Transfers objects from hand to hand	Turns to voice Polysyllabic babble	Finger feeds Fears strangers
1 y	Stands independently	Pincer grip (10 mo) Points	2–3 words Understands name	Drinks from cup Waves
15–18 mo	Walks independently and steadily	Immature grip of pencil Random scribble	6–10 words Points to two body parts	Feeds self with spoon Beginning to help with dressing
2½ y	Runs and jumps	Draws	3-word to 4-word sentences Understands two joined commands	Parallel play Clean and dry

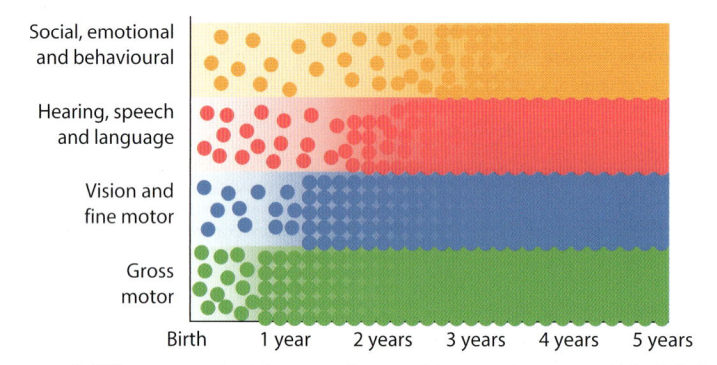

Figure 3.8 Developmental skills are acquired in a serial way. There are features of all skill domains emerging from birth, but there are ages, shown here by the colour blocks becoming more intense, when there is particularly rapid expansion of the skill area.

circumstances and specific experiences. This has been called operational thought.

It is only in the early to midteens that an adult style of abstract thought (formal operational thought) begins to develop, with the ability for abstract reasoning, testing hypotheses and manipulating abstract concepts.

Analysing developmental progress

Detailed assessment

So far, emphasis has been mainly on thinking about developmental progress in a longitudinal way, taking each skill field and its progression separately, and then relating the progress in each field to that occurring in the others, and to chronological age. This is the fundamental concept of learning how to think about developmental assessment of children. Detailed questioning and observation is required to assess children with developmental problems but is unnecessary whilst screening developmental progress in normal clinical practice, when a short-cut approach can be adopted.

The short-cut approach

This concentrates on the most actively changing skills for the child's age. The age at which developmental progress accelerates differs in each of the developmental fields. Fig. 3.8 demonstrates the age when there is

the most rapid emergence of skills in each developmental field. This means there is for:
- gross motor development: an explosion of skills during the first year of life
- vision and fine motor development: more evident acquisition of skills from 1 year onwards
- hearing, speech and language: a big expansion of skills from 18 months of age
- social, emotional and behavioural development: expansion in skills particularly from 2.5 years of age.

Understanding the time when acceleration in each skill field becomes more obvious and knowing the child's age helps guide initial developmental questioning. Thus for a child aged:
- less than 18 months – it is likely to be most useful to begin questions around gross motor abilities, acquisition of vision and hearing skills, followed by questions about hand skills
- 18 months to 2.5 years – initial developmental questioning is likely to be most usefully directed at acquisition of speech and language and fine motor (hand) skills with only brief questioning about gross motor skills (as it is likely the child would have presented earlier if these were of concern)
- 2.5 to 4 years – initial questions are best focused around speech and language and social, emotional, and behaviour development.

Developmental questioning needs to cover all areas of developmental progression but this more focused way of taking a developmental history allows a useful short-cut approach. It directs the assessment to current abilities instead of concentrating on parents trying to remember the age when their child acquired developmental milestones sometime in the past.

Observation during questioning

Of equal importance to taking the developmental history is the examiner's ability to observe the child throughout any visit. Not only will this provide an almost immediate guide to where to begin questioning but it also offers the opportunity for a rapid overview of the child's abilities, behaviour, peer group and parent–child relationships, all of which will go towards determining the overall picture about the child and his/her developmental abilities.

Equipment for developmental testing

Simple basic equipment is all that is needed for most developmental assessments. Equipment is aimed at bringing out the child's skills using play. Cubes, a ball, picture book, doll and miniature toys such as a tea set, crayons and paper allow a quick but useful screen of mobility, hand skills, play, speech and language and behaviour. These items allow the child to relax by having fun at the same time as facilitating observer assessment of his skills.

Developmental screening and assessment

Developmental screening (checks of whole populations of children at set ages by trained professionals) is a formal process within the child health surveillance and promotion programme. It is also an essential role of all health professionals to screen a young child's developmental progress opportunistically at every health contact, e.g. by the general practitioner for a sore throat, in the Accident and Emergency department for a fall, or on admission to a paediatric ward. In this way, every child contact is optimized to check that development is progressing normally.

There are a number of problems inherent in developmental screening:
- it is a subjective clinical opinion and therefore has its limitations
- a single observation of development may be limited by the child being tired, hungry, shy or simply not wishing to take part
- while much of the focus of early developmental progress in infants is centred on motor development, this is a poor predictor of cognitive function and later school performance. Development of speech and language is a better predictor of cognitive function but is less easy to assess rapidly. It is likely to manifest at an age when there is increased surveillance by health professionals.

The reliability of screening tests can be improved by adding a questionnaire completed by parents beforehand. Screening is being increasingly targeted towards children at high risk or when there are parental concerns.

Developmental assessment is the detailed analysis of particular areas of development and follows concern after screening that a child's developmental progress may be disordered in some way. It is part of the diagnostic process and includes investigation, therapy and advice on how to optimize the child's progress. Developmental assessment is by referral to a specialist service such as the local multidisciplinary child development service, which is able to offer input by a paediatrician and therapists.

A range of tests have been developed to screen or to assess development in a formal reproducible manner. These include:
- screening tests, e.g. the Schedule of Growing Skills and the Denver Developmental Screening Test
- standardized tests that assess the overall development of infants and young children, e.g. Griffiths and the Bailey Infant Development Scales,

> **Summary**
>
> **Analysing child development**
> When analysing a young child's developmental progress:
> - consider the child's age and then focus your questions on the areas of likely current developmental progress
> - offer the child suitable toys to find out about skills through play
> - observe how the child uses the toys and interacts with people.

- which are used, for instance, in follow-up studies of preterm infants
- standardized tests concentrating on assessing specific aspects of development, e.g. the Reynell Language Scale, the Gross Motor Function Measure, the Autism Diagnostic Interview and the Autism Diagnostic Observation Schedule. These tests are time consuming and require training for reliable results.

Cognitive function (higher mental function) can be assessed objectively with formal intelligence quotient (IQ) tests. However, IQ tests:

- may be affected by cultural background and linguistic skills
- do not test all skill areas
- do not necessarily reflect an individual child's ultimate potential
- may be compromised by specific disabilities, such as a motor disorder as in cerebral palsy.

'Verbal' reasoning tests, especially those for younger children, reflect general intellectual skills, particularly relating to language. 'Performance' or 'non-verbal' reasoning tests assess abilities independent of language. Verbal and performance testing together with other tests of cognitive function such as processing speed and working memory allows formulation of a verbal IQ and performance IQ, which together give an overall IQ figure. Children with disabilities may have problems with speech or hand skills that may compromise testing, so that an overall result in these situations has to be interpreted with care.

Cognitive (higher mental function) assessment of school-age children using IQ and other tests is carried out by clinical or educational psychologists.

Summary

Developmental screening and assessment

- *Developmental screening* – checks of whole populations or groups of children at set ages by trained professionals.
- *Developmental assessment* – detailed analysis of overall development or specific areas of development.

Child health surveillance

In the UK, the Healthy Child Programme spans from pregnancy to 19 years of age (Table 3.2), but the main emphasis is on ages 0–5 years.

Table 3.2 Overview of the Healthy Child Programme in UK provided by integrated local services

Age	0–2 y	2–10 y	10–19 y
Screening	Antenatal health promoting visit Newborn examination (<72 h old) Bilirubin check by 48 h if jaundiced Biochemical screening (Day 5) Repeat newborn examination (6–8 weeks)	Preschool vision and hearing screen National Child Measurement Programme (4–5 years)	National Child Measurement Programme (10–11 y)
Immunization	Hepatitis B, BCG (if at risk) Diphtheria, tetanus, pertussis, polio, Hib, PCV, rotavirus, meningococcal B and C and MMR	Children's flu, MMR Diphtheria, tetanus, pertussis, polio	Tetanus, diphtheria, polio, meningococcal ACWY, HPV (girls)
Developmental reviews	New baby review (by 14 days) 12–13-mo review	2–2½ y (Ages and Stages questionnaire) Preschool review	Health review at school transition at 10–11 y and 15–16 y (questionnaires)
Health promotion	Feeding, weaning, safety at home and in cars, passive smoke, SIDS prevention Personal child health record and *Birth to Five* book.	Nutrition, obesity prevention, injury prevention, emotional health, psychological well-being	Encourage physical activity, emotional health, psychological well-being and mental health, reduction of risk-taking behaviour, sexual health

Hib: *Haemophilus influenzae* type B; HPV: human papilloma virus; MMR: measles, mumps and rubella; PCV: pneumococcal virus; SIDS: sudden infant death syndrome.

It offers families a programme of:

- screening tests – early detection
- immunization – disease prevention
- developmental reviews
- health promotion – information and guidance to support parenting and healthy lifestyle choices.

From 0 to 5 years of age, there are a limited number of universal health visitor reviews:

- antenatal health promoting visit
- the new baby review
- 6–8-week assessment (the health visitor or family nurse-led check)
- 1-year assessment
- 2–2½-year review.

Their aim is to:

- support parents to give their child the optimal start in life and identify if families need extra help
- early identification and treatment of problems to reduce health and social care needs later in life
- review immunization status to ensure full coverage
- allow collection of specific public health data at a national level.

The programme relies on parents identifying problems with health, development, hearing and vision, rather than universal screening. Health visitor support is tailored to need, with most input reserved for families with complex needs.

Details of each review are entered into the child's personal child health record kept by parents and brought whenever the child is seen by a health professional.

> **Summary**
>
> **The child health surveillance and promotion programme**
> - Is provided in primary care.
> - Includes screening, immunization, developmental reviews and health promotion.
> - Emphasizes the role of parents in the early detection of problems with health, development, hearing and vision.

Hearing

During the later stages of pregnancy, the fetus responds to sound. At birth, a baby startles to sound, and there is a marked preference for voices. The ability to locate and turn towards sounds comes later in the first year.

Hearing tests

Newborn

Early detection and treatment of hearing impairment improves the outcome for speech and language and behaviour. In order to detect hearing impairment in the newborn period, hearing can be tested by:

- otoacoustic emission (OAE; Fig. 3.9a) – an earphone produces a sound which evokes an echo or emission from the ear if cochlear function is normal
- auditory brainstem response (ABR) audiometry (Fig. 3.9b) – computer analysis of electroencephalogram waveforms evoked in response to a series of auditory stimuli.

Universal neonatal hearing screening has been introduced in many countries. Since 2006 in the UK, OAE testing is offered as initial screening in well babies. This is often done before the child leaves the hospital after birth or within the first few weeks of life. If the test is abnormal, the infant is referred to an audiologist and ABR audiometry is carried out if necessary. Babies on the special care baby unit are usually screened with both OAE and automated ABR.

Hearing tests in older children are shown in Figs 3.10, 3.11 and 3.12.

Distraction testing

This was the mainstay of hearing screening but has been replaced by universal neonatal screening. It is now only used as a screening test for infants at 7–9 months of age who have not had newborn screening or cannot tolerate or cooperate with more complex testing. The test relies on the baby locating and turning appropriately towards sounds, but before the child develops the ability for object permanence, that is, the ability to remember that an assessor is standing behind them even without seeing them. High-frequency and low-frequency sounds are presented out of the infant's field of vision. Testing is unreliable if not carried out by properly trained staff, because it can be difficult to identify hearing-impaired infants as they are particularly adept at using non-auditory cues.

Visual reinforcement audiometry

This is particularly useful to assess hearing impairment in infants between 10 and 18 months of age, although it can be used between the ages of 6 months and 3 years. It is also used in some older children with learning disability. Hearing thresholds are established using visual rewards (illumination of toys) to reinforce the child's head turn to stimuli of different frequencies. Localisation of the stimuli is not necessary and insert earphones may be used to obtain ear-specific information, thus making it more useful than free field tests such as distraction and performance testing.

Performance and speech discrimination testing

Performance testing using high-frequency and low-frequency stimuli and speech discrimination testing

Hearing tests

Hearing screening of newborn infants

a Otoacoustic emission (OEA)

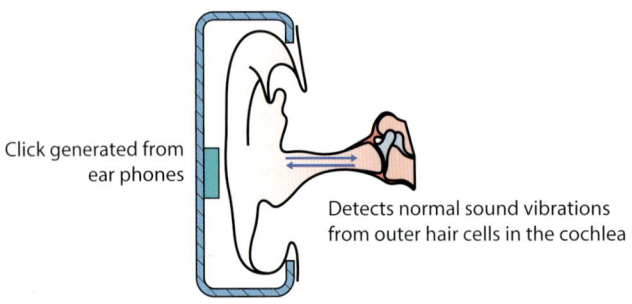

Click generated from ear phones

Detects normal sound vibrations from outer hair cells in the cochlea

Advantages:
- simple and quick to perform, though is affected by ambient noise

Disadvantages:
- misses auditory neuropathy as function of auditory nerve or brain not tested
- relatively high false-positive rate in first 24 hours after birth as vernix or amniotic fluid are still in ear canal
- not a test of hearing but a test of cochlear function

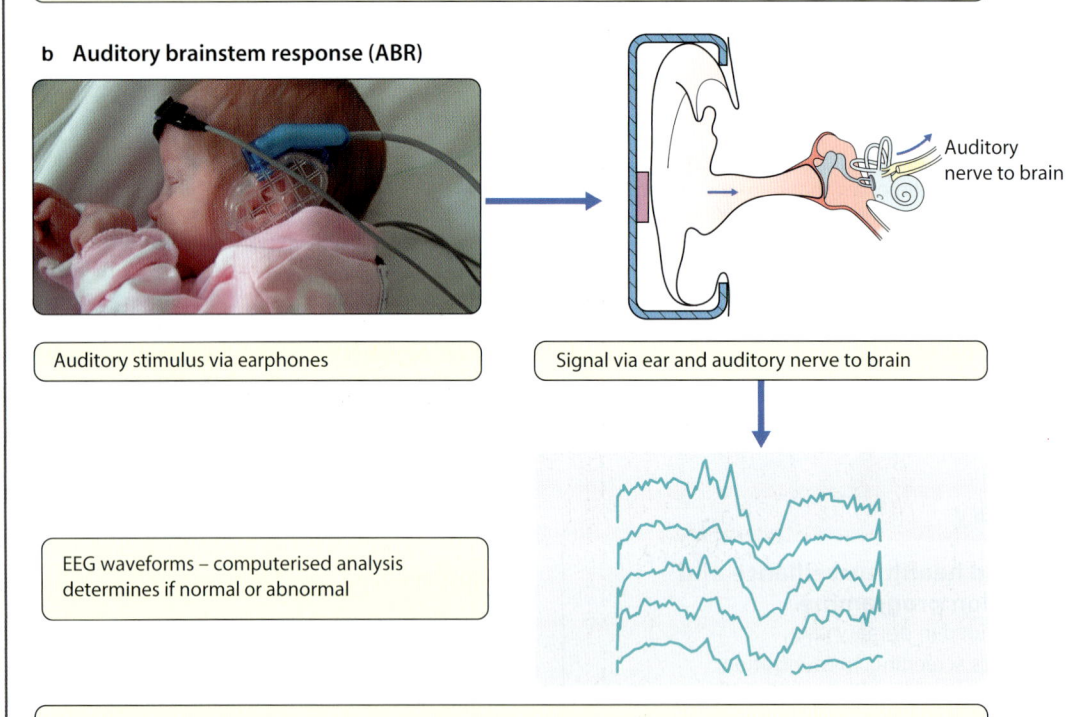

b Auditory brainstem response (ABR)

Auditory stimulus via earphones

Signal via ear and auditory nerve to brain

Auditory nerve to brain

EEG waveforms – computerised analysis determines if normal or abnormal

Advantages:
- screens hearing pathway from ear to brainstem
- low false-positive rate

Disadvantages:
- affected by movement, so infants need to be asleep or very quiet, so time consuming
- complex computerised equipment, but is mobile
- requires electrodes applied to infant's head, which parents may dislike

Figure 3.9 Universal neonatal hearing screening is usually performed using (a) otoacoustic emission testing or (b) auditory brainstem response audiometry.

Hearing tests

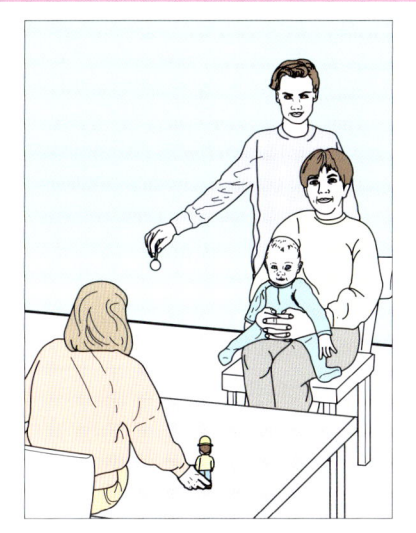

Figure 3.10 Distraction hearing test. The test is hard to perform reliably as babies with hearing difficulties learn to compensate by using shadows, smells and guesswork to locate the presenter. The test must be done by well-trained professionals.

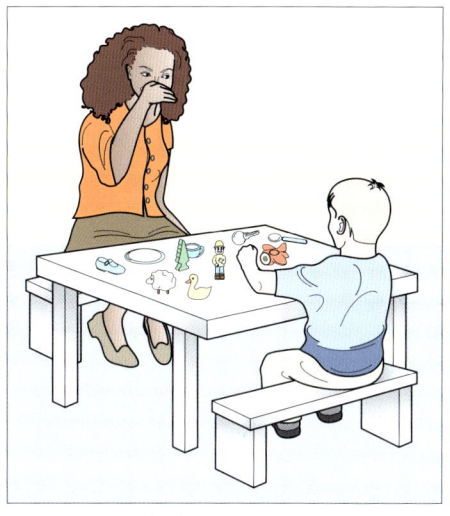

Figure 3.12 Speech discrimination testing using miniature toys to detect hearing loss in children between 18 months and 4 years of age.

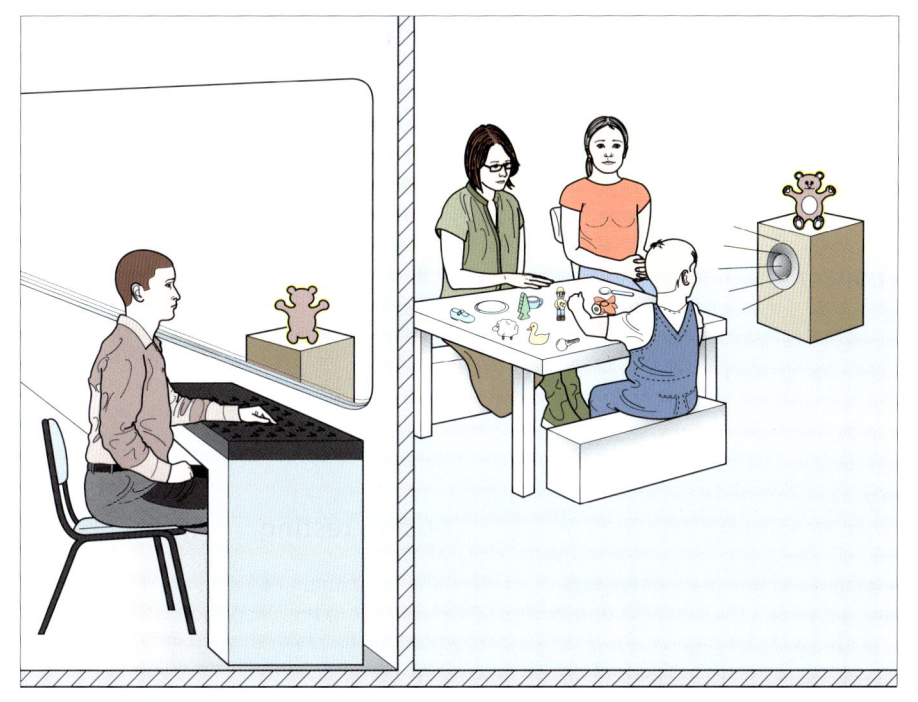

Figure 3.11 Visual reinforcement audiometry. While an assistant plays with the child, sounds of a specific frequency are emitted from a speaker. When the child turns to it, the tester lights up a toy by the speaker to reinforce the sound with a visual reward. This test is particularly useful at 10–18 months of age.

Normal child development, hearing and vision

Box 3.1 Hearing checklist for parents

Shortly after birth	Startles and blinks at a sudden noise, e.g. slamming of door
By 1 month	Notices sudden prolonged sounds, e.g. a vacuum cleaner, and pauses and listens when they begin
By 4 months	Quietens or smiles to the sound of your voice even when he/she cannot see you. May also turn the head or eyes towards you if you come up from behind and speak from the side
By 7 months	Turns immediately to your voice across the room or to very quiet noises made on each side, so long as not too occupied with other things
By 9 months	Listens attentively to familiar everyday sounds and searches for very quiet sounds made out of sight. Should also show pleasure in babbling loudly and tunefully
By 12 months	Shows some response to his/her own name and to other familiar words. May respond when you say 'no' and 'bye-bye', even when cannot see any accompanying gesture

If you suspect that your baby is not hearing normally, seek advice from your health visitor or doctor.

Used with permission from Dr Barry McCormick, Children's Hearing Assessment Centre, Nottingham, UK.

using miniature toys can be used for children with suspected hearing loss at 18 months to 4 years of age or for older children with learning disabilities.

Audiometry

Threshold audiometry using headphones, where the child responds to a pure tone stimulus, can be used to detect and assess the severity of hearing loss in children from 4 years of age.

Parental concern

At all ages, parental concern about hearing warrants further assessment. A checklist for parents of normal hearing responses during infancy is shown in Box 3.1.

> **Summary**
>
> **Hearing**
> - Early detection and treatment of hearing impairment improves the outcome of speech and language and behaviour.
> - Newborn hearing screening is performed for the early identification of hearing impairment.
> - If there is parental concern about hearing, further assessment is warranted.

Vision

A newborn infant's vision is limited; there is some visual awareness of light sources, faces and areas of high contrast. Visual acuity is low – large targets can be detected at about 30 cm distance but appear fuzzy. The peripheral retina is well developed but the fovea is immature and the optic nerve is unmyelinated. Well-focused images on the retina are required for the acquisition of visual acuity and any obstruction to this, e.g. from a cataract, will interfere with the normal development of the optic pathways and visual cortex unless corrected early in life. This type of visual loss can be permanent and is called amblyopia.

In the first few weeks of life, infants develop the capacity to maintain fixation on a moving target such as a face or dangling coloured ball, though they may have a transient squint. By 6 weeks of age most babies can perform this task. By 5 months of age a baby can fixate on a 2.5-cm block; by 12 months on a 1-mm 'hundreds-and-thousands' cake sprinkle. Clarity of vision also matures: visual acuity improves from 6/200 at birth to 6/60 at 3 months and 6/6 at 5 years of age.

Vision testing

The assessment of vision at different ages is shown in Table 3.3. In the UK, orthoptist-led screening is recommended for children aged 4–5 years to detect reduced visual acuity, primarily amblyopia.

> **Summary**
>
> **Vision**
> - Visual acuity is low at birth but gradually increases to normal adult levels by about 5 years of age.
> - Vision screening is performed at school entry or in preschool children.

Table 3.3 Testing vision at different ages[a]

Age	Test
Birth	Aware of light
	May fix and follow horizontally a face or large coloured toy
6–8 weeks	Face fixation and following large coloured toy
6 mo	Fixates 2.5-cm brick
	Visually directed reach
	Responds to preferential looking tests of acuity (e.g. Keeler or Teller cards)
12 mo	Fixates 1-mm crumb
1–2 y	Preferential looking tests of acuity (e.g. Cardiff cards)
2–3 y	Names or matches pictures in linear array (e.g. Kay pictures or Lea symbols). Distant and near
3 y +	Names or matches letters (e.g. Sonksen logMAR, or logMAR crowded). Distant and near

Note: Using single letters/pictures should not be used as these overestimate acuity and will miss significant interocular differences (i.e. miss amblyopia).
[a]At all ages: observe the child's eyes. Is eye contact established? What is the child looking at? How does the child respond to what is apparently seen?

Acknowledgements

We would like to acknowledge contributors to this chapter in previous editions, whose work we have drawn on: Angus Nicoll (1st Edition), Diane Smyth (2nd, 3rd, 4th Edition), Neil Wimalasundera (4th Edition).

Further reading

Meggitt C: *Child Development: An Illustrated Guide: Birth to 19 Years,* Harlow, 2012, Pearson Education Limited

Websites (accessed November 2016)

Birth-to-five development timeline: Available at: http://www.nhs.uk/Tools/Pages/birthtofive.aspx#close. *An interactive guide to child development, including videos*

Evidence underpinning the Healthy Child Programme 2015: Available at: https://www.gov.uk/government/publications/healthy-child-programme-rapid-review-to-update-evidence

Healthy Child Programme: Pregnancy and the first five years of life: Available at: https://www.gov.uk/government/publications/healthy-child-programme-pregnancy-and-the-first-5-years-of-life

NICE guideline 2012: *Social and emotional wellbeing: early years.* Available at: https://www.nice.org.uk/guidance/ph40

Vaccination schedule, UK: Available at: https://www.gov.uk/government/publications/the-complete-routine-immunisation-schedule

Developmental problems and the child with special needs

Abnormal development – key concepts	46	Specific learning difficulty	54
Developmental delay	47	Hearing impairment	56
Abnormal motor development	47	Abnormalities of vision and the ocular system	58
Disordered speech and language development	53	Multidisciplinary child development services	60
Abnormal development of social/communication skills (autism spectrum disorders)	53	Education	62
		Transition of care to adult services	62
Slow acquisition of cognitive skills/ general learning difficulty	54	The rights of disabled children	63

Features of developmental problems and the child with special needs are:

- developmental problems present in the perinatal period and throughout childhood
- with developmental delay, the difference with their peers increases as the child gets older
- cerebral palsy is the most common cause of motor impairment in children
- in autism spectrum disorder, there is abnormal development of social and communication skills
- attention deficit hyperactivity disorder (ADHD) needs to be differentiated from normal, boisterous children
- early detection of severe impairment of hearing or vision is important to minimize its detrimental effect on development
- their medical, social, emotional and educational requirements are complex
- are looked after by local multidisciplinary child development services.

Any child whose development is delayed or disordered needs assessment to determine the cause and management. Neurodevelopmental problems present at all ages, with an increasing number now recognized antenatally (Table 4.1). Many are identified in the neonatal period because of abnormal neurology or dysmorphic features. During infancy and early childhood, problems often present at an age when a specific area of development is most rapid and prominent (i.e. motor problems during the first 18 months of age, speech and language problems between 18 months and 3 years, and social and communication disorders between 2–4 years of age). Abnormal development may be caused not only by neurodevelopmental disorders (Table 4.2) but also by ill health or if the child's physical or psychological needs are not met. When carrying out a clinical examination on a young child with a possible developmental problem:

- ask the parent what the child's abilities are. Start at a level below what a child of that age is likely to be able to do to retain confidence of the parent and child
- *observe* the child from the first moment seen
- make it fun. The assessment should be perceived as a game by the child
- toys to use are cubes, a ball, car, doll, pencil, paper, pegboard, miniature toys, picture book. Adapt their use to the child
- formulate a developmental picture in terms of gross motor; vision and fine motor; hearing, speech and language; and social, emotional and

Table 4.1 Features that may suggest neurodevelopmental concerns by age

Prenatal	Positive family history, e.g. affected siblings or family members; ethnicity, e.g. Tay–Sachs disease in Jewish parents
	Antenatal screening tests, e.g. ultrasound including nuchal thickness, triple blood test or non-invasive prenatal testing (NIPT, cell-free DNA testing of fetal cells from maternal blood) for conditions such as Down syndrome; neural tube defects, e.g. spina bifida and hydrocephalus. Amniocentesis for suspected genetic disorders
Perinatal	Following birth asphyxia/neonatal encephalopathy
	Preterm infants with intraventricular haemorrhage/periventricular leucomalacia, post-haemorrhagic hydrocephalus
	Dysmorphic and neurocutaneous features
	Abnormal neurological behaviour – tone, feeding, movement, seizures, visual inattention
Infancy	Global developmental delay
	Delayed or asymmetric motor development
	Neurocutaneous and dysmorphic features (cataracts)
	Vision or hearing concerns by parents or after screening
Preschool	Speech and language delay
	Abnormal gait, clumsy motor skills
	Poor social communication skills
	Behaviour – stereotypical, overactivity, inattention
School age	Problems with balance and coordination
	Learning difficulties
	Attention control
	Hyperactivity
	Specific learning difficulties, e.g. dyslexia, dyspraxia
	Social communication difficulties
Any age	Acquired brain injury, e.g. after meningitis, head injury
	Loss of skills

behaviour. As you become more confident, you will screen all these skills simultaneously
- assess the child to a short level above what they appear able to do in order to establish their ceiling of skill for each developmental area
- remember to adjust developmental expectations for prematurity
- at the end of developmental screening you should be able to describe what a child is able to do and what the child cannot do, if the abilities are within normal limits for age and, if not, which developmental fields are outside the normal range
- clinical signs to look for that may aid diagnosis or guide investigation are:
  - patterns of growth: height, weight, head circumference with centile plotting
  - dysmorphic features: face, limbs, body proportions, cardiac, genitalia
  - skin: neurocutaneous stigmata, injuries, cleanliness
  - central nervous system examination: abnormal posture/symmetry, wasting, tone and power, deep tendon reflexes, clonus, plantar responses, cranial nerves
  - cardiovascular examination: abnormalities are associated with many dysmorphic syndromes
  - visual function and ocular abnormalities
  - hearing: by questioning parents about hearing and language development and checking if neonatal hearing screening was done
  - patterns of mobility, dexterity, hand dominance, communication and social skills, general behaviour
  - cognition.

Many examination findings can be predicted from *observation* of functional skills and behaviour.

Many parental concerns about their child's development are found to be variations of normal, in which case the parents should be reassured. If in doubt, observe the child's progress over a period of time.

Table 4.2 Conditions that cause abnormal development and learning difficulty

Prenatal		
	Genetic	Chromosome/DNA disorders, e.g. Down syndrome, fragile X syndrome, chromosome microdeletions or duplications
		Cerebral dysgenesis, e.g. microcephaly, absent corpus callosum, hydrocephalus, neuronal migration disorder
	Cerebrovascular	Stroke – haemorrhagic or ischaemic
	Metabolic	Hypothyroidism, phenylketonuria
	Teratogenic	Alcohol and drug abuse
	Congenital infection	Rubella, cytomegalovirus, toxoplasmosis, HIV
	Neurocutaneous syndromes	Tuberous sclerosis, neurofibromatosis, Sturge–Weber, Ito syndrome
Perinatal		
	Extreme prematurity	Intraventricular haemorrhage/periventricular leucomalacia
	Birth asphyxia	Hypoxic-ischaemic encephalopathy
	Metabolic	Symptomatic hypoglycaemia, hyperbilirubinemia
Postnatal		
	Infection	Meningitis, encephalitis
	Anoxia	Suffocation, near drowning, seizures
	Trauma	Head injury – accidental or non-accidental
	Metabolic	Hypoglycaemia, inborn errors of metabolism.
	Cerebrovascular	Stroke
	Nutritional deficiency	Maternal deficiency (breast fed), food intolerances, restrictions
Other		
Unknown (about 25%): chronic illness, physical abuse, emotional neglect		

Note: The site and severity of brain damage influence the clinical outcome, i.e. whether specific or global developmental delay, learning and/or physical disability.

Abnormal development – key concepts

The terminology can be confusing, but:

- *delay* – implies slow acquisition of all skills (global delay) or of one particular field or area of skill (specific delay), particularly in relation to developmental problems in the 0–5-year age group
- *learning difficulty* – used in relation to children of school age and may be cognitive, physical, both, or relate to specific functional skills
- *disorder* – maldevelopment of a skill.

The following are agreed definitions:

- *impairment* – loss or abnormality of physiological function or anatomical structure
- *disability* – any restriction or lack of ability due to the impairment
- *disadvantage* – this results from the disability, and limits or prevents fulfilment of a normal role. It is situationally specific; a child with a learning disability may, for example, be a good skier or enjoy swimming.

The term 'handicap' is now discouraged as it can imply a person deserves pity. Difficulty and disability are often used interchangeably, but difficulty is used particularly in an educational context. Impairment is now generally used instead of disability when describing problems such as visual impairment or hearing impairment.

The *pattern* of abnormal development (global or specific) can be categorized as (Fig. 4.1):

- slow but steady
- plateau effect
- showing regression
  - acute regression following acute brain injury with subsequent slow recovery but not to normal levels (partial recovery) or slow regression as with neurodegenerative disorders.

The *severity* can be categorized as:

- mild
- moderate

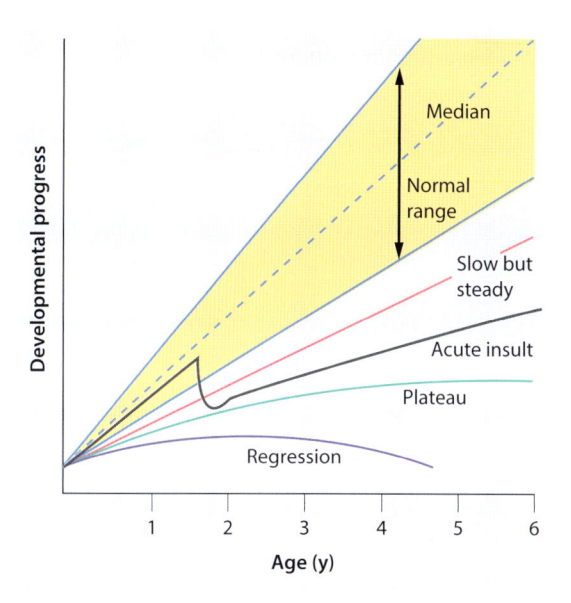

Figure 4.1 Patterns of abnormal development. These may be slow but steady, plateau, regression. They may follow an acute injury.

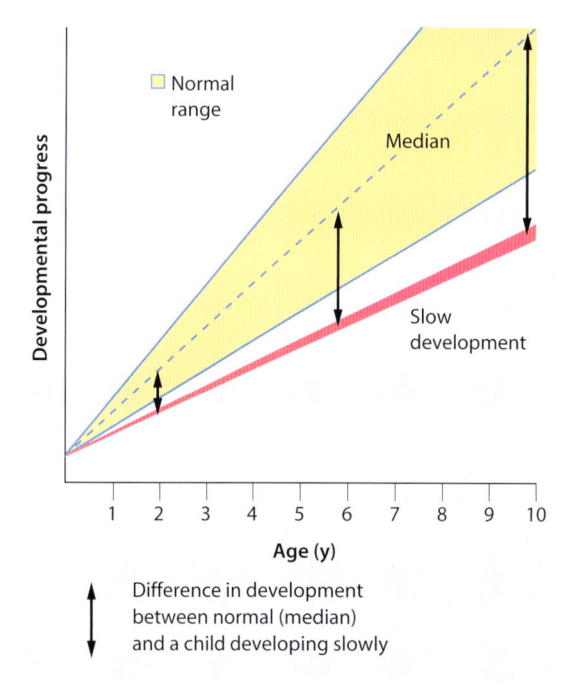

Figure 4.2 For children with abnormal development, the gap between their abilities and what is normal widens with age.

- severe
- profound.

Other features of developmental delay are:
- the gap between normal and abnormal development becomes greater with increasing age, and therefore becomes more apparent over time (Fig. 4.2)

- it may be the presentation of a wide variety of underlying conditions (Table 4.2)
- the site and severity of brain damage influences the clinical outcome, i.e. whether there will be specific or global developmental delay, learning and/or physical disability
- it may be genetic, with important implications for the family
- there is a wide age band across which it can be normal to achieve a developmental skill
- limit ages denote beyond the normal range.

The choice of investigations to identify the cause is influenced by the child's age, the history and clinical findings (Table 4.3). In some children, no cause can be identified even after extensive investigation.

Summary

Disordered development
- Incorporates global and specific delay or disorder, learning difficulty, impairment and disability.
- Varies in pattern of progression and severity.
- Becomes more apparent with age.

Developmental delay

Global developmental delay (also called early developmental impairment) implies delay in acquisition of all skill fields (gross motor, vision and fine motor, hearing and speech, language and cognition, social/emotional and behaviour). It usually becomes apparent in the first 2 years of life. Global developmental delay is likely to be associated with cognitive difficulties, although these may only become apparent several years later. The presence of global developmental delay should always generate investigation into a possible cause such as those listed in Table 4.2. When children become older and the clinical picture is clearer, it is more appropriate to describe the individual difficulties such as learning disability, motor disorder and communication difficulty, rather than using the term global developmental delay.

Specific developmental impairment is when one field of development or skill area is more delayed than others. It may also be developing in a disordered way.

☀ Global developmental delay usually presents in the first 2 years of life.

Abnormal motor development

This may present as a delay in acquisition of motor skills, e.g. head control, rolling, sitting, standing, walking or as problems with balance, an abnormal gait, asymmetry of hand use, involuntary movements or rarely loss of motor skills. Concern about motor

Table 4.3 Investigations or assessment to consider for developmental delay

Cytogenetic	Comparative genomic hybridization microarray or chromosome karyotype[a]
	Fragile X analysis[a]
	DNA fluorescence in situ hybridization analysis, e.g. for chromosome 7, 15, and 22 deletions; telomere screening; whole-exome sequencing
Metabolic	Thyroid function tests, liver function tests, bone chemistry, urea and electrolytes, plasma amino acids[a], blood film
	Creatine kinase, blood lactate, very long-chain fatty acids, ammonia, blood gases, white cell (lysosomal) enzymes, urine amino and organic acids, urine mucopolysaccharides (GAG), and oligosaccharide screen, urine reducing substances, lead levels, urate, ferritin, biotinidase, vitamin B6 and B12
	Maternal amino acids for raised phenylalanine
Infection	Congenital infection screen for cytomegalovirus, etc.
Imaging	Cranial ultrasound in newborn
	CT and MRI brain scans
	Skeletal survey, bone age
Neurophysiology	EEG – for seizures and can be diagnostic for specific neurological disorders and syndromes
	Nerve conduction studies, electromyogram, visual evoked potentials, electroretinogram
Histopathology/ histochemistry	Nerve, skin and muscle biopsy
Other	Hearing[a]
	Vision[a]
	Clinical genetics
	Cognitive and behavioural assessment (clinical and educational psychologist)
	Therapy assessment – physiotherapy, occupational therapy, speech and language therapy
	Child psychiatry
	Dietician
	Nursery/school reports[a]

[a]Basic screening tests.

development usually presents between 3 months–2 years of age when acquisition of motor skills is occurring most rapidly. Examination may reveal underlying abnormal motor signs.

Causes of abnormal motor development include:

- central motor deficit, e.g. cerebral palsy (CP)
- congenital myopathy/primary muscle disease
- spinal cord lesions, e.g. spina bifida
- global developmental delay, as in many syndromes, or of unidentified cause.

As hand dominance is not acquired until 1–2 years of age or later, asymmetry of motor skills during the first year of life is always abnormal and may suggest an underlying hemiplegia.

Late walking (>18 months old) may be caused by any of the aforementioned causes but also needs to be differentiated from children who display the normal locomotor variants of bottom-shuffling or commando crawling (see Ch. 3) where walking occurs later than with crawlers, and from children with joint hypermobility who may also achieve walking later than average.

Concern about abnormal motor development needs assessment by a neurodevelopmental paediatrician and physiotherapist. Ongoing physiotherapy input and subsequent involvement of an occupational therapist are also likely to be needed.

Cerebral palsy

CP is difficult to define, but the international group for Surveillance of Cerebral Palsy in Europe defines it as an umbrella term for a permanent disorder of movement and/or posture and of motor function due to a non-progressive abnormality in the developing brain.

The motor disorders of CP are often accompanied by disturbances of cognition, communication, vision, perception, sensation, behaviour, seizure disorder and secondary musculoskeletal problems. Although the causative lesion is non-progressive and damage to the brain is static, clinical manifestations emerge over time, reflecting the balance between normal and abnormal cerebral maturation. Motor dysfunction is usually evident early, often from birth. If the brain injury occurs after the age of 2 years, it is diagnosed as acquired brain injury.

CP is the most common cause of motor impairment in children, affecting about 2 per 1000 live births.

Causes

About 80% of CP is antenatal in origin due to cerebrovascular haemorrhage or ischaemia, cortical migration disorders or structural maldevelopment of the brain during gestation. Some of these problems are linked to gene deletions. Other antenatal causes are genetic syndromes and congenital infection.

Only about 10% of cases are thought to be due to hypoxic-ischaemic injury before or during delivery and this proportion has remained relatively constant over the last decade. About 10% are postnatal in origin.

Preterm infants are especially vulnerable to brain damage from periventricular leukomalacia secondary to ischaemia and/or severe intraventricular haemorrhage and venous infarction. The improved survival of extremely preterm infants has been accompanied by an increase in survivors with CP, although the number of such children is relatively small.

Postnatal causes are meningitis/encephalitis/encephalopathy, head trauma from accidental or non-accidental injury, symptomatic hypoglycaemia, hydrocephalus and hyperbilirubinemia.

MRI brain scans may assist in identifying the cause of the CP, in directing further investigations and in supporting explanations to the parents, but is not required to make the diagnosis.

Clinical presentation

Many children who develop CP will have been identified as being at risk in the neonatal period. Early features of CP are:

- abnormal limb and/or trunk posture and tone in infancy with delayed motor milestones (Fig. 4.3); this may be accompanied by slowing of head growth
- feeding difficulties, with oromotor incoordination, slow feeding, gagging and vomiting
- abnormal gait once walking is achieved
- asymmetric hand function before 12 months of age.

In CP, primitive reflexes, which facilitate the emergence of normal patterns of movement and which need to disappear for motor development to progress, may persist and become obligatory (see Ch. 3).

The diagnosis is made by clinical examination, with particular attention to assessment of posture and the pattern of tone in the limbs and trunk, hand function and gait.

Table 4.4 Gross motor function classification system (GMFCS)

Level	
Level I	Walks without limitations
Level II	Walks with limitations
Level III	Walks using a handheld mobility device
Level IV	Self-mobility with limitations; may use powered mobility
Level V	Transported in a manual wheelchair

Note: See http://www.canchild.ca/en/measures/gmfcs.asp for further details.

CP is now categorized according to neurological features as:

- spastic: bilateral, unilateral, not otherwise specified (90%)
- dyskinetic (6%)
- ataxic (4%)
- other.

The gross motor function level (functional ability) is described using the Gross Motor Function Classification System (Table 4.4).

In the past, the description was based on the parts of the body affected (hemiplegia, quadriplegia, diplegia).

For children with high-risk factors for brain damage such as significant prematurity or those with difficulties around the time of birth, a formal standardized assessment of general movements may identify at a very young age those at greater risk of developing CP. It is a specialized assessment usually performed by a trained therapist or clinician.

Spastic cerebral palsy

In this type, there is damage to the upper motor neurone (pyramidal or corticospinal tract) pathway. Limb tone is persistently increased (spasticity) with associated brisk deep tendon reflexes and extensor plantar responses. The tone in spasticity is velocity dependent, so the faster the muscle is stretched the greater the resistance it will have. This elicits a dynamic catch, which is the hallmark of spasticity. The increased limb tone may suddenly yield under pressure in a 'clasp knife' fashion. Limb involvement is increasingly described as unilateral or bilateral to acknowledge asymmetrical signs. Spasticity tends to present early and may even be seen in the neonatal period. Sometimes there is initial hypotonia, particularly of the head and trunk. There are three main types of spastic CP:

- unilateral (*hemiplegia*) – unilateral involvement of the arm and leg. The arm is usually affected more than the leg, with the face spared. Affected children often present at 4–12 months of age with fisting of the affected hand, a flexed arm, a pronated forearm, asymmetric reaching, hand function or toe pointing when lifting the child. Subsequently, a tiptoe walk (toe–heel gait) on the affected side may become evident. Affected limbs may initially be flaccid and hypotonic, but

Normal and abnormal motor development

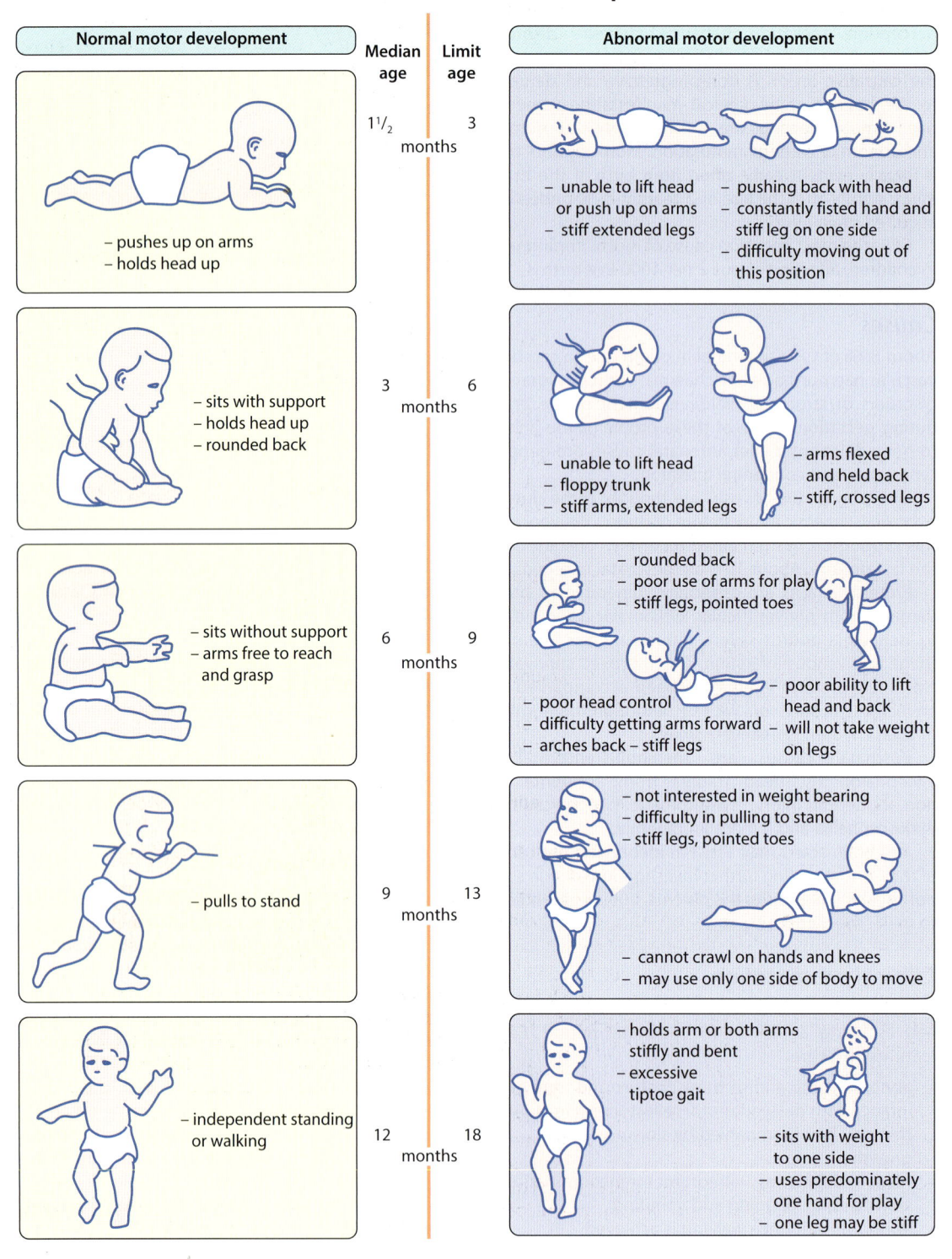

Normal motor development	Median age	Limit age	Abnormal motor development
– pushes up on arms – holds head up	1½ months	3 months	– unable to lift head or push up on arms – stiff extended legs – pushing back with head – constantly fisted hand and stiff leg on one side – difficulty moving out of this position
– sits with support – holds head up – rounded back	3 months	6 months	– unable to lift head – floppy trunk – stiff arms, extended legs – arms flexed and held back – stiff, crossed legs
– sits without support – arms free to reach and grasp	6 months	9 months	– rounded back – poor use of arms for play – stiff legs, pointed toes – poor head control – difficulty getting arms forward – arches back – stiff legs – poor ability to lift head and back – will not take weight on legs
– pulls to stand	9 months	13 months	– not interested in weight bearing – difficulty in pulling to stand – stiff legs, pointed toes – cannot crawl on hands and knees – may use only one side of body to move
– independent standing or walking	12 months	18 months	– holds arm or both arms stiffly and bent – excessive tiptoe gait – sits with weight to one side – uses predominately one hand for play – one leg may be stiff

Figure 4.3 Normal motor milestones and patterns of abnormal motor development. Cerebral palsy (hemiplegia or quadriplegia) is the most common cause of developmental problems. (Adapted from Pathways Awareness Foundation, Chicago, IL.; see also https://pathways.org/)

increased tone soon emerges as the predominant sign. The medical history may be normal, with an unremarkable birth history and no evidence of hypoxic-ischaemic encephalopathy giving rise to the possibility of a prenatal cause, which is often silent. In some children, the condition is caused by neonatal stroke. More severe vascular insults may cause a hemianopia (loss of half of visual field) of the same side as the affected limbs

- bilateral (*quadriplegia*) – all four limbs are affected, often severely. The trunk is involved with a tendency to opisthotonus (extensor posturing), poor head control and low central tone (Fig. 4.4). This more severe form of CP is often associated with seizures, microcephaly and moderate or severe intellectual impairment. There may have been a history of perinatal hypoxic-ischaemic encephalopathy
- bilateral (*diplegia*) – all four limbs, but the legs are affected to a much greater degree than the arms, so that hand function may appear to be relatively normal. Motor difficulties in the arms are most apparent with functional use of the hands. Walking is abnormal. Diplegia is one of the patterns associated with preterm birth due to periventricular brain damage. The MRI brain scan may show periventricular leukomalacia.

Dyskinetic cerebral palsy

Dyskinesia refers to movements that are involuntary, uncontrolled, occasionally stereotyped and often more evident with active movement or stress. Muscle tone is variable and primitive motor reflex patterns predominate. May be described as:

- chorea – irregular, sudden and brief non-repetitive movements
- athetosis – slow writhing movements occurring more distally such as fanning of the fingers
- dystonia – simultaneous contraction of agonist and antagonist muscles of the trunk and proximal muscles often giving a twisting appearance.

Intellect may be relatively unimpaired. Affected children often present with floppiness, poor trunk control and delayed motor development in infancy. Abnormal movements may only appear towards the end of the first year of life. The signs are due to damage or dysfunction in the basal ganglia or their associated pathways (extra-pyramidal). In the past, the most common cause was hyperbilirubinemia (kernicterus) due to rhesus disease of the newborn but it is now hypoxic-ischaemic encephalopathy at term. The MRI brain scan will often show bilateral changes predominantly in the basal ganglia.

Ataxic (hypotonic) cerebral palsy

Most are genetically determined. When due to acquired brain injury (cerebellum or its connections), the signs occur on the same side as the lesion but are usually relatively symmetrical. There is early trunk and limb hypotonia, poor balance and delayed motor development. Incoordinate movements, intention tremor and an ataxic gait may be evident later.

The different types of CP are summarized in Fig. 4.5.

Management

Parents should be given details of the diagnosis as early as possible, but prognosis is difficult during infancy until the severity and pattern of evolving signs and the child's developmental progress have become clearer over several months or years of life. Children with CP are likely to have a wide range of associated medical, psychological and social problems, making it essential to adopt a multidisciplinary approach to assessment and management, as described later in this chapter.

There are recently developed novel treatments for treating hypertonia in CP such as botulinum toxin injections to muscles, selective dorsal rhizotomy (a proportion of the nerve roots in the spinal cord are selectively cut to reduce spasticity), intrathecal baclofen (a skeletal muscle relaxant) and deep brain stimulation of the basal ganglia.

Cerebral palsy

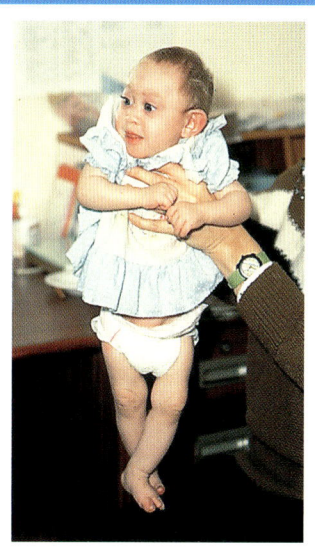

Figure 4.4 An infant with spastic bilateral (quadriplegia) cerebral palsy showing scissoring of the legs from excessive adduction of the hips, pronated forearms and 'fisted' hands.

Summary

Cerebral palsy

- Has many causes. Only about 10% follow hypoxic-ischaemic encephalopathy.
- Usually presents in infancy with abnormal tone and posture, delayed motor milestones and feeding difficulties.
- May be spastic, dyskinetic, ataxic, or a mixed pattern.

Summary

Patterns of cerebral palsy

Type of cerebral palsy	Aetiology	Clinical features
Unilateral cerebral palsy (hemiplegia) Spastic or dystonic	Often due to perinatal middle cerebral artery infarct	Spastic or dystonic tone, one side of body affected (opposite to the side of the brain lesion) Arm often more affected than leg May have visual field defect on side of hemiplegia Risk of learning difficulties and seizures Often GMFCS level 1 and 2
Bilateral spastic cerebral palsy (diplegia)	Damage to the periventricular areas of developing brain often associated with prematurity. Leg motor fibres from the homunculus are closest to the ventricles, so legs more affected than arms.	Young child – pattern with walking on their toes with scissoring of the legs. 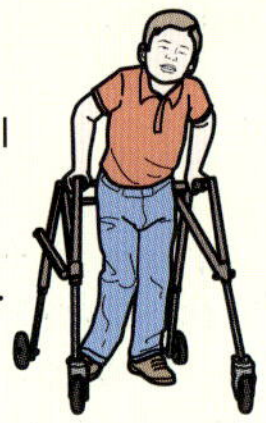 Older child – crouch gait pattern is typical when the child gets heavier and can't remain on their toes. Predominantly affects legs. Arms may be subtly affected (supination, fine motor control). Spasticity is main motor type. Usually no feeding or communication difficulties and good cognition. Often associated with squints. Frequently GMFCS level 1–3
Bilateral spastic cerebral palsy (quadriplegia, 4 limb pattern)	Extensive damage to the periventricular areas of the developing brain, including cortex.	Both arm and leg involvement – predominantly spastic but dystonia often also present. Associated with learning difficulty, feeding difficulties, problems with speech, vision and hearing. Seizures common. At increased risk of hip subluxation and dislocation and scoliosis. Usually dependent on others for activities of daily living Powered mobility a common requirement. Often GMFCS levels 4 and 5.
Dyskinetic cerebral palsy (dystonia, athetosis, chorea)	Perinatal asphyxia – particularly affecting the basal ganglia. Also kernicterus, but this is now rare.	Typical dystonic pattern with open mouth posture and internal rotation and extension of the arms. 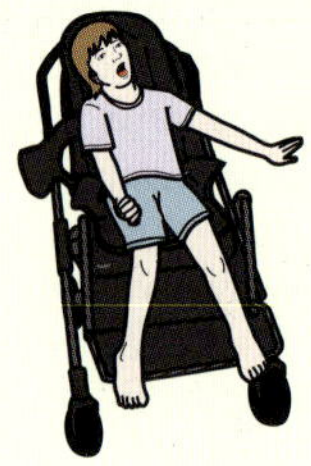 Mixture of motor patterns including dystonia, athetosis and chorea. Cognition may be preserved but feeding difficulties are common. Risk of hip deformity and scoliosis. Many are dependent on others for activities of daily living due to their severe movement difficulties even if cognitively normal. Usually GMFCS level 4–5.

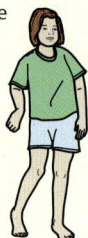

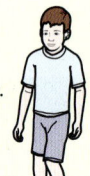

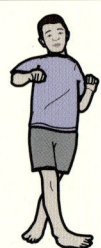

Figure 4.5 The different types of cerebral palsy.

Disordered speech and language development

A child may have a deficit in either receptive or expressive speech and language, or both. The deficit may be a delay or a disorder.

Speech and language *delay* may be due to:

- hearing loss
- global developmental delay
- difficulty in speech production from an anatomical deficit, e.g. cleft palate, or oromotor incoordination, e.g. CP
- environmental deprivation/lack of opportunity for social interaction
- normal variant/familial pattern.

Speech and language *disorders* include disorders of:

- language comprehension
- language expression – inability or difficulty in producing speech whilst knowing what is needing to be said
- intelligibility and speech production such as stammering (dysfluency), dysarthria or verbal dyspraxia
- pragmatics (difference between sentence meaning and speaker's meaning), construction of sentences, semantics, grammar
- social/communication skills (autistic spectrum disorder).

Speech and language problems are usually first suspected by parents or primary healthcare professionals. A hearing test and assessment by a speech and language therapist are the initial steps. In early years, there is considerable overlap between language and cognitive (intellectual) development. Involvement of a neurodevelopmental paediatrician and paediatric audiological physician is indicated. Speech and language therapy may be provided on a continuous, burst or review basis. The speech therapist may promote alternative methods of communication such as signing (with Makaton or the Picture Exchange Communication System). Special schooling (usually language units attached to a mainstream primary school) is available but only appropriate for a very few. Many children with early speech and language problems will need learning support at school entry.

There are many tests of language development. These include:

- the Symbolic Toy test, which assesses very early language development
- the Reynell test for receptive and expressive language, used for preschool children.

Abnormal development of social/communication skills (autism spectrum disorders)

Children who fail to acquire normal social and communication skills may have an autism spectrum disorder. The prevalence of autism spectrum disorder is 3–6 per 1000 live births. The worldwide prevalence is estimated to be 7.6 per 1000 persons. It is more common in boys. Presentation is usually between 2–4 years of age when language and social skills normally rapidly expand. The child presents with a triad of difficulties and associated comorbidities (Box 4.1).

Where only some of the behaviours are present, the child may be described as having autistic features but not the full spectrum.

Asperger syndrome refers to a child with the social impairments of an autism spectrum disorder but at the milder end, and near-normal speech development. Such children still have major difficulties with the give-and-take of ordinary social encounters, a stilted way

Box 4.1 Features of autism spectrum disorders

Impaired social interaction:

- does not seek comfort, share pleasure, form close friendships
- prefers own company, no interest or ability in interacting with peers (play or emotions)
- gaze avoidance
- lack of joint attention
- socially and emotionally inappropriate behaviour
- does not appreciate that others have thoughts and feelings
- lack of appreciation of social cues.

Speech and language disorder:

- delayed development, may be severe
- limited use of gestures and facial expression
- formal pedantic language, monotonous voice
- impaired comprehension with over-literal interpretation of speech
- echoes questions, repeats instructions, refers to self as 'you'
- can have superficially good expressive speech.

Imposition of routines with ritualistic and repetitive behaviour:

- on self and others, with violent temper tantrums if disrupted
- unusual stereotypical movements such as hand flapping and tiptoe gait
- concrete play
- poverty of imagination in play and general activities
- peculiar interests and repetitive adherence
- restriction in behaviour repertoire.

Comorbidities:

- general learning and attention difficulties (about two-thirds)
- seizures (about one-quarter, often not until adolescence)
- affective disorders – anxiety, sleep disturbance
- mental health disorders – attention deficit hyperactivity disorder.

of speaking and narrow, unusual and often intense interests which they do not share with others, and are often clumsy. In reality, autism spectrum disorders are a continuum of behavioural states ranging from the severe form of autism with or without severe learning difficulties to the milder Asperger syndrome, or to autistic features occurring secondary to other clinical problems.

Autism spectrum disorders are diagnosed by assessing for specific features and seeing if they meet a specific threshold according to the Diagnostic and Statistical manual in the US (DSM5) or International Classification of Diseases. For DSM5 diagnoses, terminologies such as Asperger syndrome and autistic disorder are no longer used, and these are replaced by the term autism spectrum disorder with a description of the particular strengths and difficulties of the child.

Autism is diagnosed by observation of behaviour, including the use of formal standardized tests (Autism Diagnostic Interview, Autism Diagnostic Observation Schedule, and Diagnostic Interview for Social and Communication Disorders). It may arise as the result of different organic processes but in many cases no specific cause can be identified. There is probably multiple aetiology with a genetic component in at least some children. The condition is not the result of emotional trauma or deviant parenting. There is no evidence for a suggested link with the measles, mumps and rubella vaccine.

Management

The condition has lifelong consequences of varying degree for the child's social/communication and learning skills. Parents need a great deal of support. They often feel initial guilt that they did not recognize the problem earlier. A wide range of interventions have been promoted over the last 10 years but with little evidence except for applied behavioural analysis, a behaviour modification approach that helps to reduce ritualistic behaviour, develop language, social skills and play, and to generalize use of all these skills. It is currently the most widely accepted treatment approach but requires 25–30 hours of individual therapy each week, so is costly and time consuming. An appropriate educational placement needs to be sought. Some schools incorporate an applied behavioural analysis approach into their teaching methods. Fewer than 10% of children with autism are able to function independently as adults.

> **Autism spectrum disorder:**
> - Presents at 2–4 years of age with impaired social interaction, speech and language disorder and imposition of routines with ritualistic and repetitive behaviour.
> - Usually managed by behaviour modification such as applied behavioural analysis.

Slow acquisition of cognitive skills/general learning difficulty

The term 'learning difficulty or disability' (reflecting cognitive learning difficulties) is now preferred to 'mental retardation' or 'mental handicap'. Medical and educational classification of intelligence quotients (IQs) can be different, with medical models having lower ranges. The educational levels briefed in the following section are useful for general use.

Children with borderline and mild (IQ 70–80) learning difficulties are usually supported by additional helpers (learning support assistants) in mainstream schools, whereas children with moderate (IQ 50–70), severe (IQ 35–50), and profound (IQ < 35) learning difficulties are likely to need the resources of special schools.

Severe or profound learning difficulties are usually apparent from infancy as marked global developmental delay, whereas moderate learning difficulties emerge only as delay in speech and language becomes apparent. Mild learning difficulties may only become apparent when the child starts school or much later.

A child with profound learning difficulties will have no significant language and be completely dependent for all of his/her needs. A child with severe learning difficulties is likely to be able to learn minimal self-care skills and acquire simple speech and language. Both will need high or total supervision and support throughout life.

The prevalence of severe learning difficulty is about 3–4 per 1000 children. Most have an organic cause irrespective of social class, in contrast to moderate learning difficulty (30 per 1000 children) in which children of parents from lower socioeconomic classes are over-represented.

Common causes of developmental delay and learning difficulty are listed in Table 4.2.

Specific learning difficulty

Specific learning difficulty implies that the skill described is more delayed than would be expected for the child's level of cognitive ability. Some examples are described below.

Developmental coordination disorder or dyspraxia

Developmental coordination disorder (developmental dyspraxia) is a disorder of motor planning and/or execution with no significant findings on standard neurological examinations. It is a disorder of the higher cortical processes and there may be associated problems of perception (how the child interprets what he/she sees and hears), use of language and putting thoughts together.

The difficulties may impact on educational progress and self-esteem and suggest the child has greater academic difficulties than may be the case. Features include problems with:

- handwriting, which is typically awkward, messy, slow, irregular and poorly spaced
- dressing (buttons, laces, clothes)
- cutting up food
- poorly established laterality
- copying and drawing
- messy eating from difficulty in coordinating biting, chewing, and swallowing (oromotor dyspraxia). Dribbling of saliva is common.

Assessment and advice are primarily from an occupational therapist and when necessary a speech and language therapist (oromotor skills/speech). A visual assessment may also be helpful. Dyspraxia in its milder form often goes undetected during the first few years of life as the child achieves gross motor milestones at the normal times. With therapy (emphasis on sensory integration, sequencing, executive planning, and where needed speech/language therapy) and maturity, the condition should improve. Verbal dyspraxia is where there are more specific difficulties related to speech production in the absence of muscle or nerve damage. It is considered part of developmental dyspraxia.

Dyslexia

Dyslexia is a disorder of reading skills disproportionate to the child's IQ. The term is often used when the child's reading age is more than 2 years behind his/her chronological age. Assessment needs to include vision and hearing and involves an educational psychologist.

Dyscalculia, dysgraphia

These are disorders in the development of calculation or writing skills.

Disorder of executive functions

Executive functions are a collection of cognitive processes that are responsible for activities such as planning and organization self-regulation, cognitive flexibility, problem solving and abstract reasoning. They are very necessary to function and interact within one's social environment. Deficits in executive function can occur as a consequence of acquired brain injury such as those following hypoxia, infection, stroke or trauma. Executive dysfunction may manifest as poor concentration, forgetfulness, volatile mood, overeating and poor social skills.

Associated comorbidities of specific learning disorders

These are:
- attention deficit disorder
- hyperactivity
- sensory processing disorder (poor sensory integration skills of touch, balance)
- depression, conduct disorders, obsessive compulsive disorder.

Management of specific learning disorders

Assessment may include vision and hearing and assessment by an occupational therapist, physiotherapist, speech and language therapist and educational psychologist. Comorbidities need to be identified. Treatment is aimed at improving skill acquisition, with educational and information technology support as appropriate.

Problems with concentration and attention

Attention deficit hyperactivity disorder

Young children are characteristically lively, some more than others, by virtue of their immaturity. When their level of motor activity exceeds that regarded as normal, they may be termed 'hyperactive' by their parents. This is a judgement that depends upon the parents' standards and expectations. The term can thus incorrectly be used as a complaint about a child who is normally active in overall terms but who can be cheeky and boisterous at times. Such a child is *not* hyperactive, but the parents need advice about how to handle unwanted behaviour.

In the true *hyperkinetic disorder* or *attention deficit hyperactivity disorder* (ADHD), the child is undoubtedly overactive in most situations and has impaired concentration with a short attention span or distractibility. Differences in diagnostic criteria and threshold mean that prevalence rates among prepubertal schoolchildren are variously estimated as between 10–50 per 1000 children, with boys exceeding girls three-fold. There is a powerful genetic predisposition and the underlying problem is a dysfunction of brain neuron circuits that rely on dopamine as a neurotransmitter and which control self-monitoring and self-regulation.

Affected children are unable to sustain attention or persist with tasks. They cannot control their impulses – they manifest disorganized, poorly regulated and excessive activity; have difficulty with taking turns or sharing; are socially disinhibited; and butt into other people's conversations and play. Their inattention and hyperactivity are worst in familiar or uninteresting situations. They also cannot regulate their activity according to the situation – they are fidgety; have excessive movements inappropriate to task completion; lose possessions; and are generally disorganized. Typically, they have short tempers and form poor relationships with other children, who find them exasperating.

The children do poorly in school and lose self-esteem. They may drift into antisocial activities for a variety of reasons, partly because their behaviour drives parents, teachers and peers to use coercion and punishment, which are ineffectual or breed resentment.

In addition to child psychiatric or paediatric evaluation, the child will usually need to be assessed by an educational psychologist.

First-line management in preschool children and school-aged children with mild-to-moderately severe disorder is the active promotion of behavioural and educational progress by offering specific advice to parents and teachers to build concentration skills, encourage quiet self-occupation, increase self-esteem and how to moderate extreme behaviour. Behavioural interventions similar to those embedded in parenting programmes are helpful. These involve having clear rules and expectations and consistent use of rewards to encourage adherence and where appropriate, consequences to discourage unacceptable behaviour.

For those children in whom this is insufficient, hyperactivity responds symptomatically to several types of medication, although this is usually reserved for children older than 6 years of age. Stimulants, such as methylphenidate or dexamphetamine, and non-stimulants, such as atomoxetine, reduce excessive motor activity and improve attention on task and focused behaviour. The usual approach is not to put the child on medication until behavioural and educational progress is actively promoted by the specific measures mentioned earlier. However, in severe cases with high degrees of impairment, simultaneous psychosocial and medical treatment may be required. It may be necessary to continue medication for several years, sometimes into adulthood. Yearly off-medication trial is recommended to evaluate the need for continuing treatment. Specialist supervision is mandatory. Close liaison with the school is required throughout the years of treatment.

The role of diet in the cause and management of hyperactivity is controversial. Current evidence indicates that the sort of diet which aims blindly to reduce sugar, artificial additives or colourants has no effect. A few children display an idiosyncratic behavioural reaction such as excitability or irritability to particular foods. If this seems likely, trying the child on an exclusion of that particular food may be useful. In general, food and drinks with caffeine are not advised. Overzealous dietary exclusion can lead to malnutrition, especially in a child on stimulant medication that may already have the side-effect of appetite reduction.

> **Summary**
>
> **Attention deficit hyperactivity disorder**
> - Affects males more than females.
> - Clinical features: cannot sustain attention, excessively active, socially disinhibited, easily distracted and impulsive, poor at relationships, prone to temper tantrums, poor school performance.
> - Management: educational psychologist assessment, behavioural programmes in school, parenting intervention, medication if necessary.

Hearing impairment

Any concern about hearing impairment should be taken seriously. Any child with delayed language or speech, learning difficulties or behavioural problems should have his/her hearing tested, as a mild hearing loss may be the underlying cause without parents or other carers realizing. Unilateral hearing loss can cause hearing difficulties when the good ear has an acute ear infection or glue ear. It can also cause difficulty with localizing sounds.

Hearing loss may be:

- sensorineural – caused by a lesion in the cochlea or auditory nerve and is usually present at birth
- conductive – from abnormalities of the ear canal or the middle ear, most often from otitis media with effusion.

The causes, natural history and management of hearing loss are listed in Table 4.5.

Hearing tests are described in Chapter 3. The typical audiogram in sensorineural and conductive hearing loss is shown in Fig. 4.6.

Sensorineural hearing loss

This type of hearing loss is uncommon. In England the incidence of permanent childhood hearing impairment (PCHI) is 0.9 per 1000 live births, with unilateral PCHI adding a further 0.7 per 1000 live births and another 0.7 per 1000 children acquire permanent hearing loss by the age of 10 years. It is usually present at birth or develops in the first few months of life. It is irreversible and can be of any severity, including profound.

The child with severe bilateral sensorineural hearing impairment will need early amplification with hearing aids for optimal speech and language development. Hearing aid use requires close supervision, beginning in the home together with the parents and continuing into school. Children often resist wearing hearing aids because background noise can be amplified unpleasantly. Children with microtia (congenital underdeveloped external ear) and meatal atresia can be helped with bone conduction hearing aids. Cochlear implants may be required where hearing aids give insufficient amplification (Fig. 4.7).

Many children with moderate hearing impairment can be educated within the mainstream school system or in partial hearing units attached to mainstream schools. Children with hearing impairment should be placed in the front of the classroom so that they can readily see the teacher. Gesture, visual context and lip movement will also allow children to develop language concepts. Speech may be delayed, but with appropriate therapy can be of good quality. Modified and simplified signing such as Makaton can be helpful for children who are both hearing-impaired and learning-disabled. Specialist teaching and support service in preschool and school years is provided by peripatetic teachers for children with hearing impairment. Those with profound hearing impairment may need to attend a school for children who are deaf.

Conductive hearing loss

Conductive hearing loss from middle ear disease is usually mild or moderate but may be severe. It is much more common than sensorineural hearing loss. In association with upper respiratory tract infections,

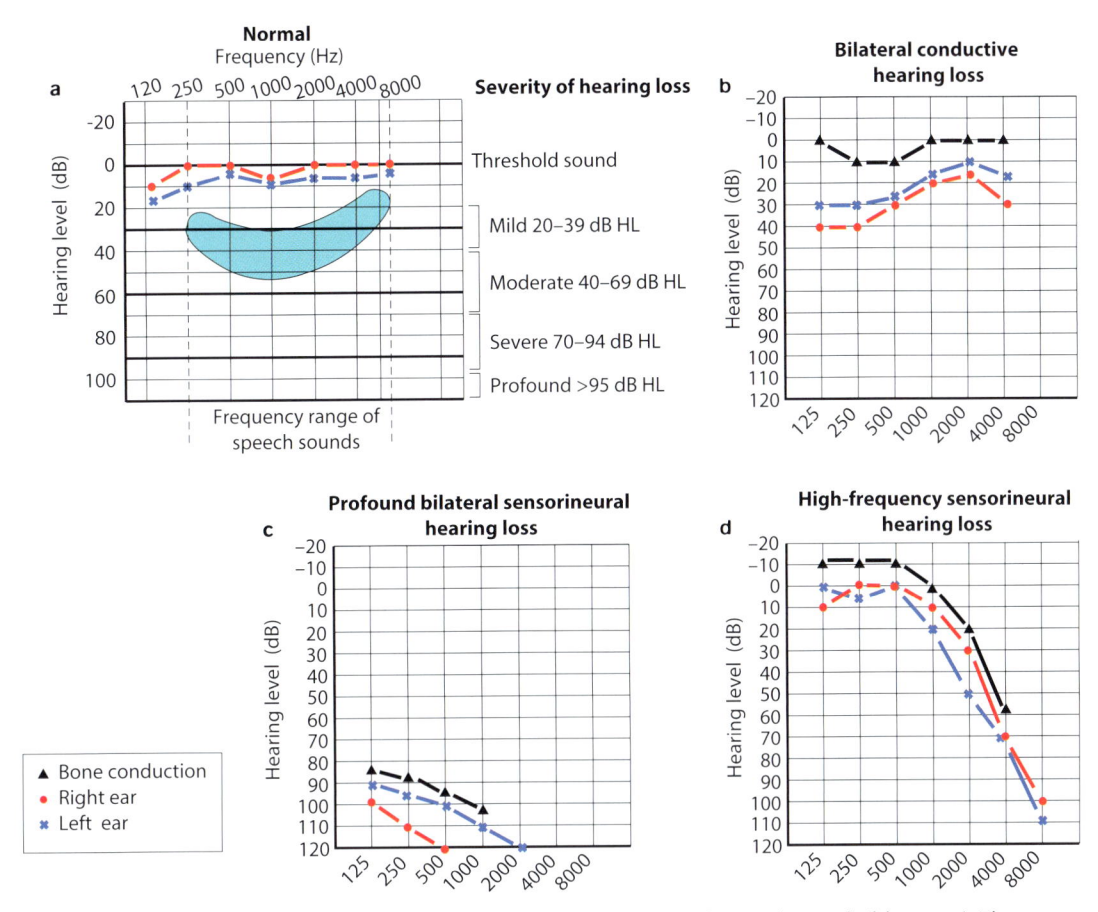

Figure 4.6 (a) Audiogram showing normal hearing and the loudness of normal speech (blue area). The consonants are high-frequency sounds, whereas the vowels are low-frequency sounds; (b) audiogram showing bilateral conductive hearing loss. There is a 30-dB to 40-dB hearing loss in both the right and left ears; (c) audiogram showing bilateral profound sensorineural hearing loss; and (d) audiogram showing bilateral high-frequency sensorineural hearing loss.

many children have episodes of hearing loss, which are usually self-limiting. In some cases of chronic otitis media with effusion, the hearing loss may last many months or years. In most affected children, there are no identifiable risk factors present but children with Down syndrome, cleft palate and atopy are particularly prone to hearing loss from middle ear disease.

Impedance audiometry tests, which measure the air pressure within the middle ear and the compliance of the tympanic membrane, determine if the middle ear is functioning normally. If the condition does not improve spontaneously, medical treatment (decongestant or a long course of antibiotics or treatment of nasal allergy) can be given. If that fails, surgery is considered, with insertion of tympanostomy tubes (grommets) with or without the removal of adenoids. Hearing aids are used in cases where problems recur after surgery.

The decision whether to intervene surgically should be based on the degree of functional disability rather than on absolute hearing loss.

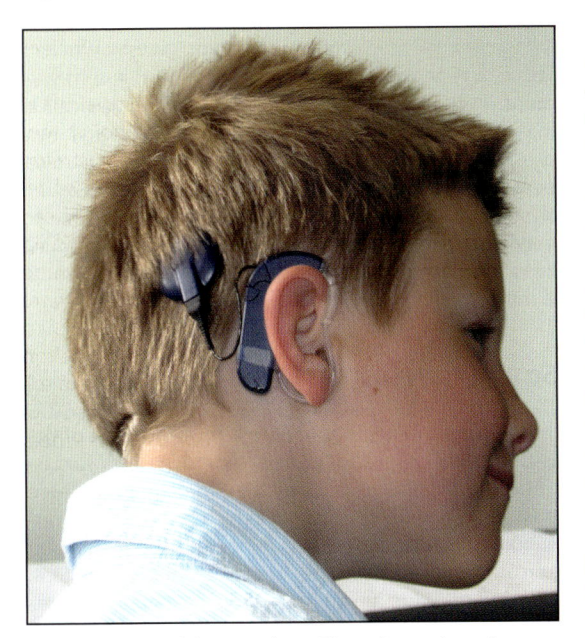

Figure 4.7 Cochlear implant. There is a microphone to detect sound, a speech processor and a transmitter and receiver/stimulator. They convert speech into electric impulses, which are conveyed to the auditory nerve, bypassing the ear. It provides a deaf person with a representation of sounds.

> Any child with poor or delayed speech or language must have his/her hearing assessed.

Table 4.5 Causes and management of hearing loss

	Sensorineural	Conductive
Causes	Genetic (the majority)	Otitis media with effusion (glue ear)
	Antenatal and perinatal: • congenital infection • preterm • hypoxic-ischaemic encephalopathy • hyperbilirubinemia	Eustachian tube dysfunction: • Down syndrome • cleft palate • Pierre Robin sequence • midfacial hypoplasia
	Postnatal: • meningitis/encephalitis • head injury • drugs, e.g. aminoglycosides, furosemide (frusemide) • neurodegenerative disorders	Wax (only rarely a cause of hearing loss)
Hearing loss	May be profound (>95-dB hearing loss)	Maximum of 60-dB hearing loss
Natural history	Does not improve and may progress	Intermittent or resolves
Management	Amplification or cochlear implant if necessary	Conservative, amplification or surgery

> **Summary**
>
> **Hearing loss**
> Sensorineural hearing loss:
> - is usually present at birth and is irreversible
> - early amplification with hearing aids or cochlear implants is needed for severe hearing impairment for optimal speech and language development
> - assistance is required from peripatetic teachers for children with moderate/severe hearing impairment.
>
> Conductive hearing loss:
> - is usually due to middle ear disease, often otitis media with effusion
> - is usually mild or moderate and transient
> - consider insertion of tympanostomy tubes (grommets) with or without the removal of adenoids if it does not resolve.

Abnormalities of vision and the ocular system

Normal visual development and tests of vision are described in Chapter 3.

Visual impairment may present in an infant or young child with:

- obvious ocular malformation (e.g. anophthalmia)
  - absent red reflex or white reflex (leukocoria), which may be due to opacification of intraocular structures, corneal abnormalities or intraocular tumour (retinoblastoma)
- not smiling responsively by 6 weeks' post-term
- concerns about poor visual responses, including poor eye contact
- roving eye movements
- nystagmus
- squint.

Any infant presenting with an ocular abnormality needs prompt referral to an ophthalmologist as some underlying conditions are sight threatening, and retinoblastoma is life threatening.

Nystagmus

This is a repetitive, involuntary, rhythmical eye movement. It is usually horizontal but can be vertical. It may be found in association with a structural eye problem (sensory defect nystagmus), but can also be a consequence of a problem at the cortical level. Nystagmus which is a manifestation of an eye problem, may improve over time. If no structural eye (or brain) problem is found, a diagnosis of idiopathic nystagmus is made.

Squint (strabismus)

In this common condition there is misalignment of the visual axes. Squint should be assessed in order for the underlying cause to be identified and treated where possible. There may be a family history. Transient misalignment is common up to 3 months of age. Marked epicanthic folds may give an appearance of a squint. Any infant with a squint should have red reflexes checked. Squints persisting beyond 3 months of age should be referred for a specialist ophthalmological opinion. The most common underlying cause is refractive error, but cataracts, retinoblastoma, and other intraocular causes must be excluded.

Squints are commonly divided into:
- *concomitant* (non-paralytic, common) – usually due to a refractive error in one or both eyes. Correction of the refractive error with glasses often corrects the squint. The squinting eye most often turns inwards (convergent), but there can be outward (divergent) or, rarely, vertical deviation
- *paralytic* (rare) – varies with gaze direction due to paralysis of the motor nerves. This can be sinister because of the possibility of an underlying space-occupying lesion such as a brain tumour.

Corneal light reflex test

Non-specialists can use this test to detect squints (Fig. 4.8). A pen torch is held at a distance to produce reflections on both corneas simultaneously. If the light reflection does not appear in the same position in the two pupils, a squint is present. However, a minor squint may be difficult to detect.

Cover test

The child is encouraged to look at a toy/light. If the fixing eye is covered, the squinting eye will move to take up fixation. (Fig. 4.9). The test should be performed with near (33 cm) and distant (at least 6 m) objects, as certain squints are present only at one distance. These tests are difficult to perform and reliable results are best obtained by an orthoptist or ophthalmologist.

Refractive errors

Hypermetropia (long sight)

This is the most common refractive error in young children. Mild hypermetropia is common in early childhood and is overcome through the process of accommodation – changing the shape of the lens in the eye. Hypermetropia can be corrected with convex (plus) lenses. These make the eye look bigger. Mild hypermetropia may not need spectacle correction.

Myopia (short sight)

This is relatively uncommon in young children, presenting usually in adolescence. However, in children born preterm it is the most common refractive error and may present at a younger age. Myopia can be corrected with concave (minus) lenses. These make the eye look smaller.

Astigmatism (abnormal corneal curvature)

Minor degrees of astigmatism are common and may not cause problems or require correction. Unilateral astigmatism can result in amblyopia.

Amblyopia

This is a potentially permanent reduction of visual acuity in an eye that has not received a clear image. It affects 2–3% of children. It is usually unilateral but can be bilateral. The most common causes of amblyopia are squint, refractive errors and obstruction to the visual pathway, e.g. cataract. Amblyopia may occur in squint when the brain is unable to combine the markedly differing images from each eye – the vision from the squinting eye is 'switched off' to avoid double vision. Treatment entails tackling the underlying condition, together with patching of the 'good' eye for specific periods of the day to force the 'lazy' eye to work, and therefore develop better vision. Early treatment is essential, as after 7 years of age improvement is unlikely. Considerable encouragement and support should to be given often to both the child and parents, as young children usually dislike having their better eye patched. Amblyopia may be asymptomatic, and is the main target condition for preschool vision screening in the UK.

Severe visual impairment

This affects 1 in 1000 live births in the UK, but is higher in developing countries. The main causes are listed in

---

Squints

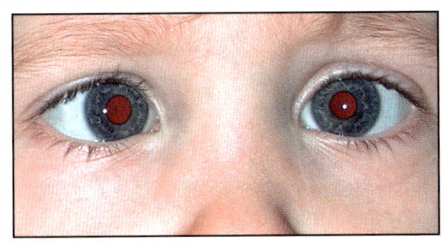

Figure 4.8 Corneal light reflex (reflection) test to detect a squint. The reflection is in a different position in the two eyes because of a small convergent squint of the right eye.

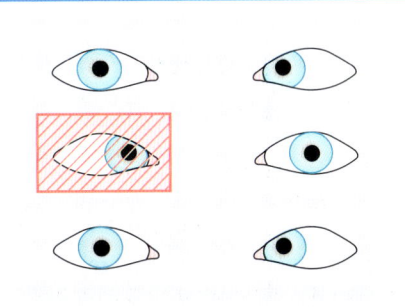

Figure 4.9 The cover test is used to identify a squint. If the fixing eye is covered, the squinting eye moves to take up fixation. This diagram shows a left convergent squint.

Box 4.2 Causes of visual impairment

Genetic	Antenatal and perinatal	Postnatal
Cataract	Congenital infection	Trauma
Albinism	Retinopathy of prematurity	Infection
Retinal dystrophy	Hypoxic-ischaemic encephalopathy	Juvenile idiopathic arthritis
Retinoblastoma	Cerebral abnormality/damage	
	Optic nerve hypoplasia	

Box 4.2. Recent epidemiological studies suggest that in the UK up to 50% of children have cerebral pathology as the underlying cause; about one-third of cases are hereditary, affecting eye structures. In developing countries, acquired causes such as infection are more prevalent.

Investigations may include an electroretinogram or visual evoked potentials. When visual impairment is of cortical origin, resulting from cerebral damage, examination of the eye, including the pupillary responses, may be normal.

Although few causes of severe visual impairment can be cured, early detection allows certain elements to be treated and timely advice can be given on supporting developmental progress. In the UK, this advice is usually provided by peripatetic teachers for children with visual impairment, who work with families from the time of diagnosis, irrespective of the child's age. Input from a paediatrician and other members of the child development team are also required. Partially sighted children may benefit from provision of low vision aids, high-powered magnifiers and small telescopic devices and computers. Although many severely visually impaired children have a visual disability alone, at least half have additional neurodevelopmental problems.

Summary

Regarding vision
- Visual impairment and ocular abnormalities including refractive errors are more common in children with neurodevelopmental problems.
- An absent red reflex or white reflex or a squint persisting after 3 months of age – refer to an ophthalmological opinion.
- Abnormal eye movements in an infant, absence of responsive smiling, or parental concern about vision at any age – consider visual impairment and refer to an ophthalmological opinion.
- Testing for squints – corneal light reflex (reflection) test for the non-specialist, cover test for the specialist.
- Amblyopia may be asymptomatic; treatment often includes patching of the 'good' eye for short periods each day.

Multidisciplinary child development services

Although children with a wide range of conditions have additional needs, the term 'special needs' is usually used for children with developmental problems and disabilities. In order to optimize the child's assessment and care on an ongoing basis, child development services in the UK are based on geographic areas and are secondary care services.

A child development service:
- is multidisciplinary with predominantly health professionals (paediatrician, physiotherapist, occupational therapist, speech and language therapist, clinical psychologist, specialist health visitor, dietician) in the team but often also includes a social worker (Fig. 4.10)
- is multiagency (Fig. 4.11) and may include health, social services, education, volunteers, voluntary agencies, parent support groups
- aims to provide a coordinated service with good inter-agency liaison to meet the functional needs of the child and optimize his/her care
- may provide multidisciplinary support and monitor children up to school-leaving age (16–19 years)
- maintains a register of children with disabilities and special needs
- has emphasis on children's needs within the community (home, nursery, school), regardless of its location.

Child development services in the UK now usually use the Common Assessment Framework to allow multidisciplinary sharing of information. The emphasis is on:
- diagnosis
- assessment of functional skills: mobility, hand function, vision, hearing, communication, behaviour, social/self-care skills and learning
- provision of therapy
- regular review
- a coordinated approach to care (multidisciplinary, multiagency).

Many children with special needs have medical problems which require investigation, treatment, and review. Good inter-professional communication is vital for well-coordinated care. This is assisted by all professionals keeping entries in the child's personal child health record up to date.

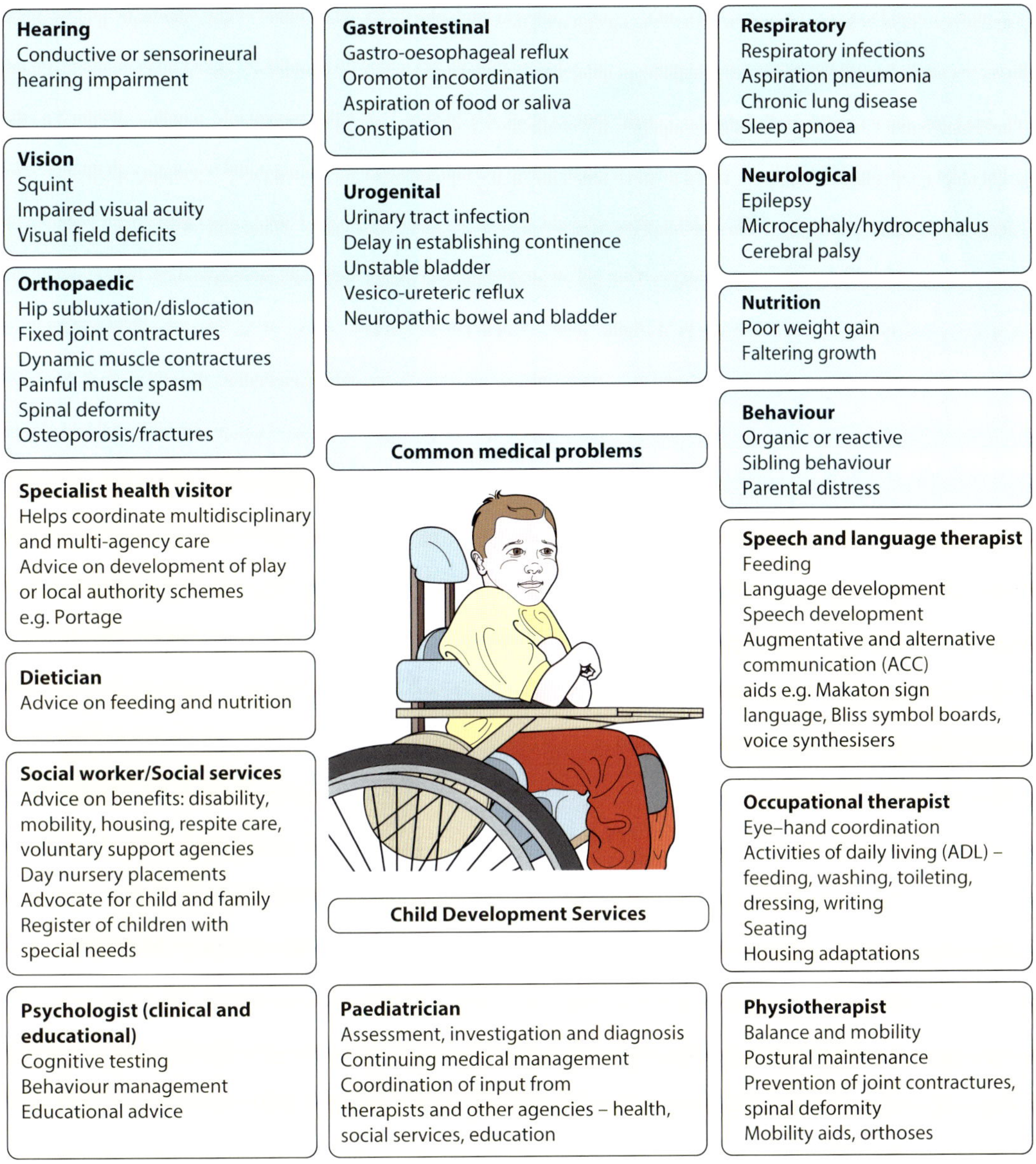

Developmental problems and the child with special needs

Common medical problems

Hearing
Conductive or sensorineural hearing impairment

Vision
Squint
Impaired visual acuity
Visual field deficits

Orthopaedic
Hip subluxation/dislocation
Fixed joint contractures
Dynamic muscle contractures
Painful muscle spasm
Spinal deformity
Osteoporosis/fractures

Gastrointestinal
Gastro-oesophageal reflux
Oromotor incoordination
Aspiration of food or saliva
Constipation

Urogenital
Urinary tract infection
Delay in establishing continence
Unstable bladder
Vesico-ureteric reflux
Neuropathic bowel and bladder

Respiratory
Respiratory infections
Aspiration pneumonia
Chronic lung disease
Sleep apnoea

Neurological
Epilepsy
Microcephaly/hydrocephalus
Cerebral palsy

Nutrition
Poor weight gain
Faltering growth

Behaviour
Organic or reactive
Sibling behaviour
Parental distress

Child Development Services

Specialist health visitor
Helps coordinate multidisciplinary and multi-agency care
Advice on development of play or local authority schemes e.g. Portage

Dietician
Advice on feeding and nutrition

Social worker/Social services
Advice on benefits: disability, mobility, housing, respite care, voluntary support agencies
Day nursery placements
Advocate for child and family
Register of children with special needs

Psychologist (clinical and educational)
Cognitive testing
Behaviour management
Educational advice

Paediatrician
Assessment, investigation and diagnosis
Continuing medical management
Coordination of input from therapists and other agencies – health, social services, education

Speech and language therapist
Feeding
Language development
Speech development
Augmentative and alternative communication (ACC) aids e.g. Makaton sign language, Bliss symbol boards, voice synthesisers

Occupational therapist
Eye–hand coordination
Activities of daily living (ADL) – feeding, washing, toileting, dressing, writing
Seating
Housing adaptations

Physiotherapist
Balance and mobility
Postural maintenance
Prevention of joint contractures, spinal deformity
Mobility aids, orthoses

Figure 4.10 Common medical conditions and the many professionals in the child development services involved in the care of children with developmental problems.

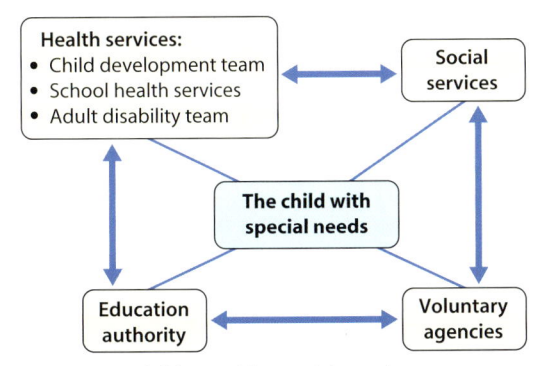

Figure 4.11 Children with special needs are supported by the integrated inputs of health and social services, local education authorities and voluntary agencies.

Health services:
- Child development team
- School health services
- Adult disability team

Social services

Education authority

Voluntary agencies

The child with special needs

In addition to locally organized child development services, specialist neurodisability services are required for:

- rehabilitation following acquired brain injury
- surgery for cerebral palsy, scoliosis
- gait analysis
- spasticity management, including botulinum toxin injections to muscles
- epilepsy unresponsive to two or more anticonvulsants or where there is severe cognitive and behavioural regression related to epilepsy
- complex communication disorders – diagnosis and therapeutic intervention
- mixed complex learning problems, often with neuropsychiatric comorbid symptoms
- provision of communication aids (Fig. 4.12)
- sensory impairments (e.g. cochlear implants)

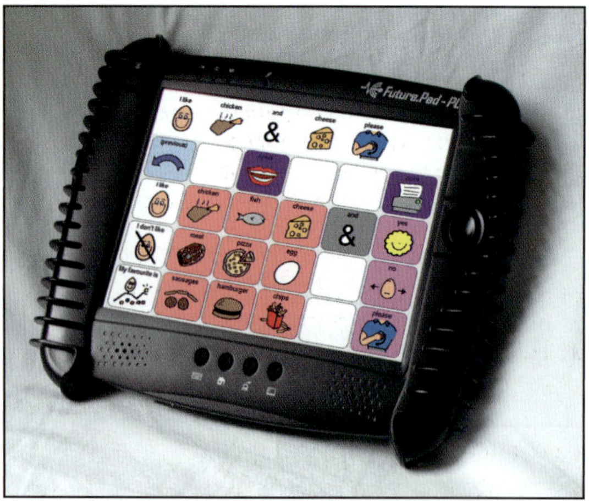

Figure 4.12 An example of a touchscreen speaking communication aid to assist children who may have speaking and movement difficulties.

- children with severe visual and hearing impairment
- specialized seating/wheelchairs and orthoses (Fig. 4.13)
- management of movement disorders (e.g. continuous infusion of intrathecal baclofen, selective dorsal rhizotomy and deep brain stimulation to basal ganglia).

Needs are likely to change over time, with key stages being at transition to school and adult services. A care plan should be developed at each stage; it may include education and social care as well as health. Care plans should be shared with the child and family and then regularly reviewed. Involvement with specialist services may be of variable frequency throughout childhood. Collaboration across services is vital in promoting a service tailored around the child and family.

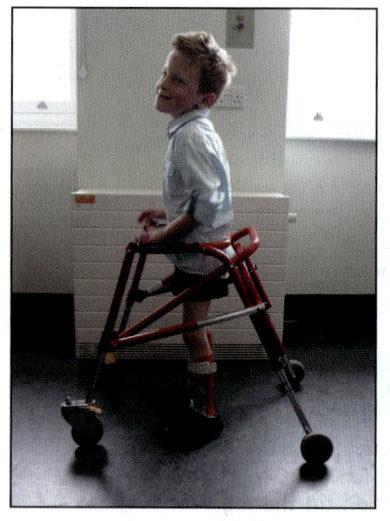

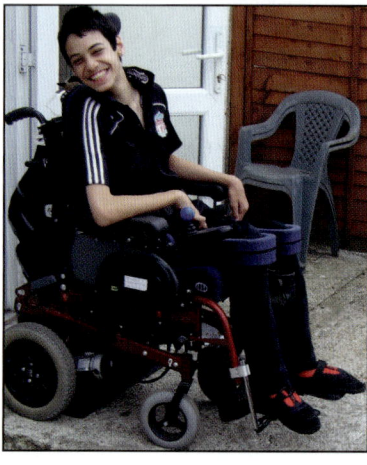

Figure 4.13 (a) A boy with spastic cerebral palsy is able to walk with the help of a frame; and (b) a motorized wheelchair that enables this young person with cerebral palsy to be mobile.

> **Summary**
>
> **Children with developmental problems and disabilities**
> - Are looked after by local multidisciplinary child development services.
> - Often have complex medical needs.
> - Need regular review, as needs change with time, as will the child's ability to participate in it.
> - Require coordination of care between the family and the many professionals involved, as well as close liaison with education and social services.

Education

Children with special educational needs should receive educational input according to their requirements, including integration into mainstream schooling whenever possible. However, there are special needs' schools for children with more significant learning and/or physical disabilities. There are also specialist educational placements for children with certain conditions such as severe visual or hearing impairment or autism spectrum disorders. These specialist educational settings have access to a higher level of therapies (physiotherapy, occupational therapy and speech and language therapy) and specialist teaching than are available through a mainstream educational placement. Assessment and support for behavioural and learning needs may come from an educational or clinical psychologist.

Transition of care to adult services

In the UK, adult disability services are, in general, still poorly developed by comparison with those provided for children. Young adults with severe learning and physical disabilities are supported by Adult Learning Disability Teams, but there is only limited national provision for those with mild or moderate learning disabilities or with a predominantly physical disability. Major problems for young adults with disabilities include social issues around care, housing, mobility, finance, leisure, employment, and genetic and sexual counselling. Health information must be properly transferred from child to adult health services if reinvestigation of already well-clarified conditions is to be avoided.

The rights of disabled children

Irrespective of their disability, the aspirations and rights of children, as affirmed by the United Nations Convention on the Rights of the Child, need to be respected. Technological advances to improve mobility, communication and emotional expression are helping enable people with disability to better achieve their full potential, rather than being held back by their disability. However, this requires skilled assistance and adequate resources. Prominent public figures who function effectively despite disabilities help to make the public appreciate what can be achieved and serve as an inspiration to those with disabilities. The World Health Organization stresses the important outcomes of activity and participation. Any health interventions for people with disability either on an individual level or in society as a whole should aim to also improve these outcomes.

Acknowledgements

We would like to acknowledge contributors to this chapter in previous editions, whose work we have drawn on: Angus Nicoll (1st Edition), Diane Smyth (2nd, 3rd, 4th Edition), Neil Wimalasundera (4th Edition).

Further reading

Hall D, Elliman D: *Health for All Children*, ed 4, Oxford, 2006, Oxford University Press.

Hall D, Williams J, Elliman D: *The Child Surveillance Handbook*, ed 3, Oxford, 2009, Radcliffe Medical Press.

Meggitt C: *Child Development: An Illustrated Guide: Birth to 19 Years*, Harlow, 2012, Pearson Education Limited.

Websites (Accessed November 2016)

Contact a family: Available at: http://www.cafamily.org.uk.
Organization supporting families of disabled children across the UK.

Disability matters: Available at: https://www.disabilitymatters.org.uk.
A fantastic Web-based learning resource for everyone involved with the care of children and young people with disability.

HemiHelp: Available at: http://www.hemihelp.org.uk/
Information about heniplegia.

NICE guidelines: Available at: http://www.nice.org.uk/.
ADHD, autism spectrum disorders, spasticity management.

SCOPE: Available at: http://www.scope.org.uk/.
About disability.

Special educational needs and disability: Available at: https://www.gov.uk/topic/schools-colleges-childrens-services/special-educational-needs-disabilities

The National Autistic Society: Available at: http://www.autism.org.uk/

International Classification of Functioning, Disability and Health (ICF), Geneva, 2001, WHO.

http://www.who.int/classifications/icf/en/

5

Care of the sick child and young person

Primary care	64	Communicating serious problems	71
Secondary care	65	Palliative and end-of-life care	71
Children in hospital	67	Ethics	72
Pain in children	69	Evidence-based paediatrics	75
Prescribing medicines for children	70		

Features of the care of the sick child and young person are:

- the number of children and young people attending and being admitted to hospital continues to increase
- the care of children and their families in hospital should include their holistic, emotional, spiritual and social needs
- pain management needs to be considered, even in patients too young to describe it
- ethical and consent issues are centred around considering their best interests; when able to understand the issues, the child or young person should also be involved
- research is vital to provide an evidence base to deliver quality care.

Sick children have different requirements of medical care from adults. This is true both in primary care and in hospital. Not only does hospital care need to be child and family centred, but also the holistic care provided needs to include the management of pain, safe prescribing and good communication. It should be based on sound ethical principles and, whenever possible, on evidence-based medicine underpinned by research. If needed, palliative and end-of-life care should be available. How these apply to paediatric practice is described in this chapter.

Primary care

The majority of acute illness in children is mild and transient (e.g. upper respiratory tract infection, gastroenteritis) or readily treatable (e.g. exacerbation of asthma) and is provided by parents at home (Fig. 5.1). When more seriously ill, e.g. a high fever, not feeding, difficulty breathing, lethargy, parents require rapid access to advice or assessment by an experienced clinician. Advice may be provided on the Internet or by telephone (e.g. NHS Direct). Medical care is initially provided by general practitioners or in some countries by primary care paediatricians in conjunction with other healthcare professionals. Ready access

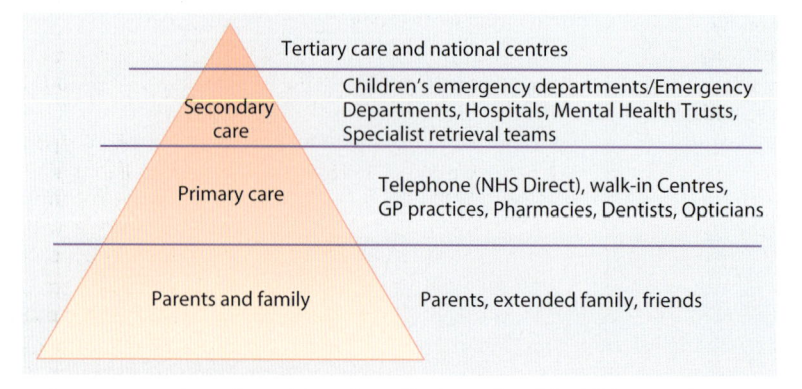

Figure 5.1 Schematic representation of provision of medical care for sick children in the UK. Most is by the family with medical support from primary care. Relatively few need secondary care, and only a very small number require tertiary or national centres.

to secondary care should be available. Although an individual general practitioner will care for relatively few children with serious chronic paediatric illnesses (e.g. cystic fibrosis, diabetes mellitus) or disability (e.g. cerebral palsy), each affected child and family are likely to require considerable input from the whole of the primary care team. The medical care of normal children, the healthy child programme of immunization, screening and developmental reviews and health promotion are provided within primary care.

Secondary care

Emergency and urgent care

Almost 5 million children and young people aged 0–19 years (1 in 4) attend an Accident and Emergency department each year in the United Kingdom. This number continues to increase. The rates of attendance are highest in preschool children (almost 2 million) and are only exceeded by those over 80 years of age. One reason for this is that young children need urgent review if they become significantly ill, often with a high fever or difficulty breathing, as their condition can deteriorate rapidly. Another common reason for attendance is injuries. Specially trained staff and special facilities are required for the urgent assessment and management of children and young people attending an Accident and Emergency department, as listed in Box 5.1. Children should be kept separate from the often unpleasant environment of adult emergency departments. Increasingly, dedicated separate emergency departments for children are being created.

Hospital admission rates

In England just over 2 million children younger than 15 years of age were admitted to hospital in 2012. This represents 11.4% of the total number of hospital admissions. Almost three quarters of acute admissions are under the care of paediatricians, and the remainder are surgical patients (although a paediatrician or paediatric surgeon is also involved in their care while they are in hospital, to oversee any medical requirements). Most paediatric admissions are of infants and young children under 5 years of age and are emergencies, whereas surgical admissions peak at 5 years of age, one-third of which are elective (Fig. 5.2). The most common reasons for medical admission are shown in Table 5.1.

> **Hospital admission of children:**
> - should be avoided whenever possible
> - most medical admissions are infants and young children; surgical admissions occur throughout childhood.

Most emergency paediactric admissions are infants and young children.

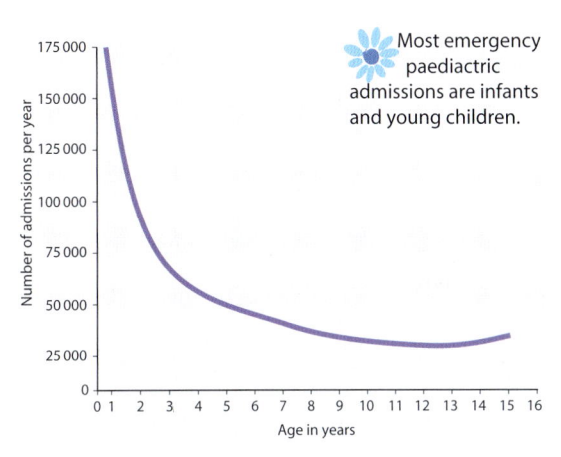

Figure 5.2 Age of hospital admission for children and young people aged 0–14 years in England, excluding births. (Data from Hospital Episode Statistics, 2013–2014. Available at: http://www.hesonline.nhs.uk.)

Box 5.1 Services that should be available for children attending an Accident and Emergency department

Environment	Staff	Medical care
Initial clinical assessment occurs within 15 min of arrival	Medical and nursing staff trained and experienced in the care and treatment of children and young adults, including mental health	Resuscitation and other equipment for children
Separate waiting area, play facilities, child friendly treatment and recovery areas	Non-paediatric staff trained in communicating with children and families	Children given priority for prompt treatment
Access for parents to examination, X-ray and anaesthetic rooms	Effective communication with other health professionals	Special priority arrangement for children with serious long-term illnesses
		Rapid transfer if inpatient admission is needed. If intensive or specialist care required, dedicated transport services available within regional critical care or specialist networks.
		Child protection advice available from experienced paediatrician
		Procedures and counselling in place following the sudden death of a child

Adapted from *Welfare of Children in Hospital*, HMSO, London, 1991 and Standards for *Children and Young People in Emergency Care Settings*, RCPCH 2012. http://www.rcpch.ac.uk/sites/default/files/page/Redbook%202012.pdf

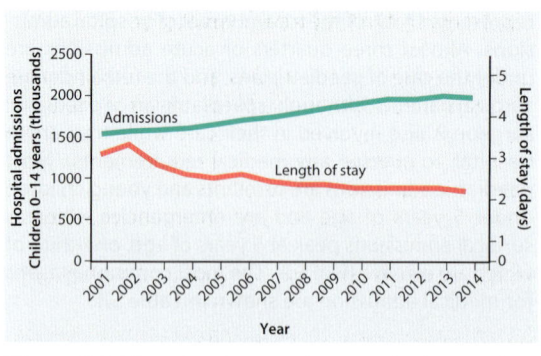

Figure 5.3 There has been an increase in the number of children and young people (0–14 years) admitted to hospital in England. This is because of a marked increase in the number of paediatric admissions, whereas surgical admissions have declined slightly. However, the average length of stay continues to fall. (Data from Hospital Episode Statistics, 2013–2014. Available at: http://www.hesonline.nhs.uk.)

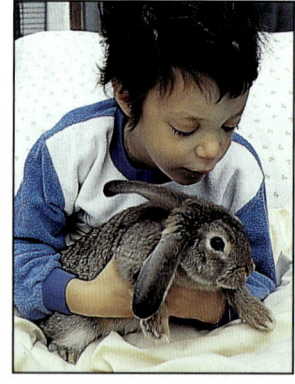

Figure 5.4 Providing palliative care in a child's home. Although this child required a subcutaneous morphine infusion to control her pain from malignant disease, she was able to remain at home and enjoyed playing with her pet rabbit. (By kind permission of her parents and Dr Ann Goldman.)

Table 5.1 Reasons for emergency admission of children under 15 years of age to hospital

System	Specific disorders
Respiratory 25%	Respiratory infections 20%
	Asthma 3%
Injuries and poisoning 17%	Head injury 5%
	Poisoning 1%
Gastroenterological 13%	Gastroenteritis 5%
Infection 6%	Viral infection 5%
Urogenital 3%	Urinary tract infection 2%
Neurological 2%	Seizures 1%
Endocrine and metabolic 2%	Diabetes mellitus 1%
Skin 2%	
Musculoskeletal 2%	
Other 28%	

Data based on 58 061 admissions, 2009–2010. ISD, Scotland.

The hospital admission rate has continued to rise over the last 20 years. Between 1999 and 2010 there was an increase of 28% in the number of emergency admissions (Fig. 5.3). The effect was most marked in younger children. The reasons for this are unclear, but probably include:

- lower threshold for admission
- the lack of an instant test to rule out serious illness
- the increasingly risk-averse nature of medical practice, which has resulted in an increase in short-stay admissions (<24 hours)
- repeated admission of children with complex conditions who survive longer, e.g. ex-preterm infants, children with cancer or organ failure.

Although the number of admissions continues to increase, strenuous efforts have been made to reduce the rate and length of hospitalization (Fig. 5.3):

- ambulatory paediatrics has developed to provide hospital care for medical problems outside inpatient paediatric wards. In addition, the subspecialty of paediatric emergency medicine has been developed to provide specialists with expertise to provide care for all acutely ill children, with an aim of preventing admission whenever possible
- dedicated children's short-stay beds within or alongside the emergency department are increasingly available to allow children to be treated or observed for a number of hours and discharged home directly, avoiding the need for admission to the ward
- day-case surgery has been instituted for many operations, and day units are used for complex investigations and procedures instead of inpatient wards
- home-care teams aim to provide care in the child's home and thereby reduce hospital attendance, admission and length of stay. This may include specialist care, e.g. for treating diabetes and asthma or providing home oxygen therapy or palliative care for terminally ill children (Fig. 5.4)
- children's hospices provide respite and palliative care for children with life-threatening conditions such as malignant and neurodegenerative disorders
- some teams provide a 'hospital-at-home' service for children who are acutely ill, in order to avoid hospitalization.

Summary

Regarding secondary care for children in the UK, each year:
- Up to half of infants aged under 12 months and one quarter of older children attend emergency departments.
- 1 in 11 children are referred to a hospital outpatient clinic.
- 1 in 10–15 children are admitted to hospital.
- 1 in 1000 children require intensive care.
- 1 in 10–15 newborn babies are admitted to a neonatal unit. Of those, about 2% need intensive care.

Children in hospital

Children should only be admitted to hospital if effective and safe care cannot be provided at home. Removing young children from their familiar environment to a strange hospital ward is stressful and frightening for the child, parents and family. Ill or injured children may regress in their behaviour, acting younger than their actual age. It places the child at risk of nosocomial infections and iatrogenic harm through medical errors, e.g. prescribing errors. It also disrupts family routines, not only of the child in hospital but also of siblings who still need to be looked after at home and transported to and from nursery or school.

Putting the family and child at the centre of care

Care in hospital should be child-centred and family-centred, with a holistic approach towards the child and family rather than simply focusing on the medical condition. This requires the child's care to be tailored to their physical and emotional maturity and needs and not having to adapt to standardized ward routines.

Parents of infants and young children should be allowed to stay with their child overnight (amazingly something not allowed in the 1950s) and continue to provide the care and support they would give at home. Parents know best about their child's usual behaviour and habits and due attention must be paid to their worries or comments, including intuition in recognizing acute deterioration in their child. Increasingly, this is recorded as part of the regular observations on children. Good communication is needed between staff and parents to arrive at a mutually agreed plan of responsibilities for looking after the child. This will avoid parents either feeling pressurized to accept responsibilities they are not confident about or feeling brushed aside and undervalued by staff. For children with chronic conditions, many parents rapidly learn some of the nursing skills, e.g. nasogastric tube feeding, if required by their child.

Child-orientated environment

Children should be cared for within a children's ward, which should be appropriate for the child's physical and emotional maturity and needs. Adolescents should be with others of their own age and not forced to accept ward arrangements designed for babies or adults. Education and facilities for play should be provided.

Information and psychosocial support

Detailed information should be provided, given personally and preferably also written and available in appropriate ethnic languages. Staff should be sensitive to the family's individual needs according to their social, educational, cultural and religious background. Emotional and psychological support should be available and all staff members should be aware of the effects illness and injury can have on children and their families.

For elective admissions, children and their families should be offered an advance visit and have details of proposed treatment and management explained at an appropriate level.

Skilled staff

Children in hospital should be cared for by specially trained medical, nursing and support staff. The care of every child admitted to hospital should be supervised by a paediatrician or paediatrically trained surgeon. As children constitute only a relatively small proportion of the workload in acute surgical specialities, surgeons and anaesthetists should treat a sufficient number of children to maintain their skills. Dedicated children's physiotherapists and occupational therapists have specialist skills that are required to optimize the outcomes for children. Play specialists are an essential part of the ward team because they can help children understand their illness and its treatment through play. Children with complex needs should have an experienced healthcare professional as a contact person to ensure care is coordinated and investigations or procedures are not duplicated.

Multidisciplinary care – coordinating care across boundaries

Successful management of paediatric conditions often relies on a network of multidisciplinary care, with all professionals working well together as a coordinated team. If this breaks down, particularly when dealing with complex issues such as child protection and long-term disability, there may be serious consequences for the child, family and professionals involved. Child psychiatrists, the community paediatric team and social services are important members of the team.

Tertiary care and networks

The number of children requiring tertiary care is relatively small, so it is concentrated in specialist centres. Tertiary care in paediatrics includes neonatal and paediatric intensive care and cardiac and oncology centres. They

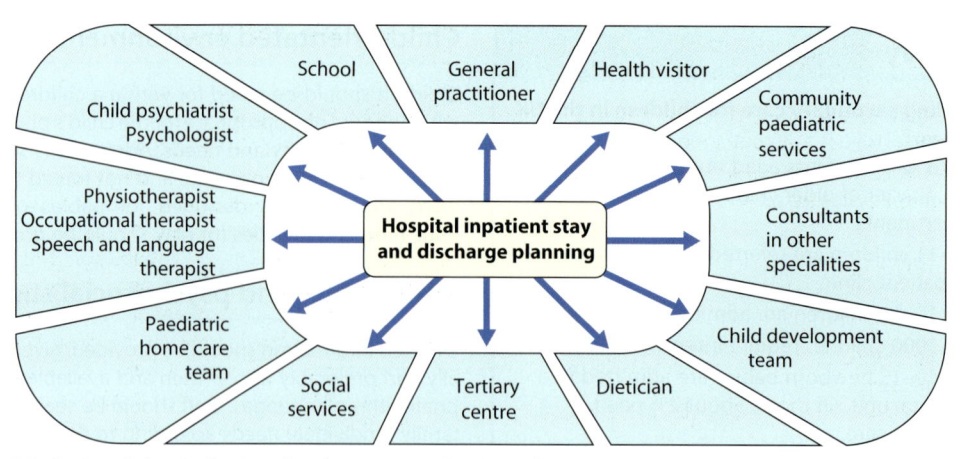

Figure 5.5 Some of the professionals who may need to be informed about the admission or discharge of a child admitted to a hospital.

have the advantage of having a wide range of specialists, not only medical and surgical staff but also nursing and other healthcare professionals, and diagnostic and other services. For critically ill neonates and children, specialist retrieval teams have been developed to provide initial resuscitation and post-resuscitation care at secondary care hospitals and then provide transport to the tertiary centre. For some rare and complex disorders (e.g. immune deficiency disorders and inborn errors of metabolism) and complex treatments (e.g. transplantation and craniofacial surgery), national centres have been developed. A disadvantage is that they are often some distance from the child's home and hospital stay may be prolonged, e.g. following a bone marrow transplant. Accommodation for parents should be provided in this situation. In order to minimize the need for the child to travel to tertiary centres, shared-care networks have been established between tertiary centres and local hospitals. For example, a child with leukaemia might attend a tertiary centre for the initial diagnostic assessment and treatment, and subsequently for specialized treatment and periodic review, but much of the maintenance therapy would be provided by the local hospital together with monitoring of their health and regular blood and other tests performed by a specialist nurse at home. Specialists from the tertiary centre may also hold periodic clinics at the shared-care centre. Such shared-care networks rely on excellent communication between all the health professionals involved.

Discharge from hospital

Children should be discharged from hospital as soon as clinically and socially appropriate. Although there is increasing pressure to reduce the length of hospital stay to a minimum, this must not allow discharge planning to be neglected. Before discharge from hospital, parents and children should be informed of:

- the reason for admission and any implications for the future
- details of medication and other treatment
- any clinical features that should prompt them to seek medical advice, and how this should be obtained (safety netting)
- problems or questions likely to be asked by other family members or in the community. These should be anticipated by the doctor and discussed. For instance, what should the nursery or school, babysitters or friends need to know? What about sports, etc.?

In addition, consider:

- suitability of home circumstances
- social support that may need to be arranged, especially in relation to child protection
- what medical information should be added to the child's personal child health record
- which professionals should be informed about the admission and what information it is relevant for them to receive.

This must be done before or at the time of discharge. The aim is to provide a seamless service of care, treatment and support with the family and ensure that all the professionals are fully informed (Fig. 5.5).

Summary

Children in hospital should be provided with:
- Family-centred care: holistic approach to family, parent of young children able to stay and provide parental care.
- Child-oriented environment: appropriate for child's age, together with education and play facilities.
- Information and psychosocial support: verbal and written information for both parents and child.
- The opportunity for children and families to express their views and fears and be listened to.
- Skilled staff, specially trained to care for children.
- Multidisciplinary care.
- Access to tertiary care, with shared-care arrangements with local hospital and primary care.

Pain in children

Pain is a major concern for children and parents across all specialties. Whilst it is easy to ignore or underestimate pain in children, it should ideally be anticipated and prevented and always taken seriously.

Acute pain

This may be caused by:

- musculoskeletal tissue or organ damage, e.g. trauma, burns or fractures
- inflammatory processes – from local infection e,g. skin, respiratory or urinary tract, joint, bone, peritonitis, meningitis
- obstruction – e.g. intussusception, renal colic, hydrocephalus
- vaso-occlusive disease, e.g. sickle cell crisis
- medical intervention, i.e. investigations e.g venepuncture or lumbar puncture or procedures e.g. change of wound dressings
- surgery.

Chronic pain

In children, chronic severe pain sometimes occurs as a result of disease such as malignant disease or juvenile idiopathic arthritis or complex regional pain syndromes. Intermittent pain of mild or moderate severity, e.g. headache or recurrent abdominal pain is more common but can be very distressing for children and their families.

Management

Pain management should be approached by recognizing, responding and reassessing.

Recognizing pain

Older children can describe the nature and severity of the pain they are experiencing. In younger children and those with developmental delay, assessing pain is more difficult. Observation and parental impression are commonly used and a number of self-assessment tools have been designed for children over 3 years of age (Fig. 5.6). Observation is a key component of pain assessment in children; the child who is extremely quiet, especially after trauma, may be in significant discomfort.

Responding to pain

The approaches to pain management are listed in Box 5.2. This should allow pain to be prevented or kept to a minimum. Age-appropriate explanation should be given when possible and the approach should be reassuring; however, it is imperative not to lie to children, otherwise they will lose trust in what they are told in the future. Distraction techniques such as blowing bubbles, telling stories, holding family toys, or playing computer games, as well as the involvement of trained play specialists, can be highly successful in ameliorating pain in children. Some children develop particular preferences for a particular venepuncture site or distraction technique, and this should be accommodated as far as possible.

Box 5.2 Approaches to pain management

Information and psychosocial support

- Psychological, by the parent, doctor, nurse or play specialist
- Behavioural
- Distraction
- Hypnosis

Medical

- Local: anaesthetic cream, local anaesthetic infiltration, nerve blocks, warmth or cold, physiotherapy, transcutaneous electrical nerve stimulation
- Analgesics:
  - mild/moderate – paracetamol, nonsteroidal anti-inflammatory drugs (NSAIDs)
  - strong – morphine
- Sedatives and anaesthetic agents:
  - ketamine, midazolam, nitrous oxide, general anaesthetic
- Antiepileptic and antidepressant drugs for neuropathic pain

Consider the route for analgesics – oral if possible, otherwise intravenous, subcutaneous or rectal. Intranasal administration is becoming increasingly popular in children as it is well tolerated.

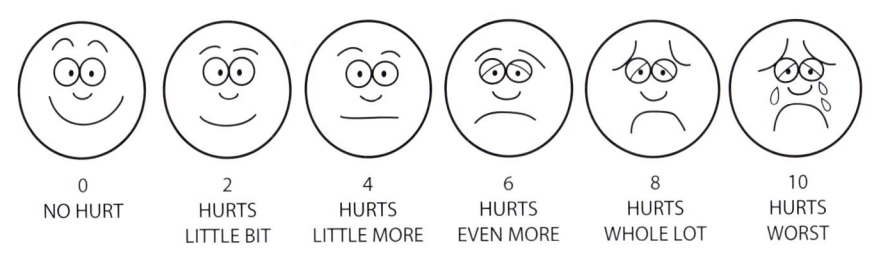

0	2	4	6	8	10
NO HURT	HURTS LITTLE BIT	HURTS LITTLE MORE	HURTS EVEN MORE	HURTS WHOLE LOT	HURTS WORST

Figure 5.6 An example of a scoring system for pain assessment in children. Wong Baker Faces scale. (From Wong DL, Winkelstein ML, Schwartz P, et al.: *Wong's Essentials of Pediatric Nursing*, St Louis, MO, 2001, Mosby with permission).

For minor medical procedures, e.g. venepuncture or inserting an intravenous cannula, pain can be alleviated by explanation and the use of a topical anaesthetic. Additional and appropriate use of inhalation agents such as nitrous oxide or the adjunctive use of mild sedatives (midazolam) or hypnotics (ketamine) alongside pain relief can be helpful for more painful procedures such as suturing a wound. For more invasive procedures, e.g. bronchoscopy, a general anaesthetic should be given.

Postoperative pain can be markedly reduced by local infiltration of the wound, nerve blocks and postoperative analgesics. Severe pain, especially from fractures and surgical procedures, should be adequately treated with opioid analgesics. In the past, there was reluctance to use morphine in children for fear of depressing breathing, but this should not occur when morphine is given in appropriate dosage under nursing supervision to children with a normal respiratory drive. Intravenous morphine can be given using a patient-controlled delivery system in older children or a nurse-controlled system in young children. Acutely, intranasal opiate agents (e.g. diamorphine) can be given, which are highly effective as they are absorbed rapidly from a child's nasal mucosa.

Reassessing pain

This is a vital part of pain management in children. Although children often have parents and carers as advocates, the child's pain scores should be regularly reviewed.

☀ **Pain should be anticipated and prevented as well as being treated promptly**

Prescribing medicines for children

There are marked differences in the absorption, biology, clearance and distribution (ABCD) of drugs between children and adults. Many doses of medicines have to be calculated using either weight, age or surface area. This added complexity means that children are at high risk of prescribing errors. Indeed, a recent survey across five London hospitals found an error in 13% of all prescriptions for children.

Young children find it difficult to take tablets and thus a liquid formulation is required. Most are glucose free. Persuading children to take medicines is often a problem, especially if the preparation has an unpleasant taste; experience and imagination help to overcome their reluctance. Adherence (compliance) is improved when medicines are only required once or twice a day and if regimens are kept simple.

A basic understanding of the pharmacology of the commonly encountered medicines in paediatrics is helpful – i.e. how it is absorbed in different age groups, how it works (its biology), how it is cleared (and how quickly), and how it is distributed. All these will affect dosing. Sometimes only limited data are available. An up-to-date reference formulary (e.g. the British National Formulary for Children) should be consulted for all prescriptions.

Absorption

In neonates and infants, oral formulations of drugs are given as liquids. However, their intake cannot be guaranteed and absorption is unpredictable as it is affected by gastric emptying and acidity, gut motility and the effects of milk in the stomach. In acutely ill neonates and infants, drugs are therefore given intravenously to ensure reliable and adequate blood and tissue concentrations. Intramuscular injections should be avoided if at all possible as there is little muscle bulk available for injection, absorption is variable and they are painful. Rectal administration can be used for some drugs; although absorption is more reliable than oral administration, this route is not popular in the UK. Significant systemic absorption can occur across the skin, particularly in preterm infants. This is a potential cause of toxicity, e.g. alcohol and iodine absorption from cleansing solutions applied to the skin for procedures.

Biology

The precise mechanism of action can vary considerably between adults and children and within children of different ages for the same drug. For instance, paracetamol is metabolized by a different and slower mechanism in neonates compared with older children and adults; this increases the risk of overdose. Some medicines should be avoided in children as they may cause idiosyncratic adverse reactions (e.g. aspirin should be avoided in children <16 years of age as it is associated with a risk of Reye syndrome, causing encephalopathy and liver failure).

Clearance

In neonates, drug biotransformation is reduced, as microsomal enzymes in the liver are immature. This leads to a prolonged half-life of drugs metabolized in the liver, e.g. theophylline. Renal excretion is reduced by the low glomerular filtration rate, which increases the half-life of some drugs, e.g. gentamicin. Measuring the plasma drug concentration is necessary under these circumstances.

Distribution

Water comprises a larger percentage of the body in the neonate (80%) than in older children and adults (55%). Drugs that distribute within extracellular fluid will require a larger dose relative to body weight in infants than in adults. As extracellular fluid correlates with body surface area, this is used when accurate drug dosage is required, e.g. cytotoxic agents. For drugs with a high margin of safety, drug dosages are expressed per kilogram body weight or based on age, with the assumption that the child is of average size. Weight-based dosages should not simply be extrapolated to older children, as the dosage will be excessively large.

In the first few months of life, plasma protein concentration is low and some drugs may be partially unbound and remain pharmacologically active. In jaundiced babies, for example, bilirubin may compete with some drugs, e.g. sulphonamides, for albumin binding sites, making such drugs unsuitable for use in this situation.

> ## Summary
>
> **Regarding medicines for children:**
> - Oral formulations need to be given as liquids in infants and young children.
> - Medicines are usually prescribed per kilogram of body weight, but check the maximum dose.
> - Intramuscular drugs should be avoided if at all possible.
> - Intravenous drug dosages can easily be miscalculated as they vary widely in children because of their different size, and drugs often need to be diluted; all dosages and dilutions must be checked independently by two trained members of staff.
> - To improve compliance, use formulations requiring the least number of times to be taken per day.
> - Always check drug dosage in the *British National Formulary for Children*.

Communicating serious problems

Doctors often face the difficult task of imparting serious issues to parents and children. In paediatric practice, it may be because there is:

- a serious congenital abnormality at birth, e.g. chromosomal disorder
- the diagnosis of a disabling condition, e.g. cerebral palsy, neurodegenerative disorder, gross intracranial abnormality seen at ultrasound in a preterm infant
- a serious illness, e.g. meningitis or malignant disease, or an accident, e.g. head injury
- sudden death of a child, e.g. sudden infant death syndrome (SIDS).

In addition, families often perceive less serious problems as being very serious, and many of the principles described in the following section will be applicable.

Initial interview

The manner in which the initial interview is conducted is very important. It may have a profound influence on the parents' ability to cope with the problem and their subsequent relationship with health professionals. Parents often continue to recall and recount for many years details of the initial interview when they were informed that their child had a serious problem. Parents of children with life-threatening illnesses have said that what they valued most was open, sympathetic, direct and uninterrupted discussion in private that allowed sufficient time for doctors to repeat and clarify information and for them to ask questions (Box 5.3).

Palliative and end-of-life care

Palliative care should begin from the time of diagnosis of a life-limiting illness and may continue for many years. It includes pain and symptom management for the child, psychosocial support for the child and family, attention to practical needs and spiritual care. It may also include respite care and bereavement support for the family after the child has died. End-of-life care is used specifically to describe the period of care when death is imminent.

Care plan

A care plan should be developed for children with a life-threatening illness. It needs to address symptom care and medical and emotional support, clarify the roles of the clinical teams involved and make management plans for potential crises. It needs regular review as the illness evolves.

Place of care

If the child is in hospital, there should be a private area for the child and family. If care is provided at home, it is essential that the family has support and information about whom to contact for routine and emergency problems, including medications, and what to expect when the child dies and afterwards. The needs of the child are paramount, but all family members must be considered. Many will not have encountered death before. Some families will have specific religious needs.

Care after death

Families should be involved in the child's end-of-life care and care after the death, according to their wishes. Their individual cultural and religious beliefs and rituals should be accommodated whenever possible. For example, some families may wish to take their child home from the hospital or hospice and some cultures have specific requirements about burial and its timing. Families are encouraged to hold the child before and afterwards, if they wish to do so. The family should be provided with information about registering a death and making funeral arrangements. Some families create memory boxes with mementos from the child. All health professionals involved should be informed when the child has died. Grief following death is normal and intense and may continue to affect families for years. The family should be informed about support that is available.

Caring for staff

Many staff will be distressed as they will have known the child for a long time. If the death was sudden and unexpected, there may be feelings of failure. Open discussion is often helpful by clarifying the events and allowing staff to express their concerns.

Box 5.3 How parents wish to be told about a serious problem

Setting
- In private
- Uninterrupted
- Unhurried
- Both parents (or friend/relative) present if possible
- Senior doctor
- Nurse or social worker present

Establish contact
- Find out what the family knows or suspects
- Respect the family's vulnerability
- Use the child's name
- Do not avoid looking at them
- Be direct, open, sympathetic

Provide information
- Flexibility is essential
- Do not protect from bad news, but pace giving it
- Name the illness/problem
- Describe symptoms relevant to child's condition
- Discuss aetiology – parents will usually want to know
- Anticipate and answer questions. Do not avoid difficult issues because parents have not thought to ask

Explain long-term prognosis
- If the child is likely to die, listen to concerns about time, place, and nature of death
- Outline the support/treatment available

Address feelings
- Be prepared to tolerate reactions of shock, especially anger or weeping
- Acknowledge uncertainty
- How is it likely to affect the family?
- What and how to tell other children, relatives and friends?

Concluding the interview
- Elicit what parents have understood
- Clarify and repeat
- Acknowledge that it may be difficult for parents to absorb all the information
- Mention sources of support
- If possible, give parents a contact telephone number
- Give address of self-help group.

Follow-up
- Offer early follow-up
- Suggest to families that they write down questions in preparation for the next appointment
- Ensure adequate communication of content of interview to:
  – other members of staff
  – general practitioner and health visitor
  – other professionals, e.g. a referring paediatrician

Adapted from Woolley H, Stein A, Forrest GC, Baum JD. Imparting the diagnosis of life-threatening illness in children. *British Medical Journal* 298:1623–1626, 1989.

Ethics

Situations arise in paediatric practice in which the course of action that should be followed is unclear. Knowledge of the ethical theories and principles that underpin medical practice may be helpful in understanding the issues involved. It is important to justify decisions to investigate or treat in accordance with these principles and in language that is clear to all concerned.

Definitions of the principles of medical ethics

- *Non-maleficence* – do no harm (psychological and/or physical).
- *Beneficence* – positive obligation to do good (these two principles have been part of medical ethics since the Hippocratic Oath).
- *Justice* – fairness for all, equity and equality of care.
- *Respect for autonomy* – respect for individuals' rights to make informed and thought-out decisions for themselves in accordance with their capabilities.
- *Truth telling and confidentiality* – important aspects of autonomy that support trust, essential in the doctor–patient relationship.
- *Duty* – the moral obligation to act irrespective of the consequences in accordance with moral laws, which are universal, apply equally to all and which respect persons as autonomous beings.
- *Utility* – the obligation to do the greatest good for the greatest number.
- *Rights* – justifiable moral claims, e.g. the right to life, respect and education, which impose moral obligations upon others.

Application of ethical principles to paediatrics

Non-maleficence

Children are more vulnerable to harm. This includes their suffering from fear of procedures, which they may be too young to express verbally. Doctors may do harm from lack of skill or knowledge, especially if they do not treat children frequently.

Beneficence

The child's interest is paramount. In the UK, this is enshrined in the Children Act 1989 and the United Nations Convention on the Rights of the Child. This may sometimes conflict with parental autonomy, such as the emergency treatment of a child where the parent is not immediately available or when details are given to social workers in suspected child abuse.

Justice

This involves ensuring a comprehensive child health service, including the prevention of illness and equal access to healthcare, even when poverty, language barriers and parental disability are present.

Autonomy

Children have restricted but developing rights in law. Parents are trusted to make decisions on their child's behalf because they will usually act in the child's best interests, but there may be circumstances, e.g. child abuse, in which this is not the case.

Truth telling

It is more difficult with children than adults to be sure that they understand what is happening to them. For example, it is easy to reassure children falsely that procedures will not hurt; when they find this is untrue, trust will be lost for future occasions.

Consent

Valid consent is required for all medical interventions other than emergencies or when urgent intervention is necessary to prevent serious risk of present or future harm. It provides the ethical and legal authority for action, which would otherwise be a common assault or interfere with the right of individuals to decide what should be done to them (autonomous choice). To be valid, consent must be sufficiently informed and freely given by a person who is competent to do so. Clinicians have a duty to provide sufficient information to enable a reasonable person to make the decision and must answer all questions honestly. Information has to be given in language that is clear and understandable.

In UK law, the legal age of consent to medical treatment is 16 years. The right of children below this age to give consent depends on their competence rather than their age. They may consent to medical examination and treatment provided they can demonstrate that they have the maturity and judgement to understand and appraise the nature and implications of the proposed treatment, including the risks and alternative courses of action. This case was tested in law (Gillick vs. West Norfolk Health Authority) and resulted in the Fraser Guidelines. These were originally devised to provide advice for healthcare professionals in determining when it would be appropriate to give oral contraceptive agents to girls without their parent's knowledge. In order to be Fraser Competent, the healthcare professional has to ensure that the girl (although under the age of 16) understands his/her advice, could not be persuaded to inform her parents or for them to be informed that she is very likely to continue having sex with or without contraception, her physical or mental health or both are likely to suffer unless she receives contraception and her best interests are served by receiving contraception. The principles of this case are now applied in other situations.

When a child lacks the maturity and judgement to give consent, this capacity is given to a person having parental responsibility – usually a natural parent, or to a court. In practice, problems occur only when there is disagreement between the child and the parents and clinicians over treatment.

Despite including children's views in consent, legal judgements have not supported children who refuse treatment which parents and clinicians feel to be in their best interests, especially if its purpose is to save life or prevent serious harm, e.g. heart transplantation for acute cardiomyopathy in an intelligent 15-year-old patient. Where disputes cannot be resolved by negotiation or mediation, or there is doubt over the legality of what is proposed, legal advice should be sought. Whatever the outcome, children should have their views heard and be given reasons as to why they are being overridden.

Confidentiality

Children are owed the same duty of confidentiality as adults, irrespective of their legal capacity. In general, personal information about them should not be shared without their consent or agreement unless it is necessary for their health or to protect them from serious harm, e.g. in actual or suspected child abuse.

Best interests

It is a general ethical and legal maxim that the best interests of the child are paramount. Doctors therefore have a duty to save life, restore health and prevent disease by treatments that confer maximum benefit and minimal harm and which respect the autonomy of the child as far as possible. Parents have the ethical and legal duty to make decisions on behalf of their child, provided that they act in their best interests. Disagreements can occur between parents and healthcare professionals over the best interests of the child especially when the withholding or withdrawing of life-sustaining treatment is involved. Under these circumstances, an independent opinion may be helpful, but sometimes legal intervention is required. Courts have generally been supportive of the position that in some circumstances the burden to the child of providing life-sustaining treatment outweighs its benefits.

Case Histories 5.1 and 5.2 demonstrate some of the ethical problems encountered in paediatrics.

The ethics of research in paediatrics

Research involving children is important in promoting children's health and well-being and in providing an evidence base for practice. However, the number of trials and other forms of research is much less than in adult medicine. This paucity of research is highly detrimental to improving care, and great effort is being made to increase research conducted in paediatrics. A particular example is our knowledge about drug therapy

Case history 5.1

Diabetes mellitus

Jack, aged 5 years, has a high blood sugar and is showing classical signs of diabetes. Jack hates needles and makes it clear that he rejects any sort of injection. 'No I don't want an injection, go away' is the message, loud and clear, when you try to take blood to confirm the diagnosis. Yet with the full and anxious approval of his parents, you go ahead and do these things anyway. If Jack was 25 years old and made it clear that he refused your interventions, while you would strongly urge him to give permission and explain that he was in real danger of dying as a result of such refusal, you would not (presumably) treat him against his will, even if his mother and father still urged you to do so.

In contrast to traditional adult medical ethics, in paediatrics the autonomy of the patient either is not present at all (as in babies and young infants) or is often not sufficiently developed to be respected if the child's decision conflicts with what other people consider to be appropriate in that child's best interests. The decisions about the child's medical care are generally entrusted to the parents.

Why the parents? They are given the privilege and responsibility of making decisions on behalf of their children largely because they are most likely to protect and promote the interests of their children. The normal assumption in paediatric practice is that doctors should work closely with parents and give advice that parents may or may not accept. Wherever possible, a mutually trusting and respectful working relationship should be developed and maintained, both because it will be in the best interests of the child and because it will tend to lead to far better experiences of medical care for all involved.

Also, consider whether your decision would have been the same about performing an extra venepuncture for a special blood test for an ethically approved research project (see the 'The ethics of research in paediatrics' section).

Case history 5.2

Acute lymphatic leukaemia, truth telling and stopping treatment

Millie, aged 10 years, has acute lymphoblastic leukaemia, which was diagnosed 4 years ago. She has relapsed, with early involvement of the central nervous system. She is well known to the staff of her local children's ward as she has had four relapses of her leukaemia and a previous bone marrow transplant. It is the opinion of her paediatric consultant that no further medical treatment is likely to be curative. Millie asks one of the junior paediatric doctors why her parents had been so upset following a recent discussion with the consultant, at which she had not been present. The parents had made it very clear to all the staff that they did not want their child to be informed of the poor prognosis, nor would they tell her why she was not having further chemotherapy.

The parents have heard of a new drug that is claimed, in some reports on the internet, to help such children. However, it is very expensive, there is evidence that it does not cross the blood–brain barrier and the doctors consider it highly unlikely to be of benefit. The parents insist on a trial of the drug.

Ethical issues to consider are:

- *Autonomy* – the parents claim the right to control the information reaching their child on the grounds that it is in her best interests as judged by them.
- *Truth telling* – the staff feel that it would be wrong to reassure her falsely.
- *Non-maleficence* – the parents wish to avoid the shock of the news and the loss of hope in their daughter.
- *Beneficence* – the staff wish to support the child effectively, which would be difficult if she were to be isolated by ignorance of what is upsetting her family and carers.
- *Justice* – should scarce resources be used on this new drug? Because her parents are desperate, should Millie be given a drug which, in the specialist's opinion, will not benefit her?
- *Best interests* – what are Millie's best interests and who should decide them? What weight should be given to Millie's own views based on her experience of her illness?

In such situations, further discussion between the parents and staff whom they trust is usually the key to resolving the situation. The parents will need to understand the mutual benefits of adopting as open a pattern of communication as possible. They may be helped by a member of staff being present or helping them talk or listen to the child, who will usually understand more than the parents suspect.

Parents almost always wish to do the best for their child. Detailed explanation is likely to help them see that the child's best interests may not be to seek further cure but to accept a change of focus towards palliative care. A second opinion from an independent specialist may be helpful, as may a specific ethical review. If, despite all efforts to reach agreement, the parents reject the doctor's advice, it is fairest to let a court of law decide whether or not to accept the parents' demands.

in children. Although they differ from adults in their anatomy, physiology, disease patterns and responses to therapy, many drugs are not licensed for use in children because they have not been specifically tested in them. Pharmaceutical companies are now being encouraged or forced by legislation to test their medications in children.

Where a child suffers from a particular disease, e.g. acute lymphoblastic leukaemia, randomized controlled trials may be used to compare treatment regimens. The ethical justification for such trials is that there is no good reason to believe that one of the treatments would be better than the other – 'therapeutic equipoise' – and that the standard treatment used for comparative purposes is the best currently available.

The situation is different when an investigation, e.g. blood test, X-ray or intervention is proposed for healthy children as part of a control group in a trial or for the purpose of establishing a normal range. Both can be ethically justified provided that the procedure in question carries no more risk than generally encountered and accepted in everyday life.

Whatever the nature of the research, a number of criteria must be met:
- appropriate research should be first carried out in adults or older children
- the project should have a sound scientific basis and be well designed
- the researchers should be competent to carry it out in the time specified
- sufficient information should be given in a form comprehensible to the child and family to enable them to give valid consent to participation, e.g. by provision of information sheets in an appropriate form and language or by the use of independent translators
- parents must have the option to withdraw their child from the research at any stage without prejudice
- the project must be reviewed and approved by an independent scientific and ethical process (Research Ethics Committee).

This is an increasing requirement for not only groups of parents and carers to be involved in considering research studies, but to also get input from groups of children and young people themselves.

Summary

Ethics in paediatrics:
- Both clinicians and parents aim to do what is in their child's best interests.
- Conflicting views can usually be resolved by good communication.
- If not resolved, help may be sought from further, wider communication or a second, truly independent opinion, or sometimes from hospital ethical committees or may go to court.
- In older children who understand the issues and have strong views as to what should or should not be done to them, there is increasing ethical and legal support for them to exercise as much autonomy as they are capable of.

Evidence-based paediatrics

Clinicians have always sought to make decisions in the best interests of their patients. However, such decisions have often been made intuitively, given as clinical opinion, which is difficult to generalize, scrutinize or challenge. Evidence-based practice provides a systematic approach to enable clinicians to use the best available evidence, usually from research, to help them solve their clinical problems. The difference between this approach and old-style clinical practice is that clinicians need to know how to turn their clinical problems into questions that can be answered by the research literature, to search the literature efficiently and to analyze the evidence using epidemiological and biostatistical rules (Figs 5.7 and 5.8). Sometimes the best available evidence will be a high-quality systematic review of randomized controlled trials, which are directly applicable to a particular patient. For other questions, lack of more valid studies may mean that the decision has to be based on previous experience with a small number of similar patients. The important factor is that, for any decision, clinicians know the strength of the evidence and therefore the degree of uncertainty. As this approach requires clinicians to be explicit about the evidence they use, others involved in the decisions (patients, parents, managers and other clinicians) can debate and judge the evidence for themselves.

Why practise evidence-based paediatrics?

There are many examples from the past where, through lack of evidence, clinicians have harmed children, for example:

- *Blindness from retinopathy of prematurity*. In the 1950s, following anecdotal reports, many neonatal units started nursing all premature infants in additional ambient oxygen, irrespective of need. This reduced mortality, but as no properly conducted trials were performed of this new therapy, it took several years for it to be realized that it was also responsible for many thousands of babies becoming blind from retinopathy of prematurity.
- *Advice that babies should sleep lying on their front (prone), which increases the risk of SIDS (Sudden Infant Death Syndrome)*. Medical advice given during the 1970s and 1980s to put babies to sleep prone, appears to have been based on physiological studies in preterm babies, which showed better oxygenation when nursed prone. Furthermore, autopsies on some infants who died of SIDS showed milk in the trachea, which was assumed to have been aspirated and this was thought to be more likely if they were lying on their back. However, an accumulation of more valid evidence from cohort and case–control studies showed that placing term infants prone was associated with an *increased* risk of SIDS.

Application of evidence-based medicine to clinical problems

Clinical problem

↓

Frame question → What evidence is needed to reach your decision? Clinical problems are often complex and the different elements (aetiology, diagnosis, therapy, prognosis) need to be tackled as separate questions. Most clinical questions can be structured into these three components:

Patient population	Intervention	Clinical outcome
A population similar to your patient	e.g. giving antibiotics compared with not giving antibiotics	The most important outcomes, good or bad

↓

Search for the evidence → Search the research literature. Use search filters for efficiency. For randomized clinical trials and systematic reviews of interventions, go to Cochrane Library.
If there is nothing which addresses your question, or if your question is about prognosis or diagnosis, you need to use an online database, such as MEDLINE.

↓

Appraise the evidence → Appraise the validity (closeness to the truth) and usefulness (relevance to your patient) of the evidence.
In intervention studies, there is a hierarchy of validity:
- A systematic view of randomized controlled trials (RCTs)
- Individual RCTs
- Cohort studies
- Case–control studies
- Case reports or anecdotal experience of respected authorities

If your question is about a *diagnostic test* or *observation*, you need a study that has made an independent, blind comparison with an adequate reference standard based on patients with a similar spectrum of disease to your patient.
If your question is about *prognosis*, you need a study that follows a group of patients similar to your patient (cohort), over an adequate period, to see what happens to them.

↓

Make a decision → Incorporate the evidence into clinical or policy decisions. This depends on judgements about the validity and relevance of the evidence, the probability of the different outcomes, and the values assigned to them by the patient, clinician and wider society. They are also heavily influenced by what is feasible within the organization. We will often agree on the validity of the evidence and the probability of the different outcomes, but decisions may differ because the people involved hold different values.

↓

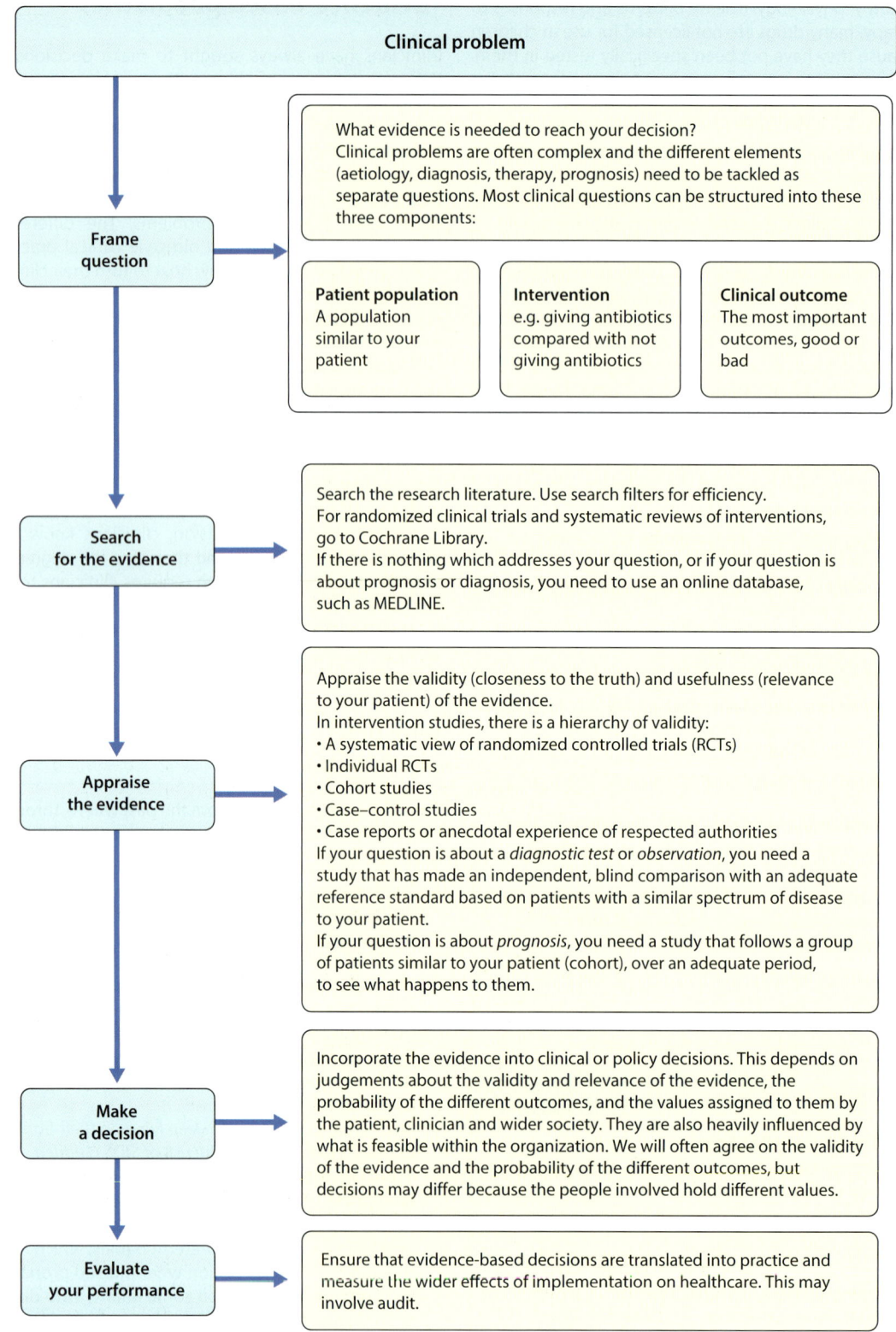

Evaluate your performance → Ensure that evidence-based decisions are translated into practice and measure the wider effects of implementation on healthcare. This may involve audit.

Figure 5.7 Application of evidence-based medicine to clinical problems.

Example of evidence-based practice in solving a clinical problem

Clinical problem:
Should you treat a 3-year-old boy with otitis media with antibiotics?

Frame question

Population	Intervention	Outcomes
Children with acute otitis media (AOM)	Antibiotics compared with none	Pain Hearing loss Adverse drug effects Other complications

Search for the evidence

Cochrane Library – 47 meta-analyses, one corresponding best to this child

Appraise the evidence

Outcome	Risk ratio (95% CI)
Pain at 24 hours	0.89 (0.78–1.01)
Pain at 2–3 days	0.70 (0.57–0.82)
Pain at 4–7 days	0.76 (0.63–0.91)
Perforation	0.82 (0.74–0.90)
Vomiting, diarrhoea, or rash	1.38 (1.19–1.59)
Deafness at 3 months	0.97 (0.76–1.24)

Reduced risk ← 0.5 — 1.0 — 1.5 → Increased risk

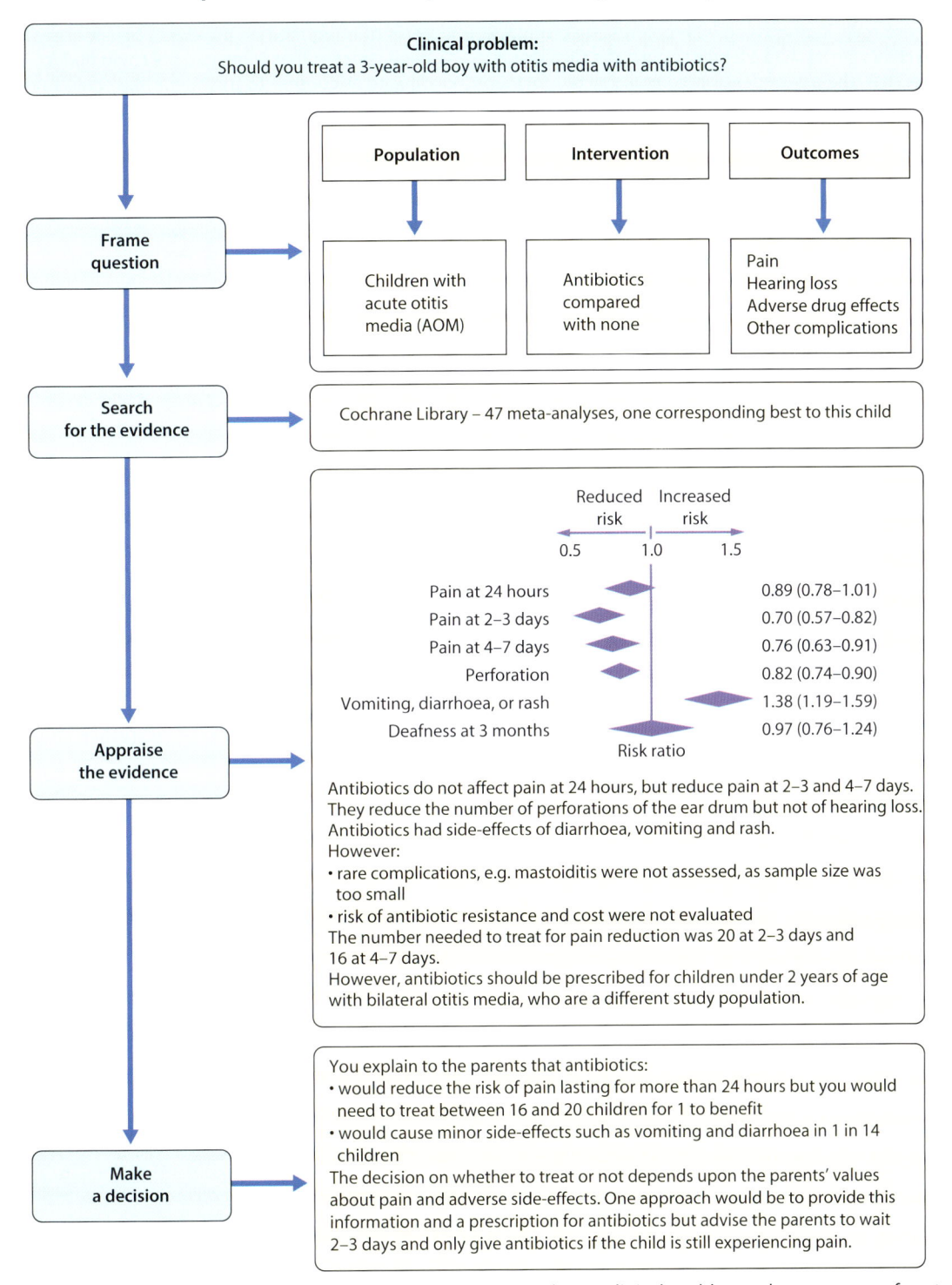

Antibiotics do not affect pain at 24 hours, but reduce pain at 2–3 and 4–7 days. They reduce the number of perforations of the ear drum but not of hearing loss. Antibiotics had side-effects of diarrhoea, vomiting and rash.
However:
- rare complications, e.g. mastoiditis were not assessed, as sample size was too small
- risk of antibiotic resistance and cost were not evaluated

The number needed to treat for pain reduction was 20 at 2–3 days and 16 at 4–7 days.
However, antibiotics should be prescribed for children under 2 years of age with bilateral otitis media, who are a different study population.

Make a decision

You explain to the parents that antibiotics:
- would reduce the risk of pain lasting for more than 24 hours but you would need to treat between 16 and 20 children for 1 to benefit
- would cause minor side-effects such as vomiting and diarrhoea in 1 in 14 children

The decision on whether to treat or not depends upon the parents' values about pain and adverse side-effects. One approach would be to provide this information and a prescription for antibiotics but advise the parents to wait 2–3 days and only give antibiotics if the child is still experiencing pain.

Figure 5.8 An example of an evidence-based medicine approach to a clinical problem – the treatment of acute otitis media with antibiotics. (From Venekamp RP, Sanders SL, Glasziou PP, Del Mar CB, Rovers MM: Antibiotics for acute otitis media in children. *Cochrane Database of Systematic Reviews* (1):CD000219, 2015 with permission).

Evidence-based medicine allows clinicians to be explicit about the probability (or risk) of important outcomes. For example, in discussing with parents the prognosis of a child who has had a febrile seizure, the clinician can state that 'the risk of developing epilepsy is 1 in 100', instead of using vague terms, such as 'he/she is unlikely to develop epilepsy'.

Explicit analysis of evidence has also become more important with the increasing delivery of healthcare by teams rather than individuals. Each team member needs to understand the rationale for decisions and the probability of different outcomes in order to contribute towards clinical decisions and to provide consistent information to patients and parents.

To what extent is paediatric practice based on sound evidence?

There are two paediatric specialities in which there is a considerable body of reliable, high-quality evidence underpinning clinical practice, namely, paediatric oncology and, to a lesser extent, neonatology. Management protocols of virtually all children with cancer are part of multicentre trials designed to identify which treatment gives the best possible results. The trials are national or, increasingly, international, and include short-term and long-term follow-up. Examples of the range of evidence available in paediatrics are given in Box 5.4. In general, the evidence base for paediatrics is poorer than in adult medicine. Reasons for this are:

- the relatively small number of children with significant illness requiring investigation and treatment. To overcome this, multicentre trials are required, which are more difficult to organize and expensive
- consent is required on the child's behalf; there has been concern that some parents could find it difficult to consent to treatment that could turn out to be inferior to the standard treatment or have previously unknown side-effects and that they had agreed to this
- consent is often required during a time of parental distress, e.g. after the birth of a preterm infants or after the acute onset of a serious illness
- as children cannot give consent themselves, it may not be possible to justify performing additional investigations or other tests, especially if they are painful or not of direct benefit to the child
- there is less of a culture of research, and of conducting randomized controlled trials in particular, in paediatrics compared with adult medicine.

For evidence-based practice to become more widespread, clinicians must recognize the need to ask questions, particularly about procedures or interventions which are common practice. However, evidence-based medicine is not cookbook medicine. Incontrovertible evidence is rare, and clinical decisions are complex, which is why clinical care is provided by skilled and experienced clinicians. Evidence-based healthcare cannot change this, but is an essential tool to help clinicians make rational, informed decisions together with their patients. In addition, evidence-based paediatrics provides a way for clinicians to articulate their priorities for research and thereby set research agendas that are relevant to service needs.

Box 5.4 Examples of the range of evidence available in paediatrics

1. Clear evidence of benefit

Therapeutic hypothermia for newborn infants with hypoxic-ischaemic encephalopathy

Meta-analysis of moderate cooling before 6 hours of age for 72 hours shows reduced death or major neurodisability at 18 months of age, with seven babies needed to be treated for benefit; there is also improved survival with normal neurological function (Fig. 11.4 in Ch. 11: Neonatal Medicine).

On the basis of animal studies, several multicentre, prospective randomized studies of term infants with perinatal asphyxia of intensive care with or without cooling were conducted.

Infants had to be identified, assessed, transferred to a treatment centre and treatment started within 6 hours of birth.

Consent had to be obtained rapidly from parents, shortly after being informed that their baby was dangerously ill. They had to understand that randomization meant their baby may not receive the new treatment, and the new treatment may have unknown side-effects.

It was only when the results of several trials were amalgamated that significant improvement was identified. This demonstrates some of the difficulties that have to be overcome when conducting trials in children, but that it is often possible to overcome them. Cooling for moderate or severe perinatal asphyxia has become standard practice in the UK and many countries.

2. Clear evidence, but need to balance benefits and harms

Antibiotic treatment for children with otitis media

As shown in Fig. 5.8, there is a balance of risk and benefits.

3. No clear evidence

Migraine in children

Although there is good evidence for the use of simple analgesic agents, prophylactic treatment of migraine with β-blockers or pizotifen is poor. (See Wöber-Bingöl Ç Pharmacological treatment of acute migraine in adolescents and children. Paediatr Drugs. 2013 Jun;15(3):235–46 (http://www.ncbi.nlm.nih.gov/pubmed/23575981?dopt=Abstract)). This causes a dilemma when choosing the best prophylaxis for a child.

> **Summary**
>
> **Evidence-based paediatrics:**
> - Requires clinical problems to be framed into questions, to search the literature and then appraise the evidence in order to make a decision.
> - Is less well developed than in adult medicine.
> - Should be adopted whenever possible. However, clinical decisions are complex and the evidence base usually informs rather than determines clinical decision making.

Acknowledgements

We would like to acknowledge contributors to this chapter in previous editions, whose work we have drawn on: Tom Lissauer (1st, 2nd, 3rd, 4th Editions), Maude Meates-Dennis (2nd, 3rd Edition), Graham Clayden (2nd Edition), Ruth Gilbert (2nd Edition), Raanon Gillon (2nd Edition), Vic Larcher (3rd Edition).

Further reading

Websites (Accessed November 2016)

Accident and Emergency Statistics: *Demand, Performance and Pressure.* House of Commons Library. 2016. www.parliament.uk
Accident and Emergency Statistics Review for UK

BMJ Clinical Evidence: Available at: http://clinicalevidence.bmj.com/ceweb.
Overview of topics in evidence-based medicine.

Centre for Evidence-Based Care (CEBM), Oxford:
Available at: http://www.cebm.net.
Details about evidence-based medicine.

Cochrane Systematic Reviews: Available at: http://www.cochrane.org.

Every Child Matters: Available at: www.education.gov.uk.
National framework for services for children and young people.

Trip Database: Available at: http://www.tripdatabase.com.
Research engine for evidence-based medicine and clinical guidelines.

Paediatric emergencies

The seriously ill child	80		Sepsis	88
Cardiopulmonary resuscitation	83		Anaphylaxis	89
The seriously injured child	83		Neurological emergencies	90
Respiratory failure	83		Apparent life-threatening events	94
Shock	87		Unexpected death of a child	94

Features of paediatric emergencies are:
- the rapid clinical assessment of the seriously ill child, including assessment of level of consciousness, should take less than 1 minute
- the management of cardiopulmonary resuscitation in children is different from adults but follows the same principles
- key to management of the seriously ill child is early recognition and intervention to prevent respiratory or circulatory failure; once present they are difficult to reverse
- management of status epilepticus and anaphylaxis is according to national guidelines.

There are few situations that provoke greater anxiety than being called to see a child who is seriously ill or injured. Although such situations in children are uncommon, it is critically important to recognize those with serious physiological deterioration and to start the correct treatment promptly.

Some children will require transfer to a paediatric intensive care unit (PICU). PICUs are usually based in children's hospitals and in the UK, children are usually transferred to the PICU by a specialized transport team.

This chapter outlines a basic approach to the emergency management of the seriously ill or injured child.

The seriously ill child

The rapid clinical assessment of the seriously ill child will identify potential respiratory, circulatory or neurological failure. This should take less than 1 minute. Normal vital signs are shown in Fig. 6.1 and a rapid assessment schema is shown in Fig. 6.2.

Resuscitation is given immediately, if necessary, followed by secondary assessment and other emergency treatment.

The seriously ill child may present with shock, respiratory distress, as a drowsy/unconscious or fitting child, or with a surgical emergency. Their causes are listed in Fig. 6.4. Early recognition of the deteriorating child is key to a successful outcome and, in the UK, paediatric early warning scores are now recommended in order to identify children who are seriously unwell. These may include measurement of heart rate, respiratory rate, oxygen saturation and temperature; a higher score than normal suggests deterioration of clinical condition requiring intervention.

Vital signs

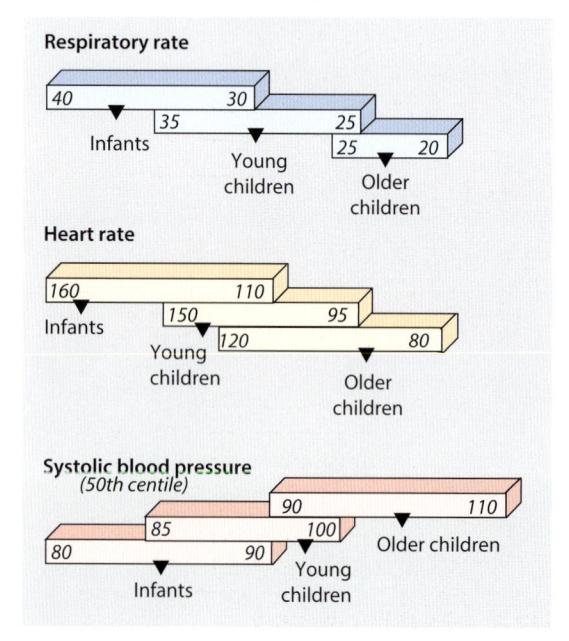

Respiratory rate
- Infants: 40–30
- Young children: 35–25
- Older children: 25–20

Heart rate
- Infants: 160–110
- Young children: 150–95
- Older children: 120–80

Systolic blood pressure (50th centile)
- Infants: 80–85
- Young children: 90–100
- Older children: 90–110

Figure 6.1 Variation in the normal range for respiratory rate, heart rate, and systolic blood pressure with age.

Assessment of the seriously ill child

The rapid clinical assessment:
ABCDE
Should take <1 min

Airway and breathing
Look, listen, and feel for:
Airway obstruction or respiratory distress
Work of breathing (respiratory effort)
Respiratory rate
Stridor, wheeze
Auscultation for air entry
Cyanosis
Oxygen saturation

Circulation
Feel and assess:
Heart rate
Pulse volume
Capillary refill time (Fig 6.3)
Blood pressure

Disability
Observe and note:
Level of consciousness (Box 6.1)
Posture – hypotonia, decorticate, decerebrate
Pupil size and reactivity

Exposure

→

Resuscitation (if necessary)

Includes basic/advanced life support
Consider:
Jaw and neck positioning
Oxygen
Suction and foreign body removal
Supporting breathing
Chest compression
Monitoring oxygen saturation and heart rate

↓

Secondary assessment

History from:
- parents
- witnesses
- general practitioner
- paramedical staff
- police

Examination including:
- evidence of trauma
- rash, e.g. meningococcal
- smell, e.g. ketones, alcohol
- scars, e.g. underlying congenital heart disease
- MedicAlert bracelet

Investigations
- blood glucose

↓

Other emergency interventions

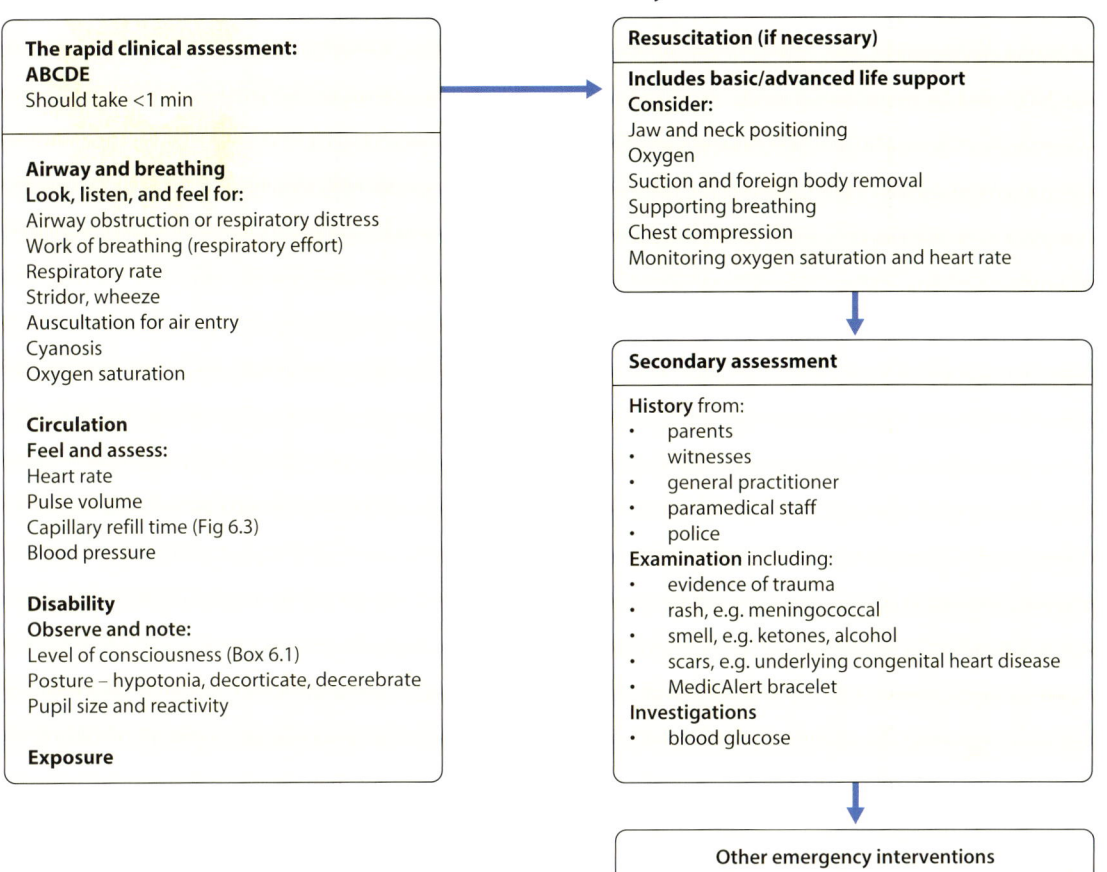

Figure 6.2 Assessment of the seriously ill child.

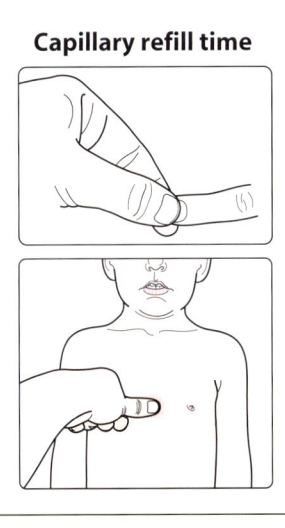

Capillary refill time

Press on the skin of the sternum or a digit at the level of the heart
Apply blanching pressure for 5 s
Measure time for blush to return
Prolonged capillary refill if >2 s

Figure 6.3 Capillary refill time.

Box 6.1 Rapid assessment of level of consciousness (AVPU) – more detailed evaluation is with the Glasgow Coma Scale (see Table 6.2)

A	ALERT
V	Responds to VOICE
P	Responds to PAIN
U	UNRESPONSIVE

A score of P means that the child's airway is at risk and will need to be maintained by a manoeuvre or adjunct.

☀ **Capillary refill time is affected by body exposure to a cold environment**

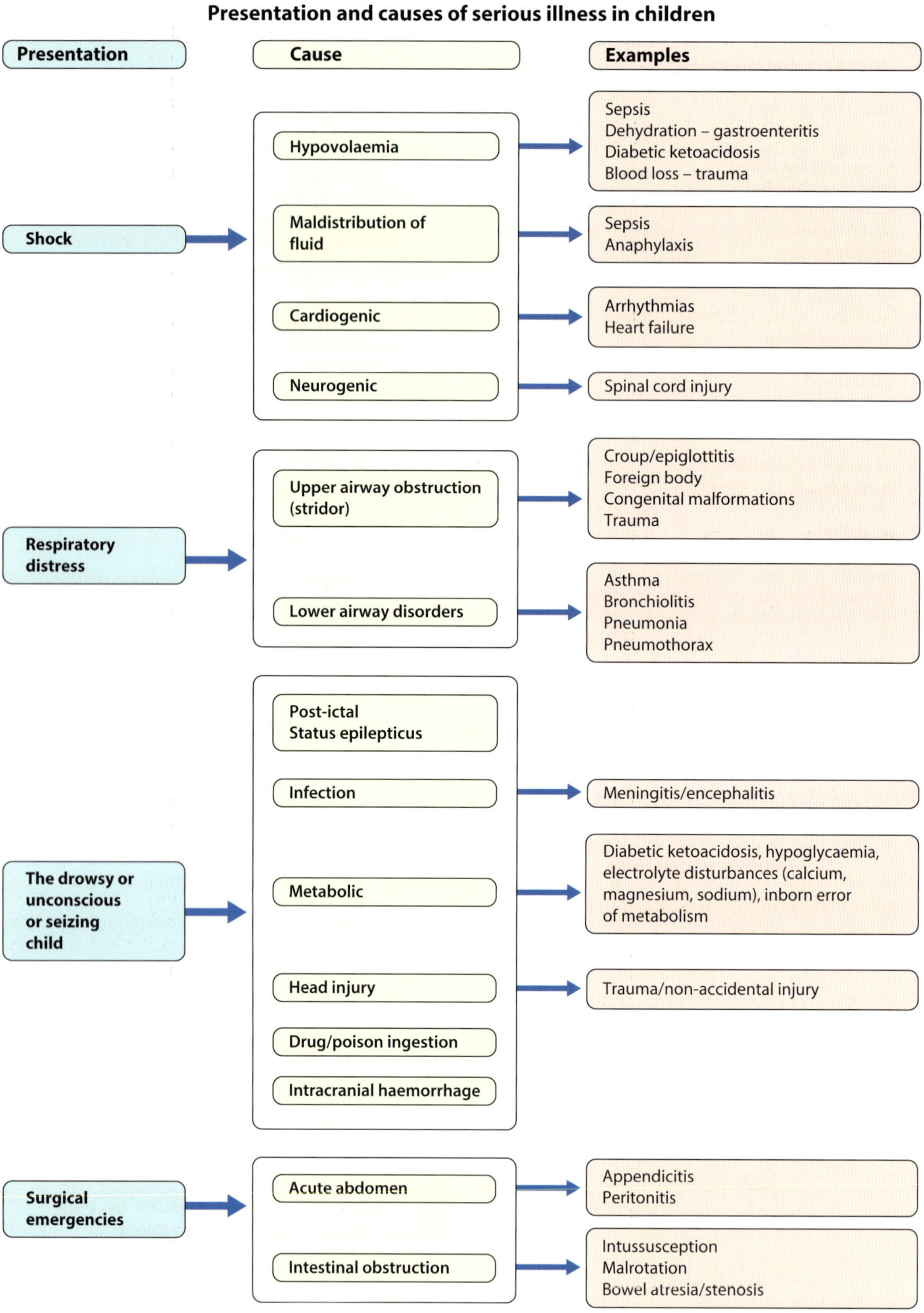

Presentation and causes of serious illness in children

Presentation	Cause	Examples
Shock	Hypovolaemia	Sepsis Dehydration – gastroenteritis Diabetic ketoacidosis Blood loss – trauma
	Maldistribution of fluid	Sepsis Anaphylaxis
	Cardiogenic	Arrhythmias Heart failure
	Neurogenic	Spinal cord injury
Respiratory distress	Upper airway obstruction (stridor)	Croup/epiglottitis Foreign body Congenital malformations Trauma
	Lower airway disorders	Asthma Bronchiolitis Pneumonia Pneumothorax
The drowsy or unconscious or seizing child	Post-ictal Status epilepticus	
	Infection	Meningitis/encephalitis
	Metabolic	Diabetic ketoacidosis, hypoglycaemia, electrolyte disturbances (calcium, magnesium, sodium), inborn error of metabolism
	Head injury	Trauma/non-accidental injury
	Drug/poison ingestion	
	Intracranial haemorrhage	
Surgical emergencies	Acute abdomen	Appendicitis Peritonitis
	Intestinal obstruction	Intussusception Malrotation Bowel atresia/stenosis

Figure 6.4 The main modes of presentation of serious illness in children and their causes.

Summary

Regarding the seriously ill child
- Prevention of cardiopulmonary arrest is by early recognition and treatment of respiratory distress and/or respiratory or circulatory failure.
- Paediatric early warning scores are recommended to help identify deterioration in clinical condition.

Cardiopulmonary resuscitation

In adults, cardiopulmonary arrest is often cardiac in origin, secondary to ischaemic heart disease. By contrast, in previously well children with healthy hearts, cardiopulmonary arrest is usually secondary to hypoxia from respiratory or neurological failure or shock. Basic life support must be started immediately.

Paediatric basic life support

See Fig. 6.5.

Paediatric advanced life support

See Fig. 6.6. Children who have been resuscitated successfully should be transferred to a paediatric high-dependency or intensive care unit.

☼ Doctors should be able to provide life support for children of all ages, from newborn to adolescents.

The seriously injured child

A structured approach to major trauma ensures that life-threatening injuries are identified and managed during the primary survey before other less serious injuries are identified during the secondary survey. Cervical spine injury should be assumed; the preferred method of immobilization is manual in-line stabilization (holding the neck in a midline neutral position) followed by head blocks and straps if necessary. Routine application of cervical collars is no longer recommended. In trauma, catastrophic haemorrhage should be dealt with immediately, before the usual airway, breathing, circulation (ABC) approach (Fig. 6.7).

Respiratory failure

Respiratory failure may be defined as failure of the lungs to maintain adequate gas exchange. It may be due to alveolar hypoventilation, diffusion impairment, intrapulmonary shunting, or ventilation–perfusion mismatch. These may occur singly or in combination depending on the clinical condition, e.g. pneumonia may be associated with both diffusion impairment and ventilation–perfusion mismatch. Respiratory failure causes hypoxaemia, which can lead to tissue hypoxia, or hypercarbia which can cause carbon dioxide narcosis, or both. In addition to these potentially life-threatening complications, when respiratory distress is prolonged, the child is at risk of becoming exhausted and having a respiratory arrest. Respiratory failure must therefore be recognized and treated promptly in order to maintain gas exchange and prevent complications.

Assessment

Assessment of the child with respiratory failure (Box 6.2) follows the standard ABC approach, with an emphasis on the work of breathing and the effects of hypoxaemia on other organ systems, particularly the heart and brain. Once an initial assessment of severity has been made and supportive measures are instituted, investigations and therapy are commenced. Specific conditions causing respiratory failure and their treatment are discussed in Chapter 17 (Respiratory disorders).

Supportive therapy

Supportive therapy can be escalated from oxygen (via face mask or nasal cannula) to noninvasive ventilation to endotracheal intubation and mechanical ventilation.

Oxygen

Children with peripheral capillary oxygen saturation (SpO_2) less than 92% should receive oxygen to achieve normal saturations. The fraction of inspired oxygen (FiO_2) can be titrated according to pulse oximetry. The maximum fractional concentration of oxygen delivered via facemask is 0.60 unless a reservoir bag is added.

Noninvasive ventilation

Noninvasive ventilation (ventilatory support without endotracheal intubation) includes continuous positive airways pressure (CPAP) or biphasic positive airways pressure via face mask or nasal mask. Recently,

---

Box 6.2 Indicators of respiratory distress in infancy

Moderate
- Tachycardia
- Respiratory rate >50 bpm
- Nasal flaring
- Use of accessory muscles
- Intercostal and subcostal recession
- Head retraction
- Unable to feed

Severe
- Cyanosis
- Getting tired
- Reduced conscious level
- Saturation <92% despite oxygen therapy
- Rising partial pressure of carbon dioxide (pCO_2)

Paediatric basic life support
(Trained resuscitator, no equipment)

SAFE approach → Approach with care / Free from danger / Get help if >1 rescuer or witnessed, sudden collapse when defibrillation may be needed.

↓

Check responsiveness:
Ask 'Are you all right?'
Stimulate gently
Do not shake infants or suspected cervical spine injury

↓ No

Shout for help

↓

Open airway:
- Head tilt, chin lift
- Jaw thrust (if unsuccessful)

↓ No breathing

Check breathing for max 10 s:
- Look – for chest movement
- Listen – for breath sounds
- Feel – for air movement
- No or abnormal breathing

↓ No or abnormal breathing

Breathe
Remove any obvious obstruction
Give 5 initial rescue breaths

↓

Assess 'signs of life' - movements, coughing, normal breathing
Check pulse for max 10 s:
>1-year old – carotid, femoral
<1-year old – brachial, femoral

↓ No 'signs of life' (unless definite pulse >60/min)

Chest compressions:
15 chest compressions: 2 breaths
Rate 100–120 compressions/min

❀ Push 'hard and fast'

❀ If alone, give 1 min of resuscitation before seeking help. It may be possible to continue CPR whilst carrying an infant or small child to summon help.

Airway
Airway opening using head tilt/chin lift manoeuvre

Chin lift in infants
- Head in **neutral** position
- Avoid overextension
- Remove secretions/foreign body under direct vision

Chin lift in children
Head in 'sniffing' position
Jaw thrust
Two fingers of each hand behind each side of the mandible and push the jaw forward

Breathing (if bag-mask not available)
Infant: mouth over infant's nose and mouth (if bag mask not available)
Child: pinch nose, mouth to mouth
The chest should rise with each breath. Blow for 1 s

Circulation
Optimal position for chest compression

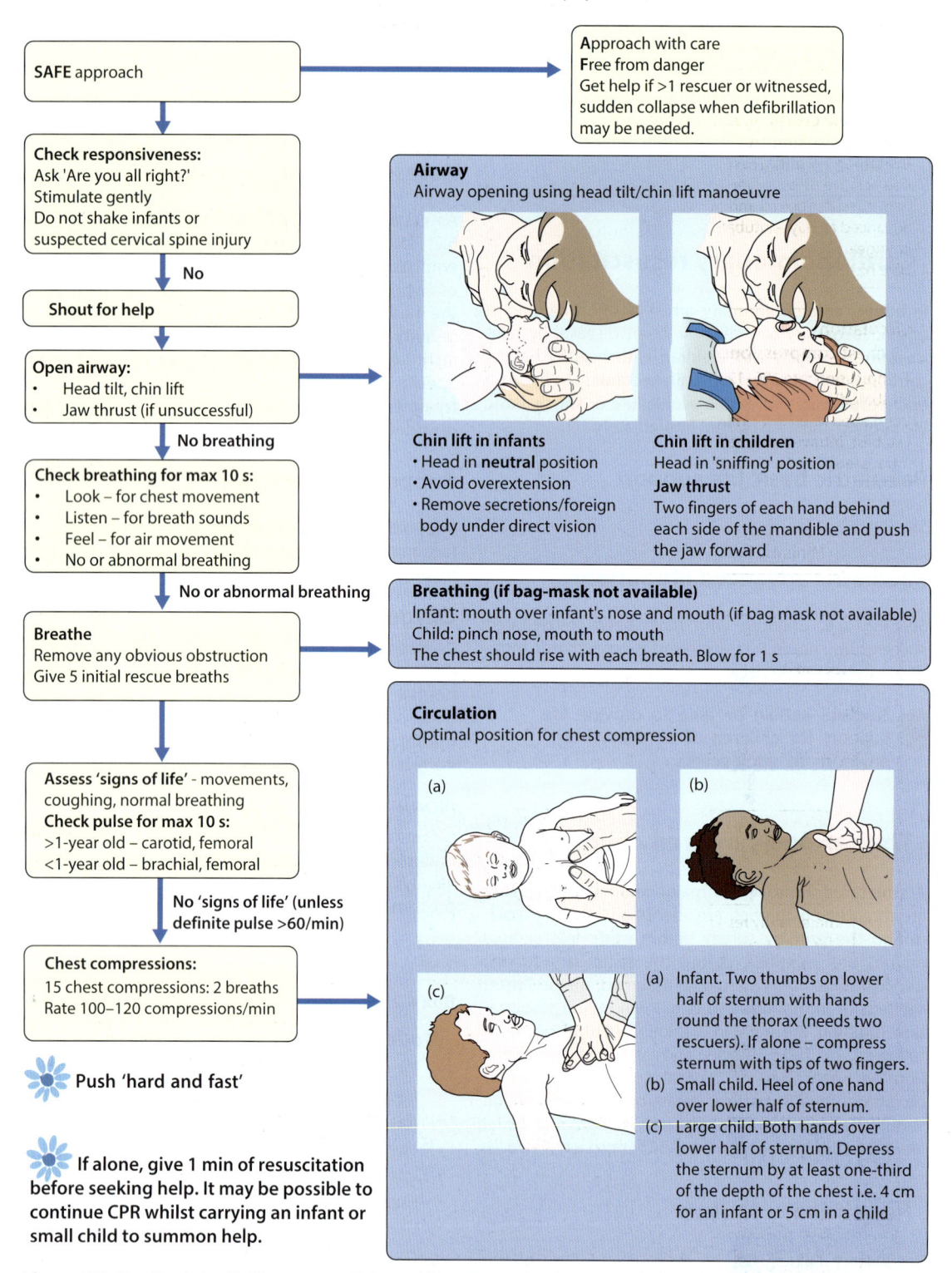

(a) Infant. Two thumbs on lower half of sternum with hands round the thorax (needs two rescuers). If alone – compress sternum with tips of two fingers.
(b) Small child. Heel of one hand over lower half of sternum.
(c) Large child. Both hands over lower half of sternum. Depress the sternum by at least one-third of the depth of the chest i.e. 4 cm for an infant or 5 cm in a child

Figure 6.5 Paediatric basic life support. (Adapted from Resuscitation Council (UK): *Guidelines on Paediatric Life Support*, London, 2015, Resuscitation Council.)

Paediatric advanced life support
(Health professional with equipment)

Unresponsive?
Not breathing or only occasional gasps? → **Call resuscitation team** (1 min CPR first, if alone)

Airway and breathing airway
– see basic life support
Breathing – 5 initial rescue breaths
Use positive pressure ventilation, preferably bag and mask. If required and skilled operator present, advanced airway – intubate and ventilate or laryngeal mask
Give high concentration O₂

Formula for endotracheal tube size by age in whole years
Internal diameter (mm) = (age/4) + 4
Length for oral tube (cm) = (age/2) + 12
Length for nasal tube (cm) = (age/2) + 15

Circulation
15 chest compressions: 2 breaths
Compression rate 100–120/min (continuously if intubated)
Ventilation rate 10–12/min
Establish intravenous access, if delay use intraosseous route

Technique to establish intraosseous infusion in the tibia
- 18-gauge trochar with needle
- Anterior surface, 2–3 cm below tibial tuberosity

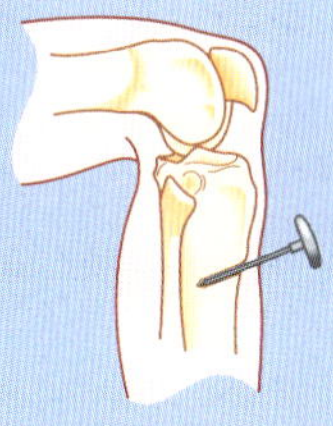

Attach defibrillator/monitor
Minimise interruption

Assess rhythm

Shockable
Ventricular fibrillation (VF) or pulseless ventricular tachycardia (VT)

Return of spontaneous circulation

Non-shockable
Pulseless electrical activity (PEA) or asystole

1 Shock 4J/kg

Post-cardiac arrest treatment
- Use ABCDE approach
- Controlled oxygenation and ventilation
- Investigations
- Treat precipitating cause
- Temperature control
- Therapeutic hypothermia?

Immediately resume CPR for 2 min Minimise interruptions

Immediately resume CPR for 2 min Minimise interruptions

Give adrenaline (epinephrine) every 3–5 min (alternate cycles) IV/IO

Give adrenaline (epinephrine) immediately, then every 3–5 min (alternate cycles)

During CPR
- Ensure high-quality CPR: rate, depth, recoil
- Plan actions before interrupting CPR
- Give oxygen
- Vascular access (intravenous, intraosseous)
- Give adrenaline (epinephrine) every 3–5 min (10 µg/kg IV or IO, i.e. 0.1 ml/kg of 1 in 10 000 solution), otherwise 100 µg/kg via tracheal tube
- Consider advanced airway and capnography (end-tidal CO₂ monitoring)
- Continuous chest compressions when advanced airway in place
- Correct reversible causes
- Consider amiodarone (5 mg/kg) after 3 and 5 shocks

Reversible causes
- Hypoxia
- Hypovolaemia
- Hypokalaemia/ hyperkalaemia, metabolic
- Hypothermia
- Tension pneumothorax
- Thrombosis (coronary or pulmonary)
- Tamponade – cardiac
- Toxic/therapeutic disturbances

Figure 6.6 Paediatric advanced life support. (Adapted from Resuscitation Council (UK): *Guidelines on Paediatric Life Support*, London, 2015, Resuscitation Council.)

Management of the seriously injured child

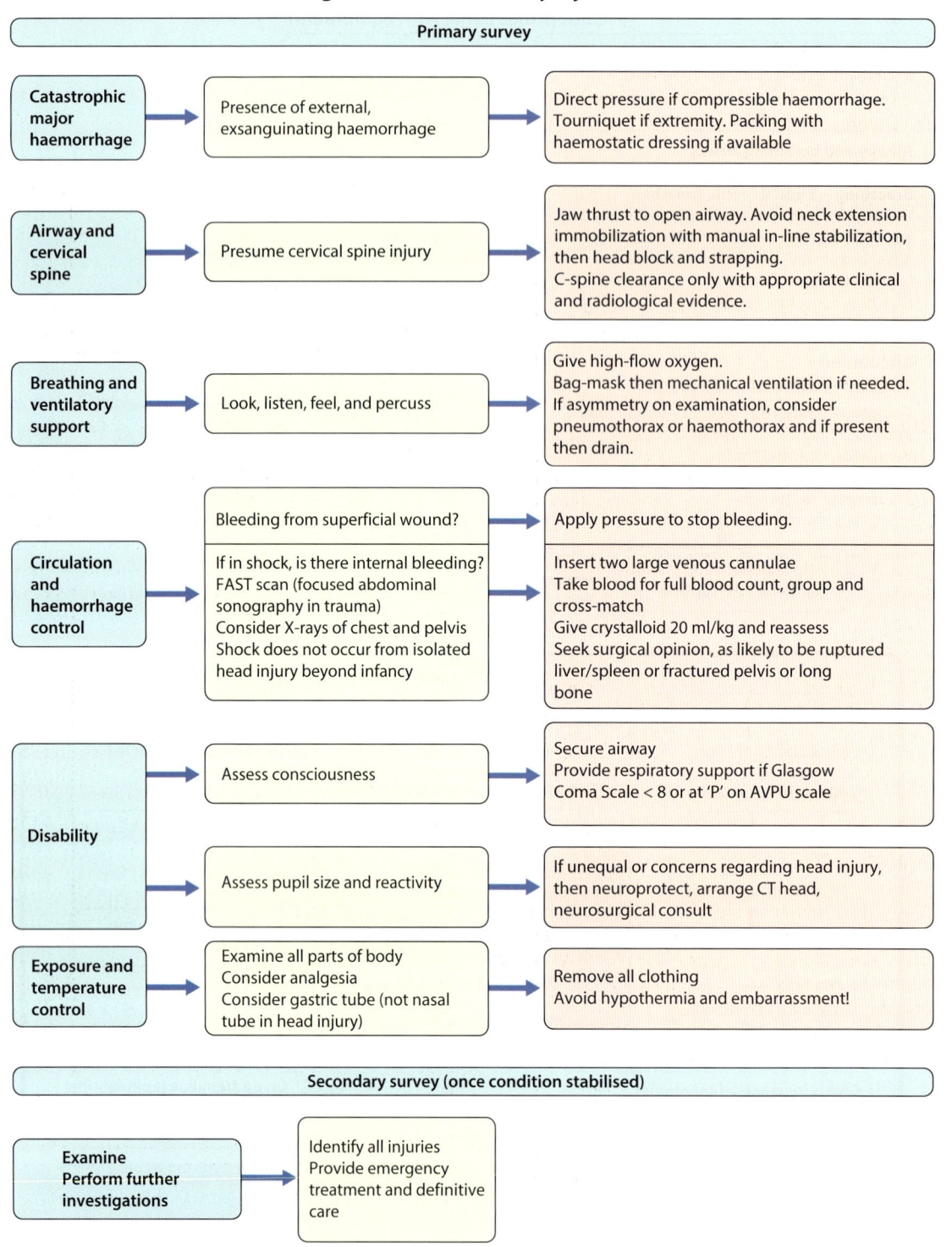

Primary survey

Step	Assessment	Action
Catastrophic major haemorrhage	Presence of external, exsanguinating haemorrhage	Direct pressure if compressible haemorrhage. Tourniquet if extremity. Packing with haemostatic dressing if available
Airway and cervical spine	Presume cervical spine injury	Jaw thrust to open airway. Avoid neck extension immobilization with manual in-line stabilization, then head block and strapping. C-spine clearance only with appropriate clinical and radiological evidence.
Breathing and ventilatory support	Look, listen, feel, and percuss	Give high-flow oxygen. Bag-mask then mechanical ventilation if needed. If asymmetry on examination, consider pneumothorax or haemothorax and if present then drain.
Circulation and haemorrhage control	Bleeding from superficial wound?	Apply pressure to stop bleeding.
	If in shock, is there internal bleeding? FAST scan (focused abdominal sonography in trauma) Consider X-rays of chest and pelvis Shock does not occur from isolated head injury beyond infancy	Insert two large venous cannulae Take blood for full blood count, group and cross-match Give crystalloid 20 ml/kg and reassess Seek surgical opinion, as likely to be ruptured liver/spleen or fractured pelvis or long bone
Disability	Assess consciousness	Secure airway Provide respiratory support if Glasgow Coma Scale < 8 or at 'P' on AVPU scale
	Assess pupil size and reactivity	If unequal or concerns regarding head injury, then neuroprotect, arrange CT head, neurosurgical consult
Exposure and temperature control	Examine all parts of body Consider analgesia Consider gastric tube (not nasal tube in head injury)	Remove all clothing Avoid hypothermia and embarrassment!

Secondary survey (once condition stabilised)

Examine Perform further investigations	Identify all injuries Provide emergency treatment and definitive care

Figure 6.7 Management of the seriously injured child.

Box 6.3 Indications for intubation and mechanical ventilation in respiratory failure

- Severe respiratory distress
- Tiring due to excessive work of breathing (may be indicated by progressive hypercarbia)
- Progressive hypoxaemia
- Reduced conscious level
- Progressive neuromuscular weakness, e.g. Guillain–Barré syndrome

high-flow nasal cannula therapy has become available. This delivers high-flow humidified gas whilst providing some CPAP with a known oxygen concentration. These techniques may be helpful in children with evolving respiratory failure.

Invasive ventilatory support

Endotracheal intubation and mechanical ventilation should be considered in any child with the clinical features listed in Box 6.3. While worsening hypoxaemia or worsening hypercarbia may confirm the imminent need for ventilation, blood gas analysis is not a substitute for clinical assessment.

Shock

Shock is present when the circulation is inadequate to meet the metabolic demands of the tissues. This is common in critically ill children although the reasons are varied. The causes can be categorized as in Fig. 6.4.

Why are children so susceptible to fluid loss?

Children normally require a much higher fluid intake per kilogram of body weight than adults. This is because they have a higher surface area-to-volume ratio and a higher basal metabolic rate. Children may therefore become dehydrated if:

- they are unable to take oral fluids
- there are additional fluid losses due to fever, diarrhoea, or increased insensible losses (e.g. due to increased sweating or tachypnoea)
- there is loss of the normal fluid-retaining mechanisms, e.g. burns, the permeable skin of premature infants, increased urinary losses or capillary leak.

Clinical features

The clinical features of shock are manifestations of compensatory physiological mechanisms to maintain the circulation and the direct effects of poor perfusion of tissues and organs (Box 6.4).

In early, compensated shock, the blood pressure is maintained by increased heart and respiratory rates, re-distribution of blood from venous reserve volume, and diversion of blood flow from nonessential tissues

Case history 6.1

Bronchiolitis

Edward, aged 6 weeks, is admitted to hospital with difficulty feeding and cough. His symptoms started 3 days ago but he has gradually deteriorated over the last 24 hours and is now struggling to breastfeed. Examination in the children's emergency department shows that he has a temperature of 38.2°C, a respiratory rate of 40 breaths/minute, moderate chest recession and a typical bronchiolitic cough. On auscultation there are bilateral widespread crepitations and wheezing. Following admission, his oxygen saturation monitor keeps alarming. He has worsening respiratory distress and a respiratory rate of 60 breaths/minute, with occasional apnoea. Blood gas analysis demonstrates an uncompensated respiratory acidosis with a partial pressure of carbon dioxide (pCO_2) of 12 kPa. Chest radiography (Fig. 6.8) is consistent with the diagnosis. He is transferred to the high dependency unit and started on CPAP. After 4 hours he is getting more tired. A decision is made to intubate and ventilate him in the operating theatre suite. Following this, he is transferred to the regional PICU by the paediatric regional transport team. He makes a full recovery after 5 days of mechanical ventilation.

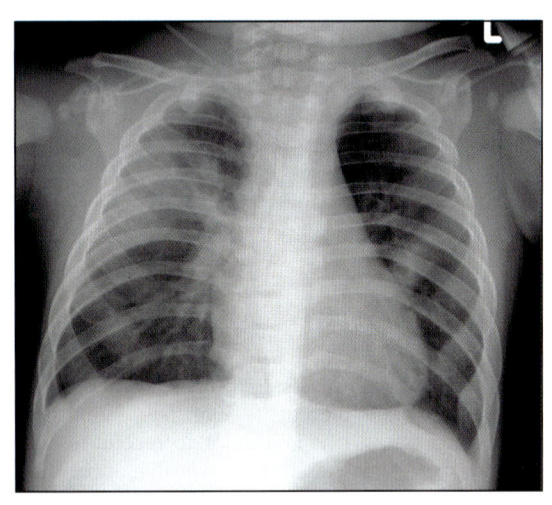

Figure 6.8 Chest radiograph in bronchiolitis, showing areas of atelectasis and collapse (right midzone) and hyperinflation (left lung). A chest radiograph is not required in uncomplicated bronchiolitis.

such as the skin in the peripheries, which become cold, to the vital organs like the brain and heart. In shock due to dehydration, there is usually over 10% loss of body weight (see Ch. 14) and a profound metabolic acidosis, which is compounded by failure to feed and drink while severely ill. After acute blood loss or redistribution of blood volume because of infection, low blood pressure is a late feature. It signifies that compensatory responses are failing.

Shock and fluid resuscitation and maintenance

Box 6.4 Clinical signs of shock

Early (compensated)	Late (decompensated)
Tachypnoea	Acidotic (Kussmaul) breathing
Tachycardia	Bradycardia
Decreased skin turgor	Confusion/depressed cerebral state
Sunken eyes and fontanelle	Blue peripheries
Delayed capillary refill (>2 s)	Absent urine output
Mottled, pale, cold skin	Hypotension
Core–peripheral temperature gap (>4° C)	
Decreased urinary output	

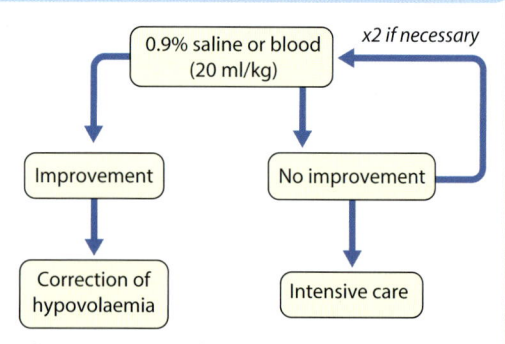

Figure 6.9 Initial fluid resuscitation in shock.

Flowchart: 0.9% saline or blood (20 ml/kg), x2 if necessary → Improvement → Correction of hypovolaemia; No improvement → Intensive care.

Table 6.1 Calculating maintenance intravenous fluid requirement in children

Body weight	Fluid requirement/24 h	Example
First 10 kg	100 ml/kg	7-kg infant: 100 × 7 = 700 ml/24 h 700/24 = 29.2 ml/h
Second 10 kg	50 ml/kg	18-kg child: (10 × 100) + (8 × 50) = 1400 ml/24 h 1400/24 = 58.3 ml/h
Subsequent kg	20 ml/kg	42-kg child: (10 × 1000) + (10 × 50) + (22 × 20) = 1940/24 = 80.8 ml/h

In late or uncompensated shock, compensatory mechanisms fail, blood pressure falls, and lactic acidosis increases. It is important to recognize early compensated shock, as this is reversible, in contrast to uncompensated shock, which may be irreversible.

Management priorities

Fluid resuscitation

Rapid restoration of the intravascular circulating volume is the priority (Fig. 6.9). This will usually be with 0.9% saline, or blood if following trauma. For shock from dehydration, the fluid deficit and maintenance and ongoing fluid losses need to be replaced. Maintenance intravenous fluids vary according to body weight, as shown in Table 6.1.

Subsequent management

If there is no improvement following initial fluid resuscitation or there is progression of shock and respiratory failure, a paediatric intensive care unit should be involved and transfer arranged as the child may need:

- tracheal intubation and mechanical ventilation
- invasive monitoring of blood pressure
- inotropic support
- correction of haematological, biochemical and metabolic derangements
- support for renal failure.

Sepsis

Bacteria may cause a focal infection or proliferate in the bloodstream, where the host response, which includes release of inflammatory cytokines and activation of endothelial cells, may lead to sepsis. The most common organisms identified from blood culture in children in the UK are coagulase-negative *Staphylococcus* (CoNS), *Staphylococcus aureus*, non-pyogenic streptococci, and *Streptococcus pneumonia* (pneumococcus). The Gram-negative organisms *Neisseria*

Box 6.5 Clinical features of septicaemia

History	Examination
Fever	Fever
Poor feeding	Tachycardia, tachypnoea, low blood pressure
Miserable, irritable, lethargy	
History of focal infection, e.g. meningitis, osteomyelitis, gastroenteritis, cellulitis	Purpuric rash (meningococcal septicaemia; Fig. 6.10)
	Shock
	Multiorgan failure
Predisposing conditions, e.g. sickle cell disease, immunodeficiency	

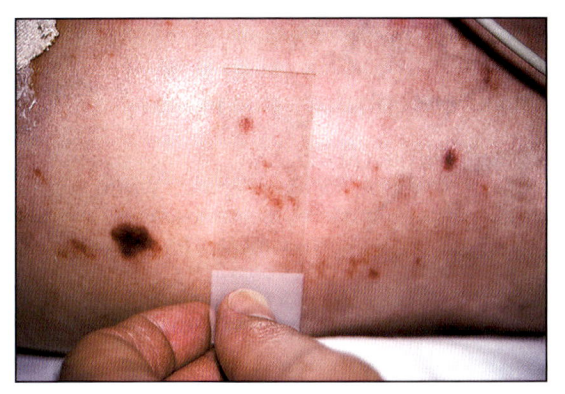

Figure 6.10 The glass test for meningococcal purpura. Parents are advised to suspect meningococcal disease if their child is febrile and has a rash that does not blanch when pressed under a glass. (Courtesy of Parviz Habibi.)

meningitidis (meningococcus) and *Escherichia coli* are also still prevalent. However, *Haemophilus influenzae*, meningococcus and pneumococcus have all declined since included in the immunization schedule. In neonates, early-onset sepsis is most commonly caused by group B *Streptococcus* and *E. coli*, whereas in late-onset sepsis CoNS predominates. Whilst CoNS is often isolated from blood culture in association with indwelling appliances, it is a common skin contaminant.

Clinical features

See Box 6.5.

Management priorities

Children with septic shock, i.e. having organ failure, need to be rapidly stabilized and may require transfer to a paediatric intensive care unit.

Antibiotics

Antibiotic therapy must be started without delay. The choice depends on the child's age and any predisposition to infection.

Fluids

Significant hypovolaemia is often present, owing to fluid maldistribution, which occurs due to the release of vasoactive mediators by host inflammatory and endothelial cells. There is loss of intravascular proteins and fluid, which may occur due to the development of 'capillary leak' caused by endothelial cell dysfunction. Circulating plasma volume is lost into the interstitial fluid. Central venous pressure monitoring and urinary catheterization may be required to guide the assessment of fluid balance. Capillary leak into the lungs causes pulmonary oedema, which may lead to respiratory failure, necessitating mechanical ventilation.

Circulatory support

Myocardial dysfunction occurs as inflammatory cytokines and circulating toxins depress myocardial contractility. Inotropic support may be required.

Disseminated intravascular coagulation

Abnormal blood clotting causes widespread microvascular thrombosis and consumption of clotting factors. If bleeding occurs, clotting derangement should be corrected with fresh frozen plasma, cryoprecipitate and platelet transfusions.

Summary

Sepsis
- Early recognition, antibiotic therapy and fluid resuscitation are life-saving.
- If very severe, the child may need admission to paediatric intensive care for management of multiorgan failure.

Anaphylaxis

Anaphylaxis is a severe, life-threatening, generalized or systemic hypersensitivity reaction. It is sudden in onset, progresses rapidly with life-threatening airway and/or breathing and/or circulation problem. Skin and/or mucosal signs of urticarial or angioedema are usually but not always present. It has an incidence of one episode every 20 000 person years, and about 1 in 1000 cases is fatal. In children, 85% of anaphylaxis is caused by food allergy; most are IgE-mediated reactions with significant respiratory or cardiovascular compromise. Other causes include insect stings, drugs, latex, exercise, inhalant allergens and idiopathic. While most paediatric anaphylaxis occurs in children under 5 years of age, when food allergy is most prevalent, the majority of fatal anaphylaxis occurs in adolescents with allergy to nuts; asthma is an additional risk factor. The acute management of anaphylaxis relies on early administration of adrenaline (epinephrine; Fig. 6.11). Long-term

Figure 6.11 — Emergency treatment of anaphylaxis

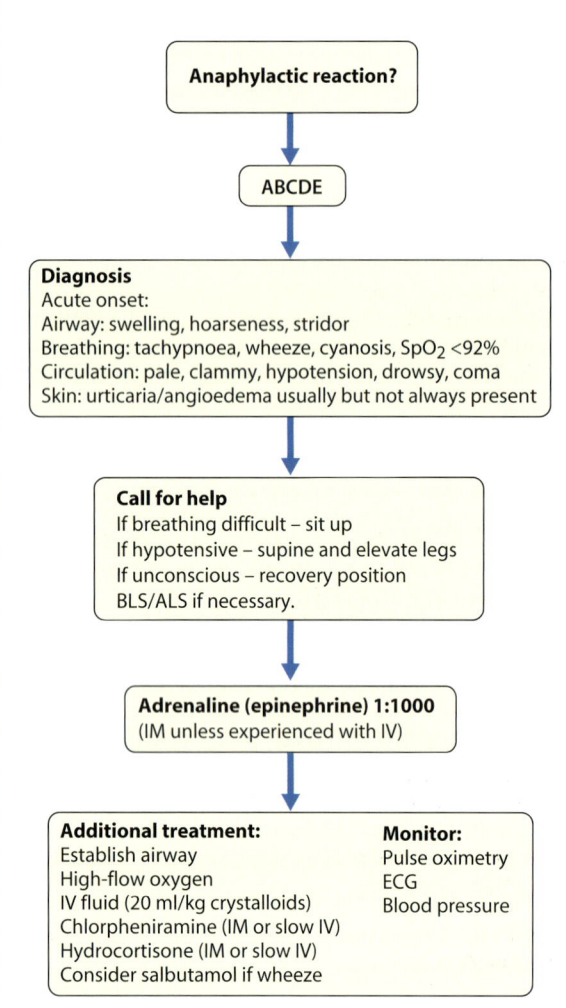

Anaphylactic reaction?
↓
ABCDE
↓
Diagnosis
Acute onset:
Airway: swelling, hoarseness, stridor
Breathing: tachypnoea, wheeze, cyanosis, SpO_2 <92%
Circulation: pale, clammy, hypotension, drowsy, coma
Skin: urticaria/angioedema usually but not always present
↓
Call for help
If breathing difficult – sit up
If hypotensive – supine and elevate legs
If unconscious – recovery position
BLS/ALS if necessary.
↓
Adrenaline (epinephrine) 1:1000
(IM unless experienced with IV)
↓
Additional treatment:
Establish airway
High-flow oxygen
IV fluid (20 ml/kg crystalloids)
Chlorpheniramine (IM or slow IV)
Hydrocortisone (IM or slow IV)
Consider salbutamol if wheeze

Monitor:
Pulse oximetry
ECG
Blood pressure

Figure 6.11 Emergency treatment of anaphylaxis. (Adapted from Resuscitation Council (UK). *Guidelines on Paediatric Life Support*, London 2015, Resuscitation Council.)

management involves detailed strategies and training for allergen avoidance, a written management plan with instructions for the treatment of allergic reactions, and the provision of an adrenaline auto-injector(s). In some cases, such as insect sting anaphylaxis, allergen immunotherapy may be effective in preventing future episodes. The experience of an anaphylactic reaction can have a significant psychological impact on the child and family.

Summary

Anaphylaxis in children/adolescents
- Reaction is mainly to foods – about 1 in 1000 episodes is fatal.
- Risk factors for fatal outcome include adolescent age group, coexistent asthma, and nut allergy.
- Acute management is ABCDE and early administration of intramuscular adrenaline.

Neurological emergencies

Convulsive status epilepticus

Status epilepticus is a common paediatric emergency and is defined as continuous seizures lasting more than 30 minutes, or intermittent clinical or electroencephalographic seizures lasting more than 30 minutes without full recovery of consciousness between seizures. It is crucial to terminate seizures as soon as possible because seizures of a longer duration are associated with a worse outcome and can be more treatment resistant. Therefore, after immediate primary assessment and resuscitation, the priority is to stop the seizure by treating any reversible causes such as hypoglycaemia or electrolyte disturbance and escalating treatment according to national guidelines as in Fig. 6.12. The aim is to prevent any seizure which is 'prolonged', i.e. lasts 5 minutes or longer, from developing into convulsive status epilepticus.

Other encephalopathic illness

Children can present with coma, psychosis, confusion, and nonconvulsive status epilepticus. Where there is an altered conscious level, this can be rapidly assessed using either the rapid assessment of level of consciousness (Box 6.1) or Glasgow Coma Scale (Table 6.2). In all cases primary assessment follows an airway, breathing, circulation, disability, exposure (ABCDE) approach (Figs 6.13 and 6.14).

For both convulsive status epilepticus and other encephalopathic illnesses, the history and secondary assessment need to focus on identification of the cause (Table 6.3). Early treatment of reversible causes, especially hypoglycaemia and infection, is paramount. Intracranial mass lesions may require neurosurgical intervention, although structural lesions are less common in children than adults.

Ongoing treatment of neurological emergencies, in particular where there is raised intracranial pressure, includes the use of neuroprotective strategies to reduce secondary brain injury. These are treated with:

- the head positioned midline and tilted up 20° to 30°
- fluid restriction with isotonic fluids
- intubation and ventilation if Glasgow Coma Scale score is less than 9
- if intubated, maintain normocapnia [partial pressure of carbon dioxide in arterial blood ($paCO_2$) 4.5–5.3 kPa]
- osmotic diuretics (e.g. mannitol) to reduce raised intracranial pressure
- maintain high normal blood pressure in order to maintain cerebral perfusion pressure
- maintain normothermia
- hypotension or hypoxaemia must be avoided during treatment.

Management protocol for status epilepticus

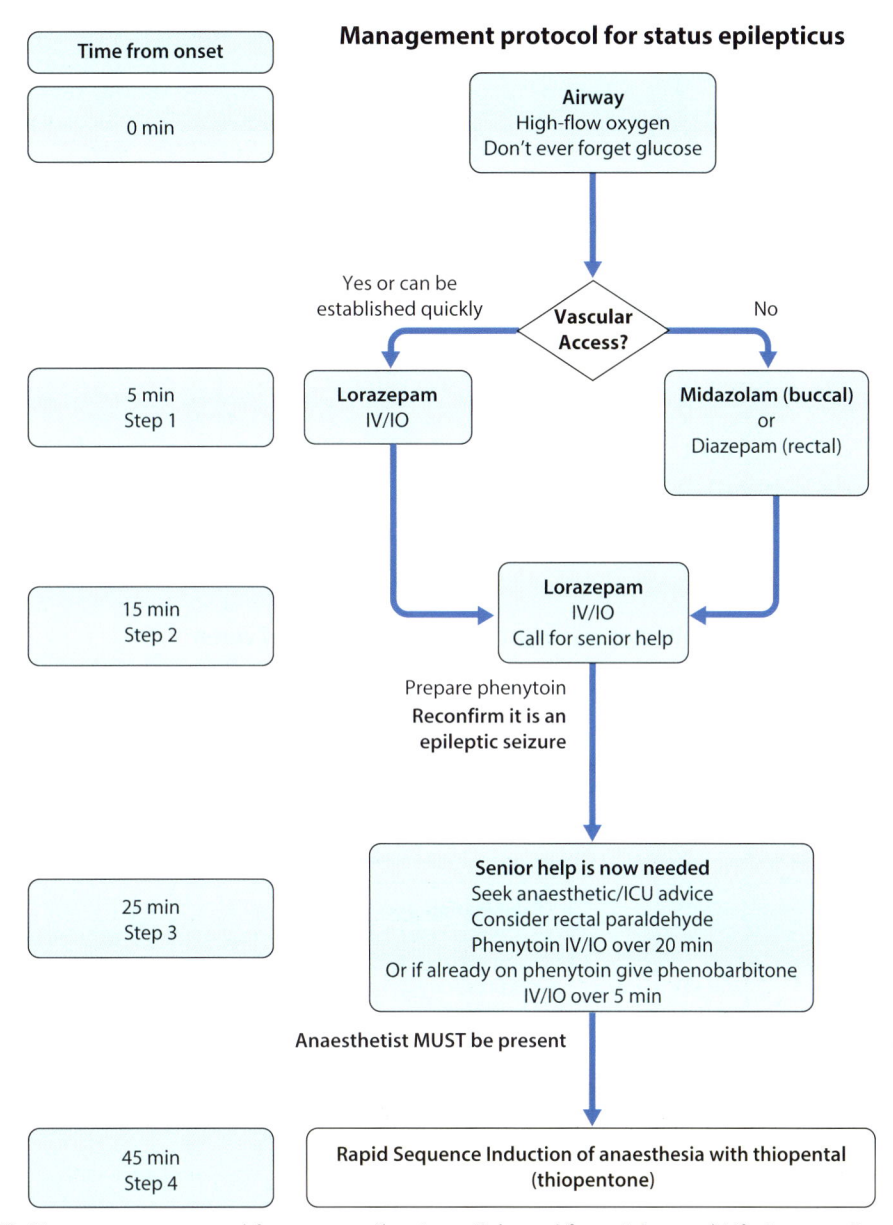

Time from onset

0 min

Airway
High-flow oxygen
Don't ever forget glucose

Vascular Access?
- Yes or can be established quickly
- No

5 min — Step 1

Lorazepam IV/IO

Midazolam (buccal) or Diazepam (rectal)

15 min — Step 2

Lorazepam IV/IO
Call for senior help

Prepare phenytoin
Reconfirm it is an epileptic seizure

25 min — Step 3

Senior help is now needed
Seek anaesthetic/ICU advice
Consider rectal paraldehyde
Phenytoin IV/IO over 20 min
Or if already on phenytoin give phenobarbitone IV/IO over 5 min

Anaesthetist MUST be present

45 min — Step 4

Rapid Sequence Induction of anaesthesia with thiopental (thiopentone)

Figure 6.12 Management protocol for status epilepticus. (Adapted from Advanced Life Support Group. 2014. *Advanced Paediatric Life Support. The Practical Approach*, 5th edition Blackwell BMJ Books, London, with permission.)

Table 6.2 Glasgow coma scale, incorporating children's coma scale

	Glasgow coma scale	**Children's coma scale (<4 years)**	
	Response	*Response*	Score
Eye opening	Spontaneous	Spontaneous	4
	To sound	To sound	3
	To pressure	To pain	2
	None	No response	1
Best verbal response	Oriented	Talks normally, interacts	5
	Confused	Words	4
	Words	Vocal sounds	3
	Sounds	Cries	2
	None	None	1
Best motor response	Obeys commands	Obeys commsnds	6
	Localising	Localises pain	5
	Normal flexion	Flexion to pain	4
	Abnormal flexion	Abnormal flexion (decorticate posture)	3
	Extension	Abnormal extension (decerebrate posture)	2
	None	No response	1

A score of <8 out of 15 means that the child's airway is at risk and will need to be maintained.

Initial assessment and management of coma

Primary assessment and resuscitation
- **A**irway – is it secure?
- **B**reathing – is respiratory effort sufficient?
- **C**irculation – treat shock
- **D**isability – check blood glucose
  – AVPU or Glasgow Coma Scale
- **E**xposure – e.g. look for meningococcal purpuric rash

Secondary assessment and emergency treatment

Examination
- Is there raised intracranial pressure – abnormal breathing, posture, pupils (Fig. 6.11), fundi (papilloedema or retinal haemorrhages)?
- Bradycardia and hypertension suggest impending brain stem herniation

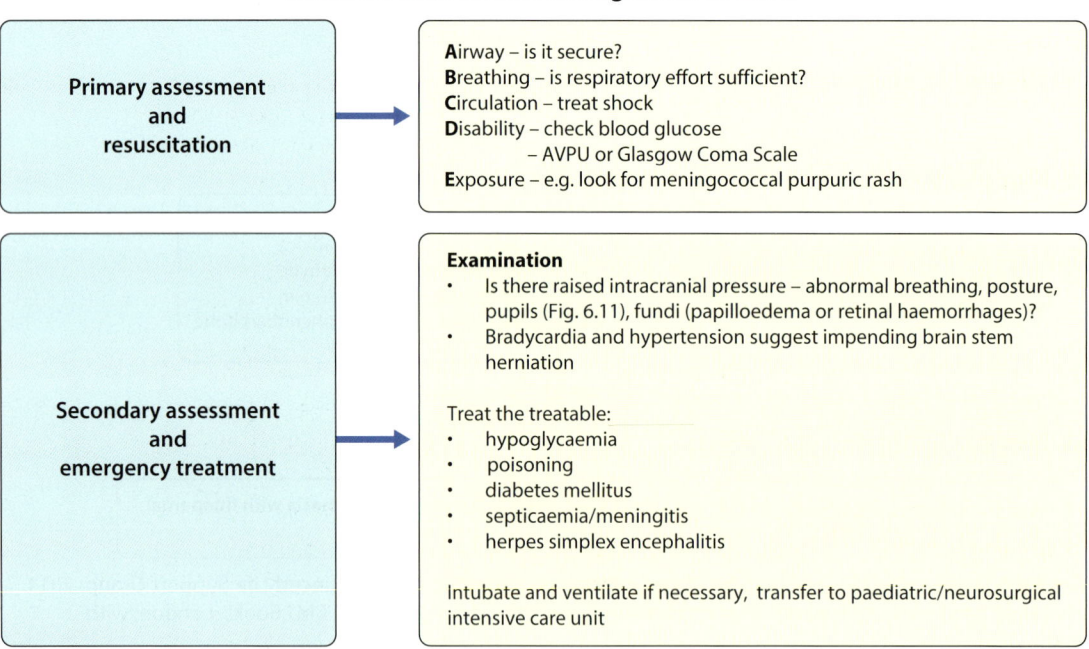

Treat the treatable:
- hypoglycaemia
- poisoning
- diabetes mellitus
- septicaemia/meningitis
- herpes simplex encephalitis

Intubate and ventilate if necessary, transfer to paediatric/neurosurgical intensive care unit

Figure 6.13 Initial assessment and management of coma.

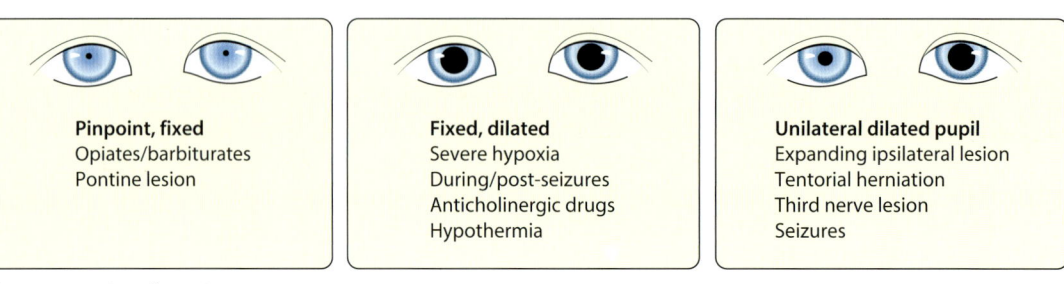

Pinpoint, fixed
Opiates/barbiturates
Pontine lesion

Fixed, dilated
Severe hypoxia
During/post-seizures
Anticholinergic drugs
Hypothermia

Unilateral dilated pupil
Expanding ipsilateral lesion
Tentorial herniation
Third nerve lesion
Seizures

Figure 6.14 Pupillary signs in coma.

Table 6.3 Causes, history and examination, and investigation of encephalopathy

Cause	History and examination	Diagnostic investigations
Infection Meningitis or meningoencephalitis	Fever Irritability, lethargy, drowsiness Poor feeding, vomiting Rash, e.g. meningococcal purpura Seizures Neck stiffness and pain; bulging fontanelle Overseas travel	Full blood count Culture of blood, urine, infected sites, and cerebrospinal fluid (unless contraindicated) for bacteria and viruses Acute-phase reactant Rapid bacterial antigen/polymerase chain reaction tests for organisms
Status epilepticus or postictal	History of seizures Neurocutaneous lesions on the skin Developmental delay Ongoing seizure activity, e.g. abnormal eye movements Focal neurological signs	Blood glucose Electrolytes – sodium, potassium, calcium, and magnesium Drug levels if on anticonvulsants EEG CT scan
Trauma – accidental/nonaccidental	History of road traffic accident, fall, etc. Bruising, haemorrhage Fractures – cervical spine, etc. Focal neurology Retinal haemorrhages	Radiological – plain X-ray or CT/MRI scans
Intracranial tumour or haemorrhage/infarct/abscess	Symptoms or signs of raised intracranial pressure Focal neurological signs, e.g. squint	Cranial CT/MRI scan Haemorrhage – coagulation screen, screen for procoagulant disorders (protein C/S deficiency)
Metabolic		
1. Diabetes mellitus	Previously diagnosed diabetes mellitus Diabetic ketoacidosis	Blood glucose, plasma electrolytes Urine for glucose and ketones Blood gas analysis
2. Hypoglycaemia	Any acutely ill child Known diabetes mellitus Sudden onset of coma	Low blood glucose
3. Inborn errors of metabolism	Previous history of loss of consciousness Sudden collapse Consanguinity, death or illness of siblings Developmental delay Hepatomegaly	Blood glucose Blood gas analysis Blood ammonia, lactate Urine amino and organic acids Plasma amino acids
4. Hepatic failure	Jaundice Abnormal bleeding	Abnormal liver function tests Prolonged prothrombin time
5. Acute renal failure	Oliguria, hypertension	Abnormal creatinine
Poisoning	Accidental – poison usually identified Deliberate – tablets may be found, also illicit drugs and alcohol	Toxicology screen Plasma level for paracetamol and salicylates
Shock	Septicaemia Dehydration Cardiac failure	Full blood count and cultures Urea, electrolytes, and blood gas
Hypertension	Symptoms and signs of raised intracranial pressure Fundoscopy – hypertensive changes	Left ventricular hypertrophy on ECG or echocardiography Creatinine and electrolytes
Respiratory failure	Severe respiratory distress, poor respiratory effort, apnoea	Chest X-ray Arterial blood gas – hypoxia, hypercarbia

Apparent life-threatening events

These are events in an infant where there is a sudden, brief and often frightening change in condition in an infant who was previously well and appears well immediately afterwards. These have been called Apparent Life Threatening Events (ALTE). The American Academy of Pediatrics has recommended this name be changed to Brief Resolved Unexplained Events in Infants (BRUE) to describe the commonest situation, where a sudden, brief and now resolved episode is observed in which there was one or more of:

- cyanosis or pallor
- absent, decreased or irregular breathing
- change in tone (increased or decreased)
- altered level of responsiveness.

Additional features are:

- no concerning features on detailed history, including a social history
- normal physical examination.

These babies require a period of observation and monitoring of vital signs. An ECG, a pernasal swab for pertussis and brief monitoring with continuous pulse oximetry are usually performed. Caregivers will need explanation about the nature of these events and basic life support training offered. Follow-up needs to be arranged.

If the clinical features are not characteristic, more detailed assessment and investigation are indicated to identify an underlying disorder. Risk factors for an underlying disorder include:

- age <60 days or gestation at birth <32 weeks
- duration of event > 1 min
- repeat event
- cardiopulmonary resuscitation (CPR) given by trained medical provider
- concerning features in history e.g. family history of cardiac death, child protection concerns, cough or breathing problems suggesting respiratory infection or abnormality, vomiting suggestive of gastro-oesophageal reflux
- Abnormalities identified on physical examination e.g. fever, respiratory distress.

Unexpected death of a child

Fortunately, the unexpected death of a child is uncommon. Most are due to accidents, mainly road traffic accidents, but during infancy the risk of death is four times greater than at any other age in childhood. Deaths that occur suddenly and unexpectedly in infancy are known as sudden unexpected death in infancy (SUDI). There were about 270 such deaths in the UK in 2013. In some, a previously undiagnosed congenital abnormality, e.g. congenital heart disease, will be found at autopsy or another condition, e.g. inborn error of metabolism, is identified. However, after 1 month of age, in most instances of sudden death in a previously well infant, no cause is identified even after a detailed autopsy, and the death is classified as sudden infant death syndrome (SIDS). The vast majority of such deaths, even when occurring more than once in the same family, are due to natural but unexplained causes. Rarely, the death may be due to suffocation or other forms of non-accidental injury.

Sudden infant death syndrome

The peak age range is 2–4 months of age (Fig. 6.15). Epidemiological studies show risk factors in the infant, parents and immediate environment (Fig. 6.16). However, the main risk factor is lying the baby to sleep in the prone position. The incidence of SIDS has fallen dramatically in the UK since the national 'Back to Sleep' campaign (Fig. 6.17). Incorporating additional risk factors from analysis of epidemiological data, parents are now advised that:

- infants should be put to sleep on their back (not their front or side)
- overheating by heavy wrapping and high room temperature should be avoided. The head should be uncovered and the blanket tucked in no higher than their shoulders
- infants should be placed in the 'feet to foot' position, i.e. feet at foot of cot
- no one should smoke near the infant
- parents should seek medical advice promptly if their infant becomes unwell
- parents should have the baby in their bedroom for the first 6 months of life
- parents should avoid bringing the baby into their bed when they are tired or have taken alcohol, sedative medicines, or drugs
- parents should avoid sleeping with their infant on a sofa, settee, or armchair
- if possible, the infant should be breastfed.

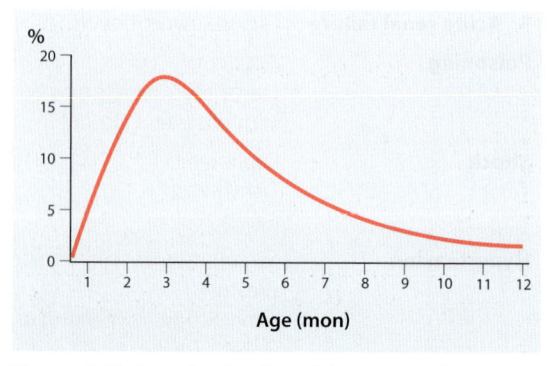

Figure 6.15 Age distribution of SIDS. (Data from Fleming P, Blair P, Bacon C, Berry PJ: *Sudden Unexpected Deaths in Infancy*, London, 2000, The Stationery Office, with permission.)

Case history 6.2

Sudden infant death syndrome

Poppy, a previously well 9-week-old baby, is found to be still and lifeless by her mother when waking her for a feed in the morning. The previous night she had fed well at midnight although she had coryzal symptoms the previous day. An ambulance is called and Poppy is rushed to hospital. Mask ventilation and cardiac compressions are performed by the paramedic ambulance crew.

The team in the children's emergency department is prepared for her arrival. A member of the nursing team is assigned to accompany her mother to a separate room. After 20 minutes of cardiopulmonary resuscitation, she still has no signs of life. The consultant paediatrician explains to her mother that the team has tried everything possible but that Poppy has died.

Poppy's partner had been called to come directly to the hospital. The paediatrician enters full details into the medical record of the medical treatment given and findings on thorough physical examination, including that there are no signs of external injury. As with any unexpected death, the police have been informed and a member of the police child protection team has arrived. The paediatrician, accompanied by the member of the child protection team, explains to the parents what has happened and takes a detailed history from them. After the discussion, the consultant paediatrician informs the local designated paediatrician for child death and the coroner. The coroner gives permission for postmortem samples and blood tests to be taken and arranges for the autopsy to be done by a paediatric pathologist.

The parents are offered the opportunity to see and hold their baby and to take photographs and gather mementoes. They are reassured that involvement of the police and social services is standard practice. Follow-up is arranged with the paediatrician. Bereavement support is offered.

The infant
- Age 1–6 months
- Low birthweight and preterm (risk 3× normal birthweight)
- Sex (boys 60%)
- Appeared ill in last 24 h

The parents
- Low income
- No maternal educational qualifications
- Poor or overcrowded housing
- Maternal age <21 years
- High maternal parity
- Maternal smoking during pregnancy
- Parental smoking after baby's birth
- Maternal alcohol or drug consumption

The environment
- The infant sleeps lying prone
- Co-sleeping
- The infant is overheated from high room temperature and too may clothes and covers, particularly when ill
- Infant pillow use
- Infant swaddling

Figure 6.16 Risk factors associated with SIDS. Presence of several risk factors increases the risk. (Data from Fleming P, Blair P, Bacon C, Berry PJ: *Sudden Unexpected Deaths in Infancy*, London, 2000, The Stationery Office.)

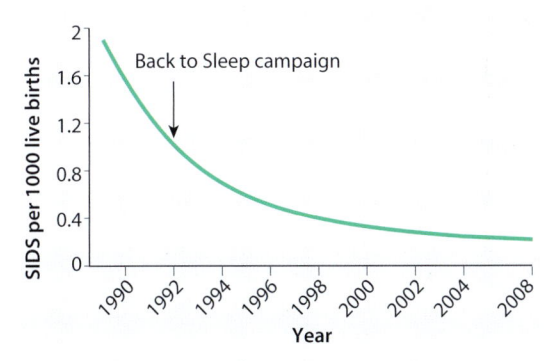

Figure 6.17 Decline in the number of deaths from SIDS in the UK from 1.9/1000 live births in 1989 to 0.31/1000 in 2012.

Following a sudden unexpected death in infancy:
- A detailed history and thorough physical examination should be performed by a paediatrician.
- The police, local designated paediatrician for child death and the coroner need to be informed.
- Parents and family should be offered the opportunity to see and hold the baby and take photographs and gather mementoes.
- Bereavement support should be offered and follow-up arranged.

> **Summary**
>
> **Sudden infant death syndrome**
> - SIDS is the most common cause of death in children aged 1 month to 1 year.
> - The peak age for the occurrence of SIDS is 2–4 months.
> - SIDS has been dramatically reduced by lying babies on their back to sleep.

Acknowledgements

We would like to acknowledge contributors to this chapter in previous editions, whose work we have drawn on: Nigel Curtis (1st Edition), Nigel Klein (1st Edition), Simon Nadel (2nd Edition). Rob Tasker (3rd Edition), Shruti Agrawal (4th Edition).

Further reading

Advanced Life Support Group: *Advanced Paediatric Life Support. A Practical Approach*, ed 6, 2016, John Wiley & Sons.

Goldman A, Hain R, Lieben S: *The Oxford Textbook of Palliative Care in Children*, ed 2, Oxford, 2011, Oxford University Press.

Goldstein B, Giroir B, Randolph A: International Consensus Conference on Pediatric Sepsis: International pediatric sepsis consensus conference: Definitions for sepsis and organ dysfunction in pediatrics. *Pediatric Critical Care Medicine* 6:2–8, 2005.

Tieder JS, Bonkowsky JL, Etzel RA, et al: Brief Resolved Unexplained Events (Formerly Apparent Life-Threatening Events) and Evaluation of Lower-Risk Infants. *Pediatrics* 137(5):e20160590, 2016.

Websites (Accessed November 2016)

Resuscitation Council (UK): *Guidelines on Paediatric Life Support*, London, 2015, Resuscitation Council. https://www.resus.org.uk

7

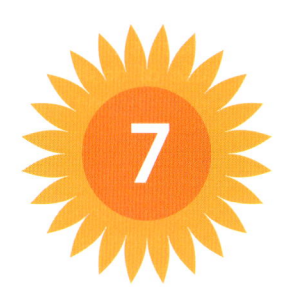

Accidents and poisoning

| Accidents | 97 | Poisoning | 103 |

Features of accidents and poisoning in children are:
- accidental injury is the most common reason for children and young people to seek emergency healthcare
- accidents are the most common cause of death in children over 1 year of age worldwide and the majority are preventable
- poisoning is a common avoidable cause of harm to children
- the features of poisoning are a demonstration of pharmacology in action.

Children need a safe, healthy, and nurturing environment to achieve their full potential. Accidents and poisoning are classified as external causes of morbidity and mortality as they are entirely dependent on the presence of an extrinsic environmental factor, for example, a motor vehicle or a swimming pool. Although the provision of a completely risk-free environment is not possible (or desirable), children and young people should be protected from external causes of serious harm. This is primarily the responsibility of parents, families, and carers, but all members of society, including health and education professionals, have important roles to play in advocating and helping to organize safe environments for children. Although external causes are the leading cause of death in 1-year-old to 14-year-old children worldwide and until recently in the UK, they have declined sufficiently to now be the second most frequent cause, after malignant diseases, in the UK (Fig. 7.1).

Accidents

Accidental injuries are extremely common in childhood. Approximately 2 million children and young people attend an emergency department with an accidental injury each year in the UK. Fortunately, the majority suffer only minor and temporary damage; however, for a small but significant proportion the consequences can be life changing. The fatal external causes in England and Wales for children aged 1-year to 14-years are shown in Fig. 7.2. Survivors of significant injuries may suffer long-term disability and disfigurement and psychological harm.

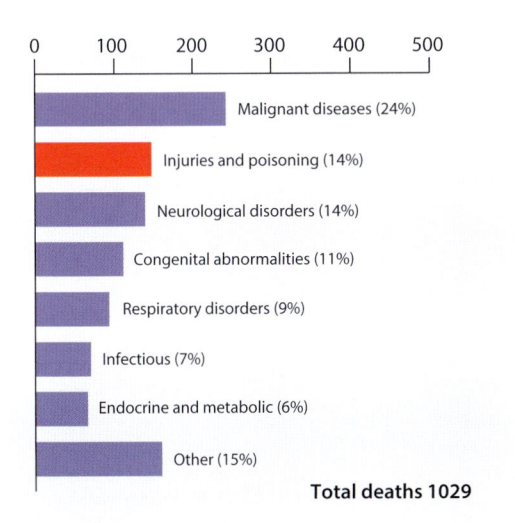

Figure 7.1 Cause of death in children aged 1 year to 15 years in England and Wales in 2013 (Data from Office of National Statistics, 2015).

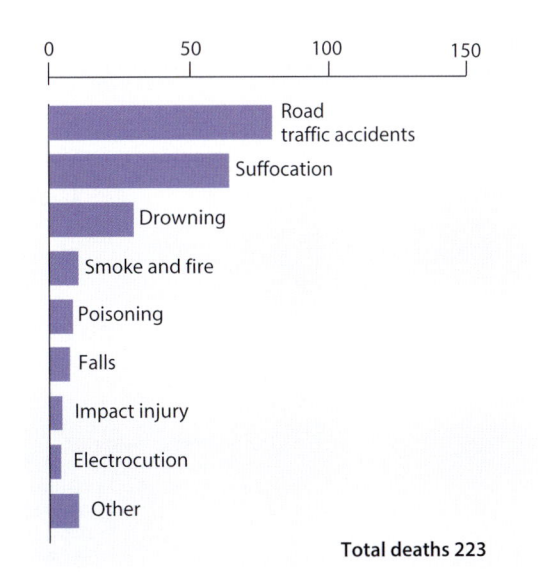

Figure 7.2 External causes of death in children aged 1 year to 14 years in England and Wales in 2010.

Accidents and poisoning

☀ **Accidents are the second most common cause of death in children over 1 year of age in England and Wales**

Different types of accidents are prevalent at different ages, relating to the child's development. Babies and preschool children sustain most accidental injuries at home as this is where they spend most of their time. These injuries result from their natural inquisitiveness combined with lack of appreciation of potential danger and poor coordination. Typical injuries are falls down steps and trapping fingers in doors. By school age, accidents are more likely to occur outside the home; in particular, injuries from road traffic collisions are the leading cause of serious injury, accounting for over half of accidental deaths in children aged 5–14 years. The majority of these children are pedestrians. Older children and young people may indulge in risk-taking behaviour and underestimate the magnitude of the associated danger.

Accident prevention

Accident prevention, or more correctly, injury control, is an important public health issue. Primary prevention strategies relate to the avoidance of the event causing the injury in the first place. Secondary prevention strategies include the provision of appropriate healthcare services for the treatment of the injured children – for example, specialized trauma and burn services, with follow-on tailored rehabilitation.

Primary accident prevention strategies typically tackle three main factors:

- modification of product design, e.g. for road traffic accidents, vehicle child restraint design, and legislation change
- alteration of the environment, e.g. reduction in speed limits or road layout design
- education of children and their carers, e.g. public service announcements and school safety campaigns.

Specific examples of these are shown in Fig. 7.3. Healthcare professionals are well placed to deliver anticipatory guidance as well as to identify and publicize risk factors. Implementation is usually more successful when supported by legislative change, rather than education alone.

☀ **The number of deaths of children in the UK due to accidental injury has declined steadily over the last 25 years**

Head and neck injuries

Head injury is common in children. Fortunately, in the vast majority it is only minor and a full recovery with no long-term adverse effects can be expected. However, it is also the most frequent cause of death and serious morbidity in children who have been injured (Fig. 7.4). Initial assessment is therefore directed at identifying the small proportion of children who are likely to have sustained an intracranial injury, and thus need neuroimaging. This assessment is based on the history and neurological condition of the patient. Various clinical

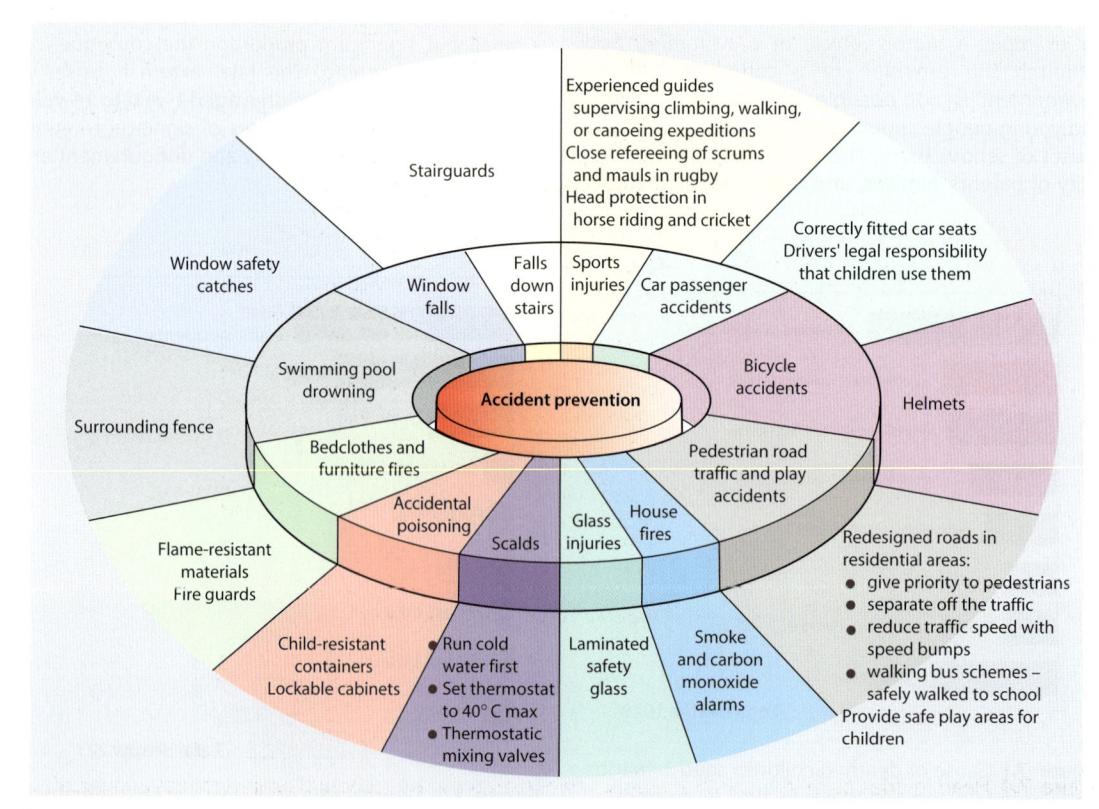

Figure 7.3 Examples of accident prevention.

Head injuries in children

Pathogenesis

Primary damage
Injury to neural tissue:
- focal cerebral contusions and lacerations
- diffuse axonal injury

Injury to blood vessels:
- Extradural, subdural, subarachnoid haemorrhage

Penetrating injury

Secondary damage
Cerebral oedema
Hypotension
Hypoxia
Seizures
Hypoglycaemia
Infection (later)

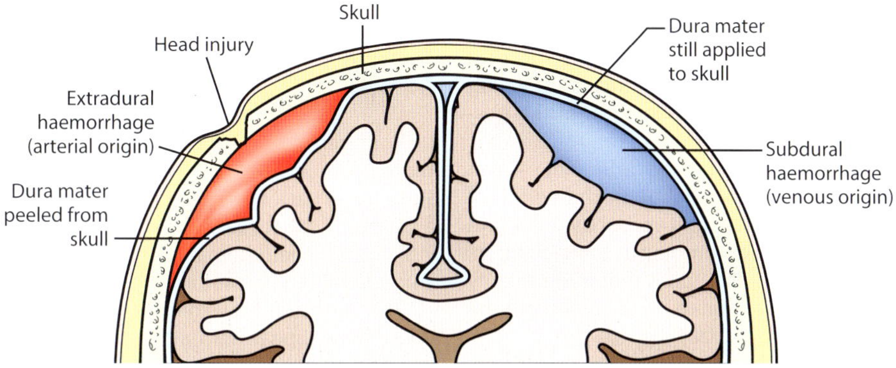

Head injury — Skull — Dura mater still applied to skull
Extradural haemorrhage (arterial origin)
Dura mater peeled from skull
Subdural haemorrhage (venous origin)

Initial assessment and management

Initial assessment:
- Airway
- Breathing
- Circulation
- Disability: conscious level, pupils
- Exposure

Is the child (any of):
- Unresponsive?
- Responsive only to pain?
- Breathing inadequately?

Yes:
- Intubate and ventilate
- Urgent CT scan
- Urgent neurosurgical and intensive care referral

No →

Are any of the following present?
- Suspicion of non-accidental injury
- Post-traumatic seizure
- Glasgow coma score <14 initially or <15 2 h after injury
- Suspected open or depressed skull fracture
- Sign of basal skull fracture (haemotympanum, 'panda eyes', Battle sign, CSF leak from nose/ears
- Focal neurological signs
- <1-y old with bruise or swelling >5 cm on the head

Yes → Urgent CT scan

No →

Are any of the following present?
- Witnessed loss of consciousness >5 min
- Abnormal drowsiness
- 3 or more discrete episodes of vomiting
- Dangerous mechanism of injury (high speed road traffic collision; fall from >3 m height)
- Amnesia lasting >5 min

Yes >1 present → Urgent CT scan

Yes only 1 present →
- Admit and observe for at least 6 h
- CT scan if further concerns

No → No imaging required. Use clinical judgment to determine if further observation is required

Figure 7.4 Head injuries in children. Pathogenesis, site of extradural and subdural haemorrhages and initial assessment and management (based on NICE guideline 2014).

guidelines have been developed to help determine which children need brain imaging (Fig. 7.4 and Case history 7.1). These decisions tend to be highly sensitive but not highly specific, resulting in many normal CT scans for every scan that identifies a significant injury.

If an intracranial injury is identified, the aim of management is to avoid secondary damage to the brain. This is achieved by maintaining the blood supply to the brain while minimizing the damage from raised intracranial pressure. This may require surgical evacuation of intracranial haemorrhage and/or intubation and ventilation to allow control of blood pressure and blood carbon dioxide levels, both of which affect cerebral perfusion.

In infants with unfused skull sutures, significant bleeding into the brain and surrounding space may occur leading to shock before neurological symptoms and signs appear. Significant head injury in young infants must always lead to consideration of the possibility of deliberately inflicted injury.

Children with severe traumatic brain injury can make a good physical recovery though the period of rehabilitation may be long. Cognitive, behavioural, and mental health problems are common in these children, however, and specialist follow-up is required for early identification and intervention to try to ameliorate the effect of these problems on daily life.

Neck injury resulting in spinal cord damage is very rare in children and is usually only associated with significant trauma associated with high-speed road traffic collisions. The most common neck injury is fracture of the upper two cervical vertebrae. The elasticity of the cervical spine can also allow damage to the spinal cord without injury to the bony structures, i.e. spinal cord injury without radiologic abnormality.

Internal injuries

Internal injuries in children are usually associated with severe trauma due to road traffic collisions and falls from significant heights. In particular, young children have less fat and a more elastic skeleton protecting tightly packed internal organs. This means that impact force is distributed widely through the body, resulting in a greater possibility of multisystem trauma compared with adolescents or adults.

Abdominal injuries are typically caused by blunt trauma due to seat belt restraints or bicycle handlebar injuries. Liver and spleen rupture may occur and become apparent rapidly, while bowel and pancreatic injuries may take longer to become apparent. Close observation and imaging are necessary. Focused abdominal sonography in a trauma scan can be useful but must be combined with clinical judgement. Contained splenic and hepatic haematomas can be managed conservatively but rapid access to paediatric surgery must be available immediately in the event of clinical deterioration.

Chest injuries, including pneumothorax and haemopericardium, are also typically due to blunt trauma. The pliable rib cage in children may allow significant injury to underlying organs with little external evidence. There must be a high index of suspicion for these injuries in the event of a significant mechanism of injury.

Case history 7.1

Head injury

Tom, a 3-year-old boy, is being carried on his uncle's shoulders when he falls 6 feet to the ground, banging his head on the concrete floor. He cries immediately but does not lose consciousness. He is taken to the emergency department where he vomits once. Clinical examination is normal apart from a 4-cm diameter firm swelling over his left temple. He is discharged home with advice to return if he:

- vomits repeatedly
- complains of a worsening headache
- becomes abnormally sleepy
- behaves abnormally
- develops weakness of one side of his body.

Tom remains well overnight but the following morning begins to vomit again and becomes lethargic. He is taken back to the emergency department where a CT brain scan reveals an extradural haematoma (Fig. 7.5). Tom's haematoma is evacuated by the neurosurgeons and he makes an uneventful recovery.

This illustrates how children with a significant head injury may appear normal at initial presentation. It is essential to provide parents and caregivers with safety net advice to ensure they know to return should symptoms evolve.

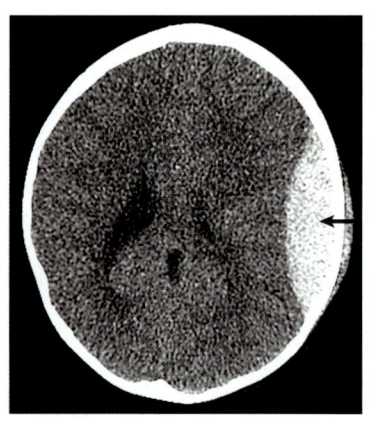

Figure 7.5 CT scan of head showing a left extradural haemorrhage (arrow).

Summary

Accidental head injury management:
- no symptoms or signs and benign mechanism of injury – discharge home with written advice
- minor symptoms or dangerous mechanism of injury – monitor for evolution of symptoms
- significant or progressive symptoms and signs – resuscitate (if necessary), CT scan, and neurosurgical referral as appropriate.

Choking, suffocation and strangulation

Choking is particularly common in young children, who frequently put things in their mouths and lack the oromotor skills to avoid choking on them or inhaling them. In addition, their airway diameter is small and more readily occluded than in adolescents and adults. Food is the most common cause of non-fatal choking, followed by toys. The emergency management of the choking child is outlined in Fig. 7.6 and 7.7.

Children may strangle themselves accidentally when clothing or bedding gets caught on furniture, particularly young children in cots. Following some tragic incidents, the possibility of strangling on blind and curtain cords has been the subject of a number of public information campaigns.

Drowning

Drowning, the respiratory impairment produced by submersion or immersion in liquid, is a significant cause of accidental death in children. Babies and toddlers tend to drown in baths, paddling pools, or garden ponds. Older children get into difficulty in canals, lakes, and the sea. Once submerged, asphyxiation occurs with or without aspiration of water. Up to 30% of fatalities can be avoided by skilled on-scene resuscitation. If the water is cold, the resulting hypothermia can have a protective effect and, even in the presence of fixed

The choking child

Management of the choking child

Assess severity

- **Severe airway obstruction** (ineffective cough)
  - **Unconscious** — Start CPR
  - **Conscious**
    Child:
    • 5 abdominal thrusts
    Infant:
    • 5 back blows
    • 5 chest thrusts
- **Mild airway obstruction** (effective cough)
  - **Encourage to cough**
    Continue to check for deterioration until obstruction cleared or cough becomes effective

Figure 7.6 Management of the choking child from an inhaled foreign body.

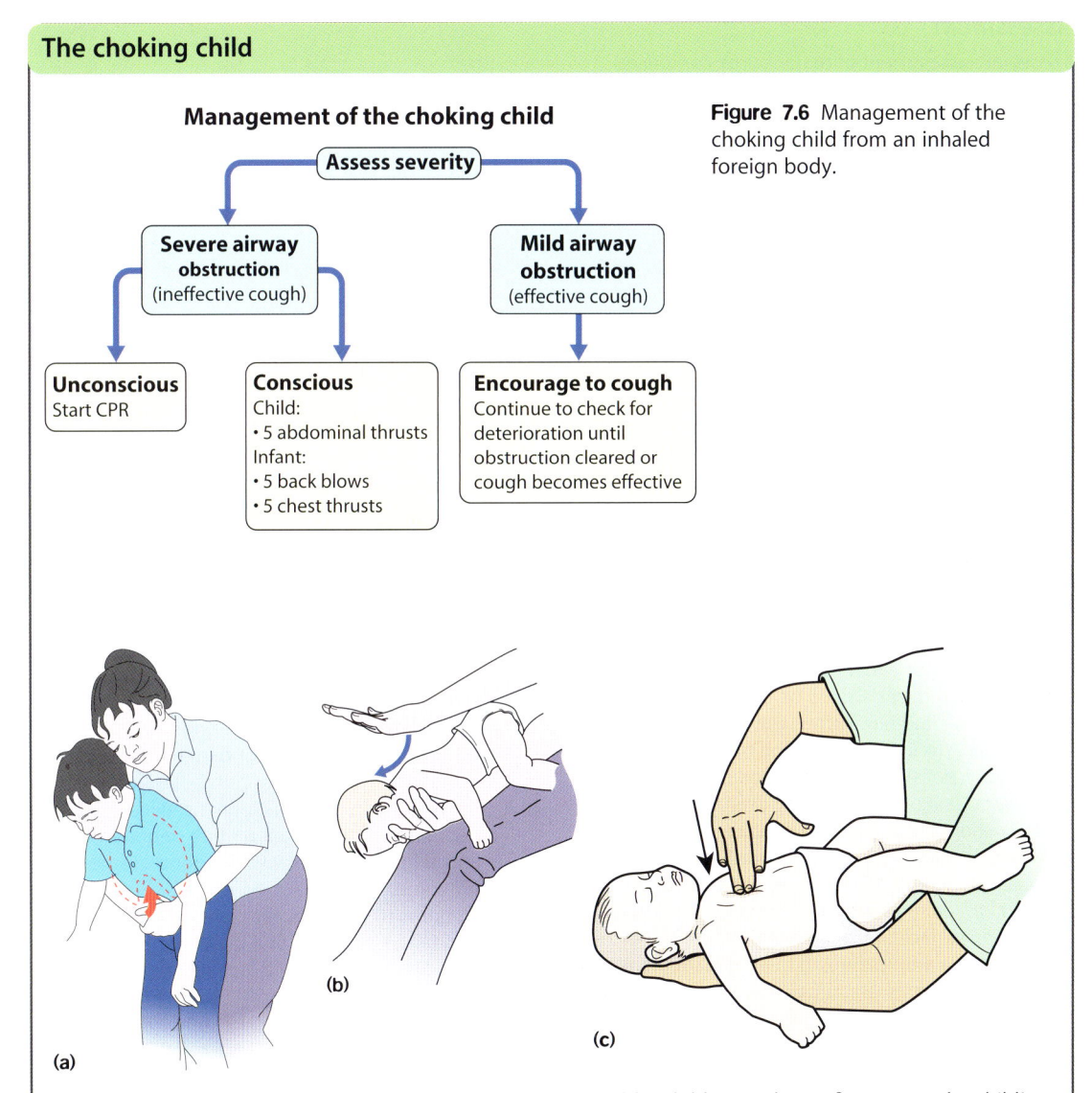

Figure 7.7 (a) Abdominal thrusts (Heimlich manoeuvre) in older children – place a fist against the child's upper abdomen in the midline and grasp with the other hand. Pull backwards and upwards to expel air from the lungs. In infants, back blows (b) and chest thrusts (c) are recommended, avoiding abdominal thrusts due to the risk of injury to the liver and spleen.

dilated pupils, resuscitation should continue until the child is warmed up as recovery may still be possible.

Burns and scalds

Burns and scalds are relatively common in children. This relates to the natural inquisitiveness and lack of sense of danger in young children and the risk-taking behaviour of older children and young people. They are a significant cause of death, although typically deaths in house fires are due to asphyxiation from gas and smoke inhalation rather than the thermal injury. Inhalation of superheated smoke or steam may also cause significant airway swelling. This can occur when steam has been inhaled directly from the spout of a kettle or teapot. Injuries from house fires may also be complicated by serious injury as a result of, for example, falls from a height during escape.

Assessment

Immediate assessment of major burns comprises:

- airway and breathing – in particular, check for evidence of airway burns:
  - soot in the nasal and oral cavities
  - cough, hoarseness, or stridor
  - coughing up black sputum
  - breathing and/or swallowing difficulty
  - blistering around or in the mouth
  - scorched eyebrows or hair
- early intubation if there is evolving airway swelling; intubation may become impossible with progressive obstruction of the airway
- circulation:
  - early circulatory compromise is rarely due to the burn injury and other sources of fluid loss should be sort (e.g. major haemorrhage)
  - in electrical burns, an ECG should be obtained.

Further assessment and initial management of burns:

- burn first aid:
  - cool the area with running water for up to 20 minutes but avoid hypothermia
  - chemical burns should be copiously irrigated
  - plastic (cling film) wraps can be used after cooling to limit evaporation from the burnt area
  - pain relief should be provided immediately; intranasal opiates are very useful
- estimation of burn surface area (Fig. 7.8):
  - a burn diagram should be used
  - as a rough measure, an area the size of the child's palm represents 1% body surface area
  - body surface area involvement determines need for admission and fluid management
  - burn depth assessment should be attempted (Fig. 7.9) but is often difficult and unreliable immediately after the event.

Further management

This should be directed at:

- relieving pain – assess with pain score; intravenous analgesia such as morphine or ketamine is often required on an ongoing basis

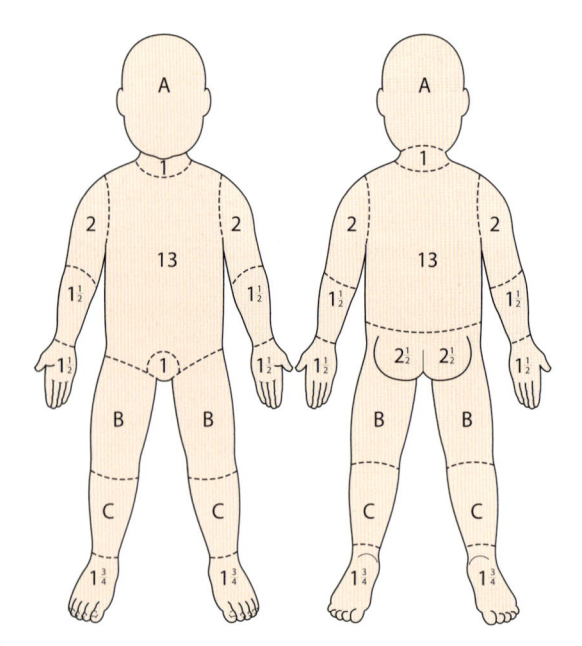

Area indicated	Surface area at			
	1 year	5 years	10 years	15 years
A	8.5	6.5	5.5	4.5
B	3.25	4.0	4.5	4.5
C	2.5	2.75	3.0	3.25

Figure 7.8 Lund and Browder chart for accurate assessment of body surface area.

- maintaining circulation – intravenous fluids are required if over 10% of the body surface area is affected. Urine output is the best measure to assess the adequacy of fluid replacement
- provision of wound care:
  - superficial burns with erythema only are treated with simple exposure
  - small superficial partial thickness burns can be cleaned and dressed. They should heal spontaneously, but require review
  - partial thickness burns covering over 5% of the body surface area, deeper partial thickness burns, and full thickness burns should be reviewed by a specialist burns service
  - deeper burns will often require débridement and skin grafting to ensure a good cosmetic outcome
  - all burns to the face, ears, eyes, hands, feet, genitalia, perineum, or a major joint, even if less than 5% to 10% should also be referred to a specialist burns service
  - signs of infection should be monitored and treated if found, as there is a risk of significant invasive infection.
- for all burns, the possibility of inflicted injury must be considered (see Fig. 8.2b)
- psychological support should be provided if required, as psychological sequelae of severe burns are often marked and long lasting.

The depth of burns

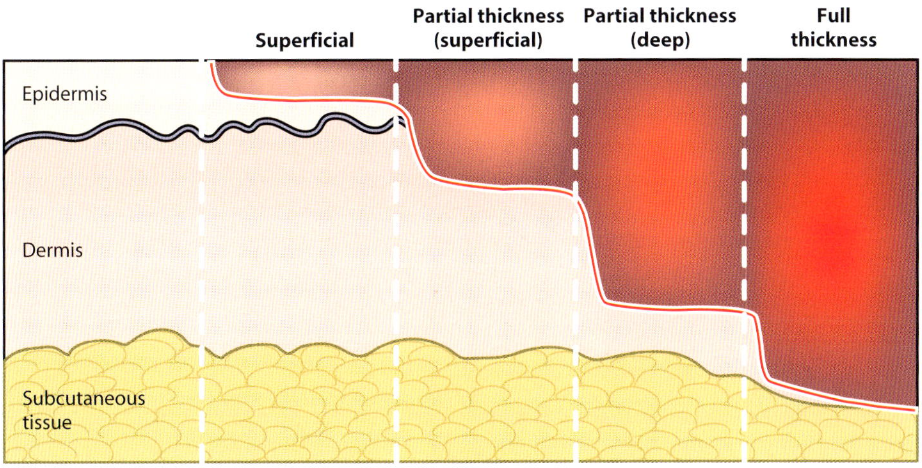

Depth	Superficial – limited to epidermis	Partial thickness (superficial)	Partial thickness (deep)	Full thickness
Possible cause	Sunburn, minor scald	Scald	Scald, brief contact with flame	Significant flame contact
Appearance	Dry and erythematous	Moist, erythematous, blistered	Moist with white slough, erythematous, mottled	Dry, charred, white
Pain sensation	Painful	Painful	Painless	Painless
Healing	Rapid – 1 week	1–3 weeks	3–4 weeks – often requires grafting	Needs skin grafting to heal

Figure 7.9 Burn depth assessment.

Summary

In burn management:
- cool the burn, not the child
- burnt children require effective analgesia
- refer deep and/or extensive burns or burns to sites where scarring would be particularly troublesome or disfiguring to specialist burns services.

Poisoning

Poisoning in children may be:
- accidental – common in young children
- due to deliberate self-harm or experimentation with recreational substances – by adolescents and young people
- iatrogenic – as a result of drug errors occasionally made by health professionals
- intentional – by parents or carers, though this is rare.

Accidental poisoning usually occurs when young children are found by parents or carers either playing with tablets or household or garden substances or with some in their mouths. The peak age is 30 months, and typically exposure occurs in the child's home. Serious harm is uncommon as many common household substances and medications are of low toxicity, and children usually ingest only small amounts. The relative toxicity of some common medicines and household and garden substances is shown in Table 7.1; a small number of medicines are potentially fatal to young children even in small doses. The most common causative agents vary from country to country due to differing availability of medications over the counter, and a variation in rural and urban lifestyles.

Table 7.1 Relative toxicity following ingestion of some common medicines and household and garden substances

Toxicity	Medicines	Household products	In the garden
Low	Oral contraceptives, most antibiotics, topical hydrocortisone	Liquid soap, lipstick, washing-up liquid, fish food, water-based glue and paint	Animal faeces, slugs, geraniums, compost
High	Opioids, beta-blockers, tricyclic antidepressants, oral hypoglycaemics, paracetamol, digoxin, iron, salicylates	Strong bleach, concentrated oven cleaner, liquid nicotine, ethylene glycol (antifreeze), petroleum distillates	Laburnum, death cap mushroom, yew, foxglove, organophosphorus pesticides, kerosene

There has been a marked reduction in the incidence of severe poisoning from accidental ingestion by young children. Reasons for this include:

- the introduction of child-resistant containers for many medicines and household products and use of blister packs for medicines
- reduction in the number of tablets available per pack in analgesics bought over the counter.

Adolescents attempting self-harm also typically ingest medications commonly found in their environment – paracetamol and ibuprofen, with their wide over-the-counter availability, are the most commonly ingested substances. However, they are likely to have ingested much larger quantities of tablets than young children and are therefore more likely to suffer significant toxicological effects.

Investigation and management

An approach to the investigation and management of the potentially poisoned patient is outlined in Fig. 7.10. Details of some of the more commonly ingested poisons with their specific management are detailed in Table 7.2. Usually, the identity of the ingested substance is known. Occasionally, poisoning is suspected but the substance is unknown; clinical signs may then help to identify the class of causative agent (Table 7.3 and Case history 7.2). These can be useful to aid further investigation and treatment.

All older children and young people who have attempted to deliberately harm themselves must be assessed for risk of a repeated attempt, irrespective of the toxicity of the ingested substance. The risk of recurrence is increased by a number of factors, including ongoing thoughts of self-harm or suicide, a lack of regret, evidence of planning, e.g. leaving a note, and a lack of protective social factors. The social circumstances of young people who inadvertently poison themselves as a result of experimentation with illicit drugs or alcohol should also be explored, with onward referral to substance misuse services, where appropriate.

Young children who have been exposed to agents of low toxicity and are asymptomatic can typically be discharged with advice to return if symptoms develop. The circumstances surrounding the exposure need to be considered to determine if there are social issues such as inadequate supervision that need to be addressed.

Chronic environmental poisoning

Young children are a high risk group for chronic environmental poisoning, because their exposure potentially occurs when they are most physiologically susceptible. Their engagement in frequent hand-to-mouth activities during play and meals leads to ingestion of more contaminants in dust and dirt than adults. Their small body size makes them more susceptible to doses that would not harm an adult and their developing brains are at greater risk of permanent damage due to neurotoxic effects of exposure.

Lead poisoning is one of the most important chronic environmental toxins affecting children worldwide. Although it is now uncommon in the UK and other developed countries, in some developing countries contamination of water supplies and the home environment by mining processes and factories remains a significant problem. The symptoms of chronic lead exposure are nonspecific but include:

- behavioural changes
- hyperactivity or decreased activity
- developmental delay or loss of developmental milestones
- chronic lead nephropathy.

More significant exposure may result in:

- abdominal pain, vomiting, constipation
- headache and ataxia
- lethargy, seizures, and coma.

The most important treatment is to prevent further exposure to lead. Chelation therapy can be effective in reversing acute symptoms such as encephalopathy but treatment is complex, particularly as lead is deposited in bone and therefore has a long half-life.

Although acute exposure to organophosphate and carbamate pesticides results in well-known acute syndromes, there is growing evidence that chronic exposure to these agents in early life can have adverse effects on neurodevelopment and behaviour. In addition, there is evidence associating some pesticides with an increased incidence of leukaemia and brain tumours.

Management of a poisoned child or young person

Outline of management

Identify the agent
- Question parents, child, or young person
- Clinical symptoms and signs may help where history is unclear (Table 7.3)

Determine toxicity of agent
Consider:
- intrinsic toxicity (use poisons information service)
- reported dose ingested
- presence of symptoms
- time since ingestion

Is reduction of absorption possible/indicated?
Activated charcoal:
- high surface area leads to adsorption of many drugs
- can be effective in reducing absorption of toxic agent if administered within 1 h of ingestion
- ineffective for iron, hydrocarbons, and pesticides

Gastric lavage and induced vomiting no longer recommended

Are investigations indicated?
- General blood tests (e.g. full blood count, renal and liver function) dependent on mechanism and likelihood of toxicity
- ECG for drugs with cardiovascular toxicity
- Specific blood concentrations only helpful for paracetamol, iron, salicylates, and alcohol
- Urine toxicology screen not helpful in the acute situation but may help to confirm diagnosis

Clinical management
Mainly determined by toxicity of agent:
- specific management including antidote as directed by poisons information service
- assessment of circumstances of ingestion important to prevent future recurrence
- assessment by child and adolescent psychiatrist or mental health services in cases of deliberate self-harm

Figure 7.10 Outline of management of poisoning.

Table 7.2 Some poisons and their treatment

Agent	Clinical symptoms	Mechanism	Management
Paracetamol	Early: • abdominal pain, vomiting Later (12 h to 24 h): • liver failure	Initial gastric irritation Toxic metabolite (NAPQI) produced by saturation of liver metabolism	Risk assessed by measuring plasma paracetamol concentration Treat with intravenous acetylcysteine if concentration is high or liver function abnormal
Button batteries	Abdominal pain Gut perforation and stricture formation	Leakage: corrosion of gut wall due to electrical circuit production	X-ray of chest and abdomen to confirm ingestion and identify position Endoscopic removal is recommended if in the oesophagus, the object fails to pass, or symptoms are present (e.g. abdominal pain or melaena)
Carbon monoxide	Early: • headache, nausea Later: • confusion, drowsiness leading to coma	Binds to haemoglobin causing tissue hypoxia	High-flow oxygen to hasten dissociation of carbon monoxide The role of hyperbaric oxygen therapy is unclear
Salicylates	Early: • vomiting, tinnitus Later: • respiratory alkalosis followed by metabolic acidosis	Direct stimulation of respiratory centre Uncouples oxidative phosphorylation leading to metabolic acidosis and hypoglycaemia	Plasma salicylate concentration 2–4 h after ingestion helps to estimate toxicity Alkalinization of urine increases excretion of salicylates. Haemodialysis also effectively removes salicylate
Tricyclic antidepressants	Early: • tachycardia, drowsiness, dry mouth Later: • arrhythmias, seizures	Anti-cholinergic effects, interference with cardiac conduction pathways	Treatment of arrhythmias with sodium bicarbonate Support ventilation
Ethylene glycol (anti-freeze)	Early: • intoxication Later: • tachycardia, metabolic acidosis leading to renal failure	Production of toxic metabolites that interfere with intracellular energy production	Fomepizole inhibits the production of toxic metabolites; alcohol may also be used but has more adverse effects Haemodialysis to remove toxic metabolites in severe cases
Alcohol (accidental or experimenting by older children)	Hypoglycaemia Coma Respiratory failure	Direct inhibitory effect on glycolysis in the liver and neurotransmission in the brain	Monitor blood glucose and correct if necessary. Support ventilation if required Blood alcohol levels may help to predict severity

Table 7.2 Some poisons and their treatment—cont'd

Agent	Clinical symptoms	Mechanism	Management
Iron	Initial: vomiting, diarrhoea, haematemesis, melaena, acute gastric ulceration Latent period of improvement 6–12 h later: drowsiness, coma, shock, liver failure with hypoglycaemia, and convulsions Long term: gut strictures	Local corrosive effect on gut mucosa Disruption of oxidative phosphorylation in mitochondria leads to free radical production, lipid peroxidation, and metabolic acidosis	Serious toxicity if >75 mg/kg elemental iron ingested Serum iron level 4 h after ingestion is the best laboratory measure of severity Intravenous desferoxamine chelates iron and should be administered in cases of moderate-to-severe toxicity
Hydrocarbons (e.g. paraffin, kerosene)	Pneumonitis Coma	Low viscosity and high volatility makes aspiration easy, resulting in direct lung toxicity Direct inhibitory effect on neurotransmission in the brain	No specific antidote – supportive treatment only
Organophosphorus pesticides	Cholinergic effects: • salivation, lacrimation, urination, diarrhoea and vomiting, muscle weakness, cramps and paralysis, bradycardia. and hypotension Central nervous system effects: • seizures and coma	Inhibition of acetylcholinesterase resulting in accumulation of acetylcholine throughout the nervous system	Supportive care Atropine (often in large doses) as an anticholinergic agent Pralidoxime to reactivate acetylcholinesterase

NAPQI, *N*-acetyl-*p*-benzoquinone imine.

Table 7.3 Physical findings that may help identify different classes of drugs in overdose

Type of effect	Heart rate and blood pressure	Respiratory rate	Temperature	Pupils	Sweating
Anticholinergic (e.g. tricyclic antidepressants, antihistamines)	Increased	No effect	Increased	Dilated	Reduced
Opioid (e.g. morphine, codeine)	Reduced	Reduced	Reduced	Constricted	Reduced
Sympathomimetic (e.g. cocaine, amphetamines)	Increased	Increased	Increased	Dilated	Increased
Sedative-hypnotic (e.g. anticonvulsants, benzodiazepines)	Reduced	Reduced	Reduced	No effect	Reduced

Case history 7.2

A 14-year-old girl with vomiting and abdominal pain

Jemima, a 14-year-old girl, is brought to the emergency department in the morning by her mother as she has been vomiting and complaining of severe abdominal pain. On examination she has a generally tender abdomen. Blood tests reveal an extremely high alanine transaminase concentration, well above normal for her age. Her clotting is also deranged with a prothrombin time of 17 seconds. An initial diagnosis of hepatitis is considered but on discussion with the consultant the lack of jaundice is considered atypical. On further direct questioning, Jemima admits to having taken 22 paracetamol tablets (500 mg) the previous afternoon following an altercation with another girl at school. Jemima is commenced on *N*-acetylcysteine and makes a full recovery.

This case highlights the need to consider a toxicological cause when the history, examination findings, and investigation results do not fit together.

Summary

Accidental poisoning in children:
- is common in toddlers and young children
- most substances do not cause serious illness
- when an ingestion has occurred, identify the agent and assess its toxicity to plan management
- poisons potentially harmful in children include alcohol, acids and alkalis, bleach, digoxin, batteries, iron, paracetamol, petroleum distillates, salicylates, and tricyclic antidepressants
- assess the social circumstances behind why it happened.

Acknowledgements

We would like to acknowledge contributors to the chapter on accidents and poisoning in previous editions, whose work we have drawn on: Jo Sibert (1st, 2nd, 3rd Edition, Environment), Barbara Phillips (2nd edition, Environment), Ian Maconochie (3rd Edition, Environment), Rebecca Salter (4th Edition, Accidents, Poisoning and Child Protection).

Further reading

Websites (Accessed November 2016)

Child Accident Prevention Trust (CAPT): Available at: www.capt.org.uk.

Making the link – working together for safer children: Available at: www.makingthelink.net.

Paediatric Trauma Manual of the Royal Children's Hospital Melbourne: Available at: www.rch.org.au/paed_trauma/manual/Paediatric_Trauma_Manual.

The Poison Review: Available at: www.thepoisonreview.com.

Toxbase: Available at: www.toxbase.org. *Requires password.*

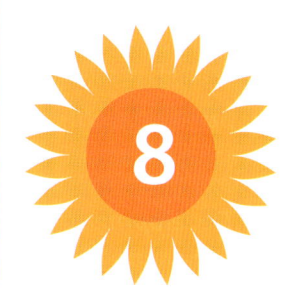

Child protection

Types of child abuse and neglect 110
Prevalence of child maltreatment 111
Safeguarding children 113

Features of child protection are:
- protecting children from harm is a duty of all health professionals
- physical and sexual abuse may dominate the media, but it also encompasses neglect, emotional abuse, sexual exploitation, fabricated illness, and female genital mutilation
- issues are often complex and difficult, so decisions usually require a multidisciplinary approach by specially trained, experienced professionals.

Children and young people require parents or carers who love, look after, provide shelter, and protect them from harm. Unfortunately, this is not the case for all children. Emotional, physical and sexual abuse and neglect of children by parents, carers and others continue to blight the lives of children and young people as it has throughout history. Recent issues in the protection of vulnerable children and adolescents have included harm from observing intimate partner violence, sexual exploitation, and female genital mutilation (FGM). Maltreatment significantly decreases the likelihood that a child will reach his or her full potential, although this is not inevitable; some resilient individuals manage despite very adverse circumstances.

Society, including the medical profession, was largely reluctant to accept that child maltreatment occurred until the second half of the twentieth century, when attention was drawn by two American paediatricians to the 'battered child'. It is now accepted that child abuse and neglect exist and legislation is in place making abuse a criminal offence.

The UN Convention on the Rights of the Child (Box 8.1) specifically refers to the right of children to be protected from maltreatment, both physical and mental. It gives governments the responsibility to ensure that children are properly cared for and protected from violence, exploitation, abuse, and neglect.

In the UK, there has been a series of high-profile cases of child abuse, starting with Maria Colwell in 1973 and followed by Victoria Climbie in 2000 and Peter Connelly (Baby P) in 2007, resulting in the death of the abused child with multiple injuries. This prompted publication of reports and initiatives highlighting the need for better information sharing and cooperative working by health professionals. More recently, there was the tragic case of Daniel Pelka (Box 8.2). The exposure of systematic sexual abuse of vulnerable young people, including abuse by a wide range of celebrity, political and other high-status figures, over many years has further highlighted the difficulties faced by all professionals with responsibility for the welfare of children. Social workers, teachers, police, healthcare professionals, and those in many spheres of public life are more aware than ever of the need to recognize and respond appropriately to the alerting signs of child abuse and neglect.

However, fear of missing child abuse has to be weighed against the damage of falsely accusing parents of abusing their children. This requires sensible judgement, excellent communication with the parents, and a professional culture in which any concern that a child is being maltreated can be readily discussed with senior members of the team.

High-profile cases of child abuse:
- can make some doctors frightened to deal with child protection or become overly suspicious from fear of missing cases
- have led to improved multiagency guidelines and procedures
- have resulted in better, regularly updated child protection training for all health professionals.

Box 8.1 Summary of the United Nations Convention on the Rights of the Child (1989)

1 Survival rights
The child's right to life and to the most basic needs – food, shelter, and access to healthcare.

2 Developmental rights
To achieve their full potential – education, play, freedom of thought, conscience, and religion. Those with disabilities to receive special services.

3 Protection rights
Against all forms of abuse, neglect, exploitation, and discrimination.

4 Participation rights
To take an active role in their communities and nations.

Summary

- Child maltreatment has existed for centuries but societies have been very slow to acknowledge it as a problem.
- Children and young people are vulnerable and cannot protect themselves – the basis of children's rights.
- Protecting children and young people from harm is a key role of parents or carers and all involved with children.
- All healthcare professionals, social workers, teachers, police, and others have a duty to ensure that they know what to do if they have concerns that a child or young person may be being abused.

Box 8.2 A recent high-profile case of child abuse in the UK

Daniel Pelka, aged 4-years, died from a head injury in March 2012. In the months before his death he was denied food, force-fed salt, held under the water in a bath until becoming unconscious, and regularly beaten and imprisoned in an unheated box room. Police received 26 reports of domestic abuse at his home. Lack of rigorous questioning and poor record-keeping meant officials never got to the bottom of what was going on. The serious case review into his death identified three main failures when the abuse could have been stopped:
- professionals believed his parents' story too readily in 2011 that he broke his arm when he fell off a sofa
- his primary school failed to act on a pattern of injuries spotted during the 4 months before his death in 2012. Teachers watched him fish half-eaten food from bins because he was so hungry. His mother convinced them that he had an eating disorder
- a paediatrician, just a month before he died, failed to spot child abuse as the key reason for Daniel's dramatic weight loss: he weighed less than 11 kg when he died.

The report said professionals needed to have much more inquiring minds and to be focused and determined in their intentions to address concerns that would have offered greater protection for Daniel. What is striking and depressing is that no professional ever asked Daniel how he was feeling and what was happening in his life that made him want to eat from bins. Talking to the child and seeking his or her view is a key component of good safeguarding practice.

Types of child abuse and neglect

Abuse and neglect are both forms of maltreatment of a child. Somebody may abuse or neglect a child by inflicting harm, or by failing to act to prevent harm. Children may be abused in a family at home or in an institution or community, usually by someone known to them or, more rarely, by a stranger. They may be abused by one or more adults or another child or other children. Conventionally, child abuse is categorized into:

- physical abuse
- emotional abuse
- sexual abuse, including sexual exploitation
- neglect
- fabricated or induced illness.

In addition to these categories, witnessing intimate partner violence is regarded as a form of child maltreatment. In the UK, the practice of FGM is also regarded as a form of child abuse.

Physical abuse

Physical abuse may involve hitting, shaking, throwing, poisoning, burning or scalding, drowning, suffocating, or otherwise causing physical harm to a child.

Emotional abuse

Emotional abuse is the persistent emotional maltreatment of a child resulting in severe and persistent adverse effects on the child's emotional development. It may involve conveying to children that they are worthless or unloved, inadequate, or valued only insofar as they meet the needs of another person. It may feature developmentally inappropriate expectations being imposed on children. These may include interactions that are beyond the child's developmental capability, as well as overprotection and abnormal social interaction. It may involve seeing or hearing the ill treatment of another child or person. It may also involve serious bullying that causes children to feel frightened or in danger, or the exploitation or corruption of children. Some level of emotional abuse is involved in all types of maltreatment of a child, although it may occur alone.

Sexual abuse and sexual exploitation

Sexual abuse involves forcing or enticing a child or young person to take part in sexual activities, including prostitution, whether or not the child is aware of what is happening. The activities may involve physical contact, including penetrative acts such as rape, buggery or oral sex, and/or noncontact activities, such as involving children in looking at or producing pornographic material or watching sexual activities or encouraging children to behave in sexually inappropriate ways.

Sexual exploitation is a type of sexual abuse in which children are sexually exploited for money, power, or status. Children or young people may be tricked into believing they are in a loving, consensual relationship. They might be invited to parties and given drugs and alcohol. They may also be groomed online. Some children and young people are trafficked into or within the UK for the purpose of sexual exploitation. Sexual exploitation can also happen to young people in gangs.

Neglect

Neglect is the persistent failure to meet a child's basic physical and/or psychological needs, likely to result in the serious impairment of the child's health or development. It may involve a parent or carer failing to provide:

- adequate food and clothing
- shelter, including exclusion from home or abandonment
- protection from physical and emotional harm or danger
- adequate supervision, including the use of inadequate caregivers
- access to appropriate medical care or treatment.

It may also include neglect or unresponsiveness to a child's basic emotional needs.

Fabricated or induced illness

This is a broad term to describe a group of behaviours by parents (or carers), but usually the mother (>80%), which cause harm to children. It fulfils the parents (or carers) own needs. It may consist of:

verbal fabrication – parents fabricate (i.e. invent) symptoms and signs in the child, telling a false story to healthcare professionals, leading them to believe the child is ill and requires investigation and treatment. Medical and nursing staff are used as the instrument to harm the child through unnecessary interventions, including medication, hospital stays, intrusive tests, and surgery. In community settings, the false stories may lead to medication, special diets, and a restricted lifestyle or special schools

induction of illness – may involve:

- suffocation of the child, which may present as an acute life-threatening event
- administration of noxious substances or poisons
- excessive or unnecessary administration of ordinary substances (e.g. excess salt)
- excess or unnecessary use of medication (prescribed for the child or others)
- the use of medically provided portals of entry (such as gastrostomy buttons, central lines).

Organic illness may coexist with fabricated or induced illness in a child, thus making the fabrication more difficult to identify. It may manifest as overprotection, imposing unwarranted restrictions, or giving treatment that is inappropriate or excessive.

The condition can be extremely difficult to diagnose, but may be suspected if the child has frequent unexplained illnesses and multiple hospital admissions with symptoms that only occur in the carer's presence and are not substantiated by clinical findings. This disorder can be very damaging to the child, as unnecessary investigations and potentially harmful treatment are likely to be given. The child also learns to live with a pattern of illness rather than health. In induced poisoning, the diagnosis may be made by identifying the drug in the blood or urine.

Intimate partner violence

Observing violence between adults who are, or have been, intimate partners or family members, irrespective of sex or sexuality, is also a form of abuse. Threatening behaviour, violence, and abuse (psychological, physical, sexual, financial, or emotional) are recognized to contribute to poor short-term and long-term outcomes for children and young people.

Female genital mutilation

This is defined by the WHO as 'all procedures that involve partial or total removal of the external female genitalia, or other injury to the female genital organs for nonmedical reasons'. It is recognized as a violation of the human rights of women and girls. Between 100–140 million women and girls are thought to be living with the consequences of FGM. It is nearly always carried out on minors. In December 2012, the United Nations general assembly unanimously voted for its elimination throughout the world. In the UK, child protection procedures are followed when there are concerns that a girl is likely to be subjected to or has undergone FGM (Fig. 8.1).

Prevalence of child maltreatment

It is only possible to estimate the size of the problem in high-income countries where there are official statistics from agencies investigating victims, e.g. child protection services or the police (investigating victims and offenders).

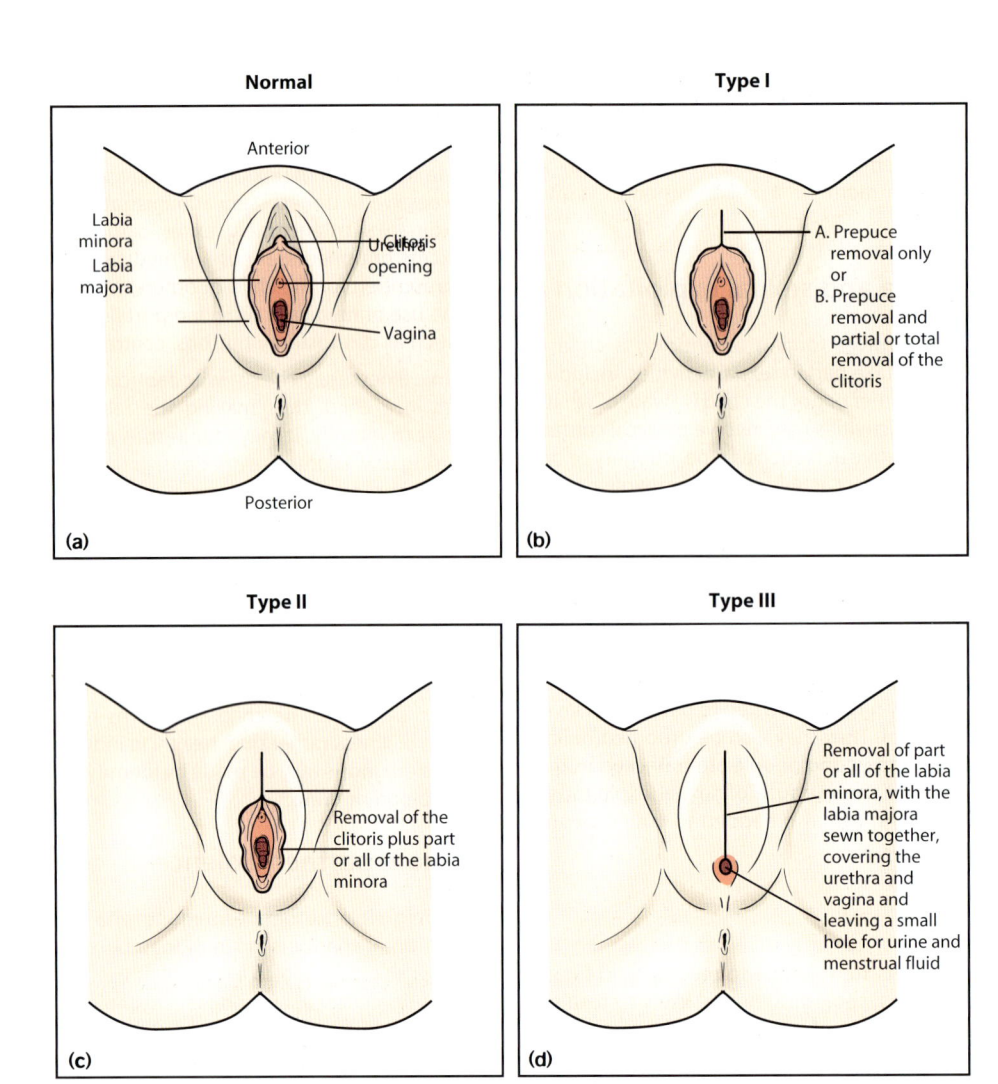

Figure 8.1 Female genital mutilation WHO Types I–III.

Table 8.1 Cumulative prevalence of abuse from self-reports (0–18 years) in high-income countries

Type of abuse	Physical	Sexual (all forms)	Emotional	Neglect	Witnessing intimate partner violence
Cumulative prevalence	5–35%	15–30% for girls 5–15% for boys	4–9%	6–12%	8–25%

From Gilbert R, Widom CS, Browne K, Fergusson D, Webb E, Janson S. Burden and consequences of child maltreatment in high-income countries. *Lancet* 373:68–81, 2009.

According to the National Society for Prevention of Cruelty to Children in England in 2013/2014:

- there were over 11.5 million children under 18 years
- almost 400 000 children received support from children's services – about 3.5% of the total child population
- over 48 000 children were identified as needing protection from abuse – about 0.4% of the total child population
- over 62 000 children and young people talked to ChildLine about abuse
- there are over 68 000 children in care (Source: http://www.nspcc.org.uk/services-and-resources/research-and-resources/statistics/).

They estimated that for every child identified as needing protection from abuse, another eight are suffering abuse. Studies based on self-reports (Table 8.1) from victims who are old enough to comply with surveys, or studies based on parents reporting severe physical punishment or patterns of care tend to confirm this. The discrepancy between 'official' agency data and those from self-reports underlines the fact that only a few children who are maltreated receive official attention.

Furthermore, evidence from several studies suggests that children who are exposed to one type of maltreatment are at high risk of other types and of repeated exposure over time, and that the frequency of exposure is correlated with the severity of maltreatment. For a few children, maltreatment is a chronic condition, not an event. Health professionals have a key role in helping children avoid the devastatingly damaging effects of maltreatment and need to be alert to the possibility that the child in front of them or the children of the adult in front of them may be being maltreated.

Safeguarding children

Safeguarding is the term used in child protection processes and procedures in the UK. It means that not only should we intervene when there are clear instances of child maltreatment as set out previously, but also vulnerabilities should be recognized and alerted to those involved in looking after the child or young person. This includes the parents or carers, teachers, social workers and the police. Providing early help is more effective in promoting the welfare of children than reacting later. The key principles of safeguarding children are:

- safeguarding is everyone's responsibility: for services to be effective each professional and organization should play their full part
- child-centred approach: for services to be effective they should be based on a clear understanding of the needs and views of children.

Safeguarding is everyone's responsibility

Risk factors

Child maltreatment occurs across socioeconomic, religious, cultural, racial, and ethnic groups. Although no specific causes have been definitively identified that lead a parent or other caregiver to abuse or neglect a child, research has recognized a number of risk factors commonly associated with maltreatment (Box 8.3). Children within families and environments in which these factors exist have a higher probability of experiencing maltreatment. It must be emphasized, however, that although certain factors are often present among families where maltreatment occurs, this does not mean that the presence of these factors will *always* result in child abuse and neglect. For example, there is a relationship between poverty and maltreatment, yet most people living in poverty do not harm their children.

Presentation

Child abuse and neglect

Child abuse may present with one or more of:
- physical symptoms and signs
- psychological symptoms and signs

Box 8.3 Risk factors for child abuse

In the child:
- failure to meet parental expectations and aspirations, e.g. disabled, 'wrong' gender, 'difficult' child
- born after forced, coercive, or commercial sex.

Parent/carer:
- mental health problems
- parental indifference, intolerance, or over-anxiousness
- alcohol, drug abuse.

In the family:
- step-parents
- domestic violence
- multiple/closely spaced births
- social isolation or lack of social support
- young parental age.

Environment:
- poverty, poor housing.

- a concerning interaction observed between the child and the parent or carer
- the child may tell someone about the abuse
- the abuse may be observed.

Identification of child abuse in children with disabilities may be more difficult; disability is also a risk factor for child abuse.

In order to diagnose child abuse or neglect, a detailed history and thorough examination are crucial. In most instances where child abuse is considered, seeking advice from colleagues, e.g. more experienced members of the team, paediatric radiologists and paediatric or orthopaedic surgeons is essential.

Factors to consider in the presentation of a physical injury are:

- the child's age and stage of development
- the history given by the child (if they can communicate)
- the plausibility and/or reasonableness of the explanation for the injury (Case History 8.1)
- any background, e.g. previous child protection concerns, multiple attendances to Accident and Emergency department or general practitioner
- delay in reporting the injury
- inconsistent histories from caregivers
- inappropriate reaction of parents or caregivers who are vague, evasive, unconcerned, or excessively distressed or aggressive.

It is often not clear whether an injury is inflicted or non-inflicted. Table 8.2 gives examples of injuries and a guide as to the likelihood that it is due to an inflicted injury. The context and observations of the family are very important in evaluating injuries that may be inflicted.

Physical injuries that can be caused by child abuse

Case history 8.1

Severe child abuse

A 2-month-old boy was brought into the Accident and Emergency department by ambulance, with sudden loss of consciousness. His mother accompanying him appeared to have learning difficulties and could not explain what had happened. His father arrived soon after and said that he had been changing the child's nappy on the floor when suddenly he 'went all floppy and asleep'.

The child was unresponsive (U on AVPU) and had shallow breathing. His pupils were dilated. He appeared well nourished and was dressed only in a nappy. There were no obvious injuries seen.

Medical management was rapidly instituted. CT head scan showed subdural haemorrhages (Fig. 8.2). A chest X-ray obtained following intubation showed old posterior rib fractures (Fig. 8.3). Subsequent ophthalmological examination showed bilateral retinal haemorrhages (Fig. 8.4).

The child was transferred to an intensive care unit, where he died. A postmortem skeletal survey showed metaphyseal fractures (Fig. 8.5).

The parents maintained their story, despite the compelling evidence of inflicted head injury and shaking. The case went to the criminal court and both were sentenced on a number of charges.

Severe physical child abuse resulting in death gains considerable attention from the media but is rare. Many more children suffer permanent injury. Most have been seen previously by health professionals. Early recognition and response to child protection concerns could prevent severe injury.

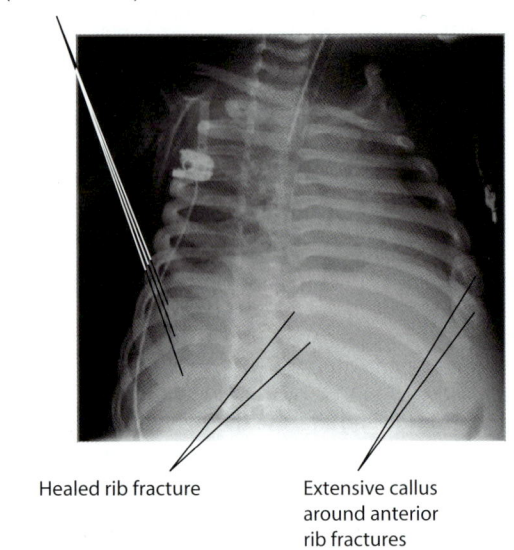

Figure 8.3 Multiple rib fractures of different ages.

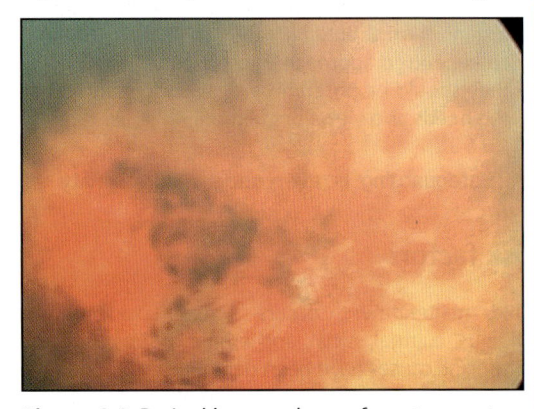

Figure 8.4 Retinal haemorrhages from trauma to the head. (Courtesy of Clare Roberts.)

Figure 8.2 Subdural haemorrhage. CSF = cerebrospinal fluid.

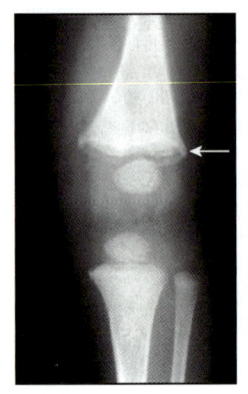

Figure 8.5 Metaphyseal fracture of distal humerus.

Table 8.2 Examples of injuries and a guide as to how likely it is due to an inflicted injury

Injury	More likely to be inflicted	May be inflicted accidental, or underlying disorder	Less likely or unlikely to be inflicted
Fractures	Any fracture in a non-mobile child (excluding fragile bones) Rib fractures Multiple fractures (unless significant accidental trauma, e.g. road traffic accident) Multiple fractures of different ages	Skull fracture in young child. Long bone fractures in a young but mobile child	Fracture in school-age child with witnessed trauma, e.g. fall from swing
Bruises	Bruising in the shape of a hand (Fig. 8.6a) or object Bruises on the neck that look like attempted strangulation Bruises around the wrists or ankles that look like ligature marks Bruise to the buttocks in a child less than 2 years or any age without a good explanation	Bruising to the trunk with a vague history	Bruises on the shins of a mobile child
Burns	Any burn in a child who is not mobile A burn in the shape of an implement – cigarette, iron A 'glove or stocking' burn consistent with forced immersion (Fig. 8.6b)		A burn to mobile toddler with splash marks, a history of pulling drink onto himself – but may indicate neglect in the form of poor supervision
Bites	Bruising in the shape of a bite thought unlikely to have been caused by a young child (Fig. 8.6c)		A witnessed biting of one toddler by another

Child protection

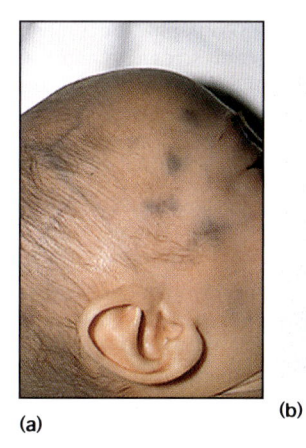

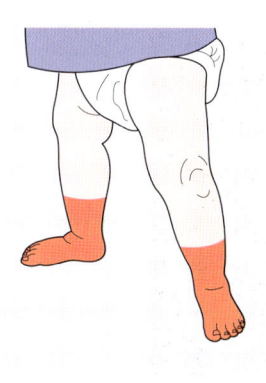

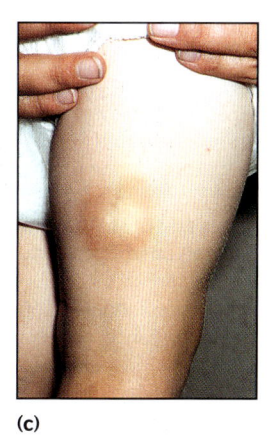

Figure 8.6 (a) Bruising from finger trauma to a baby's head; (b) scald with stocking distribution including the soles from forced immersion in hot water; and (c) a bite mark on an infant's leg. Adult bite marks may be seen in abuse, but bites from other children are not uncommon.

> **Key features of bruising**
> - The age of a bruise cannot be accurately estimated.
> - Bruising is hard to detect on children with dark skin.
> - Mongolian spots can be mistaken for bruises, as they may still be present at several years of age (see Fig. 10.14d).

Neglect

Consider the possibility of neglect when the child:

- consistently misses important medical appointments
- lacks needed medical or dental care or immunizations
- seems ravenously hungry
- is dirty
- is wearing inadequate clothing in cold weather
- is abusing alcohol or other drugs
- says there is no one at home to provide care.

Consider the possibility of neglect when the parent or other adult caregiver:

- appears to be indifferent to the child
- seems apathetic or depressed
- behaves irrationally or in a bizarre manner
- is abusing alcohol or other drugs.

Emotional abuse

This damaging form of abuse can be difficult to identify in a single brief healthcare interaction with a child and carer (Case History 8.2) but may be apparent when the observation period recurs or is longer, e.g. an inpatient or neonatal unit setting. Some clues may be found by noting how the parent or caregiver perceives the child. Is the child:

- the 'wrong' gender
- born at a time of parental separation or violence
- seen as unduly 'difficult'?

There may be clues from the behaviour of the child. This depends on the child's age:

- babies:
  - apathetic, delayed development, non-demanding
  - described by the mother as 'spoiled, attention seeking, in control, not loving her'
- toddlers and preschool children:
  - violent, apathetic, fearful
- school children:
  - wetting, soiling, relationship difficulties, nonattendance, antisocial behaviour
- adolescents:
  - self-harm, depression, oppositional, aggressive, and delinquent behaviour.

In addition to emotional abuse by a parent or carer, bullying by other children is increasingly recognized as an important form of emotional abuse. Every school should have a written bullying policy that needs to be implemented when necessary.

Sexual abuse

In suspected sexual abuse, information from different sources needs to be pieced together (Fig. 8.7).

Recognition

The child or young person may:

- tell someone about the abuse
- be identified in pornographic material
- be pregnant (by legal definition this is due to sexual abuse for a girl under the age of 13)
- have a sexually transmitted infection with no clear explanation (but some sexually transmitted infections can be passed from the mother to the baby during pregnancy or birth).

Physical symptoms

- Vaginal bleeding, itching, discharge.
- Rectal bleeding.

Behavioural symptoms

- Any of the symptoms outlined for emotional abuse in the previous section.
- Unexpected awareness or acting out of sexualized behaviour beyond what would be expected for age.
- Soiling, secondary enuresis.
- Self-harm, aggressive or sexualized behaviours, regression, poor school performance.

Signs

There are few definitive diagnostic signs of sexual abuse on examination and nearly all examinations after suspected sexual abuse show no positive findings. This is because sexual abuse of children often comprises touching or kissing or other activities that do not involve significant physical force. Furthermore, the genital area heals very quickly in young children, so signs may be absent even a few days after significant trauma. Forensic material also decays rapidly. Examination of children suspected of having been sexually abused requires a doctor with specific expertise and training, facilities for photographic documentation, sexually transmitted infection screening and management and, where indicated, forensic testing (Fig. 8.7). Forensic testing of swabs from the child or his/her clothing/bedding may reveal DNA from a body fluid of the perpetrator.

Investigation

In physical abuse, fractures in young children may not be detectable clinically and X-rays are required to identify them. Bruising overlying a fracture is rarely seen on presentation. A full radiographic skeletal survey with oblique views of the ribs should be performed in all children with suspected physical abuse under 30 months of age. Some lesions may be inconspicuous initially but, if indicated, become evident on a repeat X-ray 1–2 weeks later. Other medical conditions that

Case history 8.2

Is there emotional abuse or neglect?

A general paediatrician sees a 6-year-old boy for recurrent abdominal pain resulting in missing 20% of school this year.

The boy and his mother are accompanied by his 3 months old sister. The boy is all over the clinic room – climbing onto the examination couch, turning the ophthalmoscope on and off, crawling under the desk, trying to get hold of the computer keyboard and turning the water tap of the handbasin on and off. The baby is crying, but her mother is holding her at arm's length and not comforting her or taking any notice of her son's behaviour.

With the help of the clinic nurse, the boy is shown some toys and settles down and shows good ability to put a simple jigsaw puzzle together. The baby keeps crying until the mother eventually gives her a bottle of formula from her bag. The mother's affect is very flat and is vague about the history of abdominal pain and why so much school has been missed.

Examination shows that he is on the 50th centile for weight and height. His mother says she has lost his personal child health record. He is in school uniform and is clean but his hair is not brushed. He has dental caries but mother cannot remember when he last saw the dentist. The boy says that he cleans his teeth twice a day. He has some bruising to the shins but examination is otherwise normal.

From this description, what are the concerning features? What are the positive features (Table 8.3)?

What else do you need to know?

- Who else is at home – partner, other children, others?
- What other support is available – family, friends?
- Mother's own health and health of others in the household?
- Social work involvement previously?

Who else would be helpful to involve in order to address the concerns raised?

The main concern is about mother's flat affect – does she have significant mental health problems that are impairing her ability to be, what the child psychiatrist Donald Winnicott called a 'good enough' parent?

The general practice, health visitor and school nurse would have additional information. Children's social services need to be contacted to see if the family is known to them. Is the child known to other hospitals? A professionals meeting could enable all those involved with the family to obtain a more complete picture and plan appropriate support and monitoring.

This case history demonstrates:

- concerns about any form of abuse – in this instance possible emotional abuse and neglect – may arise in a number of settings
- once possible concerns arise, the clinician needs to know what to do next. Arranging a meeting for information sharing to obtain a detailed picture is a helpful first step
- early intervention and appropriate support to families may prevent more severe harm.

Table 8.3 Concerning and positive features relating to the family

Concerning features	Positive features
6-year-old boy	**6-year-old boy**
Has missed 20% of school	Shows good concentration
Very active, risky or inappropriate behaviour in clinic – does he have attention-deficit/hyperactivity disorder?	Is in a school uniform and is clean.
Hair is not brushed	Says that he cleans his teeth twice a day
Has dental caries	Growth is satisfactory
Baby	
Crying most of the time	
Mother	**Mother**
Affect seems very flat	Has thought to bring along a bottle of formula for the baby
Not intervening to stop inappropriate behaviour	Has dressed the 6-year-old in a clean uniform
Holding her baby at arm's length and not comforting her	
Cannot remember when her son last saw the dentist	
Has lost the personal child health record	

The assessment of sexual abuse

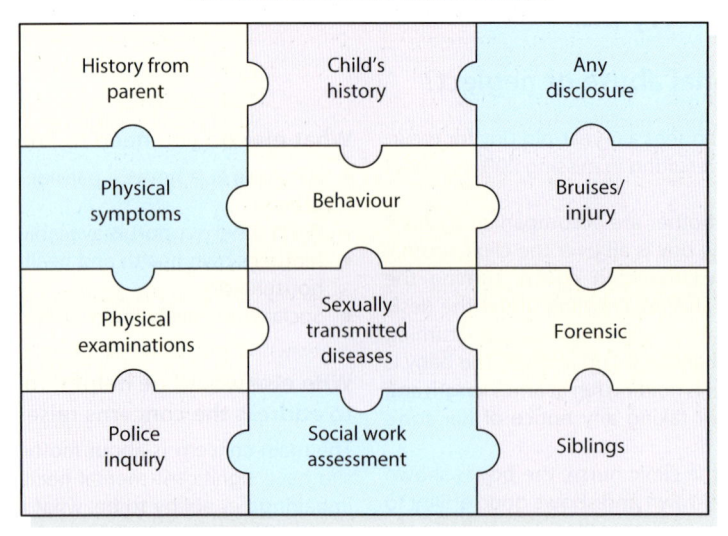

History from parent	Child's history	Any disclosure
Physical symptoms	Behaviour	Bruises/injury
Physical examinations	Sexually transmitted diseases	Forensic
Police inquiry	Social work assessment	Siblings

Figure 8.7 The assessment of sexual abuse is like a jigsaw puzzle. Many different pieces of information need to be pieced together to make an informed opinion. (From Royal College of Paediatrics and Child Health: *Child Protection Companion*, 2005. After Hobbs CJ, Wynne JM: The sexually abused battered child. *Archives of Disease in Childhood* 65:423–427, 1990. Reproduced with permission from the BMJ Publishing Group.)

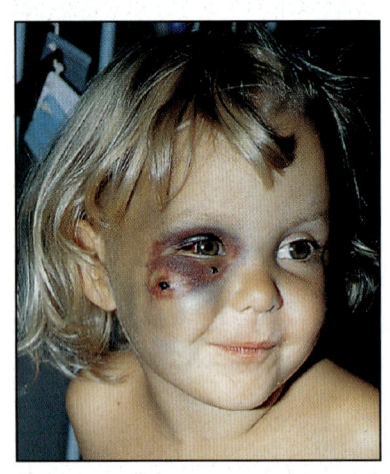

Figure 8.8 A thorough medical assessment is required in all children when non-accidental injury is suspected. This girl's large bruise followed what was said to be a minor bump. Non-accidental injury was suspected, but examination showed multiple bruises and petechiae. She had immune thrombocytopenic purpura.

need to be considered and excluded in suspected child abuse are:

- bruising – coagulation disorders (Fig. 8.8), Mongolian blue spots on the back or thighs
- fractures – osteogenesis imperfecta, commonly referred to as brittle bone disease. The type commonly involved with unexplained fractures is type I, which is an autosomal dominant disorder, so there may be a family history. Blue sclerae are a key clinical finding and there may be generalized osteoporosis and Wormian bones in the skull (extra bones within skull sutures) on skeletal survey
- scalds and cigarette burns – may be misinterpreted in children with bullous impetigo or scalded skin syndrome.

Where brain injury is suspected all children require:

- an immediate CT head scan followed later by a MRI head scan
- a skeletal survey to exclude fractures
- an expert ophthalmological examination to identify retinal haemorrhages
- a coagulation screen.

Management

Abused children may present to doctors in the hospital or to medical or nursing staff in the community. They may also be brought for a medical opinion by social services or the police. In all cases, the procedures of the local safeguarding children board should be followed. For children who are able to talk it is good practice to use a chaperone and speak to children without parents present. The medical consultation should be the same as for any medical condition, with a detailed history and full examination. It is usually most productive when this is conducted in a sensitive and concerned way without being accusatory or condemning. Any injuries or medical findings should be carefully noted, measured, recorded, and drawn on a body map and photographed (with consent). The height, weight and head circumference (where appropriate) should be recorded and plotted on a centile chart. The interaction between the child and parents should be noted. All notes must be meticulous, dated, timed, and signed on each page. Treatment of specific injuries should be instigated and blood tests and X-rays undertaken.

If abuse is suspected or confirmed, a decision needs to be made as to whether the child needs immediate protection from further harm. If this is the case, this may be achieved by admission to hospital, which also allows investigations and multidisciplinary assessment. If sympathetically handled, most parents are willing to accept medical advice for hospital admission for observation and investigation. Occasionally, this is not possible and legal enforcement is required. If medical treatment is not necessary but it is felt to be unsafe for the child to return home, a placement may be found with foster carers.

When dealing with any child suspected of having been abused, the safety of any other siblings or children at home must be considered. The police and/or social services should be alerted to any concerns.

In addition to a detailed medical assessment, evaluation by social workers and other health professionals will be required. A strategy meeting and later a child protection conference may be convened in accordance with local procedures. Members may include social workers, health visitors, police, general practitioner, paediatricians, teachers, and lawyers. Parents attend all or part of the case conference. Details of the incident leading to the conference and the family background will be discussed. Good communication and a trusting working relationship between the professionals are vital, as it can be extremely difficult to evaluate the likelihood that injuries were inflicted deliberately and the possible outcome of legal proceedings. The conference will decide:

- whether the child should be provided with a child protection plan and under what category (see Case History 8.3)

Case history 8.3

Possible child abuse

Parents brought their 8-month-old daughter into the children's emergency department. They were worried that she had not been moving her right arm for that day. The family remembered that at the evening meal two evenings before, her father was bringing dishes for the family meal to a low corner coffee table in the sitting room. Mother was sitting with baby on her knee, next to the table, trying to control the older siblings, when father had accidentally dropped a heavy serving bowl of food. Mother automatically reached out to try to catch it, dropping the baby in doing so and in the confusion, the serving bowl hit the baby's arm. The baby cried very loudly for about 10 minutes or so but then seemed to settle. The next day she did not use the right arm but the family thought this was explained by the injury causing a 'strain' as they could not see any bruising on the arm. An X-ray showed a fracture of the right radius and ulna (Fig. 8.9).

Child protection concerns
- Baby under 1-year with fracture.
- Delayed presentation.

Positive features
- Plausible, consistent story.
- Good parent–child interaction observed by medical and nursing staff.
- Well-nourished, well-cared-for appearance of baby.
- No other injuries on full examination.
- Skeletal survey showed no other fractures.
- Personal child health record showed regularly weighed, thriving baby up to date with immunizations.
- No general practitioner or home visit concerns about the family.
- Not previously known to local children's social services.

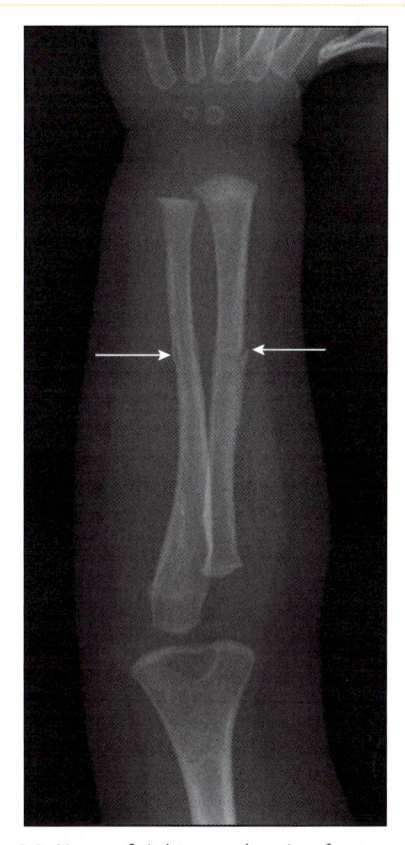

Figure 8.9 X-ray of right arm showing fracture of the radius and ulna.

Outcome
- Strategy meeting – no additional concerns identified. Decision – increased health visitor contact and parents received advice about safety in the home.

In child protection, conclusive evidence is often not available.

- whether there should be an application to the Court to protect the child
- what follow-up is needed.

Why is child protection so difficult?

Child protection:
- goes against the assumption that parents usually have their children's best interests at heart
- can involve confronting parents who may be manipulative or aggressive
- requires detailed evaluation of the history and examination to identify inconsistencies and interpret subtle findings
- depends on genuinely good multiprofessional teamwork and respect of colleagues.

Acknowledgements

We would like to acknowledge contributors to the child protection section in previous editions, whose work we have drawn on: Jo Sibert, (1st, 2nd, 3rd Edition, in Environment), Barbara Phillips (2nd Edition, Environment), Ian Maconochie (2nd, 3rd Edition, Environment), Andrea Goddard (4th Edition, (Accidents, Poisoning and Child Protection)).

> **Summary**
>
> **Child abuse**
> - Child abuse is the responsibility of all doctors, and must not be avoided or ignored because it raises difficult issues and possible appearance in Court.
> - It takes various forms – physical abuse, emotional abuse, sexual abuse, neglect, fabricated or induced illness.
> - The interests of the child should be kept uppermost to ensure protection from harm.
> - In many instances it is uncertain whether or not the problem is one of child abuse. Good communication with the parents and child is vital.

Further reading

Royal College of Paediatrics and Child Health: *Child Protection Companion*, London, 2013. Available from http://www.rcpch.ac.uk/improving-child-health/child-protection/about-child-protection-companion/about-child-protection-comp.

Websites (Accessed November 2016)

HM Government: Available at: https://www.gov.uk/government/uploads/system/uploads/attachment_data/file/419595/Working_Together_to_Safeguard_Children.pdf.
Working together to safeguard children A guide to interagency working to safeguard and promote the welfare of children March 2015.

Laming Report: 2003, 2009. http://dera.ioe.ac.uk/8646/1/12_03_09_children.pdf

Lancet Series: *Child Maltreatment*, 2008. http://www.thelancet.com/series/child-maltreatment

NICE: *NICE Guideline – Child Maltreatment*, London, 2009, NICE. https://www.nice.org.uk/guidance/cg89

9

Genetics

Chromosomal abnormalities	121	Polygenic, multifactorial		
Disorders of chromosome number	122	or complex inheritance	134	
Structural chromosome anomalies	126	Dysmorphology	135	
Mendelian inheritance	127	Gene-based therapies	137	
Unusual genetic mechanisms	132	Genetic services	138	

Features of the genetic basis of diseases are:

- the Human Genome Project resulted in the first publication of the human genome sequence in 2001
- it is now estimated that the human genome contains 20 000–25 000 genes, although the function of many of them remains unknown. Greater diversity and complexity at the protein level is achieved by alternative messenger RNA splicing and post-translational modification of gene products
- microarray techniques and high-throughput sequencing are increasing the volume and speed of genetic investigations and reducing their costs, leading to a greater understanding of the impact of genetics on health and disease
- access to genome browser databases containing DNA sequence and protein structure has greatly enhanced progress in scientific research and the interpretation of clinical test results (Fig. 9.1)
- genetic databases are available on thousands of multiple congenital anomaly syndromes, on chromosomal variations and disease phenotypes, and on all Mendelian disorders
- clinical application of these advances is available to families through specialist genetic centres that offer investigation, diagnosis, counselling and antenatal diagnosis for an ever-widening range of disorders
- gene-based knowledge is entering mainstream medical and paediatric practice, especially in diagnosis and therapeutic guidance, such as for the treatment of malignancies.

Genetic disorders are:

- common, with 2% of live-born babies having a significant congenital malformation and about 5% a genetic disorder
- burdensome to the affected individual, family, and society, as many are associated with severe and permanent disability.

Genetically determined diseases include those resulting from:

- chromosomal abnormalities
- the action of a single gene (Mendelian disorders)
- unusual genetic mechanisms
- interaction of genetic and environmental factors (polygenic, multifactorial, or complex disorders), which include epigenetic influences on gene expression from early in life.

Chromosomal abnormalities

Genes are composed of DNA that is wound around a core of histone proteins and packaged into a succession of supercoils to form the chromosomes. The human chromosome complement was confirmed as 46 in 1956. The chromosomal abnormalities in Down, Klinefelter, and Turner syndromes were recognized in 1959 and thousands of chromosome defects have now been documented.

Chromosomal abnormalities are either numerical or structural. They occur in approximately 10% of spermatozoa and 25% of mature oocytes and are a common cause of early spontaneous miscarriage. The

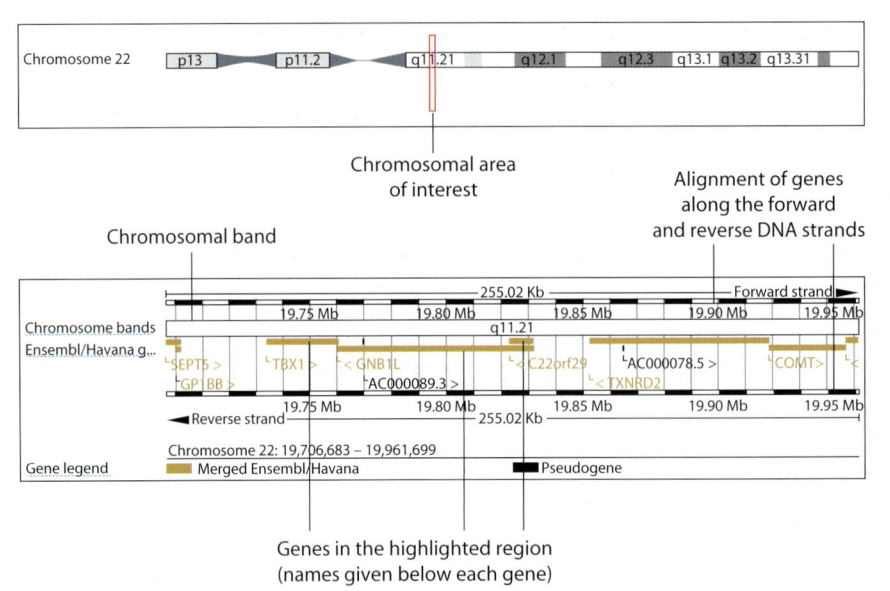

Figure 9.1 Ensembl genome browser. The image shows part of chromosome region 22q11, involved in 22q11 deletion syndrome (DiGeorge syndrome). Although only part of the commonly deleted region is shown, the image shows several genes that are deleted in 22q11 deletion syndrome. The online Ensembl browser can be used to 'zoom in' on specific areas, showing the genes present in different chromosome regions, and can also be used to show the gene sequence itself.

estimated incidence of chromosomal abnormalities in live-born infants is about 1 in 150; they often cause multiple congenital anomalies and cognitive difficulties. Acquired chromosomal changes play a significant role in carcinogenesis and tumour progression.

Disorders of chromosome number

Down syndrome (trisomy 21)

This is the most common autosomal trisomy and the most common genetic cause of severe learning difficulties. The incidence (without antenatal screening) in live-born infants is about 1 in 650, and increases with maternal age.

Clinical features

If not diagnosed antenatally, Down syndrome is usually suspected at birth because of the baby's facial appearance. Most affected infants are hypotonic and other useful clinical signs include a flat occiput, single palmar creases, incurved fifth finger, and wide 'sandal' gap between the big and second toes (Fig. 9.2a–c, Box 9.1). The diagnosis can be difficult to make when relying on clinical signs alone and a suspected diagnosis should be confirmed by a senior paediatrician. Before blood is sent for analysis, parents should be informed that a test for Down syndrome is being performed. The results may take 1–2 days, using real-time PCR (rtPCR) or rapid fluorescence in situ hybridization (FISH) techniques. Parents need information about the short-term and long-term implications of the diagnosis. They are also likely, at some stage in the future, to appreciate the opportunity to discuss how and why the condition has arisen, the risk of recurrence, and the possibility of antenatal diagnosis in future pregnancies.

It is difficult to give a precise long-term prognosis in the neonatal period, as there is great individual variation in the degree of learning difficulty and the development of complications. Over 85% of infants with trisomy 21 survive to 1 year of age. Congenital heart disease is present in about 40% and is a major cause of early mortality, particularly atrioventricular canal defects. Duodenal atresia is another problem in the newborn period. However, in the UK, at least 50% of affected individuals live longer than 50 years. Parents also need to know what assistance is available from both professionals and family support groups. Counselling may be helpful to assist the family to deal with feelings of grief, anger, or guilt.

Child development services will provide or coordinate care for the parents. This will include regular review of the child's development and health. Children with Down syndrome should be screened periodically for impairment of vision and hearing, hypothyroidism, coeliac disease, and atlantoaxial instability.

Cytogenetics

The extra chromosome 21 may result from meiotic nondisjunction, translocation, or mosaicism.

Meiotic nondisjunction (94%)

In nondisjunction trisomy 21:

- most cases result from an error at meiosis
- the chromosome 21 pair fails to separate, so that one gamete has two chromosome 21s and one has none (Fig. 9.3)

- fertilization of the gamete with two chromosome 21s gives rise to a zygote with trisomy 21
- parental chromosomes do not need to be examined.

The incidence of trisomy 21 due to nondisjunction is related to maternal age (Table 9.1). However, as the proportion of pregnancies in older mothers is small, most affected babies are born to younger mothers. Furthermore, meiotic nondisjunction can occur in spermatogenesis so that the extra copy of chromosome 21 can be of paternal origin. All pregnant women are now offered screening tests measuring biochemical markers in blood samples and nuchal thickening on ultrasound (thickening of the soft tissues at the back of the neck) to identify an increased risk of Down syndrome in the fetus. When an increased risk is identified, amniocentesis is offered to check the fetal karyotype. Noninvasive prenatal testing (NIPT) is now possible, in which cell-free fetal DNA is analyzed from maternal blood, and is becoming part of routine screening in the UK. After having one child with trisomy 21 due to nondisjunction, the risk of recurrence of Down syndrome is given as 1 in 200 for mothers under the age of 35 years, but remains similar to their age-related population risk for those over the age of 35 years.

Down syndrome

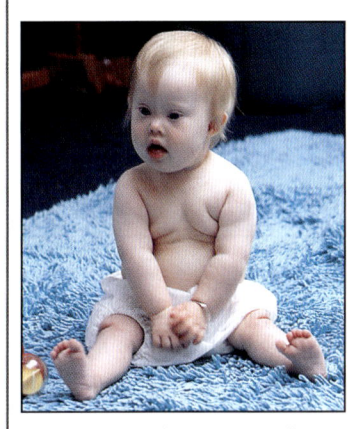

Figure 9.2a Characteristic facies seen in Down syndrome. Her posture is due to hypotonia.

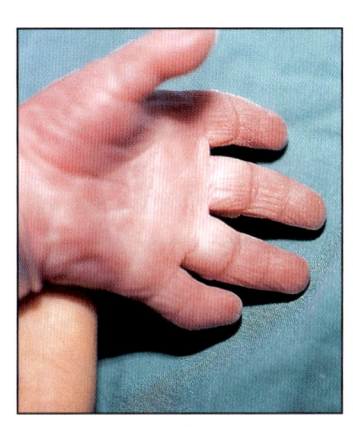

Figure 9.2b Single palmar crease.

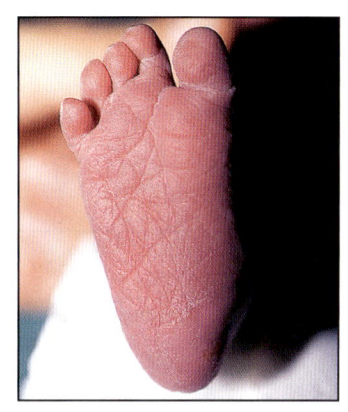

Figure 9.2c Pronounced 'sandal' gap with wide space and often a deep fissure between the big toe and second toe.

Box 9.1 Characteristic clinical manifestations of Down syndrome

Typical craniofacial appearance:
- round face and flat nasal bridge
- upslanted palpebral fissures
- epicanthic folds (a fold of skin running across the inner edge of the palpebral fissure)
- Brushfield spots in iris (pigmented spots)
- small mouth and protruding tongue
- small ears
- flat occiput and third fontanelle.

Other anomalies:
- short neck
- single palmar creases, incurved and short fifth finger, and wide 'sandal' gap between first and second toes
- hypotonia
- congenital heart defects (in 40%)
- duodenal atresia
- Hirschsprung disease (<1%).

Later medical problems:
- delayed motor milestones
- learning difficulties – severity is variable, usually mild to moderate but may be severe
- short stature
- increased susceptibility to infections
- hearing impairment from secretory otitis media (75%)
- visual impairment from cataracts (15%), squints, myopia (50%)
- increased risk of leukaemia and solid tumours (<1%)
- acquired hip dislocation and atlantoaxial instability
- obstructive sleep apnoea (50% to 75%)
- increased risk of hypothyroidism (15%) and coeliac disease
- epilepsy
- early-onset Alzheimer disease.

Inheritance of Down syndrome

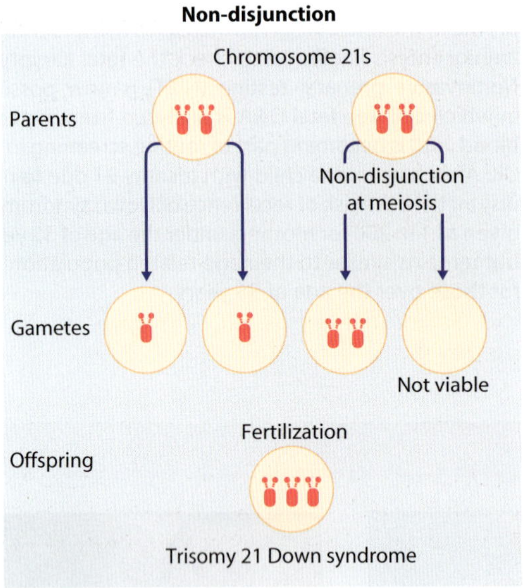

Figure 9.3 Nondisjunction Down syndrome.

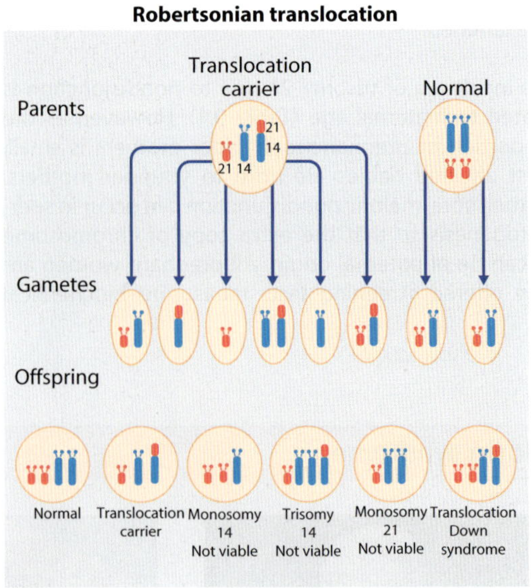

Figure 9.4 Translocation Down syndrome. There is a Robertsonian translocation involving chromosomes 21 and 14, which has been inherited from a parent.

Translocation (5%)

When the extra chromosome 21 is joined onto another chromosome (usually chromosome 14, but occasionally chromosome 15, 22, or 21), this is known as a Robertsonian translocation. This may be present in a phenotypically normal carrier with 45 chromosomes (two being 'joined together') or in someone with Down syndrome and a set of 46 chromosomes but with three copies of chromosome 21 material. In this situation, parental chromosomal analysis is recommended, because one of the parents may well carry the translocation in balanced form (in 25% of cases; Fig. 9.4).

In translocation Down syndrome:

- the risk of recurrence is 10–15% if the mother is the translocation carrier and about 2.5% if the father is the carrier
- if a parent carries the rare 21:21 translocation, all the offspring will have Down syndrome
- if neither parent carries a translocation (75% of cases), the risk of recurrence is less than 1%.

Mosaicism (1%)

In mosaicism, some of the cells are normal and some have trisomy 21. This usually arises after the formation of the chromosomally normal zygote by nondisjunction at mitosis but can arise by later mitotic nondisjunction in a trisomy 21 conception. The phenotype is sometimes milder in Down syndrome mosaicism.

Table 9.1 Risk of Down syndrome (live births) with maternal age at delivery, prior to screening in pregnancy

Maternal age (years)	Risk of Down syndrome
All ages	1 in 650
20	1 in 1530
30	1 in 900
35	1 in 385
37	1 in 240
40	1 in 110
44	1 in 37

Summary

Down syndrome (trisomy 21)
- Natural incidence – about 1.5 per 1000 infants.
- Cytogenetics – nondisjunction (most common, related to maternal age), translocation (one parent may carry a balanced translocation), or mosaicism (rare).
- Presentation – antenatal screening, prenatal diagnosis, or clinical presentation; confirmed on chromosome analysis.
- Immediate medical complications – increased risk of duodenal atresia, congenital heart disease.
- Clinical manifestations – see Box 9.1.

Edwards syndrome and Patau syndrome

Box 9.2 Clinical features of Edwards syndrome (trisomy 18)

- Low birthweight
- Prominent occiput
- Small mouth and chin
- Short sternum
- Flexed, overlapping fingers (Fig. 9.5)
- 'Rocker-bottom' feet
- Cardiac and renal malformations

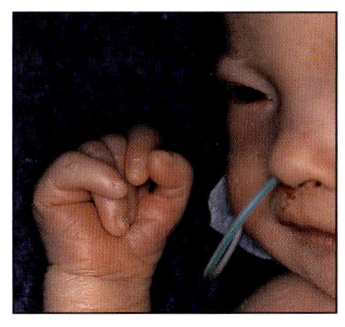

Figure 9.5 Overlapping of the fingers in Edwards syndrome.

Box 9.3 Clinical features of Patau syndrome (trisomy 13)

- Structural defect of brain
- Scalp defects
- Small eyes (microphthalmia) and other eye defects
- Cleft lip and palate
- Polydactyly
- Cardiac and renal malformations.

Edwards syndrome (trisomy 18) and Patau syndrome (trisomy 13)

Although rarer than Down syndrome (1 in 8000 and 1 in 14 000 live births respectively), particular constellations of severe multiple abnormalities suggest these diagnoses at birth; most affected babies die in infancy (Fig. 9.5, Boxes 9.2 and 9.3) but extended survival is possible. The diagnosis is confirmed by chromosome analysis. Many affected fetuses are detected by ultrasound scan during the second trimester of pregnancy and diagnosis can be confirmed antenatally by amniocentesis and chromosome analysis. Can also be diagnosed on non-invasive prenatal testing (NIPT). Recurrence risk is low, except when the trisomy is due to a balanced chromosome rearrangement in one of the parents.

Turner syndrome (45, X)

Turner syndrome usually results in early miscarriage (>95%) and is increasingly detected by ultrasound antenatally when fetal oedema of the neck, hands, or feet or a cystic hygroma may be identified. In live-born females, the incidence is about 1 in 2500. Fig. 9.6 and Box 9.4 show the clinical features of Turner syndrome,

Turner syndrome

Box 9.4 Clinical features of Turner syndrome

- Lymphoedema of hands and feet in neonate, which may persist
- Spoon-shaped nails
- Short stature – a cardinal feature
- Neck webbing or thick neck
- Wide carrying angle (cubitus valgus)
- Widely spaced nipples
- Congenital heart defects (particularly coarctation of the aorta)
- Delayed puberty
- Ovarian dysgenesis resulting in infertility, although pregnancy may be possible with in vitro fertilization using donated ova
- Hypothyroidism
- Renal anomalies
- Pigmented moles
- Recurrent otitis media
- Normal intellectual function in most cases

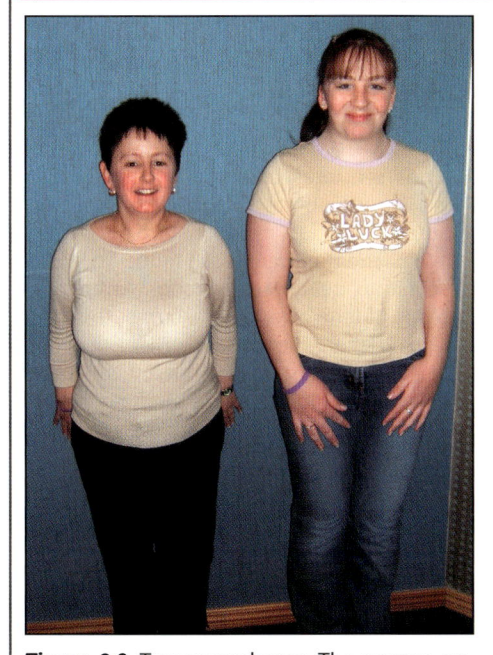

Figure 9.6 Turner syndrome. The woman on the left has marked short stature but no other clinical features; the adolescent female on the right has neck webbing and has received growth hormone and is 150 cm in height.

125

although short stature may be the only clinical abnormality in children.

Treatment is with:

- growth hormone therapy
- oestrogen replacement for development of secondary sexual characteristics at the time of puberty (but infertility persists).

In about 50% of girls with Turner syndrome, there are 45 chromosomes, with only one X chromosome. The other cases have a deletion of the short arm of one X chromosome, an isochromosome that has two long arms but no short arm, or a variety of other structural defects of one of the X chromosomes. The presence of a Y chromosome sequence may increase the risk of gonadoblastoma. The incidence does not increase with maternal age and risk of recurrence is very low.

Klinefelter syndrome (47, XXY)

This disorder occurs in about 1–2 per 1000 live-born males. For clinical features, see Box 9.5. Recurrence risk is very low.

Structural chromosome anomalies

Reciprocal translocations

An exchange of material between two different chromosomes is called a reciprocal translocation. When this exchange involves no loss or gain of chromosomal material, the translocation is 'balanced' and usually has no phenotypic effect. Balanced reciprocal translocations are relatively common, occurring in 1 in 500 of the general population. A translocation that appears balanced on conventional chromosome analysis may still involve the loss of a few genes or the disruption of a single gene at one of the chromosomal break points and result in an abnormal phenotype, often including cognitive difficulties. Studying the break points in such individuals has been one way of identifying the location of specific genes.

Unbalanced reciprocal translocations contain an 'incorrect' amount of chromosomal material and often impair both physical and cognitive development, leading to dysmorphic features, congenital malformations, developmental delay, and learning difficulties. When recognized in a newborn baby, the prognosis is difficult to predict but the effect is usually severe. The parents' chromosomes should be checked to determine whether the abnormality has arisen de novo, or as a consequence of a parental rearrangement. Finding a balanced translocation in one parent indicates a recurrence risk for future pregnancies, so that antenatal diagnosis by chorionic villus sampling or amniocentesis should be offered as well as testing relatives who might be carriers.

Deletions

Deletions are another type of structural abnormality. Loss of part of a chromosome usually results in physical

Box 9.5 Clinical features of Klinefelter syndrome

- Infertility – most common presentation
- Hypogonadism with small testes
- Pubertal development may appear normal (some males benefit from testosterone therapy)
- Gynaecomastia in adolescence
- Tall stature
- Intelligence usually in the normal range, but some have educational and psychological problems

abnormalities and cognitive impairment. The deletion may involve loss of the terminal or an interstitial part of a chromosome arm.

An example of a deletion syndrome involves loss of the tip of the short arm of chromosome 5, hence the name 5p- or monosomy 5p. Because affected babies have a high-pitched mewing cry in early infancy, it is also known as cri-du-chat syndrome. Parental chromosomes should be checked to see if one parent carries a balanced chromosomal rearrangement. The clinical severity varies greatly, depending on the extent of the deletion. It is now possible to specify the genes involved in chromosomal deletions as molecular methods are replacing standard cytogenetic investigations.

A deletion of band q11 on chromosome 22 (i.e. 22q11) can be associated with a range of phenotypes including both the DiGeorge syndrome (Fig. 15.27) and the velocardiofacial syndrome. Williams syndrome is another example of a microdeletion syndrome due to loss of chromosomal material at band q11 on the long arm of chromosome 7 (i.e. 7q11; Fig. 9.18, see also Box 9.12).

Duplications

Gain of structural material can also lead to congenital malformations and intellectual impairment, although duplications are often better tolerated than deletions.

An example of a duplication syndrome is partial trisomy of 17p. The duplication can range from being submicroscopic to being large enough to be visible on a karyotype. If it involves duplication of the *PMP22* gene at 17p12, then the patient will have a form of Charcot–Marie–Tooth disease (peripheral neuropathy) in addition to other features resulting from the abnormality.

Testing for submicroscopic copy number variants

An increasing number of syndromes are now known to be due to chromosome deletions (or duplications) too small to be seen by conventional cytogenetic analysis. Submicroscopic deletions can be detected by FISH studies using DNA probes specific to particular chromosome regions. FISH studies are useful when a specific chromosome deletion is suspected.

Newer techniques are beginning to supersede the karyotype and FISH (Table 9.2, Fig. 9.7a). Array comparative genomic hybridization (microarray) can be used to

Table 9.2 Cytogenetic analysis techniques

	Resolution	Microscopic	Submicroscopic	Rearrangements
Karyotype	3 Mb	+	–	+
Fluorescence in situ hybridization (FISH)	Specific to target	+	+	+
Comparative genomic hybridization array (microarray)	150 kB	+	+	–

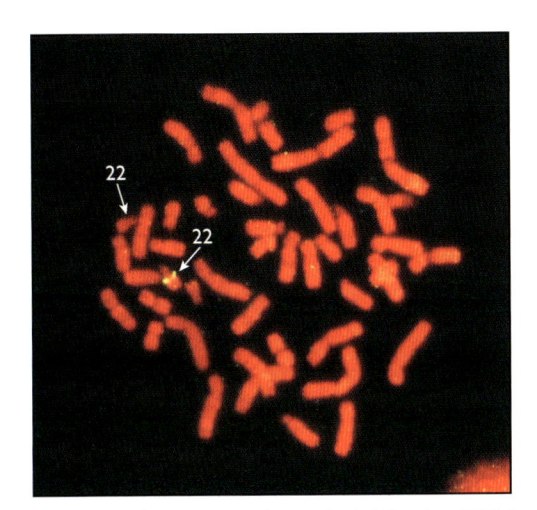

Figure 9.7a Fluorescence in situ hybridization (FISH) demonstrating a microdeletion on chromosome 22 associated with DiGeorge syndrome. Hybridization signals are seen on one chromosome 22 but not on the other because of the presence of a deletion (Courtesy of L. Gaunt, St Mary's Hospital, Manchester, UK.)

check the chromosomes for structural rearrangements larger than 150 kB in size (Fig. 9.7b).

The advantage of microarrays is that no specific target is required for the test to be effective. Many of the newly emerging submicroscopic copy number variants have overlapping clinical features, and non-targeted testing is the most effective way to identify these.

One disadvantage of array comparative genomic hybridization is that the information provided can be unhelpful if the test reveals a copy number variant of uncertain significance. In addition, microarrays only provide quantitative data, and cannot be used to check for structural rearrangements, e.g. Robertsonian translocations. The information provided by microarray often requires discussion with a clinical geneticist.

Mendelian inheritance

Mendelian inheritance, described by Mendel in 1866 from work on garden peas, is the transmission of inherited traits or diseases caused by variation in a single gene in a characteristic pattern. These Mendelian traits

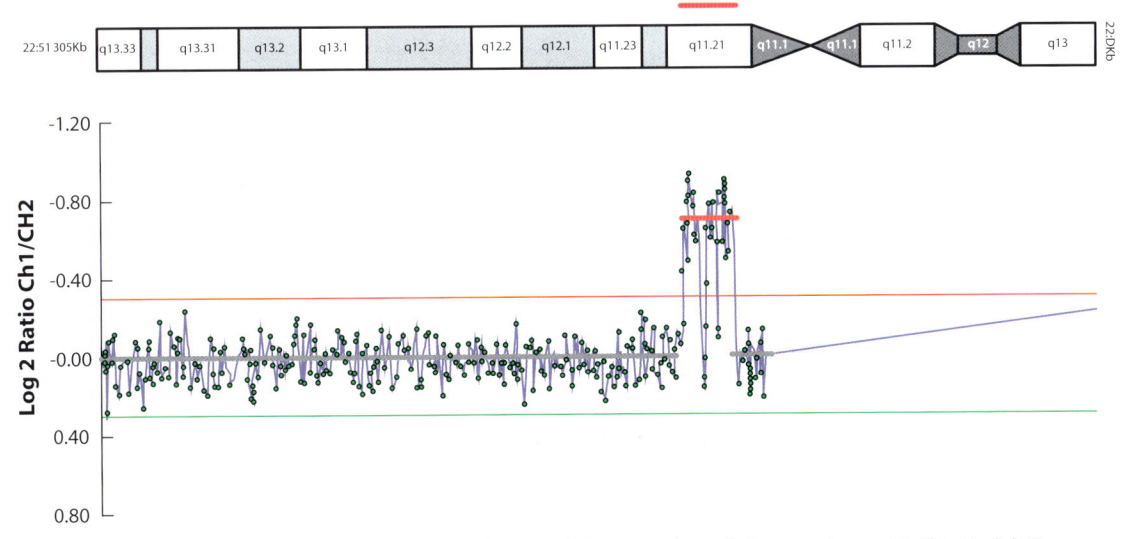

Figure 9.7b Array comparative genomic hybridization (microarray) result for a patient with 22q11 deletion. There is a reduction in the ratio of patient:control sequences from within band 22q11 on the long arm of chromosome 22.

Figure 9.8 Examples of pedigree symbols.

or disorders are individually rare but collectively numerous and important: over 6000 have been described so far. For many disorders, the Mendelian pattern of inheritance is known. If the diagnosis of a condition is uncertain, its pattern of inheritance may be evident on drawing a family tree (pedigree), which is an essential part of genetic evaluation (Fig. 9.8).

Autosomal dominant inheritance

This is the most common mode of Mendelian inheritance (Box 9.6). Autosomal dominant conditions are caused by alterations in only one copy of a gene pair, i.e. the condition occurs in the heterozygous state despite the presence of an intact copy of the relevant gene. Autosomal dominant genes are located on the autosomes (chromosomes 1–22), and so males and females are equally affected. Each child from an affected parent has a 1 in 2 (50%) chance of inheriting the abnormal gene (Fig. 9.9a,b). This appears to be straightforward, but complicating factors include the following factors.

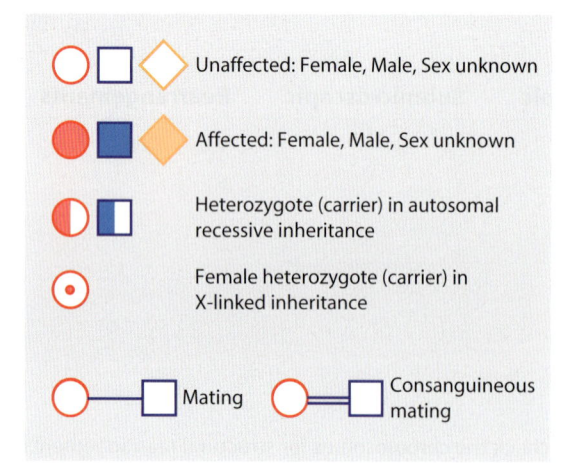

Variation in expression

Within a family, some affected individuals may manifest the disorder mildly and others more severely. This may be the result of variation at other genes, environmental effects, or sheer chance.

Non-penetrance

Refers to the lack of clinical signs and symptoms in an individual who has inherited the abnormal gene. An example of this is otosclerosis, in which only about 40% of gene carriers develop deafness (Fig. 9.10).

De novo mutation

A mutation is classed as de novo if it does not affect either parent. It may be due to:

- a new mutation in one of the gametes leading to the conception of the affected person. This is the most common reason for absence of a family history in dominant disorders, e.g. about 80% of individuals with achondroplasia have unaffected parents. The risk of new single-point mutations increases with paternal age
- parental mosaicism – very occasionally a healthy parent harbours the mutation only in some of their cells, e.g. in their gonads. This can account for recurrences of autosomal dominant disorders in siblings born to apparently unaffected parents. It has been described in congenital lethal osteogenesis imperfecta
- non-paternity – if the apparent father is not the biological father.

Homozygosity

In the rare situation where both parents are affected by the same autosomal dominant disorder, there is a 1 in 4 risk that a child will be homozygous for the altered gene. This usually causes a more severe phenotype, which may be lethal, as with achondroplasia.

Knudson two-hit hypothesis

Some autosomal dominant conditions related to cancer susceptibility follow Knudson two-hit hypothesis. Both copies of the gene need to be mutated for a malignancy to occur. If a person is born with only one working copy of the gene in every cell in his/her body, then only one further mutation event needs to occur for both copies of the gene to be inactivated. The chance of this happening is much greater than the chance of two successive mutations occurring in someone who starts life with two functional copies of the gene. The susceptibility to cancer is therefore inherited in a dominant fashion but the development of cancer within a cell can be thought of as a local event within the individual, so that not every person who inherits the susceptibility will necessarily develop a malignancy.

An example in paediatrics is mutation in the retinoblastoma (*Rb*) gene. If a child inherits the susceptibility, i.e. a mutation in one copy of the *Rb* gene, then a tumour will occur if a second hit occurs on the working copy in a cell of the relevant type, so that the child inheriting a mutation will often have a tumour in both eyes, but approximately 10% will escape with neither eye affected.

Autosomal dominant inheritance

Box 9.6 Examples of autosomal dominant disorders

- Achondroplasia
- Ehlers–Danlos syndrome (this is a family of disorders rather than a single condition)
- Familial hypercholesterolaemia
- Huntington disease
- Marfan syndrome
- Myotonic dystrophy
- Neurofibromatosis
- Noonan syndrome
- Osteogenesis imperfecta
- Otosclerosis
- Polyposis coli
- Tuberous sclerosis

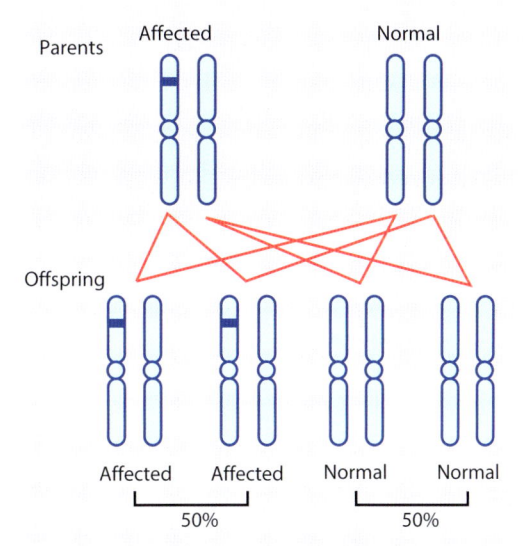

Figure 9.9a Autosomal dominant inheritance.

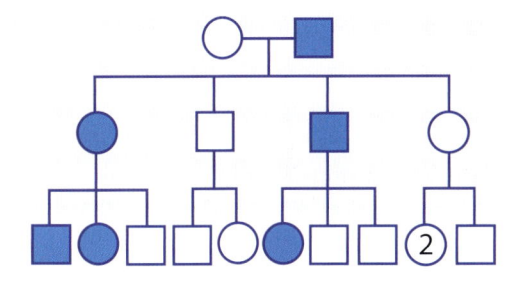

Figure 9.9b Typical pedigree of an autosomal dominant disorder.

Summary

Autosomal dominant inheritance:
- Most common mode of Mendelian inheritance.
- Affected individual carries the abnormal gene on one of a pair of autosomes.
- There is 1 in 2 chance of inheriting the abnormal gene from affected parent, but there may be variation in expression, non-penetrance, no family history (new mutation, parental mosaicism, non-paternity), or homozygosity (rare).

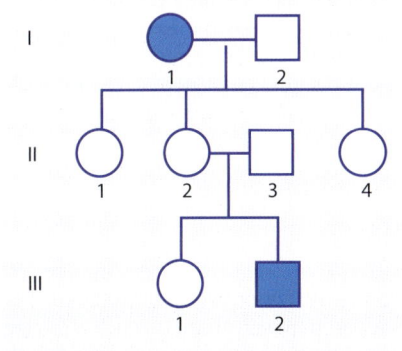

Figure 9.10 Example of nonpenetrance. I1 and III2 have otosclerosis. II2 has normal hearing but must have the gene (a new mutation event is most unlikely to arise independently for a second time in the family). The gene is nonpenetrant in II2.

Autosomal recessive inheritance

An affected individual is homozygous for the mutant allele in the gene. Sometimes, there is a different mutation on each copy of the gene, for example cystic fibrosis, and the affected individual is a compound heterozygote. In either situation, they will have inherited an abnormal allele from each parent, both of whom will usually be unaffected heterozygous carriers (Box 9.7). For a couple with both parents being carriers, the risk of any child being affected, male or female, is 1 in 4 (25%; Fig. 9.11a,b). All offspring of an affected individual will carry the condition. If an affected individual has children with an unaffected carrier, then each has a 50% chance of being affected.

Consanguinity

It is thought that we all carry six to eight abnormal recessive genes. Fortunately, our partners usually carry

Autosomal recessive inheritance

Box 9.7 Examples of autosomal recessive disorders

- Congenital adrenal hyperplasia
- Cystic fibrosis
- Friedreich ataxia
- Galactosaemia
- Glycogen storage diseases
- Hurler syndrome
- Oculocutaneous albinism
- Phenylketonuria
- Sickle cell disease
- Tay–Sachs disease
- Thalassaemia
- Werdnig–Hoffmann disease (SMA1).

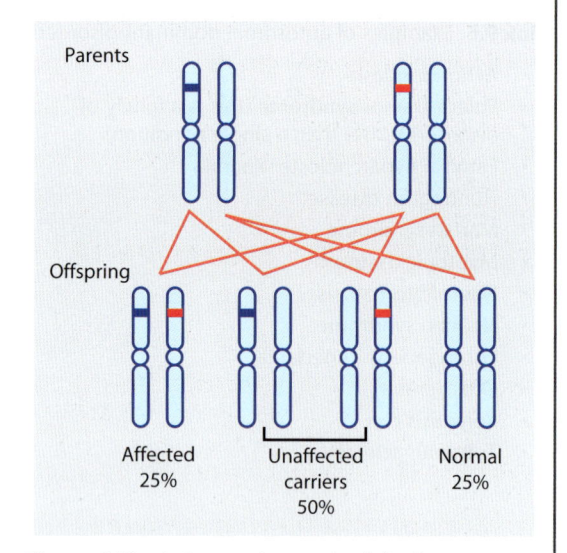

Figure 9.11a Autosomal recessive inheritance.

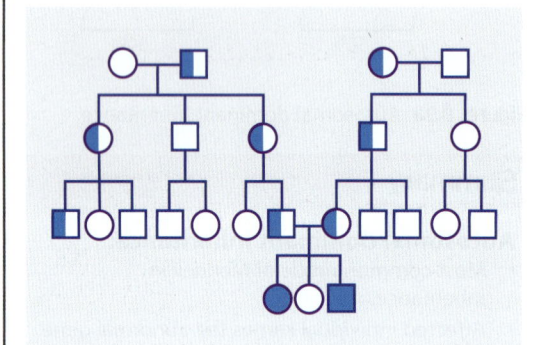

Figure 9.11b Pedigree to show autosomal recessive inheritance.

Summary

Autosomal recessive inheritance

- Affected individuals are usually homozygous for the abnormal gene; each unaffected parent will be a heterozygous carrier.
- Two carrier parents have a 1 in 4 risk of having an affected child.
- Risk of these disorders varies between populations and is increased by consanguinity.
- Autosomal recessive disorders often affect metabolic pathways, whereas autosomal dominant disorders often affect structural proteins.

---

different ones. Marrying a cousin or another relative increases the chance of both partners carrying the same autosomal recessive gene mutation. Cousins who marry have a modest increase in the risk of having a child with a serious recessive disorder: raising this for discussion with families is often a very delicate matter as it may trigger feelings of guilt, blame, and intercultural disrespect.

The frequencies of disease alleles at recessive gene loci vary between population groups. When the gene occurs sufficiently often and the gene or its effects can be detected, population-based carrier screening can be performed and antenatal diagnosis can be offered for high-risk pregnancies where both parents are carriers. Disorders that have been screened for in this way for many years include sickle cell disease in black Africans and African Americans, the thalassaemias in those from Mediterranean or Asian populations, and Tay–Sachs disease in Ashkenazi Jews. With developments in DNA-sequencing technologies, it is becoming possible for the range of disorders being screened to increase dramatically. Wealthy countries that practise customary consanguineous marriage are beginning to use these technologies to identify the genetic basis of the recessive disorders prevalent in their communities and to screen for a broad range of conditions.

X-linked inheritance

X-linked conditions are caused by alterations in genes found on the X chromosome. These may be inherited as X-linked recessive or X-linked dominant traits but the distinction between these is much less clear than in autosomal traits because of the variable pattern of X chromosome inactivation in females.

In X-linked recessive inheritance (Box 9.8, Fig. 9.12a,b):

- males are affected
- female carriers are usually healthy

X-linked recessive inheritance

Box 9.8 Examples of X-linked recessive disorders

- Colour blindness (red–green)
- Duchenne and Becker muscular dystrophies
- Fragile X syndrome
- Glucose-6-phosphate dehydrogenase deficiency
- Haemophilia A and B
- Hunter syndrome (mucopolysaccharidosis II)

Figure 9.12b Typical pedigree for X-linked (recessive) inheritance, showing Queen Victoria, a carrier for haemophilia A, and her family. It shows affected males in several generations, related through females, and that affected males do not have affected sons (contrast with autosomal dominant inheritance).

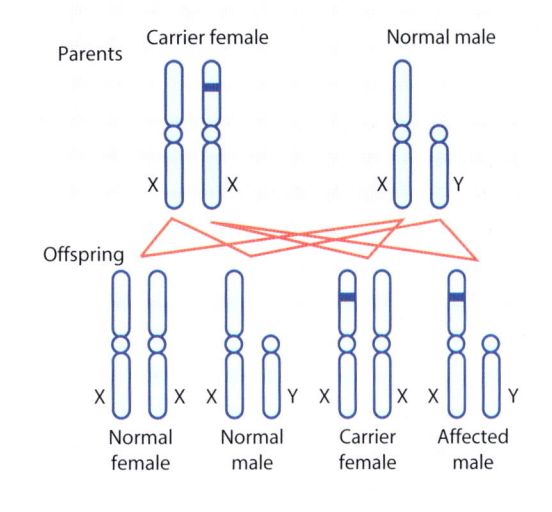

Figure 9.12a X-linked (recessive) inheritance.

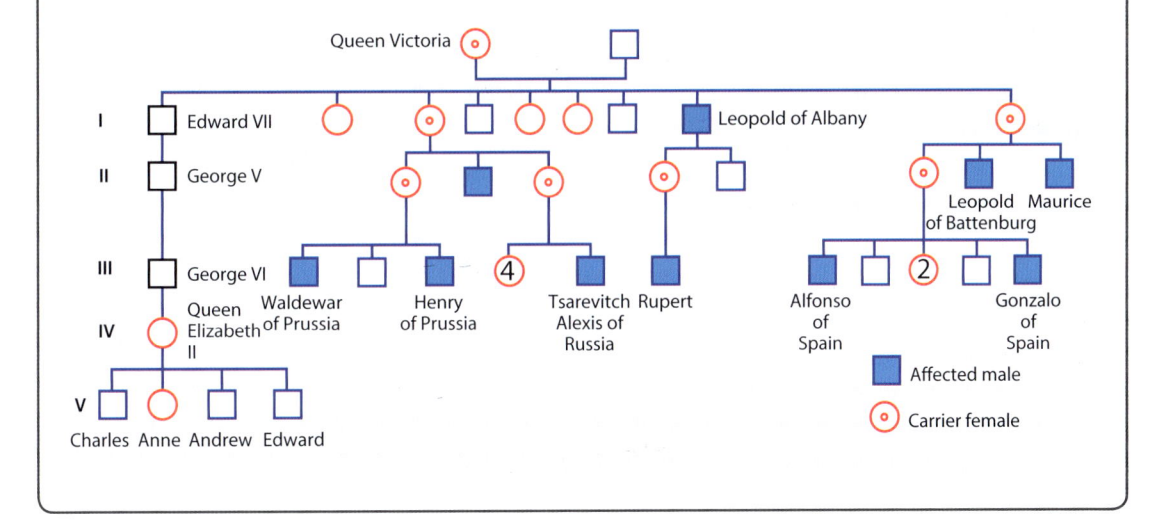

- occasionally a female carrier shows features of the disease
- each son of a female carrier has a 1 in 2 (50%) risk of being affected
- each daughter of a female carrier has a 1 in 2 (50%) risk of being a carrier
- daughters of affected males will all be carriers
- sons of affected males will not be affected, because a man passes a Y chromosome to his sons.

The family history may be negative, because new mutations and (gonadal) mosaicism are fairly common in some conditions. Identification of carrier females in a family requires interpretation of the pedigree, the search for mild clinical manifestations, and the identification of carriers through specific biochemical or molecular tests. Identifying carriers is important because a female carrier has a 50% risk of having an affected son regardless of who her partner is and X-linked recessive disorders can be very severe.

X-linked dominant disorders, where both males and females are affected, are unusual. An example is hypophosphataemic (vitamin D-resistant) rickets. In some other X-linked dominant disorders, a female carrying the mutation will be affected while the mutation-carrying males have an even more serious condition. Thus, a mutation that causes Rett syndrome (a neurodegenerative disorder) in a girl will cause a lethal, neonatal-onset encephalopathy in males. Another reason why a sex-linked condition may predominantly affect females is because it usually arises through mutations at spermatogenesis (e.g. Rett syndrome). As male offspring must inherit a Y chromosome from their father, they will not inherit any mutations on the X chromosome that arise during spermatogenesis.

> **Summary**
>
> **X-linked recessive inheritance:**
> - Males are affected; females can be carriers but are usually healthy or have mild disease.
> - Family history may be negative – many arise from new mutations or gonadal mosaicism.
> - Identifying female carriers is important to be able to provide genetic counselling.
> - All the female offspring of affected males will be carriers, but none of the male offspring can inherit the mutation.
> - Half of the male offspring of a female carrier will be affected and half of the female offspring will be carriers.

Y-linked inheritance

Y-linked traits are extremely rare. Y-linked inheritance would result in only males being affected, with transmission from an affected father to all his sons. Y-linked genes determine sexual differentiation and spermatogenesis, and mutations are associated with infertility and so are rarely transmitted.

Unusual genetic mechanisms

Trinucleotide repeat expansion mutations

This is a class of unstable mutations that consist of expansions of trinucleotide repeat sequences inherited in Mendelian fashion. Fragile X syndrome, myotonic dystrophy, and Huntington disease are among the best known of these disorders. They follow different patterns of inheritance but share certain unusual properties due to the nature of the underlying mutation. Trinucleotide repeat disorders exhibit a phenomenom known as anticipation. The triplet repeat mutation is unstable and can expand between subsequent generations. In general, a larger expansion causes a more severe form of the disease. This means that these conditions can become more severe in successive generations of the same family.

There are two major categories of triplet repeat disorder, depending on whether or not the triplet repeat is in the coding sequence of the gene. When the triplet repeat expansion is in the coding sequence, as in Huntington disease (and in a number of other neurodegenerative disorders), proteins containing an excess of the amino acid, glutamine, are produced. Glutamine can damage the cells in the central nervous system when present in excess, leading to neurodegeneration. When the triplet repeat expansion is in other regions of the gene, reduced quantities of the protein are produced. In these cases, the reduction in the amount of the available protein leads to the symptoms of the condition. One such example is myotonic dystrophy, which is described further in Chapter 29. Neurological disorders.

Most of the triplet repeat disorders are autosomal dominant but there is one autosomal recessive disorder, Friedreich ataxia, and fragile X syndrome, which is X linked.

Fragile X syndrome

The prevalence of significant learning difficulties in males due to fragile X syndrome is about 1 in 4000 (Fig. 9.13 and Box 9.9). This condition was initially diagnosed on the basis of the cytogenetic appearance of an apparent break (a fragile site) in the distal part of the long arm of the X chromosome. Diagnosis is now achieved by molecular analysis of the trinucleotide repeat expansion in the relevant gene.

Although it is inherited as an X-linked disorder, some 40% to 50% of female carriers have learning difficulties (usually mild to moderate). More puzzling is the observation that males can be unaffected but transmit the condition through their daughters to their grandsons. This is not possible in haemophilia or Becker muscular dystrophy, for example, where a male cannot inherit the condition from his family and transmit the condition to his children without himself being affected. This can occur in fragile X because the triplet repeat expansion varies in its nature with its size. The normal range of repeat numbers is up to about 45 repeats; when larger than that the block of repeats becomes increasingly unstable but continues to permit fragile X gene expression until a 'full mutation' is reached at about 200 repeats. From 55 repeats to 200 repeats is known as the 'premutation' range, and a male can inherit a premutation and transmit it to his daughters (who will all be carriers) while being intellectually normal and without the physical features of fragile X.

Because these full mutations always arise from expansion of premutations, and never directly from normal genes, the mothers of affected males have to be carriers of a premutation or full mutation. Offering referral for genetic counselling is therefore appropriate for all fragile X families, especially as there can be associated disorders for premutation carriers in adult life.

> Fragile X syndrome is the second most common genetic cause of severe learning difficulties after Down syndrome

Mitochondrial or cytoplasmic inheritance

Mitochondria are cytoplasmic organelles that function as a cellular compartment within which many different metabolic pathways are located, including most prominently the production of energy by oxidative phosphorylation. They contain their own DNA (mtDNA), but most of the proteins involved in mitochondrial metabolic reactions are encoded in the nuclear genome. The mtDNA encodes proteins involved in oxidative phosphorylation together with the RNA and proteins necessary for mitochondrial protein synthesis.

Fragile X

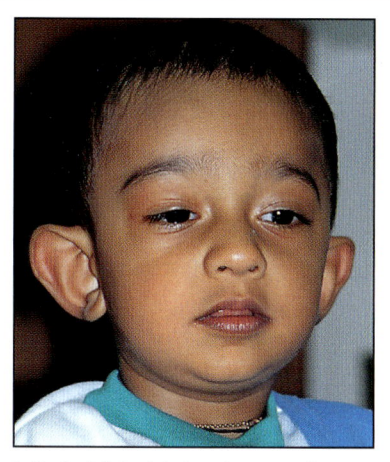

Figure 9.13 A child with fragile X syndrome. At this age, the main physical feature is often the prominent ears.

Box 9.9 Clinical findings in males in fragile X syndrome

- Moderate–severe learning difficulty (IQ 20–80, mean 50)
- Macrocephaly
- Macroorchidism – postpubertal
- Characteristic facies – long face, large everted ears, prominent mandible, and broad forehead, most evident in affected adults
- Other features – mitral valve prolapse, joint laxity, scoliosis, autism, hyperactivity

---

Each cell contains thousands of copies of the mitochondrial genome. Inherited disorders of mitochondrial function may result from mutations in the nuclear genome or, less often, from mutations in the mitochondrial genome (mtDNA). In disorders of the mtDNA, the mutation may be present in all or only some of the mitochondria, so that the tissues affected and the severity of the condition can be highly variable. Mutations in mtDNA cause overlapping clusters of disease phenotypes, with high-energy tissues such as muscle, brain, the heart, and the retina being more commonly affected (e.g. Leber hereditary optic neuropathy and various mitochondrial myopathies and encephalopathies, such as MERFF, MELAS, NARP). These conditions are described in more detail in Chapter 27 – Inborn errors of metabolism. Diseases caused by mutations in mtDNA show only maternal transmission, because only the egg contributes mitochondria to the zygote.

Imprinting and uniparental disomy

In the past, it was assumed that the activity of a gene is the same regardless of whether it is inherited from the mother or father. It has been shown that the expression of some genes is influenced by the sex of the parent who transmitted it. This phenomenon is called 'imprinting'. If one copy of a gene is said to be imprinted, that copy is switched off in at least some tissues.

An example involves Prader–Willi syndrome (PWS; hypotonia, developmental delay, hyperphagia, and obesity). The PWS chromosomal region is found at 15q11–13 (i.e. at bands 11 to 13 on the long arm of chromosome 15). Both the paternal and the maternal copies of this chromosomal region have to function for normal development. In the absence of a (functioning) paternal copy of this region, a child will develop PWS, as some genes are maternally imprinted. By contrast, the failure to inherit a (functioning) maternal copy of this chromosomal region results in an entirely different condition, Angelman syndrome, leading to severe cognitive impairment, a characteristic facial appearance, ataxia, and epilepsy because of a lack of expression of the *UBE3A* gene and the paternal copy being imprinted. There are two main ways that a child can develop one or other condition:

- deletion de novo (Fig. 9.14) – parental chromosomes are normal, and a deletion occurs as a new mutation in the child. If the deletion occurs on the paternal chromosome 15, the child has PWS. If the deletion affects the maternal chromosome 15, the child has Angelman syndrome
- uniparental disomy (Fig. 9.15) – this is when a child inherits two copies of a chromosome from one parent and none from the other parent. In PWS the affected child has no paternal (but two maternal) copies of chromosome 15q11–13. In Angelman syndrome the affected child has no maternal (but two paternal) copies of chromosome 15q11–13. This can be detected with DNA analysis
- there exist other, less common mechanisms that can lead to these conditions.

> **Imprinting is the unusual property of some genes that express only the copy derived from the parent of a given sex**

Imprinting

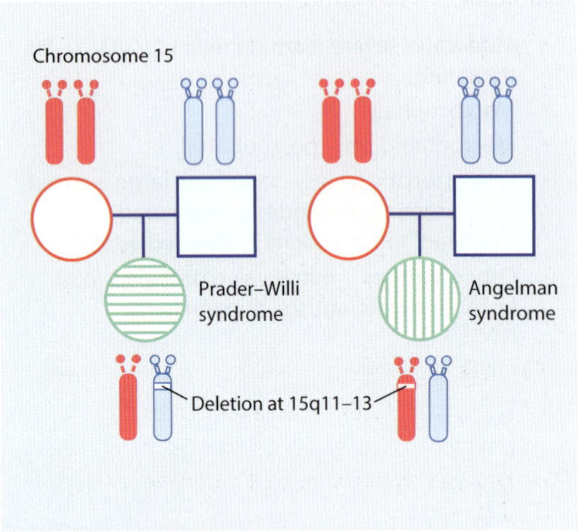

Figure 9.14 Genetic disorder resulting from deletion of an imprinted gene. If the deletion occurs on chromosome 15 inherited from the father, the child has Prader–Willi syndrome. If the deletion occurs on chromosome 15 from the mother, the child has Angelman syndrome.

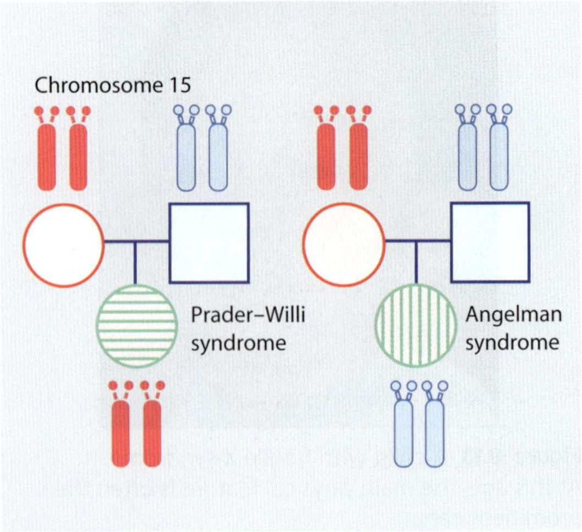

Figure 9.15 Genetic disorder resulting from uniparental disomy affecting imprinted chromosome region. A child who inherits two maternal chromosome 15s will have Prader–Willi syndrome. A child who inherits two paternal chromosome 15s will have Angelman syndrome.

Polygenic, multifactorial or complex inheritance

There is a spectrum in the aetiology of disease, from environmental factors (e.g. trauma) at one end to purely genetic causes (e.g. Mendelian disorders) at the other. Between these two extremes are many disorders that result from the interacting effects of several genes (hence the term polygenic) with or without the influence of environmental or other unknown factors, including chance (multifactorial or complex). These terms are used interchangeably (Box 9.10).

Variation in quantitative traits, such as height and intelligence, results from complex interactions between environmental factors and multiple genetic influences. The environmental factors include early-life (including intrauterine) experiences. These parameters are thought to show a Gaussian (normal) distribution in the population. Similarly, the liability of an individual to develop a disease of multifactorial or polygenic aetiology has a Gaussian distribution. The condition occurs when a certain threshold level of liability is exceeded. Relatives of an affected person show an increased liability due to inheritance of genes conferring susceptibility, and so a greater proportion of them than in the general population will fall beyond the threshold and will manifest the disorder (Fig. 9.16). The risk of recurrence of a polygenic disorder in a family is usually low and is most significant for first-degree relatives. Empirical recurrence risk data are used for genetic counselling. They are derived from family studies that have reported the frequencies at which various family members are affected. Factors that increase the risk to relatives are:

- having a more severe form of the disorder, e.g. the risk of recurrence to siblings is greater in bilateral cleft lip and palate than in unilateral cleft lip alone
- close relationship to the affected person, e.g. overall risk to siblings or children is greater than to more distant relatives
- multiple affected family members, e.g. the more siblings already affected, the greater the risk of recurrence
- sex difference in prevalence, with the recurrence risk greater in the more commonly affected sex and if the affected individual is of the less commonly affected sex.

The phenotype (clinical picture) of a disorder may have a heterogeneous (mixed) basis in different families, e.g. hyperlipidaemia leading to atherosclerosis and coronary heart disease can be due to a single gene disorder such as autosomal dominant familial hypercholesterolaemia, but some forms of hyperlipidaemia are polygenic and result from an interaction of the effect of several genes and dietary factors on various lipoproteins.

In some complex disorders, such as Hirschsprung disease, the molecular genetic basis and the important contribution of new mutations are becoming clear. In many multifactorial disorders, however, the 'environmental factors' remain obscure. Clear exceptions include dietary fat intake and smoking in atherosclerosis, and viral infection in insulin-dependent diabetes mellitus. For neural tube defects, the risk of recurrence

Multifactorial, polygenic or complex inheritance

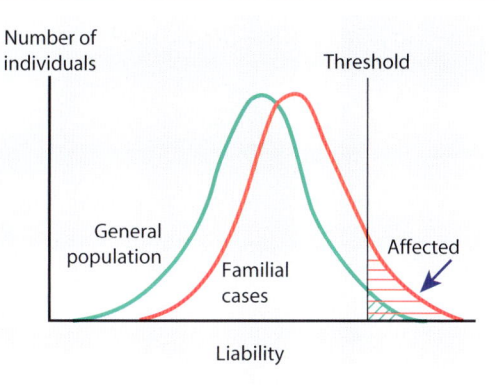

Figure 9.16 Diagram showing the increased liability to a multifactorial disorder in relatives of an affected person.

Box 9.10 Conditions often associated with multifactorial (polygenic, complex) inheritance

Congenital malformations:
- neural tube defects (anencephaly and spina bifida)
- congenital heart disease
- cleft lip and palate
- pyloric stenosis
- developmental dysplasia of the hip (DDH)
- talipes equinovarus
- hypospadias.

Childhood:
- atopy (especially asthma and eczema)
- epilepsy
- diabetes mellitus type 1 (insulin-dependent diabetes).

Adult life:
- atherosclerosis and coronary artery disease
- diabetes mellitus type 2
- Alzheimer disease
- malignancy (especially the common cancers, e.g. breast and colorectal cancer)
- hypertension
- cerebrovascular disease (especially stroke).

---

to siblings is lowered from about 4% to 1% or less in future pregnancies if the mother takes folic acid before conception and in the early weeks of pregnancy.

Dysmorphology

The term 'dysmorphology' literally means 'the study of abnormal form' and refers to the assessment of birth defects and unusual physical features that have their origin during embryogenesis.

Pathogenic mechanisms

Malformation
A primary structural defect occurring during the development of a tissue or organ, e.g. spina bifida, cleft lip, and palate.

Deformation
Implies an abnormal intrauterine mechanical force that distorts a normally formed structure, e.g. joint contractures or pulmonary hypoplasia due to fetal compression caused by severe oligohydramnios.

Disruption
Involves destruction of a fetal part that initially formed normally, e.g. amniotic membrane rupture may lead to amniotic bands that may cause limb reduction defects. Drugs such as phenytoin, warfarin, or thalidomide can cause teratogenic effects. Viruses such as rubella or cytomegalovirus may damage the normally formed embryo or fetus.

Dysplasia
Refers to abnormal cellular organization or function of specific tissue types, e.g. skeletal dysplasias, dysplastic kidney disease.

Clinical classification of birth defects

Single-system defects
These include single congenital malformations, such as spina bifida, which are often multifactorial in nature with fairly low recurrence risks.

Sequence
Refers to a pattern of multiple abnormalities occurring after one initiating defect. 'Potter syndrome' (fetal compression and pulmonary hypoplasia) is an example of a sequence in which all abnormalities may be traced to one original malformation causing failure of fetal urine excretion from renal agenesis or posterior urethral valves.

Syndromes recognized by 'Gestalt' (clinical recognition)

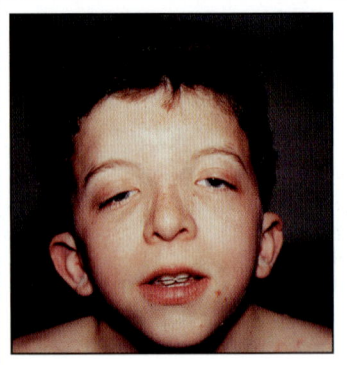

Figure 9.17 Noonan syndrome affects both males and females. There are some similarities to the phenotype in Turner syndrome, but it is caused by mutation in an autosomal dominant gene and the karyotype is normal.

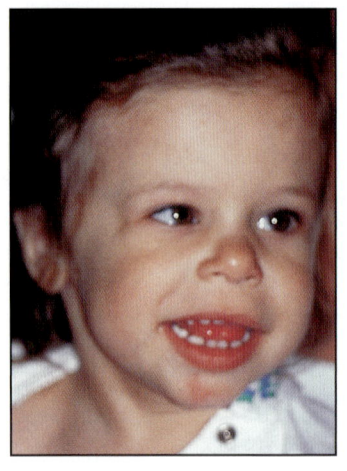

Figure 9.18 Williams syndrome is usually sporadic.

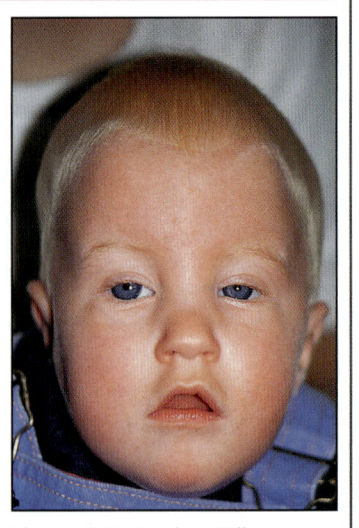

Figure 9.19 Prader–Willi syndrome.

Box 9.11 Clinical features of Noonan syndrome

- Characteristic facies
- Occasional mild learning difficulties
- Short webbed neck with trident hair line
- Pectus excavatum
- Short stature
- Congenital heart disease (especially pulmonary stenosis, atrial septal defect)

Box 9.12 Clinical features of Williams syndrome

- Short stature
- Characteristic facies
- Transient neonatal hypercalcaemia (occasionally)
- Congenital heart disease (supravalvular aortic stenosis)
- Mild-to-moderate learning difficulties

Box 9.13 Clinical features of Prader–Willi syndrome

- Characteristic facies
- Hypotonia
- Neonatal feeding difficulties
- Faltering growth in infancy
- Obesity in later childhood
- Hypogonadism
- Developmental delay
- Learning difficulties

Association

A group of malformations that occur together more often than expected by chance, but in different combinations from case to case, e.g. *v*ertebral anomalies, *a*nal atresia, *c*ardiac defects, *t*racheo-*o*esophageal fistula, *r*enal anomalies, *l*imb defects (VACTERL) association.

Syndrome

When a particular set of multiple anomalies occurs repeatedly in a consistent pattern and there is known or thought to be a common underlying causal mechanism, this is called a 'syndrome'. Multiple malformation syndromes are often associated with moderate or severe cognitive impairment and may be due to:

- chromosomal defects
- a single gene defect (dominant, recessive, or sex linked)
- exposure to teratogens such as alcohol, drugs (especially anticonvulsants such as valproate, carbamazepine, and phenytoin), or viral infections during pregnancy
- unknown cause.

Syndrome diagnosis

Although most syndromes are individually rare, recognition of a dysmorphic syndrome is worthwhile as it may give information regarding:

- risk of recurrence
- prognosis
- likely complications, which can be sought and perhaps treated successfully if detected early
- the avoidance of unnecessary investigations
- experience and information, which parents can share with other affected families through family support groups.

Examples of syndromes recognizable by facial appearance are shown in Figs 9.17–9.19 (see also Boxes 9.11–9.13). The importance and impact of syndrome diagnosis is demonstrated in Case History 9.1. Databases are available to assist with the recognition of thousands of multiple congenital anomaly syndromes (e.g. London Dysmorphology Database and Pocket Similarity Search using Multiple-Sketches).

> **Summary**
>
> **Dysmorphology**
> - Comprises birth defects and abnormal clinical features originating during embryogenesis.
> - May be a malformation, deformation, disruption, or dysplasia.
> - May be classified as a single-system defect, sequence, association, or syndrome.
> - Syndromes are recognized by 'Gestalt', which may be aided by dysmorphology databases.

Gene-based therapies

The treatment of most genetic disorders is based on conventional therapeutic approaches.

Gene therapy involves the repair, suppression, or artificial introduction of genes into genetically abnormal cells with the aim of curing the disease and is at an experimental stage for most genetic conditions being studied. There are still many technical and safety issues to be resolved. Gene therapy has been initiated in adenosine deaminase deficiency (a rare recessive immune disorder), malignant melanoma, and cystic

Case history 9.1

Syndrome diagnosis and genetic counselling

Sean, the second child of healthy parents, was born at term by emergency caesarean section for fetal distress. The pregnancy had been uneventful and no abnormalities were detected on antenatal ultrasound scan. He developed respiratory distress and investigation triggered by a cardiac murmur revealed an interrupted aortic arch and ventricular septal defect that required surgical correction in the neonatal period.

The parents asked about recurrence risk for congenital heart disease and were referred to the genetic clinic. At that time, Sean was thriving and early developmental progress appeared normal. On examination, there were minor dysmorphic features, including a short philtrum, thin upper lip, and prominent ears (Fig. 9.20). There was no family history of congenital heart disease or other significant problems and no abnormalities were detected on examination of the parents.

Because of an association between outflow tract abnormalities of the heart and deletions of chromosome 22, cytogenetic analysis was performed using FISH. A submicroscopic deletion of the long arm of one chromosome 22 (band 22q11) was detected. Other features of DiGeorge syndrome (hypocalcaemia and T-cell deficiency), which occurs with the same chromosome deletion, were excluded but could have been important in Sean's medical management.

Parental chromosome analysis showed no deletion at chromosome 22q11 in either parent, indicating a low recurrence risk for future pregnancies because gonadal mosaicism for this deletion is very rare. The older sibling was also normal on testing. Because the parents had normal karyotypes, their own brothers and sisters were not required to be tested.

Identification of a 22q11 deletion indicated that other associated problems were likely. Subsequently, Sean required assessment by a multidisciplinary child development team (for developmental delay), which led to the formal assessment of his educational needs and the recommendation for placement in an appropriate school for children with learning difficulties, input from a clinical psychologist when behavioural problems appeared (ritualistic behaviour and obsessional tendencies), input from speech therapist and plastic surgeon (indistinct speech due to velopharyngeal incompetence), and audiology review (conductive hearing loss due to recurrent otitis media).

The impact of the diagnosis and its implications was considerable for the family and the parents needed support from a variety of professionals while coming to terms with the various problems as they became apparent. Written information and details of the 22q11 support group were given to the parents. Medical care was coordinated by the paediatrician.

There was the additional worry for the family about a subsequent pregnancy. Fetal echocardiography showed no evidence of congenital heart disease, and the offer of invasive tests for cytogenetic analysis was declined because of the low chance of recurrence and the risk of miscarriage from the test. The baby was born unaffected, with chromosome studies performed on a cord blood sample revealing no abnormality.

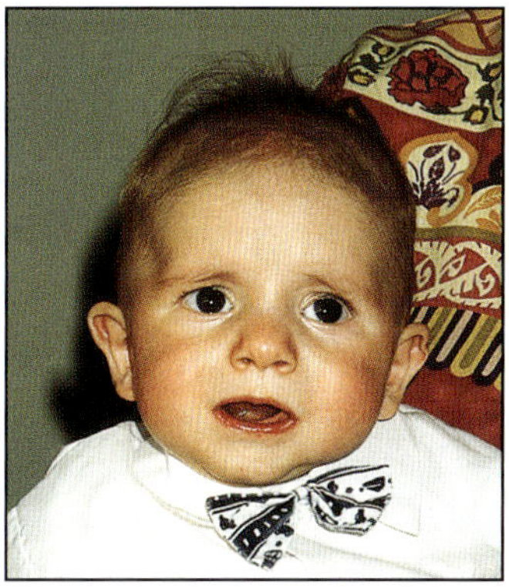

Figure 9.20 Sean's facial appearance showing the short philtrum (vertical groove in the upper lip), thin upper lip, and prominent ears.

fibrosis, and some clinical benefit has been reported in a few patients. At present, it is generally accepted that gene therapy should be limited to somatic (not germ-line) cells, so that the risk of adversely affecting future generations is minimized.

However, other treatments based on a genetic understanding of disease are being introduced into practice. Current areas of research include Duchenne muscular dystrophy, cystic fibrosis and retinitis pigmentosa.

An increasing understanding of the molecular mechanisms underlying the pathophysiology of many genetic conditions has also led to new targeted drug treatments in several condtions, including enzyme replacement therapy for certain inborn errors of metabolism and mTOR inhibitor therapy in tuberous sclerosis.

Genetic services

In the UK, all health regions have a clinical genetics centre where specialist genetic services are provided by consultants and other medical staff, genetic counsellors, and laboratory scientists. Specialist clinical genetic assessment and genetic counselling are provided at the centre and in a network of clinics throughout the region. Genetic investigations can be accessed through these clinical services as well as directly through primary and secondary care. Increased recognition of disorders antenatally has necessitated expansion of perinatal genetic services in addition to paediatric and adult services.

Genetic investigations

For many years, genetic investigation relied on determining the karyotype by visualization of the chromosomes with light microscopy. This has been transformed by the tremendous advances in molecular testing (Table 9.3).

DNA analysis using polymerase chain reaction (PCR) allows rapid analysis on small samples. Its main impact for genetic counselling is:

- confirmation of a clinical diagnosis of an increasing number of single gene disorders
- detection of female carriers in X-linked disorders, e.g. Duchenne and Becker muscular dystrophies, haemophilia A and B
- carrier detection in autosomal recessive disorders, e.g. cystic fibrosis
- presymptomatic diagnosis in autosomal dominant disorders, e.g. Huntington disease, myotonic dystrophy, familial cancer syndromes
- antenatal diagnosis of an increasing number of Mendelian conditions.

These are accomplished by the following methods.

Mutation analysis

For an increasing number of Mendelian disorders, it is possible to directly detect the actual mutation causing the disease. This provides very accurate results for confirmation of diagnosis, and presymptomatic or predictive testing. Identifying the mutation in an affected individual may be very time consuming, but once this

Table 9.3 Genetic investigations

Investigation	Application
Cytogenetic analysis – karyotype	Chromosomes stained and visualized under a microscope
	Detects alterations in chromosome number and structural rearrangements; this method is being replaced by molecular methods such as comparative genomic hybridization
Molecular cytogenetic analysis – fluorescence in situ hybridization (FISH)	Fluorescent-labelled DNA probes to detect the presence, number, and chromosomal location of specific chromosomal sequences
	Useful for microdeletion syndromes
Microarray comparative genomic hybridization	Detects chromosomal imbalances using thousands of DNA probes to investigate a whole genome with much greater sensitivity than cytogenetic methods
PCR	Amplification of a specific target site within the genome, which then permits the conventional Sanger sequencing of the amplified DNA
Next generation sequencing	Rapid sequencing of whole genomes or of selected loci within the genome
Linkage disequilibrium and genome-wide association studies	Comparing the frequency of combinations of alleles at nearby loci in a given population to identify genetic variants associated with specific diseases through a common ancestral origin

has been done, testing other relatives is usually fairly simple. Examples are:

- deletions – large deletion mutations, of at least one exon, are common in a variety of disorders including Duchenne and Becker muscular dystrophies, alpha-thalassaemia, and 21-hydroxylase deficiency (congenital adrenal hyperplasia)
- point mutations and small deletions – these can be readily identified if the same mutation causes all cases of the disorder, as in sickle cell disease. For most disorders, however, there is a spectrum of mutations. About 78% of cystic fibrosis carriers in the UK possess the ΔF508 mutation, but over 900 other mutations have been identified. Most laboratories test for a certain number of the most common mutations in the population they serve. This means that patients must be informed of the small risk that a mutation will not be detected
- trinucleotide repeat expansion mutations – these can be readily identified because the mutation in a given disease is virtually always at the same site and can be amplified from the same oligo-DNA primers used in the amplification by PCR: the only difference is the size of the repeat sequence, which can be determined from the size of the DNA fragment containing the repeat.

Next-generation sequencing

It is now possible to generate large volumes of DNA sequence data in a rapid and cost-effective fashion. These techniques of high-throughput sequencing are used to enable:

- gene panel testing – where a specific set of genes is sequenced, for example all the genes known to be relevant to a specific disease presentation (e.g. retinal degeneration, cardiomyopathy, infantile-onset epilepsy)
- whole exome sequencing – the coding regions of the genome are sequenced to determine variants, which are then analyzed to interpret the findings
- whole genome sequencing – the whole genome is sequenced, including noncoding regions. This is predominantly used as a research tool but development in this field is rapid and whole genome sequencing (WGS) has technical advantages over whole exome sequencing, so that the current use of whole exome sequencing is likely to be replaced by WGS over the next few years.

Recent studies have focused on implementation of next-generation sequencing into clinical practice. The Deciphering Developmental Disorders study utilized exome sequencing in a large cohort of undiagnosed patients with developmental delay. The results are being used to compile a database (DECIPHER) of genotypes and related phenotypes.

In the UK, the 100 000 Genomes Project is utilizing WGS to study a wide range of clinical conditions in adults and children (see Further Reading).

Genetic counselling

The main aims of genetic counselling are supportive and educational. Genetic counselling aims to support and provide information for individuals, couples, and families:

- to understand their situation
- to make their own decisions about managing the disease or risk of disease, including decisions about genetic testing and reproduction
- to adjust to their situation of being affected by or at risk of the genetic condition.

A primary goal of genetic counselling is to provide information to allow for greater autonomy and choice in reproductive decisions and other areas of personal life. Avoiding additional cases of genetic disease in a family may be a consequence of genetic counselling but is not the primary aim. The elements of genetic counselling include:

- listening to the questions and concerns of the patient, or family
- establishing the correct diagnosis – this involves detailed history, examination, and appropriate investigations that may include chromosome or DNA or other molecular genetic analysis, biochemical tests, X-rays, and clinical photographs. Despite extensive investigation, including searching databases, the diagnosis may remain unknown, e.g. in children with learning disability and normal appearance or only mild and nonspecific dysmorphic features
- risk estimation – this requires both diagnostic and pedigree information. Drawing a pedigree of three generations is an essential part of a clinical genetic assessment. The mode of inheritance may be apparent from the pedigree even when the precise diagnosis is not known. In some cases it may not be possible to define a precise recurrence risk and uncertainty may remain, e.g. conditions that only affect one member of a family and are known to follow autosomal dominant inheritance in some families and autosomal recessive inheritance in others (genetic heterogeneity)
- communication – information must be presented in an understandable and unbiased way. Families often find written information helpful to refer back to, and diagrams are often used to explain patterns of inheritance. The impact of saying 'the recurrence risk is 5% or 1 in 20' may be different from saying 'the chance of an unaffected child is 95% or 19 out of 20', and so both should be presented
- discussing options for management and prevention – if there appears to be a risk to offspring, all reproductive options should be discussed. These include not having (any more) children, reducing intended family size, taking the risk and proceeding with pregnancy or having antenatal diagnosis, and selective termination of an affected fetus. For some couples, donor insemination or ovum donation may be appropriate and for others, achieving a pregnancy

Box 9.14 Influences on decisions regarding options for genetic counselling

- Magnitude of risk
- Perceived severity of disorder
- Availability of treatment
- Person's experience of the disorder
- Family size
- Availability of a safe and reliable prenatal diagnostic test
- Parental cultural, religious, or ethical values

through in vitro fertilization and preimplantation genetic diagnosis may be possible
- putting parents in touch with appropriate sources of support, such as the charity Unique, which provides support for families affected by rare chromosomal imbalances.

Counselling should be nondirective, but should also assist in the decision-making process (Box 9.14). Information from lay support groups may also be helpful.

> Genetic counselling aims to allow parents greater autonomy and choice in reproductive decisions

Presymptomatic (predictive) testing

Children may be referred because they are at increased risk of developing a genetic disorder in childhood or adult life.

If the condition is likely to manifest in childhood (e.g. Duchenne muscular dystrophy) or if there are useful medical interventions available in childhood (e.g. screening by colonoscopy for colorectal tumours in children at risk of familial adenomatosis polyposis coli), then genetic testing is appropriate in childhood.

If the child is at risk of a late-onset and untreatable disorder (e.g. Huntington disease), then there is a very strong case for deferring genetic testing until the child becomes an adult, or at least sufficiently mature to be actively involved in seeking the test and can make the decision for himself/herself.

If the child is not at risk of developing the condition but may be a carrier at risk of transmitting the disorder to their future children, then there is also a good case for deferring testing until the young person can participate actively in the decision. There may be less at stake with these reproductive carrier tests than with predictive tests for untreatable disorders but there are still good grounds for caution and for careful discussion before proceeding with such tests.

These difficult issues are often best handled through a process of genetic counselling supporting open and sustained communication within the family and especially between parents and children.

> Presymptomatic testing of disorders which manifest in adult life should not be performed until the individual can consent on their own behalf unless there is clear clinical benefit from testing earlier

Acknowledgements

We would like to acknowledge contributors to this chapter in previous editions, whose work we have drawn on: Elizabeth Thompson (1st Edition), Helen Kingston (2nd, 3rd Edition), Angus Clarke (4th Edition). We would also like to thank Madeleine Tooley for her contribution to the current chapter.

Further reading

Clarke A: *Harper's Practical Genetic Counselling*, ed 8, 2016, CRC Press

Firth HV, Hurst JA: *Oxford Desk Reference – Clinical Genetics*, Oxford, 2005, Oxford University Press.

Harper PS: *A Short History of Medical Genetics*, New York, 2008, Oxford University Press.

Jones KL: *Smith's Recognisable Patterns of Human Malformation*, ed 7, Philadelphia, 2013, WB Saunders.

Read A, Donnai D: *The New Clinical Genetics*, ed 3, Bloxham, 2015, Scion.

Strachan T, Read AP: *Human Molecular Genetics*, ed 4, London, 2010, Garland.

Turnpenny P, Ellard S: *Emery's Elements of Medical Genetics*, ed 14, Edinburgh, 2012, Churchill Livingstone.

Website (Accessed November 2016)
Genome browsers

Decipher: Available at: http://decipher.sanger.ac.uk.

E!Ensembl: Available at: http://www.ensembl.org.

NCBI MapViewer: Available at: http://www.ncbi.nlm.nih.gov/projects/mapview.

Online resources

1000 Genomes Project: Available at: http://www.1000genomes.org.

Contact-a-family: Available at: http://www.cafamily.org.uk. UK family support group alliance. *Resource for families with disabled children.*

GeneReviews: Available at: http://www.ncbi.nlm.nih.gov/books/NBK1116/.
Resource for clinicians, with information on many rare genetic diseases.

Genomics England: Available at: http://www.genomicsengland.co.uk.
The 100 000 Genome Project.

London Medical Database: Available at: http://www.lmdatabases.com/.
Database of genetic conditions, with photographs.

Online Mendelian Inheritance in Man (OMIM): Available at: www.ncbi.nlm.nih.gov/omim.

Orphanet: Available at: www.orpha.net/. *Portal for rare diseases and orphan drugs.*

The British Society for Genetic Medicine: Available at: http://www.bsgm.org.uk.

Unique: the rare chromosome disorder support group: Includes printable information sheets about many chromosomal disorders. Available at: http://www.rarechromo.co.uk.

Your Genes, Your Health: information on some common genetic disorders and links to DNA tutorials. Available at: http://ygyh.org/.

Perinatal medicine

Pre-pregnancy care	142	Adaptation to extrauterine life	152
Antenatal diagnosis	143	Neonatal resuscitation	153
Obstetric conditions affecting the fetus	146	Size at birth	158
Maternal conditions affecting the fetus	148	Routine examination of the newborn infant	160
Maternal drugs affecting the fetus	149		
Congenital infections	150		

Features of perinatal medicine are:
- good pregnancy and neonatal outcomes depend on good maternal health and care
- non-invasive antenatal diagnosis is reducing the risk of fetal loss from invasive tests
- maternal viral infection during pregnancy can seriously affect the fetus
- worldwide, prematurity is the leading cause of mortality in children < 5 years old
- when required, newborn resuscitation can be achieved with simple measures in most instances
- newborn infants have a number of assessments shortly after birth – routine examination, hearing and biochemical screening and increasingly, oxygen saturation screening for critical congenital heart disease.

The term 'perinatal medicine' refers to medical care of the fetus and infant, particularly those with complex problems, before, during and after birth, acknowledging the continuity of fetal and neonatal life. Using modern technology, such as high-resolution ultrasound, magnetic resonance imaging and DNA analysis, detailed information about the fetus can now be obtained for a large and increasing number of conditions. Close cooperation is important between the professionals involved in the care of the pregnant mother and fetus and those caring for the newborn infant.

Some definitions used in perinatal medicine are listed in Box 10.1.

Pre-pregnancy care

The better a mother's state of health and nutrition and the higher her socioeconomic living standard and the quality of healthcare she receives, the greater the likelihood of a successful outcome to her pregnancy.

Box 10.1 Some definitions used in perinatal medicine

Commonly used terms in perinatal medicine:
- stillbirth – fetus born with no signs of life ≥24 weeks of pregnancy
- perinatal mortality rate – stillbirths + deaths within the 1st week per 1000 live births and stillbirths
- neonatal mortality rate – deaths of live-born infants within the first 4 weeks after birth per 1000 live births
- neonate – infant ≤28 days old
- preterm – gestation <37 weeks of pregnancy
- term – 37–41 weeks of pregnancy
- post-term – gestation ≥42 weeks of pregnancy
- low birthweight – <2500-g
- very low birthweight – <1500-g
- extremely low birthweight – <1000-g
- small for gestational age – birthweight <10th centile for gestational age
- large for gestational age – birthweight >90th centile for gestational age

Couples planning to have a baby often ask what they should do to optimize their chances of having a healthy child. They can be informed that for the mother:

- *smoking* reduces birthweight, which may be of critical importance if born preterm. On average, the babies of smokers weigh 170 g less than those of non-smokers, but the reduction in birthweight is related to the number of cigarettes smoked per day. Smoking is also associated with an increased risk of miscarriage and stillbirth. The infant has a greater risk of sudden infant death syndrome

- *pre-pregnancy folic acid* supplements reduce the risk of neural tube defects in the fetus. Low-dose folic acid supplementation is recommended for all women planning a pregnancy. A higher dose is recommended for women at increased risk of neural tube defects – if they have had or have a close relative with a previously affected fetus or have diabetes or are using certain anticonvulsants
- *pre-existing medical conditions*, such as diabetes, epilepsy or hypertension, must be reviewed and monitored and management changed if necessary
- *certain medications* such as retinoids, warfarin, and sodium valproate should be avoided because of teratogenic effects
- *alcohol* ingestion and *drug abuse* (opiates, cocaine) may damage the fetus
- *congenital rubella* is preventable by maternal immunization before pregnancy
- *exposure to toxoplasmosis* should be minimized by avoiding eating undercooked meat and by wearing gloves when handling cat litter
- *Listeria infection* can be acquired from eating unpasteurized dairy products, soft ripened cheeses, e.g. brie, camembert and blue veined varieties, Pâté and ready-to-eat poultry, unless thoroughly reheated
- *eating liver* during pregnancy is best avoided as it contains a high concentration of vitamin A
- avoid eating swordfish and limit tuna because of high levels of mercury. Limit oily fish intake as may contain pollutants.

Any obstetric risk factors for complications of pregnancy or delivery (e.g. recurrent miscarriage or previous preterm delivery) should be identified and treated or monitored. Maternal obesity is associated with an increased risk of miscarriage, gestational diabetes and pregnancy-induced hypertension. Babies of obese mothers are at an increased risk of stillbirth, congenital abnormalities, macrosomia and neonatal mortality. In addition, the children of obese mothers are more likely to be obese themselves and develop metabolic disorders associated with this.

Couples at increased risk of inherited disorders should receive genetic counselling before pregnancy. They can then be fully informed, decide whether or not to proceed and consider antenatal diagnosis if available. Pregnancies at increased risk of fetal abnormality include those in which:

- the mother is older (if she is >35 years old, the risk of Down syndrome is >1 in 380), although screening is now available for all mothers
- there is previous congenital abnormality
- there is a family history of an inherited disorder
- the parents are identified as carriers of an autosomal recessive disorder, e.g. thalassaemia
- a parent carries a chromosomal rearrangement
- parents are close blood relatives (consanguinity).

☀ **Pre-pregnancy folic acid supplements reduce the risk of neural tube defects in the fetus**

Antenatal diagnosis

Antenatal diagnosis has become available for an increasing number of disorders. Screening tests performed on maternal blood and ultrasound of the fetus are listed in Box 10.2. The main diagnostic techniques for antenatal diagnosis are maternal serum screening and detailed ultrasound scanning. More specialized techniques are chorionic villus sampling, fetal blood sampling, amniocentesis and non-invasive prenatal testing (Fig. 10.1). In some rare conditions, preimplantation genetic diagnosis allows genetic analysis of cells from a developing embryo before transfer to the uterus. The structural malformations and other lesions that can be identified on ultrasound are listed in Box 10.3, with an example in Fig. 10.2.

Antenatal screening for disorders affecting the mother or fetus allows:

- reassurance where disorders are not detected
- optimal obstetric management of the mother and fetus
- interventions for a limited number of fetal conditions, such as relieving bladder obstruction or draining pleural effusions to improve perinatal outcome
- counselling and neonatal management to be planned in advance
- the option of termination of pregnancy to be offered for severe disorders affecting the fetus (Case History 10.1) or compromising maternal health.

Parents require accurate medical advice and counselling to help them with these difficult decisions. Many transient or minor structural disorders of the fetus are also detected, which may cause considerable anxiety.

☀ **Antenatal diagnosis allows many congenital malformations which used to be diagnosed at birth or during infancy to be identified before birth**

Fetal medicine

The fetus can sometimes be treated by giving medication to the mother. Examples include:

- *glucocorticoid therapy* before preterm delivery accelerates lung maturity and surfactant production. This has been tested in over 15 randomized trials and markedly reduces the incidence of respiratory distress syndrome (relative risk 0.66), intraventricular haemorrhage (relative risk 0.54) and neonatal mortality (relative risk 0.69) in preterm infants. For optimal effect, a completed course needs to be given at least 24 hours before delivery
- *digoxin or flecainide* can be given to the mother to treat fetal supraventricular tachycardia.

Box 10.2 Screening tests for antenatal diagnosis

Maternal blood	Blood group and antibodies – for rhesus and other red cell incompatibilities
	Hepatitis B
	Syphilis
	Rubella
	HIV infection
	Neural tube defects – raised maternal serum alphafetoprotein with spina bifida or anencephaly, but ultrasound alone increasingly used
	Down syndrome (trisomy 21), Edwards syndrome (trisomy 18) and Patau syndrome (trisomy 13) – risk estimate calculated from maternal age and maternal and fetoplacental hormones. This is combined with ultrasound screening for nuchal translucency (back of neck) and confirmed with amniocentesis or chorionic villous sampling. Detects 90% with Down syndrome, but 3–5% false-positive rate and 1% risk of fetal loss. Alternatively, identification by non-invasive prenatal testing (NIPT) is increasingly available and scheduled as routine screening test in UK.
Ultrasound screening	Gestational age – can be estimated reliably if early in pregnancy
	Multiple pregnancies – can be identified
	Structural malformation – up to 80% of major congenital malformations can be detected. If a significant abnormality is suspected, a more detailed scan by a specialist is indicated
	Fetal growth – can be monitored by serial measurement of abdominal circumference, head circumference and femur length, supplemented with Doppler ultrasound umbilical and fetal flow velocity waveform measurements if indicated
	Amniotic fluid volume – oligohydramnios may result from reduced fetal urine production (because of dysplastic or absent kidneys or obstructive uropathy) from prolonged rupture of the membranes, or may be associated with severe intrauterine growth restriction. It may cause pulmonary hypoplasia and limb and facial deformities from pressure on the fetus (Potter syndrome)
	Polyhydramnios – this is associated with maternal diabetes and structural gastrointestinal abnormalities, e.g. atresia in the fetus

Amniocentesis
Chromosome/microarray and DNA analysis
Fetal infection – PCR

Fetal blood sampling
Fetal haemoglobin for anaemia
Fetal infection serology
Fetal blood transfusion

Chorionic villus sampling
Chromosome/microarray and DNA analysis
Fetal infection – PCR
Enzyme analysis of inborn error of metabolism

Preimplantation genetic diagnosis (PGD)
In vitro fertilization allows genetic analysis of cells from developing embryo before transfer to the uterus

Fetoscopy
Minimally invasive surgery, e.g. laser photo-coagulation of communicating vessels in twin–twin transfusion syndrome

Non-invasive prenatal testing (NIPT) – cell-free fetal DNA (cffDNA) from maternal blood
Identification of Down syndrome and other chromosomal disorders, fetal gender and rhesus status

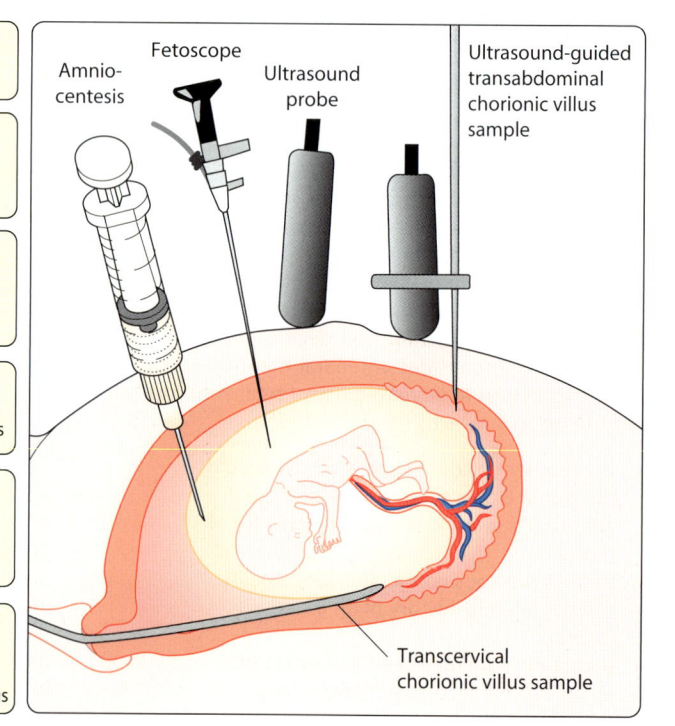

Figure 10.1 Some of the techniques used for antenatal diagnosis.

Box 10.3 Main structural malformations and other lesions detectable by ultrasound

Central nervous system	Anencephaly – always detected Spina bifida Hydrocephalus, microcephaly, encephalocele
Cardiac	About 50% of severe malformations detected on 'routine' screening, over 90% at specialist centres
Intrathoracic	Diaphragmatic hernia, congenital cystic adenomatoid lung malformation (CCAM), oesophageal atresia
Facial	Cleft lip
Gastrointestinal	Bowel obstruction, e.g. duodenal atresia Exomphalos and gastroschisis
Genitourinary	Dysplastic or cystic kidneys Obstructive disorders of kidneys or urinary tract (hydronephrosis, distended bladder)
Skeletal	Skeletal dysplasias, e.g. achondroplasia and limb reduction deformities
Hydrops	Oedema of the skin, pleural effusions, and ascites
Chromosomal	Down syndrome – suspected from thickened back of neck (nuchal translucency), duodenal atresia or an atrioventricular canal defect of the heart. Other chromosomal disorders – from identifying multiple abnormalities

Example of antenatal diagnosis – gastroschisis

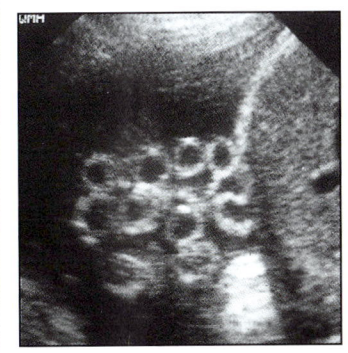

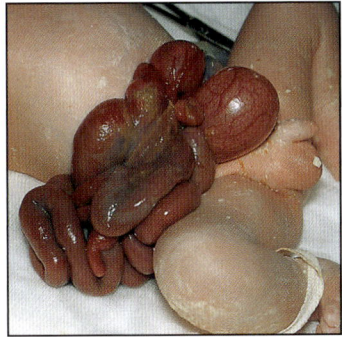

Figure 10.2 Gastroschisis on antenatal ultrasound showing free loops of small bowel in the amniotic fluid (a) and following delivery (b). Antenatal diagnosis allowed the baby to be delivered at a paediatric surgical unit and the parents to be forewarned about the need for surgery. Satisfactory surgical repair was achieved. (Courtesy of Karl Murphy.)

Case history 10.1

Antenatal diagnosis

A routine ultrasound scan at 18 weeks' gestation identified an abnormal 'lemon-shaped' skull (Fig. 10.3). This, together with an abnormal appearance of the cerebellum, is the Arnold–Chiari malformation, which is associated with spina bifida. An extensive spinal defect was confirmed on ultrasound. Dilatation of the cerebral ventricles and talipes equinovarus already present in this fetus suggested a severe spinal lesion. After counselling, the parents decided to terminate the pregnancy.

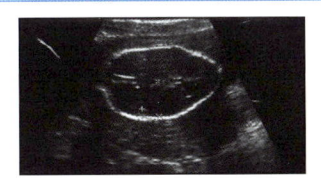

Figure 10.3 Transverse section showing a 'lemon-shaped' skull on ultrasound instead of the normal oval shape. This is associated with spina bifida. (Courtesy of Guy Thorpe-Beeston.)

There are a few conditions in which therapy can be given to the fetus directly:

- *rhesus isoimmunization* – severely affected fetuses become anaemic and may develop *hydrops fetalis*, with oedema and ascites. Infants at risk are identified by maternal antibody screening. Regular ultrasound of the fetus is performed to detect fetal anaemia noninvasively using Doppler velocimetry of the fetal middle cerebral artery. Fetal blood transfusion via the umbilical vein may be required regularly from about 20 weeks' gestation. The incidence of rhesus haemolytic disease has fallen markedly since anti-D immunization of mothers was introduced but hydrops fetalis is still seen due to other red blood cell antibodies such as Kell
- *perinatal isoimmune thrombocytopenia* – this condition is analogous to rhesus isoimmunization but involves maternal antiplatelet antibodies crossing the placenta. It is rare, affecting about 1 in 5000 births. Intracranial haemorrhage secondary to fetal thrombocytopenia occurs in up to 25% of cases. The problem may be anticipated if there was a previously affected infant, when prenatal intravenous immunoglobulin and maternal glucocorticoid therapy can be given.

> Maternal glucocorticoid therapy before preterm delivery markedly reduces morbidity and mortality in the neonate

Fetal surgery

Fetal surgery is a relatively new development with varying results. Procedures that have been performed include:

- catheter shunts inserted under ultrasound guidance. This is to drain fetal pleural effusions (pleuro-amniotic shunts), often from a chylothorax (lymphatic fluid) or congenital cystic adenomatous malformation of the lung. One end of a looped catheter lies in the chest, the other end in the amniotic cavity. Procedure works well; outcome depends on underlying problem
- laser therapy to ablate placental anastomoses, which lead to the twin–twin transfusion syndrome
- intrauterine shunting for obstruction to urinary outflow as with posterior urethral valves, but does not appear to improve outcome.

Careful case selection and follow-up are required to ensure that these novel forms of treatment are of long-term benefit.

Obstetric conditions affecting the fetus

Pre-eclampsia

Mothers with pre-eclampsia may require preterm delivery because of the maternal risks of eclampsia and cerebrovascular accident or the fetal risks associated with placental insufficiency and growth restriction. Determining the optimal time for preterm delivery requires an evaluation of the risk to the mother and fetus of allowing the pregnancy to continue compared with the neonatal complications associated with preterm birth.

Placental insufficiency and intrauterine growth restriction (IUGR)

Fetal growth may be progressively restricted because of placental insufficiency. Transfer of oxygen and nutrients is reduced. The growth-restricted fetus will need to be monitored closely to prevent intrauterine death. This is done by measuring growth parameters, the biophysical profile (amniotic fluid volume, fetal movement, fetal tone, fetal breathing movements and fetal heart activity) and Doppler blood flow velocity (umbilical and middle cerebral arteries). Absence or reversal of flow velocity during diastole carries an increased risk of morbidity from hypoxic damage to the gut or brain, or of intrauterine death. These measurements assist in deciding the optimal time for delivery of a growth-restricted fetus.

Preterm delivery

In the UK, 7.2% of births were preterm in 2012. However, only 5.9% of births in Sweden and Japan were preterm, but 11.5% in the United States.

Neonates may be born preterm following:

- spontaneous labour with intact membranes (40–50%)
- preterm premature rupture of the membranes (25–30%)
- labour induction or caesarean delivery for maternal or fetal indications (30–35%).

The main causes are shown in Fig. 10.4.

There are many epidemiological risk factors presumably responsible for the wide inter-country variation in prematurity rate, but they are poorly understood. Factors that increase the risk of preterm delivery include previous preterm infant, a short inter-pregnancy interval (<6 months), maternal age (<20 or >35 years), obesity, ethnicity (e.g. higher in Black mothers), multiple births (influenced by assisted reproduction practices), maternal infection, smoking and substance misuse and maternal psychological or social stress.

The management of preterm labour may involve:

- antenatal corticosteroids
- antibiotics to reduce risk of chorioamnionitis and neonatal infection for preterm premature rupture of the membranes
- tocolysis – to suppress uterine contractions to try and suppress labour and allow completion of the course of antenatal steroids
- magnesium sulphate – may be given as studies show it reduces the incidence of cerebral palsy; however, its mode of action is unknown
- in utero transfer to a centre appropriate for care of the preterm baby.

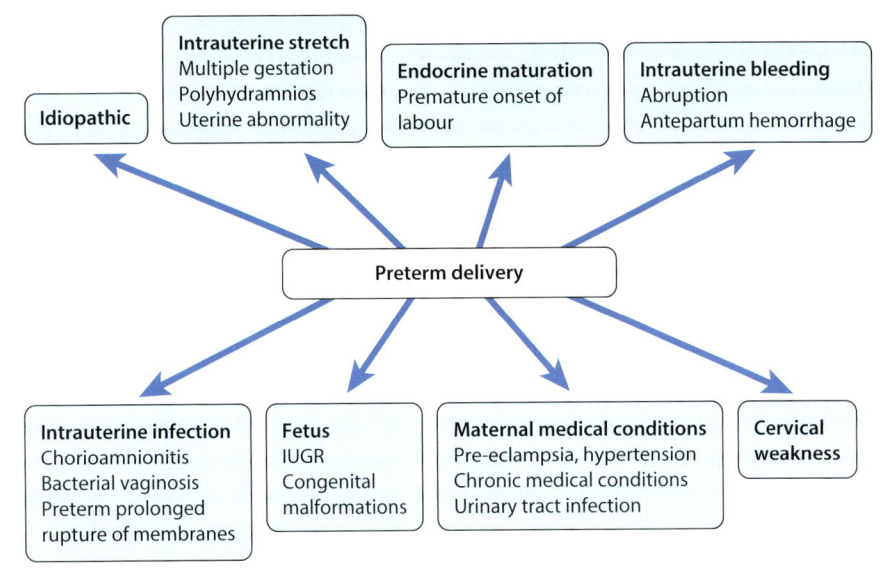

```
                    Intrauterine stretch
                    Multiple gestation    Endocrine maturation   Intrauterine bleeding
                    Polyhydramnios        Premature onset of     Abruption
       Idiopathic   Uterine abnormality   labour                 Antepartum hemorrhage

                                    Preterm delivery

   Intrauterine infection   Fetus          Maternal medical conditions   Cervical
   Chorioamnionitis         IUGR           Pre-eclampsia, hypertension   weakness
   Bacterial vaginosis      Congenital     Chronic medical conditions
   Preterm prolonged        malformations  Urinary tract infection
   rupture of membranes
```

Figure 10.4 Causes of prematurity. (IUGR, intrauterine growth restriction). (From Lissauer T, Fanaroff A, Miall L, et al.: *Neonatology at a Glance,* 3rd edition, Oxford, 2015, Wiley Blackwell, with permission).

The aim is to prolong pregnancy for as long as possible whilst ensuring that the condition of the mother and fetus is not compromised. The mode of delivery needs to be planned, and arrangements made for the infant to receive the required level of care. The care of preterm infants is described in Chapter 11 (Neonatal medicine).

Multiple births

Twins occur naturally in the UK in about 1 in 90, triplets in 1 in 8000, and quadruplets in 1 in 700 000 deliveries. In recent years, the number of triplets and higher-order births has more than doubled, mainly from assisted reproduction programmes and advancing maternal age; 1 in 64 births is now a multiple birth, although the number multiple births has recently declined in the UK mainly as a result of limiting embryo transfers following in vitro fertilization.

The main problems for the infant associated with multiple births are:

- preterm labour – the median gestation for twins is 37 weeks, for triplets 34 weeks and for quads 32 weeks. Preterm delivery is the most important cause of the greater perinatal mortality of multiple births, especially for triplets and higher-order pregnancies. When a higher-order pregnancy is identified, embryo reduction may be offered
- intrauterine growth restriction (IUGR) – fetal growth in one or more fetuses may deteriorate and needs to be monitored regularly
- congenital abnormalities – these occur twice as frequently as in a singleton, but the risk is increased four-fold in monochorionic twins (shared placenta)
- twin–twin transfusion syndrome in monochorionic twins. May cause extreme preterm delivery, fetal death and discrepancy in growth
- complicated deliveries – e.g. due to malpresentation of the second twin at vaginal delivery.

Finding sufficient intensive care cots in the same neonatal intensive care unit for preterm multiple births can be problematic.

Although multiple births may look endearing, the families may need additional assistance and support:

- feeding – often possible to breastfeed twins, usually not possible for higher-order births
- practical – with their care and housework (requires about 200 h/week for triplets in infancy) and going out
- emotional and physical exhaustion
- loss of privacy as a couple; increased rate of separation and divorce
- additional financial costs
- increased behavioural problems in the infants and their siblings. While being a multiple birth may provide companionship, affection, and stimulation between each other, it may also engender domination, dependency, and jealousy.

There are local and national support groups for parents of multiple births.

> **Summary**
>
> **Multiple births**
> - Have markedly increased over the last 20 years.
> - Are associated with an increased risk of prematurity, IUGR, congenital malformations, and twin–twin transfusion syndrome (in monochorionic twins).
> - Are responsible for 30% of very low birthweight infants (<1.5 kg birthweight).
> - Provide many additional difficulties for their parents to care for them.

Maternal conditions affecting the fetus

Diabetes mellitus

Women with insulin-dependent diabetes find it more difficult to maintain good diabetic control during pregnancy and have an increased insulin requirement. Poorly controlled maternal diabetes is associated with polyhydramnios and preeclampsia, increased rate of early fetal loss, congenital malformations and late unexplained intrauterine death. Ketoacidosis carries a high fetal mortality rate. With meticulous attention to diabetic control, the perinatal mortality rate is now only slightly greater than in non-diabetics. The National Institute for Health and Care Excellence (NICE) has produced guidance on the management of diabetes and its complications from preconception to the postnatal period. The emphasis is on aiming for good control of blood glucose.

Fetal problems associated with maternal diabetes are:

- *congenital malformations* – overall, there is a 6% risk of congenital malformations, a three-fold increase compared with the non-diabetic population. The range of anomalies is similar to that for the general population, apart from an increased incidence of cardiac malformations, sacral agenesis (caudal regression syndrome) and hypoplastic left colon, although the latter two conditions are rare. Studies show that good diabetic control periconceptionally reduces the risk of congenital malformations
- *IUGR* – there is a three-fold increase in growth restriction in mothers with long-standing microvascular disease
- *macrosomia* (Fig. 10.5) – maternal hyperglycaemia causes fetal hyperglycaemia as glucose crosses the placenta. As insulin does not cross the placenta, the fetus responds with increased secretion of insulin, which promotes growth by increasing both cell number and size. About 25% of such infants have a birthweight greater than 4 kg compared with 8% of non-diabetics. The macrosomia predisposes to cephalopelvic disproportion, birth asphyxia, shoulder dystocia and brachial plexus injury.

Neonatal problems include:

- *hypoglycaemia* – transient hypoglycaemia is common during the 1st day of life from fetal hyperinsulinism, but can often be prevented by early feeding. The infant's blood glucose should be closely monitored during the first 24 hours and hypoglycaemia treated
- *respiratory distress syndrome* – more common as lung maturation is delayed
- *hypertrophic cardiomyopathy* – hypertrophy of the cardiac septum occurs in some infants. It regresses over several weeks but may cause heart failure from reduced left ventricular function
- *polycythaemia* (venous haematocrit >0.65) – makes the infant look plethoric. Treatment with partial exchange transfusion to reduce the haematocrit and normalise viscosity may be required if symptomatic.

Gestational diabetes is when carbohydrate intolerance occurs only during pregnancy. It is more common in women who are obese and in those of Black and Asian ethnicity. The incidence of macrosomia and its complications is similar to that of the insulin-dependent diabetic mother, but the incidence of congenital malformations is not increased. However, there are an increasing number of mothers with type 2 non-insulin-dependent diabetes associated with the increase in obesity in the population. Their fetuses are also at increased risk of congenital malformations.

> **Summary**
>
> **Maternal diabetes**
> - Meticulous control preconceptually and during pregnancy markedly reduces fetal and neonatal morbidity and mortality.
> - The fetus may be macrosomic because of fetal hyperglycaemia resulting in hyperinsulinism, or growth restricted secondary to maternal microvascular disease, and is at an increased risk of congenital malformations.
> - The macrosomic infant is at an increased risk of birth asphyxia and birth trauma from obstructed labour or delivery.
> - The newborn infant is prone to hypoglycaemia and polycythaemia.

Hyperthyroidism

If mothers have or have had Graves disease, 1–2% of their newborn infants are hyperthyroid. This is due to circulating thyroid stimulating immunoglobulin (also called TSH receptor antibody, TSHR-Ab), which crosses the placenta and binds to TSH receptors, stimulating fetal thyroid hormone production. Hyperthyroidism in the fetus is suggested by fetal tachycardia on the CTG (cardiotocography) trace, and fetal goitre may be evident on ultrasound. In the neonate it is suggested by irritability, weight loss, tachycardia, heart failure,

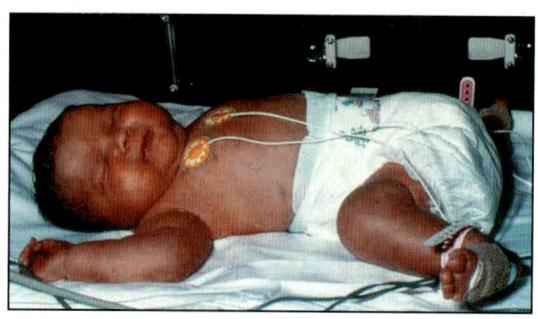

Figure 10.5 Infant of a diabetic mother showing macrosomia and plethora. Born vaginally at 36 weeks' gestation, she weighed 5.5 kg and suffered a right-sided brachial plexus injury.

diarrhoea and exophthalmos in the first 2 weeks of life. Treatment with anti-thyroid drugs may be necessary for several months until the condition resolves.

Systemic lupus erythematosus

Systemic lupus erythematosus (SLE) with antiphospholipid syndrome is associated with recurrent miscarriage, IUGR, pre-eclampsia, placental abruption and preterm delivery. Some of the infants born to mothers with antibodies to the Ro (SS-A) or La (SS-B) antigens develop neonatal lupus syndrome, in which there is a self-limiting rash and rarely, heart block.

Autoimmune thrombocytopenic purpura

In maternal autoimmune thrombocytopenic purpura (AITP), the fetus may become thrombocytopenic because maternal IgG antibodies cross the placenta and damage fetal platelets. Severe fetal thrombocytopenia places the fetus at risk of intracranial haemorrhage following birth trauma. Infants with severe thrombocytopenia or petechiae at birth should be given intravenous immunoglobulin. Platelet transfusions may be required to reduce the risk of intracranial haemorrhage or if there is acute bleeding.

Maternal drugs affecting the fetus

Relatively few drugs are known definitely to damage the fetus (Table 10.1), but it is clearly advisable for pregnant women to avoid taking medicines unless it is essential. While the teratogenicity of a drug may be recognized if it causes severe and distinctive malformations, as with limb shortening following thalidomide ingestion, milder and less distinctive abnormalities may go unrecognized. Selective serotonin reuptake inhibitors (SSRIs) are an example of this; they have been found to be associated with an increased risk of persistent pulmonary hypertension of the newborn (see Ch. 11). Caution must be taken with all new drugs; studies on pregnant women may be limited, and the recognition or emergence of teratogenic effects may be delayed.

Alcohol and smoking

Excessive alcohol ingestion during pregnancy is sometimes associated with the 'fetal alcohol syndrome'. Its clinical features are growth restriction, characteristic face (Fig. 10.6), developmental delay and cardiac defects (up to 70%). The effects of less severe ingestion and binge-drinking remain uncertain but may affect growth and development, and mothers are advised to avoid alcohol (Department of Health, UK). Maternal cigarette smoking is associated with an increased risk

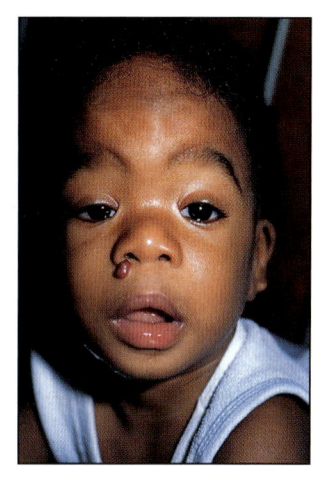

Figure 10.6 Characteristic facies of fetal alcohol syndrome with: a saddle-shaped nose; maxillary hypoplasia; absent philtrum between the nose and upper lip; and short, thin upper lip. This child also has a strawberry naevus below the right nostril.

Table 10.1 Maternal medication that may adversely affect the fetus

Medication	Adverse effect on fetus
Anticonvulsant therapy with carbamazepine, valproic acid (sodium valproate) or hydantoins (phenytoin)	Fetal carbamazepine/valproate/hydantoin syndrome – midfacial hypoplasia, central nervous system, limb and cardiac malformations, and developmental delay
Cytotoxic agents	Congenital malformations
Iodides/propylthiouracil	Goitre, hypothyroidism
Lithium	Congenital heart disease
Selective serotonin reuptake inhibitors (SSRIs)	Persistent pulmonary hypertension of the newborn
Tetracycline	Enamel hypoplasia of the teeth
Thalidomide	Limb shortening (phocomelia)
Vitamin A and retinoids	Increased spontaneous abortions, abnormal face
Warfarin	Interferes with cartilage formation (nasal hypoplasia and epiphyseal stippling); cerebral haemorrhages and microcephaly

Drug abuse

Maternal drug abuse with opiates is associated with an increased risk of prematurity and growth restriction. Many narcotic abusers take multiple drugs. Infants of mothers abusing heroin, methadone and other opiates during pregnancy often show evidence of drug withdrawal, with jitteriness, sneezing, yawning, poor feeding, vomiting, diarrhoea, weight loss and seizures during the first 2 weeks of life. Cocaine abuse is associated with placental abruption and preterm delivery, but rarely with withdrawal in the infant, although it may result in irritability and tremor in the few days of life. Amphetamine abuse is also associated with gastrointestinal and cerebral infarction. Mothers who abuse drugs and their infants are also at increased risk of hepatitis B and C and HIV infections. Hepatitis B vaccine is given to babies when indicated. Social and child protection aspects must be considered and social services involved.

Infants who develop significant features of drug withdrawal require treatment, usually with an oral opiate, morphine sulphate, and often need to be admitted to the neonatal unit. One of the major problems in managing these infants is that the parents' lifestyle and temperament are often not conducive to the needs of babies and young children. Close supervision or alternative caregivers are often required.

> If there are unexplained clinical signs in an infant, consider drug withdrawal

Drugs given during labour

Potential adverse effects of drugs given during labour on the fetus are:

- *opioid analgesics/anaesthetic agents* – may suppress respiration at birth
- *epidural anaesthesia* – may cause maternal pyrexia during labour. It is often difficult to differentiate this from fever caused by an infection. There is an increase in the rate of assisted deliveries
- *sedatives, e.g. diazepam* – may cause sedation, hypothermia and hypotension in the newborn
- *oxytocin and prostaglandin F2* – may cause hyperstimulation of the uterus leading to fetal hypoxia. It is also associated with a small increase in bilirubin levels in the neonate
- *intravenous fluids* – may cause neonatal hyponatraemia unless they contain an adequate concentration of sodium.

Congenital infections

Intrauterine infection is usually from maternal primary infection during pregnancy. Those that can damage the fetus are:

- rubella
- cytomegalovirus (CMV)

Congenital infections

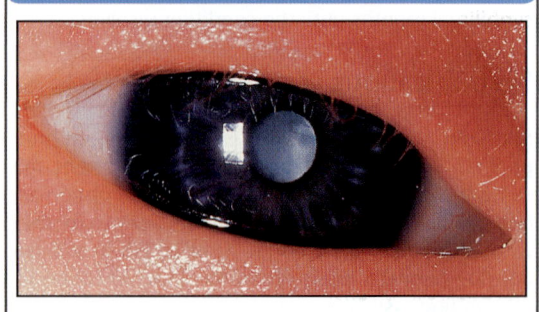

Figure 10.7a Cataract from congenital rubella. Congenital heart disease and deafness are the other common defects.

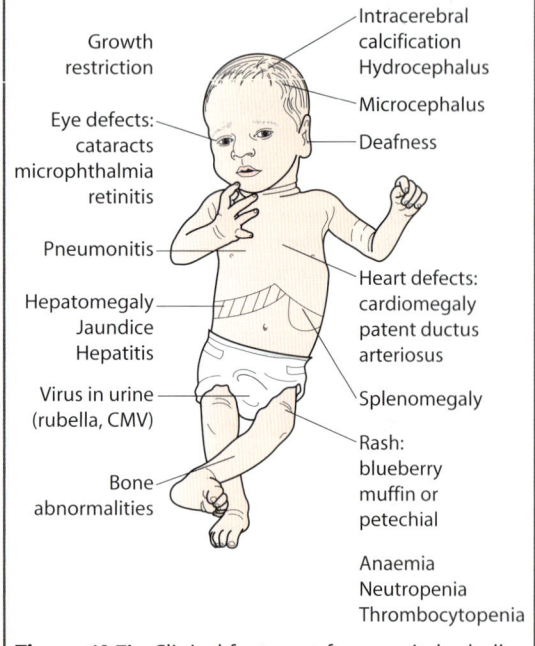

Figure 10.7b Clinical features of congenital rubella, cytomegalovirus, toxoplasmosis, and syphilis.

- *Toxoplasma gondii*
- parvovirus
- varicella zoster
- syphilis.

Rubella

The diagnosis of maternal infection must be confirmed serologically as clinical diagnosis is unreliable. The risk and extent of fetal damage are mainly determined by the gestational age at the onset of maternal infection. Infection before 8 weeks' gestation causes deafness, congenital heart disease, and cataracts in over 80% of cases (Fig. 10.7a). About 30% of fetuses of mothers infected at 13–16 weeks' gestation have impaired hearing; beyond 18 weeks' gestation, the risk to the fetus is minimal. Viraemia after birth continues to damage the infant. Tests used to confirm the diagnosis

Box 10.4 Confirmation of diagnosis of congenital rubella, cytomegalovirus, *Toxoplasma* infection and syphilis

Mother	Seroconversion on screening serology
Fetus	Amniocentesis or chorionic villus sample, polymerase chain reaction (PCR)
Placenta	Microscopy for syphilis, PCR
Urine from infant	Rubella, CMV – culture, PCR
Blood, cerebrospinal fluid, and other samples from infant	Culture, PCR
Blood serology	Rubella-specific IgM, CMV-specific IgM, *Toxoplasma*-specific IgM and persistently raised *Toxoplasma* IgG

are shown in Box 10.4. The range of clinical features characteristic of congenital infections is shown in Fig. 10.7b.

Congenital rubella is preventable. In the UK, it has become extremely rare since the measles/mumps/rubella vaccine was introduced into the childhood immunization programme, but this is dependent on the maintenance of a high vaccine uptake rate.

Cytomegalovirus

CMV is the most common congenital infection, affecting 0.5/1000 to 1/1000 live births in the UK. In Europe, 50% of pregnant women are susceptible to CMV. About 1% of susceptible women will have a primary infection during pregnancy, and in about 40% of them the infant becomes infected. The infant may also become infected following an episode of recurrent infection in the mother, but this is much less likely to damage the fetus. When an infant is infected:

- 90% are normal at birth and develop normally
- 5% have clinical features at birth, such as hepatosplenomegaly and petechiae (Fig. 10.7b), most of whom will have neurodevelopmental disabilities such as sensorineural hearing loss, cerebral palsy, epilepsy and cognitive impairment
- 5% develop problems later in life, mainly sensorineural hearing loss.

Infection in the pregnant woman is usually asymptomatic or causes a mild nonspecific illness. There is no CMV vaccine and pregnant women are not screened for CMV. Early treatment with antiviral therapy, e.g. ganciclovir, for infants with sensorineural hearing loss or central nervous system involvement can reduce the adverse impact on sensorineural hearing loss and long-term neurodevelopment.

Toxoplasmosis

Acute infection with *T. gondii*, a protozoan parasite, may result from the consumption of raw or undercooked meat and from contact with the faeces of recently infected cats. In the UK, fewer than 20% of pregnant women have had past infection, in contrast to 80% in France and Austria. Transplacental infection may occur during the parasitaemia of a primary infection, and about 40% of fetuses become infected. In the UK, the incidence of congenital infection is only about 0.1/1000 live births. Most infected infants are asymptomatic. About 10% have clinical manifestations (Fig. 10.7b), of which the most common are:

- retinopathy, an acute fundal chorioretinitis, which sometimes interferes with vision
- cerebral calcification
- hydrocephalus.

These infants usually have long-term neurological disabilities. Infected newborn infants are usually treated (pyrimethamine and sulfadiazine) for 1 year. Asymptomatic infants remain at risk of developing chorioretinitis into adulthood.

Varicella zoster

A total of 15% of pregnant women are susceptible to varicella (chickenpox). Usually, the fetus is unaffected but will be at risk if the mother develops chickenpox:

- in the first half of pregnancy (<20 weeks), when there is a less than 2% risk of the fetus developing severe scarring of the skin and possibly ocular and neurological damages and digital dysplasia
- within 5 days before or 5 days after delivery, when the fetus is unprotected by maternal antibodies and the viral dose is high. About 25% develop a vesicular rash. The illness has a mortality as high as 30%.

Exposed susceptible mothers can be protected with varicella zoster immune globulin and treated with aciclovir. Infants born in the high-risk period should also receive zoster immune globulin and are closely monitored and given aciclovir if any signs of infection develop.

> **If a mother develops chickenpox shortly before or after delivery, the infant needs protection from infection**

Syphilis

Congenital syphilis is rare in the UK. The clinical features are shown in Fig. 10.7b. Those specific to congenital syphilis include a characteristic rash on the soles of the feet and hands and bone lesions. If mothers with syphilis identified on antenatal screening are fully treated 1 month or more before delivery, the infant does not require treatment and has an excellent prognosis. If there is any doubt about the adequacy of maternal treatment, the infant should be treated with penicillin.

Adaptation to extrauterine life

In the fetus, the lungs are filled with fluid. The fetus therefore relies on the delivery of nutrients and oxygen from the placenta. The blood vessels that supply and drain the lungs are constricted (high pulmonary vascular resistance), so most blood from the right side of the heart bypasses the lungs and flows through the ductus arteriosus into the aorta, and some flows across the foramen ovale (Fig. 10.8). As a consequence of the fetal circulation, fetal oxygen saturations are about 65% (upper body) to 35% (lower body). To compensate for the low oxygen saturations, oxygen delivery to the tissues is enhanced by the high haemoglobin concentration (typically 160 g/L at term), along with the shift to the left of the oxygen dissociation curve of fetal haemoglobin compared with adult haemoglobin (see Fig. 23.1).

Shortly before and during labour, lung liquid production is reduced. During descent through the birth canal, the infant's chest is squeezed and some lung liquid drained. Multiple stimuli, including thermal (cold), tactile and hormonal (with a particularly dramatic increase in catecholamine levels) initiate breathing. The high catecholamine levels also stimulate reabsorption of alveolar fluid. It is normal practice now to delay cord clamping (typically 2–5 minutes) in term babies, as this increases the circulating blood volume by about 30% and reduces later anaemia. On average, the first breath occurs 6 seconds after delivery. Lung expansion is generated by intrathoracic negative pressure and a functional residual capacity is established. The mean time to establish regular breathing is 30 seconds. Once the infant breathes, the majority of the remaining lung fluid is absorbed into the lymphatic and pulmonary circulation.

Pulmonary expansion at birth is associated with a rise in oxygen tension, and with falling pulmonary vascular resistance the pulmonary blood flow increases. Increased left atrial filling results in a rise in the left atrial pressure with closure of the foramen ovale. The flow of oxygenated blood through the ductus arteriosus causes physiological and eventual anatomical ductal closure. After an elective caesarean section, when the mother has not been in labour, it may take several hours for the lung fluid to be completely absorbed, causing rapid, laboured breathing [transient tachypnoea of the newborn, see Ch. 11 (Newborn medicine)]. The delay in absorption of lung liquid is not only because the infant's chest has not been squeezed through the birth canal, but also because of the absence of the surge in maternal catecholamines during labour and delivery, which stimulates reabsorption of alveolar fluid.

Some infants do not breathe at birth. This may be due to asphyxia, when the fetus experiences a lack of oxygen during labour and/or delivery. It does not necessarily mean that the brain has been injured but asphyxia can lead to brain injury or death. A fetus deprived of oxygen in utero will attempt to breathe, often termed gasping, but if this is unsuccessful (as it will be if still in utero), it will then become apnoeic

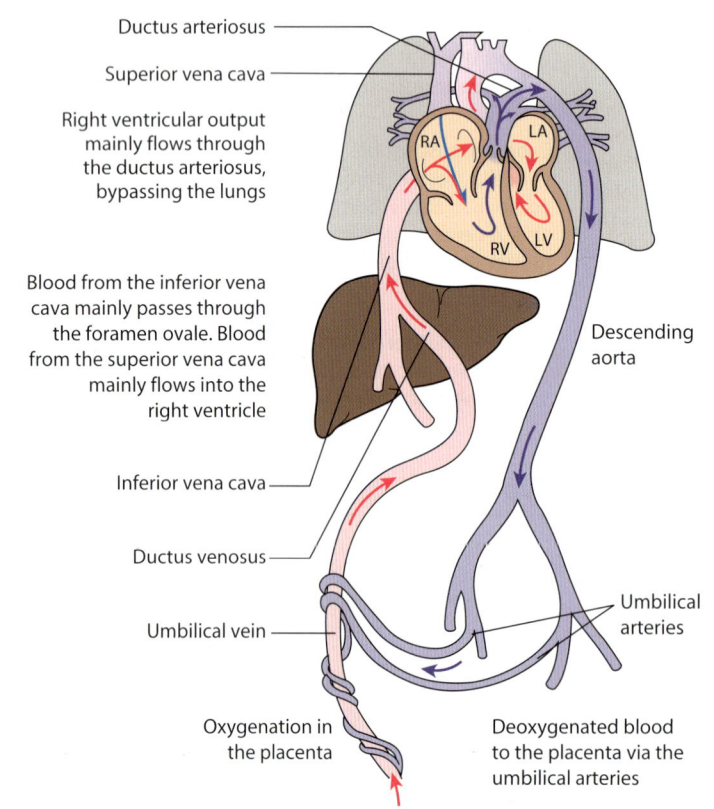

Figure 10.8 The fetal circulation.

Table 10.2 The Apgar score

	Score		
	0	**1**	**2**
Heart rate	Absent	<100 beats/min	≥100 beats/min
Respiratory effort	Absent	Gasping or irregular	Regular, strong cry
Muscle tone	Flaccid	Some flexion of limbs	Well flexed, active
Reflex irritability	None	Grimace	Cry, cough
Colour	Pale/blue	Body pink, extremities blue	Pink

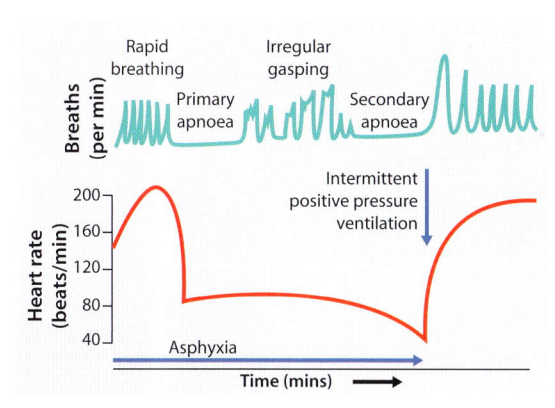

Figure 10.9 Changes in respiration and heart rate with continuous asphyxia. Once the infant has stopped gasping in secondary apnoea, resuscitation with lung expansion is required to establish regular respiration and restore the circulation.

(primary apnoea), during which time the heart rate is maintained. If oxygen deprivation continues, primary apnoea is followed by irregular gasping and then a second period of apnoea (secondary apnoea), when the heart rate and blood pressure fall. If delivered at this stage, the infant will only recover if help with lung expansion is provided, e.g. by positive pressure ventilation using a face mask or directly to the lungs via a tracheal tube (Fig. 10.9).

The human fetus rarely experiences a continuous asphyxial insult, except after placental abruption or complete occlusion of umbilical blood flow in a cord prolapse. More commonly, asphyxia which occurs during labour and delivery is intermittent, e.g. from prolonged and frequent uterine contractions. Although birth asphyxia is an important cause of failure to establish breathing requiring resuscitation at birth, there are other causes, including birth trauma, maternal analgesic or anaesthetic agents, retained lung fluid, preterm infant, or a congenital malformation, which interfere with breathing.

The Apgar score is used to describe a baby's condition at 1 minute and 5 minutes after delivery (Table 10.2). It is also measured at 5-minute intervals thereafter if the infant's condition remains poor. The most important components are the heart rate and respiration.

Neonatal resuscitation

Most infants do not require any resuscitation. Shortly after birth, the baby will take a breath or cry, establish regular breathing and become pink. The baby can be handed directly to his or her mother, dried, and covered to maintain a normal body temperature (36.5–37.5°C). The need for resuscitation can usually be anticipated e.g. preterm delivery, and preparations made before delivery (Fig. 10.10a). A newborn infant who does not establish normal respiration directly will need to be transferred to a resuscitation table for further assessment. There should be an overhead radiant heater and the infant should be dried and partially covered and kept warm. Suction of the mouth and nose is usually unnecessary and vigorous suction of the back of the throat may provoke bradycardia from vagal stimulation and should be avoided. If the infant's breathing in the 1st minute of life is irregular or shallow, but the heart rate is satisfactory (>100 beats/min), breathing is encouraged with airway opening manoeuvres.

If the infant does not start to breathe, or if the heart rate drops below 100 beats/minute, airway positioning and lung inflation by mask ventilation should be started (Fig. 10.10b–d). If the baby's condition does not improve promptly, or if the infant is clearly in very poor condition at birth, additional assistance should be summoned immediately while continuing to maintain ventilation. Oxygen saturation and ECG monitoring should be considered.

If the heart rate drops below 60 beats/minute after five effective inflation breaths and 30 seconds of effective ventilation, chest compressions should be given (Fig. 10.10k). If the response to ventilation and chest compression remains inadequate, drugs should be given, but are rarely required (Fig. 10.10o). Evidence for their efficacy is very poor.

If the infant does not respond to airway manoeuvres and mask ventilation or the infant is in very poor condition, tracheal intubation may need to be performed (Fig. 10.10j). This should result in a rapid rise in heart rate and breathing should be established. If this is not the case, the reasons listed in Box 10.5 should be considered.

> **Providing effective lung inflation, shown by good chest wall movement, is the key to successful neonatal resuscitation**

a) Newborn Life Support – Preparation

- All health professionals dealing with newborn infants should be proficient in basic resuscitation i.e. **A**irway, **B**reathing with mask ventilation, **C**irculation with cardiac compressions
- Additional skilled assistance is needed if the baby does not respond rapidly and should be called without delay
- The need for resuscitation can usually be anticipated and a person proficient in advanced resuscitation should be in attendance at all high-risk deliveries
- A clock should be started at birth for accurate timing of changes in the infant's condition
- Keep the infant warm. Dry the infant, remove the wet towel and replace with dry one. This will also provide stimulation. Can place directly on mother's chest and covered if crying, good tone and colour and desired by the mother
- Resuscitation should be performed under a radiant warmer
- If preterm and <32 weeks' gestation, to avoid heat loss, place the infant in a plastic bag without drying but under a radiant warmer and on a warm mattress. Leave the head exposed and cover with a hat.
- Assess the infant's condition. Is the baby breathing or crying, good heart rate (>100 beats/min, best assessed by listening with a stethoscope), good colour and muscle tone?
- If not, commence neonatal resuscitation

b) Newborn life support – overview

Always needed →

- Start the clock
- Dry the baby
- **Assess** – breathing, heart rate (tone)

Airway
Breathing – 5 inflation breaths

Check airway and breathing
Repeat inflation breaths

Chest compressions

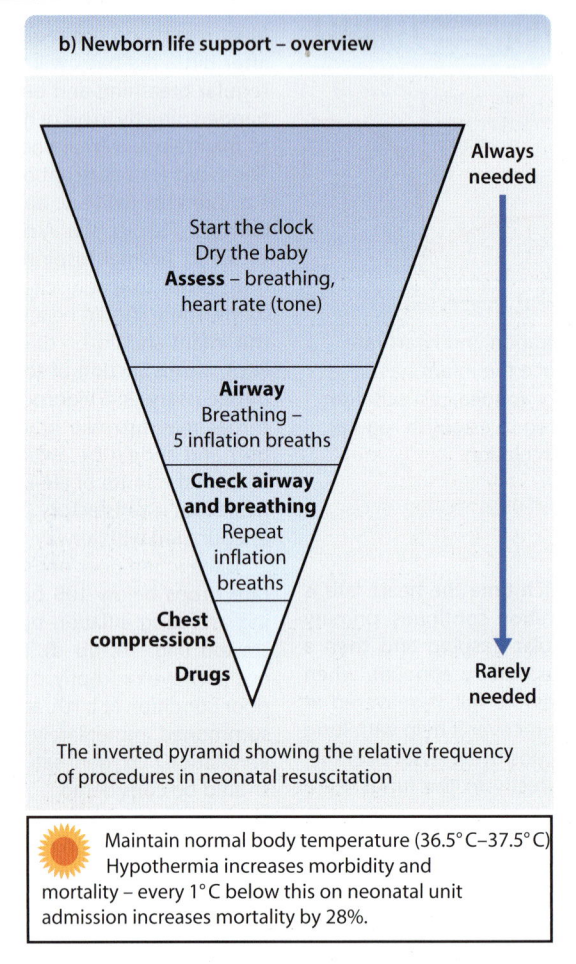

Drugs

← Rarely needed

The inverted pyramid showing the relative frequency of procedures in neonatal resuscitation

> Maintain normal body temperature (36.5°C–37.5°C) Hypothermia increases morbidity and mortality – every 1°C below this on neonatal unit admission increases mortality by 28%.

Figure 10.10 Neonatal resuscitation. (From *Newborn Life Support*, 2015, Resuscitation Council (UK) with permission)

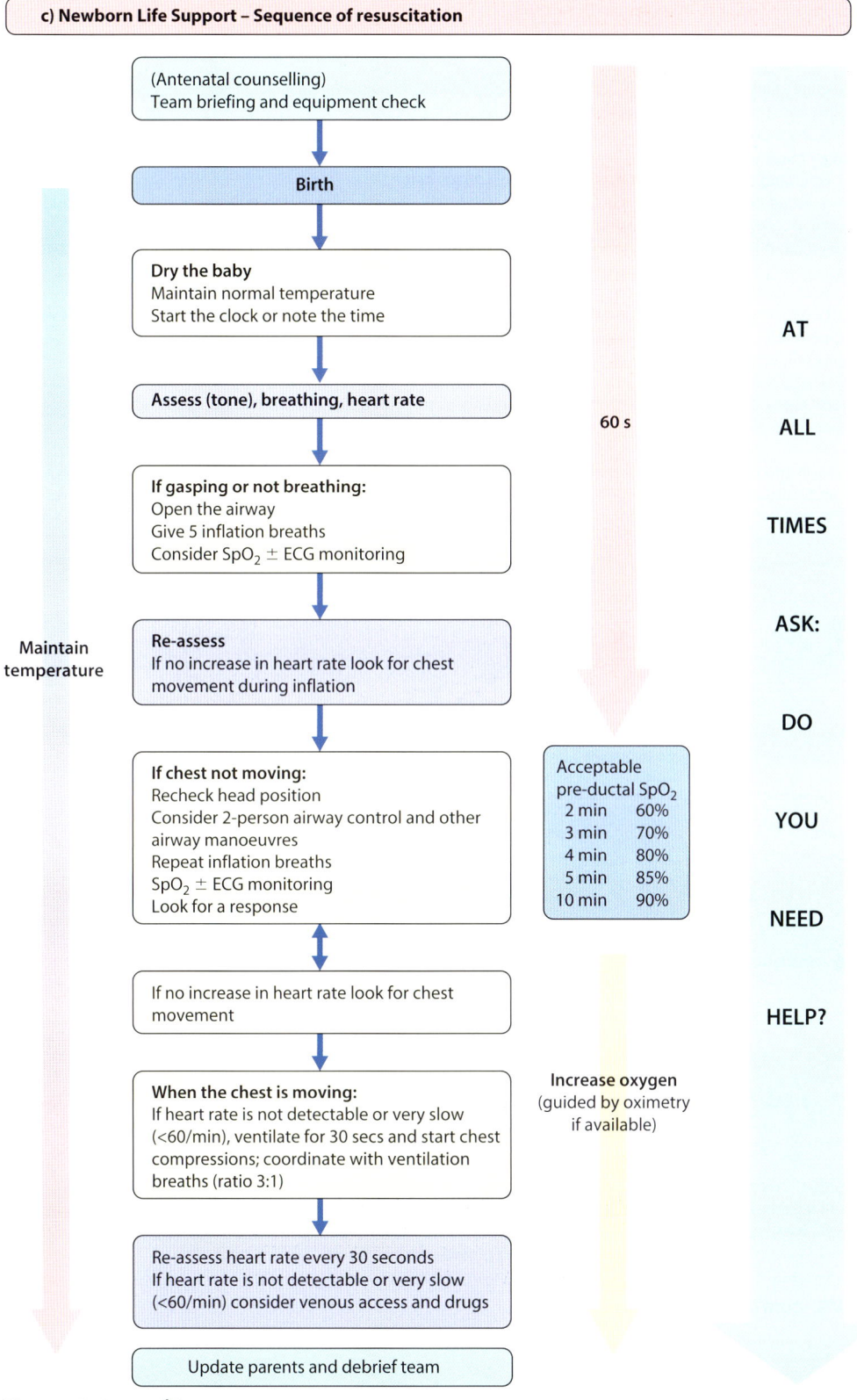

c) Newborn Life Support – Sequence of resuscitation

```
(Antenatal counselling)
Team briefing and equipment check
            ↓
          Birth
            ↓
Dry the baby
Maintain normal temperature
Start the clock or note the time
            ↓
Assess (tone), breathing, heart rate
            ↓
If gasping or not breathing:
Open the airway
Give 5 inflation breaths
Consider SpO₂ ± ECG monitoring
            ↓
Re-assess
If no increase in heart rate look for chest
movement during inflation
            ↓
If chest not moving:
Recheck head position
Consider 2-person airway control and other
airway manoeuvres
Repeat inflation breaths
SpO₂ ± ECG monitoring
Look for a response
            ↕
If no increase in heart rate look for chest
movement
            ↓
When the chest is moving:
If heart rate is not detectable or very slow
(<60/min), ventilate for 30 secs and start chest
compressions; coordinate with ventilation
breaths (ratio 3:1)
            ↓
Re-assess heart rate every 30 seconds
If heart rate is not detectable or very slow
(<60/min) consider venous access and drugs
            ↓
Update parents and debrief team
```

Maintain temperature

60 s

Acceptable pre-ductal SpO₂	
2 min	60%
3 min	70%
4 min	80%
5 min	85%
10 min	90%

Increase oxygen
(guided by oximetry
if available)

AT ALL TIMES ASK: DO YOU NEED HELP?

Figure 10.10, cont'd.

Continued

d) Newborn Life Support – Airway and Breathing

Airway
- Opened by placing the infants's head in a neutral position (e). Place some support under shoulders if necessary
- Provide chin lift or jaw thrust if necessary (f)
- Suction any blood or secretions under direct vision if blocking airway.

Breathing – mask ventilation
- If not breathing adequately, start mask ventilation. Call for help
- Mask is placed over mouth and nose (g) and connected to flow-controlled pressure-limited circuit (e.g. mechanical ventilator or Neopuff) or self-inflating bag (h)
- Give 5 inflation breaths, inflation time 2–3 seconds at inspiratory pressure of 30 cmH$_2$O in term infants to expand lungs
- Monitor heart rate with ECG and oxygen saturation with pre-ductal (right hand) pulse oximeter if indicated
- If heart rate increases, but breathing does not start, continue with peak inspiratory pressure to achieve chest wall movement (15–25 cmH$_2$O, 0.5 second inflation time) and rate of 30–40 breaths/min
- Begin ventilatory resuscitation in air to avoid excessive tissue oxygenation. Titrate additional oxygen with oxygen saturation.
- Reassess every 30 seconds. If heart rate not responding, ensure adequate chest movement. Consider using two-person airway control (i).

Intubation
- Intubation and mechanical ventilation (j) are indicated if: mask ventilation is ineffective, tracheal suction needed to clear an obstructed airway or congenital upper airway abnormality. Intubation may also be performed to give surfactant to extremely preterm infants.
- Limit intubation attempts to 20–30 seconds.

(e) Head position, vital for airway management

i) Head in correct, neutral airway position – incorrect iii) Head flexed – incorrect ii) Head over-extended

(f) Chin lift   Jaw thrust

(g) Correct size and position of the face mask. It should cover the mouth, nose, and chin

Correct
Covers mouth, nose, and chin but not eyes

Incorrect
Too large – covers eyes and extends over chin

Incorrect
Too small – does not cover nose and mouth completely

(h) Mask ventilation

Pressure-limited air/oxygen

Mask ventilation delivered with pressure-limited circuit via T-piece (as shown), Neopuff or self-inflating bag.

(i) Two-person airway control

Consider if mask inflation ineffective. One person holds the head in the correct position, applies jaw thrust and holds the mask in place. The assistant operates the T-piece to provide lung inflation.

(j) Tracheal intubation

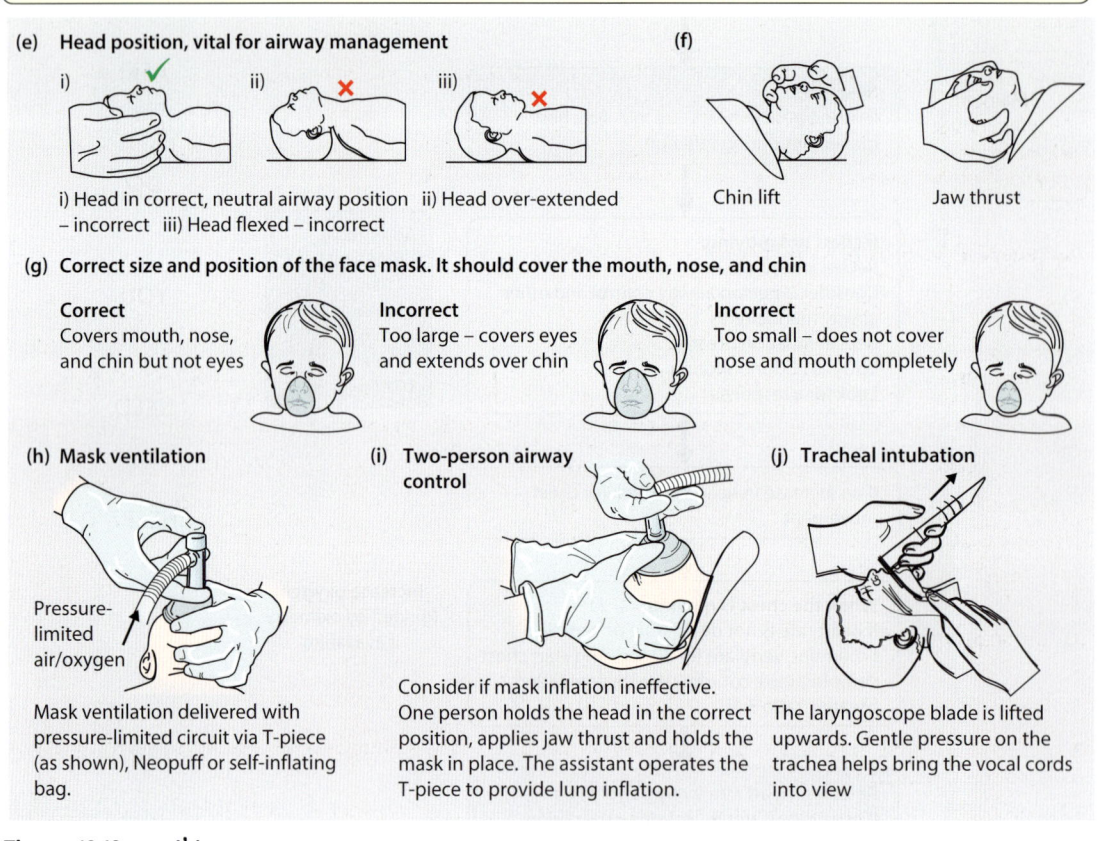

The laryngoscope blade is lifted upwards. Gentle pressure on the trachea helps bring the vocal cords into view

Figure 10.10, cont'd.

k) Circulation

Chest compression (l, m and n)
- Start if heart rate <60 beats/min in spite of effective lung inflation
- Ratio of compression: lung inflation of 3:1, rate of 90 compressions: 30 breaths/min (120 events/min) – avoid compressing chest during a ventilation breath.
- Recheck heart rate every 30 seconds; stop when heart rate >60 beats/min

(l) Chest compression
Landmarks for chest compression

Apply pressure to lower third of sternum, just below imaginary line joining the nipples. Depress to reduce antero-posterior diameter by one-third (1–1.5 cm).

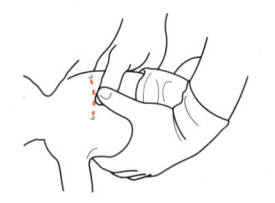

(m) Thumb technique, with hands encircling the chest. In larger infants thumbs can be placed side by side.

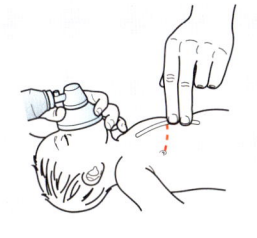

(n) Two-finger technique – less effective but easier if alone.

o) Volume and drugs

Consider drugs (p) if heart rate <60 beats/min in spite of adequate ventilation and chest compression, though evidence for their efficacy is lacking and they are rarely needed.
Drugs should ideally be given centrally via an umbilical venous catheter, or, if not possible, via an intraosseous needle.
If hypovolaemic, 0.9% sodium chloride or blood transfusion with Group O rhesus negative blood may be required; there may be a history of antepartum haemorrhage or acute twin-to-twin transfusion

(q) Drugs used in neonatal resuscitation

Drug	Concentration	Route/dosage	Indications
Epinephrine (adrenaline)	1:10 000	IV: 0.1 ml/kg (10 µg/kg), then 0.1–0.3 ml/kg (10–30 µg/kg) ET: 0.5–1ml/kg (50–100 µg/kg), i.e. 5–10 times the IV dose, whilst IV access is obtained	Heart rate <60 beats/min in spite of adequate ventilation and external cardiac compression
Sodium bicarbonate	4.2%	2–4 ml/kg (1–2 mmol/kg)	Severe lactic acidosis
Dextrose	10%	2.5 ml/kg (250 mg/kg)	Hypoglycaemia
Volume expander	0.9% Sodium chloride Blood	10 ml/kg, repeat if necessary	Blood loss

Figure 10.10, cont'd.

Box 10.5 Conditions to consider if, after tracheal intubation, the heart rate does not increase and good chest movement is not achieved

For this purpose, the mnemonic 'DOPE' may be used:
- **d**isplaced tube: often in the oesophagus or right main bronchus
- **o**bstructed tube: especially meconium
- **p**atient:
  - tracheal obstruction
  - lung disorders: lung immaturity or respiratory distress syndrome, pneumothorax, diaphragmatic hernia, lung hypoplasia, pleural effusion
  - shock from blood loss
  - perinatal asphyxia or trauma
  - upper airways obstruction: choanal atresia.
- **e**quipment failure: gas supply exhausted or disconnected

If there is any uncertainty about the adequacy of ventilation in an intubated baby, consider removing the tracheal tube, give mask ventilation, and then re-intubate if necessary.

Meconium aspiration

The passage of meconium becomes increasingly common the greater the infant's gestational age, particularly when post-term. Infants who become acidotic may inhale thick meconium and develop meconium aspiration syndrome. Attempting to aspirate meconium from the nose and mouth while the infant's head is on the perineum is not recommended, as it is ineffective. If the infant cries at birth and establishes regular respiration, no resuscitation is required. If respiration is not established, initiating lung inflation within the 1st minute of life is the priority. If the baby was born through thick meconium, it is reasonable to inspect the oropharynx rapidly and remove any thick meconium by suctioning with a large-bore suction catheter, but if the infant becomes bradycardic, positive pressure ventilation to aerate the lungs is indicated despite the presence of meconium.

Resuscitation of the preterm infant

Preterm infants are particularly liable to hypothermia, and every effort must be made to keep them warm during resuscitation. Infants of less than 30 weeks' gestation should, with the exception of the face, be placed into a plastic bag or wrapped in clear plastic sheeting without drying to allow the plastic to cling to the skin. A radiant heat source from the resuscitation table and/or thermal mattress can then warm the baby in the bag/wrap, which acts almost like another layer of skin by avoiding evaporative heat loss. Excessive tissue oxygenation may cause tissue damage to the brain, lungs and eyes from oxygen-free radicals. Whereas air is used for initial resuscitation in term infants, a low concentration (21–30%) should be used for preterm infants. An air/oxygen mixer should be used and any additional oxygen given should be titrated against oxygen saturation, thus avoiding exceeding a preductal saturation of 95%. Preterm infants less than 30 weeks' gestation may benefit from non-invasive respiratory support in the form of CPAP (continuous positive airways pressure) to avoid the need for intubation. Very premature infants may develop respiratory distress syndrome, and early tracheal administration of artificial surfactant may be indicated. Resuscitation of infants at the threshold of viability, at 22–24 weeks' gestation, raises particularly difficult ethical and management issues. An experienced paediatrician should be responsible for counselling the parents before delivery, if possible, and lead the management of the baby after birth.

Post-resuscitation care

If, following resuscitation, the baby is significantly preterm or ill, the infant will need to be stabilized before transfer to the neonatal unit [see Ch. 11 (Newborn medicine)]. Particular attention needs to be paid to provide adequate respiratory support and to the prevention of hypothermia and hypoglycaemia.

Failure to respond to resuscitation

The decision to stop resuscitation is always difficult and should be made by a senior paediatrician. The longer it takes a baby to respond to resuscitation, the less likely is survival. If there is no breathing or cardiac output after 10 minutes of effective resuscitation, further efforts are likely to be unproductive and consideration should be given to stop resuscitation. If prolonged resuscitation has been required, the infant should be transferred to the neonatal unit for assessment and monitoring.

Size at birth

An infant's gestation and birthweight influence the nature of the medical problems likely to be encountered in the neonatal period. In the UK, 7% of babies are of low birthweight (<2.5 kg). However, they account for approximately 70% of neonatal deaths.

Definitions

Babies with a birthweight below the 10th centile for their gestational age are called small for gestational age or small-for-dates (Fig. 10.11). The majority of these infants are normal, but small. The incidence of congenital abnormalities and neonatal problems is higher in those whose birthweight falls below the second centile (approximately two standard deviations below the mean), and some authorities restrict the term to this group of babies. An infant's birthweight may also be low because of preterm birth, or because the infant is both preterm and small for gestational age.

Small for gestational age infants may have grown normally but are small, or they may have experienced IUGR, i.e. they have failed to reach their full genetically determined growth potential and appear thin and malnourished. Babies with a birthweight above the 10th centile may also be malnourished, e.g. a fetus growing along the 80th centile that develops growth failure and whose weight falls to the 20th centile.

Patterns of growth restriction

Growth restriction in both the fetus and infant has traditionally been classified as symmetrical or asymmetrical. In the more common asymmetrical growth restriction, the weight or abdominal circumference lies on a lower centile than that of the head. This occurs when the placenta fails to provide adequate nutrition late in pregnancy but brain growth is relatively spared at the expense of liver glycogen and skin fat (Fig. 10.12). This form of growth restriction is associated with uteroplacental dysfunction secondary to maternal pre-eclampsia, multiple pregnancies, maternal smoking or it may be idiopathic. These infants rapidly put on weight after birth. However, this is associated with an increased risk of obesity and type 2 diabetes in later life.

In symmetrical growth restriction, the head circumference is equally reduced. It suggests a prolonged

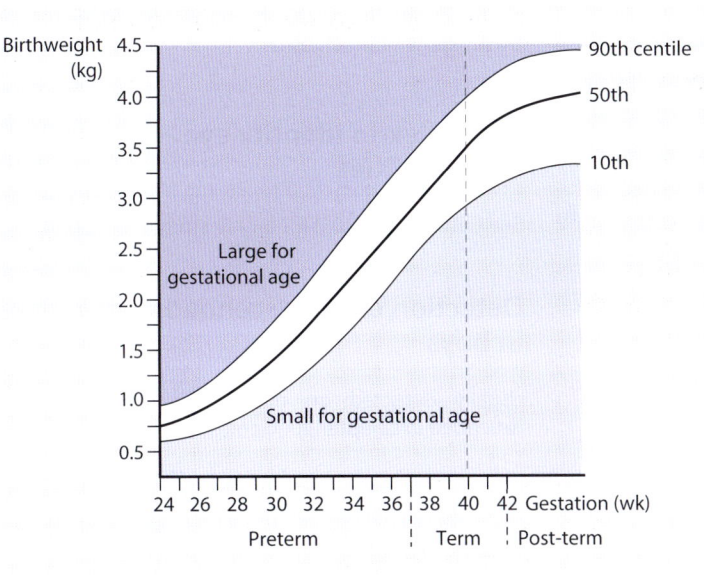

Figure 10.11 The birthweight of small for gestational age infants is below the 10th centile for their gestation. Small for gestational age infants may be preterm, term, or post-term.

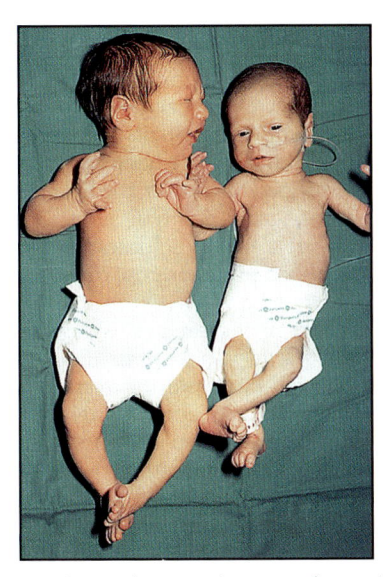

Figure 10.12 Severe intrauterine growth restriction in a twin.

period of poor intrauterine growth starting in early pregnancy (or that the gestational age is incorrect). It is usually due to a small but normal fetus, but may be due to a fetal chromosomal disorder or syndrome, a congenital infection, maternal drug and alcohol abuse, a maternal chronic medical condition or malnutrition. These infants are more likely to remain small permanently.

In practice, distinction between asymmetrical and symmetrical growth restriction often cannot be made.

Monitoring the growth-restricted fetus

The fetus with IUGR is at risk from:
- intrauterine hypoxia and 'unexplained' intrauterine death
- asphyxia during labour and delivery.

The growth-restricted fetus will need to be monitored closely to determine the optimal time for delivery. Progressive uteroplacental failure results in:
- reduced growth in femur length and abdominal circumference
- oligohydramnios from reduced fetal urine production
- abnormal umbilical artery Doppler waveforms – absent or reversed end-diastolic flow velocity, due to increased placental impedance
- redistribution of blood flow in the fetus – increased flow to the brain, reduced flow to the gastrointestinal tract, liver, skin and kidneys
- abnormal ductus venosus Doppler waveform from cardiac dysfunction
- reduced fetal breathing and movements
- abnormal fetal heart rate trace.

The growth-restricted infant

After birth, these infants are liable to:
- hypothermia because of their relatively large surface area (especially their head)
- hypoglycaemia from poor fat and glycogen stores
- hypocalcaemia
- polycythaemia (venous haematocrit >0.65).

> **Summary**
>
> **Size at birth**
> - Small for gestational age – birthweight <10th centile.
> - IUGR – fails to reach genetically determined growth potential.
> - Growth restriction – symmetrical or asymmetrical, but often mixed.

Perinatal medicine

159

Large for gestational age infants

Large-for-gestational-age infants are those above the 90th weight centile for their gestation. Most are normal, large infants, but is a feature of infants of mothers with either type 1 or gestational diabetes or a baby with certain congenital syndromes (e.g. Beckwith–Wiedemann syndrome). The problems associated with being large for gestational age are:

- birth trauma, especially from shoulder dystocia at delivery (difficulty delivering the shoulders from impaction behind maternal symphysis pubis)
- birth asphyxia from a difficult delivery
- hypoglycaemia due to hyperinsulinism
- polycythaemia
- breathing difficulty from an enlarged tongue in Beckwith–Wiedemann syndrome.

Routine examination of the newborn infant

Immediately after a baby is born, parents are naturally anxious to know if their baby is alright and appears normal. To answer this, the midwife (or the paediatrician or obstetrician, if present) will briefly but carefully check that the baby is pink, breathing normally and has no major abnormalities. If a significant problem is identified, an experienced paediatrician must explain the situation to the parents. If the baby is markedly preterm, small or ill, admission to a neonatal unit will be required. Should there be any uncertainty about the child's sex, it is important not to guess but to explain to the parents that further tests are necessary. Babies are given vitamin K at birth to prevent haemorrhagic disease of the newborn unless parents will not give consent.

Within 72 hours of birth every baby should have a full and thorough examination, the 'routine examination of the newborn infant'. Its purpose is to:

- detect congenital abnormalities not already identified at birth, e.g. eye abnormalities, congenital heart disease, undescended testis or developmental dysplasia of the hip (DDH)
- check for potential problems arising from maternal disease or familial disorders
- provide an opportunity for the parents to discuss any questions about their baby.

Before approaching the mother and baby, the obstetric and neonatal notes must be checked to identify relevant information. The examination (Box 10.6) should be performed with the mother or ideally both parents present. Many findings in the newborn resolve spontaneously (Box 10.7). Common significant abnormalities detectable at birth are listed in Box 10.8. A serious congenital anomaly is present at birth in about 10/1000–15/1000 live births (Table 10.3). In addition, many congenital anomalies, especially of the heart, present clinically at a later age. In the UK, the newborn examination is repeated at 6–8-weeks of age, usually by the general practitioner.

Red reflex to identify eye abnormalities

See Case History 10.2 for a case study on red reflex.

Detection of undescended testes in boys

Usually detected on newborn examination. It is described in Chapter 20 (Genital disorders).

Checking for developmental dysplasia of the hip (DDH)

To check for DDH, (previously called congenital dislocation of the hip), the infant needs to be relaxed, as kicking or crying results in tightening of the muscles around the hip and prevents satisfactory examination. The pelvis is stabilized with one hand. With the other hand, the examiner's middle finger is placed over the greater trochanter and the thumb around the distal medial femur. In the Barlow manoeuvre, the hip is held flexed and the femoral head is gently adducted and pushed downwards. If the hip is dislocatable, the femoral head will be pushed posteriorly out of the acetabulum (Fig. 10.18a).

The next part of the examination is the Ortolani manoeuvre to see if the hip can be returned from its dislocated position back into the acetabulum. While gently abducting the hip, upward leverage is applied (Fig. 10.18b). A dislocated hip will return with a 'clunk' into the acetabulum. Ligamentous clicks without any movement of the head of femur are of no significance. It should also be possible to abduct the hips fully, but this may be restricted if the hip is dislocated. Clinical examination does not identify some infants who have hip dysplasia from lack of development of the acetabular shelf. DDH is more common in girls (six-fold increase), if there is a positive family history (20% of affected infants), if the birth is a breech presentation (30% of affected infants) or if the infant has a neuromuscular disorder.

Early recognition of DDH is important as early splinting in abduction reduces long-term morbidity. A specialist orthopaedic opinion should be sought in the management of this condition. Ultrasound examination of the hip joint is performed increasingly in many hospitals, either following an abnormal hip examination, the presence of neuromuscular disorder in the lower legs or talipes equinovarus, or to screen babies at increased risk (breech presentation or positive family history). Ultrasound examination can be performed to screen all babies, but is not currently recommended in the UK as it is expensive, requires considerable expertise and there are many false positives. It will, however, identify some babies missed on clinical examination.

Routine examination of the newborn infant

Box 10.6 Routine examination of the newborn infant

- **Birthweight, gestational age, and birthweight centile** are noted (Fig. 10.13).
- **General observation of the baby's appearance, posture, and movements** provides valuable information about many abnormalities. The baby must be fully undressed during the examination.
- **The head circumference** is measured with a paper tape measure and its centile noted. This is a surrogate measure of brain size.
- **The fontanelle** and sutures are palpated. The fontanelle size is very variable. The sagittal suture is often separated and the coronal sutures may be overriding. A tense fontanelle when the baby is not crying may be due to raised intracranial pressure and cranial ultrasound should be performed to check for hydrocephalus. A tense fontanelle is also a late sign of meningitis.
- **The face** is observed. If abnormal, this may represent a syndrome, particularly if other anomalies are present. Down syndrome is the most common, but there are hundreds of syndromes. When the diagnosis is uncertain, a book or a computer database may be consulted and advice should be sought from a senior paediatrician or geneticist.
- **If plethoric or pale**, the haematocrit should be checked to identify polycythaemia or anaemia. Central cyanosis, which always needs urgent assessment, is best seen on the tongue.
- **Jaundice** within 24 hours of birth requires further evaluation.
- **The eyes** are checked for red reflex with an ophthalmoscope. If absent, may be from cataracts (see Case History 10.2), retinoblastoma and corneal opacity. This reflex can be hard to illicit in darker skinned infants but the retinal vessels can be visualized.
- **The palate** needs to be visually inspected, including posteriorly to exclude a posterior cleft palate, and palpated to detect an indentation of the posterior palate from a submucous cleft.
- **Breathing and chest wall movement** are observed for signs of respiratory distress.
- **On auscultating the heart**, the normal rate is 110–160 beats/minute in term babies, but may drop to 85 beats/minute during sleep.
- **On palpating the abdomen**, the liver normally extends 1 cm to 2 cm below the costal margin, the spleen tip may be palpable, as may the kidney on the left side. Any intraabdominal masses, which are usually renal in origin, need further investigation.
- **The femoral pulses** are palpated. Their pulse pressure is:
  - reduced in coarctation of the aorta. This can be confirmed by measuring the blood pressure in the arms and legs
  - increased if there is a patent ductus arteriosus.
- **The genitalia and anus** are inspected on removing the nappy. Patency of the anus is confirmed. In boys, the presence of testes in the scrotum is checked by palpation.
- **Muscle tone** is assessed by observing limb movements. Most babies will support their head briefly when the trunk is held vertically.
- **The whole of the back and spine** is observed, looking for any midline defects of the skin.
- **Primitive reflexes** are checked including the grasp and Moro reflexes (Table 3.1) for asymmetric or reduced movements.
- **The hips** are checked for DDH. This is left until last as the procedure is uncomfortable.

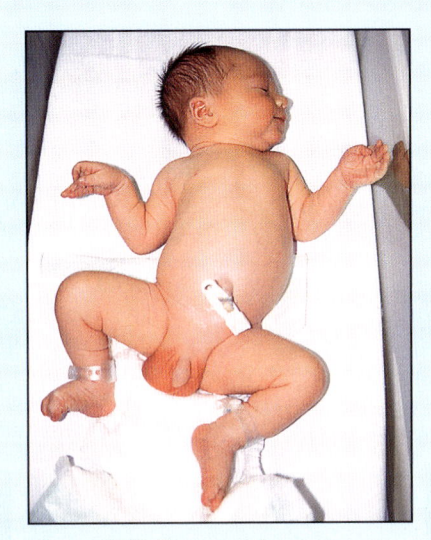

Figure 10.13 Term newborn.

Vitamin K therapy

Vitamin K deficiency may result in haemorrhagic disease of the newborn, a rare condition with an incidence of 0.6/100 000 births. This disorder can occur early, during the 1st week of life, or late, from 1–8-weeks of age. In most affected infants, the haemorrhage is mild, such as bruising, haematemesis and melaena, or prolonged bleeding of the umbilical stump or after circumcision. However, some suffer from intracranial haemorrhage, half of whom are permanently disabled or die.

Breast milk, which has many benefits to both the mother and her baby, is a poor source of vitamin K, whereas infant formula milk has much higher vitamin K content. Haemorrhagic disease of the newborn may occur in infants who are wholly breastfed but not if fed with an infant formula. Infants of mothers taking anticonvulsants, which impair the synthesis of vitamin

Lesions in newborn infants that resolve spontaneously

Box 10.7 Lesions in newborn infants that resolve spontaneously

Peripheral cyanosis of the hands and feet – common in the 1st day.

Traumatic cyanosis from a cord around the baby's neck or from a face or brow presentation – causes blue discolouration of the skin, petechiae over the head and neck or affected part but not the tongue.

Swollen eyelids and distortion of shape of the head from the delivery.

Subconjunctival haemorrhages – occur during delivery but should be documented to avoid confusion with non-accidental injury when older.

Small white pearls along the midline of the palate (Epstein pearls).

Cysts of the gums (epulis) or floor of the mouth (ranula).

Breast enlargement – may occur in newborn babies of either sex (Fig. 10.14a). A small amount of milk may be discharged.

White vaginal discharge or small withdrawal bleed in girls. There may be a prolapse of a ring of vaginal mucosa.

Capillary haemangioma or 'stork bites' – pink macules on the upper eyelids, midforehead, and nape of the neck are common and arise from distension of the dermal capillaries. Those on the eyelids gradually fade over the 1st year; those on the neck become covered with hair.

Neonatal urticaria (erythema toxicum) – a common rash appearing at 2–3-days of age, consisting of white pinpoint papules at the centre of an erythematous base (Fig. 10.14b). The fluid contains eosinophils. The lesions are concentrated on the trunk; they come and go at different sites.

Milia – white pimples on the nose and cheeks, from retention of keratin and sebaceous material in the pilosebaceous follicles (Fig. 10.14c).

Mongolian blue spots – blue/black macular discolouration at the base of the spine and on the buttocks (Fig. 10.14d); occasionally occur on the legs and other parts of the body. Usually but not invariably in Afro-Caribbean or Asian infants. They fade slowly over the first few years. They are of no significance unless misdiagnosed as bruises.

Umbilical hernia – common, particularly in Afro-Caribbean infants. No treatment is indicated as it usually resolves within the first 2–3-years.

Positional talipes – the feet often remain in their in utero position. Unlike true talipes equinovarus, the foot can be fully dorsiflexed to touch the front of the lower leg (Fig. 10.14e and f).

Caput succedaneum (see Fig. 11.6) and **cephalhaematoma** (Figs. 11.6 and 11.7).

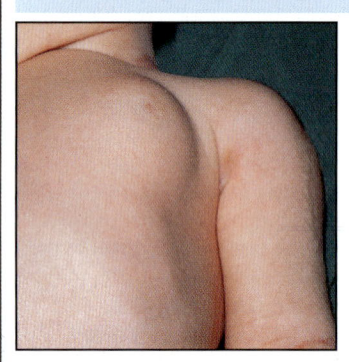

Figure 10.14a Breast enlargement in a newborn infant.

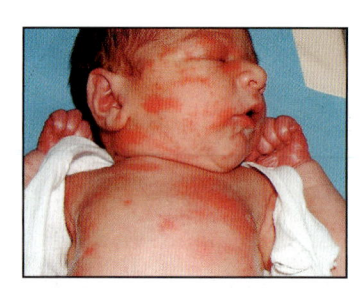

Figure 10.14b Erythema toxicum (neonatal urticaria) often has a raised pale centre (Courtesy of Nim Subhedar.)

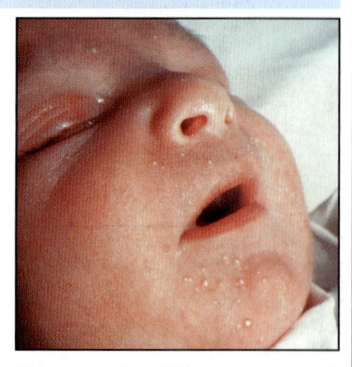

Figure 10.14c Milia (Courtesy of Rodney Rivers.)

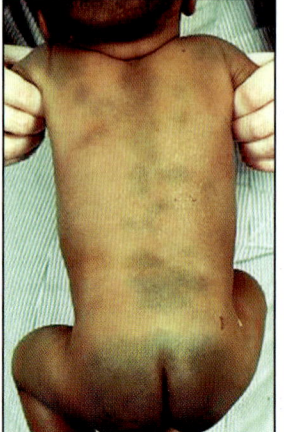

Figure 10.14d Mongolian blue spot.

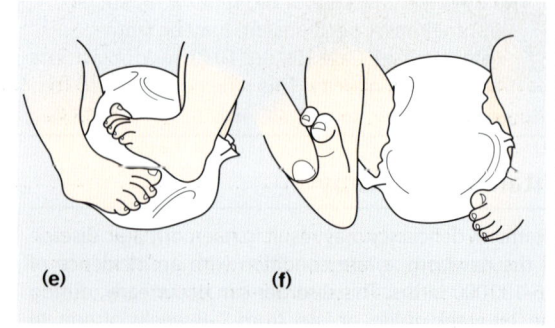

Figure 10.14e Positional talipes. Appearance at birth.

Figure 10.14f The foot can be fully dorsiflexed to touch the front of the lower leg. In true talipes equinovarus this is not possible.

Some significant abnormalities detected on routine examination

Box 10.8 Some significant abnormalities detected on routine examination

- **Port-wine stain (naevus flammeus).** Present from birth and usually grows with the infant (Fig. 10.15a). It is due to a vascular malformation of the capillaries in the dermis. Rarely, if along the distribution of the trigeminal nerve, it may be associated with intracranial vascular anomalies (Sturge–Weber syndrome), or severe lesions on the limbs with bone hypertrophy (Klippel–Trenaunay syndrome). Disfiguring lesions can now be improved with laser therapy.
- **Strawberry naevus (cavernous haemangioma).** Usually not present at birth, but appear in the 1st month of life and may be multiple (Fig. 10.15b). They are more common in preterm infants. Increase in size until 3–15-months of age, then gradually regress. No treatment is indicated for small lesions, but topical propranolol may speed regression. Large lesions or if interferes with vision or the airway are treated with oral propranolol. Ulceration or haemorrhage may occur.
- **Natal teeth consisting of the front lower incisors** – may be present at birth. If loose, they should be removed to avoid the risk of aspiration.
- **Extra digits** – are sometimes connected by a thin skin tag but may be completely attached containing bone (Fig. 10.15c) and should ideally be removed by a plastic surgeon or else tied off at its base. Skin tags anterior to the ear and accessory auricles should be removed by a plastic surgeon.
- **Heart murmur** – poses a difficult problem, as most murmurs audible in the first few days of life resolve shortly afterwards. However, some are caused by congenital heart disease. If there are any features of a significant murmur (see Ch. 18), upper and lower limb blood pressures, and pre-ductal and post-ductal pulse oximetry should be checked followed by an echocardiogram. Otherwise, a follow-up examination is arranged and the parents warned to seek medical assistance if their baby feeds poorly, develops laboured breathing, or becomes cyanosed.
- **Midline abnormality over the spine or skull**, such as a tuft of hair, swelling, or naevus – requires further evaluation as it may indicate an underlying abnormality of the vertebrae, spinal cord, or brain.
- **Palpable and large bladder** – if there is urinary outflow obstruction, particularly in boys with posterior urethral valves. Requires prompt evaluation with ultrasound. Usually diagnosed on antenatal ultrasound.
- **Talipes equinovarus** – cannot be corrected as in positional talipes.

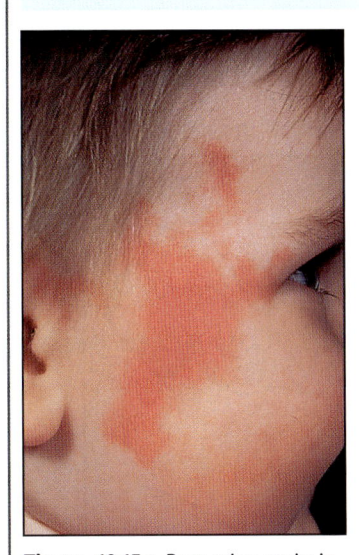

Figure 10.15a Port-wine stain in an infant.

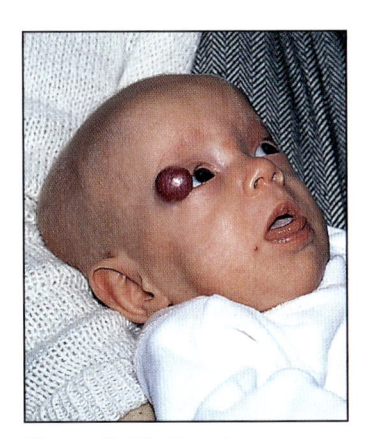

Figure 10.15b Strawberry naevus.

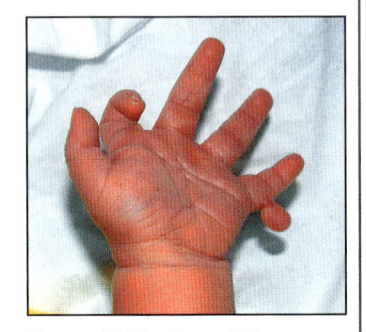

Figure 10.15c Extra digits.

K-dependent clotting factors, are at increased risk of haemorrhagic disease, both during delivery and soon after birth. Infants with liver disease are also at increased risk.

The disease can be prevented if vitamin K is given by intramuscular injection, and in the UK, it was widely given to all newborn infants immediately after birth. In the early 1990s, one study suggested a possible association between vitamin K given intramuscularly and the development of cancer in childhood, but this has not been found in other much larger studies. It is recommended that all newborn infants are given intramuscular vitamin K. However, parents may request oral vitamin K as an alternative. As absorption via the

Case history 10.2

Congenital cataract

On checking for red reflexes (Fig. 10.16) during the routine newborn examination, bilateral absent red reflexes were noted in a male term baby (see Fig. 10.7a). The remainder of the examination was normal. Urgent ophthalmology review confirmed bilateral congenital cataracts (presumed idiopathic, but many are genetic). These occur in about 3–4/10,000 live births and is responsible for about 10% of blindness in children worldwide. Early surgical treatment in the first few weeks of life improves long-term visual function. Other eye abnormalities that may be detected are congenital glaucoma (Fig. 10.17a) and coloboma (Fig. 10.17b).

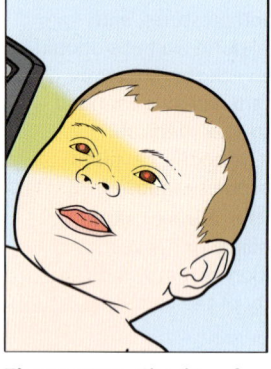

Figure 10.16 Checking for red reflex. Done by examining the eyes through a direct ophthalmoscope 15–20 cm from the eyes.

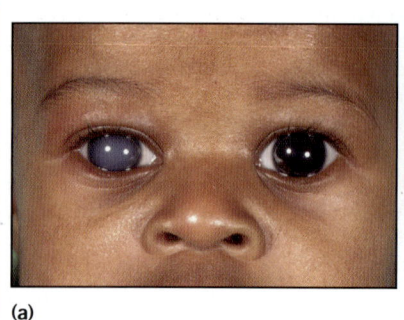

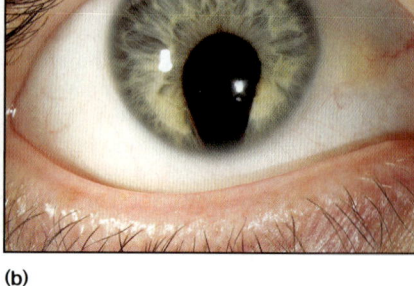

Figure 10.17 Eye abnormalities on newborn examination. (**a**) Congenital glaucoma of right eye (Courtesy of Alistair Fielder. And (**b**) iris coloboma. Keyhole-shaped pupil due to defect of the iris inferiorly (Courtesy of Louise Allen)

Checking for developmental dysplasia of the hip (DDH)

Barlow manoeuvre

(a)

(b)

Femoral head dislocated posteriorly out of acetabulum

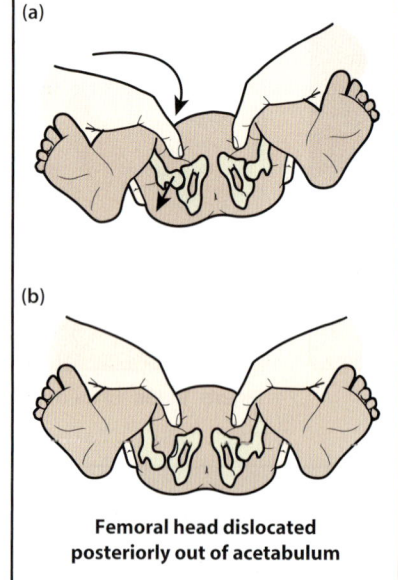

Figure 10.18a The hip is dislocated posteriorly out of the acetabulum (Barlow manoeuvre).

Ortolani manoeuvre

(a)

(b)

Dislocated femoral head relocated back into acetabulum

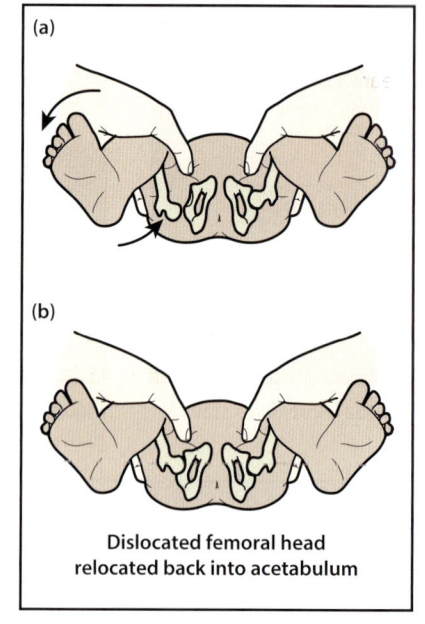

Figure 10.18b The dislocated hip is relocated back into the acetabulum (Ortolani manoeuvre).

Table 10.3 Prevalence of serious congenital anomalies per 1000 live births (England and Wales)

Anomaly	Prevalence
Congenital heart disease	6–8 (0.8 on the 1st day of life)
DDH	1.5 (but about 6/1000 have an abnormal initial clinical examination)
Talipes	1.0
Down syndrome	1.0
Cleft lip and palate	0.8
Urogenital (hypospadias, undescended testes)	1.2
Spina bifida/anencephaly	0.1

oral route is variable, three doses are needed over the first 4 weeks of life to achieve adequate liver storage. Mothers on anticonvulsant therapy should receive oral prophylaxis from 36 weeks' gestation and the baby should be given intramuscular vitamin K.

> Vitamin K should be given to all newborn infants to prevent haemorrhagic disease of the newborn

Newborn hearing screening

Universal screening has been introduced in the UK to detect severe hearing impairment in newborn infants. Early detection and intervention improves speech and language. Otoacoustic emission (OAE) testing, in which an earphone is placed over the ear and a sound is emitted, which evokes an echo or emission from the ear if cochlear function is normal, is used as the initial screening test. If a normal test result is not achieved, referral is made to a paediatric audiologist. Testing with auditory brainstem response (ABR) audiometry, using computer analysis of electroencephalogram waveforms evoked in response to a series of clicks, may be performed [see Ch. 3 (Normal child development, hearing, and vision) for further details].

> Newborn hearing screening is performed on all infants to detect severe hearing impairment

Oxygen saturation screening for critical congenital heart disease

Is increasingly performed in the first 24 hours of life to identify duct-dependent congenital heart disease as early diagnosis and treatment can prevent collapse when the duct closes at 24–48-hours after birth. A low post-ductal oxygen saturation or an abnormally large difference between pre-ductal (right hand) and post-ductal measurement prompts medical review and echocardiography. A low oxygen saturation may also occur with respiratory disease or sepsis.

Biochemical screening

Biochemical newborn screening (previously called the Guthrie test) is performed on every baby. A blood sample, usually a heel prick, is taken when feeding has been established on days 5–7 of life. In the UK, all infants are screened for:

- congenital hypothyroidism
- haemoglobinopathies (sickle cell and thalassaemia)
- cystic fibrosis
- six inherited metabolic diseases:
  - phenylketonuria
  - MCAD (Medium-chain acyl-coenzyme A dehydrogenase deficiency)
  - maple syrup urine disease
  - isovaleric acidaemia
  - glutaric aciduria type 1
  - homocystinuria.

Details about the inborn errors of metabolism are described in Chapter 27 (Inborn errors of metabolism). Screening for cystic fibrosis is performed by measuring the serum immunoreactive trypsin, which is raised if there is pancreatic duct obstruction. If raised, DNA analysis is also performed to reduce the false-positive rate [see Ch. 17 (Respiratory disorders)].

> In the UK, biochemical screening is performed on all babies to identify congenital hypothyroidism, haemoglobinopathies, cystic fibrosis and six inborn errors of metabolism

Acknowledgements

We would like to acknowledge contributors to this chapter in previous editions, whose work we have drawn on: Tom Lissauer (1st, 2nd, 3rd, 4th Editions), Karen Simmer (1st Edition), Michael Weindling (2nd Edition), Andrew Whitelaw (3rd Edition), Andrew Wilkinson (4th Edition).

Further reading

Lissauer T, Fanaroff A, Miall L, et al.: *Neonatology at a Glance*, ed 3, Oxford, 2015, Wiley Blackwell.

Rennie JM: *Roberton's Textbook of Neonatology*, Edinburgh, 2012, Churchill Livingstone.

Websites (Accessed November 2016)

Newborn Life Support: Available at: www.resus.org.uk. *Resuscitation Council, UK.*

11

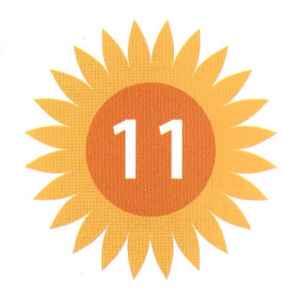

Neonatal medicine

Hypoxic-ischaemic encephalopathy	167	Hypoglycaemia	189
Birth injuries	169	Neonatal seizures	189
Stabilizing the preterm or sick infant	171	Perinatal stroke	190
The preterm infant	171	Craniofacial disorders	190
Jaundice	181	Gastrointestinal disorders	191
Respiratory distress in term infants	185	Child protection and the newborn	192
Infection	187		

Features of neonatal medicine are:

- hypoxic-ischaemic encephalopathy is a major cause of death and neurodevelopmental disability worldwide
- the premature infant, especially those born at very early gestations (23–28 weeks), have many short and long-term problems
- jaundice is common in newborn infants; the aim of its management is to identify any underlying cause and prevent kernicterus
- newborn infants are particularly susceptible to group B streptococcal and other infections in the first 3 months of life

- although craniofacial and serious gastrointestinal abnormalities are usually detected on antenatal ultrasound screening, they may present in the neonatal period.

The dramatic reduction in neonatal mortality throughout the developed world has resulted from advances in the management of newborn infants together with improvements in maternal health and obstetric care. Neonatal intensive care became increasingly available in the UK from 1975, and since then the mortality of very low birthweight infants has fallen (Fig. 11.1).

Most babies do not require any additional medical care after birth and are nursed alongside their mothers

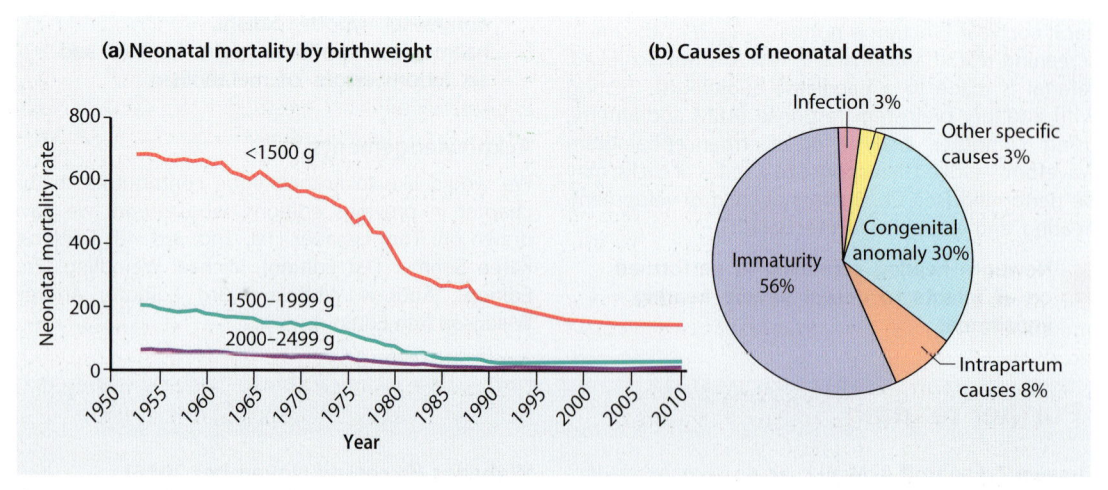

Figure 11.1 (**a**) The dramatic fall in neonatal mortality rate in England and Wales in the second half of the twentieth century, according to birthweight. In very low birthweight infants (<1500 g), the marked fall in the mortality occurred after the introduction of intensive care in the 1970's (**b**) Causes of neonatal deaths in England and Wales, 2012. (Data from ONS 2014.)

in the maternity unit. Some babies require transitional care, where some additional monitoring or care is required, e.g. if the baby is born at 33–37 weeks' gestation, this is usually provided with the baby nursed alongside his/her mother on the postnatal ward in the maternity unit. About 8–10% of babies born in the UK are admitted to a neonatal unit for special medical and nursing care, although whenever possible babies should remain on the postnatal wards to avoid separating mothers from their babies. In the UK, neonatal units are organized as networks, with units providing either:

- special care (level 1)
- short-term intensive care (level 2, local neonatal units)
- long-term intensive care (level 3, neonatal intensive care), usually linked to specialist fetal and obstetric care to form a specialist tertiary perinatal centre. About 1–3% of babies require intensive care.

Modern technology allows even tiny preterm infants to benefit from the full range of intensive care, anaesthesia, and surgery. If it is anticipated during pregnancy that the infant is likely to require long-term intensive care or surgery, it is preferable for the transfer to the tertiary centre to be made in utero. When a baby requires transfer postnatally, transport should be by an experienced team of doctors and nurses; this is often organized to serve a number of neonatal units in a regional network. Arrangements should also be made for parents to be close to their infant during this stressful time.

Hypoxic-ischaemic encephalopathy

In perinatal asphyxia, gas exchange, either placental or pulmonary, is compromised or ceases altogether, resulting in cardiorespiratory depression. Hypoxia, hypercarbia and metabolic acidosis follow. Compromised cardiac output diminishes tissue perfusion, causing hypoxic-ischaemic injury to the brain and other organs (Fig. 11.2). The neonatal condition is called hypoxic-ischaemic encephalopathy (HIE). It remains an important cause of brain damage, resulting in disability or death, and its prevention is one of the key aims of modern obstetric care. In high-income countries, approximately 0.5–1/1000 live-born term infants develop HIE and 0.3/1000 have significant neurologic disability. The incidence is higher in low and middle-income countries.

Most cases of HIE follow a significant hypoxic event immediately before or during labour or delivery. These include:

- failure of gas exchange across the placenta – excessive or prolonged uterine contractions, placental abruption, ruptured uterus
- interruption of umbilical blood flow – cord compression including shoulder dystocia, cord prolapse
- inadequate maternal placental perfusion, maternal hypotension or hypertension
- compromised fetus – intrauterine growth restriction, anaemia
- failure of cardiorespiratory adaptation at birth – failure to breathe.

The clinical manifestations start immediately or up to 48 hours after asphyxia, and can be graded:

- mild – the infant is irritable, responds excessively to stimulation, may have staring of the eyes, hyperventilation, hypertonia and has impaired feeding
- moderate – the infant shows marked abnormalities of movement, is hypotonic, cannot feed and may have seizures
- severe – there are no normal spontaneous movements or response to pain; tone in the limbs may fluctuate between hypotonia and hypertonia; seizures are prolonged and often refractory to treatment; multi-organ failure is present.

The neuronal damage may be immediate from primary neuronal death or may be delayed from reperfusion injury causing secondary neuronal death from secondary energy failure. This delay offers the opportunity for neuroprotection with mild therapeutic hypothermia. Recording of amplitude-integrated electroencephalogram (aEEG, cerebral function monitor) may be used to detect abnormal background brain activity to confirm early encephalopathy. It is also used to identify seizures.

Management

Skilled resuscitation and stabilization will minimize neuronal damage.

Infants with HIE may need (Fig. 11.2):

- respiratory support
- treatment of clinical seizures with anticonvulsants
- fluid restriction because of transient renal impairment
- treatment of hypotension by volume and inotrope support
- monitoring and treatment of hypoglycaemia and electrolyte imbalance, especially hypocalcaemia.

Recent randomized clinical trials have shown that mild hypothermia (cooling to a rectal temperature of 33°C to 34°C for 72 hours by wrapping the infant in a cooling blanket) for infants 36 weeks' gestation and over with moderate or severe HIE reduces brain damage if started within 6 hours of birth (Fig. 11.3). Analysis of these trials has demonstrated that for every eight babies cooled, one extra baby will survive without disability. Whilst cooling has become the standard therapy in the UK and many high-income countries, it requires neonatal intensive care facilities and is not available in most low and middle-income countries. Fig. 11.4 presents the outcomes of therapeutic hypothermia trials compared with standard care for the treatment of term/near-term babies with hypoxic-ischaemic encephalopathy.

Prognosis

When HIE is mild, complete recovery can be expected. Infants with moderate HIE who have recovered fully on clinical neurological examination and are feeding

Hypoxic-ischaemic encephalopathy

Figure 11.2 Pathogenesis and clinical features of severe hypoxic-ischaemic encephalopathy.

```
Hypoxia-ischaemia from failure of oxygenation across
placenta, umbilicus or postnatal respiratory depression
                    │
        ┌───────────┴────────────┐
        ▼                        ▼
   Hypoxaemia              Low cardiac output
   Hypercarbia             Decreased tissue perfusion
   Respiratory acidosis    Ischaemia
                           Metabolic acidosis
                           Capillary leak, oedema
        └───────────┬────────────┘
                    ▼
Hypoxic-ischaemic encephalopathy with multi-organ dysfunction
```

Encephalopathy	Respiratory failure	Myocardial dysfunction	Metabolic	Other organ dysfunction
• Abnormal neurological signs • Seizures	• Persistent pulmonary hypertension of the newborn	• Hypotension	• Hypoglycaemia • Hypocalcaemia • Hyponatraemia	• Renal failure • DIC (Disseminated intravascular coagulation)

Figure 11.3 Therapeutic hypothermia for moderate or severe hypoxic-ischaemic encephalopathy.

- aEEG monitor — useful to confirm encephalopathy and identify seizures
- ☀ Start cooling within 6 hours of birth. Avoid hyperthermia (>37.5°C)
- Infant wrapped in cooling mattress to maintain rectal temperature of 33–34°C for 72 hours
- ☀ Mild hypothermia for moderate and severe HIE reduces death and severe disability and increases the likelihood of survival with normal neurological function

Figure 11.4 Outcomes of therapeutic hypothermia trials compared with standard care for the treatment of term/near-term babies with hypoxic-ischaemic encephalopathy. The figure shows reduction of death or major disability. Reduction in seizures is not demonstrated and there may be an increase in persistent pulmonary hypertension of the newborn (PPHN). (Data from Jacobs SE, Berg M, Hunt R, Tarnow-Mordi WO, Inder TE, et al.: Cooling for newborns with hypoxic-ischaemic encephalopathy. *The Cochrane Database of Systematic Reviews* CD003311, 2013.)

	Risk ratio
Death or major disability	0.75 (0.68–0.83)
Mortality only	0.75 (0.64–0.88)
Major neurodisability	0.77 (0.63–0.94)
Cerebral palsy in survivors	0.66 (0.54–0.82)
Persistent pulmonary hypertension (PPHN)	1.36 (0.94–1.97)
Seizures	0.91 (0.83–1.00)

Favours hypothermia ← | → Favours standard care

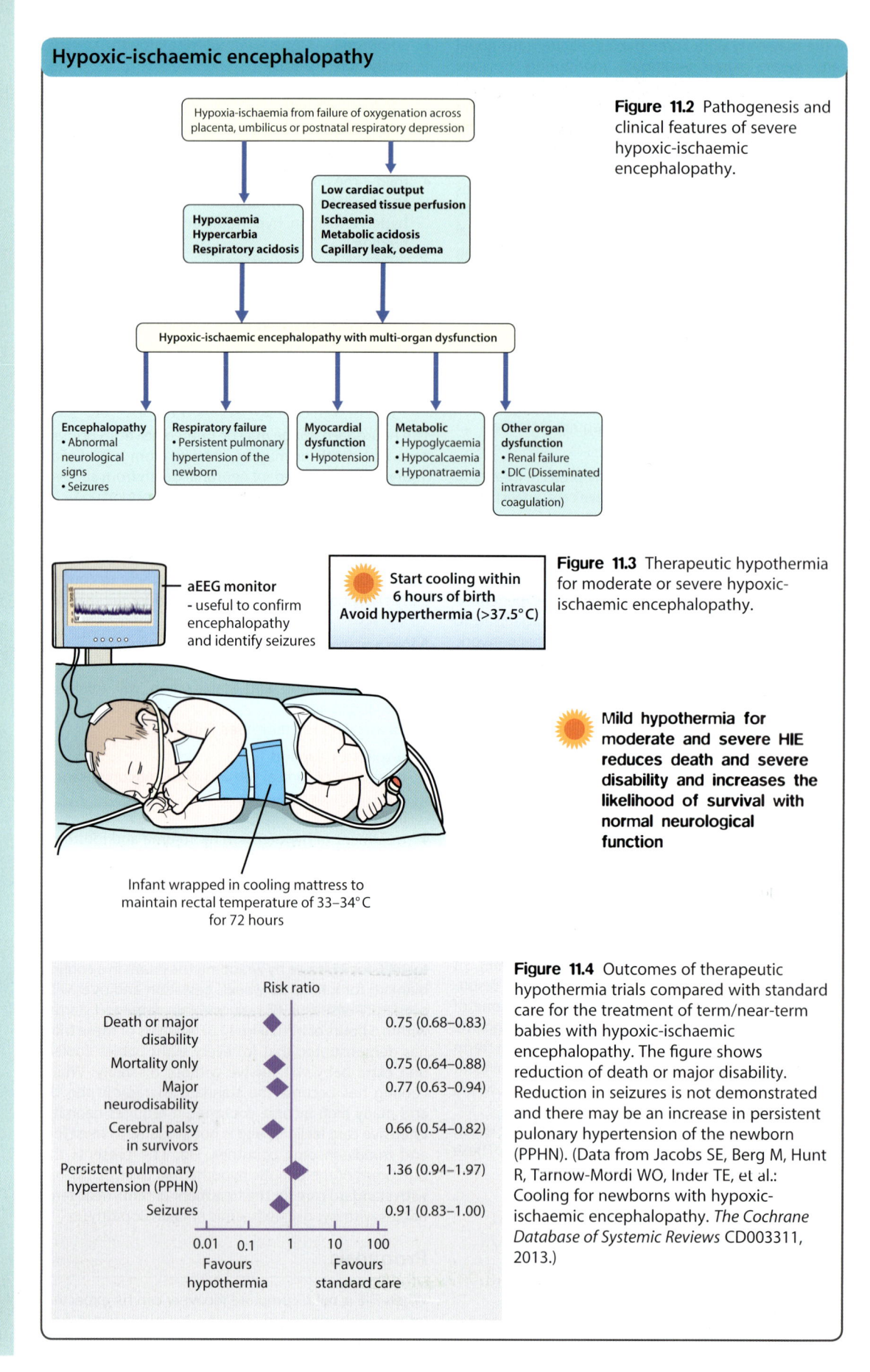

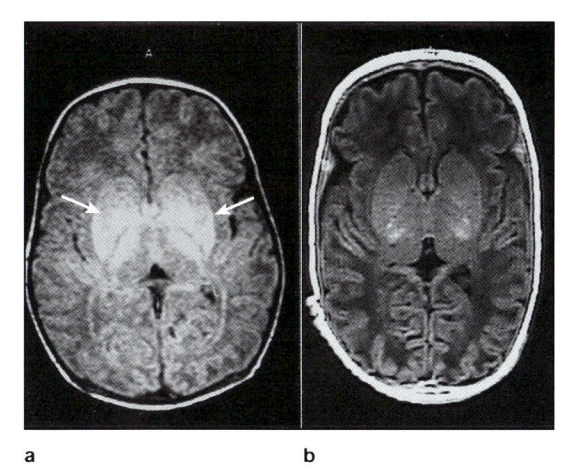

Figure 11.5 Magnetic resonance image of the brain at 14 days in term infant. (**a**) abnormal (white) signal in the basal ganglia and thalami (arrows) and absence of signal in the internal capsule bilaterally carries high risk of cerebral palsy (**b**) normal scan for comparison showing grey basal ganglia and a white signal from myelin in the posterior limb of the internal capsule.

normally by 2 weeks of age have a good long-term prognosis, but if clinical abnormalities persist beyond that time, full recovery is unlikely. Severe HIE has a mortality of 30–40%, and, of survivors without cooling, over 80% have neurodevelopmental disabilities, particularly cerebral palsy. Even with cooling, mortality and long-term neurodevelopmental disability rates are high. If magnetic resonance imaging (MRI) of the brain at 5–14 days in a term infant shows significant abnormalities, there is a high risk of later cerebral palsy (Fig. 11.5).

Hypoxic-ischaemic injury causing encephalopathy usually occurs antenatally or during labour or delivery, or may occur postnatally, but the encephalopathy may sometimes be caused by another neonatal condition, e.g. inborn error of metabolism or kernicterus. The diagnosis 'birth asphyxia' has potentially serious medicolegal implications; it has been recommended that infants who have the clinical features of HIE should only be considered to have birth asphyxia if there is:

- evidence of severe hypoxia antenatally or during labour or at delivery
- resuscitation needed at birth
- features of encephalopathy
- evidence of hypoxic damage to other organs such as liver, kidney or heart
- no other prenatal or postnatal cause identified.

Summary

Hypoxic-ischaemic encephalopathy
- Is an important cause of morbidity and mortality worldwide.
- If severe, causes encephalopathy and multi-organ dysfunction.
- Therapeutic hypothermia has become standard therapy in the UK and many countries if moderate or severe.

Birth injuries

Infants may be injured at birth, particularly if they are malpositioned or too large for the pelvic outlet. Injuries may also occur during manual manoeuvres, from forceps blades or at Ventouse deliveries. Fortunately, now that caesarean section is available in every maternity unit, heroic attempts to achieve a vaginal delivery with resultant severe injuries to the infant have become extremely rare.

Soft-tissue injuries

These include:

- caput succedaneum (Fig. 11.6) – bruising and oedema of the presenting part extending beyond the margins of the skull bones; resolves in a few days
- cephalhaematoma (Figs 11.6, 11.7) – haematoma from bleeding below the periosteum, confined within the margins of the skull sutures. It usually involves the parietal bone. The centre of the haematoma feels soft. It resolves over several weeks
- chignon (Fig. 11.8) – oedema and bruising from Ventouse delivery
- bruising to the face after a face presentation and to the genitalia and buttocks after breech delivery. Preterm infants bruise readily from even mild trauma
- abrasions to the skin from scalp electrodes applied during labour or from accidental scalpel incision at caesarean section
- forceps marks to face from pressure of blades – transient
- subaponeurotic haemorrhage (Fig. 11.6; very uncommon) – diffuse, boggy swelling of scalp on examination, blood loss may be severe and can lead to hypovolaemic shock and coagulopathy.

Nerve palsies

Brachial nerve palsy results from traction to the brachial plexus nerve roots. They may occur at breech deliveries or with shoulder dystocia. Upper nerve root (C5 and C6) injury results in an Erb palsy (Fig. 11.9). It may be accompanied by phrenic nerve palsy causing an elevated diaphragm. Erb palsy usually resolves completely, but should be referred to an orthopaedic or plastic surgeon if not resolved by 2–3 months. Most recover by 2 years. A facial nerve palsy may result from compression of the facial nerve against the mother's ischial spine or pressure from forceps. It is unilateral, and there is facial weakness on crying but the eye remains open. It is usually transient, but methylcellulose drops may be needed for the eye. Rarely, nerve palsies may be from damage to the cervical spine, when there is lack of movement below the level of the lesion.

Birth injuries

Soft-tissue injuries:
- caput succedaneum, cephalhaematoma, chignon, bruises, and abrasions
- subaponeurotic haemorrhage

Nerve palsies:
- brachial plexus – Erb palsy
- facial nerve palsy

Fractures:
- clavicle, humerus, femur

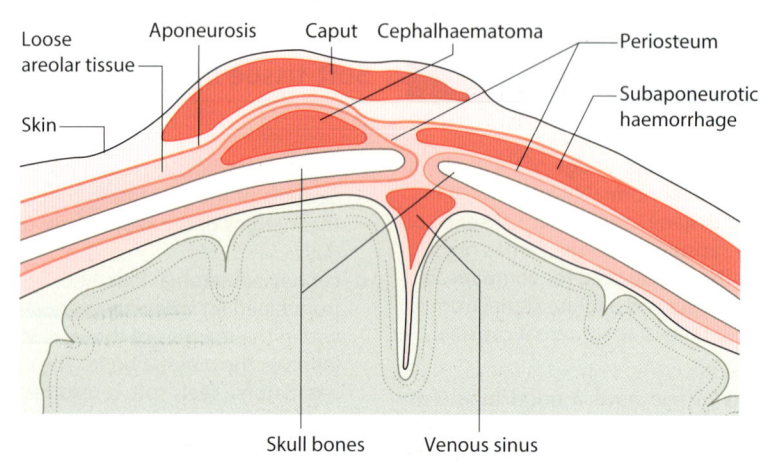

Figure 11.6 Location of extracranial haemorrhages.

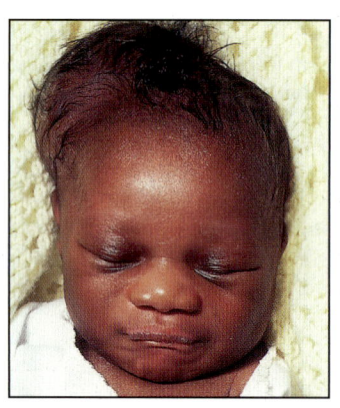

Figure 11.7 A large cephalhaematoma.

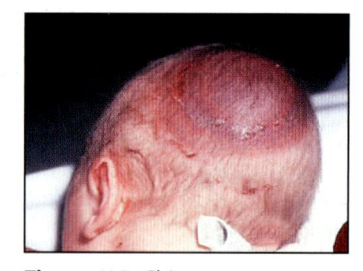

Figure 11.8 Chignon.

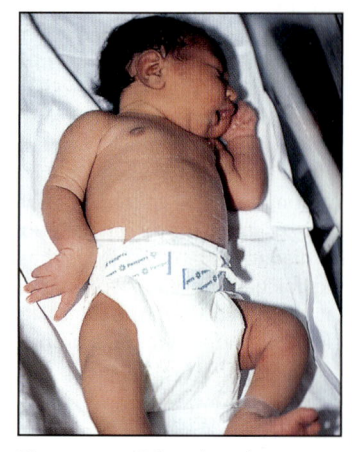

Figure 11.9 Erb palsy. The affected arm lies straight, is limp, and with the hand pronated and the fingers flexed (waiter's tip position).

Fractures

Clavicle

Usually from shoulder dystocia. A snap may be heard at delivery or the infant may have reduced arm movement on the affected side, or a lump from callus formation may be noticed over the clavicle at several weeks of age. The prognosis is excellent and no specific treatment is required.

Humerus/femur

Usually midshaft, occurring at breech deliveries, or fracture of the humerus at shoulder dystocia. There is deformity, reduced movement of the limb and pain on movement. They heal rapidly with immobilization.

Stabilizing the preterm or sick infant

Preterm infants of less than 34 weeks' gestation and newborn infants who become seriously ill require their condition to be stabilized and monitored (Fig. 11.10). Many of them will need respiratory, circulatory and nutritional support.

The preterm infant

The appearance, the likely clinical course, chances of survival, and long-term prognosis depend on the gestational age at birth. The appearance and maturational changes of very preterm infants are described in Table 11.1 (also see Fig. 11.11) and the importance of parental involvement is shown in Figs 11.12a and b. The external appearance and neurological findings can be scored to provide an estimate of an infant's gestational age if not known from ultrasound scanning (see Appendix).

The rate and severity of problems associated with prematurity decline markedly with increasing gestation. Infants born at 23–25 weeks' gestation encounter many problems (Box 11.1), require many weeks of intensive and special care in hospital, and have a high overall mortality. With modern neonatal care, the prognosis is excellent after 30 weeks' gestational age.

Respiratory distress syndrome

In respiratory distress syndrome (RDS, also called hyaline membrane disease), there is a **deficiency of surfactant, which lowers surface tension**. Surfactant is a mixture of phospholipids and proteins excreted by the type II pneumocytes of the alveolar epithelium. Surfactant deficiency leads to **widespread alveolar collapse** and **inadequate gas exchange**. The more preterm the infant, the higher the incidence of RDS. It is very common in infants born before 28 weeks' gestation and tends to be more severe in boys than girls. Surfactant deficiency is rare at term but may occur in infants of diabetic mothers and very rarely from genetic mutations in the surfactant genes. The term hyaline membrane disease derives from a proteinaceous exudate seen in the airways on histology. **Glucocorticoids**, given antenatally to the mother, stimulate fetal surfactant production and are given if preterm delivery is anticipated (see Ch. 10.). The evidence of their benefit is substantial; it significantly **reduces RDS, bronchopulmonary dysplasia**, and **intraventricular haemorrhage (IVH)** in infants less than 34 weeks' gestation.

At delivery or within 4 hours of birth, babies with RDS develop clinical signs of:

- tachypnoea over 60 breaths/minute
- laboured breathing with chest wall recession (particularly sternal and subcostal indrawing) and nasal flaring

Box 11.1 Medical problems of preterm infants

- Need for resuscitation and stabilization at birth
- Respiratory:
  - respiratory distress syndrome
  - pneumothorax
  - apnoea and bradycardia
- Hypotension
- Patent ductus arteriosus
- Temperature control
- Metabolic:
  - hypoglycaemia
  - hypocalcaemia
  - electrolyte imbalance
  - osteopenia of prematurity
- Nutrition
- Infection
- Jaundice
- Intraventricular haemorrhage/periventricular leukomalacia
- Necrotizing enterocolitis
- Retinopathy of prematurity
- Anaemia of prematurity
- Iatrogenic
- Bronchopulmonary dysplasia (BPD)
- Inguinal hernias.

- expiratory grunting in order to try to create positive airway pressure during expiration and maintain functional residual capacity
- cyanosis if severe.

The characteristic chest X-ray appearance is shown in Fig. 11.13. Treatment with raised ambient oxygen is required (Box 11.2), and surfactant therapy may be given by instilling surfactant directly into the lungs via a **tracheal tube** or **catheter**. Additional respiratory support may be provided non-invasively with continuous positive airway pressure (CPAP) or high-flow nasal cannula therapy or invasively with mechanical ventilation via a tracheal tube. Mechanical ventilation (with intermittent positive pressure ventilation or high-frequency oscillation) is adjusted according to the infant's oxygenation (which is measured continuously), chest wall movements and blood gas analyses. Non-invasive respiratory support is used in preference to mechanical ventilation whenever possible as it has fewer complications.

> **Surfactant therapy reduces morbidity and mortality of preterm infants with respiratory distress syndrome**

Pneumothorax

In RDS, air from the overdistended alveoli may track into the interstitium, resulting in pulmonary interstitial emphysema. In up to 10% of infants ventilated for RDS, air leaks into the pleural cavity and causes a pneumothorax. When this occurs, the infant's oxygen

Stabilizing preterm or sick infants

Airway, breathing:
- respiratory distress – tachypnoea, laboured breathing with chest wall recession, nasal flaring, expiratory grunting, cyanosis
- apnoea.

Management, as required:
- clear the airway
- oxygen
- continuous positive airway pressure (CPAP) or high-flow nasal cannula therapy
- mechanical ventilation.

Monitoring:
- oxygen saturation (maintain at 91–95% if preterm)
- heart rate
- respiratory rate
- temperature
- blood pressure
- blood glucose
- blood gases
- weight.

Temperature control:
- place in plastic bag at birth to keep warm if extremely preterm
- perform stabilization under a radiant warmer with or without a heated mattress or in a humidified incubator to avoid hypothermia.

Venous and arterial lines

Peripheral intravenous line:
- required for intravenous fluids, antibiotics, and other drugs.

Umbilical venous catheter:
- may be used for intravenous access at resuscitation, in extremely preterm infants for the first few days or to administer high osmolality fluids (e.g. high-concentration dextrose) or medications needing central delivery (e.g. inotropes).

Arterial line:
- inserted if frequent blood gas analysis, blood tests, and continuous blood pressure monitoring are required. Usually umbilical artery catheter, sometimes peripheral cannula if for short period or no umbilical artery catheter possible
- the arterial oxygen tension is maintained at 8–12 kPa (60–90 mmHg) and the CO_2 tension at 4.5–6.5 kPa (35–50 mmHg).

Peripherally inserted central (PIC) line for parenteral nutrition, if indicated:
- inserted peripherally when infant is stable.

Chest X-ray with or without abdominal X-ray
Assists in the diagnosis of respiratory disorders and to confirm the position of the tracheal tube and central lines.

Investigations:
- haemoglobin, neutrophil count, platelet count
- blood urea, creatinine, electrolytes, and lactate
- culture – blood ± cerebrospinal fluid ± urine
- blood glucose
- C-reactive protein/acute phase reactant
- coagulation screen if indicated.

Antibiotics
Broad-spectrum antibiotics are given.

Minimal handling
All procedures, especially painful ones, adversely affect oxygenation and the circulation. Handling the infant is kept to a minimum and done as gently, rapidly and efficiently as possible. Analgesia should be provided to prevent pain as necessary.

Parents
Although medical and nursing staff are usually fully occupied stabilizing the baby, time must be found for parents and immediate relatives to allow them to see and touch their baby and to be kept fully informed.

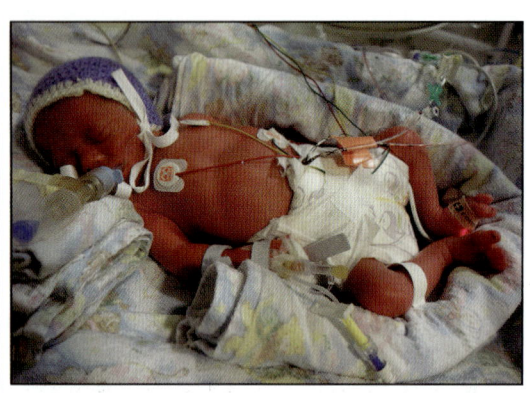

Figure 11.10 Stabilizing preterm or sick infants is important to prevent complications. This preterm infant has leads on his limbs for monitoring heart rate and respiratory rate, temperature and oxygen saturation. There are arterial and intravenous cannulae and an endotracheal tube for artificial ventilation.

The preterm infant: Maturational changes in appearance and development

Figure 11.11 (**a**) Preterm infant at 23–27 weeks, (**b**) term infant.

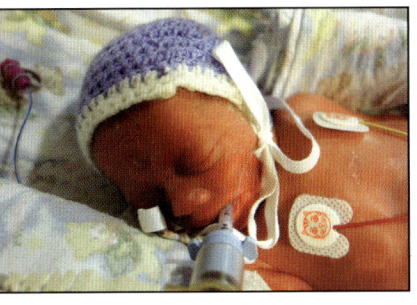

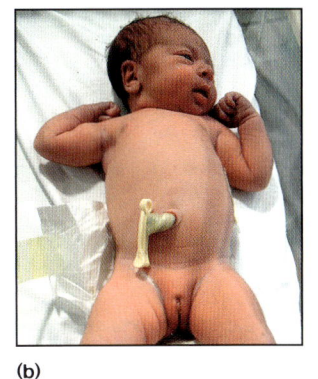

Table 11.1 The preterm infant compared with the term infant

Gestation	23–27 weeks	Term (37–42 weeks)
Birthweight (50th centile)	At 24 weeks – male 700 g, female 620 g	At 40 weeks – male 3.55 kg, female 3.4 kg
Skin	Very thin (Fig. 11.11a)	Thick skin (Fig. 11.11b)
	Dark red colour all over body	Pale pink colour
Ears	Pinna soft, no recoil	Pinna firm, cartilage to edge, immediate recoil
Breast tissue	No breast tissue palpable	One or both nodules >1 cm
Genitalia	Male – scrotum smooth, no testes in scrotum	Male – scrotum has rugae, testes in scrotum
	Female – prominent clitoris, labia majora widely separated, labia minora protruding	Female – labia minora and clitoris covered
Breathing	Needs respiratory support. Apnoea common	Rarely needs respiratory support. Apnoea rare
Sucking and swallowing	No coordinated sucking	Coordinated (from 34–35 weeks)
Feeding	Usually needs parenteral nutrition and tube feeding	Cries when hungry. Feeds on demand
Cry	Faint	Loud
Vision, interaction	Eyelids may be fused. Infrequent eye movements. Not available for interaction	Makes eye contact, alert wakefulness
Hearing	Startles to loud noise	Responds to sound
Posture	Limbs extended, jerky movements	Flexed posture, smooth movements

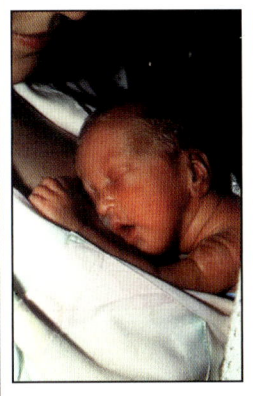

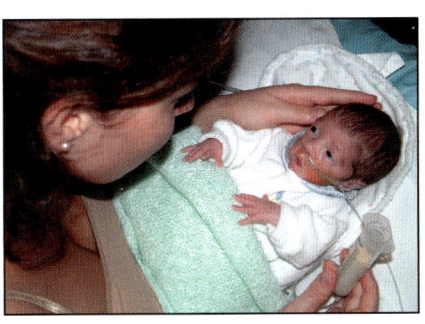

Figure 11.12a Parental involvement in neonatal care. Skin-to-skin contact between infant and parent (Kangaroo care) promotes bonding.

Figure 11.12b Parental involvement in neonatal care. Mother giving her baby expressed breast milk (in syringe) via nasogastric tube, allowing close eye and skin contact between mother and baby.

Neonatal medicine

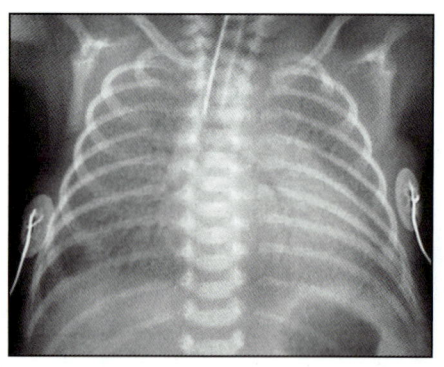

Figure 11.13 Chest X-ray in respiratory distress syndrome showing a diffuse granular or 'ground glass' appearance of the lungs and an air bronchogram, where the larger airways are outlined. The heart border is indistinct. A tracheal tube is present. (From Lissauer T, Fanaroff AA, Miall L, et al.: *Neonatology at a Glance*, 3rd edition, Oxford, 2015, Wiley Blackwell with permission.)

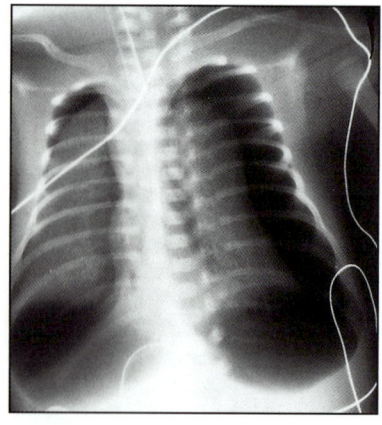

Figure 11.14 Chest X-ray showing bilateral pneumothoraces in a preterm infant with respiratory distress syndrome.

Box 11.2 Oxygen therapy in preterm infants

Oxygen therapy should be provided to correct hypoxaemia.
However:
- there is increasing evidence that excess oxygen leading to hyperoxia is damaging from excess free radicals
- for neonatal resuscitation, it is now recommended to start with 21–30% oxygen in preterm infants, avoiding oxygen saturation over 95%; in term infants air should be used
- in preterm infants avoid low saturations (<91%) – increased risk of necrotizing enterocolitis and death
- in preterm infants avoid high saturation (>95%) – increased risk of retinopathy of prematurity.

requirement usually increases and the breath sounds and chest movement on the affected side are reduced, although this can be difficult to detect clinically. A pneumothorax may be demonstrated by transillumination with a bright fibre-optic light source applied to the chest wall or on a chest X-ray (Fig. 11.14). A tension pneumothorax is treated urgently with decompression by inserting a chest drain. In order to try and prevent pneumothoraces, infants are ventilated with the lowest pressures that provide adequate chest movement and satisfactory blood gases.

Apnoea and bradycardia and desaturation

Episodes of apnoea and bradycardia and desaturation are common in very low birthweight infants until they reach about 32-weeks' gestational age. Bradycardia may occur either when an infant stops breathing for over 20–30 seconds or when breathing continues but against a closed glottis. An underlying cause (hypoxia, infection, anaemia, electrolyte disturbance, hypoglycaemia, seizures, heart failure or aspiration due to gastro-oesophageal reflux) needs to be excluded, but in many instances the cause is immaturity of central respiratory control. Breathing will usually start again after gentle physical stimulation. Treatment with the respiratory stimulant caffeine often helps and has been demonstrated to improve outcomes. CPAP or mechanical ventilation may be necessary if apnoeic episodes are frequent.

Temperature control

Hypothermia causes increased energy consumption and may result in hypoxia and hypoglycaemia, failure to gain weight and is an independent risk factor for mortality soon after birth. Preterm infants are particularly vulnerable to hypothermia, as:

- they have a large surface area relative to their mass, so there is greater heat loss (related to surface area) than heat generation (related to mass)
- their skin is thin and heat permeable, so transepidermal water loss is important in the 1st week of life
- they have little subcutaneous fat for insulation
- they are often nursed naked and cannot conserve heat by curling up or generate heat by shivering.

There is a neutral temperature range in which an infant's energy consumption is at a minimum level. In the very immature baby, this neutral temperature is highest during the first few days of life and subsequently declines. The temperature of these small babies is maintained using incubators (Fig. 11.15) or initially with overhead radiant heaters. Incubators also allow ambient humidity to be provided, which reduces transepidermal heat loss.

Patent ductus arteriosus

The ductus arteriosus remains patent in many preterm infants. Shunting of blood across the ductus, from the

Temperature control

Prevention of heat loss in newborn infants:

1. **Convection:**
   - raise temperature of ambient air in incubator
   - clothe, including covering head
   - avoid draughts
2. **Radiation:**
   - cover baby
   - double walls for incubators
3. **Evaporation:**
   - dry and wrap at birth; if extremely preterm, place baby's body directly into plastic bag at birth without drying
   - humidify incubator
4. **Conduction:**
   - nurse on heated mattress

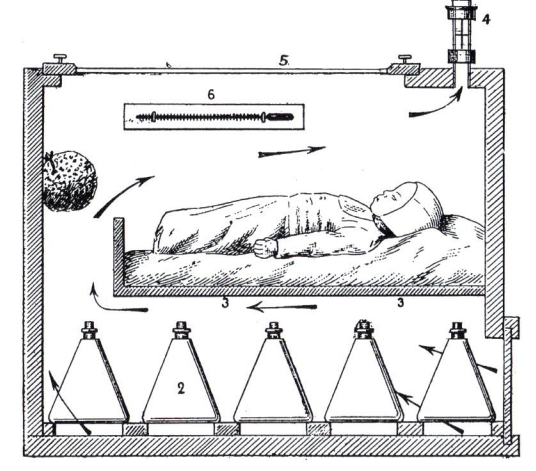

Figure 11.15 The importance of avoiding hypothermia in newborn infants has long been recognised. This incubator was used in the late nineteenth century to keep newborn infants warm. The sponge is to increase ambient humidity.

---

left to the right side of the circulation, is most common in infants with RDS. It may produce no symptoms or it may cause apnoea and bradycardia, increased oxygen requirement and difficulty in weaning the infant from artificial ventilation. The pulses are 'bounding' from an increased pulse pressure, the precordial impulse becomes prominent and a systolic murmur may be audible. With increasing circulatory overload, signs of heart failure may develop. More accurate assessment of the infant's circulation can be obtained on echocardiography. If the infant is symptomatic, pharmacological closure with a prostaglandin synthetase inhibitor, indomethacin or ibuprofen, is used. If these measures fail to close a symptomatic duct, surgical ligation will be required.

Fluid balance

A preterm infant's fluid requirements will vary with gestational and chronological age. It is adjusted according to the infant's clinical condition, plasma electrolytes, urine output, and weight change. On the 1st day of life, about 60–90 ml/kg is usually required, which increases by 20–30 ml/kg per day to 150–180 ml/kg per day by about day 5 of life.

Nutrition

Preterm infants have a high nutritional requirement because of their rapid growth. Preterm infants at 28 weeks' gestation double their birthweight in 6 weeks and treble it in 12 weeks, whereas term babies double their weight in only 4.5 months and treble it in a year.

Infants of 35–36 weeks' gestational age are mature enough to suck and swallow milk. Less mature infants will need to be fed via an orogastric or nasogastric tube. Even in very preterm infants, enteral feeds, preferably breast milk, are introduced as soon as possible. In these infants, breast milk needs to be supplemented with phosphate and may need supplementation with protein and calories (in breast milk fortifier) and calcium. In some neonatal units, extremely preterm infants are initially fed on donor breast milk if maternal breast milk is not available. If formula feeding is required, special infant formulas are available, which are designed to meet the increased nutritional requirements of preterm infants but, in contrast to breast milk, do not provide protection against infection or other benefits of breast milk. In the very immature or sick infant (typically <1 kg birthweight), parenteral nutrition is often required. This is usually given through a peripherally inserted central line (PIC or long line), or an umbilical venous catheter, paying strict attention to aseptic technique both during insertion and when lines are accessed. Central lines carry a significant risk of septicaemia; other risks include thrombosis of a major vein. For this reason, parenteral nutrition may sometimes be given via a peripheral vein, but extravasation may cause skin damage with scarring. Because of the significant risk of septicaemia from parenteral nutrition and the increased risk of necrotizing enterocolitis with cow's milk-based formula, mothers should be encouraged and supported to provide breast milk.

Poor bone mineralization (osteopenia of prematurity) was previously common but is prevented by provision of adequate phosphate, calcium and vitamin D. Because iron is mostly transferred to the fetus during the last trimester, preterm babies have low iron stores and are at a risk of iron deficiency. This is in addition to loss of blood from sampling and an inadequate erythropoietin response. Iron supplements

Necrotizing enterocolitis

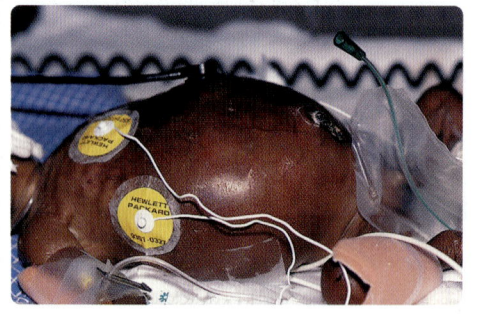

Figure 11.16a Necrotizing enterocolitis showing gross abdominal distension and tense and shiny skin over the abdomen.

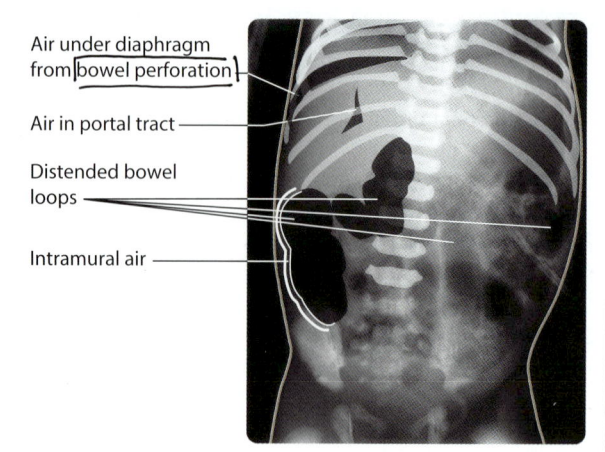

Figure 11.16b Diagram of characteristic features of necrotizing enterocolitis on abdominal X-ray.

Labels: Air under diaphragm from bowel perforation; Air in portal tract; Distended bowel loops; Intramural air.

are started at several weeks of age and continued after discharge home.

Infection

Preterm infants are at an increased risk of infection, as IgG is mostly transferred across the placenta in the last trimester and no IgA or IgM is transferred. In addition, infection in or around the cervix is often a reason for preterm labour and may cause infection shortly after birth. Most infections in preterm infants occur after several days of age and are nosocomial (hospital derived); they are often associated with indwelling catheters or mechanical ventilation. Infection is considered in more detail later in this chapter.

> Infection in preterm infants is a major cause of death and contributes to bronchopulmonary dysplasia, brain injury and later disability

Necrotizing enterocolitis

Necrotizing enterocolitis is a serious illness and one of the greatest challenges facing modern neonatal medicine today. The incidence increases with increasing prematurity and it is typically seen in the first few weeks of life. The bowel of the preterm infant is vulnerable to ischaemic injury and bacterial invasion, both key risk factors for necrotizing enterocolitis. Preterm infants fed cow's milk formula are more likely to develop this condition than if they are fed only breast milk. Supplementing milk feeds with prebiotics and probiotics may also be beneficial.

Early signs of necrotizing enterocolitis include feed intolerance and vomiting, which may be bile stained. The abdomen becomes distended (Fig. 11.16a) and the stool sometimes contains fresh blood. The infant may rapidly become shocked and require mechanical ventilation because of abdominal distension and pain. The characteristic X-ray features are distended loops of bowel and thickening of the bowel wall with intramural gas, and there may be gas in the portal venous tract (Fig. 11.16b). The disease may progress to bowel perforation, which can be detected by X-ray or by transillumination of the abdomen.

Treatment is to stop oral feeding and give broad-spectrum antibiotics to cover both aerobic and anaerobic organisms. Parenteral nutrition is always needed and mechanical ventilation and circulatory support are often required. Surgery is performed for bowel perforation. The disease has significant morbidity and a mortality of about 20%. Long-term sequelae include the development of strictures and malabsorption if extensive bowel resection has been necessary, as well as a greater risk of a poor neurodevelopmental outcome.

Preterm brain injury

Haemorrhages in the brain occur in 20% of very low birthweight infants and are easily recognised on cranial ultrasound scans (Fig. 11.17a). Typically, they occur in the germinal matrix above the caudate nucleus, which contains a fragile network of blood vessels. Most intraventricular haemorrhages (IVHs) occur within the first 72 hours of life. They are more common following perinatal asphyxia and in infants with severe RDS. Pneumothorax is a significant risk factor. Antenatal glucocorticoids prior to preterm delivery is associated with a reduction in the incidence and severity of RDS, and therefore of IVH.

Small haemorrhages are confined to the germinal matrix, but larger haemorrhage extends into the ventricles. The most severe haemorrhage is unilateral haemorrhagic infarction involving the parenchyma of the brain; this usually results in hemiplegia (Fig. 11.17b).

Cranial ultrasound in preterm infants

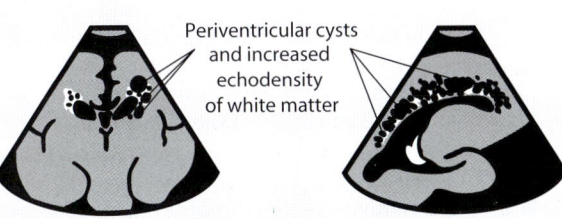

Figure 11.17a Cranial ultrasound in preterm infants.

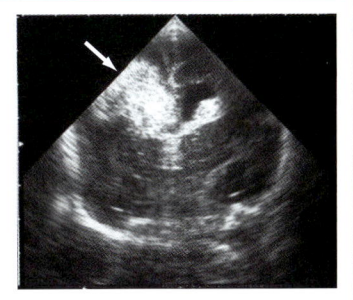

Figure 11.17b Large intraventricular haemorrhage with parenchymal haemorrhagic infarct on the right (arrow).

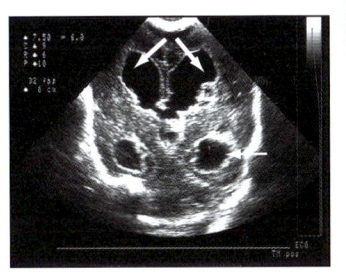

Figure 11.17c Dilatation of lateral ventricles following intraventricular haemorrhage.

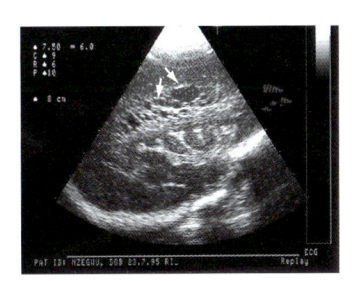

Figure 11.17d Widespread cysts in periventricular leukomalacia.

A large IVH may impair the drainage and reabsorption of cerebrospinal fluid (CSF), thus allowing CSF to build-up under pressure. This dilatation (Fig. 11.17c) may resolve spontaneously or progress to hydrocephalus, which may cause the cranial sutures to separate, the head circumference to increase rapidly and the anterior fontanelle to become tense. A ventriculoperitoneal shunt may be required, but initially symptomatic relief may be provided by removal of CSF by lumbar puncture or ventricular tap. About half of infants with progressive post-haemorrhagic ventricular dilatation have cerebral palsy, a higher proportion if parenchymal infarction is also present.

Periventricular white matter brain injury may occur following ischaemia or inflammation even in the absence of haemorrhage. It is more difficult to detect by cranial ultrasound. Initially, there may be an echo-dense area or 'flare' within the brain parenchyma. This may resolve within a week (in which case the risk of cerebral palsy is not increased), but if cystic lesions become visible on ultrasound 2–4 weeks later, there is definite loss of white matter. Bilateral multiple cysts, called periventricular leukomalacia (PVL), have an 80–90% risk of spastic diplegia, often with cognitive impairment, if posteriorly sited (Fig. 11.17d).

Both IVH and periventricular leukomalacia may occur in the absence of abnormal clinical signs. Similarly, although cranial ultrasound abnormalities are associated with later disability, about a third of premature infants <32 weeks' gestation who go onto to have cerebral palsy have a normal cranial ultrasound, which suggests that more subtle neuronal injury can cause long-term disability.

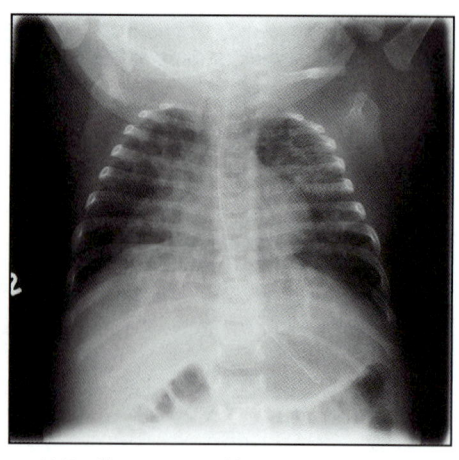

Figure 11.18 Chest X-ray of bronchopulmonary dysplasia (BPD) showing fibrosis and lung collapse, cystic changes and over-distension of the lungs.

Retinopathy of prematurity

Retinopathy of prematurity affects developing blood vessels at the junction of the vascularized and non-vascularized retina. There is vascular proliferation, which may progress to retinal detachment, fibrosis and blindness. It was initially recognised that the risk is increased by uncontrolled use of high concentrations of oxygen. Now, even with careful monitoring of the infant's oxygenation, retinopathy of prematurity is still identified in about 35% of all very low birthweight infants. The eyes of susceptible preterm infants (≤1500 g birthweight or <32 weeks' gestation) are screened by an ophthalmologist. Laser therapy reduces visual impairment, and intravitreal anti-VEFG (anti-vascular endothelial growth factor) therapy is being investigated. Severe bilateral visual impairment occurs in about 1% of very low birthweight infants, mostly in infants <28 weeks' gestation.

Bronchopulmonary dysplasia

Infants who still have an oxygen requirement at a postmenstrual age of 36 weeks are described as having bronchopulmonary dysplasia (BPD) (previously called chronic lung disease). The lung damage is now thought to be mainly from delay in lung maturation, but may also be from pressure and volume trauma from artificial ventilation, oxygen toxicity and infection. The chest X-ray characteristically shows widespread areas of opacification, sometimes with cystic changes (Fig. 11.18). Some infants need prolonged artificial ventilation, but most are weaned onto CPAP or high-flow nasal cannula therapy followed by additional ambient oxygen, sometimes over several months. Corticosteroid therapy may facilitate earlier weaning from the ventilator and often reduces the infant's oxygen requirements in the short term, but concern about increased risk of abnormal neurodevelopment including cerebral palsy limits use to those at highest risk and only short, low-dose courses are given. Some babies go home while still receiving additional oxygen. A few infants with severe disease may die of intercurrent infection or pulmonary hypertension. Subsequent pertussis and respiratory viral infection (e.g. respiratory syncytial virus or rhinovirus) may cause respiratory failure necessitating intensive care.

Problems following discharge

Some of the medical problems likely to be encountered on discharge from hospital are summarised in Case History 11.1.

About 5–10% of very low birthweight infants develop cerebral palsy, but the most common impairments are learning difficulties. The prevalence of cognitive impairment and of other associated difficulties increases with decreasing gestational age at birth, and is greatest if born at very early gestational age (<26 weeks' gestation; Fig. 11.20). It becomes increasingly evident when the individual child is compared with their peers at nursery or school. In addition, children may have difficulties with:

- fine motor skills, e.g. threading beads
- concentration, with short attention span
- behaviour problems, especially attention deficit disorders
- abstract reasoning, e.g. mathematics
- processing several tasks simultaneously.

A small proportion also have hearing impairment, with 1–2% requiring amplification, or visual impairment, with 1% blind in both eyes. A greater proportion have refraction errors and squints, and therefore require glasses.

Follow-up studies of very preterm infants who are now adults indicate that they are less socially engaged, are poor in communication, and easily become worried compared with their peers. This impacts adversely on relationships and careers.

> **During infancy, extremely preterm infants, especially those who had bronchpulmonary dysplasia, are at increased risk of respiratory failure from brochiolitis and other lower respiratory tract infections**

Case history 11.1

The ex-preterm infant going home

Mohammed was born at 24 weeks' gestation. The care pathway showing the potential problems and their timing for an infant born at this gestation is shown in Fig. 11.19. He is about to be discharged from the neonatal unit at 41 weeks' gestational age. His discharge planning meeting identified his needs when going home, which included:

- Home oxygen for his bronchopulmonary dysplasia – he will have respiratory reviews to allow him to wean safely off his oxygen with growth.
- Respiratory syncytial virus prophylaxis during the winter months – to reduce the risk of readmission and need for respiratory support.
- Cardiac monitoring – to make sure he is not developing pulmonary hypertension.
- Dietician input – he is breastfeeding and taking preterm formula. His phosphate, iron and vitamin needs will need to be considered.
- He has already had two sets of primary immunizations at the normal time and this course needs completing.
- He is at a greater risk of inguinal hernias.
- Ophthalmology review – will monitor his early retinopathy of prematurity and decide if any treatment is required.
- Low threshold for hospital readmission – rate increased four-fold, mainly for respiratory disorders.
- In addition to the healthy child programme for all children, his growth and neurodevelopment will be monitored, especially during the early years of life.

Care pathway for 24-week gestation infant showing potential problems and their timing

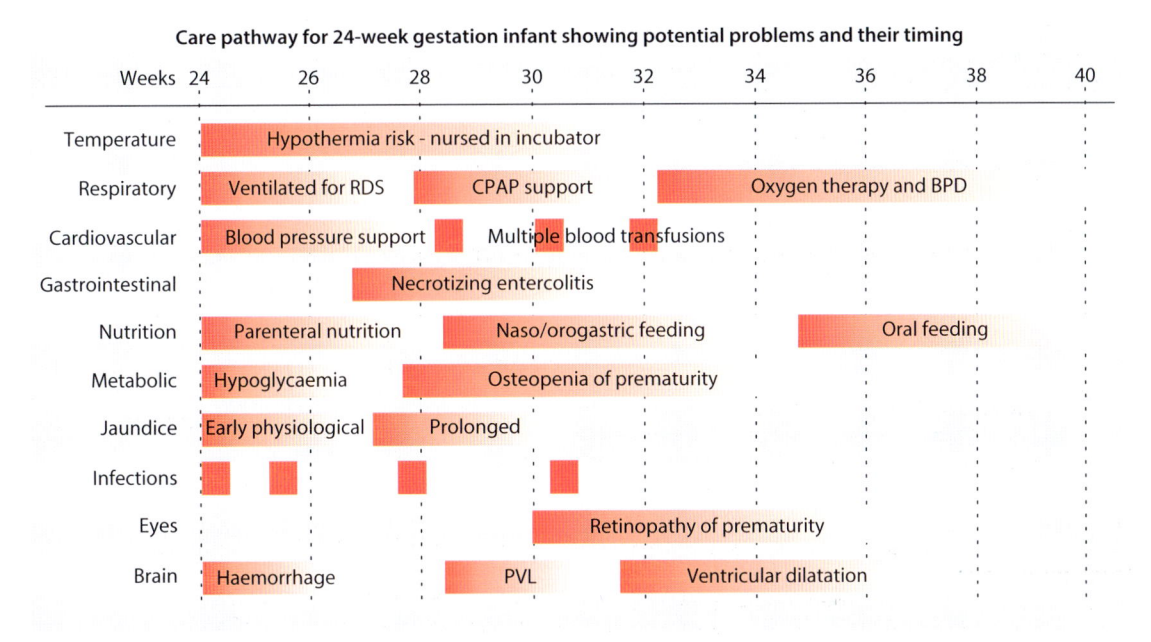

Weeks	24	26	28	30	32	34	36	38	40
Temperature	Hypothermia risk - nursed in incubator								
Respiratory	Ventilated for RDS		CPAP support			Oxygen therapy and BPD			
Cardiovascular	Blood pressure support			Multiple blood transfusions					
Gastrointestinal			Necrotizing enterocolitis						
Nutrition	Parenteral nutrition			Naso/orogastric feeding			Oral feeding		
Metabolic	Hypoglycaemia			Osteopenia of prematurity					
Jaundice	Early physiological		Prolonged						
Infections									
Eyes					Retinopathy of prematurity				
Brain	Haemorrhage		PVL		Ventricular dilatation				

Figure 11.19 Typical care pathway for a 24-week gestation infant showing potential complications and their timing. (RDS, respiratory distress syndrome; CPAP, continuous positive airway pressure; BPD, bronchopulmonary dysplasia; PVL, periventricular leukomalacia).

Summary

Summary of problems of very low birthweight infants (<1.5 kg)

Respiratory

Respiratory distress syndrome (surfactant deficiency)(74%)
- respiratory distress within 4 hours of birth
- antenatal corticosteroids and surfactant therapy reduce morbidity and mortality
- oxygen therapy, but excess may damage the retina
- nasal CPAP (continuous positive airway pressure) (67%) and mechanical ventilation (64%) - often required to expand lungs and prevent lung collapse; high-flow nasal cannula therapy may also be used (51%)

Pneumothorax (4%)
Apnoea and bradycardia and desaturations
Bronchopulmonary dysplasia (BPD) – O_2 requirement at 36 weeks post-menstrual age (27%)

Circulation
Hypotension – may require volume support, intropes or corticosteroids
Patent ductus arteriosus – needing medical treatment (34%) or surgical ligation (8%)

Nutrition
Nasogastric tube feeding – until 35–36 weeks post-menstrual age
Feeding intolerance - PN (parenteral nutrition) often required

Gastrointestinal
Necrotizing enterocolitis (6%)
– serious, management is medical or surgery for bowel necrosis or perforation

Metabolic
Hypoglycaemia – common
Electrolyte disturbances
Osteopenia of prematurity from phosphate deficiency

Hearing
Checked before discharge

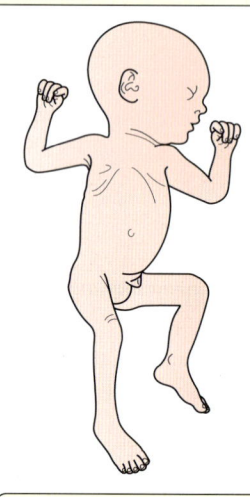

Temperature control
Avoid hypothermia
Nurse in neutral thermal environment
Nurse in incubator or under radiant warmer
Clothe if possible
Humidity reduces evaporative heat loss

Infection
Common and potentially serious (25%)
Increased risk of early-onset infection – group B streptococcus
Main problem is nosocomial infection – mainly coagulase-negative staphylococcus, also fungal and other infections

Jaundice
Jaundice – common, low treatment threshold

Anaemia
Often need blood transfusions

Eyes
Retinopathy of prematurity – may need laser therapy (4%)

Brain injury
Haemorrhage (20%)
- germinal layer, intraventricular, parenchymal
Ventricular dilatation – may need ventriculo-peritoneal shunt
Periventricular leukomalacia (3%) – ischaemic white matter injury

Following discharge
Specialist community nursing support helpful, if available
Increased risk of respiratory infection and wheezing – especially from bronchiolitis (caused by respiratory syncitial virus, RSV) and pertussis; may need intensive care
Consider prophylaxis against RSV infection
Increased rehospitalisation – respiratory disorders, inguinal hernias
Monitor growth, development (for learning disorders, co-ordination, cerebral palsy), behaviour, attention, vision, hearing – increased risk of impairment

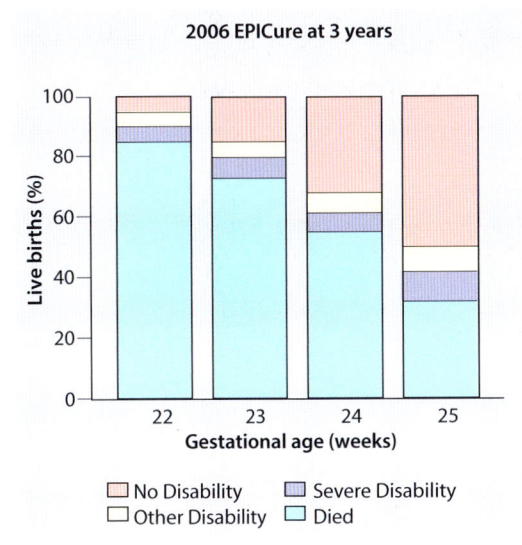

Figure 11.20 Outcome data at 3 years of age, a population-based study of all preterm infants <26 weeks' gestation born in England in 2006 (EPICure 2). Compared with babies born in 1995 (EPICure study), there have been improvements in survival but disability remains similar. (Data from Moore T, Hennessy EM, Myles J, Johnson SJ, Draper ES, et al.: Neurological and developmental outcome in extremely preterm children born in England in 1995 and 2006: the EPICure studies. *British Medical Journal* 345:e7961, 2012.)

Jaundice

Over 50% of all newborn infants become visibly jaundiced (Fig. 11.21). This is because:

- there is marked physiological release of haemoglobin from the breakdown of red cells because of the high haemoglobin concentration at birth
- the red cell lifespan of newborn infants (70 days) is markedly shorter than that of adults (120 days)
- hepatic bilirubin metabolism is less efficient in the first few days of life.

Neonatal jaundice is important as:

- it may be a sign of another disorder, e.g. haemolytic anaemia, infection, inborn error of metabolism, liver disease
- unconjugated bilirubin can be deposited in the brain, particularly in the basal ganglia, causing kernicterus.

Kernicterus

This is the encephalopathy resulting from the deposition of unconjugated bilirubin in the basal ganglia and brainstem nuclei (Fig. 11.22). It may occur when the level of unconjugated bilirubin exceeds the albumin-binding capacity of bilirubin of the blood. As this free bilirubin is fat soluble, it can cross the blood–brain barrier. The neurotoxic effects vary in severity from transient disturbance to severe damage and death. Acute manifestations are lethargy and poor feeding. In severe cases, there is irritability, increased muscle tone causing the baby to lie with an arched back (opisthotonos), seizures and coma. Infants who survive may develop choreoathetoid cerebral palsy (due to damage to the basal ganglia), learning difficulties and sensorineural deafness. Kernicterus used to be an important cause of brain damage in infants with severe rhesus haemolytic disease, but has become rare since the introduction of prophylactic anti-D immunoglobulin for rhesus-negative mothers. However, a few cases of kernicterus continue to occur, especially in slightly preterm infants (35–37 weeks) and dark-skin toned infants in whom jaundice is more difficult to detect; this has led NICE (National Institute for Health and Care Excellence) to issue guidelines on the management of neonatal jaundice.

Clinical evaluation

Babies become clinically jaundiced when the bilirubin level reaches about 80 µmol/l. Management varies according to the infant's gestational age, age at onset, bilirubin level and rate of rise, and the overall clinical condition.

Age at onset

The age of onset is a useful guide to the likely cause of the jaundice (Table 11.2).

Jaundice <24 hours of age

Jaundice starting within 24 hours of birth usually results from haemolysis. This is particularly important to identify as the bilirubin is unconjugated and can rise very rapidly and reach extremely high levels.

Haemolytic disorders

Rhesus haemolytic disease

Affected infants are usually identified antenatally and monitored and treated if necessary (see Ch. 10). The birth of a severely affected infant, with anaemia, hydrops and hepatosplenomegaly with rapidly developing severe jaundice has become rare. Antibodies may develop to rhesus antigens other than D and to the Kell and Duffy blood groups, but haemolysis is usually less severe.

ABO incompatibility

This is now more common than rhesus haemolytic disease. Most ABO antibodies are IgM and do not cross the placenta, but some group O women have an IgG anti-A-haemolysin in their blood, which can cross the placenta and haemolyse the red cells of a group A infant. Occasionally, group B infants are affected by anti-B haemolysins. Haemolysis can cause severe jaundice but it is usually less severe than in rhesus disease. The infant's haemoglobin level is usually normal or only slightly reduced and, in contrast to rhesus disease, hepatosplenomegaly is absent. The direct antibody test (Coombs' test), which demonstrates antibody on the surface of red cells, is positive. The jaundice usually peaks in the first 12 hours to 72 hours.

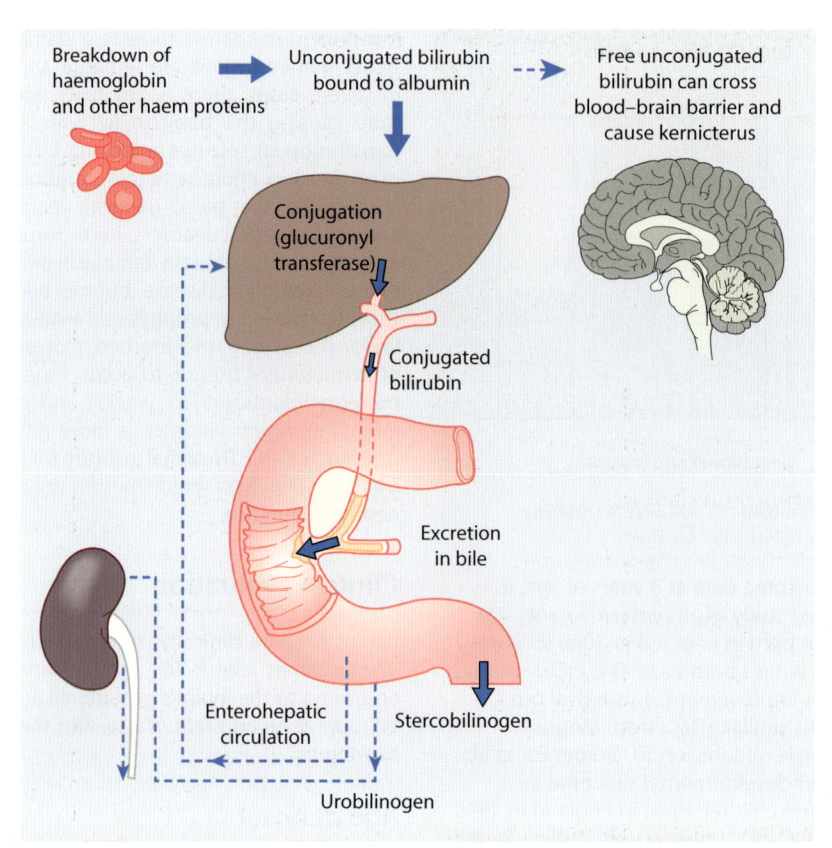

Figure 11.21 The breakdown product of haemoglobin is unconjugated bilirubin (indirect bilirubin), which is insoluble in water but soluble in lipids. It is carried in the blood bound to albumin. When the albumin binding is saturated, free unconjugated bilirubin can cross the blood–brain barrier, as it is lipid soluble. Unconjugated bilirubin bound to albumin is taken up by the liver and conjugated by glucuronyl transferase to conjugated bilirubin (direct bilirubin), which is water soluble and excreted in bile into the gut and then as stercobilinogen and urobilinogen. Some bilirubin in the gut is converted to unconjugated bilirubin and reabsorbed via the enterohepatic circulation and matabolised in the liver.

Table 11.2 Causes of neonatal jaundice

Jaundice starting at <24 h of age	Haemolytic disorders: 　Rhesus incompatibility 　ABO incompatibility 　G6PD deficiency 　Spherocytosis, pyruvate kinase deficiency Congenital infection	**Jaundice at >2 weeks of age**	Unconjugated: 　Physiological or breast milk jaundice 　Infection (particularly urinary tract) 　Hypothyroidism 　Haemolytic anaemia, e.g. G6PD deficiency 　High gastrointestinal obstruction, e.g. pyloric stenosis Conjugated (>25 µmol/l): 　Bile duct obstruction 　Neonatal hepatitis
Jaundice at 24 h to 2 weeks of age	Physiological jaundice Breast milk jaundice Infection, e.g. urinary tract infection Haemolysis, e.g. G6PD deficiency, ABO incompatibility Bruising Polycythaemia Crigler–Najjar syndrome		

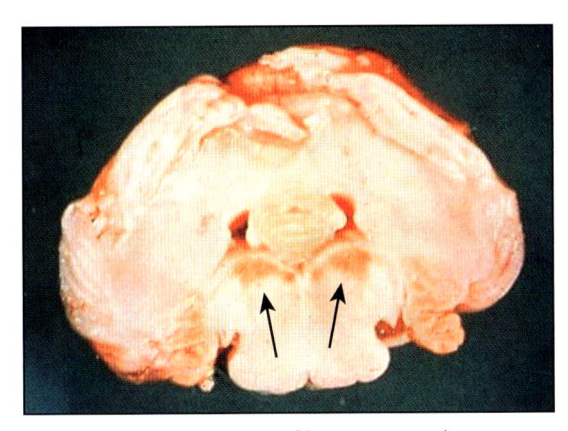

Figure 11.22 Postmortem of brainstem and cerebellum showing kernicterus with yellow bilirubin staining of brainstem nuclei (arrows).

G6PD (glucose-6-phosphate dehydrogenase) deficiency (see Ch. 23)
Mainly in people originating in the Mediterranean, Middle-East and Far East or in Africa. Mainly affects male infants, but some females develop significant jaundice. Parents of affected infants should be given a list of drugs to be avoided, as they may precipitate haemolysis.

Spherocytosis
This is considerably less common than G6PD deficiency (see Ch. 23). There is often, but not always, a family history. The disorder can be identified by recognising spherocytes on the blood film.

Congenital infection
Jaundice at birth can also be from congenital infection. In this case, the bilirubin is conjugated and the infants have other abnormal clinical signs, such as growth restriction, hepatosplenomegaly and thrombocytopenic purpura.

Jaundice at 2 days–2 weeks of age
Physiological jaundice
Most babies who become mildly or moderately jaundiced during this period have no underlying cause and the bilirubin has risen as the infant is adapting to the transition from fetal life. The term 'physiological jaundice' can only be used after other causes have been considered.

Breast milk jaundice
Jaundice is more common and more prolonged in breastfed infants. The hyperbilirubinaemia is unconjugated. The cause is multifactorial but may involve increased enterohepatic circulation of bilirubin.

Dehydration
In some infants, the jaundice is exacerbated if milk intake is poor from a delay in establishing breastfeeding and the infant becomes dehydrated (>10% weigh loss from birthweight). Breastfeeding should be continued, although supplemental feeding is sometimes needed to reverse the dehydration. In some infants, intravenous fluids are needed to correct dehydration.

Infection
An infected baby may develop an unconjugated hyperbilirubinaemia from poor fluid intake, haemolysis, reduced hepatic function and an increase in the enterohepatic circulation. If infection is suspected, appropriate investigations and treatment should be instigated. In particular, urinary tract infection may present in this way.

Other causes
Although jaundice from haemolysis usually presents in the 1st day of life, it may occur during the 1st week. Bruising and polycythaemia (venous haematocrit is >0.65) will exacerbate the infant's jaundice. The very rare Crigler–Najjar syndrome, in which glucuronyl transferase is deficient or absent, may result in extremely high levels of unconjugated bilirubin.

The causes and management of jaundice at over 2 weeks (term infants) or over 3 weeks (preterm infants) of age (persistent or prolonged neonatal jaundice) are different and are considered separately below.

Severity of jaundice
Jaundice can be observed most easily by blanching the skin with one's finger. The jaundice tends to start on the head and face and then spreads down the trunk and limbs. If the baby is clinically jaundiced, the bilirubin should be checked with a transcutaneous bilirubin meter or blood sample. It is easy to underestimate in dark-skin toned and preterm babies, and a low threshold should be adopted for measuring the bilirubin of these infants. A high transcutaneous bilirubin level must be checked with a blood laboratory measurement. It is now recommended in the UK that all babies should be checked clinically for jaundice in the first 72 hours of life, whether at hospital or home, and if clinically jaundiced a transcutaneous measurement should be obtained.

Rate of change
The rate of rise tends to be linear until a plateau is reached, so serial measurements can be plotted on a chart and used to anticipate the need for treatment before it rises to a dangerous level.

Gestation
Preterm infants are more susceptible to damage from raised bilirubin, so the intervention threshold is lower.

Clinical condition
Infants who experience severe hypoxia, hypothermia or any serious illness may be more susceptible to damage from severe jaundice. Drugs that may displace bilirubin from albumin, e.g. sulphonamides and diazepam, are avoided in newborn infants.

Management
Poor milk intake and dehydration will exacerbate jaundice and should be corrected, but studies have failed to show that routinely supplementing breastfed infants with water or dextrose solution reduces jaundice.

Case history 11.2

Jaundice needing phototherapy

A term male infant was noted to be markedly jaundiced at 10 hours of age. His bilirubin was 170 micromol/l, direct antibody test positive, maternal blood group O rhesus positive, and his blood group was A rhesus positive. A diagnosis of ABO incompatibility was made. He was started on intensive phototherapy and his bilirubin closely monitored and plotted on a bilirubin chart for term infants (Fig. 11.23). His bilirubin resolved with phototherapy, so Ig therapy and exchange transfusion were not required.

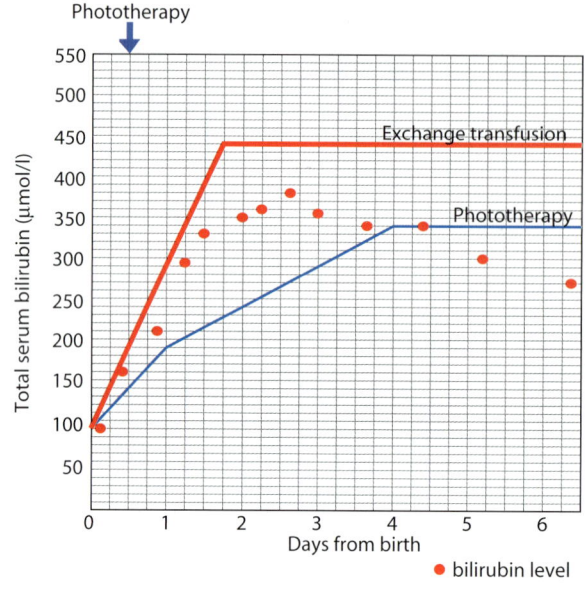

Figure 11.23 Bilirubin chart of bilirubin level and time from birth. It also shows the threshold for starting phototherapy and need to perform an exchange transfusion. Plotting the bilirubin values, as shown for this infant with ABO incompatibility, allows the rate of rise to be readily determined and if preparation needs to be made for an exchange transfusion. (Adapted from NICE: *National Institute for Health and Care Excellence guideline: Jaundice in newborn babies under 28 days*. March 2014 https://www.nice.org.uk/guidance/qs57/chapter/introduction)

Phototherapy is the most widely used therapy, with exchange transfusion for severe cases.

Phototherapy

Light (wavelength 450 nm) from the blue–green band of the visible spectrum converts unconjugated bilirubin into a harmless water-soluble pigment excreted predominantly in the urine. It is delivered with an overhead light source placed at an optimal distance above the infant to achieve high irradiance. Although no long-term sequelae of phototherapy from overhead light have been reported, it is disruptive to normal care of the infant and should not be used indiscriminately. The infant's eyes are covered, as bright light is uncomfortable. Phototherapy can result in temperature instability as the infant is undressed, a macular rash, and bronze discoloration of the skin if the jaundice is conjugated.

Continuous multiple (intensive) phototherapy is given if the bilirubin is rising rapidly or has reached a high level (Case History 11.2).

Exchange transfusion

Exchange transfusion is required if the bilirubin rises to levels that are considered potentially dangerous. Blood is removed from the baby in small aliquots (usually from an arterial line or the umbilical vein) and replaced with donor blood (via peripheral or umbilical vein). Usually, twice the infant's blood volume (2 × 90 ml/kg) is exchanged. Donor blood should be as fresh as possible and screened to exclude cytomegalovirus, hepatitis B and C and HIV infections. The procedure does carry some risk of morbidity and mortality.

Phototherapy has been very successful in reducing the need for exchange transfusion. In infants with rhesus haemolytic disease or ABO incompatibility unresponsive to intensive phototherapy, intravenous immunoglobulin reduces the need for exchange transfusion.

There is no bilirubin level known to be safe or which will definitely cause kernicterus. In rhesus haemolytic disease, it was found that kernicterus could be prevented if the bilirubin was kept below 340 μmol/l (20 mg/dl).

Summary

Assessment of neonatal jaundice

Severity? → Clinical assessment – press skin to assess jaundice, which progresses from head to limbs, may underestimate if dark skin or preterm
If clinically jaundiced – check bilirubin with transcutaneous meter or blood sample

Gestation? → Lower treatment threshold if preterm

Age? → If <24 hours old – likely to be haemolysis and potentially serious
If > 2 weeks (3 weeks if preterm) – persistent neonatal jaundice. Need to check if unconjugated or conjugated.

Well or unwell? → Check for clinical evidence of sepsis and if dehydrated

Risk factors? → Haemolysis – check for antenatal antibodies, if mother is blood group O (ABO incompatability), if Mediterranean, Far-Eastern or African origin (G6PD deficiency)
Sepsis, unwell, acidosis, low serum albumin (if measured)

Needing treatment? → Plot bilirubin on gestation specific chart according to age since birth
Plot rate of change of bilirubin to identify potentially high levels

---

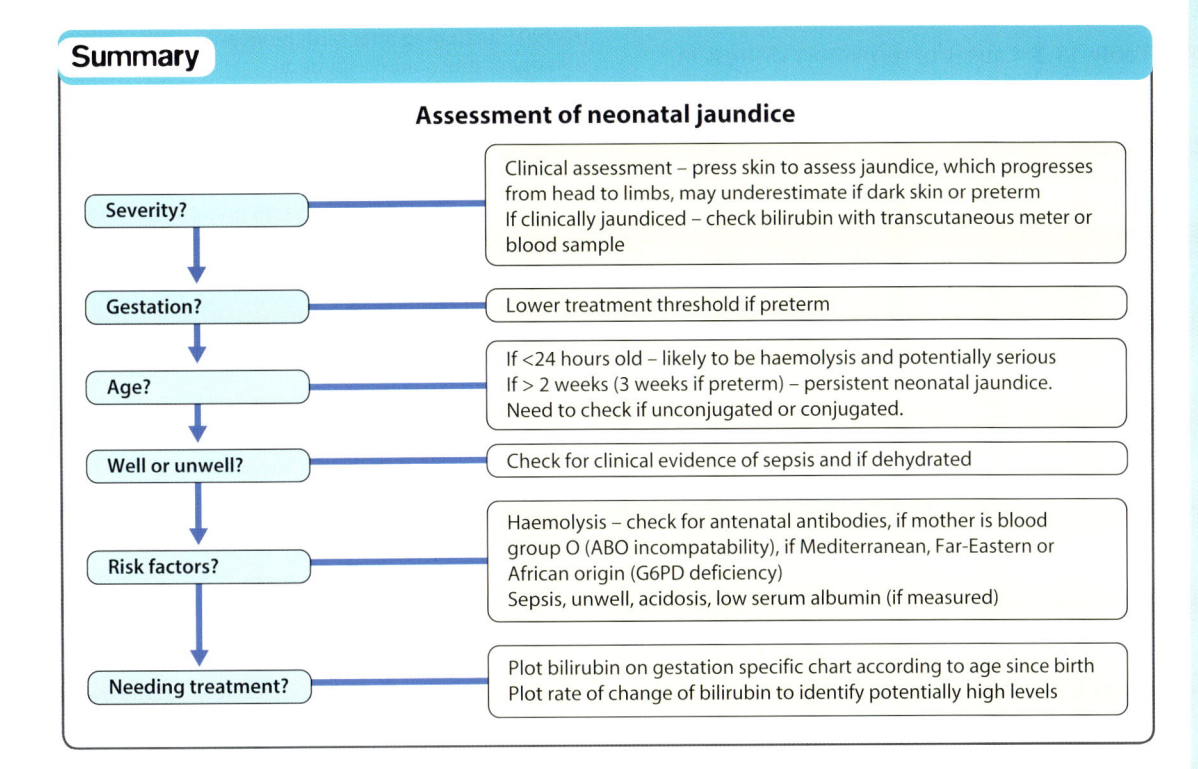

As there is no consensus among paediatricians on the bilirubin levels for phototherapy and exchange transfusion, guidelines have been published by NICE (National Institute for Health and Care Excellence) to ensure uniform practice in the UK.

Jaundice at >2 weeks of age

Jaundice in babies >2 weeks old (3 weeks if preterm) is called persistent or prolonged neonatal jaundice. The key feature is that it may be caused by biliary atresia, and it is important to diagnose biliary atresia promptly, as delay in surgical treatment adversely affects outcome (see Ch. 21 for further details).

However, in most infants with persistent neonatal jaundice, the hyperbilirubinaemia is unconjugated, but this needs to be confirmed on laboratory testing.

In prolonged unconjugated hyperbilirubinaemia:

- 'breast milk jaundice' is the most common cause, affecting up to 15% of healthy breastfed infants; the jaundice gradually fades and disappears by 4–5 weeks of age
- infection, particularly of the urinary tract, needs to be considered
- congenital hypothyroidism may cause prolonged jaundice before the clinical features of coarse facies, dry skin, hypotonia and constipation become evident. Affected infants should be identified on routine neonatal biochemical screening (Guthrie test).

Conjugated hyperbilirubinaemia (>25 µmol/l) is suggested by the baby passing dark urine and unpigmented pale stools. Hepatomegaly and poor weight gain are other clinical signs that may be present. Its causes include neonatal hepatitis syndrome and biliary atresia, with improved prognosis of biliary atresia with early diagnosis (see Ch. 21 for further details).

Respiratory distress in term infants

Newborn infants with respiratory problems develop the following signs of respiratory distress:

- tachypnoea (>60 breaths/min)
- laboured breathing, with chest wall recession (particularly sternal and subcostal indrawing) and nasal flaring
- expiratory grunting
- cyanosis if severe.

The causes in term infants are listed in Table 11.3.

Affected infants should be admitted to the neonatal unit for monitoring of heart and respiratory rates, oxygenation and circulation. A chest X-ray will be required to help identify the cause, especially those causes that may need immediate treatment, e.g. pneumothorax or diaphragmatic hernia. Additional ambient oxygen, respiratory support that may be non-invasive, e.g. CPAP or high-flow nasal cannula therapy, or else mechanical ventilation and circulatory support are given as required.

Transient tachypnoea of the newborn

This is by far the most common cause of respiratory distress in term infants. It is caused by delay in the resorption of lung liquid and is more common after birth by caesarean section. The chest X-ray may show fluid in the horizontal fissure. Additional ambient oxygen may be required. The condition usually settles within

Table 11.3 Causes of respiratory distress in term infants

Pulmonary	
Common	Transient tachypnoea of the newborn
Less common	Meconium aspiration
	Pneumonia
	Respiratory distress syndrome
	Pneumothorax
	Persistent pulmonary hypertension of the newborn
	Milk aspiration
Rare	Diaphragmatic hernia
	Tracheo-oesophageal fistula
	Pulmonary hypoplasia
	Airways obstruction, e.g. choanal atresia
	Pulmonary haemorrhage
Non-pulmonary	
	Congenital heart disease
	Hypoxic-ischaemic/neonatal encephalopathy
	Severe anaemia
	Metabolic acidosis

the 1st day of life but can take several days to resolve completely. This is a diagnosis made after consideration and exclusion of other causes such as infection.

Meconium aspiration

Meconium is passed before birth by 8–20% of babies. It is rarely passed by preterm infants, and occurs increasingly the greater the gestational age, affecting 20–25% of deliveries by 42 weeks. It may be passed in response to fetal hypoxia. Asphyxiated infants may start gasping and aspirate meconium before or at delivery. Meconium is a lung irritant and results in both mechanical obstruction and a chemical pneumonitis, as well as predisposing to infection. In meconium aspiration the lungs are overinflated, accompanied by patches of collapse and consolidation. There is a high incidence of air leak, leading to pneumothorax and pneumomediastinum. Mechanical ventilation is often required. Infants with meconium aspiration may develop persistent pulmonary hypertension of the newborn, which may make it difficult to achieve adequate oxygenation despite high-pressure ventilation (see the following section for management). Severe meconium aspiration is associated with significant morbidity and mortality. There is no evidence that aspiration of meconium from an infant's oropharynx immediately after delivery of the head or removal of meconium by intubation and tracheal suctioning after birth reduces the incidence or severity of meconium aspiration.

Pneumonia

Prolonged rupture of the membranes, chorioamnionitis and low birthweight predispose to pneumonia. Infants with respiratory distress will usually require investigation to identify any infection. Broad-spectrum antibiotics are started early until the results of the infection screen are available.

Pneumothorax

A pneumothorax may occur spontaneously in up to 2% of deliveries. It is usually asymptomatic but may cause respiratory distress. Pneumothoraces also occur secondary to meconium aspiration, respiratory distress syndrome or as a complication of mechanical ventilation. (Management is described earlier in this chapter.)

Milk aspiration

This occurs more frequently in preterm infants and those with respiratory distress or neurological damage. Babies with bronchopulmonary dysplasia often have gastro-oesophageal reflux, which predisposes to aspiration. Infants with a cleft palate are prone to aspirate respiratory secretions or milk.

Persistent pulmonary hypertension of the newborn

This life-threatening condition is usually associated with birth asphyxia, meconium aspiration, septicaemia or RDS. It sometimes occurs as a primary disorder. As a result of the high pulmonary vascular resistance, there is right-to-left shunting within the lungs and at atrial and ductal levels. Cyanosis occurs soon after birth. Heart murmurs and signs of heart failure are often absent. A chest X-ray shows that the heart is of normal size and there may be pulmonary oligaemia. An urgent echocardiogram is required to exclude congenital heart disease and identify the signs of pulmonary hypertension such as raised pulmonary pressures and tricuspid regurgitation.

Most infants require mechanical ventilation and circulatory support in order to achieve adequate oxygenation. Inhaled nitric oxide, a potent vasodilator, is often beneficial. Another vasodilator, sildenafil (Viagra), is also a treatment option for some babies. High-frequency or oscillatory ventilation is sometimes helpful. Extracorporeal membrane oxygenation (ECMO) where the infant is placed on heart and lung bypass for several days is indicated for severe but reversible cases, but is only performed in a few specialist centres.

Diaphragmatic hernia

This occurs in about 1 in 4000 births. Many are now diagnosed on antenatal ultrasound screening. In the newborn period, it usually presents with failure to respond to resuscitation or as respiratory distress. In

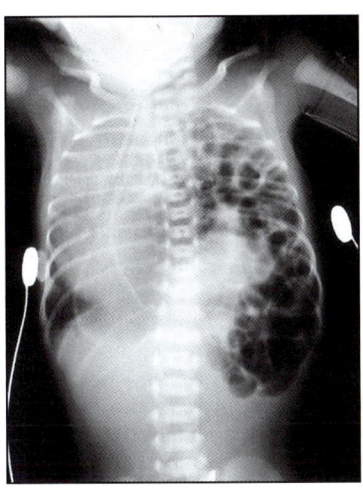

Figure 11.24 Chest X-ray of diaphragmatic hernia showing loops of bowel in the left chest and displacement of the mediastinum.

> **Box 11.3** Clinical features of neonatal sepsis
>
> - Fever or temperature instability or hypothermia
> - Poor feeding
> - Vomiting
> - Apnoea and bradycardia
> - Respiratory distress
> - Abdominal distension
> - Jaundice
> - Neutropenia
> - Hypoglycaemia/hyperglycaemia
> - Shock
> - Irritability
> - Seizures
> - Lethargy, drowsiness
>
> ***In meningitis:***
>
> - tense or bulging fontanelle
> - head retraction (opisthotonos)

most cases, there is a left-sided herniation of abdominal contents through the posterolateral foramen of the diaphragm. The apex beat and heart sounds will then be displaced to the right side of the chest, with poor air entry in the left chest. Vigorous resuscitation may cause a pneumothorax in the normal lung, thereby aggravating the situation. The diagnosis is confirmed by X-ray of the chest and abdomen (Fig. 11.24). Once the diagnosis is suspected, a large nasogastric tube is passed and suction is applied to prevent distension of the intrathoracic bowel. After stabilization, the diaphragmatic hernia is repaired surgically, but in most infants with this condition the main problem is pulmonary hypoplasia – where compression by the herniated viscera throughout pregnancy has prevented development of the lung in the fetus. If the lungs are hypoplastic, mortality is high.

Other causes

Other causes of respiratory distress are listed in Table 11.3. When due to heart failure, abnormal heart sounds and/or heart murmurs may be present on auscultation. An enlarged liver from venous congestion is a helpful sign. The femoral arteries must be palpated in all infants with respiratory distress, as coarctation of the aorta and interrupted aortic arch are important causes of heart failure in newborn infants.

Infection

The time of highest risk in childhood for acquiring a serious invasive bacterial infection is the neonatal period. Infections fall into two broad categories, early-onset and late-onset sepsis.

Early-onset infection

In early-onset sepsis (<48 hours after birth), bacteria have ascended from the birth canal and invaded the amniotic fluid. The fetus is secondarily infected because the fetal lungs are in direct contact with infected amniotic fluid. These infants have pneumonia and secondary bacteraemia/septicaemia. By contrast, in congenital viral infections and early-onset infection with *Listeria monocytogenes*, fetal infection is acquired via the placenta following maternal infection.

The risk of early-onset infection is increased if there has been prolonged or premature rupture of the amniotic membranes, and when chorioamnionitis is clinically evident such as when the mother has fever during labour. Presentation is with respiratory distress, temperature instability and the other clinical features which may be present which are listed in Box 11.3. A chest X-ray is performed, together with a septic screen. A full blood count analysis is performed to detect neutropenia, as well as blood cultures. An acute-phase reactant (C-reactive protein) is helpful but takes 12–24 hours to rise, so one normal result does not exclude infection, but two consecutive normal values are strong evidence against infection. Antibiotics are started immediately without waiting for culture results. Intravenous antibiotics are given to cover group B streptococci, *L. monocytogenes* and other Gram-positive organisms (usually benzylpenicillin or amoxicillin), combined with cover for Gram-negative organisms (usually an aminoglycoside such as gentamicin). If cultures and C-reactive protein are negative and the infant has no clinical indicators of infection, antibiotics can be stopped after 36–48 hours. If the blood culture is positive or if there are neurological or generalised signs, CSF must be examined and cultured.

Late-onset infection

In late-onset infection (>48 hours after birth), the source of infection is often the infant's environment. The presentation is usually non-specific (Box 11.3). Nosocomially acquired infections are an inherent risk in a neonatal unit, and all staff must adhere strictly to effective hand hygiene measures to prevent cross-infection. In neonatal intensive care, the main sources of infection are indwelling central venous catheters for parenteral nutrition, invasive procedures that break the protective barrier of the skin and tracheal tubes. Coagulase-negative staphylococcus (*Staphylococcus epidermidis*) is the most common pathogen, but the range of organisms is broad, and includes Gram-positive bacteria (*Staphylococcus aureus* and *Enterococcus faecalis*) and Gram-negative bacteria (*Escherichia coli* and *Pseudomonas*, *Klebsiella*, and *Serratia* species). Initial therapy (e.g. with flucloxacillin and gentamicin) is aimed to cover most staphylococci and Gram-negative bacilli. If the organism is resistant to these antibiotics or the infant's condition does not improve, specific antibiotics (e.g. vancomycin for coagulase-negative staphylococci or enterococci) or broad-spectrum antibiotics (e.g. meropenem) may be indicated. Use of prolonged or broad-spectrum antibiotics predisposes to invasive fungal infections (e.g. *Candida albicans*) in premature babies. Serial measurements of an acute-phase reactant (C-reactive protein) are useful to monitor response to therapy.

Neonatal meningitis, although uncommon, has a mortality of 20–50%, with one-third of survivors having serious sequelae. Presentation is nonspecific (Box 11.3); a bulging fontanelle and hyperextension of neck and back (opisthotonos) are late signs and rarely seen in newborn infants. If meningitis is thought likely, ampicillin or penicillin and a third-generation cephalosporin (e.g. cefotaxime, which has CSF penetration) are given. Complications include cerebral abscess, ventriculitis, hydrocephalus, hearing loss and neurodevelopmental impairment.

Some specific infections

Group B streptococcal infection

Around 10–30% of pregnant women have faecal or vaginal carriage of group B streptococci. The organism causes early-onset and late-onset sepsis. In early-onset sepsis, the newborn baby has respiratory distress and pneumonia. In the UK, approximately 0.5–1/1000 babies have early-onset infection; most have pneumonia only, but it may cause septicaemia and meningitis. Mortality in babies with positive blood or CSF cultures is up to 10%.

Up to half of infants born to mothers who carry group B streptococcus are colonized on their mucous membranes or skin. Some of these babies develop late-onset disease, up to 3 months of age. It usually presents with meningitis or occasionally with focal infection (e.g. osteomyelitis or septic arthritis).

In colonised mothers, risk factors for infection are preterm, prolonged rupture of membranes, maternal fever during labour (>38°C), maternal chorioamnionitis or previously infected infant. Prophylactic intrapartum antibiotics given intravenously to the mother can prevent group B streptococcus infection in the newborn baby. There are two approaches to the use of intrapartum antibiotics – universal screening at 35–38 weeks to identify mothers who carry the organism (as practiced in the USA and Australia) and a risk-based approach, in which mothers with risk factors for infection are offered antibiotics (as in the UK).

> Group B streptococcal infection is a serious bacterial infection in term as well as preterm infants, from birth to 3 months

L. monocytogenes infection

Fetal or newborn *Listeria* infection is uncommon but serious. The organism is transmitted to the mother in food, such as unpasteurized milk, soft cheeses and undercooked poultry. It causes a bacteraemia, often with mild, influenza-like illness in the mother and passage to the fetus via the placenta. Maternal infection may cause spontaneous abortion, preterm delivery or fetal/neonatal sepsis. Characteristic features are meconium staining of the liquor amnii, unusual in preterm infants, a widespread rash, septicaemia, pneumonia and meningitis. The mortality is 30%.

Gram-negative infections

Early-onset infection is acquired in the same way as group B streptococcal infection. Late-onset infection is usually from infected central venous lines, but occasionally from translocation from the intestines to the circulation.

Conjunctivitis

Sticky eyes are common in the neonatal period, starting on the 3rd or 4th day of life. Cleaning with saline or water is all that is required and the condition resolves spontaneously. A more troublesome discharge with redness of the eye may be due to staphylococcal or streptococcal infection and can be treated with a topical antibiotic eye ointment, e.g. chloramphenicol or neomycin.

Purulent discharge with conjunctival injection and swelling of the eyelids within the first 48 hours of life may be due to gonococcal infection. The discharge should be Gram-stained urgently, as well as cultured, and treatment started immediately, as permanent loss of vision can occur. In countries such as the UK and the USA where penicillin resistance is a problem, a third-generation cephalosporin is given intravenously. The eye needs to be cleansed frequently.

Chlamydia trachomatis eye infection usually presents with a purulent discharge, together with swelling of the eyelids (Fig. 11.25), at 1–2 weeks of age, but may also present shortly after birth. The organism can be identified with immunofluorescent staining. Treatment is with oral erythromycin for 2 weeks. The mother and partner also need to be checked and treated.

Umbilical infection

The umbilicus dries and separates during the first few days of life. If the skin surrounding the umbilicus becomes inflamed, systemic antibiotics are indicated. Sometimes the umbilicus continues to be sticky, as it is prevented from involuting by an umbilical granuloma. This can be removed by applying silver nitrate while protecting the surrounding skin to avoid chemical burns, or by applying a ligature around the base of the exposed stump.

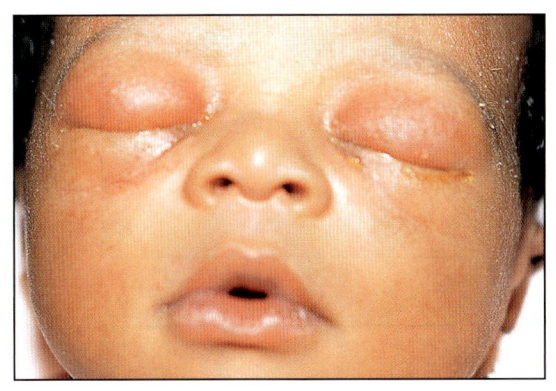

Figure 11.25 Purulent discharge, together with swollen eyelids, in an 8-day-old infant. This is the characteristic presentation of conjunctivitis from *Chlamydia trachomatis*. *Neisseria gonorrhoeae* was absent.

Herpes simplex virus infections

Neonatal herpes simplex virus (HSV) infection is uncommon, occurring in 1 in 3000 to 1 in 20 000 live births. HSV infection is usually transmitted during passage through an infected birth canal or occasionally by ascending infection. The risk to an infant born to a mother with a primary genital infection is high, about 40%, whereas the risk from recurrent maternal infection is less than 3%. In most infants who develop HSV infection, the condition is unexpected as the mother does not know that she is infected (asymptomatic or non-specific illness).

Infection is more common in preterm infants. Presentation is at any time up to 4 weeks of age, with localised herpetic lesions on the skin or eye, or with encephalitis or disseminated disease. Mortality due to localised disease is low, but, even with aciclovir treatment, disseminated disease has a high mortality with considerable morbidity after encephalitis. If the mother is recognised as having primary disease or develops genital herpetic lesions at the time of delivery, elective caesarean section is indicated. Women with a history of recurrent genital infection can be delivered vaginally as the risk of neonatal infection is low and maternal treatment before delivery minimizes the presence of virus at delivery. Aciclovir can be given prophylactically to the baby during the at-risk period, but its efficacy is unproven.

Hepatitis B

Infants of mothers who are hepatitis B surface antigen (HBsAg)-positive should receive hepatitis B vaccination shortly after birth to prevent vertical transmission. The vaccination course needs to be completed during infancy and antibody response checked. Babies are at highest risk of becoming chronic carriers when their mothers are 'e' antigen-positive but have no 'e' antibodies. Infants of 'e' antigen-positive mothers should also be given passive immunization with hepatitis B Ig soon after birth and definitely within 24 hours of birth.

☀ **Infants of HBsAg-positive mothers should be vaccinated against hepatitis B**

Hypoglycaemia

Hypoglycaemia is particularly likely in the first 24 hours of life in babies with intrauterine growth restriction, who are preterm, born to mothers with diabetes mellitus, are large-for-dates, hypothermic, polycythaemic or ill for any reason. Growth-restricted and preterm infants have poor glycogen stores, whereas the infants of a diabetic mother have sufficient glycogen stores, but hyperplasia of the islet cells in the pancreas causes high insulin levels. Symptoms are jitteriness, irritability, apnoea, lethargy, drowsiness and seizures.

There is no agreed definition of hypoglycaemia in the newborn. Many babies tolerate low blood glucose levels in the first few days of life, as they are able to utilise lactate as energy stores. Some studies suggest that blood glucose levels above 2.6 mmol/l are desirable for optimal neurodevelopmental outcome, although during the first 24 hours after birth many asymptomatic infants transiently have blood glucose levels below this level. There is good evidence that prolonged, symptomatic hypoglycaemia can cause permanent neurological disability.

Hypoglycaemia can usually be prevented by early and frequent milk feeding. In infants at increased risk of hypoglycaemia, blood glucose is regularly monitored at the bedside. If an asymptomatic infant has two low glucose values (i.e. below 2.6 mmol/l) in spite of adequate feeding or one very low value (<1.6 mmol/l) or becomes symptomatic, glucose is given by intravenous infusion aiming to maintain the glucose level over 2.6 mmol/l. The concentration of the intravenous dextrose may need to be increased from 10% to 15% or even 20%. Abnormal blood glucose results should be confirmed in the laboratory. High-concentration intravenous infusions of glucose should be given via a central venous catheter to avoid extravasation into the tissues, which may cause skin necrosis and reactive hypoglycaemia. If there is difficulty or delay in starting the infusion, or a satisfactory response is not achieved, glucagon can be given.

Neonatal seizures

Many babies startle or have tremors when stimulated or make strange jerks during active sleep. By contrast, seizures are unstimulated. Typically, there are repetitive, rhythmic (clonic) movements of the limbs that persist despite restraint and are often accompanied by eye movements and changes in respiration. Many neonatal units now use continuous single-channel electroencephalogram (amplified-integrated electroencephalogram, aEEG, also called a cerebral function monitor) to be able to confirm changes in electrical discharges in the brain. The causes of seizures are listed in Box 11.4.

Whenever seizures are observed, hypoglycaemia and meningitis need to be excluded or treated urgently. A cerebral ultrasound is performed to identify haemorrhage or cerebral malformation. Identification of some cerebral ischaemic lesions or cerebral malformations will require MRI scans of the brain. Treatment

Box 11.4 Causes of neonatal seizures

- Hypoxic-ischaemic encephalopathy
- Cerebral infarction
- Septicaemia/meningitis
- Metabolic:
  - hypoglycaemia
  - hyponatraemia/hypernatraemia
  - hypocalcaemia
  - hypomagnesaemia
  - inborn errors of metabolism
  - pyridoxine dependency
- Intracranial haemorrhage
- Cerebral malformations
- Drug withdrawal, e.g. maternal opiates
- Congenital infection
- Kernicterus

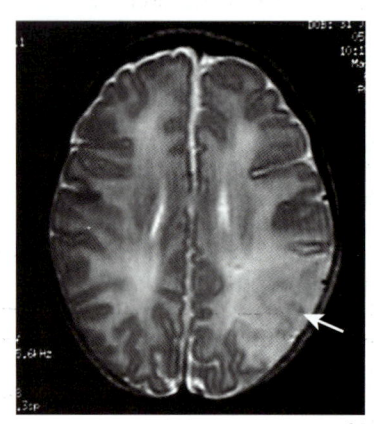

Figure 11.26 Magnetic resonance imaging scan showing infarction in the territory of a branch of the left middle cerebral artery.

is directed at the cause, whenever possible. Ongoing or repeated seizures are treated with an anticonvulsant, although their efficacy in suppressing seizures is much poorer than in older children. The prognosis depends on the underlying cause.

Perinatal stroke

These result from cerebral vascular injury in the fetus or neonate. The commonest cause is ischaemia of the middle cerebral artery. Other causes are haemorrhage or venous thrombosis in the dural venous sinuses. They present with seizures at 12–48 hours in a term infant. The seizures may be focal or generalized. In contrast to infants with HIE, there are no other abnormal clinical features. The diagnosis is confirmed by MRI (Fig. 11.26). The mechanism of perinatal arterial ischaemic strokes is thought to be thrombotic, either thromboembolism from placental vessels or sometimes secondary to inherited thrombophilia. Nearly 50% develop motor disability, usually a hemiplegia of the contralateral side presenting in infancy or childhood, and some cognitive dysfunction. Large lesions may result in epilepsy.

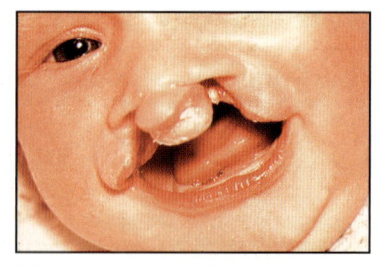

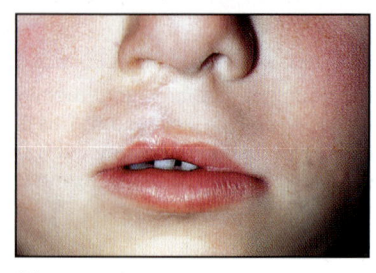

Figure 11.27 Before (**a**) and after (**b**) operation for cleft lip. Photographs showing the impressive results of surgery help many patients cope with the initial distress at having an affected infant. (Courtesy of Mr N. Waterhouse.)

Craniofacial disorders

Cleft lip and palate

A cleft lip (Fig. 11.27a) may be unilateral or bilateral. It results from failure of fusion of the frontonasal and maxillary processes. In bilateral cases the premaxilla is anteverted. Cleft palate results from failure of fusion of the palatine processes and the nasal septum. Cleft lip and palate affect about 0.8 per 1000 babies. Most are inherited polygenically, but they may be part of a syndrome of multiple abnormalities, e.g. chromosomal disorders. Some are associated with maternal anticonvulsant therapy. They may be detected on antenatal ultrasound scanning.

Surgical repair of the lip (Fig. 11.27b) usually takes place at about 3 months of age. The palate is usually repaired at 6–12 months of age. A cleft palate may make feeding more difficult, but some affected infants can still be breastfed successfully. In bottle-fed babies, if milk is observed to enter the nose and cause coughing and choking, special teats and feeding devices may be helpful. Orthodontic advice and a dental prosthesis may help with feeding. Secretory otitis media is relatively common and should be sought on follow-up. Infants are also prone to acute otitis media. Adenoidectomy is best avoided, as the resultant gap between the abnormal palate and nasopharynx will exacerbate feeding problems and the nasal quality of speech. A multidisciplinary team approach is required, involving plastic and ENT surgeons, paediatrician, orthodontist, audiologist and speech therapist. Parent support groups can provide valuable support and advice for families (Cleft Lip and Palate Association).

Pierre Robin sequence

The Pierre Robin sequence is an association of micrognathia (Fig. 11.28), posterior displacement of the tongue (glossoptosis) and midline cleft of the soft palate. There may be difficulty feeding and, as the tongue falls back, there is obstruction to the upper airways, which may result in cyanotic episodes. The infant is at risk of growth faltering during the first few months. If there is upper airways obstruction, the infant may need to lie prone, allowing the tongue and small mandible to fall forward. Persistent obstruction can be treated using a nasopharyngeal airway. Eventually, the mandible grows and these problems resolve. The cleft palate can then be repaired.

Gastrointestinal disorders

Oesophageal atresia

Oesophageal atresia is usually associated with a tracheo-oesophageal fistula (Fig. 11.29). It occurs in 1 in 3500 live births and is associated with polyhydramnios during pregnancy or an absent stomach bubble on antenatal ultrasound screening. If suspected, a wide-calibre feeding tube is passed after birth and checked by X-ray to see if it reaches the stomach. If not suspected before birth, clinical presentation is with persistent salivation and drooling from the mouth. If the diagnosis is not made at this stage, the infant will cough and choke when fed, and have cyanotic episodes. There may be aspiration into the lungs of saliva (or milk) from the upper airways and acid secretions from the stomach. Almost half of the babies have other congenital malformations, e.g. as part of the *v*ertebral, *a*norectal, *c*ardiac, *t*racheo-*o*esophageal, *r*enal, and radial *l*imb anomalies (VACTERL) association. Continuous suction is applied to a tube passed into the oesophageal pouch to reduce aspiration of saliva and secretions pending transfer to a neonatal surgical unit for correction. Following surgery there are a number of know later complications including gastro-oesophageal reflux, chronic cough, and sometimes oesophageal dilation is required in infancy or childhood.

Small bowel obstruction

This may be recognised antenatally on ultrasound scanning. Otherwise, small bowel obstruction presents with persistent vomiting, which is bile stained unless the obstruction is above the ampulla of Vater. Meconium may initially be passed, but subsequently its passage is usually delayed or absent with no transition to normal stool. Abdominal distension becomes increasingly prominent the more distal the bowel obstruction. High lesions will present soon after birth, but lower obstruction may not present for some days.

Small bowel obstruction may be caused by:

- atresia or stenosis of the duodenum (Fig. 11.30) – one-third have Down syndrome and it is also associated with other congenital malformations
- atresia or stenosis of the jejunum or ileum – there may be multiple atretic segments of bowel
- malrotation with volvulus – a dangerous condition as it may lead to infarction of the entire midgut

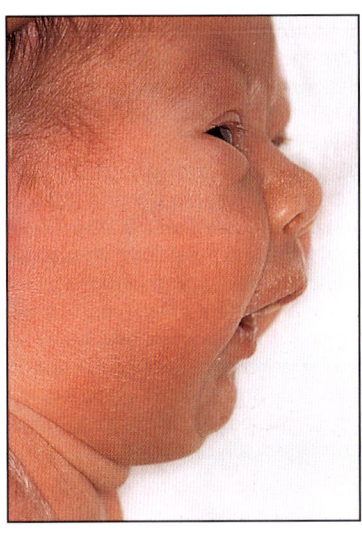

Figure 11.28 Micrognathia in Pierre Robin sequence.

Figure 11.29 Oesophageal atresia and tracheo-oesophageal fistula.

86% Atresia with fistula between distal oesophagus and trachea

8% Atresia without fistula

4% H-type fistula without atresia

Neonatal medicine

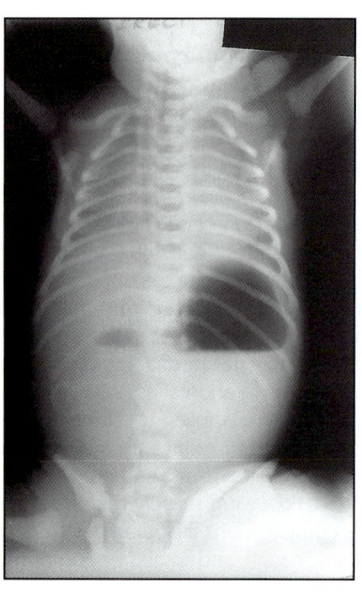

Figure 11.30 Abdominal X-ray in duodenal atresia showing a 'double bubble' from distension of the stomach and duodenal cap. There is absence of air distally.

- meconium ileus – thick inspissated meconium, of puttylike consistency, becomes impacted in the lower ileum; almost all affected neonates have cystic fibrosis
- meconium plug – a plug of inspissated meconium causes lower intestinal obstruction.

The diagnosis is made on clinical features and abdominal X-ray showing intestinal obstruction. Atresia or stenosis of the bowel and malrotation are treated surgically, after correction of fluid and electrolyte depletion. A meconium plug will usually pass spontaneously. Meconium ileus may be dislodged using Gastrografin contrast medium but otherwise will require surgery.

Large bowel obstruction

This may be caused by:

- *Hirschsprung disease* – absence of the myenteric nerve plexus in the rectum, which may extend along the colon. It is more common in boys and in infants with Down syndrome. The baby often does not pass meconium within 48 hours of birth and subsequently the abdomen distends. About 15% present as an acute enterocolitis (see Ch. 14)
- *rectal atresia* – absence of the anus at the normal site. Lesions are high or low, depending on whether the bowel ends above or below the levator ani muscle. In high lesions, there is a fistula to the bladder or urethra in boys, or adjacent to the vagina or to the bladder in girls. Treatment is surgical.

> Bile-stained vomiting is from intestinal obstruction until proven otherwise

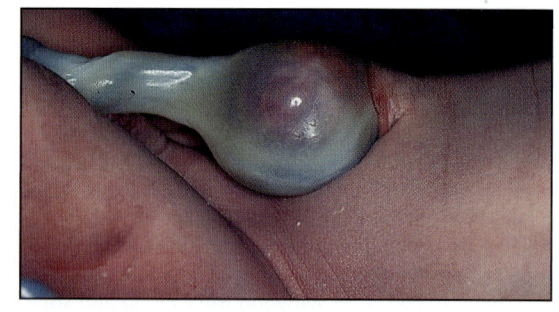

Figure 11.31 Small exomphalos with loops of bowel confined to the umbilicus. Care needs to be taken not to put a cord clamp across these lesions.

Exomphalos/gastroschisis

These lesions are often diagnosed antenatally (see Ch. 10). In exomphalos (also called omphalocele), the abdominal contents protrude through the umbilical ring, covered with a transparent sac formed by the amniotic membrane and peritoneum (Fig. 11.31). It is often associated with other major congenital abnormalities. In gastroschisis, the bowel protrudes through a defect in the anterior abdominal wall adjacent to the umbilicus, and there is no covering sac (see Fig. 10.2). It is not associated with other congenital abnormalities.

Gastroschisis carries a much greater risk of dehydration and protein loss, so the abdomen of affected infants should be covered with a clear occlusive wrap to minimize fluid and heat loss. A nasogastric tube is passed and aspirated frequently and intravenous fluids given. Replacement of fluid loss is often required early on to prevent hypovolaemia. Many lesions can be repaired by primary closure of the abdomen. With large lesions, the intestine is enclosed in a silastic sac sutured to the edges of the abdominal wall and the contents gradually returned into the peritoneal cavity.

Child protection and the newborn

Already during pregnancy there is a need to consider if there are any child protection issues that may arise when the baby is born. This may be because the mother is abusing alcohol or drugs, or due to maternal mental health problems or where the family background, e.g. of violence or previous child protection problems, could compromise the health and well-being of the newborn. Premature infants may be especially difficult to manage at home after discharge and are at an increased risk from child abuse.

To avoid potential child protection concerns later in childhood in normal infants, any abnormalities found during the routine examination of the newborn must be fully described and documented, e.g. Mongolian blue spots as they may be mistaken for bruising and subconjunctival haemorrhages following delivery, which may be mistaken for non-accidental injury.

Acknowledgements

We would like to acknowledge contributors to this chapter in previous editions, whose work we have drawn on: Tom Lissauer (1st, 2nd, 3rd, 4th Editions), Karen Simmer (1st Edition), Michael Weindling (2nd Edition), Andrew Whitelaw (3rd Edition), Andrew Wilkinson (4th Edition).

Further reading

Lissauer T, Fanaroff AA, Miall L, et al.: *Neonatology at a Glance*, ed 3, Oxford, 2015, Wiley Blackwell. *Short, illustrated textbook.*

Rennie JM: *Roberton's Textbook of Neonatology*, ed 4, Edinburgh, 2011, Elsevier/Churchill Livingstone. *Comprehensive textbook.*

Websites (Accessed November 2016)

BLISS: Available at: http://www.bliss.org.uk/.
For parents of infants born too early, too small or too sick.

Population screening programme UK: Available at: https://www.gov.uk/topic/population-screening-programmes

Sands: Available at: http://www.uk-sands.org/. *Stillbirth and neonatal death charity.*

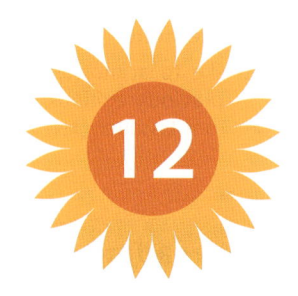

Growth and puberty

Normal growth	194		Tall stature	204
Measurement	194		Abnormal head growth	204
Puberty	196		Premature sexual development	206
Short stature	199		Delayed puberty	209

Features of growth and puberty are:
- growth is a key element of child health, and should be considered whenever children are seen
- the growth of all children should be monitored regularly, especially during the first months of life, and recorded on the growth charts in the parent-held personal child health record
- knowledge about normal growth and pubertal development is required for deviation from the norm to be recognized
- deviation of growth from expected centiles or the normal sequence of pubertal development requires further assessment.

Normal growth

There are four phases of normal human growth (Fig. 12.1).

Fetal

This is the fastest period of growth, accounting for about 30% of eventual height. Size at birth is determined by the size of the mother and by placental nutrient supply, which in turn modulates fetal growth factors [insulin-like growth factor 2 (IGF-2), human placental lactogen, and insulin]. Optimal placental nutrient supply is dependent on an adequate maternal diet. Size at birth is largely independent of the father's height and of growth hormone (GH). Severe intrauterine growth restriction and extreme prematurity when accompanied by poor postnatal growth can result in permanent short stature. Paradoxically, low birthweight increases the later metabolic risk of childhood obesity.

Infantile phase

Growth during infancy to around 18 months of age is also largely dependent on adequate nutrition. Good health and normal thyroid function are also necessary. This phase is characterized by a rapid but decelerating growth rate, and accounts for about 15% of eventual height. By the end of this phase, children have changed from their fetal length, largely determined by the uterine environment, to their genetically determined height. An inadequate rate of weight gain during this period is called 'faltering growth' (see Ch. 13).

Childhood phase

This is a slow, steady but prolonged period of growth that contributes 40% of final height. Pituitary GH secretion acting to produce IGF-1 at the epiphyses is the main determinant of a child's rate of growth, provided there is adequate nutrition and good health. Thyroid hormone, vitamin D, and steroids also affect cartilage cell division and bone formation. Profound chronic unhappiness can decrease GH secretion and accounts for psychosocial short stature.

Pubertal growth spurt

Sex hormones, mainly testosterone and oestradiol, cause the back to lengthen and boost GH secretion. This adds 15% to final height. The same sex steroids cause fusion of the epiphyseal growth plates and a cessation of growth. If puberty is early, which is not uncommon in girls, the final height is reduced because of early fusion of the epiphyses.

Measurement

Growth must be measured accurately, with attention to correct technique and accurate plotting of the data:
- weight – readily and accurately determined with electronic scales but must be performed on a naked infant or a child dressed only in underclothing as an entire month's or year's weight gain can be represented by a wet nappy or heavy jeans, respectively

Determinants of childhood growth

Infant (15% of adult height)
- Nutrition
- Good health and happiness
- Thyroid hormones

Childhood (40% of adult height)
- Genetics
- Good health and happiness
- Growth hormone
- Thyroid hormones

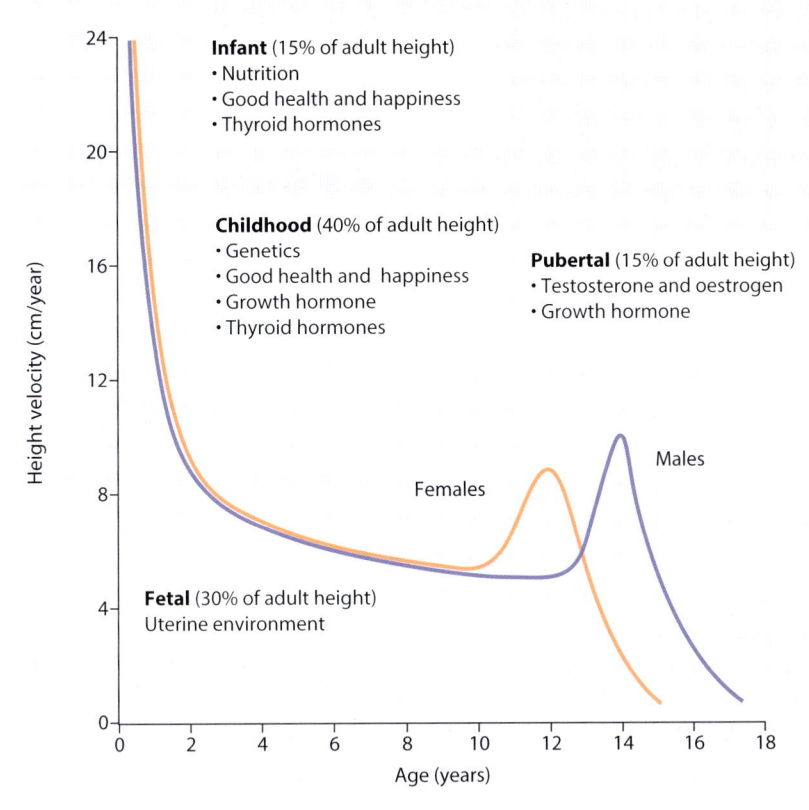

Pubertal (15% of adult height)
- Testosterone and oestrogen
- Growth hormone

Fetal (30% of adult height)
Uterine environment

Figure 12.1 Male and female height velocity charts (50th percentile) showing the determinants of childhood growth. The fetal and infantile phases are mainly dependent on adequate nutrition, whereas the childhood and pubertal phases are dependent on general health, growth hormone, and other hormones. Adult males are taller than females as they have a longer childhood growth phase, their peak height velocity is higher, and their growth ceases later.

- height – the equipment must be regularly calibrated and maintained. In children over 2 years of age, the standing height is measured as illustrated in Fig. 12.2. In children under 2 years, length is measured lying horizontally (Fig. 12.3), using the parent to assist. Accurate length measurement in infants can be difficult to obtain, as the legs need to be held straight and infants often dislike being held still. For this reason, routine measurement of length in infancy is often omitted from child surveillance, but it should always be performed whenever there is doubt about an infant's growth
- head circumference – the occipitofrontal circumference is a measure of head and hence brain growth. Plot the maximum of three measurements. It is of particular importance in developmental delay or suspected hydrocephalus
- body mass index – calculate this using height in square metres/weight in kilogram and plot on a gender-specific body mass index centile chart to assess underweight or obese children.

These measurements should be plotted as a simple dot on an appropriate growth centile chart. Standards for a population should be constructed and updated every generation to allow for the trend towards earlier puberty and taller adult stature from improved childhood

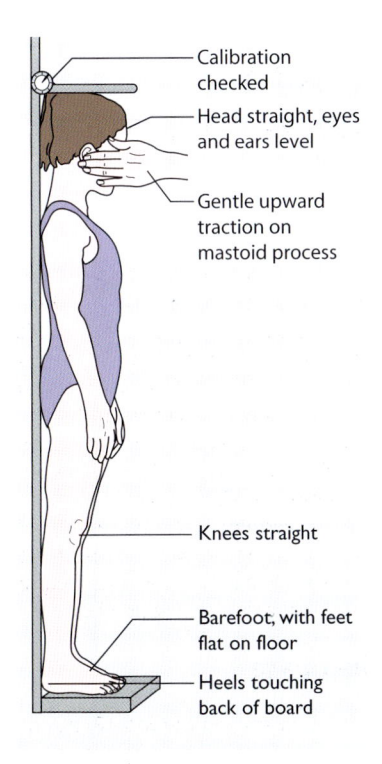

Figure 12.2 Measuring height accurately in children.

Growth and puberty

nutrition. In 2009, the UK adopted the World Health Organization new global Child Growth Standards for infants and children 0–4 years old (see Appendix Fig. A1). The new charts are based on the optimal growth of healthy children exclusively breastfed up to the age of 6-months. These charts allow for the lower weight of exclusively breastfed infants and therefore reduce the number of breastfed babies labelled as underweight and may also allow earlier identification of formula-fed babies gaining weight too rapidly.

Height in a population is normally distributed and the deviation from the mean can be measured as a centile or standard deviation (SD; Fig. 12.4). The bands on the growth reference charts have been chosen to be two-thirds of an SD apart and correspond approximately to the 25th, 9th, 2nd, and 0.4th centiles below the mean, and the 75th, 91st, 98th, and 99.6th centiles above the mean. The further these centiles lie from the mean, the more likely it is that a child has a pathological cause for his/her short or tall stature. For instance, values below the 0.4th or above the 99.6th centile will occur by chance in only 4 per 1000 children and can be used as a criterion for referral from primary to specialist care. A single growth parameter should not be assessed in isolation from the other growth parameters, e.g. a child's low weight may be in proportion to the height if short, but abnormal if tall. Serial measurements are used to show the pattern and determine the rate of growth. This is helpful in diagnosing or monitoring many paediatric conditions. The child's growth should be assessed in the context of his/her family size. Heights from both biological parents should be used to calculate midparental height and the child's target range.

Summary

Measurement of children
- Measurement must be accurate for meaningful monitoring of growth.
- Growth parameters should be plotted on charts.
- Significant abnormalities of height are:
  - measurements below the 0.4th or above the 99.6th centiles or outside the midparental height range
  - if markedly discrepant from weight
  - serial measurements, which cross growth centile lines after the 1st year of life.
- The pattern of growth is essential information when assessing the health of a child; consider genetics, nutrition, general health, and hormones as potential causes of abnormal growth.

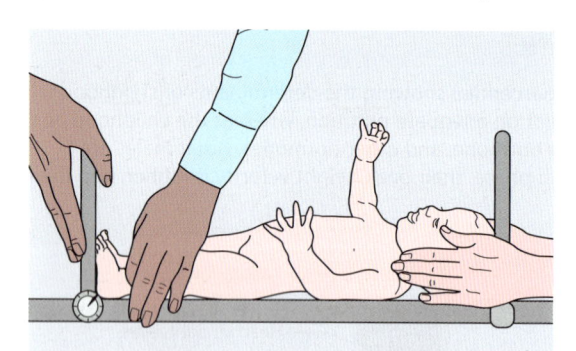

Figure 12.3 Measuring length in infants and young children. An assistant is required to hold the legs straight.

Puberty

Puberty follows a well-defined sequence of changes that may be assigned stages, as shown in Figs 12.5 and 12.6. Over the last 20 years, the mean age at which puberty starts in girls has lowered. However, the age at which menarche occurs has remained stable. Therefore, females now remain in puberty for longer.

In *females* the features of puberty are:

- breast development – a palpable breast disc is the first sign, usually starting between 8.5 and 12.5 years
- pubic hair growth and rapid height growth – occur almost immediately after breast development

Figure 12.4 Interpretation of the UK growth reference charts. The lines show the mean and bands, which are two-thirds of a standard deviation (SD) apart. The centiles are shown in the diagram.

| 0.4th centile −2.6 SD | 2nd centile −2 SD | 9th centile −1.3 SD | 25th centile −0.66 SD | 50th centile Mean | 75th centile +0.66 SD | 91st centile +1.3 SD | 98th centile +2 SD | 99.6th centile +2.6 SD |

Stages of puberty

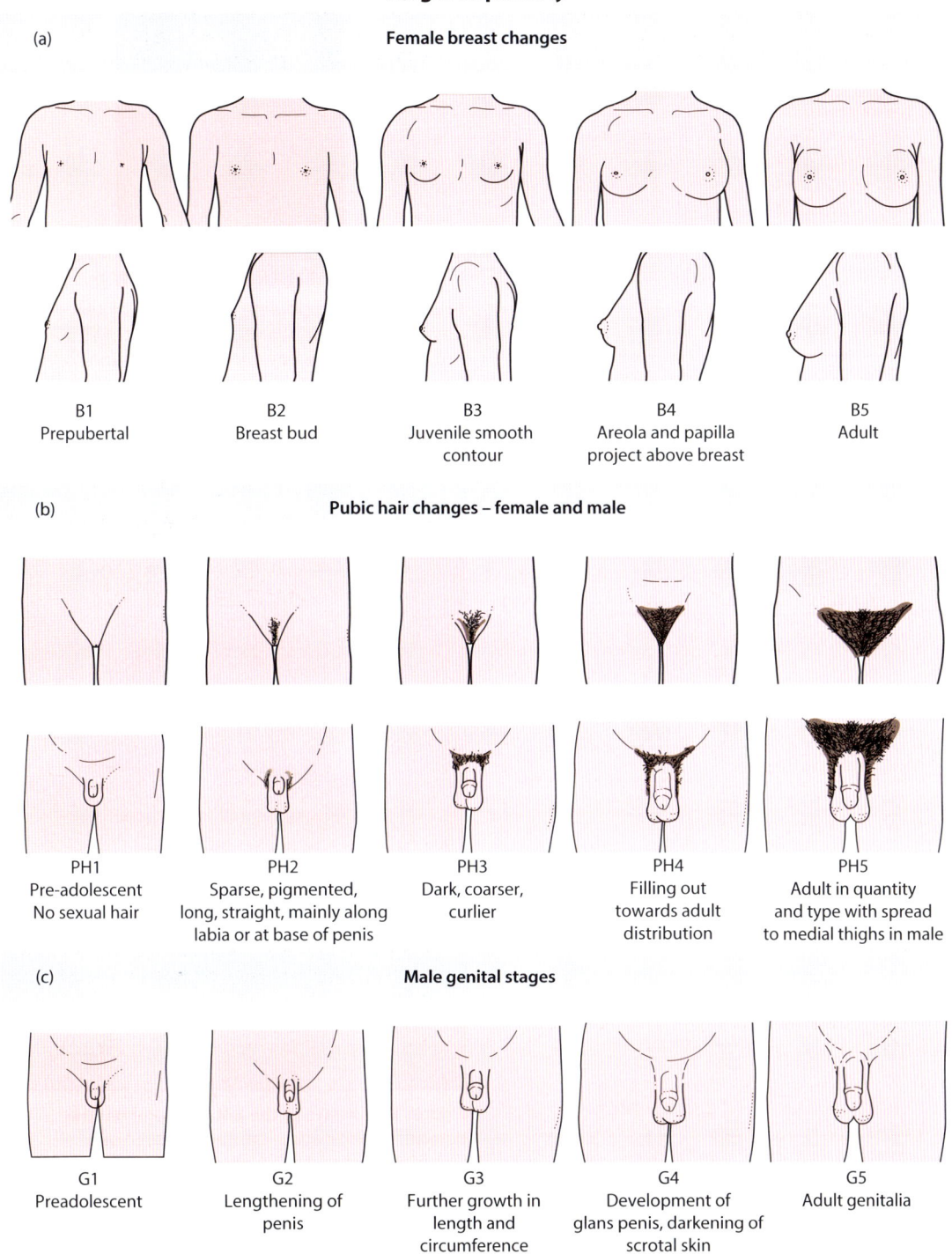

(a) Female breast changes

| B1 Prepubertal | B2 Breast bud | B3 Juvenile smooth contour | B4 Areola and papilla project above breast | B5 Adult |

(b) Pubic hair changes – female and male

| PH1 Pre-adolescent No sexual hair | PH2 Sparse, pigmented, long, straight, mainly along labia or at base of penis | PH3 Dark, coarser, curlier | PH4 Filling out towards adult distribution | PH5 Adult in quantity and type with spread to medial thighs in male |

(c) Male genital stages

| G1 Preadolescent | G2 Lengthening of penis | G3 Further growth in length and circumference | G4 Development of glans penis, darkening of scrotal skin | G5 Adult genitalia |

Figure 12.5 Schematic drawings of male and female stages of puberty. Pubertal changes are shown according to the Tanner stages of puberty.

- menarche – occurs on average 2.5 years after the start of puberty and signals that growth is coming to an end, with only around 5-cm height gain remaining.

In *males*:
- testicular enlargement to over 4-mL volume measured using an orchidometer (Fig. 12.7) – the first clinical sign of puberty
- pubic hair growth – follows testicular enlargement, usually between 10-years and 14-years of age
- rapid height growth – when the testicular volume is 12 mL to 15 mL, after a delay of around 18 months
- The growth spurt in males occurs later and is of greater magnitude than in females, accounting for the greater final average height of males than females.

Timing of puberty

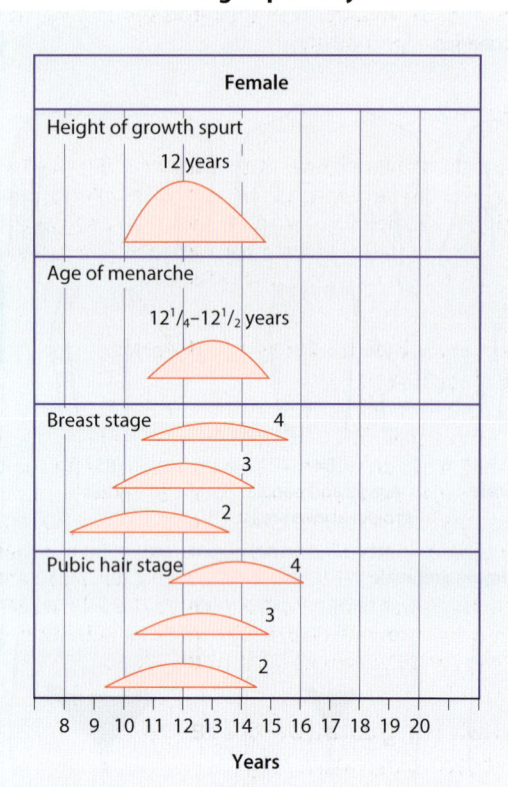

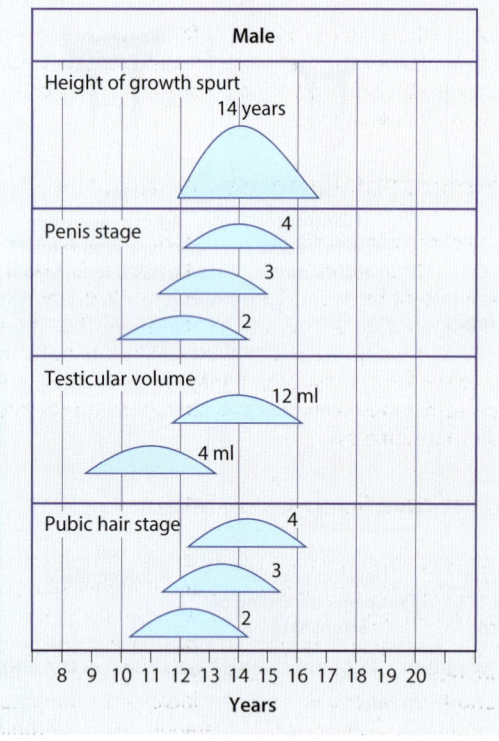

Figure 12.6 Timing of puberty. Pubertal changes are shown according to the Tanner stages of puberty. (Adapted from Zitelli BJ, Davis HW: *Atlas of Pediatric Physical Diagnosis*, ed 2, Philadelphia, 1992, Lippincott; Johnson TR, Moore WM, Jeffries JE: *Children are Different*, ed 2, Columbus, 1978, Ross Laboratories (Division of Abbot Laboratories.))

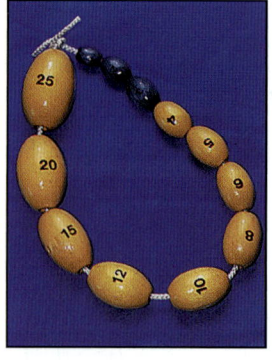

Figure 12.7 Orchidometer to assess testicular volume (in millilitre). (From Wales JKH, Rogol AD, Wit JM: *Pediatric Endocrinology and Growth,* London, 2003, Saunders with permission.)

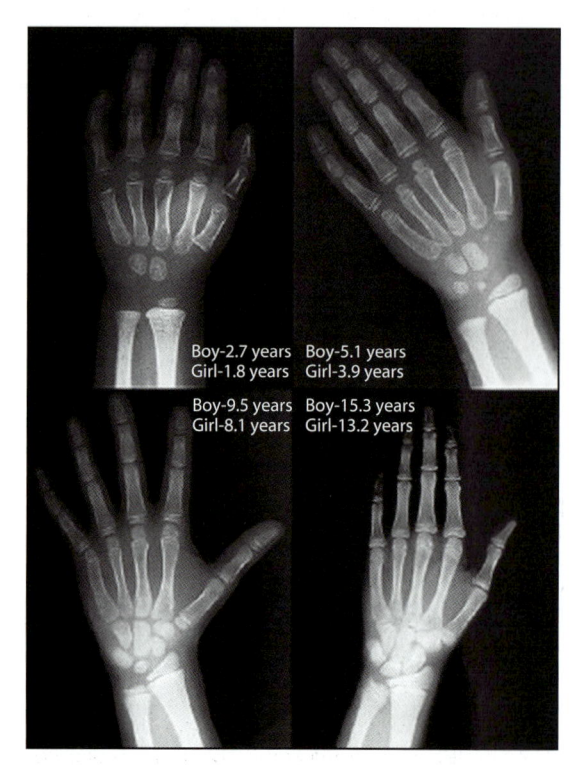

Figure 12.8 X-rays of the left wrist and hand to determine bone ages. This technique allows assessment of skeletal maturation from the time of appearance or maturity of the epiphyseal centres, using a standardized rating system. The child's height can be compared with skeletal maturation and an adult height prediction made. The ages show bone age of each X-ray.

In *both sexes*, there will be development of acne, axillary hair, body odour, and mood changes.

If puberty is abnormally early or late, it can be further assessed by:

- bone age measurement from a hand and wrist X-ray to determine skeletal maturation (Fig. 12.8)
- in females, pelvic ultrasound can be used to assess uterine size and endometrial thickness.

Menstruation has a wide range of normal variation. The normal cycle length varies between 21 days and 45 days. The length of blood loss varies between 3 days and 7 days and the average blood loss/cycle is less than 80 mL – passage of blood clots or the use of more than six pads/day implies heavy bleeding, which needs evaluation. Rarely, it can indicate clotting disorders such as von Willebrand disease.

> **Summary**
>
> **Puberty**
> - The first sign of female puberty is a palpable breast bud; the first sign of male puberty is testicular volume over 4 ml.
> - In females, the height spurt occurs shortly after breast development; in males, it starts almost 18 months after the first signs of puberty.

Short stature

Short stature is usually defined as a height below the second centile (i.e. 2 SDs below the mean). Most of these 1 in 50 children will be normal, though short, with short parents. However, the further the child is below these centiles, the more likely it is that there will be a pathological cause. Only 1 in 250 (4 in 1000) children are shorter than the 0.4th centile (−2.6 SD) and these should be assessed for a cause. However, the rate of growth may be abnormal a long time prior to the child's height being below these values. This growth failure can be identified from the child's height falling across centile lines plotted on a height velocity chart (Fig. 12.1). This allows growth failure to be identified whilst the child's height is still above the 2nd centile.

Measuring height velocity is a sensitive indicator of growth failure. Two *accurate* measurements at least 6 months but preferably a year apart allow calculation of height velocity in cm/year (Fig. 12.1). This is plotted at the midpoint in time on a height velocity chart. A disadvantage of using height velocity calculations is that they are highly dependent on the accuracy of the height measurements and so tend not to be used outside specialist growth clinics.

The height centile of a child must be compared with the weight centile and an estimate of his/her genetic expected height calculated from the height of his/her parents. This is calculated as the mean of the father's and mother's height with 7 cm added for the midparental target height of a boy, and 7 cm subtracted for a girl. The 9th to 91st centile range of this estimate is given by ±10 cm in a boy and ±8.5 cm in a girl (see Fig. 12.9a).

Most short children are psychologically well adjusted to their size. However, there may be problems from being teased or bullied at school, poor self-esteem, and they are likely to be at a considerable disadvantage in most competitive sport. They are also assumed by adults to be younger than their true age and may be treated inappropriately.

Familial

Most short children have short parents and fall within the centile target range allowing for midparental height. Care needs to be taken, though, that both the child and a parent do not have an inherited growth disorder, such as a skeletal dysplasia.

Constitutional delay in growth and puberty

Constitutional delay in growth and puberty is a variation of normal growth, which presents with short stature in teenage years because of a delay in the onset of puberty. Growth during childhood is usually within the lower limits of normal, bone age is somewhat delayed, and onset of secondary sexual development is delayed but final height is normal. There is usually a family history of delayed growth and puberty but normal height as adults (Case History 12.5).

Small for gestational age and extreme prematurity

About 10% of children born small for gestational age or who were extremely premature remain short. GH treatment may be indicated if there is insufficient catch-up growth by 4 years of age.

Chromosomal disorder/syndromes

Many chromosomal disorders and syndromes are associated with short stature. Down syndrome is usually diagnosed at birth, but Turner (see Fig. 12.10 and Ch. 9), Noonan (Fig. 9.17), and Russell–Silver (Fig. 12.9) syndromes may present with short stature and minimal symptoms. Turner syndrome may be particularly difficult to diagnose clinically and should be considered in all short females.

Nutritional/long-term illness

This is a relatively common cause of abnormal growth. These children are usually short and underweight, i.e. their weight is on the same or a lower centile than their height. Inadequate nutrition may be due to insufficient food, restricted diets or poor appetite associated with a long-term illness, or from the increased nutritional requirement from a raised metabolic rate. Chronic illnesses that may present with short stature include:

- coeliac disease, which usually presents in the first 2 years of life, but can present late with faltering growth. Coeliac disease may result in short stature without gastrointestinal symptoms
- Crohn's disease
- chronic kidney disease – may be present in the absence of a history of renal disease

Causes & evaluation of short stature

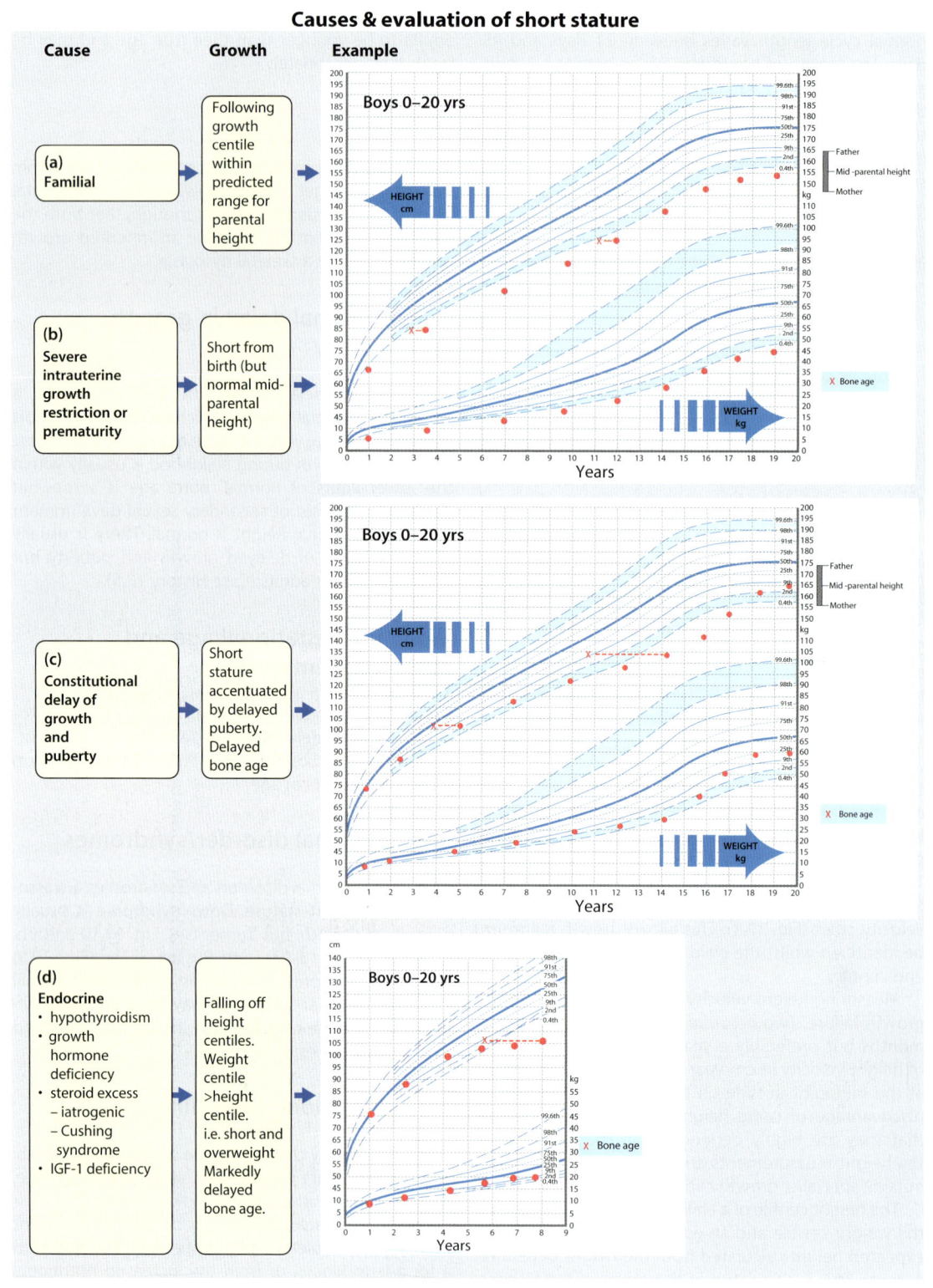

Cause	Growth	Example
(a) Familial	Following growth centile within predicted range for parental height	Boys 0–20 yrs
(b) Severe intrauterine growth restriction or prematurity	Short from birth (but normal mid-parental height)	
(c) Constitutional delay of growth and puberty	Short stature accentuated by delayed puberty. Delayed bone age	Boys 0–20 yrs

(d) Endocrine
• hypothyroidism
• growth hormone deficiency
• steroid excess
  – iatrogenic
  – Cushing syndrome
• IGF-1 deficiency
	Falling off height centiles. Weight centile >height centile. i.e. short and overweight Markedly delayed bone age.	Boys 0–20 yrs

Figure 12.9 Causes of short stature. (Charts © Child Growth Foundation. Further supplies and information from www.healthforallchildren.co.uk. Reproduced with permission.)

Causes & evaluation of short stature

Cause → **Growth** → **Example**

(e) **Nutrition/long-term illness**
- gastrointestinal – coeliac, Crohn's disease
- chronic kidney disease

(f) **Psychosocial**
- emotional deprivation/neglect

→ Falling off height centiles. Weight centile < height centile. Delayed bone age.

→ Crohn's disease (Boys 0–20 yrs growth chart, with Diagnosis and treatment marked; × = Bone age)

(g) **Syndromes**
- Turner
- Noonan
- Down
- Russell–Silver

→ Dysmorphic features.

→ Russell–Silver syndrome

(h) **Extreme short stature** → Rare

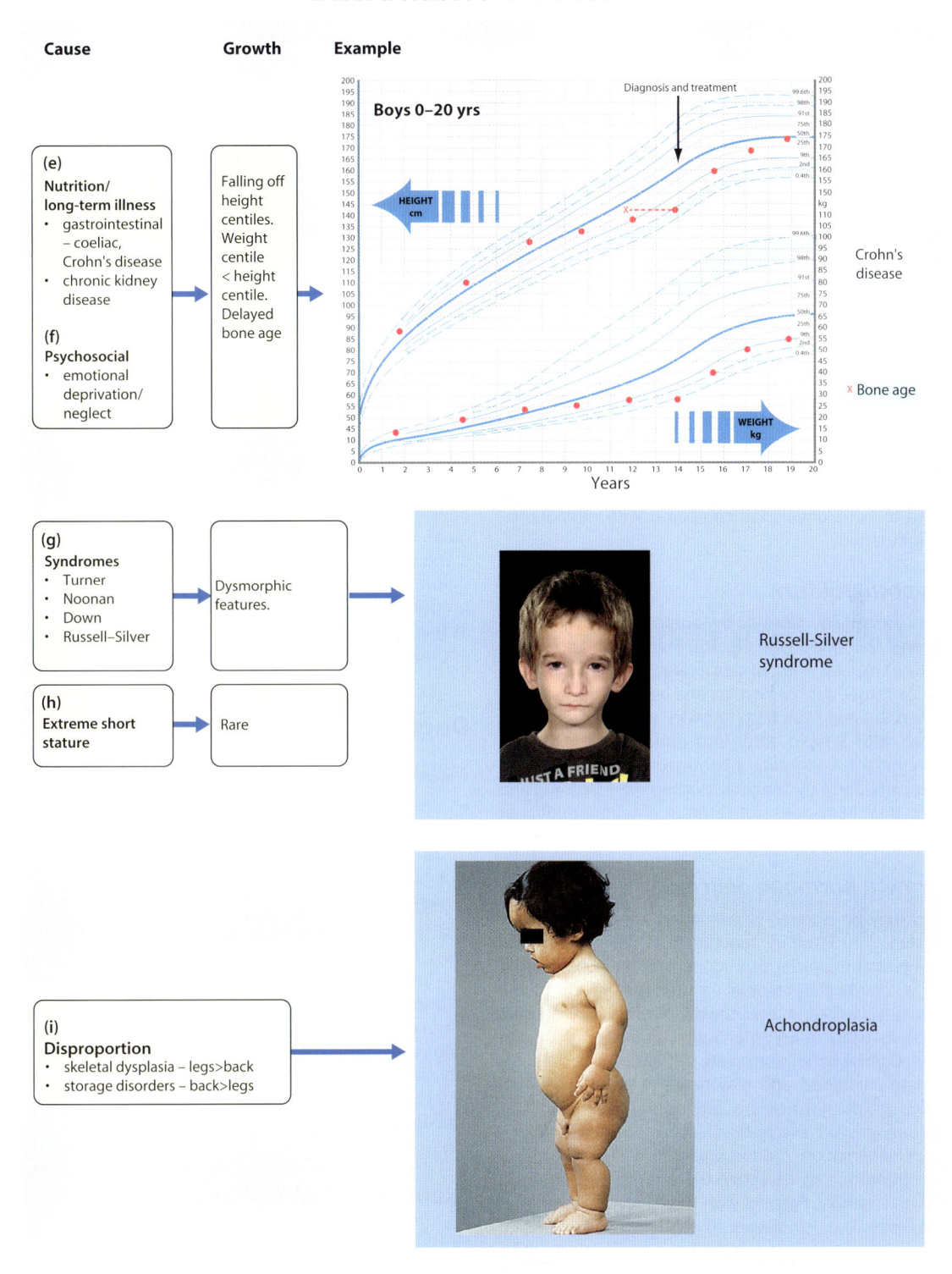

(i) **Disproportion**
- skeletal dysplasia – legs>back
- storage disorders – back>legs

→ Achondroplasia

Figure 12.9, cont'd

- cystic fibrosis – malabsorption, recurrent infections, increased work of breathing, and reduced appetite
- congenital heart disease – increased work of breathing.

Psychosocial deprivation

Children subjected to physical and emotional deprivation may be short and underweight and show delayed puberty. This condition may be extremely difficult to identify, but affected children show catch-up growth if placed in a nurturing environment.

Endocrine

Hypothyroidism, GH deficiency, IGF-1 deficiency, and steroid excess are uncommon causes of short stature. They are associated with children being relatively overweight, i.e. their weight on a higher centile than their height. By contrast, children with nutritional obesity tend to be relatively tall compared with midparental height range.

Hypothyroidism

This is usually caused by autoimmune thyroiditis during childhood (see Ch. 26). This produces growth failure, usually with excess weight gain. It may go undiagnosed for many years and lead to short stature. When treated, catch-up growth rapidly occurs but often with a rapid entry into puberty that can limit final height. Congenital hypothyroidism is diagnosed soon after birth by neonatal biochemical screening and with treatment does not result in any abnormality of growth.

Growth hormone deficiency

This may be isolated or secondary to wider pituitary dysfunction. Pituitary function may be abnormal in congenital midfacial or midline defects or as a result of a craniopharyngioma (a tumour affecting the pituitary region), a hypothalamic tumour, or trauma such as head injury, meningitis, and cranial irradiation. Craniopharyngioma (see Ch. 22) usually presents in late childhood and may result in abnormal visual fields (characteristically a bitemporal hemianopia as it impinges on the optic chiasm), optic atrophy, or papilloedema on fundoscopy. Laron syndrome is a condition due to defective GH receptors resulting in GH insensitivity. Patients with this condition have high GH levels but low levels of the downstream active product of GH known as IGF-1 produced at the growth plate and in the liver. Rare abnormalities in the gene producing IGF-1 have recently been discovered in children.

Corticosteroid excess, Cushing syndrome

This is usually iatrogenic, as corticosteroid therapy is a potent growth suppressor and a number of chronic conditions are treated with corticosteroids. This effect is reduced by alternate day therapy, but some growth suppression may be seen even with relatively low doses of inhaled or topical steroids in susceptible individuals. Noniatrogenic Cushing syndrome is very unusual in childhood and may be caused by pituitary or adrenal pathology. Growth failure may be very severe, and is accompanied by excess weight gain, although normalization of body shape and height occurs on withdrawal of corticosteroid therapy or treatment of the underlying steroid excess. Cushing syndrome during puberty can result in permanent loss of height (see Ch. 26).

Extreme short stature

There are a few rare conditions that cause extreme short stature in children. Idiopathic short stature refers to short stature that does not have a diagnostic explanation. In addition, abnormalities in a gene called short stature homeobox (*SHOX*) located on the X chromosome lead to severe short stature with skeletal abnormalities when present on both copies of the gene. Absence of one *SHOX* gene in Turner syndrome is thought to be the cause of short stature in this condition (and additional copies in Klinefelter syndrome produce taller than normal stature). Polymorphisms in this gene probably account for a proportion of idiopathic short stature.

Disproportionate short stature

This is confirmed by measuring:

- sitting height – base of spine to top of head
- subischial leg length – subtraction of sitting height from total height
- limited radiographic skeletal survey to identify the skeletal abnormality.

Charts exist to assess the normality of body proportions. Conditions with abnormal body proportions are rare and may be caused by disorders of the formation of bone (skeletal dysplasias). They include achondroplasia and other short-limbed dysplasias. If the legs are extremely short, treatment by surgical leg lengthening may be appropriate. The back may be short from severe scoliosis or some storage disorders, such as the mucopolysaccharidoses.

Examination and investigation

Plotting present and previous heights and weights on appropriate growth charts, together with the clinical features, usually allows the cause to be identified without any investigations (Fig. 12.9a–i). Previous height and weight measurements should be available from the parent-held personal child health record. The bone age may be helpful, as it is markedly delayed in some endocrine disorders, e.g. hypothyroidism and GH deficiency, and is used to estimate adult height potential. Investigations that may be indicated are shown in Table 12.1.

Table 12.1 Investigations considered for short stature

Investigation	Significance
X-ray of the left hand and wrist for bone age	Some delay in constitutional delay of growth and puberty. Marked delay for hypothyroidism or growth hormone deficiency
Full blood count	Anaemia in coeliac or Crohn's disease
Creatinine and electrolytes	Creatinine raised in chronic kidney disease
Calcium, phosphate, alkaline phosphatase	Renal and bone disorders
Thyroid-stimulating hormone	Raised in primary hypothyroidism
Karyotype	Turner syndrome shows 45,XO, other chromosomal disorders
Anti-endomysial (EMA) and anti-tissue transglutaminase (anti-TTGa) immunoglobulin A antibodies	Usually present in coeliac disease
C-reactive protein (acute-phase reactant) and erythrocyte sedimentation rate	Raised in Crohn's disease
Growth hormone provocation tests (using insulin, glucagon, clonidine, or arginine in specialist centres)	Growth hormone deficiency
IGF-1	Disorders of the growth hormone axis, including IGF-1 deficiency
0900 h cortisol and dexamethasone suppression test	Cushing syndrome
MRI scan if neurological symptoms/signs	Craniopharyngioma or intracranial tumour
Limited skeletal survey	Skeletal dysplasia, scoliosis

Growth hormone treatment of short stature

GH deficiency is treated with biosynthetic GH, which is given by subcutaneous injection, usually daily. It is expensive and the management of GH deficiency is undertaken at specialist centres. The best response is seen in children with the most severe hormone deficiency. Other indications include Turner syndrome (Case history 12.1), Prader–Willi syndrome (Fig. 9.19), chronic kidney disease, *SHOX* deficiency, and intrauterine growth restriction or small for gestational age with failure of catch-up growth. In Prader–Willi syndrome (an imprinting disorder resulting in early hypotonia and feeding difficulties followed by short stature, obesity, and learning difficulties), GH improves muscular strength and body composition as well as modestly improving final height. Recently, recombinant IGF-1 has been used to treat children with GH resistance (e.g. Laron syndrome) and IGF-1 deficiency who would have previously not responded to GH treatment. Recombinant IGF-1 therapy is still very expensive and is confined to a few specialized centres.

Case history 12.1

Turner syndrome

This girl (Fig. 12.10), presented when 10 years old with short stature. She had a history of recurrent ear infections, but was otherwise well. She had always been very short, and her height was 126.4 cm, well below the 0.4th centile on the standard growth chart. Her chromosomes were checked, which confirmed Turner syndrome 45,XO. She was started on growth hormone injections and on ethinyl oestradiol (oestrogens) for pubertal induction at 14 years of age. At 15 years of age her height was 150 cm.

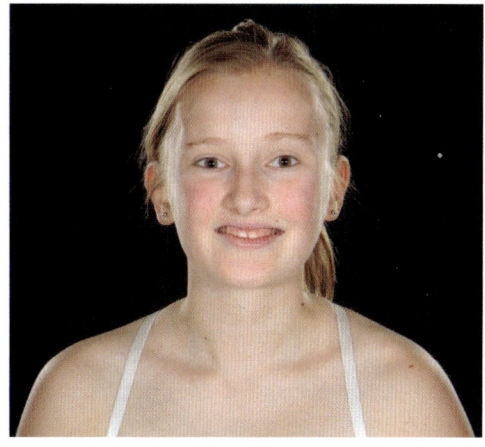

Figure 12.10 At 15 years, she has few clinical features of Turner syndrome, demonstrating the need to check the karyotype of females with marked short stature.

Summary

Assessment of a child with short stature

Examination of the growth chart:
- Following growth centile lines for length/height, weight and head circumference?
  Consider familial, low birthweight, constitutional delay of growth and puberty, syndromes and skeletal dysplasias
- Faltering growth with crossing of centile lines?
  Consider endocrine (including therapeutic corticosteroids), nutrition/chronic illness, psychosocial deprivation

Determine the mid-parental height
- For genetic target range

History
- Birth length, weight, head circumference and gestational age
- Pregnancy history: infection, intrauterine growth restriction, drug use, alcohol/smoking
- Feeding history
- Developmental milestones
- Family history of constitutional delay of growth and puberty or other diseases?
- Consanguinity pertaining to inherited conditions
- Features of chronic illness, endocrine causes, e.g. hypothyroidism, pituitary tumour, Cushing syndrome or psychosocial deprivation?
- Medications, e.g. corticosteroids?

Examination
- Dysmorphic features – chromosome/syndrome present? (But in Turner syndrome other stigmata may be absent)
- Chronic illness, e.g. Crohn's, cystic fibrosis, coeliac disease?
- Evidence of endocrine causes?
- Disproportionate short stature from skeletal dysplasia?
- Pubertal stage?

Diagnosis
Cause can usually be determined from the above and no tests are required

Tall stature

This is a less common presenting complaint than short stature, as many parents are proud that their child is tall. However, some adolescents become concerned about excessive height during their pubertal growth spurt. The causes are presented in Table 12.2. Most tall stature is inherited from tall parents. Obesity in childhood 'fuels' early growth and may result in tall stature; however, because puberty is often somewhat earlier than average, it does not increase final height.

Secondary endocrine causes are rare. Both congenital adrenal hyperplasia and precocious puberty (PP) lead to early epiphyseal fusion so that eventual height is reduced after an early excessive growth rate.

Marfan (a disorder of loose connective tissue) and Klinefelter (XXY – an excess of *SHOX* dose) syndromes both cause long-legged tall stature, and in XXY there is also infertility and learning difficulties.

Tall children may be disadvantaged by being treated as older than their chronological age. Excessive height in prepubertal or early pubertal adolescent females and males can be treated with oestrogen therapy and testosterone therapy, respectively, to induce premature fusion of the epiphyses, but as it produces variable results and has potentially serious side-effects, it is seldom undertaken. Surgical destruction of the epiphyses in the legs may also be considered in extreme cases.

Abnormal head growth

Most head growth occurs in the first 2 years of life and 80% of adult head size is achieved before the age of 5 years. This largely reflects brain growth, but small

Table 12.2 Causes of excessive growth or tall stature

Familial	Most common cause
Obesity	Puberty is advanced, so final height centile is less than in childhood
Secondary	Hyperthyroidism
	Excess sex steroids – precocious puberty from whatever cause
	Excess adrenal androgen steroids – congenital adrenal hyperplasia
	True gigantism (excess growth hormone secretion)
Syndromes	Long-legged tall stature: • Marfan syndrome • Homocystinuria • Klinefelter syndrome (47,XXY karyotype)
	Sotos syndrome – associated with large head, characteristic facial features, and learning difficulties
Excessive growth at birth	Proportionate tall stature at birth: • maternal diabetes • primary hyperinsulinism • Beckwith syndrome

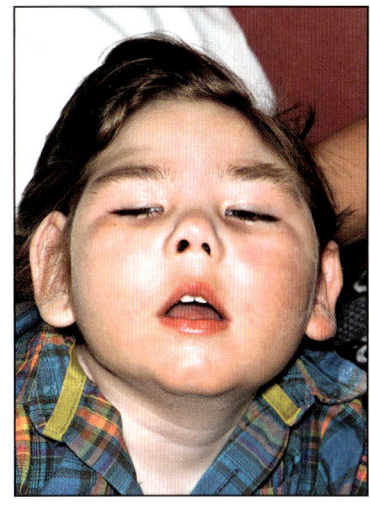

Figure 12.11 This boy has microcephaly. He has cerebral palsy. (Courtesy of Dr Gabby Chow.)

Box 12.1. Most are normal children and often the parents have large heads. A rapidly increasing head circumference, even if the head circumference is still below the 98th centile, suggests raised intracranial pressure and may be due to hydrocephalus, subdural haematoma, or brain tumour. It must be investigated promptly by cranial ultrasound if the anterior fontanelle is still open, otherwise by computed tomography or magnetic resonance imaging (MRI) scan.

or large heads may be familial, so comparison with measurements of parents' heads should be made. At birth, the sutures and fontanelle are open. During the first few months of life, the head circumference may increase across centiles, especially if small for gestational age. The posterior fontanelle has closed by 8 weeks, and the anterior fontanelle by 12 months to 18 months. If there is a rapid increase in head circumference, raised intracranial pressure should be excluded.

Microcephaly

Microcephaly, a head circumference below the 2nd centile (Fig. 12.11), may be:

- familial – when it is present from birth and development is usually normal
- an autosomal recessive condition – when it is associated with developmental delay
- caused by a congenital infection
- acquired after an insult to the developing brain, e.g. perinatal hypoxia, hypoglycaemia, or meningitis, when it is often accompanied by cerebral palsy and seizures (Case History 12.2).

Macrocephaly

Macrocephaly is a head circumference above the 98th centile. The causes of a large head are listed in

> If an infant's head circumference is enlarging and crossing centile lines, check for raised intracranial pressure

Asymmetric heads

Skull asymmetry may result from an imbalance of the growth rate at the coronal, sagittal, or lambdoid sutures, although the head circumference increases normally. Occipital plagiocephaly, a parallelogram-shaped head with flattening of the back of the skull, is seen with increased frequency since the advice to parents that babies should sleep lying on their back to reduce the risk of sudden infant death syndrome. It improves with time as the infant becomes more mobile. Plagiocephaly is also seen in infants with hypotonia. Preterm infants may develop long, flat heads from lying on their sides for long periods on the hard surface of incubators. This can be moderated by providing the infant with a soft surface to lie on and changing their head position frequently (Fig. 12.13). Under these circumstances, it is not associated with abnormal development.

Craniosynostosis

The sutures of the skull bones start to fuse during infancy but do not finally fuse until late childhood.

Case history 12.2

Microcephaly

Fig. 12.12 shows the head circumference chart of Tim, who was healthy and was developing normally. At 9-months of age, he was rushed to hospital as he was unrousable from profound hypoglycaemia secondary to the deliberate administration of insulin by his mother, who had diabetes. Although Tim was taken into care and had no further hypoglycaemic episodes, his head circumference shows cessation of growth. He has developed moderate learning difficulties and mild cerebral palsy.

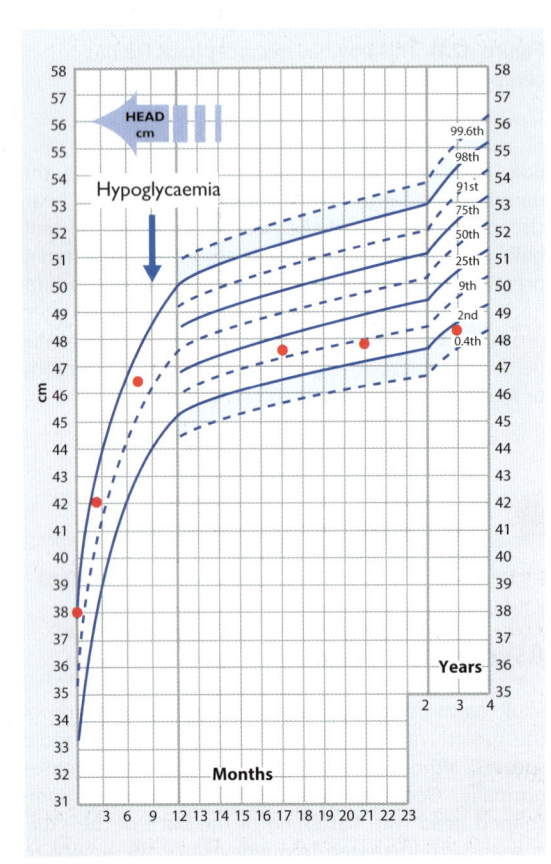

Figure 12.12 Tim's head circumference chart. (Chart © Child Growth Foundation. Further supplies and information from www.healthforallchildren.co.uk. Reproduced with permission.)

Premature fusion of one or more sutures (craniosynostosis) may lead to distortion of the head shape. Craniosynostosis is usually localized (Box 12.2). It most often affects the sagittal suture, when it results in a long narrow skull (Fig. 12.14). Rarely, it affects the lambdoid suture to result in skull asymmetry, which needs to be differentiated from plagiocephaly, where there is asymmetric flattening of one side of the skull from positional moulding.

Box 12.1 Causes of a large head

- Tall stature
- Familial macrocephaly
- Raised intracranial pressure (in an infant):
  - chronic subdural haematoma
  - brain tumour
  - neurofibromatosis
- Cerebral gigantism (Sotos syndrome)
- Central nervous system storage disorders, e.g. mucopolysaccharidosis (Hurler syndrome)

Craniosynostosis may be generalized (Box 12.2), when it may be a feature of a syndrome (Fig. 12.15). The fused suture may be felt or seen as a palpable ridge and confirmed on skull X-ray or cranial computed tomography scan. If necessary, the condition can be treated surgically because of raised intracranial pressure or for cosmetic reasons. Such operations are performed in specialist centres for craniofacial reconstructive surgery.

Premature sexual development

The development of secondary sexual characteristics before 8 years of age in females and 9 years of age in males is defined as outside the normal range in the UK. There are several recognized patterns of premature sexual development:

- precocious puberty
- premature breast development (thelarche)
- premature pubic hair development (pubarche or adrenarche)
- isolated premature menarche.

Precocious puberty

May be categorized according to the levels of the pituitary-derived gonadotrophins, follicle-stimulating hormone, and luteinizing hormone (Fig. 12.16) as:

- gonadotrophin dependent (central, 'true' precocious puberty) from premature activation of the hypothalamic–pituitary–gonadal axis. The sequence of pubertal development would be normal, described as 'consonant'
- gonadotrophin independent (pseudo, 'false' precocious puberty) from excess sex steroids outside the pituitary gland. The sequence of pubertal development would be abnormal, described as 'dissonant'.

Females

The ovaries are very sensitive to secretion of gonadotrophins from the pituitary gland, so gonadotrophin-dependent precocious puberty is fairly common in girls. It is usually idiopathic or familial. Pathological causes of precocious puberty in girls are rare and can be secondary to either:

- gonadotrophin-independent causes such as excess androgens from congenital adrenal hyperplasia or adrenal tumours, presenting with pubic and

Abnormal head shape

Box 12.2 Forms of craniosynostosis

Localized
- Sagittal suture – long narrow skull
- Coronal suture – asymmetrical skull
- Lambdoid suture – flattening of skull

Generalized
- Multiple sutures resulting in microcephaly and developmental delay
- Genetic syndromes, e.g. with syndactyly in Apert syndrome, with exophthalmos in Crouzon syndrome

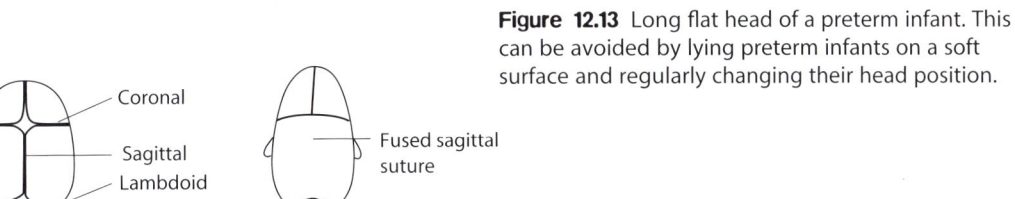

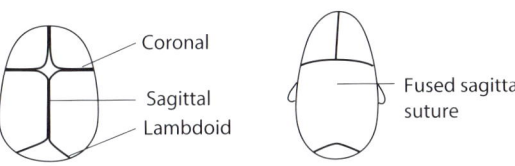

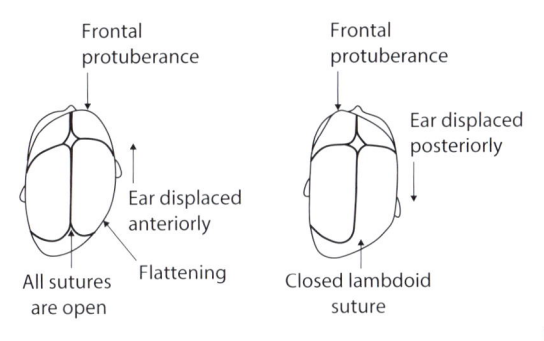

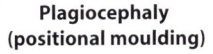

Figure 12.13 Long flat head of a preterm infant. This can be avoided by lying preterm infants on a soft surface and regularly changing their head position.

Figure 12.14 Differentiating craniosynostosis from plagiocephaly.

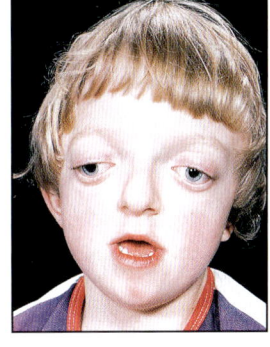

Figure 12.15 Crouzon syndrome showing the typical shallow orbits and exophthalmos. Craniofacial reconstructive surgery is required to prevent visual loss and cerebral damage from raised intracranial pressure and for cosmetic appearance.

---

axillary hair, adult body odour, acne, and virilization of the genitalia before breast development
- gonadotrophin-dependent causes such as pituitary adenoma, where pubertal development will be consonant, but perhaps rapid.

Ultrasound examination of the ovaries and uterus is helpful in assessing the progress of puberty. The uterus will change from an infantile 'tubular' shape to 'pear' shape with the progression of puberty and the endometrial lining can be identified close to menarche.

> **Precocious puberty in females is usually due to the premature onset of normal puberty**

Males

The testes are relatively insensitive to secretion of gonadotrophins from the pituitary gland, so gonadotrophin-dependent PP is uncommon in boys (Case History 12.3). It is important to exclude a pathological cause. Examination of the testes may be helpful:

- bilateral enlargement of the testes, with testicular volumes greater than 4-ml, suggests gonadotrophin-dependent PP. This can be caused by an intracranial tumour and rarely by secretion of beta-human chorionic gonadotropin from a liver tumour
- prepubertal testes suggest a gonadotrophin-independent cause, e.g. adrenal pathology such as a tumour or congenital adrenal hyperplasia
- a unilateral enlarged testis suggests a gonadal tumour.

Tumours in the hypothalamic region are best investigated by cranial MRI scan.

Causes of precocious puberty

Gonadotrophin dependent (↑LH >↑FSH)

- Pituitary
- LH ++, FSH +
- Gonad enlarges
- Oestrogen from ovary ++
  Testosterone from:
  – testis ++
  – adrenal +
- Breast enlargement
- Pubic hair growth, acne, body odour

Gonadotrophin independent (↓FSH, ↓LH)

- Pituitary
- LH↓ FSH↓
- Negative feedback
- Gonad shrinks or enlarges
- Gonadal or extra-gonadal source
- Oestrogen
- Testosterone
- Breast enlargement
- Pubic hair growth, acne, body odour

Gonadotrophin dependent (↑LH >↑FSH)
Signs of puberty are consonant.
Idiopathic/familial
CNS abnormalities
  Congenital anomalies, e.g. hydrocephalus
  Acquired, e.g. post-irradiation, infection, surgery, brain injury
  Tumours, e.g. craniopharyngioma, neurofibromatosis
Hypothyroidism

Gonadotrophin independent (↓FSH, ↓LH). Rare and signs of puberty often not consonant
Adrenal disorders – tumours, congenital adrenal hyperplasia
Ovarian – tumour (granulosa cell)
Testicular – tumour (Leydig cell)
Exogenous sex steroids

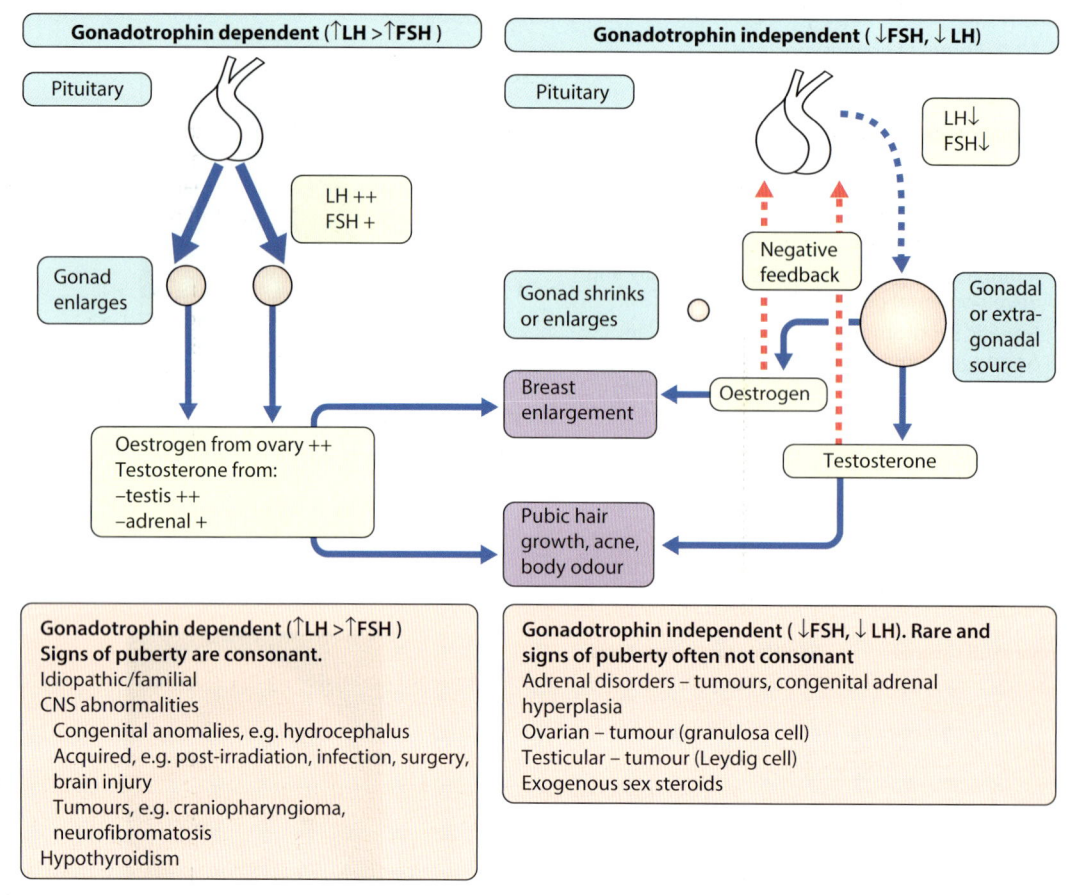

Figure 12.16 Causes of precocious puberty. (Courtesy of Emma Rhodes.)

> Gonadotrophin-dependent precocious puberty in males often has a pathological cause

Management

The management of precocious puberty is directed towards:

- detection and treatment of any underlying pathology, e.g. using MRI scan to identify an intracranial tumour, particularly in males
- reducing the rate of skeletal maturation, which is assessed by bone age. An early growth spurt may result in early cessation of growth and a reduction in adult height
- addressing psychological/behavioural difficulties associated with early progression through puberty.

Deciding whether to treat a girl who is simply going through puberty early needs further consideration. If treatment is required to delay the onset of menarche, gonadotrophin-releasing hormone analogues are the treatment of choice. In gonadotrophin-independent cases, the source of excess sex steroids needs to be identified. Inhibitors of androgen or oestrogen production or action (e.g. medroxyprogesterone acetate, cyproterone acetate, testolactone, ketoconazole) may be used.

Premature breast development (thelarche)

This usually affects females between 6 months and 2 years of age. The breast enlargement may be asymmetrical and fluctuate in size, rarely progressing beyond stage 3 of puberty. It is differentiated from gonadotrophin-dependent precocious puberty by the absence of axillary and pubic hair and of a significant growth spurt. It is nonprogressive and self-limiting. Investigations are not usually required (Case History 12.4).

Premature pubarche (adrenarche)

This occurs when pubic hair develops before 8-years of age in females and before 9-years in males but with no other signs of sexual development. It is most commonly caused by an accentuation of the normal maturation of androgen production by the adrenal gland between the age of 6 years and 8 years. It is more common in Asian and Black children. There may be a slight increase in growth rate and bone age (by 12–15 months). It is usually self-limiting. A more aggressive

Case history 12.3

Gonadotrophin-dependent precocious puberty in a boy

This 6-year-old boy presented with precocious puberty (Fig. 12.17a,b). He was noted to have multiple café-au-lait spots consistent with a diagnosis of neurofibromatosis type 1. An MRI scan showed a mass in the hypothalamus, which proved to be an optic glioma. He was treated with radiotherapy, although full remission was not possible to achieve. The site of injection of gonadotrophin super-agonist treatment to suppress his sexual development is covered by the plaster.

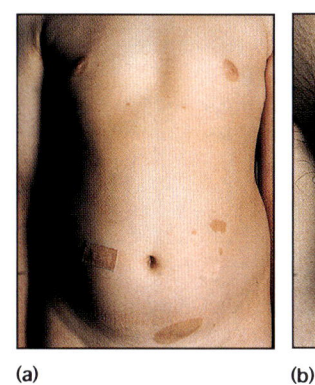

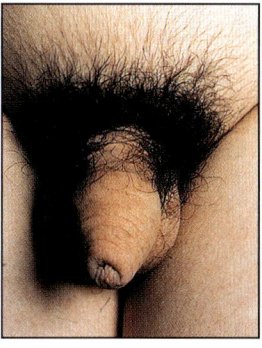

Figure 12.17 (**a**) Multiple café-au-lait spots. Neurofibromatosis type 1 was diagnosed; and (**b**) genitalia showing stage 3 genitalia and pubic hair with 12-mL testicles bilaterally. He also had adult body odour. (From Wales JKH, Rogol AD, Wit JM: *Pediatric Endocrinology and Growth,* London, 2003, Saunders with permission.)

(a) (b)

Case history 12.4

Premature thelarche

This 18-month-old female developed enlargement of both breasts (Fig. 12.18). There was no pubic hair growth, sweatiness, or body odour and her height was in the midparental range. Her bone age was only mildly advanced (21 months). Her subsequent growth rate was normal. A diagnosis of premature thelarche was made.

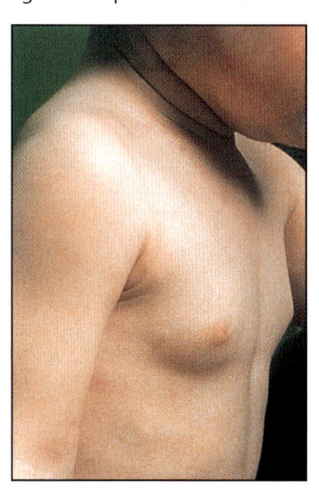

Figure 12.18 Premature breast development in an 18-month-old girl. The absence of a growth spurt and axillary and pubic hair differentiates it from precocious puberty. It is self-limiting and usually resolves. (From Wales JKH, Rogol AD, Wit JM: *Pediatric Endocrinology and Growth,* London, 2003, Saunders, with permission.)

course of virilization would suggest nonclassical congenital adrenal hyperplasia (see Ch. 26) or an adrenal tumour. Obtaining a urinary steroid profile, evaluating levels of androgens in the blood, and measuring bone age help differentiate premature pubarche from nonclassical congenital adrenal hyperplasia or an adrenal tumour. Girls who develop premature pubarche are at an increased risk of developing polycystic ovarian syndrome in later life.

Delayed puberty

Delayed puberty is often defined as the absence of pubertal development by 14 years of age in females and 15 years in males. The causes of delayed puberty are listed in Box 12.3.

In contrast to PP, delayed puberty is more common in males due to relative insensitivity of the testes to gonadotrophin secretion. Most commonly, this is constitutional delay in growth and puberty, often with a family history of delayed puberty (Case History 12.5). It is a variation of the normal timing of puberty rather than a pathological condition. It may also be induced by dieting or excessive physical training. An affected child will have delayed sexual changes compared with his/her peers, and bone age would show moderate delay. The legs will be long in comparison to the back. Eventually, the target height will be reached as growth in affected children will continue for longer than in their peers. The condition may cause psychological upset from teasing, poor self-esteem, and disadvantage in competitive sport.

In boys, assessment includes:

- pubertal staging, especially testicular volume
- identification of long-term systemic disorders.

Box 12.3 Causes of delayed puberty

Constitutional delay of growth and puberty/familial
- By far the most common

Low gonadotrophin secretion (hypogonadotropic hypogonadism)
- Systemic disease:
  - cystic fibrosis, severe asthma, Crohn's disease, organ failure, anorexia nervosa, starvation, excess physical training
- Hypothalamo-pituitary disorders:
  - pituitary dysfunction
  - isolated gonadotrophin or growth hormone deficiency
  - intracranial tumours (including craniopharyngioma)
  - Kallmann syndrome (luteinizing hormone-releasing hormone deficiency and inability to smell)
- Acquired hypothyroidism

High gonadotrophin secretion (hypergonadotropic hypogonadism)
- Chromosomal abnormalities:
  - Klinefelter syndrome (47,XXY)
  - Turner syndrome (45,XO)
- Steroid hormone enzyme deficiencies
- Acquired gonadal damage:
  - postsurgery, chemotherapy, radiotherapy, trauma, torsion of the testis, autoimmune disorder

Case history 12.5

Constitutional delay in growth and puberty

A 15-year-old boy is concerned that he is short. He is well, but gets teased at school about his height. His mother had menarche at 13 years of age and his father recalls that he was still growing when he left school at the age of 16 years. Examination reveals stage 1 pubic hair and testicular volumes of 4 mL bilaterally. His bone age is delayed by 18 months. As his mood has been significantly affected by his delayed puberty, he is treated with testosterone for 8 months with good effect on his growth rate and confidence. He then continues to make pubertal progress independently and reaches a final adult height of 179 cm (Fig. 12.9c).

Following reassurance that puberty will occur, treatment is usually not required. Should treatment be wanted, oral oxandrolone can be used in young males. This weakly androgenic anabolic steroid will induce some catch-up growth but not secondary sexual characteristics. In older boys, low-dose intramuscular testosterone will accelerate growth as well as inducing secondary sexual characteristics.

In girls, as the ovaries are sensitive to gonadotrophins, delayed puberty is less common and an organic cause should be excluded. Karyotyping should be performed to identify Turner syndrome, and thyroid and sex steroid hormones should be measured. Consider the possibility of an eating disorder and pituitary pathology. The aims of management are to:

- identify and treat any underlying pathology
- ensure normal psychological adaptation to puberty and adulthood
- accelerate growth and induce puberty if necessary.

Females may be treated with oestradiol for several months to induce puberty.

Summary

Delayed puberty
- Delayed puberty is common in boys and usually due to constitutional delay in growth and puberty.
- Delayed puberty is uncommon in girls and a cause should be sought.

Acknowledgements

We would like to acknowledge contributors to this chapter in previous editions, whose work we have drawn on: Tony Hulse (1st Edition), Jerry Wales (2nd, 3rd, 4th Edition), Paul Dimitri (4th Edition).

Further reading

Brook C, Clayton P, Brown R: *Brook's Clinical Paediatric Endocrinology*, ed 6, Oxford, 2009, Blackwell

Butler GE, Kirk J: *Paediatric Endocrinology and Diabetes*, Oxford, 2011, Oxford University Press.

Wales JKH, Rogol AD, Wit JM: *Pediatric Endocrinology and Growth*, London, 2003, Saunders.

Websites (Accessed November 2016)

NICE guideline: Available at: https://www.nice.org.uk/guidance/ta188.

Human growth hormone (somatropin) for the treatment of growth failure in children TA188.

13

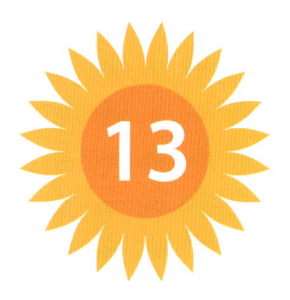

Nutrition

The nutritional vulnerability of infants and children	211	Malnutrition	221
Infant feeding	213	Vitamin D deficiency	225
Weight faltering	217	Other vitamin deficiencies	227
		Obesity	227
		Early childhood caries	232

Features of nutrition in children are:

- they are particularly vulnerable to suffer from poor nutrition, whether inadequate in quality or quantity, for short or long periods, because of their additional requirements for growth and development
- early nutrition affects the risk of developing a range of adult diseases
- there are many reasons why breastfeeding is the optimal form of feeding for newborn infants
- it is now possible to provide nutritional support to children unable to eat normal food with specialized feeds, enteral tube feeding, or by parenteral nutrition
- malnutrition contributes to over one-third of global deaths of children under 5 years of age, with about 800 million, i.e. 1 in 9 people, in the world not having enough food to lead an active and healthy life
- vitamin D deficiency is problematic in the UK
- over one-third of 11–15-year-olds in the UK are overweight or obese.

The nutritional vulnerability of infants and children

Infants and children are more likely to suffer adverse consequences from poor nutrition than are adults. There are a number of reasons for this.

Low nutritional stores

Newborn infants, particularly those born prematurely or who have experienced poor fetal growth (intra-uterine growth restriction), have poor stores of fat and protein (Fig. 13.1). The smaller the child, the less the calorie reserve and the shorter the period the child will be able to withstand starvation.

High nutritional demands for growth

Rapid growth during infancy means that nutritional requirements are high during this period (Table 13.1). The proportion of dietary energy intake used for growth is 35% in the first 3 months of life, 5% at 1 year of age, 2% by 3 years of age, and 1% to 2% until midadolescence. The risk of growth failure

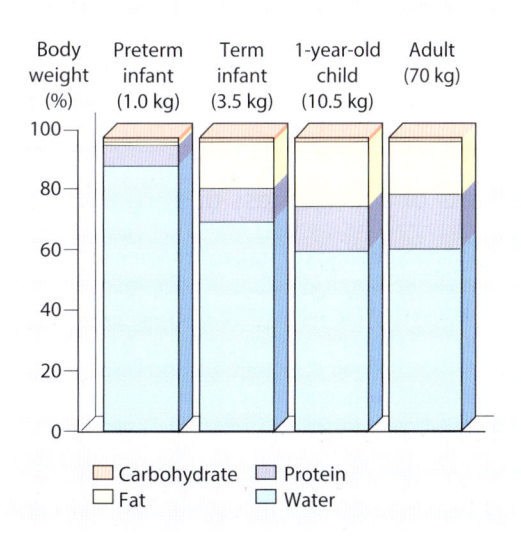

Figure 13.1 Body composition of preterm and term infants, children, and adults. Newborn infants, particularly the preterm, have poor stores of fat and protein.

Table 13.1 Reference values for energy and protein requirements

Age	Energy (kcal/kg per 24 h)	Protein (g/kg per 24 h)
0–6 months	115	2.2
6–12 months	95	2.0
1–3 years	95	1.8
4–6 years	90	1.5
7–10 years	75	1.2
Adolescence	**(male/female)**	
11–14 years	65/55	1.0
15–18 years	60/40	0.8

from restricted energy intake is therefore greater in the first 6 months of life than in later childhood. Even small but recurrent nutritional deficits in early childhood will lead to a cumulative deficit in weight and height.

Rapid brain growth and development

The brain grows rapidly during the last trimester of pregnancy and throughout the first 2 years of life. The complexity of interneuronal connections also increases substantially during this time. This process appears to be sensitive to undernutrition and is particularly important in the premature newborn. Even modest energy deprivation during periods of rapid brain growth and differentiation leads to an increased risk of adverse neurodevelopmental outcome. This is not surprising when one considers that at birth the brain accounts for approximately two-thirds of basal metabolic rate, and at 1 year of age for about 50% (Fig. 13.2). Many studies have drawn attention to the delayed development seen in children suffering from protein-energy malnutrition due to inadequate food intake, although adverse psychosocial factors in food-poor environments are also likely to contribute.

Effects of acute illness or surgery

During an acute illness or surgery, children may not be able to eat. Recurrent infections are common in infancy, and reduce food intake while increasing nutritional demands. Following surgery, after a brief anabolic phase, catecholamine secretion is increased, causing the metabolic rate and energy requirement to increase. Urinary nitrogen losses may become so great that it is impossible to achieve a positive nitrogen balance and weight is lost. After uncomplicated surgery, this phase may last for a week, but it can be much longer after extensive burns, complicated surgery, or severe sepsis. Thereafter, previously lost tissue is replaced and a positive energy and nitrogen balance can be achieved. However, infants may not show catch-up growth unless their energy intake is as high as 150–200 kcal/kg per day (normal requirements are 95–115 kcal/kg per day). In small infants with very marked growth faltering (e.g. post-surgery), it can be impossible for them to tolerate the feed volumes needed for catch-up growth and a period of partial parenteral nutrition (PN) may be necessary to achieve growth recovery and re-establish full enteral feeding.

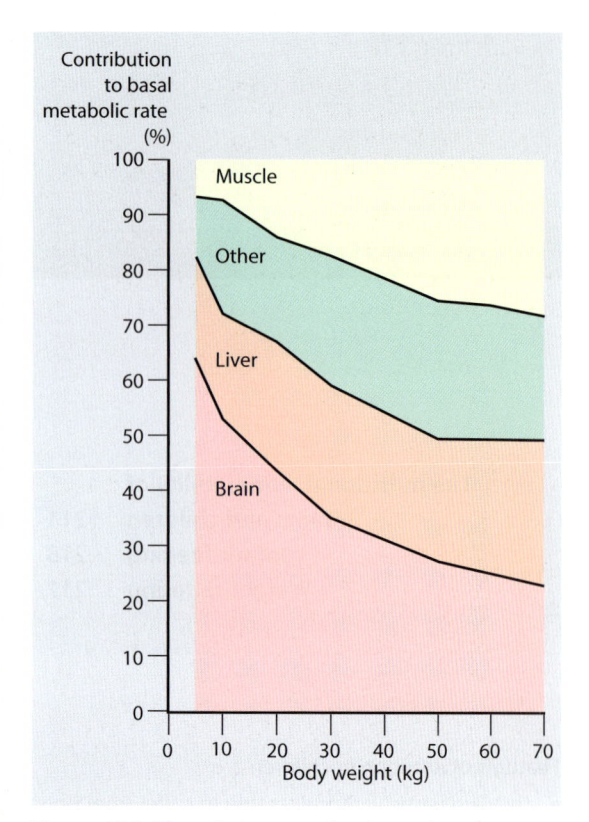

Figure 13.2 The relative contribution to basal metabolic rate derived from brain, liver, and muscle changes with growth. The brain accounts for two-thirds of the basal metabolic rate at birth, but this falls to 25% in adults. (Data from Holliday MA Metabolic rate and organ size during growth from infancy to maturity and during late gestation and early infancy. *Pediatrics* 47:169,1971.)

Long-term outcome of early nutritional deficiency

Linear growth of populations

Growth and nutrition are closely related, such that the mean height of a population reflects its nutritional status. As living conditions have improved in high-income countries, people have become taller. In the Netherlands, for example, average male height has increased by 20 cm over the last 150 years. Natural selection may also be a factor in this instance, as taller Dutch adults have been found to have greater numbers of children. Height is adversely affected by lower socioeconomic status with increasing numbers of children in a family.

Disease in adult life

There is considerable epidemiological evidence suggesting that early nutrition and lifestyle have long-term effects on later health and risk of illness (developmental programming) including coronary heart disease (Fig. 13.3), stroke, noninsulin-dependent diabetes and hypertension. Currently, three hypotheses are proposed: the 'fuel-mediated' in utero hypothesis, the accelerated postnatal weight gain hypothesis and the mismatch hypothesis (Fig. 13.4) These are not mutually exclusive and could have a greater or lesser impact in different circumstances.

> **Summary**
>
> **Nutritional vulnerability**
> Infants are more vulnerable to poor nutrition because of:
> - poor stores of fat and protein
> - extra nutritional demands for growth (the weight of a term infant doubles by 4 months and trebles by 1 year of age)
> - periods of reduced food intake and increased nutritional demands during illnesses or surgery.

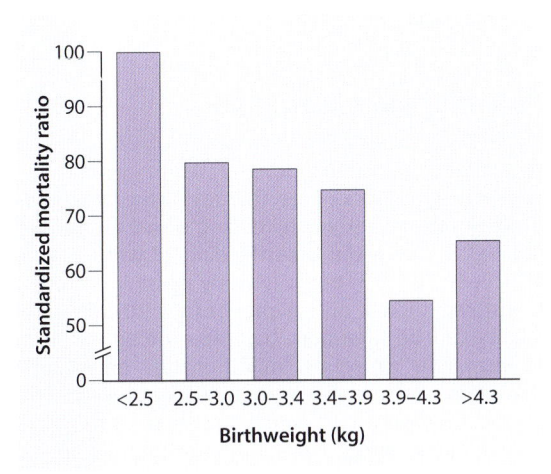

Figure 13.3 Death rates from coronary heart disease according to birthweight showing increased rate in low birthweight babies. (Data from Barker DJ: Fetal origins of adult disease. In *Growing up in Britain: ensuring the healthy future for our children. A study of 4–5 year olds.* London, 1999, BMJ Books.)

Infant feeding

Breastfeeding

Breast milk is the natural food for infants. The popularity of breastfeeding (and who should perform this task) has reflected fashion and social class. In Europe, until the middle of the seventeenth century, the aristocracy would generally favour a wet nurse. The development of infant formulas resulted in a marked decline in the popularity of breastfeeding, but breastfeeding is now universally advocated. Exclusive breastfeeding for the first 6 months is the current World Health Organization (WHO) recommendation, which has been endorsed by the Department of Health in the UK. Shorter periods of breastfeeding are also advantageous. In 2010, in the UK, 81% of babies were breastfed at birth, which is steadily rising (Fig. 13.5). A higher proportion of mothers from a managerial and professional background start breastfeeding, compared with mothers from routine and manual occupations, although this gap is closing.

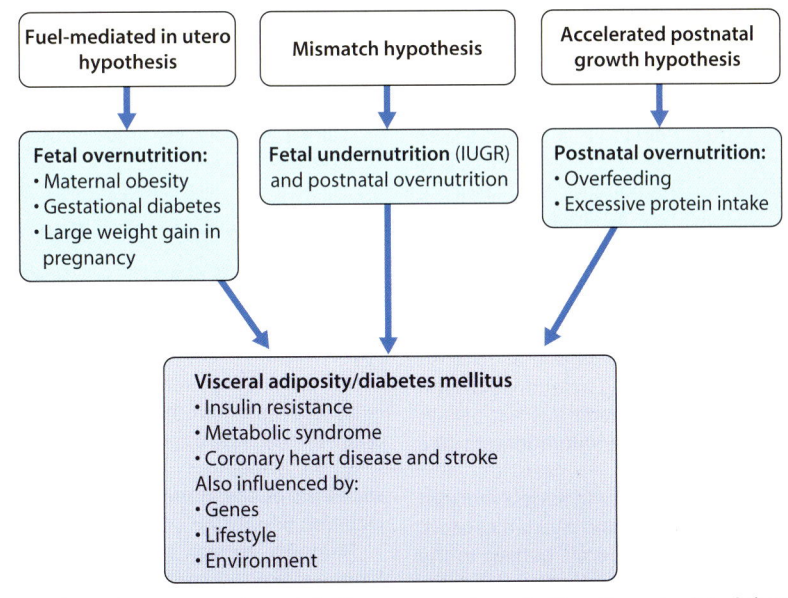

Figure 13.4 Current hypotheses on early metabolic programming of adiposity and related disease. (Adapted from Koletzko B, Symonds M, Olsen SF. Early Nutrition Programming Project; Early Nutrition Academy: Programming research – where are we and where do we go from here? *Am J Clin Nutr* 94:2036S-2043S, 2011 with permission.)

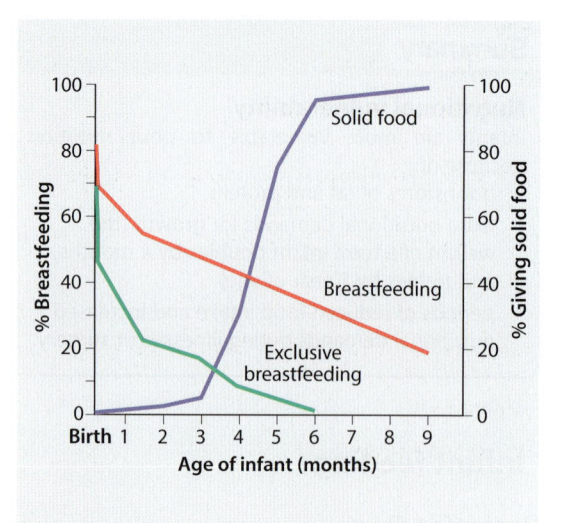

Figure 13.5 Prevalence of breastfeeding, exclusive breastfeeding (no formula milk), and proportion of infants given solid feeds during the first 9 months of life in the UK. Over the last 10 years, there has been a marked increase in the prevalence of breastfeeding and delay in weaning onto solid food (Data from Infant Feeding Survey, 2010).

Advantages

In low-income countries, breastfeeding dramatically improves survival during infancy, mainly by reducing gastrointestinal infection (see Box 13.1). It is estimated that 1.3 million to 1.45 million deaths could be prevented in 42 low-income countries by increased levels of breastfeeding. It is therefore one of WHO's four main strategies to reduce child mortality.

In developed countries, there is no convincing evidence of reduced mortality associated with breastfeeding, but gastrointestinal, lower respiratory tract infection and otitis media are reduced. Breast milk also has a protective effect against necrotizing enterocolitis in premature infants. Breastfeeding is associated with a reduced incidence of obesity, diabetes mellitus and hypertension in later life. The benefits of breastfeeding are difficult to demonstrate, as studies comparing breast milk and formula feeds cannot generally be randomized and are almost always observational, with potential confounders such as social class, education and smoking.

Many mothers who breastfeed find that it helps them establish an intimate, loving relationship with their baby (bonding), but breastfeeding is not always straightforward and help and encouragement are often required.

Health advantages to the mother include a reduced risk of type 2 diabetes and breast and ovarian cancers. Breastfeeding may also be of economic benefit to the country, from reduced infections in infants and lifetime breast cancer risk for mothers.

☀ **Exclusive breastfeeding in early infancy is life-saving in developing countries**

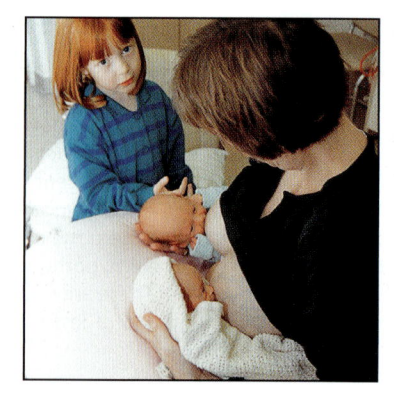

Figure 13.6 Breastfeeding of preterm twins.

Potential complications

It is difficult to know if a baby is getting enough milk except by demonstrating normal weight gain through regular weight checks, every few days in the first couple of weeks, then weekly until feeding is well established (Box 13.2). Successful breastfeeding of twins can be achieved (Fig. 13.6) but it is rarely possible to totally breastfeed triplets and higher-order births. Preterm infants can be breastfed, but the mother will need to learn how to express milk from the breast until the infant can suck. Obtaining sufficient milk can be a problem; donor breast milk has made a return to neonatal units and is collected from the non-feeding breast during suckling by mothers of well babies in the community and donated to a 'milk bank'.

Breastfeeding is restrictive for the mother, as others cannot take charge of her baby for any length of time. This is particularly important if she goes to work and may delay her return, which may cause financial hardship for the family. Facilities for breastfeeding in public places remain limited. Failure to establish breastfeeding will sometimes cause significant emotional upset in the mother.

☀ **Plotting growth on a centile growth chart helps identify inadequate nutrition or other problems**

Establishing breastfeeding

Colostrum, rather than milk, is produced for the first few days. Colostrum differs from mature milk in that the content of protein and immunoglobulin is much higher. Volumes are low, but water or formula supplements are not required while the supply of breast milk is becoming established. The first breastfeed should take place as soon as possible after birth. Subsequently, frequent suckling is beneficial as it enhances the secretion of the hormones initiating and promoting lactation (Fig. 13.7).

Primates appear not to breastfeed instinctively. Monkeys bred in captivity have to be taught how to care for their young and do not learn this skill when denied the normal social opportunity in the wild to observe child rearing. It is therefore important that breastfeeding should have as high a public profile

Box 13.1 Why 'breast is best' – the advantages of breast milk

Advantages of breastfeeding for the infant are that it:
- provides the ideal nutrition for infants during the first 4 months to 6 months of life
- is life-saving in developing countries
- reduces the risk of gastrointestinal and respiratory infection, otitis media, and necrotizing enterocolitis
- enhances the mother–child relationship
- reduces the risk of insulin-dependent diabetes, hypertension and obesity in later life.

Advantages for the mother are that it:
- promotes close attachment between mother and baby
- increases the time interval between children, which is important in reducing birth rate in developing countries
- reduces risk of breast and ovarian cancer and type 2 diabetes.

Scientific explanation of some of the properties of breast milk
Anti-infective properties
Humoral

Secretory IgA	Comprises 90% of immunoglobulin in human milk. Provides mucosal protection, but of uncertain benefit
Bifidus factor	Promotes growth of *Lactobacillus bifidus*, which metabolizes lactose to lactic and acetic acids. The resulting low pH may inhibit growth of gastrointestinal pathogens
Lysozyme	Bacteriolytic enzyme
Lactoferrin	Iron-binding protein. Inhibits growth of *Escherichia coli*
Interferon	Antiviral agent

Cellular

Macrophages	Phagocytic. Synthesize lysozyme, lactoferrin, C3, C4
Lymphocytes	T cells may transfer delayed hypersensitivity responses to infant. B cells synthesize IgA

Nutritional properties

Protein quality	More easily digested curd (whey-to-casein ratio: 60:40)
Lipid quality	Rich in oleic acid. Improved digestibility and fat absorption
Fat metabolism	Enhanced lipolysis, from breast milk lipase
Calcium-to-phosphorus ratio of 2:1	Reduces hypocalcaemic tetany and promotes calcium absorption
Renal solute load	Low
Iron content	Bioavailable (40% to 50% absorption)
Long-chain polyunsaturated fatty acids	Structural lipids; important in retinal development

---

as possible. Women who have never seen an infant being breastfed are less likely to want to breastfeed themselves. Education in schools and during pregnancy about the advantages of breastfeeding is likely to have a positive effect. Advice and support from other women who have breastfed may be important in dealing with early problems such as engorgement or cracked nipples. The WHO recommends continuing breastfeeding until 2 years of age, the American Pediatric Association until 1 year of age.

> Newborn infants of mothers planning to breastfeed should ideally not be given any formula feeds

Formula feeding

Infants who are not breastfed require a formula feed. Most are based on cow's milk, but unmodified cow's milk is unsuitable for feeding in infancy as it contains too much protein and electrolytes and inadequate iron and vitamins. Even after considerable modification, differences remain between formula feeds and breast milk (Table 13.2).

All infant formula feeds currently available in the UK have been modified to make their mineral content and renal solute load comparable with that of mature human milk. Since these changes were introduced in

Box 13.2 Potential complications of breastfeeding

Unknown intake	Volume of milk intake not known; monitor weight gain
Transmission of infection	Maternal CMV, hepatitis B and HIV – risk of transmission to the baby
Breast milk jaundice	Mild, self-limiting, unconjugated hyperbilirubinaemia; continue breastfeeding
Transmission of drugs	Antimetabolites and some other drugs contraindicated. Check formulary
Nutrient inadequacies	Breastfeeding beyond 6 months without timely introduction of appropriate solids may lead to poor weight gain and rickets
Vitamin K deficiency	Insufficient vitamin K in breast milk to prevent haemorrhagic disease of the newborn. Supplementation is required
Potential transmission of environmental contaminants	Nicotine, alcohol, caffeine, etc.
Less flexible	Other family members cannot help or take part. More difficult in public places
Emotional upset	If difficulties or lack of success, can be upsetting

Physiology of breastfeeding

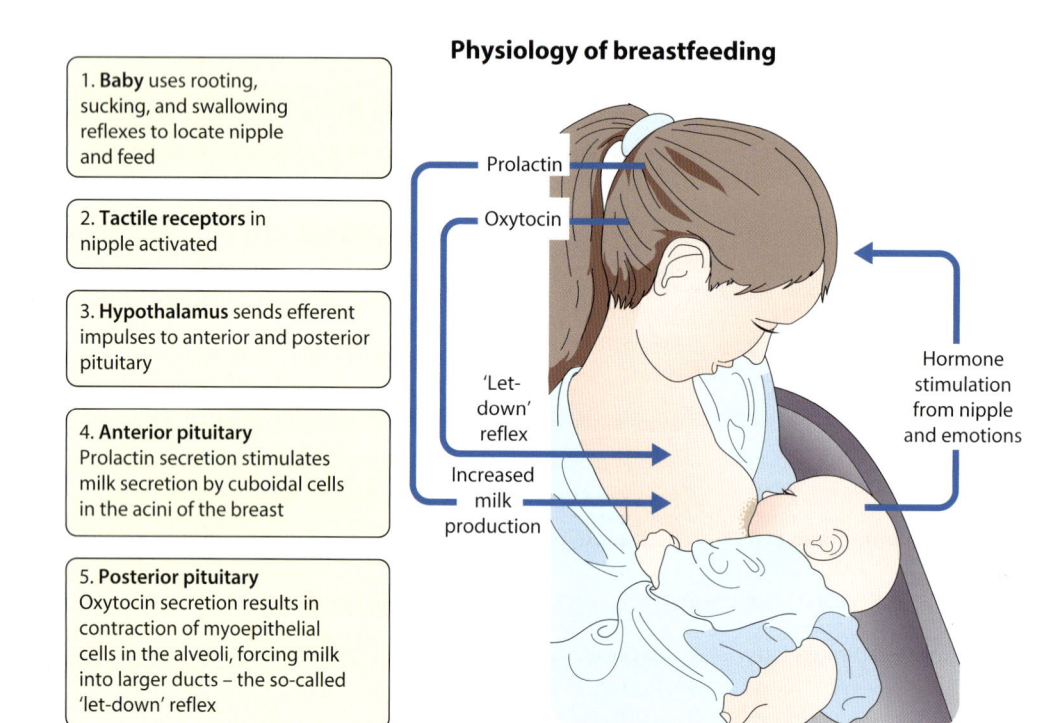

1. **Baby** uses rooting, sucking, and swallowing reflexes to locate nipple and feed

2. **Tactile receptors** in nipple activated

3. **Hypothalamus** sends efferent impulses to anterior and posterior pituitary

4. **Anterior pituitary** Prolactin secretion stimulates milk secretion by cuboidal cells in the acini of the breast

5. **Posterior pituitary** Oxytocin secretion results in contraction of myoepithelial cells in the alveoli, forcing milk into larger ducts – the so-called 'let-down' reflex

Figure 13.7 Physiology of breastfeeding.

the UK in the 1970s, there has been a marked reduction in the incidence of hypernatraemic dehydration in infants with gastroenteritis. Over time, additional modifications have been made to formula feeds, including the addition of polyunsaturated fatty acids, nucleotides, prebiotics and probiotics. Whether or not these provide additional clinical benefit is often uncertain, and it seems unlikely that an artificial feed will ever mimic the complexity of breast milk. There is no evidence that any one of the many brands of formula milk is superior to any other.

In 1981, the WHO introduced a code of marketing breast milk substitutes. This came out of concern that aggressive marketing of formula milk was associated with an increase in mortality, malnutrition and diarrhoea in young infants in developing countries. The Code prohibits any advertising of infant formula, bottles and teats and gifts to mothers or inducements to health workers.

Introduction of whole, pasteurized cow's milk

Breastfeeding or formula feeding is recommended until the age of 12 months, and there are advantages in continuing to 18 months of age. Pasteurized cow's milk given before 12 months of age is associated with

Table 13.2 A comparison of human milk, cow's milk and recommended content of infant formula (per 100 kcal).

	Mature breast milk	Cow's milk	Infant formula (modified cow's milk)
Energy (kcal)	66	65	60–70/100 ml
Protein (g)	1.0	3.4	1.8–3.0
Carbohydrate (g)	7.0	4.6	9.0–14.0
Casein:whey	40:60	80:20	40:60 to 80:20
Fat (g)	3.8	3.7	4.4–6.0
Sodium (mmol)	0.65	1.9	0.87–2.6
Calcium (mmol)	0.85	3.0	1.25–3.5
Phosphorus (mmol)	0.48	3.0	0.8–2.9
Iron (µmol)	1.2	0.36	5.4–23

Data from Koletzko B, editor: *Pediatric Nutrition in Practice*, 2nd edition, Basel, 2015, Karger. Formula content is recommended composition by expert group coordinated by ESPGHAN.

increased risk of iron deficiency, but may be given from 1 year of age. It is deficient in vitamins A, C, and D and in iron, and supplementation will be required unless the infant is having a good diet of mixed solids. Alternatively, a 'follow-on' formula can be used. These contain more protein and sodium than infant formula and, in contrast to cow's milk, are fortified with iron and vitamins. Children on cow's milk should receive full fat milk up to the age of 5 years.

Infants should not be given unmodified cow's milk in the 1st year of life

Specialized infant formula

A specialized formula may be used for the preterm infant (higher energy and mineral content), in infants with cow's milk protein allergy, lactose intolerance (primary lactase deficiency or postgastroenteritis intolerance), cystic fibrosis, neonatal cholestatic liver disease and following neonatal intestinal resection.

In a cow's milk-based formula, the protein is derived from cow's milk protein, the carbohydrate is lactose, and the fat is mainly long-chain triglycerides. In a specialized formula, the protein is derived from hydrolyzed cow's milk protein, amino acids or from soya. The carbohydrate is glucose polymer, and the fat is a combination of medium-chain and long-chain triglycerides. Medium-chain triglycerides are directly absorbed into the small intestine and need neither pancreatic enzymes nor bile salts for this process.

A soya formula should not be used for infants under 6 months of age as it has a high aluminium content and contains phytoestrogens (plant substances that mimic the effects of endogenous oestrogens). There is no compelling evidence that the use of a specialized formula prevents the development of allergic or autoimmune diseases (asthma, eczema or cow's milk protein allergy). Formula containing rice starch that becomes more viscous in the stomach with fall in pH can be used for uncomplicated gastro-oesophageal reflux; these are known as anti-reflux milks. Details of the different formula feeds can be found in the British National Formulary for Children.

Weaning

After 6 months of age, breast milk becomes increasingly nutritionally inadequate as a sole feed, as it does not provide sufficient energy, vitamins or iron. Solid foods are recommended to be introduced from around 6 months of age, not before 17 weeks and no later than 26 weeks. This is done gradually, initially with small quantities of pureed fruit, root vegetables or rice. Foods high in salt and sugar should be avoided and honey should not be given until 1 year of age because of risk of infantile botulism. Currently, there is no strong evidence that delayed introduction of more allergenic foods delays or prevents the development of food allergy. On the contrary, research has shown that early introduction of peanut in infancy significantly reduces the risk of peanut allergy in childhood.

Weight faltering

Weight faltering is suboptimal weight gain in infants or young children. If prolonged and severe, it will result in reduction in height or length (stunting) and reduction in head growth and may be associated with delayed development. This was often described as 'failure to thrive', but the term has fallen out of favour in the UK as it is regarded as somewhat pejorative, but is still used in other countries.

There is no agreed definition, and identification is often problematic. Growth is determined by plotting serial measurements of weight, length or height, and head circumference, using the WHO growth charts for boys or girls [see Ch. 12 (Growth and puberty) about their derivation and use, Appendix Fig. A1 for the charts].

Healthy children's weight will fluctuate, but it will usually progress within one centile space (the distance between two major centile lines on the growth chart). However, size at birth is determined not only by genes but also by the intrauterine environment. Over the first few weeks, infants who are large at birth will often cross down centiles (catch-down growth), whereas small babies will move up centiles (catch-up growth) to find their genetic centile growth lines. Infants who become acutely ill will often lose weight, but will regain their weight centile within 2 weeks to 3 weeks.

Identifying weight faltering

Weight faltering describes a sustained drop down two centile spaces. After the first 4 months only around 0.5% of children in the UK will do this. A single observation of weight is difficult to interpret unless markedly discrepant from the head circumference or length. All babies should be weighed during the 1st week to assess feeding, and then at around 8, 12, and 16 weeks, and at 1 year, and whenever concerns are raised. In addition, the further the weight is below the second centile, the more likely the child is 'weight faltering'. Any child whose weight crosses two centile lines or is below the 0.4th centile or has a body mass index (BMI) less than the second centile should be evaluated. The infant with growth faltering needs to be differentiated from a normal but small or thin baby (Fig. 13.8). If the child was born preterm, this should be allowed for when plotting growth during the first 1–2 years of age, depending on the degree of prematurity. Some infants with severe intrauterine growth restriction remain small, though most exhibit catch-up growth.

Causes of weight faltering

The causes of faltering growth are listed in Fig. 13.9. In most, the cause is inadequate intake of food, but the reason for this is often multifactorial. Traditionally, the causes have been divided into 'organic' and 'nonorganic' causes. However, organic causes are only found in 5% to 10%, and there are almost always symptoms and signs pointing to the underlying disease. Although weight faltering is often considered to be a manifestation of poverty (and is certainly true in poorer societies), studies in the UK have not found an association with low socioeconomic status or poor educational attainment. While neglect and child abuse must always be considered, it is relatively unusual and true in perhaps only 5% of cases. Evidence for the role of maternal depression is conflicting, with some studies suggesting an association and others being unable to demonstrate a link.

Conversely, in children without symptoms and signs of disease, investigations are likely to be negative.

Clinical features and investigation

If weight faltering is confirmed, a dietary history should be taken to include:

- history of milk feeding
- age at weaning

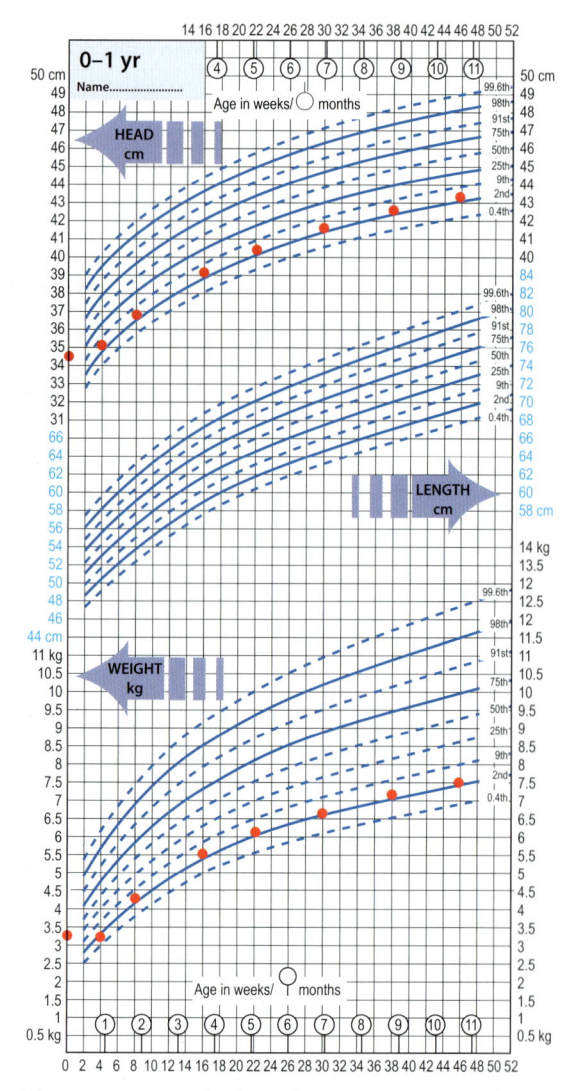

Figure 13.8 Growth chart showing normal weight gain and growth in a constitutionally small infant. The further below the 2nd, and especially the 0.4th, centile, the more likely it is that there will be an organic cause. (Chart © RCPCH, WHO, Department of Health.)

- range and type of foods now taken
- mealtime routine and eating and feeding behaviours
- a 3-day food diary will provide a more detailed and accurate picture of intake
- if possible, observe a meal being taken.

Consider also:

- was the child born preterm or had intrauterine growth restriction?
- is the child well with lots of energy or does the child have other symptoms such as diarrhoea, vomiting, cough, or lethargy?
- the growth of other family members and any illnesses in the family
- is the child's development normal?
- are there psychosocial problems at home?

Causes of growth faltering

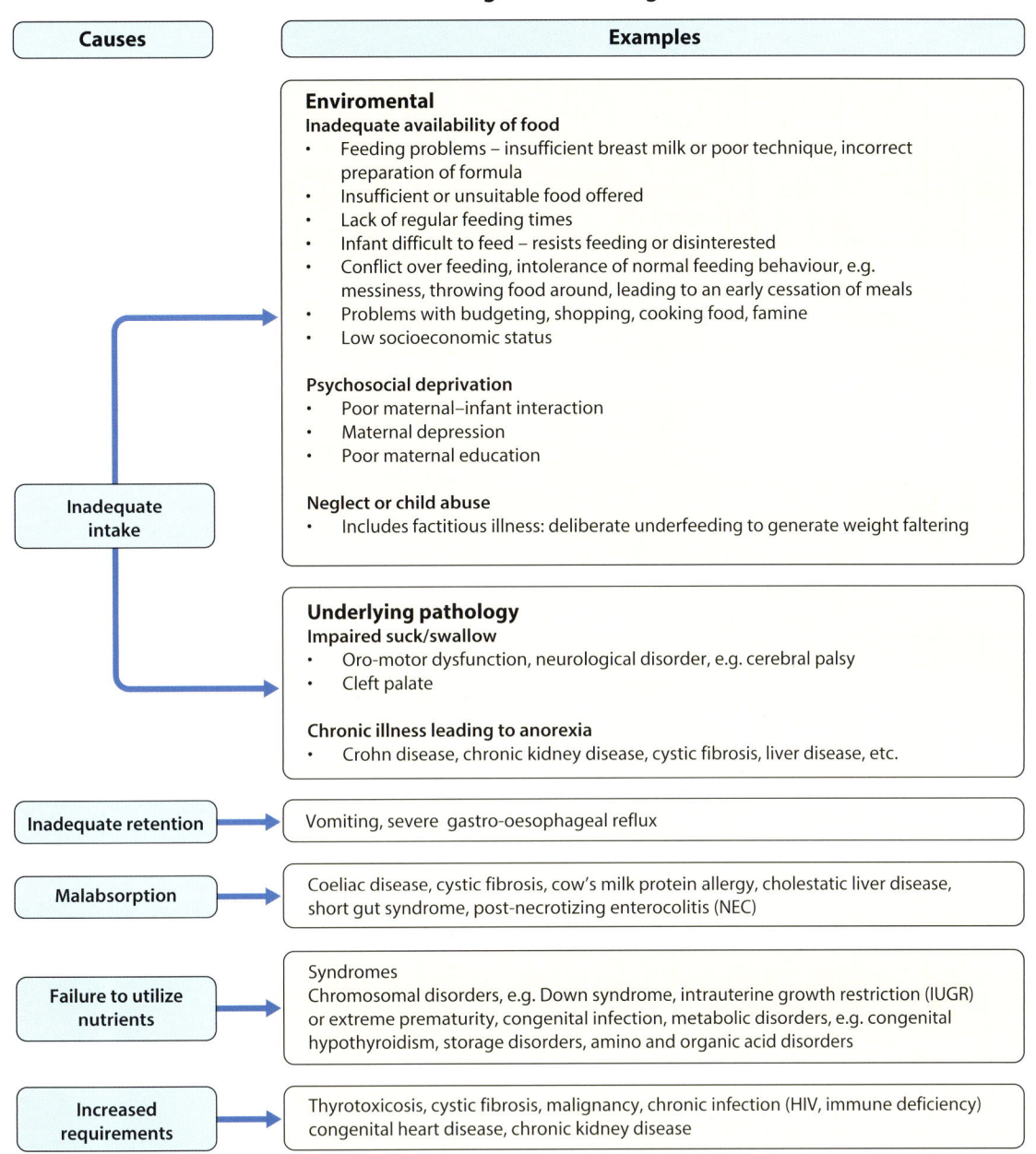

Causes	Examples
Inadequate intake	**Environmental** **Inadequate availability of food** • Feeding problems – insufficient breast milk or poor technique, incorrect preparation of formula • Insufficient or unsuitable food offered • Lack of regular feeding times • Infant difficult to feed – resists feeding or disinterested • Conflict over feeding, intolerance of normal feeding behaviour, e.g. messiness, throwing food around, leading to an early cessation of meals • Problems with budgeting, shopping, cooking food, famine • Low socioeconomic status **Psychosocial deprivation** • Poor maternal–infant interaction • Maternal depression • Poor maternal education **Neglect or child abuse** • Includes factitious illness: deliberate underfeeding to generate weight faltering **Underlying pathology** **Impaired suck/swallow** • Oro-motor dysfunction, neurological disorder, e.g. cerebral palsy • Cleft palate **Chronic illness leading to anorexia** • Crohn disease, chronic kidney disease, cystic fibrosis, liver disease, etc.
Inadequate retention	Vomiting, severe gastro-oesophageal reflux
Malabsorption	Coeliac disease, cystic fibrosis, cow's milk protein allergy, cholestatic liver disease, short gut syndrome, post-necrotizing enterocolitis (NEC)
Failure to utilize nutrients	Syndromes Chromosomal disorders, e.g. Down syndrome, intrauterine growth restriction (IUGR) or extreme prematurity, congenital infection, metabolic disorders, e.g. congenital hypothyroidism, storage disorders, amino and organic acid disorders
Increased requirements	Thyrotoxicosis, cystic fibrosis, malignancy, chronic infection (HIV, immune deficiency) congenital heart disease, chronic kidney disease

Figure 13.9 The main causes of growth faltering.

If organic disease is the cause, suggestive symptoms and signs are usually present. Examination should focus on identifying signs of organic disease, such as dysmorphic features, signs suggestive of malabsorption (distended abdomen, thin buttocks, misery), signs suggestive of chronic respiratory disease, signs of heart failure and evidence of nutritional deficiencies (koilonychia, angular stomatitis). In some children with growth faltering, a full blood count and serum ferritin may be helpful to identify iron-deficiency anaemia. This is usually secondary to inadequate iron intake and correcting it may improve appetite. In most instances, no investigations are required. Further information about the child and family from the health visitor, general practitioner or other professionals involved with the family can be particularly helpful. Investigations to be considered are listed in Box 13.4.

Management

The management of most weight faltering is carried out in primary care. Using mealtime observations and food diaries, health visitors can assess and support families to improve feeding and increase calorie intake. Access to specialist support may be required. A paediatric dietician is helpful in assessing the quantity and composition of food intake, recommending strategies for increasing energy intake and a speech and language therapist has specialist skills with feeding

Case history 13.1

Weight faltering

Jamie, aged 11 months, was causing concern to his health visitor as he was not putting on any weight (Fig. 13.10). She arranged for him to be assessed by his general practitioner, who found that he was otherwise well. His mother was a single parent who left school at 16 years of age and had Jamie at the age of 18. They lived in a high-rise flat and Jamie's mother received income support. Her own mother lived on the other side of the city.

On visiting the home, the health visitor found Jamie's mother to be tense and anxious. In particular, she was worried about making ends meet. She fed Jamie the same food as she ate herself, together with cow's milk, which she had started at 6 months of age. The meals were chaotic and there was no dining table. After a few mouthfuls, Jamie stopped eating and his mother did not coax him but became frustrated and angry.

Jamie's health visitor suggested strategies for increasing Jamie's food intake (Box 13.3). She continued to provide support and encouragement to his mother and arranged a nursery placement for Jamie. By 2 years of age, he had crossed one centile space upwards, but still ate erratically.

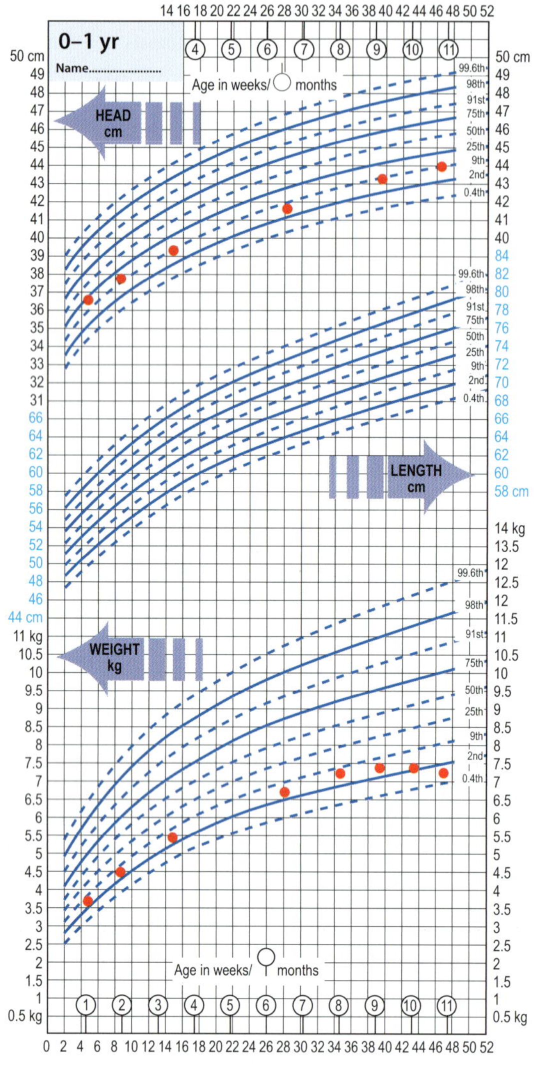

Figure 13.10 Jamie's growth chart. (Chart © RCPCH, WHO, Department of Health.)

Box 13.3 Strategies for increasing energy intake

Dietary

- Three meals and two snacks each day
- Increase number and variety of foods offered
- Increase energy density of foods (e.g. add cheese, margarine, cream)
- Limit milk intake to 500 ml/day
- Avoid excessive intake of fruit juice and squash

Behavioural

- Offer meals at regular times with other family members
- Praise when food is eaten, ignore when not
- Limit mealtime to 30 minutes
- Eat at same time as child
- Avoid mealtime conflict
- Never force feed

From: Shields B, Wacogne I, Wright CM: Weight faltering and failure to thrive in infancy and early childhood. *BMJ* 245:e5931,2012.

---

disorders. Input from a clinical psychologist and from social services may also be needed. Nursery placement can be helpful in alleviating stress at home and assisting with feeding. The key outcome measure is a rise up the weight centiles; this usually begins 4 weeks to 8 weeks after intervention.

In children under 6 months of age with severe weight faltering, hospital admission may occasionally be necessary for active refeeding and multidisciplinary team involvement. While being on a children's ward may offer the opportunity to observe and improve the parent's method and skill in feeding, this rarely transfers back to home. As children's wards are busy and focused on acute illness, admission is unlikely to be helpful unless there is a clear and agreed preadmission plan. In extreme circumstances, hospital admission can be used to demonstrate that the child will gain weight when fed appropriately.

Box 13.4 Investigations to be considered in weight faltering in a child with worrying signs or symptoms of disease

Investigation	Interpreting result
Full blood count and differential white cell count	Anaemia, neutropenia, lymphopenia (immune deficiency)
Serum creatinine, urea, electrolytes, acid–base status, calcium, phosphate	Renal failure, renal tubular acidosis, metabolic disorders, William syndrome
Liver function tests	Liver disease, malabsorption, metabolic disorders
Thyroid function tests	Hypothyroidism or hyperthyroidism
Acute phase reactant, e.g. CRP (C-reactive protein)	Inflammation
Ferritin	Iron-deficiency anaemia
Immunoglobulins	Immune deficiency
IgA tTG (IgA tissue transglutaminase antibodies)	Coeliac disease
Urine microscopy, culture, and dipsticks	Urinary tract infection, renal disease
Stool microscopy, culture, and elastase	Intestinal infection, parasites, elastase decreased in pancreatic insufficiency
Karyotype in girls	Turner syndrome
Sweat test, chest X-ray	Cystic fibrosis, other respiratory disorders

Outcome

Weight faltering appears to have a long-term effect on growth, with children remaining on a low centile. However, a randomized controlled trial of primary care intervention has shown that, at 4 years of age, children who received intervention were heavier and taller than untreated controls. Weight faltering also appears to have an adverse effect on cognition, although this is small. Some children continue to undereat (see Case History 13.1).

Summary

Weight faltering
- Is a description, not a diagnosis.
- Weights of infants are only helpful if measured accurately and plotted on an appropriate centile growth chart.
- Is present if an infant's weight falls across two centile spaces.
- Is more likely to be present the further the weight is below the second centile.
- Although complex in origin and multifactorial, the final common pathway is inadequate food intake.
- If there is underlying pathology, it is almost always accompanied by abnormal symptoms or signs.
- Most affected infants and toddlers do not require any investigations and are managed in primary care by dietary and behavioural modification designed to increase energy intake and monitoring growth.

Malnutrition

Worldwide, malnutrition is responsible directly or indirectly for about a third of all deaths of children under 5 years of age. Malnutrition from inadequate food intake also continues to occur in developed countries as a result of poverty, parental neglect or poor education. Specific nutritional deficiencies, particularly of iron, remain common in developed countries. Restrictive diets may be iatrogenic as a result of exclusion diets or parental food fads, or may be self-inflicted.

Moderate/mild malnutrition also occurs in 20–40% of children in specialist children's hospitals. At particular risk are those with long-term illness, e.g. the preterm, congenital heart disease, malignant disease during chemotherapy or bone marrow transplantation, chronic gastrointestinal conditions such as short gut syndrome following extensive bowel resection or inflammatory bowel disease, chronic kidney disease or cerebral palsy. Malnutrition results from a combination of anorexia, malabsorption and increased energy requirements because of infection or inflammation. Malnutrition in older children and adolescents may also result from eating disorders.

Assessment of nutritional status

Evaluation is divided into assessment of past and present dietary intake, anthropometry and laboratory assessments (Fig. 13.11).

Dietary assessment

Parents are asked to record the food the child eats during several days. This gives a more objective guide to food intake.

Nutritional assessment

Nutritional assessment

Anthropometry
- Weight
- Height
- Mid-upper-arm circumference (MUAC)
- Skinfold thickness

Laboratory
- Low plasma albumin
- Low concentration of specific minerals and vitamins

Food intake
- Dietary recall
- Dietary diary

Immunodeficiency
- Low lymphocyte count
- Impaired cell-mediated immunity

Figure 13.11 Assessment of nutritional status. This cannot be determined by a single measurement but is a composite of a number of variables.

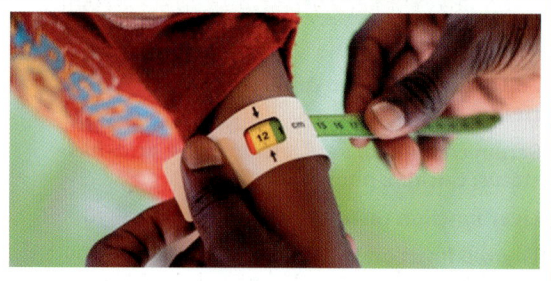

Figure 13.12 Mid-upper-arm circumference (MUAC) measurement to identify malnutrition. It is colour-coded; amber is moderate malnutrition, red is severe (<115 mm).

Anthropometry

Weight and height are key measurements. Skinfold thickness of the triceps reflects subcutaneous fat stores and can be measured with calipers. While it is difficult to measure skinfold thickness accurately in young children, mid-upper-arm circumference, which is related to skeletal muscle mass, can be measured easily and repeatedly and is independent of age in children aged 6 months to 5 years. It is especially useful for screening children for malnutrition in the community.

Laboratory investigations

These can be used in the detection of early physiological adaptation to malnutrition, but clinical history, examination and anthropometry are of greater value than any single biochemical or immunological measurement.

Consequences of malnutrition

Malnutrition is a multisystem disorder. When severe, immunity is impaired, wound healing is delayed and operative morbidity and mortality increased. Malnutrition worsens the outcome of illness, e.g. respiratory muscle weakness may delay a child being weaned from mechanical ventilation. Malnourished children are less active and more apathetic. These behavioural abnormalities are rapidly reversed with proper feeding, but prolonged and profound malnutrition can cause permanent delay in intellectual development.

The role of intensive nutritional support

Children with long-term disorders who are malnourished will grow better if given supplemental nutritional support, which may be provided by the enteral or parenteral route.

Enteral nutrition

Enteral nutrition is used when the digestive tract is functioning, as it maintains gut function and is safe. Feeds are given nasogastrically, by gastrostomy or occasionally via a feeding tube in the jejunum (e.g. if there are problems with vomiting). Feeds are often given continuously overnight, allowing the child to feed normally during the day. Gastrostomies can either be created endoscopically (Fig. 13.13) or surgically. If

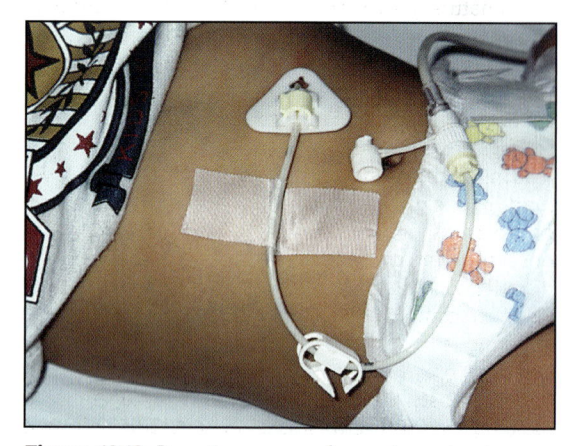

Figure 13.13 Percutaneous endoscopic gastrostomy (PEG) tube for enteral feeding in a child with severe neurodisability and unable to eat by mouth. Unlike nasogastric tubes, the PEG tube is not usually visible to others and is much less likely to be accidentally displaced. Tubes can last for several years before needing to be replaced.

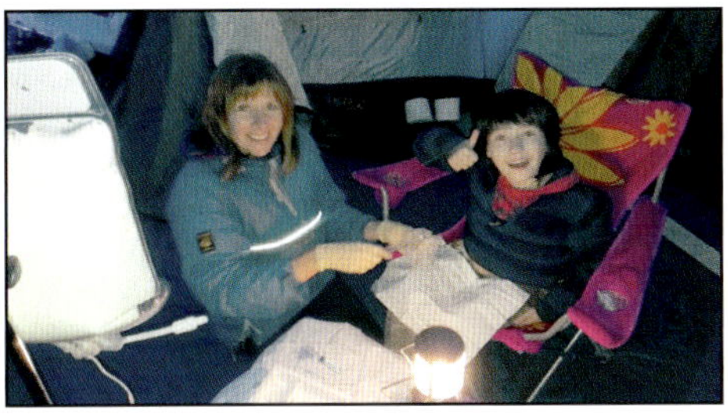

Figure 13.14 Home parenteral nutrition for patients with intestinal failure is associated with good quality of life. This boy has remained well on parenteral nutrition (now 5 nights a week), since he was a newborn infant. His parenteral nutrition is being set up whilst on a camping holiday.

long-term supplemental enteral nutrition is required (>6 weeks), a gastrostomy is preferred as it avoids repeated replacement of nasogastric tubes which is distressing for the child.

Parenteral nutrition (PN)

Can be used exclusively or as an adjunct to enteral feeds to maintain and/or enhance nutrition. The aim is to provide a nutritionally complete feed in an appropriate volume of intravenous fluid. Energy is given as glucose together with a fat emulsion (usually derived from soya bean oil, sometimes combined with fish oil, medium chain triglycerides and olive oil), whereas nitrogen is supplied as synthetic amino acids in a combination resembling egg protein. Electrolytes and a full range of vitamins, micronutrients, and trace elements are also given. Clinical deficiencies (such as zinc deficiency, causing erythematous rash around the mouth and anus) may occur and monitoring is required.

Many patients, such as the preterm newborn with an immature gastrointestinal tract, require PN for only a few weeks until they are able to tolerate full enteral feeds. Some children depend on long-term PN and if their condition is stable can be managed at home, with PN being given overnight so that they are not tied to an infusion pump during the day (Fig. 13.14). Common reasons for needing long-term PN are short bowel syndrome (e.g. major loss of bowel from complicated gastroschisis, or a volvulus), enteropathies (often with onset of severe diarrhoea in very early life), or a motility disorder such as long-segment Hirschsprung disease. PN is a complex and expensive form of therapy, requiring a multidisciplinary team incorporating the skills not only of medical and nursing staff but also of pharmacists, dieticians, surgeons and interventional radiologists. Short term, it is possible to deliver it via a cannula in a peripheral vein; long term it is delivered via a central venous catheter (CVC) as this allows infusion of hyperosmolar solutions and reliable venous access. The CVC may be inserted surgically or under radiological guidance. Complications include CVC sepsis or blockage, venous thrombosis and intestinal failure-associated liver disease.

Severe malnutrition

Severe malnutrition continues to be a major problem in many low and middle-income countries. The WHO recommends that nutritional status is expressed as:

- weight for height – a measure of wasting and an index of acute malnutrition. The weight is plotted against height on a WHO standard growth chart, and the number of standard deviations (described as z-scores) below the median is determined.
- mid-upper-arm circumference (MUAC) – colour coding of tape measures allows ready identification of moderate and severe malnutrition
- height for age – a measure of stunting and an index of chronic malnutrition.

Severe protein-calorie malnutrition is classified as:

- marasmus
- kwashiorkor
- marasmic kwashiorkor.

In marasmus, the child has a wasted, wizened appearance (Fig. 13.15). Oedema is not present. Affected children are often withdrawn and apathetic.

In kwashiorkor, there is generalized oedema as well as severe wasting (Fig. 13.15). Because of the oedema, the weight may not be as severely reduced as in marasmus. In addition, there may be:

- a 'flaky-paint' skin rash with hyperkeratosis (thickened skin) and desquamation
- a distended abdomen and enlarged liver (usually due to fatty infiltration)
- angular stomatitis
- hair that is sparse and depigmented
- diarrhoea, hypothermia, bradycardia and hypotension
- low plasma albumin, potassium, glucose and magnesium levels.

It is unclear why some children with protein-energy malnutrition develop kwashiorkor and others develop marasmus. There is some evidence that kwashiorkor is a manifestation of primary protein deficiency with energy intake relatively well maintained. It often occurs in communities where infants are not weaned from the breast until about 12 months of age and the subsequent diet is relatively high in starch. Kwashiorkor often develops after an acute intercurrent infection, such as measles or gastroenteritis. In practice, it is sometimes difficult to clearly separate the two, when the term 'marasmic kwashiorkor' is used.

Severe acute malnutrition is defined as the presence of any of the following:

- weight for height – more than 3 standard deviations (more than −3 z-score) below the median on the standard WHO growth chart.
- mid-upper-arm circumference (MUAC) – less than 115 mm in children 6 months – 5 years old.
- bilateral oedema.

Both weight for height and mid-upper-arm circumference are measured as they identify slightly

Malnutrition

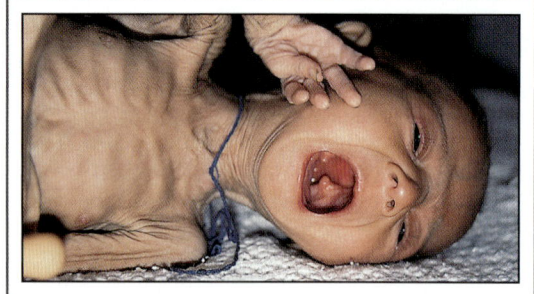

Figure 13.15 Marasmus in a 3-month-old baby who was unable to establish breastfeeding because of a cleft palate.

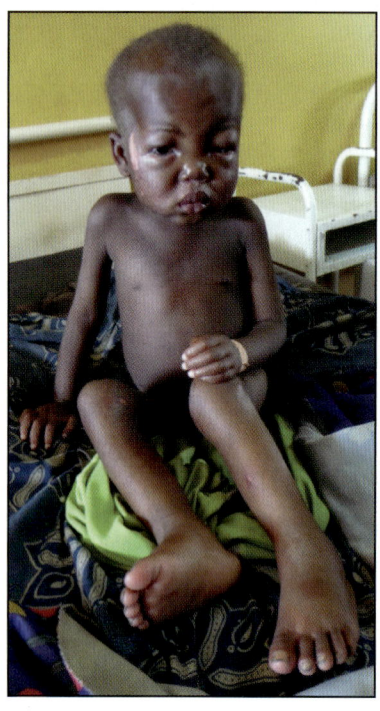

Figure 13.16 Kwashiorkor, a particular manifestation of severe protein-energy malnutrition in some developing countries, where infants are weaned late from the breast and the young child's diet is high in starch. There is oedema around the eyes and feet and legs, hyperkeratosis and depigmentation of the skin and redness of the hair.

different groups of children. Oedema identifies severe kwashiorkor.

Management

Most children with severe acute malnutrition have an appetite and are alert and can be managed within the community with ready-to-use therapeutic food (RUTF), which has revolutionized its treatment. It is based on peanut butter mixed with dried skimmed milk and vitamins and minerals and is consumed directly by the child.

Children with no appetite, severe oedema, a medical complication or are less than 6 months old have complicated severe acute malnutrition and require hospital in-patient care; it has a high mortality, up to 30%. In addition to protein and energy deficiency, there is electrolyte and mineral deficiency (potassium, zinc and magnesium) as well as micronutrient and vitamin deficiency (vitamin A).

Acute management comprises the WHO's 10 essential steps. Stabilization is to:

- treat or prevent hypoglycaemia urgently
- treat or prevent hypothermia
- treat or prevent dehydration – but avoid fluid overload as it may lead to heart failure. The standard WHO oral rehydration solution contains too much sodium (Na^+ 75 mmol/l) and too little potassium for severe acute malnutrition; they should be given a special rehydration solution (ReSoMal). Rehydration should be provided orally, by nasogastric tube if necessary. Intravenous fluids are given only for shock
- correct electrolyte imbalance – especially potassium and magnesium. Although plasma sodium may be low, they have excess body sodium
- treat infection – give broad-spectrum antibiotics; fever and other signs may be absent. Treat oral *Candida* if present
- correct micronutrient deficiency – vitamin A and other vitamins; contained in specialized feeds. Introduction of iron is delayed to 2nd week
- initiate feeding – small volumes, frequently, including through the night. Too rapid feeding may result in diarrhoea. Specialized feeds are widely available: initially Formula 75 (75 kcal/100 ml) which is low in protein and sodium and high in carbohydrate is used, subsequently Formula 100 (100 kcal/100 ml) or ready-to-use therapeutic food.

The remaining three steps are provided during rehabilitation:

- achieve catch-up growth
- provide sensory stimulation and emotional support
- provide for follow-up after recovery.

Stunting

It is estimated that in 2015 about 156 million children under 5 were stunted (height for age more than −2 SD (more than −2 z-scores) below median). This makes them more susceptible to illness and more likely to fall behind at school. As adults, they have an increased risk of becoming obese and developing non-communicable diseases. The World Health Assembly endorsed in 2012 a target of a 40% reduction in the number of children who are stunted by 2025, and many multifaceted initiatives are underway.

Summary

Malnutrition
- Worldwide – contributes to about a third of all childhood deaths; often a consequence of war and social disruption, as well as famine and natural disasters.
- In developed countries – results from poverty, parental neglect or poor education, restrictive diets, and in children with feeding disorders, chronic illness, or anorexia nervosa.
- Can be identified by anthropometric measurement.
- Marasmus – wasted, wizened appearance, apathetic.
- Kwashiorkor – generalized oedema, sparse and depigmented hair, skin rash, angular stomatitis, distended abdomen, enlarged liver, and diarrhoea.

Vitamin D deficiency

Vitamin D is derived from two main sources: synthesis in the skin (vitamin D_3) following exposure to ultraviolet light or the diet (vitamin D_2 or D_3). The main functions of vitamin D are the regulation of calcium and phosphate metabolism, making it essential for bone health, but it also has functions in regulation of the immune system. If not supplied in adequate amounts in childhood, rickets and osteomalacia will develop. Vitamin D deficiency usually results from inadequate UVB exposure, deficient intake or defective metabolism of vitamin D, causing a low serum calcium (Fig. 13.17). This triggers the secretion of parathyroid hormone and normalizes the serum calcium but demineralizes the bone. Parathyroid hormone causes renal losses of phosphate and consequently low serum phosphate levels, further reducing the potential for bone calcification.

Vitamin D deficiency usually presents with bony deformity and the classical picture of rickets. It can also present without bone abnormalities but with symptoms of hypocalcaemia, e.g. seizures, neuromuscular

Vitamin D metabolism

Variation in Vitamin D production with time of year and day
When the sun's rays enter the atmosphere at an acute angle, the atmosphere blocks the UVB part of the rays, so the skin does not convert 7-dehydrocholesterol to vitamin D_3. This is the situation during the early and late parts of the day in spring and autumn and for the entire day in winter if located away from the equator. As a rule of thumb, if your shadow is longer than you are tall, you are unlikely to produce much vitamin D_3.

Parathyroid hormone (PTH)
↑ bone resorption
↑ renal calcium reabsorption
↑ 1,25 dihydroxyvitamin D synthesis.

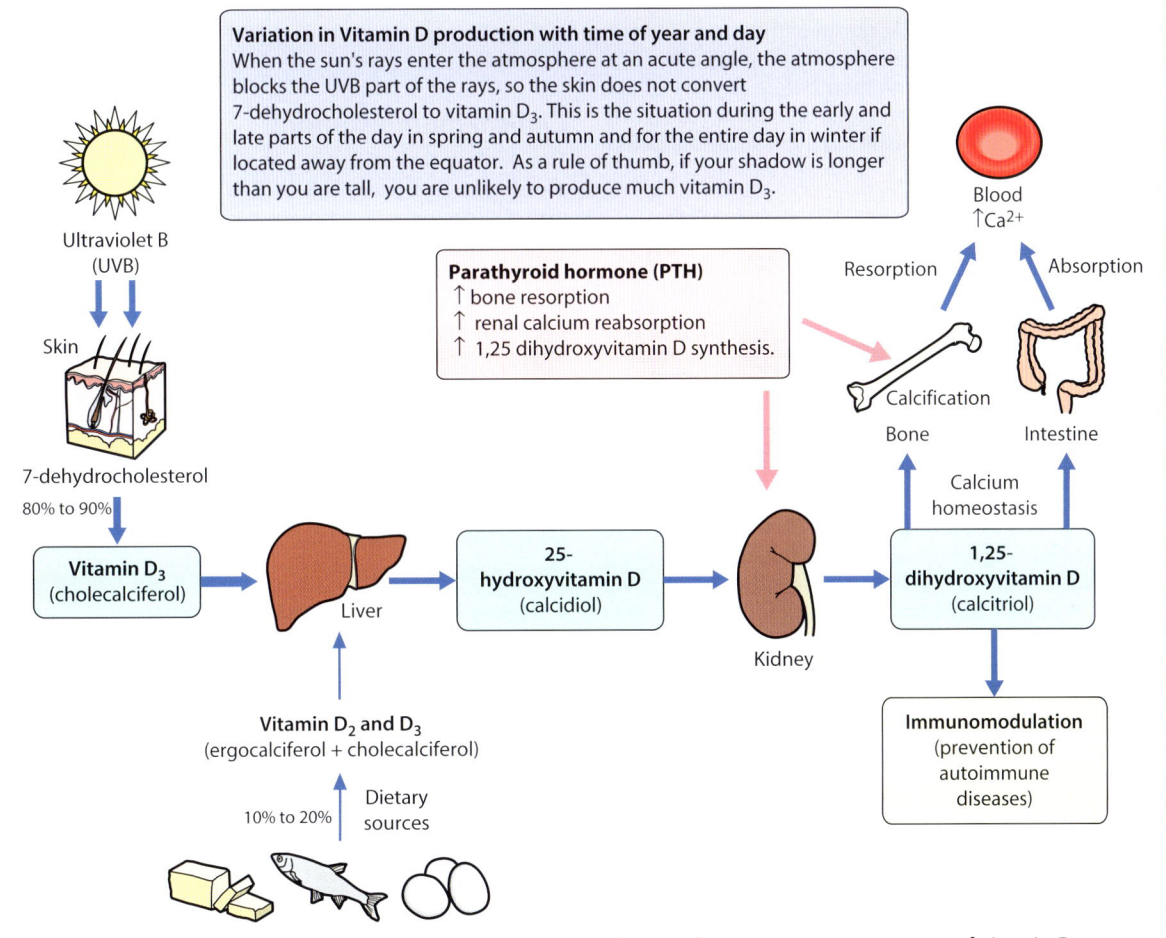

Ultraviolet B (UVB) → Skin → 7-dehydrocholesterol (80% to 90%) → Vitamin D_3 (cholecalciferol) → Liver → 25-hydroxyvitamin D (calcidiol) → Kidney → 1,25-dihydroxyvitamin D (calcitriol)

Vitamin D_2 and D_3 (ergocalciferol + cholecalciferol), Dietary sources 10% to 20%

Blood ↑Ca^{2+} — Resorption (Bone), Absorption (Intestine), Calcification, Calcium homeostasis

Immunomodulation (prevention of autoimmune diseases)

Figure 13.17 Vitamin D metabolism. In most countries, sunlight is the most important source of vitamin D. Vitamin D is not abundant naturally in food, except in fish liver oil, fatty fish, and egg yolk. Vitamin D_2 (ergocalciferol) is the form used to fortify food such as margarine. Vitamin D is hydroxylated in the liver and again in the kidney to produce 1,25-dihydroxyvitamin D, the most active form of the vitamin. It is produced following parathyroid hormone secretion in response to a low plasma calcium.

> **Box 13.5** Causes of rickets
>
> **Nutritional (primary) rickets – risk factors**
> - Living in northern latitudes
> - Dark skin
> - Decreased exposure to sunlight, e.g. in some Asian children living in the UK
> - Maternal vitamin D deficiency
> - Diets low in calcium, phosphorus, and vitamin D, e.g. exclusive breastfeeding into late infancy or, rarely, toddlers on unsupervised 'dairy-free' diets
> - Macrobiotic, strict vegan diets
> - Prolonged parenteral nutrition in infancy
>
> **Intestinal malabsorption**
> - Small bowel enteropathy (e.g. coeliac disease)
> - Pancreatic insufficiency (e.g. cystic fibrosis)
> - Cholestatic liver disease
> - High phytic acids in diet (e.g. chapattis)
>
> **Defective production of 25-hydroxyvitamin D**
> - Chronic liver disease
>
> **Increased metabolism of 25-hydroxyvitamin D**
> - Enzyme induction by anticonvulsants (e.g. phenobarbital)
>
> **Defective production of 1,25-dihydroxyvitamin D**
> - Chronic kidney disease
> - Fanconi syndrome (renal loss of phosphate)
> - Inherited disorders (rare)

irritability causing muscle spasm of the hands and feet (tetany), apnoea, stridor, and cardiomyopathy. This presentation is more common before 2 years of age and in adolescence, when a high demand for calcium in rapidly growing bone results in hypocalcaemia before rickets develops.

Rickets

Rickets signifies a failure in mineralization of the growing bone or osteoid tissue. Failure of mature bone to mineralize is osteomalacia.

Aetiology

The causes of rickets are listed in Box 13.5. The predominant cause of rickets during the early twentieth century was nutritional vitamin D deficiency due to inadequate intake or insufficient exposure to direct sunlight. Nutritional rickets remains the major cause in low and middle-income countries. In high-income countries, nutritional rickets has become rare, as formula milk and many foods such as breakfast cereals are supplemented with vitamin D. However, nutritional rickets has re-emerged in high-income countries in black or Asian infants totally breastfed in late infancy. It is also seen in extremely preterm infants from dietary deficiency of phosphorus, together with low stores of calcium and phosphorus.

Children with malabsorptive conditions such as cystic fibrosis, coeliac disease and pancreatic insufficiency can develop rickets due to deficient absorption of vitamin D or calcium, or both. Drugs, especially anticonvulsants such as phenobarbital and phenytoin, interfere with the metabolism of vitamin D and may also cause rickets. Rickets can also result from impaired metabolic conversion or activation of vitamin D (as in hepatic and renal disease) and some rare genetic disorders.

Clinical manifestations

The earliest sign of rickets is a sensation similar to pressing a ping-pong ball elicited by pressing firmly over the occipital or posterior parietal bones (craniotabes). The costochondral junctions may be palpable (rachitic rosary), wrists (especially in crawling infants) and ankles (especially in walking infants) may be widened, and there may be a horizontal depression on the lower chest corresponding to attachment of the softened ribs with the diaphragm (Harrison's sulcus; Fig. 13.18). The legs may become bowed (Fig. 13.19). The clinical features are listed in Box 13.6 (see also Case History 13.2).

Diagnosis

This is made from:
- Dietary history (prolonged breastfeeding).
- Blood tests – serum calcium is low or normal, phosphorus low, plasma alkaline phosphatase activity high, 25-hydroxyvitamin D may be low, and parathyroid hormone elevated.
- X-ray of the wrist joint – shows cupping and fraying of the metaphyses and a widened epiphyseal plate.

Management

Nutritional rickets is managed by advice about a balanced diet, correction of predisposing risk factors, and by the daily administration of vitamin D_3 (cholecalciferol). If compliance is an issue, a single oral high dose of vitamin D_3 can be given, followed by the daily maintenance dose. Foods rich in vitamin D include

Rickets

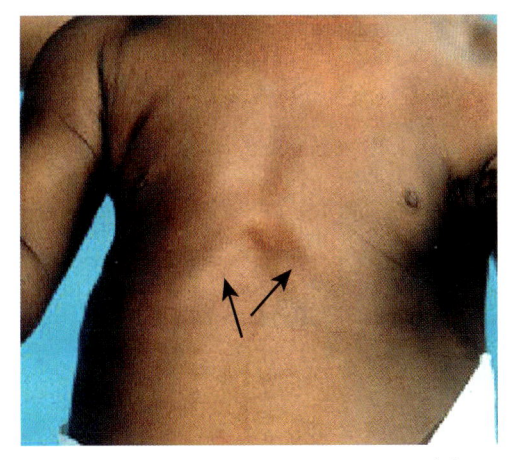

Figure 13.18 Harrison's sulcus, indentation of the softened lower ribcage at the site of attachment of the diaphragm. (Courtesy of Nick Shaw.)

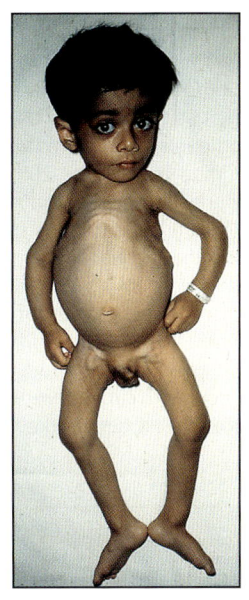

Figure 13.19 Severe rickets in a 3 year old boy secondary to coeliac disease. He has frontal bossing, a Harrison's sulcus and bowing of the legs. (Courtesy of Ian Booth.)

Box 13.6 Clinical features of hypocalcaemia and rickets

- Misery
- Poor growth/short stature
- Frontal bossing of skull
- Craniotabes
- Delayed closure of anterior fontanelle
- Delayed dentition
- Rickety rosary
- Harrison's sulcus
- Expansion of metaphyses (especially wrist)
- Bowing of weight-bearing bones
- Hypotonia
- Seizures
- Cardiomyopathy/heart failure

oily fish and egg yolk; in Europe, milk, dairy products, margarine, breakfast cereals and fruit juice are usually supplemented with vitamin D. Healing occurs in 2–4 weeks and can be monitored from the lowering of alkaline phosphatase, increasing vitamin D levels, and healing on X-rays, but complete reversal of bony deformities may take years.

Summary

Rickets
- Nutritional – has re-emerged in the UK in Asian and black infants exclusively breastfed into late infancy.
- Diagnosis – serum calcium is low or normal, phosphorus low, plasma alkaline phosphatase greatly increased, 25-hydroxyvitamin D low and parathyroid hormone elevated.
- X-ray features – cupping and fraying of the metaphyses and widened epiphyseal plate.

Other vitamin deficiencies

These are shown in Table 13.3.

Obesity

Obesity is the most common nutritional disorder affecting children and adolescents in high-income countries and is rapidly becoming a major problem in low and middle-income countries in children of more affluent families. Its importance is in its short-term and long-term complications (Box 13.7) and that obese children are likely to become obese adults.

Definitions

In children, the Body Mass Index (BMI) is (weight in kg/(height in m)^2) and is expressed as a BMI centile in relation to age-matched and sex-matched population. By convention in the UK, data from 1990 are

Case history 13.2

Seizures and rickets

Mohammed, a 13-month-old Somalian boy, was admitted to the Accident and Emergency department with a generalized afebrile seizure. This was initially controlled with per rectum diazepam. Some 20 minutes later he had another generalized seizure and needed an intravenous anticonvulsant to control his seizure.

His mother said that he was a healthy child. He was born at term, birthweight 3.1 kg, and was still breastfed. Some weaning foods were started at 7–8 months of age, but he preferred feeding at the breast. He had only recently begun to sit without support.

His weight and head circumference were on the second to ninth centile. He had marked frontal bossing, widened wrist (Fig. 13.20) and other epiphyses, Harrison's sulci, wide anterior fontanelle, craniotabes and a rachitic rosary. He would not take his weight on standing.

Investigations showed a low plasma calcium and phosphate concentration, a high alkaline phosphatase and parathyroid hormone, and a very low vitamin D, confirming rickets. Liver and renal function tests were normal and coeliac serology was negative. His wrist X-ray showed characteristic features (Fig. 13.21). A detailed dietary history revealed a diet deficient in calcium and vitamin D, confirming nutritional rickets as the cause.

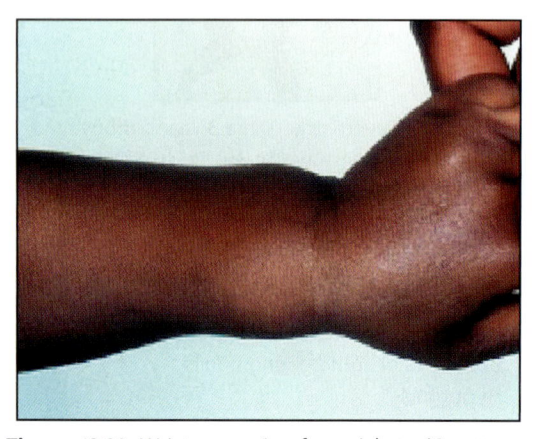

Figure 13.20 Wrist expansion from rickets. (Courtesy of Nick Shaw.)

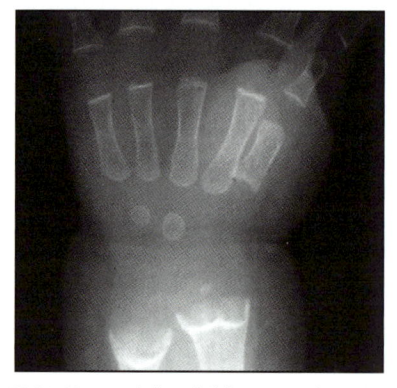

Figure 13.21 X-ray of the child's wrist showing rickets. The ends of the radius and ulna are expanded, rarefied, and cup-shaped, and the bones are poorly mineralized.

Box 13.7 Complications of obesity

- Orthopaedic – slipped upper femoral epiphysis, tibia vara (bow legs), abnormal foot structure and function
- Idiopathic intracranial hypertension (headaches, blurred optic disc margins)
- Hypoventilation syndrome (daytime somnolence, sleep apnoea, snoring, hypercapnia, heart failure)
- Non-alcoholic fatty liver disease
- Gall bladder disease/gallstones
- Polycystic ovarian syndrome
- Type 2 diabetes mellitus
- Hypertension
- Abnormal blood lipids
- Other medical sequelae, e.g. asthma, changes in left ventricular mass, increased risk of certain malignancies (endometrial, breast, and colon cancer)
- Psychological sequelae – low self-esteem, teasing, depression

used (Fig. 13.22). For clinical use, overweight is a BMI over the 91st centile, and obese is a BMI over the 98th centile.

In the UK, the National Child Measurement Programme measures height and weight of children in reception class at school (aged 4–5 years) and in year 6 (aged 10–11 years) to assess overweight and obesity at primary school. The prevalence of overweight (including obesity) between 1994 and 2013 in England is shown in Fig. 13.23. It has risen over the last 20 years, and is highest among 11–15-year-olds. In the UK, more than a third of children are overweight or obese, although the trend may have stabilized over the last decade.

> BMI is not a direct measure of adiposity – it does not distinguish lean from fat mass

Aetiology

The reasons for this marked increase in prevalence are unclear but are due to changes in the environment and

Table 13.3 Vitamin deficiencies affecting children

Fat-soluble vitamins	Dietary/environmental sources	When deficiency is encountered	Clinical consequences
A	Vitamin A in butter, eggs Provitamin A in spinach, carrots, mango, papaya Breastfeeding	Children with fat malabsorption Children in developing countries who do not receive supplements	Increased susceptibility to infection, especially measles; vitamin A supplementation recommended. Impaired adaptation to dark light, dry eyes, excessive blinking, blindness due to xerophthalmia
D	90% from ultraviolet B exposure Egg yolk and fish oil added to infant formula and margarine	Children who live further from the Equator, as ultraviolet B levels are low outside summer months Children with darker skin	Rickets (see above)
E	Vegetable oils	Children with fat malabsorption Preterm infants	Haemolytic anaemia, retinopathy, progressive neuropathy
K	Green vegetables, gut flora. Added to infant formula. Given intramuscularly or orally at birth [see Ch. 10 (Perinatal medicine)]	Newborn infants are relatively vitamin K deficient Seen in children with fat malabsorption, e.g. cystic fibrosis	Clotting abnormalities that lead to bruising/bleeding from vitamin K deficient bleeding (haemorrhagic disease of the newborn)
Water-soluble vitamins			
Thiamine B$_1$	Cereals, pulses, yeast	Children from South East Asia with a 'polished rice diet' or those with malnutrition (beriberi)	Cardiomyopathy in infants, also hoarseness, aphonia, encephalopathy, apathy, drowsiness, seizures
B$_2$ (riboflavin)	Liver, milk, eggs, vegetables	Malnutrition	Angular stomatitis, fissuring of lips
Vitamin C	Fresh fruit and vegetables	Rare but can occur in children with very restrictive diets and neurodisability	Petechiae, poor growth, irritability; painful joints may be mistaken for rickets on X-ray
Folic acid	Green vegetables, yeast extracts, liver	Children taking antifolate medications or those with haemolytic conditions Malnutrition	Macrocytic anaemia, neutropenia, thrombocytopenia

behaviour relating to diet and activity. Energy-dense foods are now widely consumed, including high-fat fast foods and processed foods. However, there is no conclusive evidence that obese children eat more than children of normal weight. The National Food Survey showed that UK household energy intake has fallen since the 1970s, the amount of fruit purchased has increased by 75% and the intake of full fat milk decreased by 80%. Children's energy expenditure has undoubtably decreased. Fewer children walk to school; transport in cars has increased; less time at school is spent doing physical activities; and children spend more time in front of small screens (video games, mobile phones, computers, and television), rather than playing outside. Children from low socioeconomic homes are more likely to be obese; females from the lowest socioeconomic quintile are 2.5 times more likely to be overweight when compared with the highest quintile.

Prevention

There are few randomized controlled trials and most involve complex packages of interventions including decreased fat intake, increased fruit and vegetables,

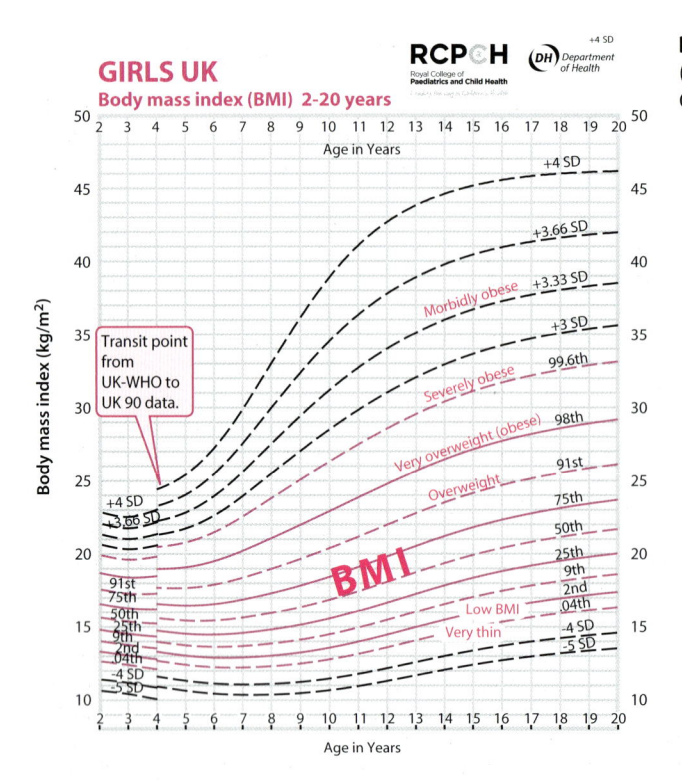

Figure 13.22 Body mass index centile chart (© 2012/13 Royal College of Paediatrics and Child Health, reproduced with permission).

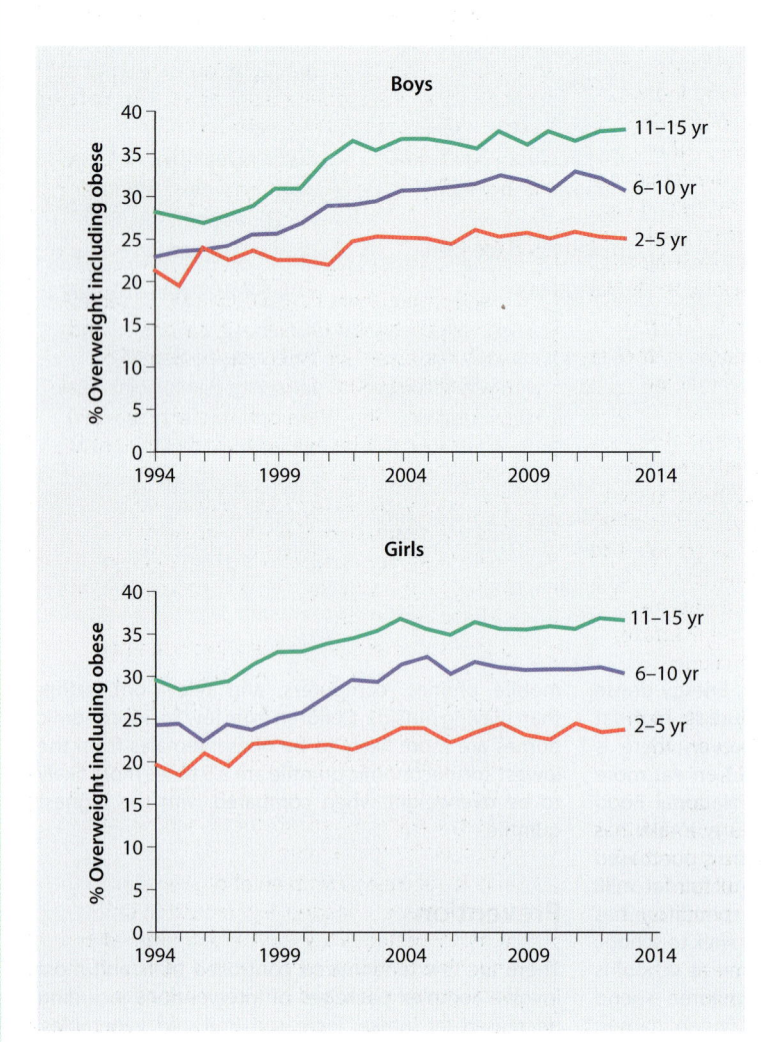

Figure 13.23 Prevalence of overweight and obesity by year and age in boys and girls. (Data from van Jaarsveld CH, Gulliford MC: Childhood obesity trends from primary care electronic health records in England between 1994 and 2013: population-based cohort study. *Arch Dis Child* 100:214–219, 2015.)

reduction in time spent in front of small screens, increased physical activity and education. Of these, a reduction in time spent on small screens appears to be the most effective single factor.

Endogenous causes

Overnutrition accelerates linear growth and puberty. Obese children are therefore relatively tall and will usually be above the 50th centile for height. Therefore, if a child is obese and short, an endogenous cause, i.e. hypothyroidism and Cushing syndrome, should be considered. In children who are obese with learning disabilities or who are dysmorphic, an underlying syndrome may be present. The most common of these is Prader–Willi (obesity, hyperphagia, poor linear growth, dysmorphic facial features, hypotonia, and undescended testes in males; see Ch. 9 and Fig. 9.19). In severely obese children under the age of 3 years, gene defects, e.g. leptin deficiency, are possible causes.

Management

Most obese children are managed in primary care. Specialist paediatric assessment is indicated in any child with complications (Box 13.7) or if an endogenous cause is suspected.

In the absence of evidence from randomized controlled trials, a pragmatic approach in any individual child, based on consensus criteria, has to be adopted. Treatment should be considered when the child is above the 98th centile for BMI and the family are willing to make the necessary difficult lifestyle changes. Weight maintenance is a more realistic goal than weight reduction and will result in a demonstrable fall in BMI on their centile chart as height increases. It can only be achieved by sustained changes in lifestyle:

- healthier eating – regular meals; eating together as a family; choosing nutrient-rich foods that are lower in energy and glycaemic index (the glycaemic index is a ranking of carbohydrate-containing foods based on the overall effect on blood glucose level; slowly absorbed foods have a low glycaemic index rating and those more rapidly absorbed a higher rating); increased vegetable and fruit intake; healthier snack food options; decreased portion sizes; drinking water as the main beverage; reduction in sugary drink intake; involvement of the entire family in making sustainable dietary changes
- physical activity can be increased by walking or cycling for transport, undertaking household chores and playing. Organized exercise programmes have a role, with children and adolescents being encouraged to choose activities that they enjoy and are sustainable (e.g. football, dancing, swimming). At least 60 minutes of moderate or greater intensity physical activity is recommended each day
- limiting television and other small screen recreational activity to less than 2 hours per day.

Drug treatment and surgery

Drug treatment has a part to play in children over the age of 12 years who have extreme obesity (BMI > 40 kg/m^2) or have a BMI over 35 kg/m^2 and complications of obesity.

Orlistat is a lipase inhibitor which reduces the absorption of dietary fat and thus produces steatorrhoea. It should not be used for children under 12 years, but may be indicated if there are comorbidities (e.g. orthopaedic, sleep apnoea) or severe psychological disturbance.

Bariatric surgery is generally not considered appropriate in children or young people unless they have almost achieved maturity, have very severe or extreme obesity with complications, e.g. type 2 diabetes or hypertension and all other interventions have failed to achieve or maintain weight loss. American data would suggest that laparoscopic adjustable gastric banding is the most appropriate operation.

Drug and surgical interventions should only be used in conjunction with a dietary, exercise and behavioural weight management programme and be restricted to specialist centres with multidisciplinary expertise in managing severe obesity. Reducing the prevalence of obesity is a major public health issue. There is recognition in the UK that there needs to be a more 'joined-up' approach to obesity, with integration between health services, local government and other key partners based on the needs of the local population.

Summary

Obesity

- An increasing major health issue for children, predisposing them to a wide range of medical and psychological problems in childhood and adult life, especially type 2 diabetes mellitus and cardiovascular disease.
- Defined as a BMI >98th centile of the UK 1990 reference chart for age and sex; overweight is BMI >91st centile.
- Exogenous causes (hypothyroidism and Cushing syndrome) of obesity are rare, and more likely in a child who is also short with falling height velocity; there are also some rare genetic syndromes.
- Successful management requires sustained changes in lifestyle, with healthier eating, increased physical activity and reduction in physical inactivity.
- Drug treatment and surgical intervention are only appropriate in a small number of children.
- Lifestyle changes are difficult to achieve and even harder to maintain.
- A cultural change from an obesogenic environment is needed, e.g. reduction or removal of unhealthy food and drinks and a more integrated approach involving health, local government and other key partners.

Early childhood caries

What is the most common reason for primary school-aged children (5–9 years old) to be admitted to hospital in England? The answer is dental caries, with 500 admissions a week. Dental decay can cause pain and discomfort and absence from school. Dental caries (Fig. 13.24) is the most common chronic infectious disease of childhood, caused by the interaction of bacteria and sugary foods on tooth enamel. The highest caries prevalence is in Africa and South-East Asia, with a range from 1–12% in infants from high-income countries.

The term 'early childhood caries' (ECC) has been adopted to focus attention on the multiple factors that contribute to caries at such early ages, rather than ascribing sole causation to inappropriate feeding methods. It is frequently associated with a poor diet and poor oral health habits. *Streptococcus mutans* and *Streptococcus sobrinus* are the main cariogenic micro-organisms. Infants acquire these organisms from their mothers. *S. mutans* can spread from mother to baby during infancy and can inoculate even predentate infants.

Salivary amylase splits fermentable carbohydrates (e.g. lactose, fructose, sucrose, galactans, fructans, polyols) into components that can be metabolized by plaque bacteria leading to acidic end products with subsequent demineralization and increased risk for caries on susceptible teeth. Inappropriate use of a baby bottle has a central role in the aetiology and severity of ECC. Increasing the time per day that fermentable carbohydrates are available is the most significant factor in shifting the remineralization equilibrium toward demineralization. Feeding through the night means there is less protection to teeth because of reduced nocturnal salivary flow.

The relationship between diet and dental caries has become weaker, which has been attributed to the widespread use of fluoride. ECC is more commonly found in children who live in poverty or in poor economic conditions, belong to ethnic and racial minorities, are born to single mothers or whose parents have low educational level.

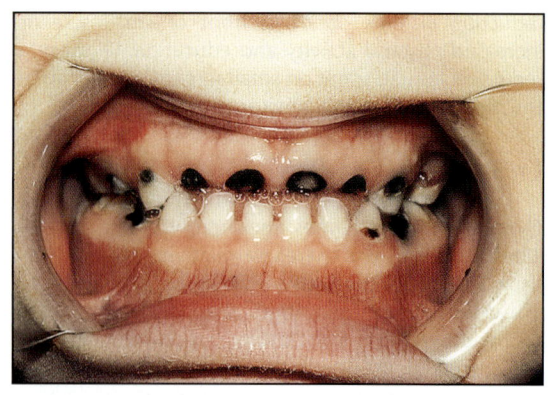

Figure 13.24 Dental caries. Prop-feeding infants when put to sleep with a bottle containing milk or other fermentable liquids places them at high risk of severe dental caries and should be discouraged.

Prevention of early childhood caries

This includes:

- reduce the bacteria in the mouth of the mother or primary caregiver – chemical suppression using chlorhexidine gluconate in the form of mouth rinses, gels, powder or paste has been shown to reduce oral microorganisms
- minimize the transmission of bacteria that cause tooth decay – avoid the sharing of utensils, food and drinks; discourage a child from putting his/her hand in the caregiver's mouth; not licking a pacifier before giving it to the child and not sharing toothbrushes
- oral health education – stimulation of tooth brushing has been among the most successful initiatives
- infants should not be put to sleep with a bottle containing fermentable carbohydrates
- breastfeeding for pleasure should be avoided after the first primary tooth begins to erupt and other dietary carbohydrates are introduced
- children should be encouraged to drink from a cup from their 1st birthday
- wean from the bottle at 12–14 months of age
- avoid repetitive consumption of any liquid containing fermentable carbohydrates
- avoid between-meal snacks and prolonged exposures to foods and juice or other beverages containing fermentable carbohydrates
- fluoridated drinking water – has been shown to be effective in reducing the severity of dental decay in entire populations. In England only 10% of the population's water has a fluoride level optimal for dental health; water fluoridation schemes are in place in 25 countries
- daily tooth brushing with fluoride-containing toothpaste – is the most cost-effective, self-applied method to prevent caries at all ages.

Acknowledgements

We would like to acknowledge that this chapter has used material from the previous chapter on Nutrition from Ian Booth (1st, 2nd, 3rd Editions). It was updated by: Jonathan Bishop (4th Edition) and Stephen Hodges (4th Edition).

Further reading

Beattie M, Dhawan A, Puntis J: *Paediatric Gastroenterology, Hepatology and Nutrition (Oxford Specialist Handbooks in Pediatrics)*, Oxford, 2009, Oxford University Press.

Koletzko B, editor: *Pediatric Nutrition in Practice*, ed 2, Basel, 2015, Karger.

Websites (Accessed November 2016)

British Dietetic Association: Available at: www.bda.uk.com.

British Nutrition Foundation: Available at: www.nutrition.org.uk.

Coeliac UK: Available at: www.coeliac.co.uk.

Details of formula feeds: Available at: https://www.evidence.nhs.uk/formulary/bnfc/current/9-nutrition-and-blood/94-oral-nutrition/942-enteral-nutrition.

Infant Feeding Survey 2010: Available at: http://www.hscic.gov.uk/catalogue/PUB08694

National Institute for Health and Care Excellence: Available at: https://www.nice.org.uk/guidance/cg189. *Guideline 189.*
Obesity: identification, assessment and management of obesity and overweight in children, young people and adults.

NHS guidance on healthy eating for children and families: Available at: http://www.nhs.uk/Livewell/Goodfood/Pages/Goodfoodhome.aspx.

Nutrition programming: Available at: http://www.project-earlynutrition.eu.

Practical information on breastfeeding: Available at: http://www.unicef.org.uk/BabyFriendly/.

Scientific Advisory Committee on Nutrition: Available at: https://www.gov.uk/government/groups/scientific-advisory-committee-on-nutrition.

Up-to-date reviews on a selection of child nutrition topics: Available at: http://www.espghan.org/guidelines/nutrition/.

World Food Programme: Available at: www.wfp.org.

World Health Organization: Available at: http://www.who.int/nutrition/topics/malnutrition/en/ *Guidelines for malnutrition in developing countries.*

World Health Organization: Available at http://apps.who.int/iris/bitstream/10665/204176/1/9789241510066_eng.pdf?ua=1 Report of Commission. 2016

14

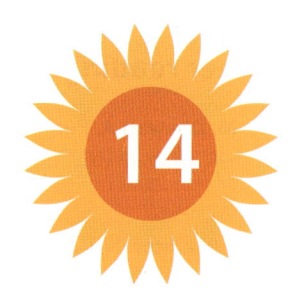

Gastroenterology

Vomiting	234	Malabsorption	249
Crying	237	Chronic non-specific diarrhoea	251
Acute abdominal pain	238	Inflammatory bowel disease	252
Recurrent abdominal pain	243	Constipation	253
Gastroenteritis	244		

Features of gastrointestinal disorders in children are:

- vomiting, abdominal pain and diarrhoea are common and usually transient; serious causes are uncommon but important to identify
- worldwide, gastroenteritis is responsible for 530 000 deaths per year, one of the most common causes of death in children under 5 years of age
- the number of children and adolescents developing inflammatory bowel disease is increasing
- in contrast to adults, bowel cancer is extremely rare.

Vomiting

Posseting and *regurgitation* are terms used to describe the non-forceful return of milk, but differ in degree. Posseting describes the small amounts of milk that often accompany the return of swallowed air (wind), whereas regurgitation describes larger, more frequent losses. Posseting occurs in nearly all babies from time to time, whereas regurgitation may indicate the presence of more significant gastro-oesophageal reflux.

Vomiting is the forceful ejection of gastric contents. It is a common problem in infancy and childhood (Fig. 14.1 and Box 14.1).

Box 14.1 'Red flag' clinical features in the vomiting child

Bile-stained vomit	Intestinal obstruction [see Ch. 11 (Neonatal medicine)]
Haematemesis	Oesophagitis, peptic ulceration, oral/nasal bleeding, and oesophageal variceal bleeding
Projectile vomiting, in first few weeks of life	Pyloric stenosis
Vomiting at the end of paroxysmal coughing	Whooping cough (pertussis)
Abdominal tenderness/abdominal pain on movement	Surgical abdomen
Abdominal distension	Intestinal obstruction, including strangulated inguinal hernia
Hepatosplenomegaly	Chronic liver disease, inborn error of metabolism
Blood in the stool	Intussusception, bacterial gastroenteritis
Severe dehydration, shock	Severe gastroenteritis, systemic infection (urinary tract infection, meningitis), diabetic ketoacidosis
Bulging fontanelle or seizures	Raised intracranial pressure
Faltering growth	Gastro-oesophageal reflux disease, coeliac disease and other chronic gastrointestinal conditions

Causes of vomiting

Infants

Gastro-oesophageal reflux
Feeding problems
Infection:
- Gastroenteritis
- Respiratory tract/otitis media
- Whooping cough (pertussis)
- Urinary tract
- Meningitis

Food allergy and food intolerance
Eosinophilic oesophagitis
Intestinal obstruction:
- Pyloric stenosis
- Atresia – duodenal, other sites
- Intussusception
- Malrotation
- Volvulus
- Duplication cysts
- Strangulated inguinal hernia
- Hirschsprung disease

Inborn errors of metabolism
Congenital adrenal hyperplasia
Renal failure

Preschool children

Gastroenteritis
Infection:
- Respiratory tract/otitis media
- Urinary tract
- Meningitis
- Whooping cough (pertussis)

Appendicitis
Intestinal obstruction:
- Intussusception
- Malrotation
- Volvulus
- Adhesions
- Foreign body – bezoar

Raised intracranial pressure
Coeliac disease
Renal failure
Inborn errors of metabolism
Torsion of the testis

School age and adolescents

Gastroenteritis
Infection – including pyelonephritis, septicaemia, meningitis
Peptic ulceration and *H. pylori* infection
Appendicitis
Migraine
Raised intracranial pressure
Coeliac disease
Renal failure
Diabetic ketoacidosis
Alcohol/drug ingestion or medications
Cyclical vomiting syndrome
Bulimia/anorexia nervosa
Pregnancy
Torsion of the testis

Figure 14.1 Causes of regurgitation/vomiting.

It is usually benign and is often caused by feeding disorders or mild gastro-oesophageal reflux or gastroenteritis. Potentially serious disorders need to be excluded if the vomiting is bilious or prolonged, or if the child is systemically unwell or has faltering growth. In infants, vomiting may be associated with infection outside the gastrointestinal tract, especially in the urinary tract and central nervous system. In intestinal obstruction, the more proximal the obstruction, the more prominent the vomiting and the sooner it becomes bile stained (unless the obstruction is proximal to the ampulla of Vater). Intestinal obstruction is associated with abdominal distension, more marked in distal obstruction. 'Red flag' clinical features suggesting significant organic pathology are listed in Box 14.1.

Gastro-oesophageal reflux

Gastro-oesophageal reflux is the involuntary passage of gastric contents into the oesophagus. It is extremely common in infancy. It is caused by inappropriate relaxation of the lower oesophageal sphincter as a result of functional immaturity. A predominantly fluid diet, a mainly horizontal posture and a short intra-abdominal length of oesophagus all contribute. While common in the 1st year of life, nearly all symptomatic reflux resolves spontaneously by 12 months of age. This is probably due to a combination of maturation of the lower oesophageal sphincter, assumption of an upright posture and more solids in the diet.

Most infants with gastro-oesophageal reflux have recurrent regurgitation or vomiting but are putting on weight normally and are otherwise well, although the mess, smell, and frequent changes of clothes (5% of those affected have 6 or more episodes each day) is frustrating for parents and carers.

Gastro-oesophageal reflux is usually a benign, self-limited condition but when it becomes a significant

> **Summary**
>
> **Vomiting in infants**
> - Common chronic cause is gastro-oesophageal reflux.
> - Feed volumes should be calculated as overfeeding is common in bottle-fed infants.
> - If transient, with other symptoms, e.g. fever, diarrhoea or runny nose and cough, most likely to be gastroenteritis or respiratory tract infection, but consider urine infection, sepsis or meningitis.
> - If projectile at 2–8 weeks of age, exclude pyloric stenosis.
> - If bile stained, potential emergency – exclude intestinal obstruction, especially intussusception, malrotation and a strangulated inguinal hernia. Assess for dehydration and shock.

problem (Box 14.2) it becomes gastro-oesophageal reflux disease and needs treatment.

Gastro-oesophageal reflux disease is more common in:

- children with cerebral palsy or other neurodevelopmental disorders
- preterm infants, especially in those with bronchopulmonary dysplasia
- following surgery for oesophageal atresia or diaphragmatic hernia.

Box 14.2 Complications of gastro-oesophageal reflux (i.e. gastro-oesophageal reflux disease)

- Faltering growth from severe vomiting
- Oesophagitis – haematemesis, discomfort on feeding or heartburn, iron-deficiency anaemia
- Recurrent pulmonary aspiration – recurrent pneumonia, cough or wheeze, apnoea in preterm infants
- Dystonic neck posturing (Sandifer syndrome)
- Apparent life-threatening events

Investigation

Gastro-oesophageal reflux is usually diagnosed clinically and no investigations are required. However, they may be indicated if the history is atypical, complications are present, or there is failure to respond to treatment. Investigations include:

- 24-hour oesophageal pH monitoring to quantify the degree of acid reflux (see Case History 14.1)
- 24-hour impedance monitoring which is available in some centres. Weakly acidic or nonacid reflux, which may cause disease, is also measured
- endoscopy with oesophageal biopsies to identify oesophagitis and exclude other causes of vomiting.

Case history 14.1

Gastro-oesophageal reflux disease

This infant (Fig. 14.2a) had a history of frequent regurgitation from the first few days of life. He developed two chest infections. Some of the vomits contained altered blood. A 24-hour oesophageal pH study showed severe gastro-oesophageal reflux disease (Fig. 14.2b,c). Endoscopy showed oesophagitis. He had probably had episodes of aspiration pneumonia. Symptoms resolved on treatment with feed thickeners and omeprazole. His parents also commented on how much better he slept at night. Treatment was reduced from 14 months of age and the symptoms did not recur.

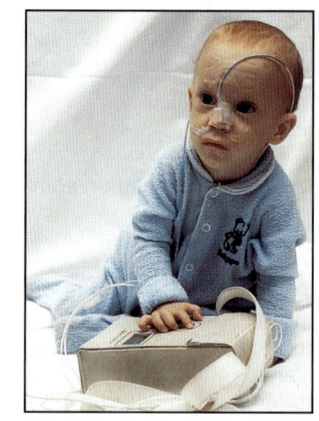

Figure 14.2a A pH sensor has been placed in the lower oesophagus. (Courtesy of Ian Booth.)

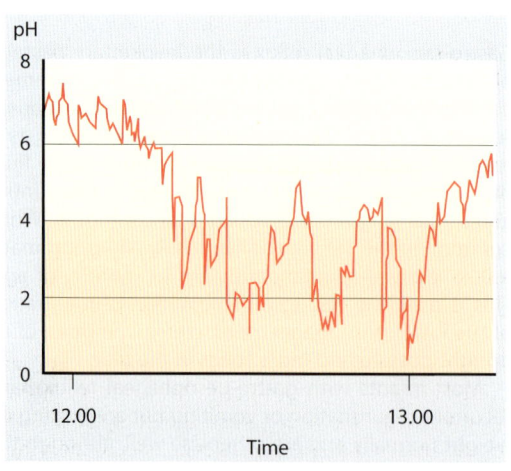

Figure 14.2b A section of the 24-hour oesophageal pH study showing severe reflux, with frequent drops in pH below 4. (Courtesy of Ian Booth.)

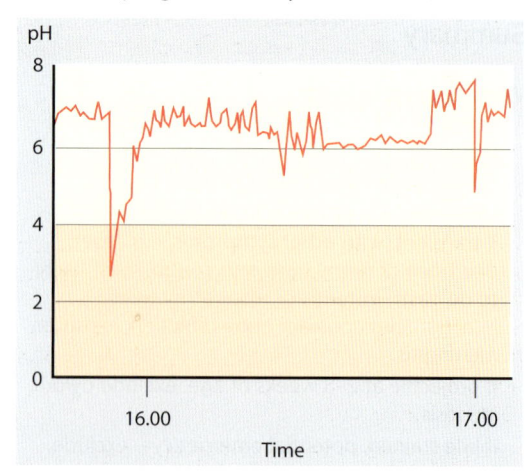

Figure 14.2c A section of a normal oesophageal pH study. The lower oesophageal pH is above 4 for most of the time. (Courtesy of Ian Booth.)

Contrast studies of the upper gastrointestinal tract may support the diagnosis but are neither sensitive nor specific. They may be required in gastro-oesophageal disease to exclude underlying anatomical abnormalities in the oesophagus, stomach, and duodenum, and to identify malrotation.

Management

Uncomplicated gastro-oesophageal reflux has an excellent prognosis and can be managed by parental reassurance, adding inert thickening agents to feeds (e.g. Carobel), and smaller, more frequent feeds.

Significant gastro-oesophageal reflux disease is managed with acid suppression with either hydrogen receptor antagonists (e.g. ranitidine) or proton-pump inhibitors (e.g. omeprazole). These drugs reduce the volume of gastric contents and treat acid-related oesophagitis. The evidence for the use of drugs that enhance gastric emptying (e.g. domperidone) is poor and as they are associated with significant side-effects their use should be discouraged. If the child fails to respond to these measures, other diagnoses such as cow's milk protein allergy should be considered and further investigations performed.

Surgical management is reserved for children with complications unresponsive to intensive medical treatment or oesophageal stricture. A Nissen fundoplication, in which the fundus of the stomach is wrapped around the intra-abdominal oesophagus, is performed either as an abdominal or as a laparoscopic procedure.

Summary

Gastro-oesophageal reflux
- Occurs in otherwise normal infants, but risk is increased if the infant has neuromuscular problems or has had surgery to the oesophagus or diaphragm.
- Is treated if troublesome with feed thickening, medication, and rarely fundoplication.
- Investigations are performed if diagnosis is unclear or complications occur (gastro-oesophageal reflux disease).

Pyloric stenosis

In pyloric stenosis, there is hypertrophy of the pyloric muscle causing gastric outlet obstruction. It presents at 2–8 weeks of age, irrespective of gestational age. It is more common in boys (4 : 1), particularly firstborn, and there may be a family history, especially on the maternal side.

Clinical features are:
- vomiting, which increases in frequency and forcefulness over time, ultimately becoming projectile
- hunger after vomiting until dehydration leads to loss of interest in feeding
- weight loss if presentation is delayed.

A hypochloraemic metabolic alkalosis with a low plasma sodium and potassium occurs as a result of vomiting stomach contents.

Diagnosis

Unless immediate fluid resuscitation is required, a test feed is performed. The baby is given a milk feed, which will calm the hungry infant, allowing examination. Gastric peristalsis may be seen as a wave moving from left to right across the abdomen (Fig. 14.3a). The pyloric mass, which feels like an olive, is usually palpable in the right upper quadrant (Fig. 14.3b). If the stomach is overdistended with air, it will need to be emptied by a nasogastric tube to allow palpation. Ultrasound examination may be helpful (Fig. 14.3c) to confirm the diagnosis prior to surgery.

Management

The initial priority is to correct any fluid and electrolyte disturbance with intravenous fluids. Once hydration and acid–base and electrolytes are normal, definitive treatment by pyloromyotomy can be performed. This involves division of the hypertrophied muscle down to, but not including, the mucosa (Fig. 14.3d). The operation can be performed either as an open procedure via a periumbilical incision or laparoscopically. Postoperatively, the child can usually be fed within 6 hours and discharged within 2 days of surgery.

Summary

Pyloric stenosis
- More common in boys and in those with a family history.
- Signs are visible gastric peristalsis, palpable abdominal mass on test feed, and possible dehydration.
- Associated with hyponatraemia, hypokalaemia, and hypochloraemic alkalosis.
- Diagnosis may be confirmed by ultrasound.
- Treated by surgery after rehydration and correction of electrolyte imbalance.

Crying

The time healthy babies cry for is highly variable. In most, it represents the baby's response to hunger and discomfort. Reassurance and advice on appropriate feeding will usually suffice.

Some babies cry for prolonged periods in spite of feeding and comforting and this is distressing for all concerned. It can engender a feeling of anxiety, helplessness and depression in parents and carers, particularly if they are inexperienced or poorly supported. It has also been suggested that the emotional climate within a home may be transmitted to a baby, and that in some instances, tense, anxious, or irritable caregivers are more likely to have fretful babies. The complaint

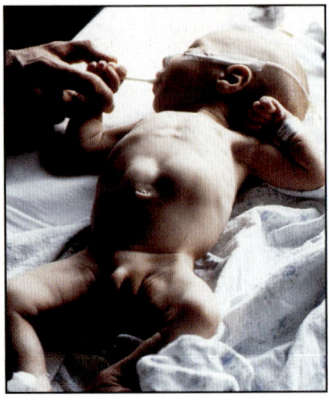

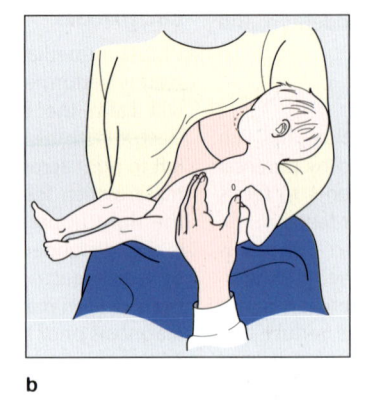

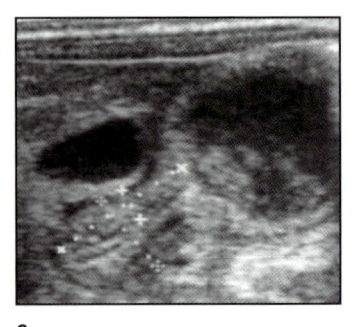

Pyloric stenosis

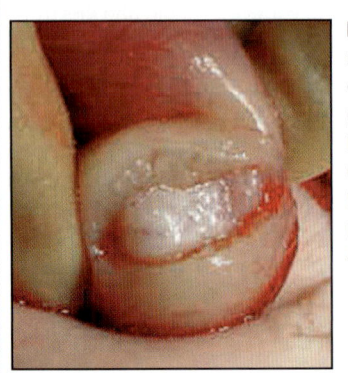

Figure 14.3 (**a**) Visible gastric peristalsis in an infant with pyloric stenosis; (**b**) Diagram showing a test feed being performed to diagnose pyloric stenosis. The pyloric mass feels like an 'olive' on gentle, deep palpation halfway between the midpoint of the anterior margin of the right ribcage and the umbilicus; (**c**) ultrasound examination showing gastric contents in the antrum and an elongated pylorus (dotted line); and. (**d**) pyloric stenosis at operation showing pale, thick pyloric muscle, and pyloromyotomy incision. (Courtesy of Anthony Lander)

that a baby is 'always crying' may also be a pointer to potential or actual non-accidental injury.

A cause for the crying is identified in a minority of infants. If of sudden onset, it may be due to a urinary tract, middle ear or meningeal infection; pain from an unrecognized fracture; oesophagitis; or torsion of the testis. Severe nappy rash and constipation may produce a miserable, crying infant. Preterm infants who have spent several weeks in hospital can be difficult to settle, as can infants with a chronic neurological disorder, e.g. cerebral palsy. On the basis of countless reports of parents, eruption of teeth is painful in some infants. However, teething does not cause vomiting, diarrhoea, high fever or seizures.

Acknowledging that troublesome crying is extremely distressing is part of the management. Reducing overstimulation from jigging and winding and encouraging a quiet environment and holding the baby close until the crying stops appear to help many babies. Parental support through follow-up by health professionals is helpful.

Infant 'colic'

The term 'colic' is used to describe a common symptom complex that occurs during the first few months of life. Paroxysmal, inconsolable crying or screaming often accompanied by drawing up of the knees and passage of excessive flatus takes place several times a day. There is no firm evidence that the cause is gastrointestinal, but this is often suspected. The condition occurs in up to 40% of babies. It typically occurs in the first few weeks of life and resolves gradually from 3–12 months of age. The condition is benign but it is very frustrating and worrying for parents and may precipitate non-accidental injury in infants already at risk. Support and reassurance should be given. 'Gripe water' is often recommended but is of unproven benefit. If severe and persistent, it may be due to a cow's milk protein allergy and an empirical 2-week trial of a protein hydrolysate formula (cow's milk protein free) may be considered and continued if symptoms improve. If they do not, then a trial of gastro-oesophageal reflux treatment may be considered.

Acute abdominal pain

Assessment of the child with acute abdominal pain requires considerable skill. The differential diagnosis of acute abdominal pain in children is extremely wide, encompassing non-specific abdominal pain, surgical causes and medical conditions (Fig. 14.4). In nearly half of the children admitted to hospital, the pain resolves undiagnosed. In young children it is essential not to delay the diagnosis and treatment of acute

```
                    Causes of acute abdominal pain
                              │
        ┌─────────────────────┼─────────────────────┐
    Surgical ◄── Intra-abdominal ──► Medical    Extra-abdominal
```

Surgical:
- Acute appendicitis
- Intestinal obstruction including intussusception
- Inguinal hernia
- Peritonitis
- Inflamed Meckel diverticulum
- Pancreatitis
- Trauma

Medical:
- Non-specific abdominal pain
- Gastroenteritis
- Urinary tract:
  - urinary tract infection
  - acute pyelonephritis
  - hydronephrosis
  - renal calculus
- Henoch–Schönlein purpura
- Diabetic ketoacidosis
- Sickle cell disease
- Hepatitis
- Inflammatory bowel disease
- Constipation
- Recurrent abdominal pain of childhood
- Gynaecological in pubertal females
- Psychological
- Lead poisoning
- Acute porphyria (rare)
- Unknown

Extra-abdominal:
- Upper respiratory tract infection
- Lower lobe pneumonia
- Torsion of the testis
- Hip and spine

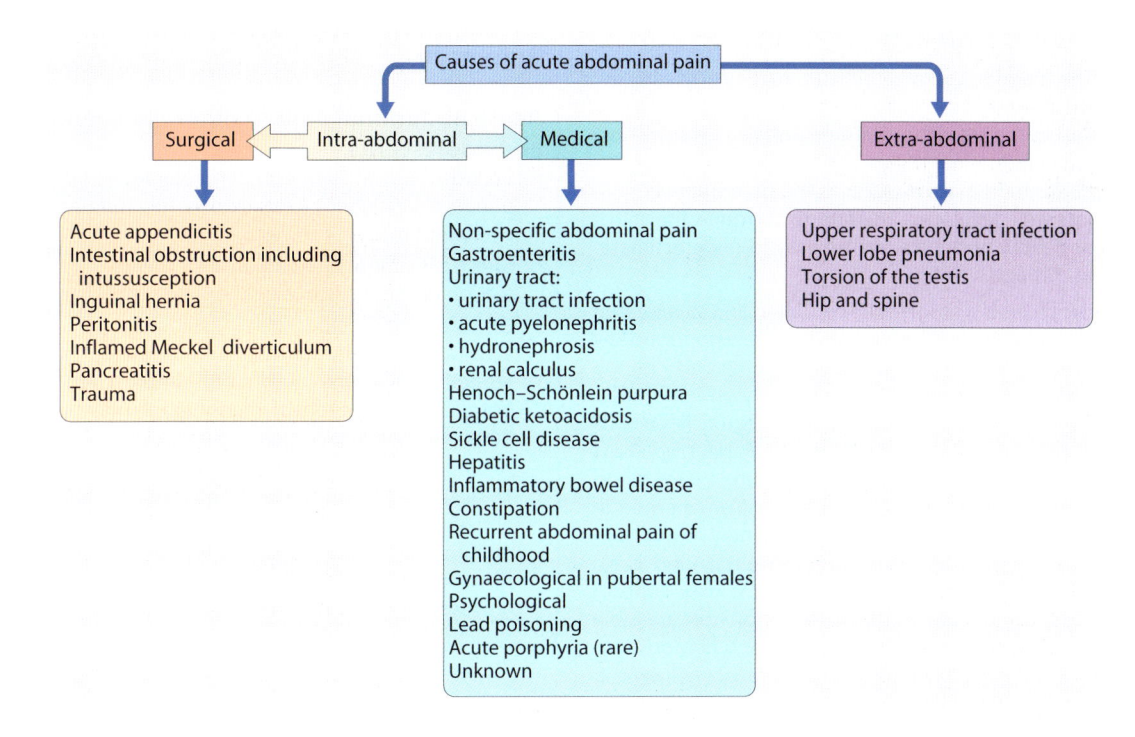

Figure 14.4 Causes of acute abdominal pain.

---

appendicitis, as progression to perforation can be rapid. It is easy to belittle the clinical signs of abdominal tenderness in young children. Of the surgical causes, appendicitis is by far the most common. The testes, hernial orifices and hip joints must always be checked. It is noteworthy that:

- lower lobe pneumonia may cause pain referred to the abdomen
- primary peritonitis is seen in patients with ascites from nephrotic syndrome or liver disease
- diabetic ketoacidosis may cause severe abdominal pain
- urinary tract infection, including acute pyelonephritis, is a relatively uncommon cause of acute abdominal pain, but must not be missed. It is important to test a urine sample, in order to identify not only diabetes mellitus but also conditions affecting the liver and urinary tract
- pancreatitis may present with acute abdominal pain and serum amylase should be checked.

Acute appendicitis

Acute appendicitis is the most common cause of abdominal pain in childhood requiring surgical intervention (Fig. 14.5). Although it may occur at any age, it is very uncommon in children under 3 years of age. The clinical features of acute uncomplicated appendicitis are:

- Symptoms
  - Anorexia
  - Vomiting

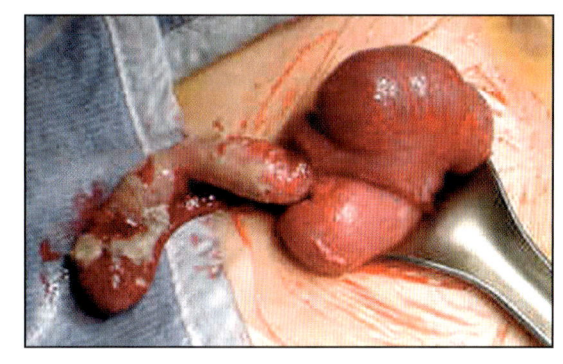

Figure 14.5 Appendicitis at operation showing a perforated acutely inflamed appendix covered in fibrin. (Courtesy of Anthony Lander.)

  - Abdominal pain, initially central and colicky (appendicular midgut colic), but then localizing to the right iliac fossa (from localized peritoneal inflammation)
- Signs
  - Fever
  - Abdominal pain aggravated by movement, e.g. on walking, coughing, jumping, bumps on the road during a car journey
  - Persistent tenderness with guarding in the right iliac fossa (McBurney's point). However, with a retrocaecal appendix, localized guarding may be absent, and in a pelvic appendix there may be few abdominal signs.

In preschool children:
- The diagnosis is more difficult, particularly early in the disease.
- Faecoliths are more common and can be seen on a plain abdominal X-ray.
- Perforation may be rapid, as the omentum is less well developed and fails to surround the appendix, and the signs are easy to underestimate at this age.

Appendicitis is a progressive condition and so repeated observation and clinical review every few hours are key to making the correct diagnosis, avoiding delay on the one hand and unnecessary laparotomy on the other.

No laboratory investigation or imaging is consistently helpful in making the diagnosis. A neutrophilia is not always present on a full blood count. White blood cells or organisms in the urine are not uncommon in appendicitis as the inflamed appendix may be adjacent to the ureter or bladder. Although ultrasound is no substitute for regular clinical review, it may support the clinical diagnosis (thickened, non-compressible appendix with increased blood flow), and demonstrate associated complications such as an abscess, perforation or an appendix mass, and may exclude other pathology causing the symptoms. In some centres, laparoscopy is available to see whether or not the appendix is inflamed.

Appendicectomy is straightforward in uncomplicated appendicitis. Complicated appendicitis includes the presence of an appendix mass, an abscess, or perforation. If there is generalized guarding consistent with perforation, fluid resuscitation and intravenous antibiotics are given prior to laparotomy. If there is a palpable mass in the right iliac fossa and there are no signs of generalized peritonitis, it may be reasonable to elect for conservative management with intravenous antibiotics, with appendicectomy being performed after several weeks. If symptoms progress, laparotomy is indicated.

Non-specific abdominal pain and mesenteric adenitis

Non-specific abdominal pain is abdominal pain which resolves in 24–48 hours. The pain is less severe than in appendicitis, and tenderness in the right iliac fossa is variable. It is often accompanied by an upper respiratory tract infection with cervical lymphadenopathy. In some of these children, the abdominal signs do not resolve and an appendicectomy is performed. Mesenteric adenitis is often diagnosed in those children in whom large mesenteric nodes are seen at laparoscopy and whose appendix is normal, but there are doubts whether this condition truly exists as a diagnostic entity.

Intussusception

Intussusception describes the invagination of proximal bowel into a distal segment. It most commonly involves ileum passing into the caecum through the ileocaecal valve (Fig. 14.6a). Intussusception is the most

> **Summary**
>
> **Acute abdominal pain in older children and adolescents**
> - Exclude medical causes, in particular lower lobe pneumonia, diabetic ketoacidosis, hepatitis, and pyelonephritis.
> - Check for strangulated inguinal hernia or torsion of the testis in boys.
> - On palpating the abdomen in children with acute appendicitis, guarding and rebound tenderness are often absent or unimpressive, but pain from peritoneal inflammation may be demonstrated on coughing, walking or jumping.
> - To distinguish between acute appendicitis and non-specific abdominal pain may require close monitoring, joint management between paediatricians and paediatric surgeons and repeated evaluation in hospital.

common cause of intestinal obstruction in infants after the neonatal period. Although it may occur at any age, the peak age of presentation is 3 months – 2 years of age. The most serious complication is stretching and constriction of the mesentery resulting in venous obstruction, causing engorgement and bleeding from the bowel mucosa, fluid loss, and subsequently bowel perforation, peritonitis and gut necrosis. Prompt diagnosis, immediate fluid resuscitation and urgent reduction of the intussusception are essential to avoid complications.

Presentation is typically with:

- Paroxysmal, severe colicky pain with pallor – during episodes of pain, the child becomes pale, especially around the mouth, and draws up the legs. There is recovery between the painful episodes but subsequently the child may become increasingly lethargic.
- May refuse feeds, may vomit, which may become bile stained depending on the site of the intussusception.
- A sausage-shaped mass – often palpable in the abdomen (Fig. 14.6b).
- Passage of a characteristic redcurrant jelly stool comprising blood-stained mucus – this is a characteristic sign but tends to occur later in the illness and may be first seen after a rectal examination.
- Abdominal distension and shock.

Usually, no underlying intestinal cause for the intussusception is found, although there is some evidence that viral infection leading to enlargement of Peyer's patches may form the lead point of the intussusception. An identifiable lead point such as a Meckel diverticulum or polyp is more likely to be present in children over 2 years of age. Intravenous fluid resuscitation is likely to be required immediately, as there is often pooling of fluid in the gut, which may lead to hypovolaemic shock.

Intussusception

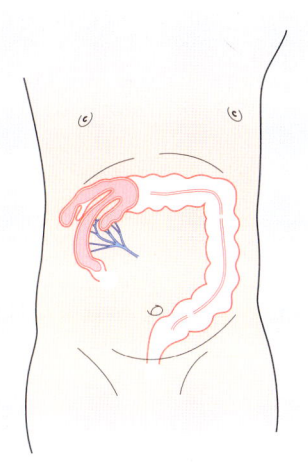

Figure 14.6a Intussusception, showing why the blood supply to the gut rapidly becomes compromised, making relief of this form of obstruction urgent.

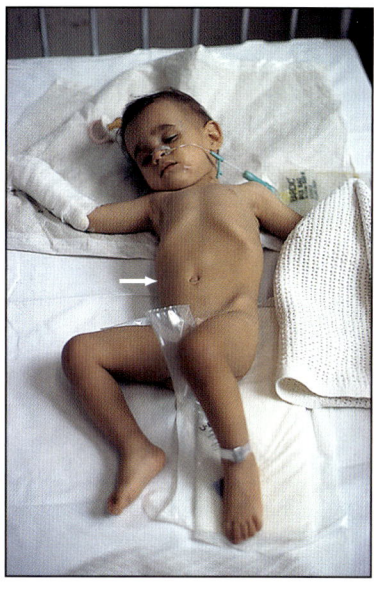

Figure 14.6b A child with an intussusception. The mass can be seen in the upper abdomen. The child has become shocked.

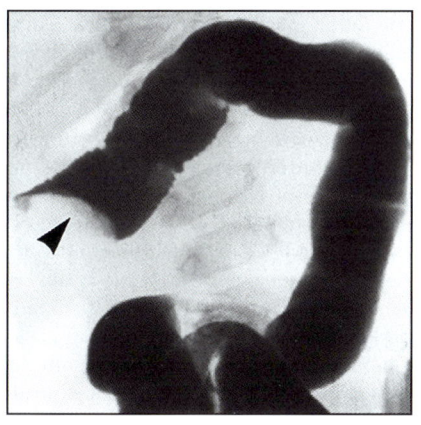

Figure 14.6c An abdominal X-ray demonstrating an intussusception (see arrowhead), with contrast.

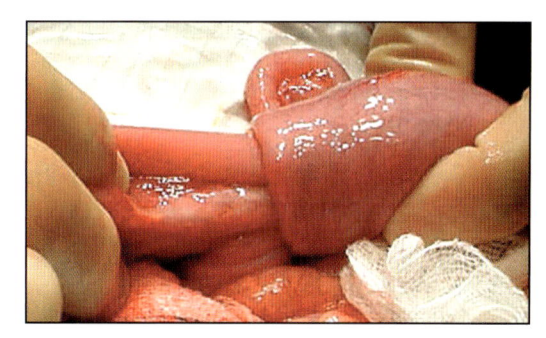

Figure 14.6d Intussusception at operation showing the ileum entering the caecum. The surgeon is squeezing the colon to reduce the intussusception. (Courtesy of Anthony Lander.)

An X-ray of the abdomen may show distended small bowel and absence of gas in the distal colon or rectum. Sometimes the outline of the intussusception itself can be visualized. Abdominal ultrasound is helpful both to confirm the diagnosis (the so-called target/doughnut sign) and to check response to treatment. Unless there are signs of peritonitis, reduction of the intussusception by rectal air insufflation is usually attempted by a radiologist (Fig. 14.6c). This procedure should only be carried out once the child has been resuscitated and is under the supervision of a paediatric surgeon in case the procedure is unsuccessful or bowel perforation occurs. The success rate of this procedure is about 75%. The remaining 25% require operative reduction (Fig. 14.6d). Recurrence of the intussusception occurs in less than 5% but is more frequent after hydrostatic reduction.

Summary

Intussusception
- Usually occurs between 3 months and 2 years of age.
- Clinical features are paroxysmal, colicky pain with pallor, abdominal mass and redcurrant jelly stool.
- Shock is an important complication and requires urgent treatment.
- Reduction is attempted by rectal air insufflation unless peritonitis is present.
- Surgery is required if reduction with air is unsuccessful or for peritonitis.

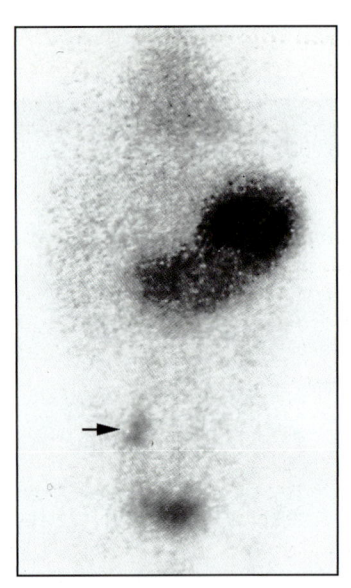

Figure 14.7 Technetium scan showing uptake by ectopic gastric mucosa in a Meckel diverticulum in the right iliac fossa.

Meckel diverticulum

Around 2% of individuals have an ileal remnant of the vitello-intestinal duct, a Meckel diverticulum, which contains ectopic gastric mucosa or pancreatic tissue. Most are asymptomatic but they may present with severe rectal bleeding, which is classically neither bright red nor true melaena. There is usually an acute reduction in haemoglobin. Other forms of presentation include intussusception, volvulus (twisting of the bowel), or diverticulitis, when inflammation of the diverticulum mimics appendicitis. A technetium scan will demonstrate increased uptake by ectopic gastric mucosa in 70% of cases (Fig. 14.7). Treatment is by surgical resection.

> **Summary**
>
> **Meckel diverticulum**
> - Occurs in 2% of individuals.
> - Generally asymptomatic, but may present with bleeding (which may be life-threatening) or intussusception or volvulus.
> - Treatment is by surgical resection.

Malrotation

During rotation of the small bowel in fetal life, if the mesentery is not fixed at the duodenojejunal flexure or in the ileocaecal region, its base is shorter than normal, and is predisposed to volvulus. Ladd bands are peritoneal bands that may cross the duodenum, often anteriorly (Fig. 14.8).

There are two presentations:
- obstruction
- obstruction with a compromised blood supply.

Obstruction with bilious vomiting is the usual presentation in the first few days of life but can be seen at a later age. Any child with dark green vomiting needs an urgent upper gastrointestinal contrast study to assess intestinal rotation, unless signs of vascular compromise are present, when an urgent laparotomy is needed. This is a surgical emergency as, when a volvulus occurs, the superior mesenteric arterial blood supply to the small intestine and proximal large intestine is compromised and unless it is corrected will lead to infarction of these areas.

At operation, the volvulus is untwisted, the duodenum mobilized, and the bowel placed in the non-rotated position with the duodenojejunal flexure on the right and the caecum and appendix on the left. The malrotation is not 'corrected', but the mesentery broadened. The appendix is generally removed to avoid diagnostic confusion should the child subsequently have symptoms suggestive of appendicitis.

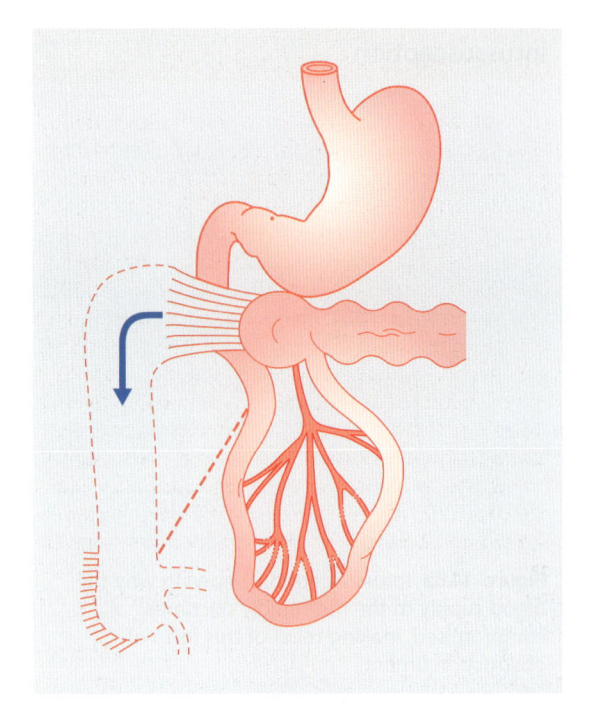

Figure 14.8 The most common form of malrotation, with the caecum remaining high and fixed to the posterior abdominal wall. There are Ladd bands obstructing the duodenum. Dotted lines show normal anatomy.

> **Summary**
>
> **Malrotation**
> - Uncommon but important to diagnose.
> - Usually presents in the first 1–3 days of life with intestinal obstruction from Ladd bands obstructing the duodenum or volvulus.
> - May present at any age with volvulus causing obstruction and ischaemic bowel.
> - Clinical features are bilious vomiting, abdominal pain and tenderness from peritonitis or ischaemic bowel.
> - An urgent upper gastrointestinal contrast study is indicated if there is bilious vomiting.
> - Treatment is urgent surgical correction.

Recurrent abdominal pain

Recurrent abdominal pain is a common childhood problem. It is often defined as pain sufficient to interrupt normal activities and lasts for at least 3 months. It occurs in about 10% of school-age children. An organic cause (see Summary box) is identified in less than 10% of cases. The pain is characteristically periumbilical and the children are otherwise entirely well. Constipation is a frequent cause of recurrent abdominal pain and must be excluded. The widely held belief that they have psychogenic pain is without foundation, with a number of studies having failed to show a difference between such children and their families and controls. In some children, it may however be a manifestation of stress (see Ch. 24) or it may become part of a vicious cycle of anxiety with escalating pain leading to family distress and demands for increasingly invasive investigations. There is evidence that anxiety may lead to altered bowel motility, which may be perceived by the child as pain.

It is increasingly recognized that many will have distinct symptom constellations resulting from functional abnormalities of gut motility – irritable bowel syndrome (most common), constipation, and less commonly coeliac disease, abdominal migraine and functional dyspepsia.

Management

The aim is to identify any serious cause without subjecting the child to unnecessary investigation, while providing reassurance to the child and parents. To do this, a full history and thorough examination is required, which includes inspection of the perineum for anal fissures. The child's growth should be checked.

A urine microscopy and culture is mandatory as urinary tract infections may cause pain in the absence of other symptoms or signs. An abdominal ultrasound is particularly helpful in excluding gall stones and pelvi-ureteric junction obstruction.

Although there are many potential organic causes, most are rare. Coeliac antibodies and thyroid function tests should be checked, but further investigations should be performed only if clinically indicated.

With irritable bowel syndrome and functional dyspepsia, it can be helpful to explain to both the child and parents that 'sometimes the insides of the intestine become so sensitive that some children can feel the food going round the bends'. It is also necessary to make a distinction between 'serious' and 'dangerous'. These disorders can be serious, if, for example, they lead to substantial loss of schooling, but they are not dangerous.

The long-term prognosis is that:

- about half of affected children rapidly become free of symptoms
- in one-quarter, the symptoms take some months to resolve
- in one-quarter, symptoms continue or return in adulthood as migraine, irritable bowel syndrome or functional dyspepsia.

Abdominal migraine

Abdominal migraine is often associated with abdominal pain in addition to headaches, and in some children the abdominal pain predominates. The attacks of abdominal pain are midline associated with vomiting and facial pallor. There is usually a personal or family history of migraine. The history is characteristic with long periods (often weeks) of no symptoms and then a shorter period (12–48 hours) of non-specific abdominal pain and pallor, with or without vomiting. Treatment with anti-migraine medication may be of benefit if the problem causes school absence.

Irritable bowel syndrome

This disorder, also common in adults, is associated with altered gastrointestinal motility and an abnormal sensation of intra-abdominal events. Symptoms may be precipitated by a gastro-intestinal infection. Studies of pressure changes within the small intestine of children with irritable bowel syndrome suggest that abnormally forceful contractions occur. It has also been shown that affected adults experience pain on inflation of balloons in the intestine at substantially lower volumes than do controls. There is therefore an inter-play between these two factors, both of which are modulated by psychosocial factors such as stress and anxiety.

There is often a positive family history and a characteristic set of symptoms, although not all patients experience every symptom:

- non-specific abdominal pain, often peri-umbilical, may be worse before or relieved by defaecation
- explosive, loose, or mucousy stools
- bloating
- feeling of incomplete defecation
- constipation (often alternating with normal or loose stools).

Some children and adults with irritable bowel symptoms have coeliac disease, which is why coeliac antibody serology must be checked.

Peptic ulceration, gastritis, and functional dyspepsia

The greater use of endoscopy in children and the identification of the Gram-negative organism *Helicobacter pylori* in association with antral gastritis have focused attention on it as a potential cause of abdominal pain in children. In adults and probably in children, there is substantial evidence that *H. pylori* is a strong predisposing factor to duodenal ulcers. Duodenal ulcers are uncommon in children but should be considered in those with epigastric pain, particularly if it wakes them at night, if the pain radiates through to the back, or when there is a history of peptic ulceration in a first-degree relative.

H. pylori causes a nodular antral gastritis, which may be associated with abdominal pain and nausea. It is usually identified in gastric antral biopsies. The organism produces urease, which forms the basis for a laboratory test on biopsies and the ^{13}C breath test

> **Summary**
>
> **Causes and assessment of the child with recurrent abdominal pain**
>
> **>90% no structural cause identified**
>
> **Gastrointestinal**
> - Irritable bowel syndrome
> - Constipation
> - Non-ulcer dyspepsia
> - Abdominal migraine
> - Gastritis and peptic ulceration
> - Eosinophilic oesophagitis
> - Inflammatory bowel disease
> - Malrotation
>
> **Gynaecological**
> - Dysmenorrhoea
> - Ovarian cysts
> - Pelvic inflammatory disease
>
> **Psychosocial** – bullying, abuse, stress, etc. – a small proportion
>
> **Hepatobiliary/pancreatic**
> - Hepatitis
> - Gall stones
> - Pancreatitis
>
> **Urinary tract**
> - Urinary tract infection
> - Pelvi-ureteric junction (PUJ) obstruction
>
> **Symptoms and signs that suggest organic disease:**
> - Epigastric pain at night, haematemesis (duodenal ulcer)
> - Diarrhoea, weight loss, growth failure, blood in stools (inflammatory bowel disease)
> - Vomiting (pancreatitis)
> - Jaundice (liver disease)
> - Dysuria, secondary enuresis (urinary tract infection)
> - Bilious vomiting and abdominal distension (malrotation)

following the administration of ^{13}C-labelled urea by mouth. Stool antigen for *H. pylori* may be positive in infected children. Serological tests are less reliable in young children but may be helpful in older children.

Children in whom peptic ulceration is suspected should be treated with proton-pump inhibitors, e.g. omeprazole, and if investigations suggest they have an *H. pylori* infection, eradication therapy should be given (amoxicillin and metronidazole or clarithromycin). Those who fail to respond to treatment or whose symptoms recur on stopping treatment should have an upper gastrointestinal endoscopy and, if this is normal, functional dyspepsia is diagnosed. Functional dyspepsia is probably a variant of irritable bowel syndrome.

As well as having symptoms of peptic ulceration, children with functional dyspepsia have rather more non-specific symptoms, including early satiety, bloating, and postprandial vomiting and may have delayed gastric emptying as a result of gastric dysmotility. Treatment is difficult but some children respond to a hypoallergenic diet.

Eosinophilic oesophagitis

Eosinophilic oesophagitis is an inflammatory condition affecting the oesophagus caused by activation of eosinophils within the mucosa and submucosa. It can present with vomiting, discomfort on swallowing or bolus dysphagia, when food "sticks in the upper chest". It is probably an allergic phenomenon although the precise pathophysiology is unclear. It is more common in children with other features of atopy (asthma, eczema, and hay fever). Diagnosis is by endoscopy where macroscopically, linear furrows and tracheaization of the oesophagus may be seen, and microscopically, eosinophilic infiltration is identified. Treatment is with swallowed corticosteroids in the form of fluticasone or viscous budesonide. Exclusion diets may be of benefit in young children.

Gastroenteritis

In developing countries, gastroenteritis remains a major cause of child mortality. In developed countries, it is a cause of significant morbidity, particularly in younger children. In the UK, approximately 10% of children under 5 years of age annually present to health services with gastroenteritis and it remains a common reason for hospital admission in young children.

The most frequent cause of gastroenteritis in developed countries is rotavirus infection, which accounts for up to 60% of cases in children under 2 years of age, particularly during the winter and early spring. An

Box 14.3 Conditions that can mimic gastroenteritis

Systemic infection	Septicaemia, meningitis
Local infections	Respiratory tract infection, otitis media, hepatitis A, urinary tract infection
Surgical disorders	Pyloric stenosis, intussusception, acute appendicitis, necrotizing enterocolitis, Hirschsprung disease
Metabolic disorder	Diabetic ketoacidosis
Renal disorder	Haemolytic uraemic syndrome
Other	Coeliac disease, cow's milk protein allergy, lactose intolerance, adrenal insufficiency

effective vaccine against rotavirus is available; it has not been adopted into the national immunization programme in the UK but is given in many other countries. Other viruses, particularly adenovirus, norovirus, calicivirus, coronavirus and astrovirus may cause outbreaks.

Bacterial causes are less common in developed countries but may be suggested by the presence of blood in the stools. *Campylobacter jejuni* infection, the most common of the bacterial infections in developed countries, is often associated with severe abdominal pain. *Shigella* and some salmonellae produce a dysenteric type of infection, with blood and pus in the stool, pain and tenesmus. *Shigella* infection may be accompanied by high fever. Cholera and enterotoxigenic *Escherichia coli* infection are associated with profuse, rapidly dehydrating diarrhoea. However, clinical features act as a poor guide to the pathogen.

The third cause of gastroenteritis is protozoan parasite infection such as *Giardia* and *Cryptosporidium*.

In gastroenteritis there is a sudden change to loose or watery stools often accompanied by vomiting. There may be contact with a person with diarrhoea and/or vomiting or recent travel abroad. A number of disorders may masquerade as gastroenteritis (Box 14.3) and, when in doubt, hospital referral is essential. Dehydration leading to shock is the most serious complication and its prevention or correction is the main aim of treatment.

The following children are at increased risk of dehydration:

- infants, particularly those under 6 months of age or those born with low birthweight
- if they have passed six or more diarrhoeal stools in the previous 24 hours
- if they have vomited three or more times in the previous 24 hours
- if they have been unable to tolerate (or not been offered) extra fluids
- if they have malnutrition.

Infants are at particular risk of dehydration because they have a greater surface area-to-weight ratio than older children, leading to greater insensible water losses (300 ml/m^2 per day, equivalent in infants to 15–17 ml/kg per day). They also have higher basal fluid requirements (100–120 ml/kg per day, i.e. 10% to 12% of bodyweight) and immature renal tubular reabsorption. In addition, they are unable to obtain fluids for themselves when thirsty.

Assessment

Clinical assessment of dehydration is important but difficult. The most accurate measure of dehydration is the degree of weight loss during the diarrhoeal illness. A recent weight measurement is useful but is often not available and may be misleading if the child had clothes on or the different measuring scales are not accurate. The history and examination are used to assess the degree of dehydration as:

- no clinically detectable dehydration (usually <5% loss of body weight)
- clinical dehydration (usually 5% to 10% loss of body weight)
- shock (usually >10% loss of body weight; Fig. 14.9 and Table 14.1). Shock must be identified without delay.

Isonatraemic and hyponatraemic dehydration

In dehydration, there is a total body deficit of sodium and water. In most instances, the losses of sodium and water are proportional and plasma sodium remains within the normal range (isonatraemic dehydration). When children with diarrhoea drink large quantities of water or other hypotonic solutions, there is a greater net loss of sodium than water, leading to a fall in plasma sodium (hyponatraemic dehydration). This leads to a shift of water from extracellular to intracellular compartments. The increase in intracellular volume leads to an increase in brain volume, which may result in seizures, whereas the marked extracellular depletion leads to a greater degree of shock per unit of water loss. This form of dehydration is more common in poorly nourished infants in developing countries.

Hypernatraemic dehydration

Infrequently, water loss exceeds the relative sodium loss and plasma sodium concentration increases (hypernatraemic dehydration). This usually results from high insensible water losses (high fever or hot, dry environment) or from profuse, low-sodium diarrhoea. The extracellular fluid becomes hypertonic with respect to the intracellular fluid, which leads to a shift of water into the extracellular space from the intracellular compartment. Signs of extracellular fluid depletion are therefore less per unit of fluid loss, and depression of the fontanelle, reduced tissue elasticity, and sunken eyes are less obvious. This makes this form of dehydration more difficult to recognize clinically, particularly in an obese infant. It is a particularly dangerous form of dehydration as water is drawn out of the brain and cerebral shrinkage within a

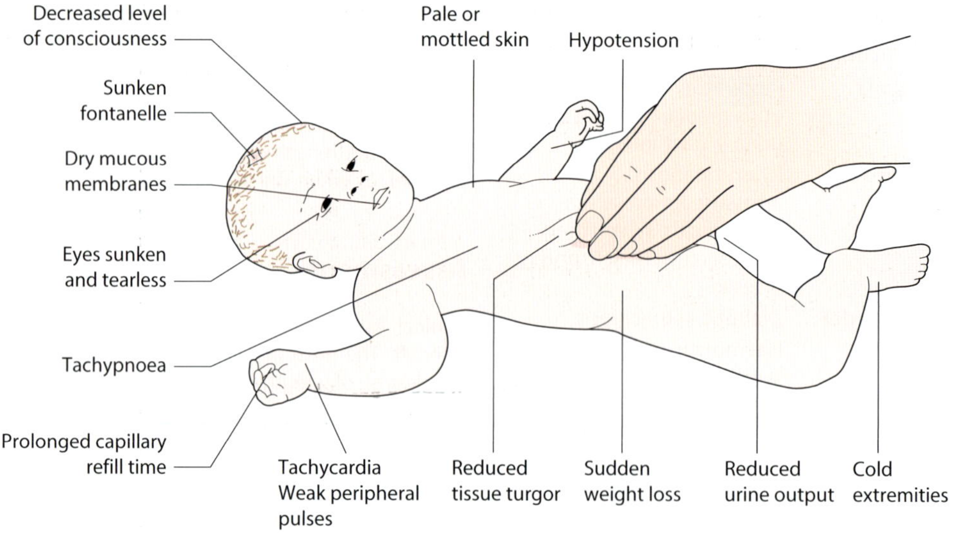

Figure 14.9 Clinical features of shock from dehydration in an infant.

Labels: Decreased level of consciousness; Sunken fontanelle; Dry mucous membranes; Eyes sunken and tearless; Tachypnoea; Prolonged capillary refill time; Tachycardia, Weak peripheral pulses; Reduced tissue turgor; Sudden weight loss; Reduced urine output; Cold extremities; Pale or mottled skin; Hypotension.

Table 14.1 Clinical assessment of dehydration

	No clinical dehydration	**Clinical dehydration**	**Shock**
General appearance	Appears well	Appears unwell or deteriorating 🚩	Appears unwell or deteriorating
Conscious level	Alert and responsive	Altered responsiveness, e.g. irritable, lethargic 🚩	Decreased level of consciousness
Urine output	Normal	Decreased	Decreased
Skin colour	Normal	Normal	Pale or mottled
Extremities	Warm	Warm	Cold
Eyes	Normal	Sunken 🚩	Grossly sunken
Mucous membranes	Moist	Dry	Dry
Heart rate	Normal	Tachycardia 🚩	Tachycardia
Breathing	Normal	Tachypnoea 🚩	Tachypnoea
Peripheral pulses	Normal	Normal	Weak
Capillary refill time	Normal	Normal	Prolonged (>2 s)
Skin turgor	Normal	Reduced 🚩	Reduced
Blood pressure	Normal	Normal	Hypotension (indicates decompensated)

The more numerous and more pronounced the symptoms and signs, the greater the severity of dehydration.
(Adapted from National Institute for Health and Clinical Excellence (NICE): *Guideline. Diarrhoea and Vomiting in Children under 5*, London, 2009, NICE.)
🚩 'Red flag' sign – helps to identify children at risk of progression to shock.

rigid skull may lead to jittery movements, increased muscle tone with hyperreflexia, altered consciousness, seizures, and multiple, small cerebral haemorrhages. Transient hyperglycaemia occurs in some patients with hypernatraemic dehydration; it is self-correcting and does not require insulin.

Investigation

Usually, no investigations are indicated. Stool culture is required if the child appears septic, if there is blood or mucus in the stools, or the child is immunocompromised. It may be indicated following recent foreign travel, if the diarrhoea has not improved by day 7, or if the diagnosis is uncertain. Plasma electrolytes, urea, creatinine, and glucose should be checked if intravenous fluids are required or there are features suggestive of hypernatraemia. If antibiotics are started, a blood culture should be taken.

Management

This is shown in Fig. 14.10. Where clinical dehydration is not present, the aim is its prevention. If there is clinical dehydration, oral rehydration solution is the mainstay of therapy (see Case History 14.2); it may also be used as an adjunct in its prevention. Intravenous fluids are only indicated for shock or deterioration or persistent vomiting.

Hypernatraemic dehydration

The management of hypernatraemic dehydration can be particularly difficult. Oral rehydration solution should be used to rehydrate hypernatraemic children with clinical dehydration. If intravenous fluids are required,

Fluid management of dehydration due to gastroenteritis

No clinical dehydration
↓
Prevent dehydration
- Continue breastfeeding and other milk feeds
- Encourage fluid intake to compensate for increased gastrointestinal losses
- Discourage fruit juices and carbonated drinks
- Oral rehydration solution (ORS) as supplemental fluid if at increased risk of dehydration

Clinical dehydration
↓
Oral rehydration solution
- Give fluid deficit replacement (50 ml/kg) over 4 hours as well as maintenance fluid requirement. Give ORS often and in small amounts
- Continue breastfeeding
- Consider supplementing ORS with usual fluids if inadequate intake of ORS
- If inadequate fluid intake or vomits persistently, consider giving ORS via nasogastric tube

↓ Deterioration or persistent vomiting

Shock
↓
Intravenous therapy
Give bolus of 0.9% sodium chloride solution. Repeat if necessary. If remains shocked, consider consulting paediatric intensive care specialist

↓ Symptoms/signs of shock improve

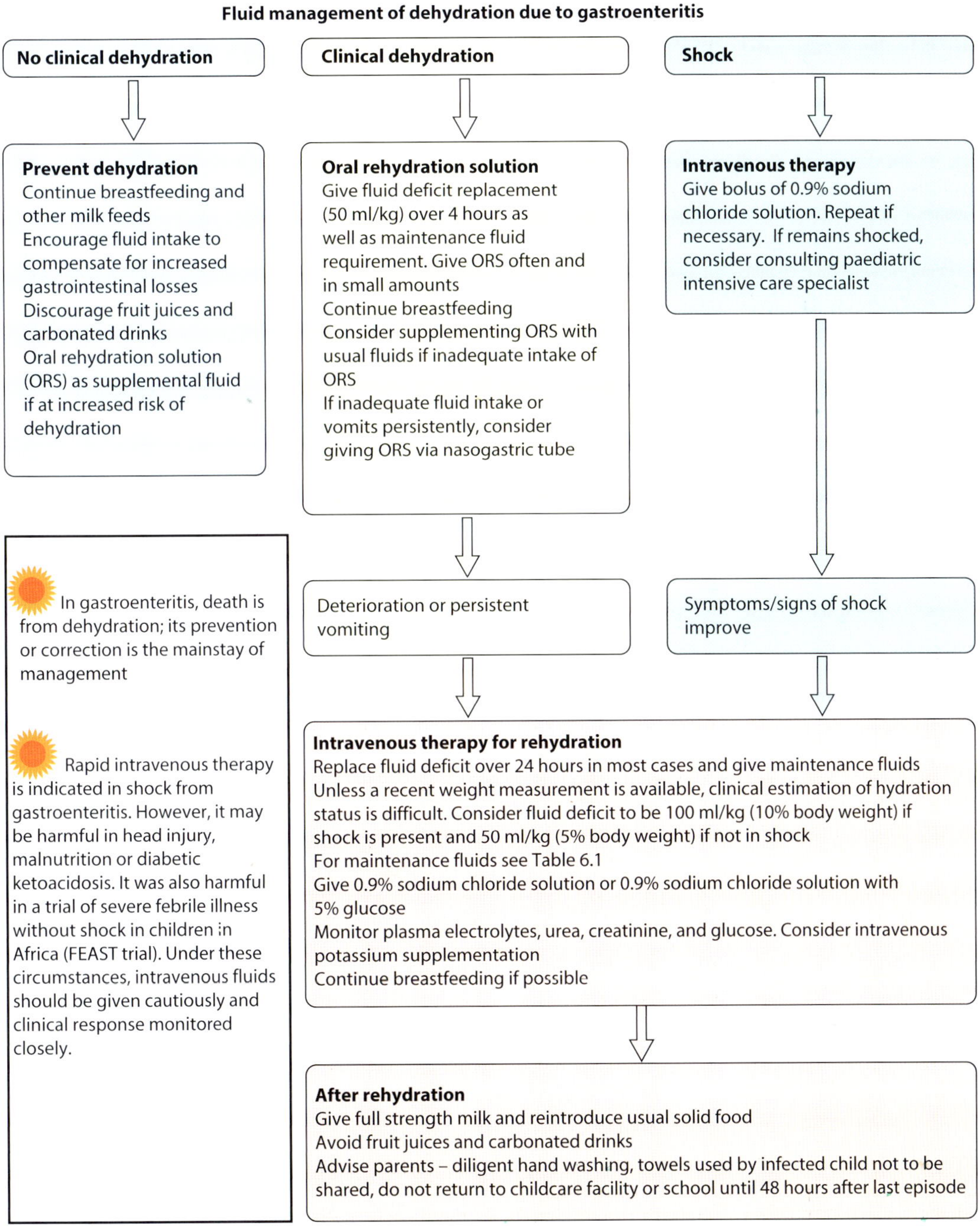

☀ In gastroenteritis, death is from dehydration; its prevention or correction is the mainstay of management

☀ Rapid intravenous therapy is indicated in shock from gastroenteritis. However, it may be harmful in head injury, malnutrition or diabetic ketoacidosis. It was also harmful in a trial of severe febrile illness without shock in children in Africa (FEAST trial). Under these circumstances, intravenous fluids should be given cautiously and clinical response monitored closely.

Intravenous therapy for rehydration
- Replace fluid deficit over 24 hours in most cases and give maintenance fluids
- Unless a recent weight measurement is available, clinical estimation of hydration status is difficult. Consider fluid deficit to be 100 ml/kg (10% body weight) if shock is present and 50 ml/kg (5% body weight) if not in shock
- For maintenance fluids see Table 6.1
- Give 0.9% sodium chloride solution or 0.9% sodium chloride solution with 5% glucose
- Monitor plasma electrolytes, urea, creatinine, and glucose. Consider intravenous potassium supplementation
- Continue breastfeeding if possible

After rehydration
- Give full strength milk and reintroduce usual solid food
- Avoid fruit juices and carbonated drinks
- Advise parents – diligent hand washing, towels used by infected child not to be shared, do not return to childcare facility or school until 48 hours after last episode

Figure 14.10 Management of dehydration. (Adapted from National Institute for Health and Clinical Excellence (NICE): *Guideline. Diarrhoea and Vomiting in Children under 5*, London, 2009, NICE.)

Case history 14.2

Gastroenteritis

Darpana is 14 months old and has had a mild fever, a runny nose, and is not interested in playing. She has been drinking only small volumes of milk, vomited four times over the last 2 days but now has increasing loose stools, with 9 or 10 watery nappies changed over the last 24 hours. On examination, she has a temperature of 37.8°C, is irritable, and has clinical dehydration. Oral rehydration solution is prescribed and her diarrhoea and vomiting settle over the next day. Why does the diarrhoea resolve with oral rehydration solution?

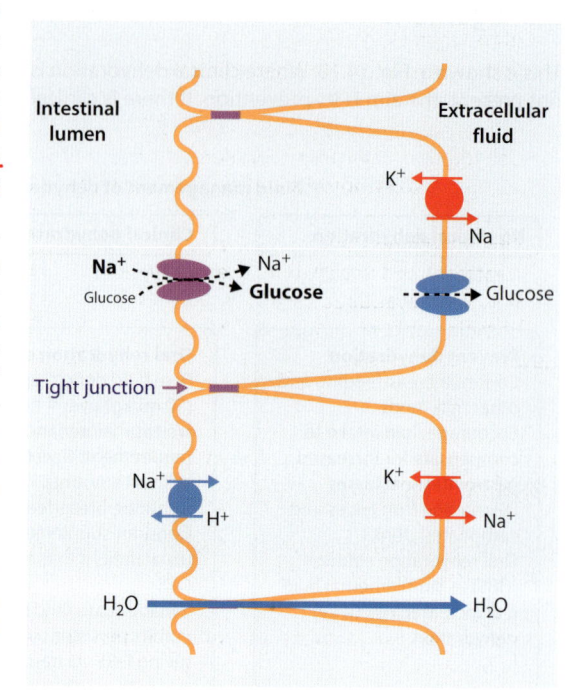

The mechanism of action of oral rehydration solution is shown in Fig. 14.11. Large quantities of sodium are excreted into the intestine, but nearly all is reabsorbed. The primary mechanism of sodium absorption is by a glucose–sodium transporter, with the active absorption of sodium allied to the absorption of glucose. The sodium is then actively pumped from epithelial cells into the circulation via sodium/potassium adenosine triphosphatase, creating an electrochemical gradient that water moves down. A second mechanism is via an active, linked sodium–hydrogen exchanger.

If an oral solution contains both sodium and glucose, sodium and passive water absorption is increased. This works effectively even in the presence of inflammation of the gut, and is therefore effective in diarrhoeal illness. The oral rehydration solution does not 'stop' the diarrhoea, which often continues, but the absorption of water and solutes exceeds secretion and keeps the child hydrated until the infective organism is eradicated. Coca-Cola and apple juice have a much lower sodium content and higher osmolarity than oral rehydration solution and are unsuitable as oral rehydration solutions.

Figure 14.11 Mechanism of action of oral rehydration solution.

---

a rapid reduction in plasma sodium concentration and osmolality will lead to a shift of water into cerebral cells and may result in seizures and cerebral oedema. The reduction in plasma sodium should therefore be slow. The fluid deficit should be replaced over at least 48 hours (with 0.9% or 0.45% saline) and the plasma sodium measured regularly, aiming to reduce it at less than 0.5 mmol/l per hour.

Antidiarrhoeal drugs (e.g. loperamide, Lomotil) and antiemetics

There is no place for medications for the vomiting or diarrhoea of gastroenteritis in children as they:
- are ineffective
- may prolong the excretion of bacteria in stools
- can be associated with side-effects
- add unnecessarily to cost
- focus attention away from oral rehydration.

Antibiotics

Antibiotics are not routinely required to treat gastroenteritis, even if there is a bacterial cause. They are only indicated for suspected or confirmed sepsis, extraintestinal spread of bacterial infection, for salmonella gastroenteritis if aged under 6 months, in malnourished or immunocompromised children, or for specific bacterial or protozoal infections (e.g. *Clostridium difficile* associated with pseudomembranous colitis, cholera, shigellosis, giardiasis).

Nutrition

In developing countries, multiple episodes of diarrhoea are a major contributing factor to the development of malnutrition. Following diarrhoea, nutritional intake should be increased. Diarrhoea may be associated with zinc deficiency and supplementation may be helpful in both acute diarrhoea and as prophylaxis.

> **In gastroenteritis, death is from dehydration; its prevention or correction is the mainstay of treatment**

Postgastroenteritis syndrome

Infrequently, following an episode of gastroenteritis, the introduction of a normal diet results in a return of watery diarrhoea. In such cases, oral rehydration therapy should be restarted.

> **Summary**
>
> **Gastroenteritis**
> - Results in death from dehydration of hundreds of thousands of children worldwide every year.
> - Is mostly viral, but it can be caused by *Campylobacter*, *Shigella*, and *Salmonella* and other organisms.
> - Infants are particularly susceptible to dehydration.
> - Dehydration is assessed as no clinical dehydration, clinical dehydration or shock according to symptoms and signs, but clinical assessment of severity is problematic.
> - Oral rehydration solution is the mainstay of treatment and usually effective; intravenous fluid is only required for shock or ongoing vomiting or clinical deterioration.

Malabsorption

Disorders affecting the digestion or absorption of nutrients manifest as:

- abnormal stools
- poor weight gain or faltering growth in most but not all cases
- specific nutrient deficiencies, either singly or in combination.

In general, parents know when their children's stools have become abnormal. The true malabsorption stool is difficult to flush down the toilet and has an odour that pervades the whole house. In general, colour is a poor guide to abnormality. Reliable dietetic assessment is important. It is inappropriate to investigate children for malabsorption as a cause of their faltering growth when dietary energy intake is demonstrably low and other symptoms are absent. Some disorders affecting the small intestinal mucosa or pancreas (chronic pancreatic insufficiency) may lead to the malabsorption of many nutrients (pan-malabsorption), whereas others are highly specific, e.g. zinc malabsorption in *acrodermatitis enteropathica*.

Coeliac disease

Coeliac disease is an enteropathy in which the gliadin fraction of gluten and other related prolamines in wheat, barley, and rye provoke a damaging immunological response in the proximal small intestinal mucosa. As a result, the rate of migration of absorptive cells moving up the villi (enterocytes) from the crypts is massively increased but is insufficient to compensate for increased cell loss from the villous tips. Villi become progressively shorter and then absent, leaving a flat mucosa. It is a relatively common disorder occurring in 1% of the population.

The incidence of 'classical' coeliac disease, diagnosed in childhood on the basis of characteristic clinical symptoms, has been about 1 in 3000 in Europe, including the UK. The age at presentation is partly influenced by the age of introduction of gluten into the diet.

The classical presentation is of a profound malabsorptive syndrome at 8–24 months of age after the introduction of wheat-containing weaning foods. There is faltering growth, abdominal distension and buttock wasting, abnormal stools, and general irritability (see Case History 14.3). However, this 'classical' form is no longer the most common presentation and children are now more likely to present less acutely in later childhood. The clinical features of coeliac disease can be highly variable and include mild, non-specific gastrointestinal symptoms, anaemia (iron and/or folate deficiency) and growth faltering. Alternatively, it is identified on screening of children at increased risk (type 1 diabetes mellitus, autoimmune thyroid disease, Down syndrome) and first-degree relatives of individuals with known coeliac disease.

The introduction of highly sensitive and specific serological screening tests, anti-tTG (immunoglobulin A tissue transglutaminase antibodies) and EMA (endomysial antibodies)) has provided evidence that coeliac disease is much more common than previously thought and as many as 1 in 100 UK school-age children may be antibody positive, but a large proportion of these children will be asymptomatic.

Diagnosis

Although the diagnosis is strongly suggested by positive serology, confirmation depends upon the demonstration of mucosal changes (increased intraepithelial lymphocytes and a variable degree of villous atrophy and crypt hypertrophy) on small intestinal biopsy performed endoscopically followed by the resolution of symptoms and catch-up growth upon gluten withdrawal.

Although there is no place for the empirical use of a gluten-free diet as a diagnostic test for coeliac disease, strongly positive serological tests such as anti-tTG and EMA in symptomatic individuals may make the need for biopsy confirmation unnecessary in a small proportion of children following assessment by a paediatric gastroenterologist.

Management

All products containing wheat, rye, and barley are removed from the diet and this results in resolution of symptoms. Supervision by a dietician is essential. In children in whom the initial biopsy or the response to gluten withdrawal is doubtful, a gluten challenge may be required in later childhood to demonstrate continuing susceptibility of the small intestinal mucosa to damage by gluten. The gluten-free diet should be adhered to for life. Non-adherence to the diet risks the development of micronutrient deficiency, especially osteopenia, and there is a small but definite increased risk in bowel malignancy, especially small bowel lymphoma.

Case history 14.3

'Classical' coeliac disease

This 2-year-old boy (Fig. 14.12a) had a history of poor growth from 12 months of age (Fig. 14.12b). His parents had noticed that he tended to be irritable and grumpy and had three or four foul-smelling stools a day. A duodenal biopsy at 2 years of age showed subtotal villous atrophy (Fig. 14.12c, d) and he was started on a gluten-free diet. Within a few days, his parents commented that his mood had improved and within a month he was a 'different child'. He subsequently exhibited good catch-up growth.

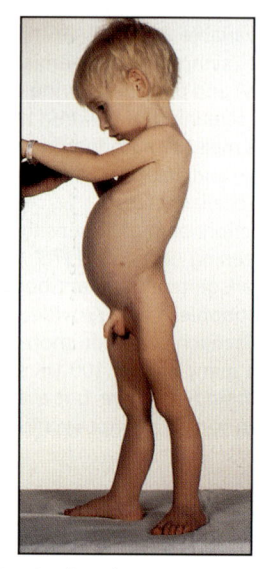

Figure 14.12a Coeliac disease causing wasting of the buttocks and distended abdomen.

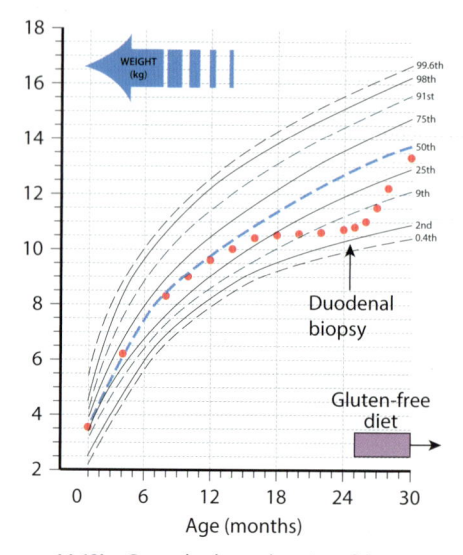

Figure 14.12b Growth chart showing faltering growth and response to a gluten-free diet. (Adapted from Growth Chart © 2012/13 Royal College of Paediatrics and Child Health.)

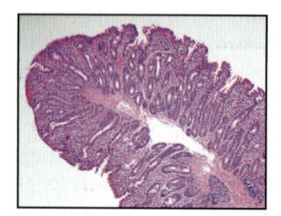

Figure 14.12c Histology of a duodenal biopsy showing lymphocytic infiltration and villous atrophy confirming coeliac disease. (Courtesy of Marie-Anne Brundler.)

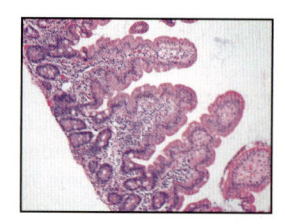

Figure 14.12d Normal duodenal histology is shown for comparison. (Courtesy of Marie-Anne Brundler.)

Summary

Coeliac disease

- A gluten-sensitive enteropathy.
- Classical presentation is at 8–24 months of age with abnormal stools, faltering growth, abdominal distension, muscle wasting, and irritability (now rare).
- Other, more subtle, modes of presentation – e.g. short stature, anaemia, abdominal pain and screening, e.g. children with diabetes mellitus, are now much more common.
- Diagnosis – positive serology (immunoglobulin A tissue transglutaminase and endomysial antibodies), flat mucosa on duodenal biopsy (usually but not always performed), and resolution of symptoms and catch-up growth upon gluten withdrawal.
- Treatment – gluten-free diet for life.

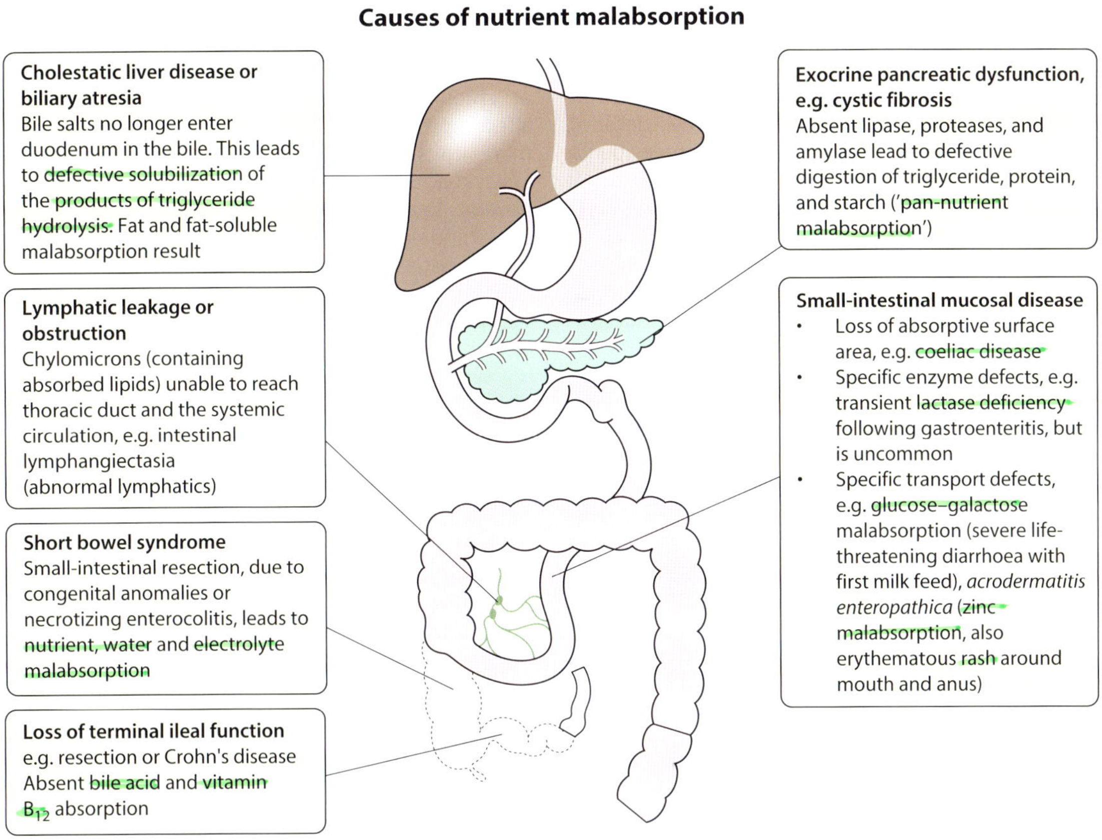

Causes of nutrient malabsorption

Cholestatic liver disease or biliary atresia
Bile salts no longer enter duodenum in the bile. This leads to defective solubilization of the products of triglyceride hydrolysis. Fat and fat-soluble malabsorption result

Lymphatic leakage or obstruction
Chylomicrons (containing absorbed lipids) unable to reach thoracic duct and the systemic circulation, e.g. intestinal lymphangiectasia (abnormal lymphatics)

Short bowel syndrome
Small-intestinal resection, due to congenital anomalies or necrotizing enterocolitis, leads to nutrient, water and electrolyte malabsorption

Loss of terminal ileal function
e.g. resection or Crohn's disease
Absent bile acid and vitamin B$_{12}$ absorption

Exocrine pancreatic dysfunction, e.g. cystic fibrosis
Absent lipase, proteases, and amylase lead to defective digestion of triglyceride, protein, and starch ('pan-nutrient malabsorption')

Small-intestinal mucosal disease
- Loss of absorptive surface area, e.g. coeliac disease
- Specific enzyme defects, e.g. transient lactase deficiency following gastroenteritis, but is uncommon
- Specific transport defects, e.g. glucose–galactose malabsorption (severe life-threatening diarrhoea with first milk feed), *acrodermatitis enteropathica* (zinc malabsorption, also erythematous rash around mouth and anus)

Figure 14.13 Causes of nutrient malabsorption. They are uncommon.

Food allergy and intolerance

This is described in Chapter 16 (Allergy).

Other causes of nutrient malabsorption

These are summarized in Fig. 14.13.

Short bowel syndrome usually occurs when an infant or child has had a large surgical resection. This may be due to congenital atresia, necrotizing enterocolitis, malrotation with volvulus, or a traumatic event such as a road traffic accident. Depending on the length and type of residual bowel (ileum or jejunum) and presence of ileocaecal valve, these children may develop malabsorption diarrhoea and malnutrition. If severe, they may require supplemental parenteral nutrition for their intestinal failure. They are at risk from nutritional deficiencies, intestinal failure-associated liver disease, and central line-associated bloodstream infections, and need to be managed by specialist multidisciplinary teams.

Chronic non-specific diarrhoea

This condition, previously known as toddler diarrhoea, is the most common cause of persistent loose stools in preschool children. Characteristically, the stools are of varying consistency, sometimes well formed, sometimes explosive and loose. The presence of undigested vegetables in the stools is common. Affected children are well and thriving. In a proportion of children the diarrhoea may result from undiagnosed coeliac disease or excessive ingestion of fruit juice, especially apple juice. Occasionally the cause is temporary cow's milk allergy following gastroenteritis, when a trial of a cow's milk protein free diet may be helpful. Once possible underlying causes have been excluded, in the majority of cases the loose stools probably result from dysmotility of the gut (a form of irritable bowel syndrome) and fast-transit diarrhoea; it almost always improves with age.

Summary

Chronic diarrhoea
- In an infant with faltering growth, consider coeliac disease and cow's milk protein allergy.
- Following bowel resection, cholestatic liver disease or exocrine pancreatic dysfunction, consider malabsorption.
- In an otherwise well toddler with undigested vegetables in the stool, consider chronic non-specific diarrhoea.

Inflammatory bowel disease

The incidence of inflammatory bowel disease in children has increased markedly in the last two decades. The reason for this is unclear, but recent evidence suggests a complex interplay between genetics, gut microbiome and mucosal immunity is responsible. A number of genes have been identified that give an increased risk, but this is often in association with increased risks of other autoimmune diseases that do not always coexist with inflammatory bowel disease. Approximately a quarter of patients present in childhood or adolescence, and in contrast with the adult population, Crohn's disease is more common than ulcerative colitis. Crohn's disease can affect any part of the gastrointestinal tract from mouth to anus, whereas in ulcerative colitis the inflammation is confined to the colon. Inflammatory bowel disease may cause poor general health, restrict growth, and have an adverse effect on psychological well-being. Management requires a specialist multidisciplinary team.

Crohn's disease

The clinical features of Crohn's disease are summarized in Fig. 14.14. Lethargy and general ill health without gastrointestinal symptoms can be the presenting features, particularly in older children. There may be considerable delay in diagnosis as it may be mistaken for psychological problems. It may also mimic anorexia nervosa. The presence of raised inflammatory markers (platelet count, erythrocyte sedimentation rate, and C-reactive protein), iron-deficiency anaemia, and low serum albumin are helpful in both making a diagnosis and confirming a relapse.

Crohn's disease is a transmural, focal, subacute, or chronic inflammatory disease, most commonly affecting the distal ileum and proximal colon. Initially, there are areas of acutely inflamed, thickened bowel. Subsequently, strictures of the bowel and fistulae may develop between adjacent loops of bowel, between bowel and skin or to other organs (e.g. vagina, bladder).

Diagnosis is based on endoscopic and histological findings on biopsy. Upper gastrointestinal endoscopy, ileocolonoscopy and small bowel imaging are required. The histological hallmark is the presence of non-caseating epithelioid cell granulomata, although this is not identified in up to 30% at presentation. Small bowel imaging may reveal narrowing, fissuring, mucosal irregularities and bowel wall thickening.

Remission is induced with nutritional therapy, when the normal diet is replaced by whole protein modular feeds (polymeric diet) for 6–8 weeks. This is effective in 75% of cases. Systemic steroids are required if ineffective.

Relapse is common and immunosuppressant medication (azathioprine, mercaptopurine or methotrexate) is almost always required to maintain remission. Anti-tumour necrosis factor agents (infliximab or adalimumab) may be needed when conventional treatments have failed. Long-term supplemental enteral nutrition (often with overnight nasogastric or gastrostomy feeds) may be helpful in correcting growth failure. Surgery is necessary for complications of Crohn's disease – obstruction, fistulae, abscess formation or severe localized disease unresponsive to medical treatment, often manifesting as growth failure. In general, the long-term prognosis for Crohn's disease beginning

Presentation of Crohn's disease in children and adolescents

Growth failure
Puberty delayed

Classical presentation (25%):
- abdominal pain
- diarrhoea
- weight loss

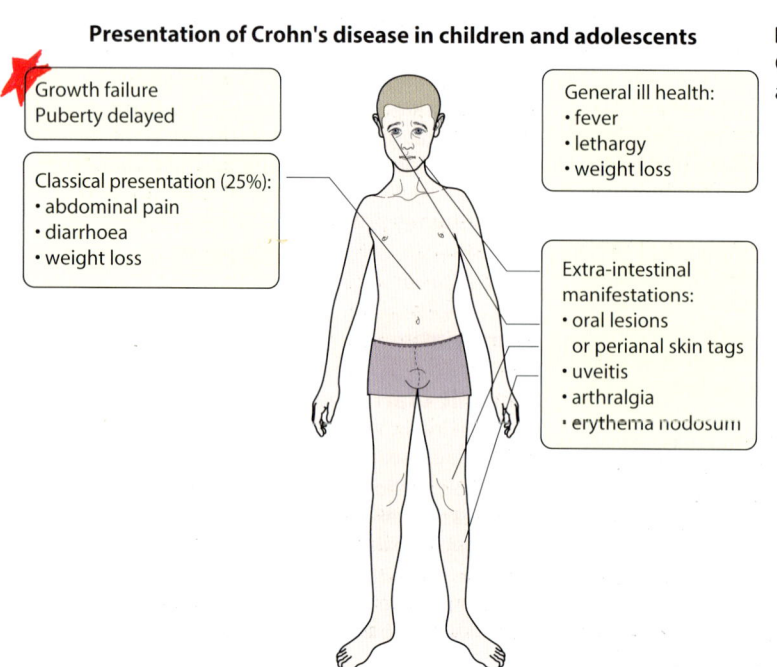

General ill health:
- fever
- lethargy
- weight loss

Extra-intestinal manifestations:
- oral lesions or perianal skin tags
- uveitis
- arthralgia
- erythema nodosum

Figure 14.14 Presentation of Crohn's disease in children and adolescents.

in childhood is good and most patients lead normal lives, despite occasional relapsing disease.

☀ **Growth failure and delayed puberty are features of Crohn's disease in children**

Ulcerative colitis

Ulcerative colitis is a recurrent, inflammatory and ulcerating disease involving the mucosa of the colon. Characteristically, the disease presents with rectal bleeding, diarrhoea and colicky pain. Weight loss and growth failure may occur, although this is less frequent than in Crohn's disease. Extra-intestinal complications include erythema nodosum and arthritis.

The diagnosis is made on endoscopy (upper and ileocolonoscopy) and on the histological features, after exclusion of infective causes of colitis. There is a confluent colitis extending from the rectum proximally for a variable length. In contrast to adults, in whom the colitis is usually confined to the distal colon, 90% of children have pancolitis. Histology reveals mucosal inflammation, crypt damage (cryptitis, architectural distortion, abscesses and crypt loss), and ulceration. Small bowel imaging is required to check that extra-colonic inflammation suggestive of Crohn's disease is not present.

In mild disease, aminosalicylates (e.g. mesalazine) are used for induction and maintenance therapy. Disease confined to the rectum and sigmoid colon (rare in children) may be managed with topical steroids. More aggressive or extensive disease requires systemic steroids for acute exacerbations and immunomodulatory therapy, e.g. azathioprine alone to maintain remission or in combination with low-dose corticosteroid therapy. There is a role for biological therapies such as infliximab or ciclosporin in patients with resistant disease, but if ineffective, surgery should not be delayed.

Severe fulminating disease is a medical emergency and requires treatment with intravenous fluids and steroids. If this fails to induce remission, ciclosporin may be used.

Colectomy with an ileostomy or ileorectal pouch is undertaken for severe fulminating disease, which may be complicated by a toxic megacolon, or for chronic poorly controlled disease. There is an increased incidence of adenocarcinoma of the colon in adults (1 in 200 risk for each year of disease between 10–20 years from diagnosis). Regular colonoscopic screening is performed after 10 years from diagnosis.

Constipation

Constipation is an extremely common reason for consultation in children. Parents may use the term to describe decreased frequency of defecation, the degree of hardness of the stool or painful defecation. The 'normal' frequency of defecation is highly variable and varies with age. Infants have an average of four stools per day in the 1st week of life, but this falls to an average of two per day by 1 year of age. Breastfed infants may not pass stools for several days and be entirely healthy. After 1 year of age, most children have a daily bowel action. A pragmatic definition of constipation is the infrequent passage of dry, hardened faeces often accompanied by straining or pain and bleeding associated with hard stools. There may be abdominal pain, which waxes and wanes with passage of stool or overflow soiling [see Ch. 24 (Child and Adolescent Mental Health)]. The constipation may have been precipitated by dehydration or reduced fluid intake or an anal fissure causing pain. In older children, it may relate to problems with toilet training, refusal and anxieties about opening bowels at school or in unfamiliar toilets.

Examination usually reveals a well child whose growth is normal, the abdomen is soft and any abdominal distension is normal for age. The back and perianal area are normal in appearance and position. A soft faecal mass may sometimes be palpable in the lower abdomen, but is not necessary for the diagnosis. A primary underlying cause for constipation is rare, but a number of underlying conditions should be considered: Hirschsprung disease, lower spinal cord problems, anorectal abnormalities, hypothyroidism, coeliac disease and hypercalcaemia. 'Red flag' symptoms and signs indicative of more significant pathology are detailed in Box 14.4. Digital rectal examination should not be performed; it may sometimes be considered by a paediatric specialist to help identify anatomical abnormalities or Hirschsprung disease. Investigations are not usually required to diagnose idiopathic constipation, but are carried out as indicated by history or clinical findings.

Box 14.4 'Red flag' symptoms or signs in the child with constipation

'Red flag' symptom/signs	Diagnostic concern
Failure to pass meconium within 24 hours of life	Hirschsprung disease
Faltering growth/growth failure	Hypothyroidism, coeliac disease, other causes
Gross abdominal distension	Hirschsprung disease or other gastrointestinal dysmotility
Abnormal lower limb neurology or deformity, e.g. talipes or secondary urinary incontinence	Lumbosacral pathology
Sacral dimple above natal cleft, over the spine – naevus, hairy patch, central pit, or discoloured skin	Spina bifida occulta
Abnormal appearance/position/patency of anus	Abnormal anorectal anatomy
Perianal bruising or multiple fissures	Sexual abuse
Perianal fistulae, abscesses, or fissures	Perianal Crohn's disease

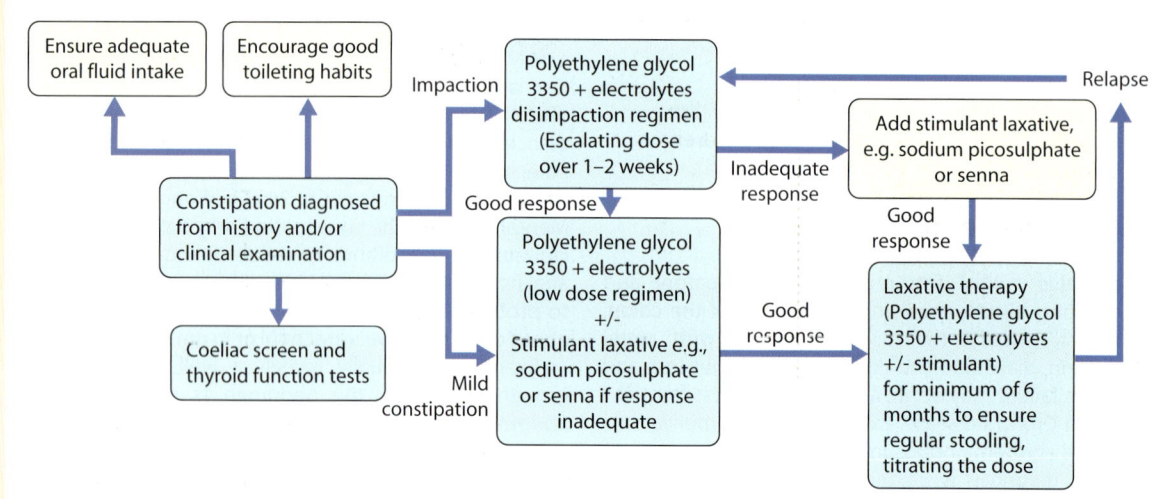

Figure 14.15 Summary of the management of constipation. (Adapted from National Institute for Health and Clinical Excellence (NICE): *Guideline. Constipation in Children and Young People*, London, 2010, NICE.)

Constipation arising acutely in young children, e.g. after an acute febrile illness, usually resolves spontaneously or with the use of maintenance laxative therapy and extra fluids.

In more long-standing constipation, the rectum becomes overdistended, with a subsequent loss of feeling the need to defecate. Involuntary soiling may occur as contractions of the full rectum inhibit the internal sphincter, leading to overflow. Management of these children is likely to be more difficult and protracted and often requires a multidisciplinary approach (Fig. 14.15). Children of school age are frequently teased as a result and secondary behavioural problems are common.

It should be explained to the child and the parents that the soiling is involuntary and that recovery of normal rectal size and sensation can be achieved but may take a long time. The initial aim is to evacuate the overloaded rectum completely. This can generally be achieved using a disimpaction regimen of stool softeners, initially with a macrogol laxative, e.g. polyethylene glycol 3350 + electrolytes (Movicol Paediatric Plain). An escalating dose regimen is administered over 1–2 weeks or until impaction resolves. If this proves unsuccessful, a stimulant laxative, e.g. senna, or sodium picosulphate, may also be required. If the polyethylene glycol + electrolytes is not tolerated, an osmotic laxative (e.g. lactulose) can be substituted.

Disimpaction must be followed by maintenance treatment to ensure ongoing regular, pain-free defecation. Polyethylene glycol (with or without a stimulant laxative) is generally the treatment of choice. The dose should be gradually reduced over a period of months in response to improvement in stool consistency and frequency.

Dietary interventions alone are of little or no benefit in managing constipation in this situation, although the child should receive sufficient fluid and a balanced diet. The addition of extra fibre to the diet is not helpful, and may make stools larger and more difficult to pass. The child should be encouraged to sit on the toilet after mealtimes to utilize the physiological gastrocolic reflex and improve the likelihood of success.

The outcome is more likely to be successful if the child is engaged in the treatment process. This requires exploring the child's concerns and motivation to change. Sometimes use of behavioural interventions, e.g. a star chart, is helpful to record and reward progress, as well as to motivate the child.

Encouragement by family and health professionals is essential, as relapse is common and psychological support is sometimes required. The mainstay of treatment is the early, aggressive and prolonged use of laxative medication in a dose that allows the passage of a large, soft stool at least once a day. One needs to emphasise that the use of laxatives is safe, even long-term, as underuse is the commonest reason for treatment failure. Occasionally, the faecal retention is so severe that evacuation is only possible using enemas or by manual evacuation under an anaesthetic. They should only be performed under specialist supervision, paying particular attention to avoiding distress and embarrassment for the child.

Hirschsprung disease

The absence of ganglion cells from the myenteric and submucosal plexuses of part of the large bowel results in a narrow, contracted segment. The abnormal bowel extends from the rectum for a variable distance proximally, ending in a normally innervated, dilated colon. In 75% of cases, the lesion is confined to the rectosigmoid, but in 10% the entire colon is involved. Presentation is usually in the neonatal period with intestinal obstruction heralded by failure to pass meconium within the first 24 hours of life. Abdominal distension and later bile-stained vomiting develop (Fig. 14.16). Rectal examination may reveal a narrowed segment and withdrawal of the examining finger often releases a gush of liquid stool and flatus. Temporary improvement in the obstruction following the dilatation caused by the rectal examination can lead to a delay in diagnosis.

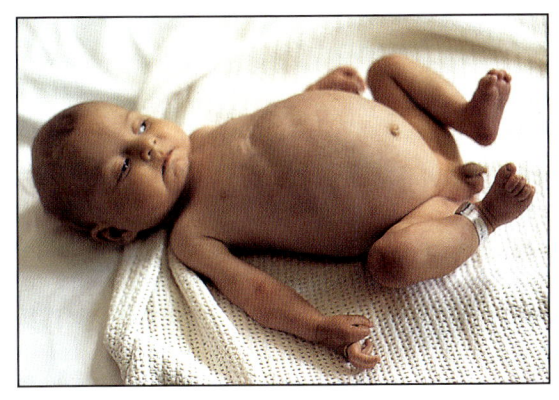

Figure 14.16 Abdominal distension from Hirschsprung disease.

> **Summary**
>
> **Hirschsprung disease**
> - Absence of myenteric plexuses of rectum and variable distance of colon.
> - Presentation – usually intestinal obstruction in the newborn period following delay in passing meconium. In later childhood – profound chronic constipation, abdominal distension, and growth failure.
> - Diagnosis – suction rectal biopsy.

Occasionally, infants present with severe, life-threatening Hirschsprung enterocolitis during the first few weeks of life. In later childhood, presentation is with chronic constipation, usually profound, and associated with abdominal distension but usually without soiling. Growth failure may also be present.

Diagnosis is made by demonstrating the absence of ganglion cells, together with the presence of large, acetylcholinesterase-positive nerve trunks on a suction rectal biopsy. Anorectal manometry or barium studies may be useful in giving the surgeon an idea of the length of the aganglionic segment but are unreliable for diagnostic purposes. Management is surgical and usually involves an initial colostomy followed by anastomozing normally innervated bowel to the anus.

Acknowledgements

We would like to acknowledge that this chapter is based on the previous chapter on Gastroenterology from the following contributors: Ian Booth (1st, 2nd, 3rd Editions) and Mr Anthony Lander (2nd, 3rd Editions). The chapter was updated by: Jonathan Bishop (4th Edition) and Stephen Hodges (4th Edition).

Further reading

Beattie M, Dhawan A, Puntis J: *Paediatric Gastroenterology, Hepatology and Nutrition (Oxford Specialist Handbooks in Paediatrics)*, Oxford, 2009, Oxford University Press.
Short handbook

Kleinman RE, Goulet OJ, Mieli-Vergani G, et al.: *Walker's Pediatric Gastrointestinal Disease*, ed 6, Ontario, 2015, Decker.
Comprehensive two-volume textbook.

Websites (Accessed November 2016)

Coeliac UK: Available at: www.coeliac.co.uk.

National Institute for Health and Clinical Excellence (NICE): *Guideline. Coeliac Disease*, London, 2009, NICE.

National Institute for Health and Clinical Excellence (NICE): *Guideline. Diarrhoea and Vomiting in Children under 5*, London, 2009, NICE.

National Institute for Health and Clinical Excellence (NICE): *Guideline. Constipation in Children and Young People*, London, 2010, NICE.

Up-to-date reviews on a selection of paediatric gastroenterology topics: Available at: http://www.espghan.org/guidelines/

15

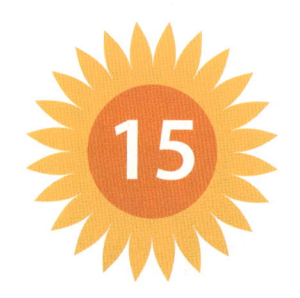

Infection and immunity

The febrile child	256		Tuberculosis	275
Serious life-threatening infections	259		Tropical infections	277
Specific bacterial infections	263		HIV infection	279
Common viral infections	265		Lyme disease	281
Uncommon viral infections	271		Immunization	281
Prolonged fever	273		Immunodeficiency	284

Infections are the most common cause of acute illness in children.

Features of infection and immunity in children are:

- worldwide, acute respiratory infections, diarrhoea, neonatal infection, malaria, measles, and HIV infection, often accompanied by undernutrition, are responsible for the deaths of more than 2.3 million children under 5 years of age annually (Fig. 15.1)
- in high-income countries, deaths caused by infections are now uncommon. However, infections are the most common cause of acute illness in children, and serious infections still occur, e.g. pneumonia, sepsis, and meningitis, and require early recognition and treatment
- some diseases that were rare in high-income countries have re-emerged, e.g. tuberculosis (TB)
- there has been a rise of multidrug-resistant pathogens over the last two decades, including methicillin-resistant *Staphylococcus aureus* and extended-spectrum beta-lactamase-producing Gram-negative bacteria
- with air travel, imported 'tropical diseases' are now encountered in all countries. Air travel has also contributed to epidemics spreading more rapidly and more widely, e.g. severe acute respiratory syndrome (SARS, caused by SARS coronavirus) and H1N1 influenza virus
- immunization has played a major role in reducing morbidity and mortality of infections throughout the world.

The febrile child

Most febrile children have a brief, self-limiting viral infection. Mild localized infections, e.g. otitis media or tonsillitis, may be diagnosed clinically. The clinical problem lies in identifying the relatively small proportion of children with a serious infection which needs prompt treatment.

Clinical features

When assessing a febrile child, consider the following
(i) How is fever identified in children?
Parents usually know if their child has been febrile. In hospital, it is measured:

- if less than 4 weeks of age, by an electronic thermometer in the axilla
- if aged 4 weeks to 5 years, by an electronic or chemical dot thermometer in the axilla or infrared tympanic thermometer.

A fever in children is a temperature over 37.5°C. In general, axillary temperatures underestimate body temperature by 0.5°C.

(ii) How old is the child?
Febrile infants less than 3 months of age can present with nonspecific clinical features [see Box 11.3] and have a bacterial infection, which cannot be identified reliably on clinical examination alone. During the first few months of life infants are relatively protected against common viral infections because of passive immunity acquired by transplacental transfer of antibodies from their mothers (Fig. 15.2). Unless a clear cause for the fever is identified, they require urgent investigation with a septic screen (Box 15.1) and broad-spectrum intravenous antibiotic therapy given immediately to avoid the illness becoming more severe and to prevent spreading of the infection to other sites of the body. This is considered in more detail in the section on neonatal infection [Ch. 11 (Neonatal medicine)].

Worldwide causes of death in children <5 years

☀ In 2015, 40% the 5.9 million deaths of children under 5 years of age were due to infection

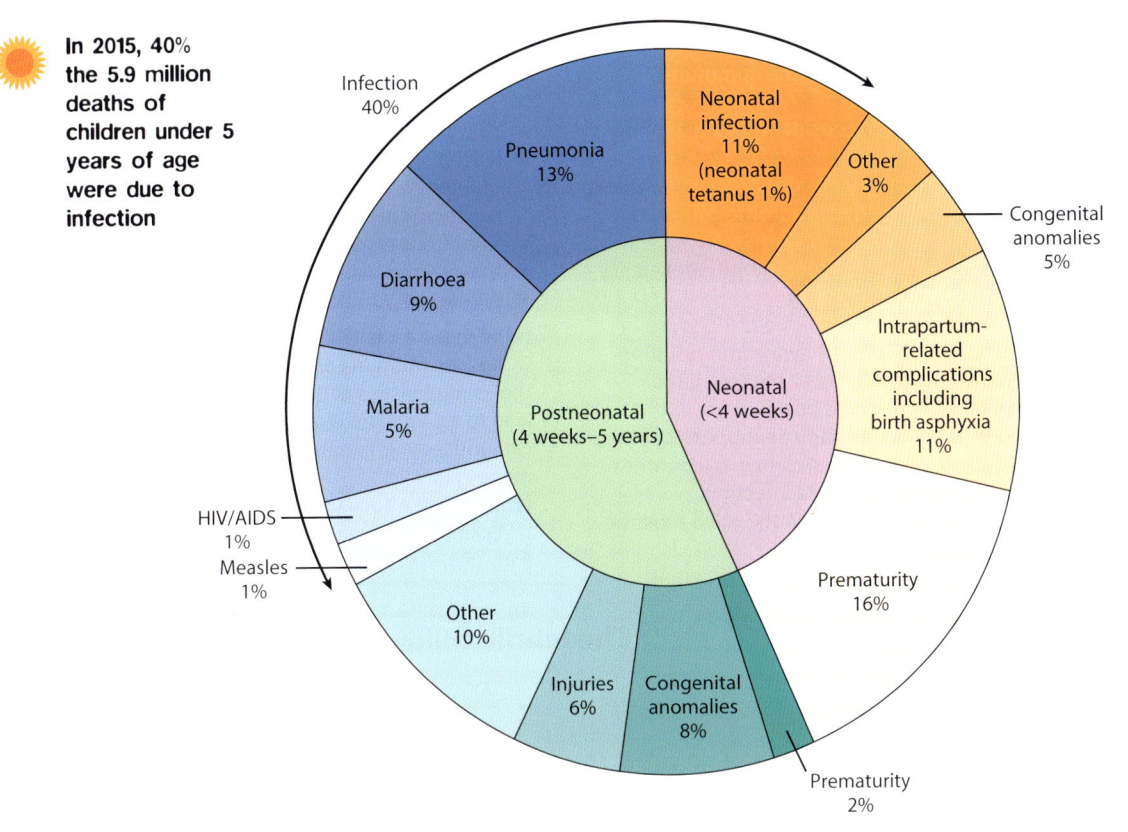

Figure 15.1 Globally, infection is responsible for 40% of the 5.9 million deaths in children under 5 years of age, 2015. (Data from http://www.who.int/gho/child_health/mortality/causes/en/, Accessed November 2016.)

Box 15.1 Septic screen

- Blood culture
- Full blood count including differential white cell count
- Acute phase reactant, e.g. C-reactive protein
- Urine sample

Consider if indicated:

- Chest X-ray
- Lumbar puncture (unless contraindicated)
- Rapid antigen screen on blood/cerebrospinal fluid (CSF)/urine
- Meningococcal and pneumococcal polymerase chain reaction (PCR) on blood/CSF samples
- PCR for viruses in CSF (especially herpes simplex virus and enteroviruses).

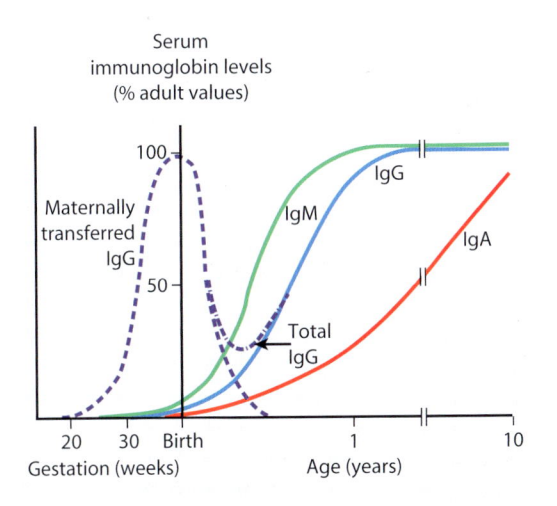

Figure 15.2 Serum immunoglobulin (antibody) levels in the fetus and infant. When maternal immunoglobulin levels decline, infants become susceptible to viral infections.

Infection and immunity

(iii) Are there risk factors for infection?
These include:

- illness of other family members
- specific illness prevalent in the community
- lack of immunizations
- recent travel abroad (consider malaria, typhoid, and viral hepatitis)
- contact with animals (consider brucellosis, Q fever, and haemolytic uraemic syndrome caused by *Escherichia coli* O157)
- increased susceptibility from immunodeficiency. This is usually secondary, e.g. post-autosplenectomy in sickle cell disease or splenectomy or nephrotic syndrome resulting in increased susceptibility to encapsulated organisms (*Streptococcus pneumoniae*, *Haemophilus influenzae*, and *Salmonella* species), or rarely, primary immunodeficiency. In countries with high prevalence of HIV infection, undiagnosed HIV infection in the child must be considered.

(iv) How ill is the child?
Red flag features suggesting serious illness and the need for urgent investigation and treatment are:

- fever over 38°C if aged less than 3 months, or over 39°C if 3 months to 6 months of age
- colour – pale, mottled, or cyanosed
- level of consciousness is reduced, neck stiffness, bulging fontanelle, status epilepticus, focal neurological signs, or seizures
- significant respiratory distress
- bile-stained vomiting
- severe dehydration or shock.

(v) Is there a rash?
Rashes often accompany febrile illnesses. In some, the characteristics of the rash and other clinical features lead to a diagnosis, e.g. a purpuric rash in meningococcal septicaemia; in many, a specific diagnosis cannot be made clinically.

(vi) Is there a focus for infection?
Examination may identify a focus of infection (Fig. 15.3). If identified, investigations and management

The febrile child

Upper respiratory tract infection
Very common, may be coincidental with another more serious illness

Otitis media
Always examine tympanic membranes in febrile children

Tonsillitis
Erythema or exudate on the tonsils?

Viral croup?
Bacterial tracheitis?

Pneumonia
Fever, cough, raised respiratory rate, chest recession, abnormal auscultation. In infants, auscultation may be normal – diagnosis may require chest X-ray

Septicaemia
Can be difficult to recognize in absence of rash before shock develops
Early signs are tachycardia, tachypnoea, and poor perfusion
Need to start antibiotics on clinical suspicion without waiting for culture results

Meningitis/encephalitis
Lethargy, loss of interest in surroundings, drowsiness or coma, seizures
Older children - headache, photophobia, neck stiffness, positive Kernig sign (pain on leg straightening)
Younger children and infants - non-specific symptoms and signs
Raised intracranial pressure - reduced concious level, abnormal pupillary responses, abnormal posturing, Cushing triad (bradycardia, hypertension, abnormal pattern of breathing)
Late signs – papilloedema, bulging fontanelle in infants, opisthotonus (hyperextension of head and back)

Seizure
Febrile seizure?
Meningitis?
Encephalitis?

Periorbital cellulitis
Redness and swelling of the eyelids
May spread to orbit of the eye

Rash
Viral exanthem?
Purpura from meningococcal infection (Fig. 6.10)

Urinary tract infection
Urine sample needed for any seriously ill young child or any febrile illness that does not settle

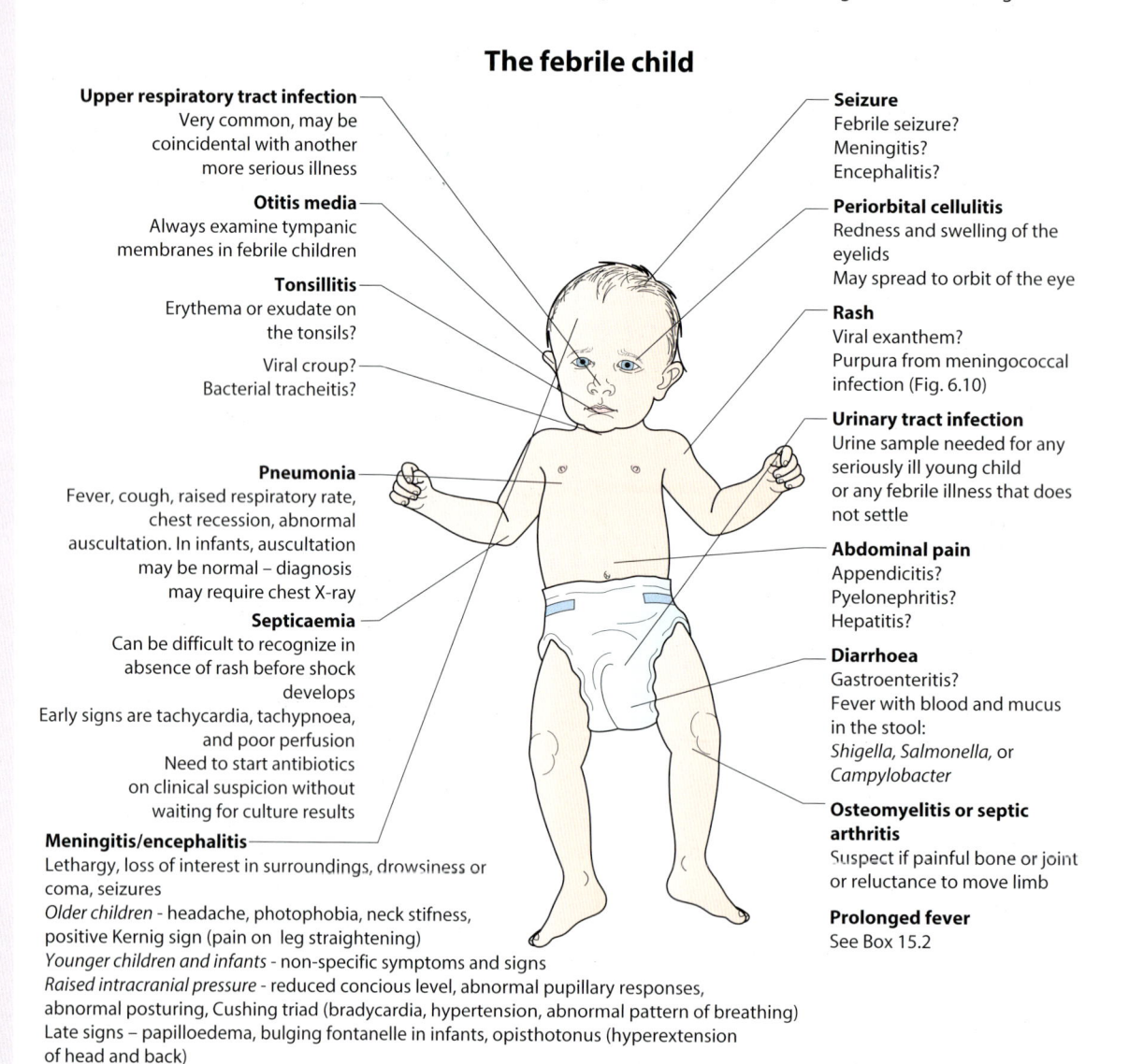

Abdominal pain
Appendicitis?
Pyelonephritis?
Hepatitis?

Diarrhoea
Gastroenteritis?
Fever with blood and mucus in the stool:
Shigella, Salmonella, or *Campylobacter*

Osteomyelitis or septic arthritis
Suspect if painful bone or joint or reluctance to move limb

Prolonged fever
See Box 15.2

Figure 15.3 Diagnostic clues to evaluating the febrile child.

will be directed towards its treatment. However, if no focus is identified, this is often because it is the prodromal phase of a viral illness, but may indicate a potentially serious bacterial infection, especially urinary tract infection or septicaemia.

Management

Children who are not seriously ill can be managed at home with regular review by the parents, as long as they are given clear instructions (e.g. what clinical features should prompt reassessment by a doctor). Children who are significantly unwell, particularly if there is no focus of infection, will require investigations and observation or treatment in a paediatric assessment unit, accident and emergency department, or children's ward. A septic screen will be required (Box 15.1).

Parenteral antibiotics should be given immediately to seriously unwell children, e.g. a third-generation cephalosporin such as cefotaxime (<1 month old who have been discharged from hospital) or high-dose ceftriaxone (>1 month old). In infants under 1 month of age, ampicillin is added to cover for *Listeria* infection. Aciclovir is given if herpes simplex virus (HSV) encephalitis is suspected. Supportive care is given as indicated.

The use of antipyretic agents should be considered in children with fever who appear distressed or unwell. Either paracetamol or ibuprofen can be used. They can be given sequentially if a single agent achieves only limited response. Evidence that antipyretics prevent febrile seizures is lacking. There are detailed National Institute for Health and Care Excellence guidelines for the management of the child under 5 years of age with fever.

> **Summary**
>
> **The febrile child**
> - Upper respiratory tract infection is a very common cause.
> - Check for otitis media.
> - Serious bacterial infection must be considered if there is no focus of infection, especially urinary tract infection or septicaemia, or there are red flag features of potentially life-threatening illness.
> - The younger the child, the lower the threshold for performing a septic screen and starting antibiotics.

Serious life-threatening infections

Sepsis

This is considered in Chapter 6 (Paediatric Emergencies).

Meningitis

Meningitis occurs when there is inflammation of the meninges covering the brain. This can be confirmed by finding white blood cells in the cerebrospinal fluid (CSF). Viral infections are the most common cause of meningitis, and most are self-resolving. Bacterial meningitis may have severe consequences. Tuberculous meningitis is rare in countries with low TB prevalence. TB meningitis mainly affects children under 5 years of age. Fungal and parasitic meningitis are rare in children and predominately affect immunocompromised individuals. Causes of noninfectious meningitis include malignancy and autoimmune diseases.

Bacterial meningitis

Over 80% of patients with bacterial meningitis in the UK are younger than 16 years of age. Bacterial meningitis remains a serious infection in children, with 5% to 10% mortality. Over 10% of survivors are left with long-term neurological impairment.

Pathophysiology

Bacterial infection of the meninges usually follows bacteraemia. Much of the damage caused by meningeal infection results from the host response to infection and not from the organism itself. The release of inflammatory mediators and activated leucocytes, together with endothelial damage, leads to cerebral oedema, raised intracranial pressure, and decreased cerebral blood flow. The inflammatory response below the meninges causes a vasculopathy resulting in cerebral cortical infarction, and fibrin deposits may block the resorption of CSF by the arachnoid villi, resulting in hydrocephalus.

Organisms

The organisms that commonly cause bacterial meningitis vary according to the child's age (Table 15.1). These have changed over time with the introduction of conjugate vaccines [against *H. influenzae* type b (Hib), meningococcal group C (and recently A, C, Y, and W), and multiple pneumococcal serotypes]. The effect of the introduction of a new recombinant group B meningococcal vaccine remains to be seen on both the individual and at the population level.

Presentation

The clinical features are listed in Fig. 15.4. The early signs and symptoms of meningitis are nonspecific, especially in infants and young children. Only children

Table 15.1 Organisms causing bacterial meningitis according to age

Neonatal to 3 months	Group B streptococcus
	Escherichia coli and other coliforms
	Listeria monocytogenes
1 month to 6 years	*Neisseria meningitides*
	Streptococcus pneumoniae
	Haemophilus influenza
>6 years	*Neisseria meningitides*
	Streptococcus pneumoniae

Assessment & investigation of meningitis/encephalitis

History	Examination	Investigations
Fever	Fever	Full blood count and differential count
Headache	Purpuric rash (meningococcal disease)	Blood glucose and blood gas (for acidosis)
Photophobia	Neck stiffness (not always present in infants)	Coagulation screen, C-reactive protein
Lethargy	Bulging fontanelle in infants	Urea and electrolytes, liver function tests
Poor feeding/vomiting	Opisthotonus (arching of back)	Culture of blood, throat swab, urine, stool for bacteria
Irritability	Positive Brudzinski/Kernig signs	Rapid antigen test for meningitis organisms (can be done on blood, CSF, or urine)
Hypotonia	Signs of shock	Samples for viral PCRs (e.g. throat swab, nasopharyngeal aspirate, conjunctival swab, stool sample)
Drowsiness	Focal neurological signs	Lumbar puncture for CSF unless contraindicated (see below for tests on CSF)
Loss of consciousness	Altered conscious level	Serum for comparison of convalescent titres
Seizures	Papilloedema (rare)	PCR of blood and CSF for possible organisms
		If TB suspected: chest X-ray, Mantoux test and/or interferon-gamma release assay, gastric aspirates or sputum for microscopy and culture (and PCR if available)
		Consider CT/MRI brain scan and EEG

Signs associated with neck stiffness

Brudzinski sign – flexion of the neck with the child supine causes flexion of the knees and hips

Kernig sign – with the child lying supine and with the hips and knees flexed, there is back pain on extension of the knee

Contraindications to lumbar puncture:

- Cardiorespiratory instability
- Focal neurological signs
- Signs of raised intracranial pressure, e.g. coma, high BP, low heart rate or papilloedema
- Coagulopathy
- Thrombocytopenia
- Local infection at the site of LP
- If it causes undue delay in starting antibiotics

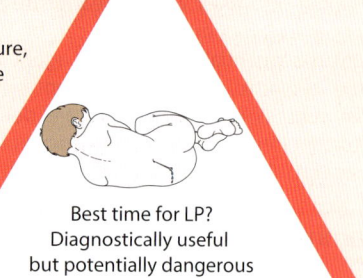

Best time for LP? Diagnostically useful but potentially dangerous

Typical changes in the CSF in meningitis or encephalitis, beyond the neonatal period

	Aetiology	Appearance	White blood cells	Protein	Glucose
Normal	—	Clear	0–5/mm^3	0.15–0.4 g/L	≥50% of blood
Meningitis	Bacterial	Turbid	Polymorphs:↑↑	↑↑	↓↓
	Viral	Clear	Lymphocytes:↑ (initially may be polymorphs)	Normal/↑	Normal/↓
	Tuberculosis	Turbid/clear/viscous	Lymphocytes:↑	↑↑↑	↓↓↓
Encephalitis	Viral/unknown	Clear	Normal/↑ lymphocytes	Normal/↑	Normal/↓

Figure 15.4 Assessment and investigation of meningitis and encephalitis.

old enough to talk are likely to describe the classical meningitis symptoms of headache, neck stiffness, and photophobia. However, neck stiffness may also be seen in some children with tonsillitis and cervical lymphadenopathy. As children with meningitis may also have sepsis, signs of shock, such as tachycardia, tachypnoea, prolonged capillary refill time and hypotension, should be sought. Purpura in a febrile child of any age should be assumed to be due to meningococcal sepsis, even if the child does not appear unduly ill at the time; meningitis may or may not be present in this situation.

Investigations

The essential investigations are listed in Fig. 15.4. A lumbar puncture is performed to obtain CSF to confirm the diagnosis, identify the organism responsible, and its antibiotic sensitivities. Characteristic findings are shown in Fig. 15.4. However, exceptions can occur, e.g. lymphocytes can predominate in bacterial meningitis, e.g. in Lyme disease, and glucose levels can be low in viral meningitis, e.g. enterovirus meningitis. If any of the contraindications for performing a lumbar puncture are present, as listed in Fig. 15.4, it should not be performed, as under these circumstances, the procedure carries a risk of coning of the cerebellum through the foramen magnum. In these circumstances, a lumbar puncture can be postponed until the child's condition has stabilized. Even without a lumbar puncture, bacteriological diagnosis can be achieved in about half of the cases from the blood by culture or polymerase chain reaction (PCR), and rapid antigen screens can be performed on blood and urine samples. Throat swabs should also be obtained for bacterial culture and viral PCRs. A serological diagnosis can be made on convalescent serum 4 weeks to 6 weeks after the presenting illness if necessary.

Management

It is imperative that there is no delay in the administration of antibiotics and supportive therapy in a child with meningitis. The choice of antibiotics will depend on the likely pathogen. A third-generation cephalosporin, e.g. ceftriaxone, is the preferred choice to cover the most common bacterial causes. Although still relatively rare in the UK, pneumococcal resistance to penicillin and cephalosporins is increasing rapidly in certain parts of the world. The length of the course of antibiotics given depends on the causative organism and clinical response. Beyond the neonatal period, there is some evidence suggesting that dexamethasone administered with the antibiotics reduces the risk of long-term complications such as deafness.

Cerebral complications

These include:

- *hearing impairment* – inflammatory damage to the cochlear hair cells may lead to deafness. All children who have had meningitis should have an audiological assessment done promptly, as children with hearing impairment may benefit from hearing amplification or a cochlear implant
- *local vasculitis* – this may lead to cranial nerve palsies or other focal neurological lesions
- *local cerebral infarction* – this may result in focal or multifocal seizures, which may subsequently result in epilepsy
- *subdural effusion* – particularly associated with *H. influenzae* and pneumococcal meningitis. This is confirmed by cranial CT or MRI scan. Most resolve spontaneously, but some require neurosurgical intervention
- *hydrocephalus* – may result from impaired resorption of CSF (communicating hydrocephalus) or blockage of the cerebral aqueduct or ventricular outlets by fibrin (noncommunicating hydrocephalus). A ventricular shunt may be required
- *cerebral abscess* – the child's clinical condition deteriorates with or without the emergence of signs of a space-occupying lesion. The temperature will continue to fluctuate. It is confirmed on cranial CT or MRI scan. Drainage of the abscess is required.

Prophylaxis

Prophylactic treatment with rifampicin or ciprofloxacin to eradicate nasopharyngeal carriage is given to all household contacts for meningococcal meningitis and Hib infection. It is not required for the patient if given a third-generation cephalosporin, as this will eradicate nasopharyngeal carriage. Household contacts of patients who have had group C meningococcal meningitis should be vaccinated with the meningococcal group C vaccine.

Partially treated bacterial meningitis

Children are frequently given oral antibiotics for a nonspecific febrile illness. If they have early meningitis, this partial treatment with antibiotics may cause diagnostic problems. CSF examination shows a markedly raised number of white cells, but cultures are usually negative. Rapid antigen screens and PCR are helpful in these circumstances. Where the diagnosis is suspected clinically, a full course of antibiotics should be given.

Viral meningitis

More than two-thirds of central nervous system (CNS) infections are viral. Causes include enteroviruses, Epstein–Barr virus (EBV), adenoviruses, and mumps. Mumps meningitis is now rare in the UK due to the measles, mumps, and rubella (MMR) vaccine. Viral meningitis is usually much less severe than bacterial meningitis and most cases make a full recovery. Diagnosis of viral meningitis can be confirmed by culture or PCR of CSF, stool, urine, nasopharyngeal aspirate, and throat swabs, as well as serology.

Uncommon pathogens and other causes

Where the clinical course is atypical or there is failure to respond to antibiotic and supportive therapy, unusual organisms, e.g. *Mycoplasma* species or *Borrelia burgdorferi* (Lyme disease), TB, or fungal infections need to be considered. Uncommon pathogens are particularly likely in children who are immunocompromised (i.e. with immunodeficiency or receiving chemotherapy or immunosuppressive medication). Recurrent bacterial meningitis may occur in the immunodeficient children or in those with structural abnormalities of the skull or meninges that facilitate bacterial access. Aseptic meningitis may be seen in malignancy or autoimmune disorders.

Neonatal meningitis

See Chapter 11.

Encephalitis/encephalopathy

In meningitis there is inflammation of the meninges, whereas in encephalitis there is inflammation of the

> **Summary**
>
> **Meningitis**
> - Predominantly a disease of infants and children.
> - Incidence has been reduced by immunization.
> - Clinical features: nonspecific in children under 12 months – fever, poor feeding, vomiting, irritability, lethargy, drowsiness, seizures, or reduced consciousness; late signs – bulging fontanelle, neck stiffness, and arched back (opisthotonos).
> - Septicaemia can kill in hours; good outcome requires prompt resuscitation and antibiotics.
> - Any febrile child with a purpuric rash should be given intramuscular benzylpenicillin immediately and transferred urgently to hospital.
> - The meningococcal vaccines now included in the infant and adolescent immunization schedule in the UK should further reduce the incidence of meningococcal sepsis and meningitis.

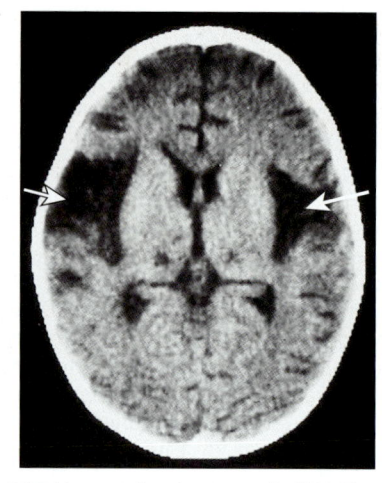

Figure 15.5 Herpes simplex encephalitis. The computed tomography scan shows gross atrophy from loss of neural tissue in the temporoparietal regions (arrows).

brain substance, although the meninges are often also affected. Encephalitis may be caused by:

- direct invasion of the brain by a neurotoxic virus (such as HSV)
- delayed brain swelling following a dysregulated neuroimmunological response to an antigen, usually a virus (postinfectious encephalopathy), e.g. following chickenpox
- a slow virus infection, such as HIV infection or subacute sclerosing panencephalitis (SSPE) following measles.

In encephalopathy from a noninfectious cause, such as a metabolic abnormality, the clinical features may be similar to infectious encephalitis.

The clinical features and investigation of encephalitis are described in Fig. 15.4. Most children present with fever, altered consciousness, and often seizures. Initially, it may not be possible to clinically differentiate encephalitis from meningitis, and treatment for both should be started. The underlying causative organism is only detected in fewer than half of the cases. In the UK, the most common causes of encephalitis are enteroviruses, respiratory viruses (influenza viruses), and herpesviruses [e.g. HSV, varicella zoster virus (VZV), and human herpesvirus 6 (HHV-6)]. Worldwide, microorganisms causing encephalitis include *Mycoplasma*, *B. burgdorferi* (Lyme disease), *Bartonella henselae* (cat scratch disease), rickettsial infections (e.g. Rocky Mountain spotted fever), and arboviruses.

HSV is a rare cause of childhood encephalitis but it can have devastating long-term consequences. All children with encephalitis should therefore be treated initially with high-dose intravenous aciclovir (acyclovir) until this diagnosis has been ruled out, because this is a very safe treatment. Most affected children do not have outward signs of herpes infection, such as cold sores, gingivostomatitis, or skin lesions. PCR is used in the majority of laboratories to detect HSV in CSF. As HSV encephalitis is a destructive infection, the electroencephalogram and CT/MRI scan may show focal changes, particularly within the temporal lobes either unilaterally or bilaterally (Fig. 15.5). These tests may be normal initially and need to be repeated after a few days if the child is not improving. Later confirmation of the diagnosis may be made from HSV antibody production in the CSF. Proven cases of HSV encephalitis or cases where there is a high index of suspicion should be treated with intravenous aciclovir for 3 weeks, as relapses may occur after shorter courses. Untreated, the mortality rate from HSV encephalitis is over 70% and survivors usually have severe neurological sequelae.

> **Summary**
>
> **Encephalitis**
> - Onset can be insidious and includes behavioural change.
> - Consider if HSV could be the cause.
> - Treat potential HSV with parenteral high-dose aciclovir until this diagnosis is excluded.

Toxic shock syndrome

Toxin-producing *S. aureus* and group A streptococci can cause this rare syndrome, which is characterized by:

- fever over 39°C
- hypotension
- diffuse erythematous, macular rash.

The toxin can be released from infection at any site, including small abrasions or burns, which may look minor. The toxin acts as a superantigen and, in addition to the aforementioned features, causes organ dysfunction, including:

- mucositis (Fig. 15.6): conjunctivae, oral mucosa, genital mucosa

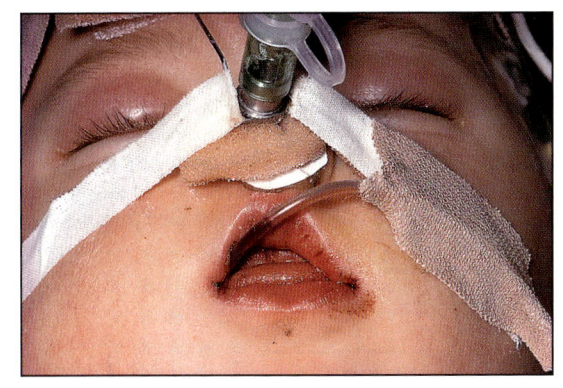

Figure 15.6 A child with toxic shock syndrome receiving intensive care, including mechanical ventilation via a nasotracheal tube. The lips are red and the eyelids are oedematous from capillary leak. (Courtesy of Professor Mike Levin.)

- gastrointestinal dysfunction: vomiting/diarrhoea
- renal impairment
- liver impairment
- clotting abnormalities and thrombocytopenia
- CNS: altered consciousness.

Intensive care support is required to manage the shock. Areas of infection should be surgically débrided. Antibiotics often include a third-generation cephalosporin (such as ceftriaxone) together with clindamycin, which acts on the bacterial ribosome to switch off toxin production. Intravenous immunoglobulin may be given to neutralize the circulating toxin. About 1 week to 2 weeks after the onset of the illness, there is desquamation of the palms, soles, fingers, and toes.

A strain of *S. aureus* has emerged in the UK and other countries that produces a toxin called Panton–Valentine leukocidin (PVL). PVL is produced by fewer than 2% of *S. aureus* strains (both methicillin-sensitive *S. aureus* and methicillin-resistant *S. aureus*). PVL-producing *S. aureus* causes recurrent skin and soft-tissue infections, but can also cause necrotizing fasciitis and a necrotizing haemorrhagic pneumonia following an influenza-like illness, both of which carry a high mortality rate. In children, the procoagulant state induced by the toxin frequently results in venous thrombosis.

Necrotizing fasciitis/cellulitis

This is a rare, severe subcutaneous infection, often involving tissue planes from the skin down to fascia and muscle. The area involved may enlarge rapidly, leaving poorly perfused necrotic areas of tissue, usually at the centre. There is severe pain and systemic illness, which usually requires intensive care. The invading organism may be *S. aureus* or a group A streptococcus, with or without another synergistic anaerobic organism. Intravenous antibiotic therapy alone is not sufficient to treat this condition. Without surgical intervention and débridement of necrotic tissue, the infection will continue to spread. Clinical suspicion of necrotizing fasciitis warrants urgent surgical consultation and intervention. Intravenous immunoglobulin (IVIG) may also be given.

Specific bacterial infections

Meningococcal infection

Meningococcal infection is a disease that strikes fear into both parents and doctors, as it can kill previously healthy children within hours (Case History 15.1). However, of the three main causes of bacterial meningitis, meningococcal infection has the lowest risk of long-term neurological sequelae, with most survivors recovering fully. The septicaemia is usually accompanied by a purpuric rash, which may start anywhere on the body and then spreads. The rash may or may not be present in cases with meningococcal meningitis. Characteristic lesions are nonblanching on palpation, irregular in size and outline, and may have a necrotic centre (Fig. 15.8a,b). Any febrile child who develops a purpuric rash should be treated immediately, at home or in the general practitioner's surgery, with intramuscular penicillin or intravenous third-generation cephalosporin before urgent admission to hospital. Following the inclusion of the meningococcus C vaccine into the routine immunization schedule in the UK,

Case history 15.1

Meningococcal septicaemia

This 7-month-old boy presented with a 12-hour history of lethargy and a spreading purpuric rash. In hospital, he required immediate resuscitation and transfer to a paediatric intensive care unit for multiorgan failure (Fig. 15.7a). The gross oedema is from leak of capillary fluid into the tissues. He required colloid and inotropic support and peritoneal dialysis for renal failure. He made a full recovery (Fig. 15.7b).

> Meningococcal septicaemia can kill children in hours. Optimal outcome requires immediate recognition, prompt resuscitation and antibiotics

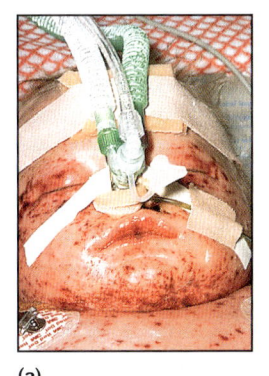

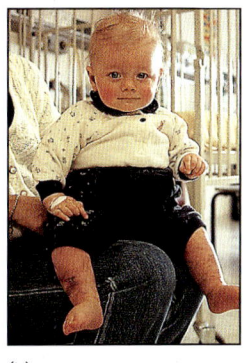

(a)   (b)

Figure 15.7 (a) A boy with meningococcal septicaemia receiving intensive care. (b) After full recovery. (Courtesy of Dr Parviz Habibi.)

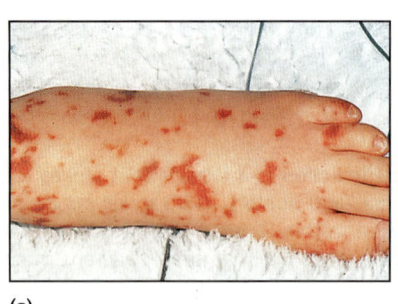

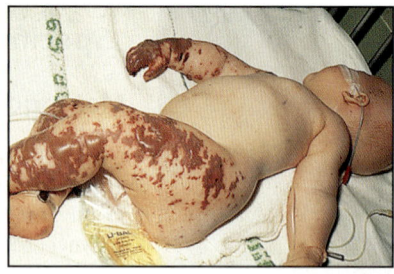

Figure 15.8 Rash of meningococcal infection. (**a**) Characteristic purpuric skin lesions, irregular in size and outline and with a necrotic centre; and (**b**) the lesions may be extensive, when it is called *purpura fulminans*.

group B meningococci causes the majority of disease. As polysaccharide conjugate vaccines against group A, B, and C meningococci have now been developed and incorporated into the immunization schedule, the incidence of meningococcal disease should decline further.

> Any febrile child with a purpuric rash should be given intramuscular benzylpenicillin immediately and transferred urgently to hospital

Pneumococcal infections

S. pneumoniae is often carried in the nasopharynx of healthy children. Asymptomatic carriage is particularly prevalent among young children and may be responsible for the transmission of pneumococcal disease to other individuals by respiratory droplets. The organism may cause pharyngitis, otitis media, conjunctivitis, sinusitis, as well as 'invasive' disease (pneumonia, bacterial sepsis, and meningitis). Invasive disease, which carries a high burden of morbidity and mortality, mainly occurs in young infants as their immune system responds poorly to encapsulated pathogens such as pneumococci. With the inclusion of the 13-valent pneumococcal vaccine (covering 13 different serotypes) into the routine immunization schedule in the UK, the incidence of invasive disease has declined. Children at increased risk, e.g. due to hyposplenism or asplenism, should also be given daily prophylactic penicillin to prevent infection by strains not covered by the vaccine.

Summary

Pneumococcal infection
- Causes not only minor infections such as otitis media but also severe invasive disease.
- Susceptibility is increased in hyposplenism (e.g. sickle cell disease) and nephrotic syndrome.
- A 13-valent pneumococcal vaccine is included in the UK standard immunization schedule.

H. *influenzae* infection

Hib was an important cause of systemic illness in children, including otitis media, pneumonia, epiglottitis, cellulitis, osteomyelitis, and septic arthritis, and was the second most common cause of meningitis in the UK. Immunization has been highly effective and Hib now rarely causes systemic disease.

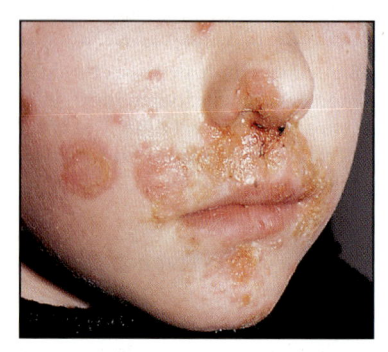

Figure 15.9 Impetigo showing characteristic confluent honey-coloured crusted lesions. (Courtesy of Dr Paul Hutchins.)

Summary

H. *influenzae* infection
- Can cause severe invasive infections, including sepsis and meningitis.
- Hib disease is now rare following the introduction of the Hib vaccine.

Staphylococcal and group A streptococcal infections

Staphylococcal and streptococcal infections are usually caused by direct invasion of the organisms. They may also cause disease by releasing toxins, which act as superantigens. Whereas conventional antigens stimulate only a small subset of T cells, which have a specific antigen receptor, superantigens bind to a part of the T-cell receptor which is shared by many T cells and therefore stimulates massive T-cell proliferation and cytokine release. Other diseases following streptococcal infections, such as poststreptococcal glomerulonephritis and rheumatic fever, are immune-mediated.

Impetigo

This is a localized, highly contagious, staphylococcal or streptococcal skin infection, most commonly occurring in infants and young children. It is more common in children with preexisting skin disease, e.g. atopic eczema. Lesions are usually on the face, neck, and hands and begin as erythematous macules that may become vesicular/pustular or even bullous (Fig. 15.9).

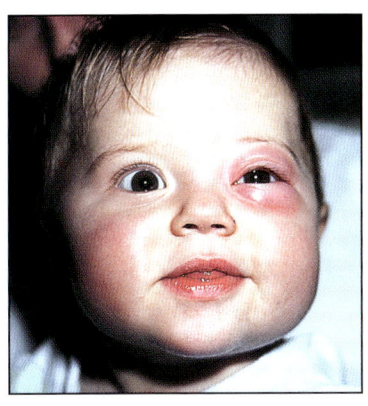

Figure 15.10 Periorbital cellulitis. It should be treated promptly with intravenous antibiotics to prevent spread into the orbit.

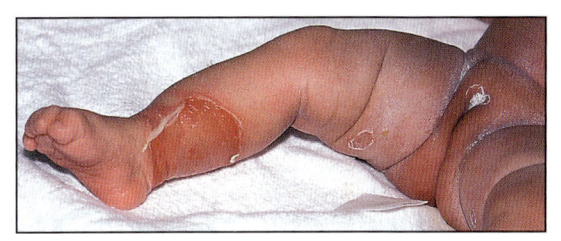

Figure 15.11 Staphylococcal scalded skin syndrome. Its appearance must not be mistaken for a scald from nonaccidental injury.

Rupture of the vesicles with exudation of fluid leads to the characteristic confluent honey-coloured crusted lesions. Infection is readily spread to adjacent areas and other parts of the body by autoinoculation of the infected exudate. Topical antibiotics (e.g. mupirocin) are sometimes effective for mild cases. Narrow-spectrum systemic antibiotics (e.g. flucloxacillin) are generally needed for more severe infections, although more broad-spectrum antibiotics such as co-amoxiclav or cefaclor have simpler oral administration regimens, taste better, and therefore have better adherence. Affected children should not go to nursery or school until the lesions are dry.

Boils

These are infections of hair follicles or sweat glands, usually caused by *S. aureus*. Treatment is with systemic antibiotics and occasionally surgical incision. Recurrent boils are usually from persistent nasal carriage in the child or family acting as a reservoir for reinfection. Only rarely are they a manifestation of an underlying immunodeficiency.

Periorbital cellulitis

In periorbital cellulitis there is fever with erythema, tenderness, and oedema of the eyelid or other skin adjacent to the eye (Fig. 15.10). It is almost always unilateral. It may follow local trauma to the skin. In older children, it may spread from a paranasal sinus infection or dental abscess. Periorbital cellulitis should be treated promptly with intravenous antibiotics such as high-dose ceftriaxone to prevent posterior spread of the infection causing orbital cellulitis. In orbital cellulitis, there is proptosis, painful or limited ocular movement with or without reduced visual acuity. It may be complicated by abscess formation, meningitis, or cavernous sinus thrombosis. Where orbital cellulitis is suspected, a CT or MRI scan should be performed to assess the posterior spread of infection.

Staphylococcal scalded skin syndrome

This is caused by an exfoliative staphylococcal toxin, which causes separation of the epidermal skin through the granular cell layers. It mainly affects infants and young children, who develop fever and malaise and may have a purulent, crusting, and localized infection around the eyes, nose, and mouth with subsequent widespread erythema and tenderness of the skin. Areas of epidermis separate on gentle pressure (Nikolsky sign), leaving denuded areas of skin (Fig. 15.11), which subsequently dry and heal, generally without scarring. Management is with an intravenous antistaphylococcal antibiotic (e.g. flucloxacillin), analgesia, and monitoring of hydration and fluid balance.

> **Summary**
>
> **Staphylococcal and streptococcal infections**
> - Symptoms are caused by direct invasion of bacteria or by release of toxins.
> - Can cause a broad range of diseases, including toxic shock syndrome.
> - Immune-mediated diseases following streptococcal infections include glomerulonephritis and rheumatic fever.
> - Impetigo is highly contagious.
> - Periorbital cellulitis should be treated aggressively with intravenous antibiotics to prevent spread to the orbit or brain.
> - Scalded skin syndrome is a rare but serious disease.

Common viral infections

Many of the common childhood infections present with a fever and rash (Table 15.2). Incubation periods vary from 24 hours to 48 hours for viral gastroenteritis to about 2 weeks for chickenpox, but for some diseases, such as HIV, the length of time between exposure and the development of symptomatic illness may extend to many years.

The infectious period characteristically begins a day or two before the rash appears and, for purposes of nursery/school exclusion, is generally considered to last until the rash has resolved or the lesions have

Table 15.2 Causes of fever and a rash

Maculopapular rash:			Vesicular, bullous, pustular	
Viral	Human herpes virus-6 (HHV-6) or HHV-7 (roseola infantum) – *<2 years old*		Viral	Varicella zoster virus – chickenpox, shingles
	Enterovirus rash			Herpes simplex virus
	Parvovirus (slapped cheek) – *usually school age*			Coxsackie virus – hand, foot and mouth
	Measles – *uncommon if immunized*		Bacterial	Impetigo – *characteristic crusting*
	Rubella – *uncommon if immunized*			Boils
Bacterial	Scarlet fever (group A streptococcus)			Staphylococcal bullous impetigo
	Rheumatic fever – erythema marginatum			Staphylococcal scalded skin
	Salmonella typhi (typhoid fever) – *classically rose spots*		Other	Erythema multiforme; Stevens–Johnson syndrome; toxic epidermal necrolysis
	Lyme disease – erythema migrans		**Petechial, purpuric**	
Other	Kawasaki disease		Bacterial	Meningococcal, other bacterial sepsis
	Systemic onset juvenile idiopathic arthritis			Infective endocarditis
			Viral	Enteroviruses, adenoviruses, and other viral infections
			Other	Henoch–Schönlein purpura
				Thrombocytopenia
				Vasculitis
				Malaria

dried up, although this varies depending on the infectious agent. For details about incubation and exclusion periods, see the Public Health England website.

The human herpesviruses

There are currently eight known HHVs: HSV-1 and HSV-2, VZV, cytomegalovirus (CMV), EBV, HHV-6, HHV-7, and HHV-8. HHV-8 is associated with Kaposi sarcoma in HIV-infected individuals. The other herpesviruses will be discussed in this section, in order of their prevalence.

The hallmark of most herpesviruses is that, after primary infection, latency is established and there is long-term persistence of the virus within the host, usually in a dormant state. After certain stimuli, re-activation of infection may occur.

Herpes simplex virus infections

HSV usually enters the body through the mucous membranes or skin, and the site of the primary infection may be associated with intense local mucosal damage. HSV-1 is usually associated with lip and skin lesions, and HSV-2 more commonly with genital lesions, but both viruses can cause both types of disease. The wide variety of clinical manifestations are described in the following sections. Treatment is with aciclovir, a viral DNA polymerase inhibitor, which may be used to treat severe symptomatic skin, ophthalmic, cerebral, and systemic infections.

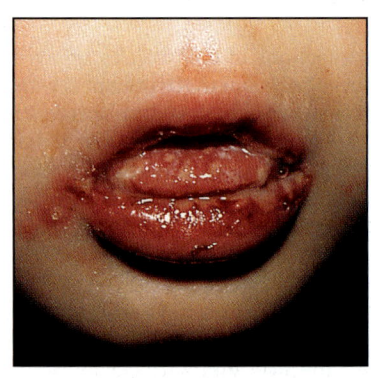

Figure 15.12 Vesicles with ulceration in gingivostomatitis.

Asymptomatic

Herpes simplex infections are very common and are mostly asymptomatic.

Gingivostomatitis

This is the most common form of primary HSV illness in children. It usually occurs from 10 months to 3 years of age. There are vesicular lesions on the lips, gums, and anterior surfaces of the tongue and hard palate, which often progress to extensive, painful ulceration with bleeding (Fig. 15.12). There is a high fever and the child is very miserable. The illness may persist for up to 2 weeks. Eating and drinking are painful, which may lead to dehydration. Management is symptomatic, but severe disease may necessitate intravenous fluids and aciclovir.

Skin manifestations

Mucocutaneous junctions and damaged skin are particularly prone to infection. 'Cold sores' are recurrent HSV lesions on the gingival/lip margin.

Eczema herpeticum – In this serious condition, widespread vesicular lesions develop on eczematous skin (Fig. 15.13). This may be complicated by secondary bacterial infection, which may result in septicaemia.

Herpetic whitlows – These are painful, erythematous, oedematous white pustules on the site of broken skin, typically on fingers. Spread is by autoinoculation from gingivostomatitis and infected adults kissing their children's fingers. A less common cause is contact with genital herpetic lesions.

Eye disease

HSV may cause blepharitis or conjunctivitis. It may extend to involve the cornea, producing dendritic ulceration. This can lead to corneal scarring and ultimately loss of vision. Any child with herpetic lesions near or involving the eye requires urgent ophthalmic assessment involving examination of the cornea by slit lamp examination.

Disseminated infection

Neonatal HSV infection (see Ch. 11) – The infection may be focal, affecting the skin or eyes, or encephalitis, or may be disseminated. Its morbidity and mortality are high.

Infection in the immunocompromised host – Infection may be severe. Cutaneous lesions may spread to involve adjacent sites, e.g. oesophagitis and proctitis. Pneumonia and disseminated infections involving multiple organs are serious complications.

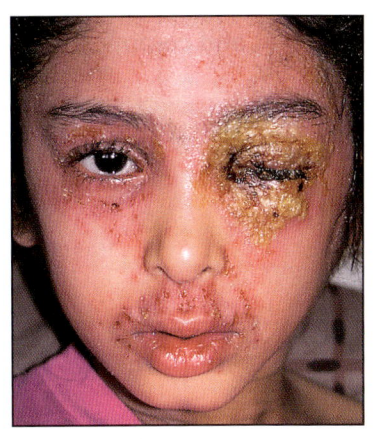

Figure 15.13 Eczema herpeticum.

Chickenpox (primary varicella zoster infection)

Clinical features

These are shown in Fig. 15.14.

There are a number of rare but serious complications that can occur in previously healthy children

- *Secondary bacterial infection* with staphylococci, group A streptococci, or other organisms. May lead to further complications such as toxic shock syndrome or necrotizing fasciitis. Secondary bacterial infection should be considered where there is onset of a new fever or persistent high fever after the first few days.
- *Encephalitis* – this may be generalized, usually occurring early during the illness. In contrast to the encephalitis caused by HSV, the prognosis is good. Most characteristic is a VZV-associated cerebellitis. This usually occurs about a week after the onset of rash. The child is ataxic with cerebellar signs. It usually resolves within a month.
- *Purpura fulminans* – this is the consequence of vasculitis in the skin and subcutaneous tissues. It is best known in relation to meningococcal disease and can lead to loss of large areas of skin by necrosis. It may rarely occur after VZV infection due to production of antiviral antibodies, which cross-react and inactivate the inhibitory coagulation factors protein C or protein S. This results in an increased risk of clotting, which most often manifests as purpuric skin rash.

In the immunocompromised host, primary varicella infection may result in severe progressive disseminated disease, which has a mortality of up to 20%. The vesicular eruptions persist and may become haemorrhagic. The disease in the neonatal period is described in Chapter 10.

Treatment and prevention

Oral aciclovir has highly variable absorption and therefore limited benefit, and is not recommended in the UK. Immunocompromised children should be treated with intravenous aciclovir initially. Oral valaciclovir can be substituted at a later point if organ dissemination has not occurred. Human varicella zoster immunoglobulin

---

Summary

Herpes simplex virus infections
- Most are asymptomatic.
- Gingivostomatitis – may necessitate intravenous fluids and aciclovir.
- Skin manifestations – mucocutaneous junctions, e.g. lips and damaged skin.
- Eczema herpeticum – may result in secondary bacterial infection and septicaemia.
- Herpetic whitlows – painful pustules on the fingers.
- Eye disease – blepharitis, conjunctivitis, and corneal ulceration.
- CNS – aseptic meningitis, encephalitis.
- Pneumonia and disseminated infection in the immunocompromised.

Clinical features and complications of chickenpox

Exposure
Spread by respiratory droplets
Highly infectious during viral shedding

Illness

Viral shedding

Days: incubation 10–23 (median 14)   −2 −1 0 1 2 3 4 5 6 7

Temp (°C): 40°C – 37°C

Papules
Vesicles
Pustules
Crusts

Rash comes in crops for 3–5 days

Complications

Bacterial superinfection
Staphylococcal
Streptococcal
May lead to toxic shock syndrome or necrotizing fasciitis

Central nervous system
Cerebellitis
Generalized encephalitis
Aseptic meningitis

Immunocompromised
Haemorrhagic lesions
Pneumonitis
Progressive and disseminated infection
Disseminated intravascular coagulation

Typical vesicular rash
50–500 lesions start on head and trunk, progress to peripheries. (But may be just a few lesions.)
Appear as crops of papules, vesicles with surrounding erythema **(Fig. 15.14a)** and pustules at different times for up to one week.
Lesions may occur on the palate.
Itchy and scratching; may result in permanent, depigmented scar formation or secondary infection.
New lesions appearing beyond 10 days suggest defective cellular immunity

(a)

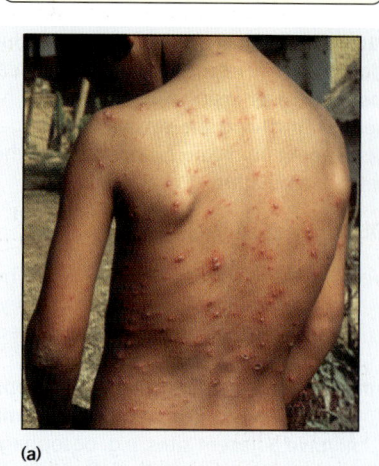

Figure 15.14 Clinical features and complications of chickenpox. (**a**) Vesicles ith surrounding erythema appearing in crops are characteristic of chickenpox.

> Watch for the child with chickenpox whose fever initially settles, but then recurs a few days later – this is likely to be due to secondary bacterial infection

> Beware of admitting a chickenpox contact to a clinical area with immunocompromised children, in whom it can disseminate and cause potentially fatal disease

is recommended for high-risk immunocompromised individuals with deficient T-cell function following contact with chickenpox. Protection from infection with human varicella zoster immunoglobulin is not absolute, and depends on how soon after contact with chickenpox it is given.

Shingles (herpes zoster)

Shingles is uncommon in children. It is caused by reactivation of latent VZV, causing a vesicular eruption in the dermatomal distribution of sensory nerves. It occurs most commonly in the thoracic region, although any dermatome can be affected (Fig. 15.15). Children, unlike adults, rarely suffer neuralgic pain with shingles. Shingles in childhood is more common in those who had primary varicella zoster infection in the 1st year of life. Recurrent or multidermatomal shingles is strongly associated with underlying immunocompromise, e.g. HIV infection. In the immunocompromised individuals, reactivated infection can also disseminate to cause severe disease.

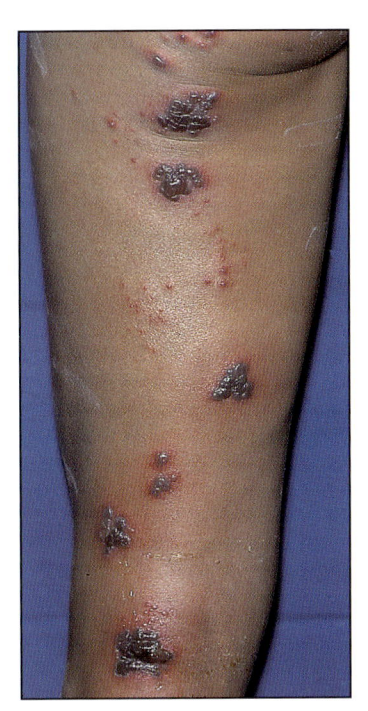

Figure 15.15 Herpes zoster (shingles) in a child. Distribution is along the S1 dermatome. (Courtesy of Dr Sam Walters.)

☼ **Recurrent or multidermatomal shingles suggests a primary or secondary T-cell immune defect**

Summary

Chickenpox
- Clinical features – fever and itchy, vesicular rash, which crops for up to 7 days.
- Complications – secondary bacterial infection, encephalitis; disseminated disease in the immunocompromised.
- Human varicella zoster immunoglobulin – if immunocompromised and in contact with chickenpox or if there is maternal chickenpox shortly before or after delivery.
- Treatment is mainly supportive; intravenous aciclovir for severe chickenpox and for immunocompromised children.

Epstein–Barr virus: infectious mononucleosis (glandular fever)

EBV is the causative agent of infectious mononucleosis, but it is also involved in the pathogenesis of Burkitt lymphoma, lymphoproliferative disease in immunocompromised hosts, and nasopharyngeal carcinoma. The virus has a particular tropism for B lymphocytes and epithelial cells of the oropharynx. Transmission usually occurs by oral contact and the majority of infections are subclinical.

Older children, and occasionally young children, may develop a syndrome with:

- fever
- malaise
- tonsillitis/pharyngitis – often severe, limiting fluid and food intake; rarely, breathing may be compromised
- lymphadenopathy – prominent cervical lymph nodes, often with diffuse lymphadenopathy elsewhere.

Other possible features include:

- petechiae on the soft palate
- splenomegaly (50%), hepatomegaly (10%)
- a maculopapular rash (5%)
- jaundice.

Diagnosis is supported by:

- atypical lymphocytes (numerous large T cells seen on blood film)
- a positive monospot test (the presence of heterophile antibodies, i.e. antibodies that agglutinate sheep or horse erythrocytes, but which are not absorbed by guinea pig kidney extracts – this test is often negative in young children with the disease)
- seroconversion with production of three antibodies: viral capsid antigen antibodies (VCA) IgG and IgM, and EB nuclear antigen (EBNA) antibodies.

Symptoms may persist for 1 month to 3 months but ultimately resolve. Fatigue is often a prominent feature in adolescents and adults.

Treatment is symptomatic. When the airway is severely compromised, corticosteroids may be considered. In 5% of infected individuals, group A streptococcus is grown from the tonsils. This may be treated with penicillin. Ampicillin or amoxicillin can cause a florid maculopapular rash in children infected with EBV and should therefore be avoided.

Cytomegalovirus

CMV is usually transmitted via saliva, genital secretions, or breastmilk, and more rarely via blood products and organ transplants as well as transplacentally. The virus causes mild or subclinical infection in normal paediatric and adult hosts. In high-income countries, about half of the adult population show serological evidence of past infection. In low-income countries, most children have been infected by 2 years of age, often via breastmilk. In the immunocompromised host and the developing fetus, CMV is an important pathogen that can cause considerable morbidity.

CMV may cause a mononucleosis-like syndrome. Pharyngitis and lymphadenopathy are not usually as prominent as in EBV infections. Patients may have atypical lymphocytes on the blood film but are heterophile antibody negative. Maternal CMV infection may result in congenital CMV infection (see Ch. 10), which may be present at birth or manifest at an older age. In the immunocompromised host, CMV can cause retinitis, pneumonitis, bone marrow failure, encephalitis, hepatitis, oesophagitis, and enterocolitis. It is a very important pathogen following bone marrow and organ transplantation. Transplant recipients are closely monitored for evidence of CMV reactivation by sensitive tests such as blood PCR. Interventions used to reduce the risk of transmission of CMV include the use of CMV-negative blood for transfusions and antiviral prophylaxis (ganciclovir); also, if possible, transplant of CMV-positive organs into CMV-negative recipients is avoided.

CMV disease may be treated with intravenous ganciclovir, oral valganciclovir, or foscarnet, but each of these drugs can cause serious side-effects.

Human herpesvirus 6 and human herpesvirus 7

HHV-6 and HHV-7 are closely related and have similar presentations, although HHV-6 is more prevalent. Most children are infected with HHV-6 or HHV-7 by the age of 2 years, usually from the oral secretions of a family member. They classically cause exanthema subitum (also known as roseola infantum), characterized by a high fever with malaise lasting a few days, followed by a generalized macular rash, which appears as the fever wanes. Many children have a febrile illness without rash, and many have a subclinical infection. Exanthema subitum is frequently clinically misdiagnosed as measles or rubella; these infections are rare in the UK and if suspected should be confirmed serologically. Another frequent occurrence in primary HHV-6 infection is that infants seen by a doctor during the febrile stage are prescribed antibiotics, and when the rash appears, it is erroneously attributed to an 'allergic' reaction to the drug. Rarely, they may cause aseptic meningitis, encephalitis, hepatitis, or a mononucleosis-like syndrome.

Human parvovirus B19

Human parvovirus B19 (HPV-B19) causes erythema infectiosum or fifth disease (so-named because it was the fifth disease to be described of a group of illnesses with similar rashes), also referred to as 'slapped-cheek syndrome'. Infections can occur at any time of the year, although outbreaks are most common during the spring. Transmission is via respiratory secretions from affected patients, by vertical transmission from mother to fetus and by transfusion of infected blood products. HPV-B19 infects the erythroblastoid red cell precursors in the bone marrow.

HPV-B19 causes a range of clinical syndromes:

- asymptomatic infection – common; about 5% to 10% of preschool children and 65% of adults have antibodies
- erythema infectiosum – the most common illness, with a viraemic phase of fever, malaise, headache, and myalgia followed by a characteristic rash on the face (slapped-cheek) a week later, progressing to a maculopapular, 'lace'-like rash on the trunk and limbs; complications are rare in children, although arthralgia or arthritis are relatively common in adults
- aplastic crisis – the most serious consequence of HPV-B19 infection; it occurs in children with chronic haemolytic anaemias, where there is an increased rate of red cell turnover (e.g. sickle cell disease or thalassaemia); and in immunocompromised children (e.g. with malignancy) who are unable to produce an antibody response to neutralize the infectious agent
- fetal disease – transmission of maternal HPV-B19 infection may lead to fetal hydrops and death due to severe anaemia, although the majority of infected fetuses will recover.

> **Summary**
>
> **Parvovirus**
> - Usually asymptomatic or erythema infectiosum.
> - Can cause aplastic crisis in patients with haemolytic anaemia (e.g. sickle cell disease and thalassaemia) or the fetus (fetal hydrops).

Enteroviruses

Human enteroviruses, of which there are many (including the coxsackie viruses, echoviruses, and polioviruses), are a common cause of childhood infection. Transmission is primarily by the faecal–oral and respiratory droplet routes. Following replication in the pharynx and gut, the virus spreads to infect other organs. Infections occur most commonly in the summer and autumn. Over 90% of infections are asymptomatic or cause a nonspecific febrile illness, sometimes with a rash usually over the trunk that is blanching or consists of fine petechiae. Some children have a history of loose stools or vomiting, or a contact history. The child is not usually systemically unwell, but if the rash is non-blanching, admission for observation and parenteral antibiotics (such as ceftriaxone) until negative blood cultures have ruled out sepsis is indicated.

Other characteristic clinical syndromes exist and are listed in the following sections. (For polioviruses, see the 'Immunization' section.)

Hand, foot, and mouth disease

Painful vesicular lesions on the hands, feet, mouth, and tongue, and often also on the buttocks. Systemic features are generally mild. The disease subsides within a few days.

Herpangina

Vesicular and ulcerated lesions on the soft palate and uvula causing anorexia, pain on swallowing, and fever. Severe cases may require intravenous fluids and appropriate analgesia.

Meningitis/encephalitis

In high-income countries, enteroviruses are the most common cause of viral meningitis. Long-term neurological sequelae are rare; the majority of cases make a full recovery.

Pleurodynia (Bornholm disease)
An acute illness with fever, pleuritic chest pain, and muscle tenderness. There may be a pleural rub, but examination is otherwise normal. Recovery occurs within a few days.

Myocarditis and pericarditis
Both manifestations are rare. Affected children may present with chest pain and/or heart failure associated with a febrile illness and evidence of myocarditis on ECG.

Enteroviral neonatal sepsis syndrome
This rare syndrome occurs in the first few weeks of life, and predominately results from transplacental or intrapartum infection of the infant. It is thought that transplacental infection results in very high viral loads, and the symptoms are consequently often very severe, mimicking bacterial sepsis. Affected infants may present with hypotension and multiorgan failure, requiring intensive care support. Currently, there are no antiviral drugs that are effective against enteroviruses; the use of intravenous immunoglobulin remains controversial.

> **Summary**
>
> **Enterovirus infection**
> - Mostly asymptomatic or self-limiting illness with rash, which may be petechial.
> - Can cause hand, foot, and mouth disease; herpangina; meningitis/encephalitis; myocarditis/pericarditis; and neonatal sepsis syndrome.

Uncommon viral infections

Measles
Health practitioners in the UK need to be aware of measles due to the rise in cases following public anxiety about the MMR vaccination, which resulted in low immunization coverage (see the 'Immunization' section), as well as it continuing to be a major cause of morbidity and death worldwide. As with chickenpox and HPV-B19, older children and adults tend to have more severe disease than the very young. For epidemiological tracking of infection, PCR-based or serological confirmation of clinical cases of measles should be undertaken by testing either blood or saliva.

Clinical features
These are shown in Fig. 15.16. There are a number of serious complications that can occur in previously healthy children

- *Encephalitis* occurs in about 1 in 5000 cases, a few days after the onset of the illness. Initial symptoms are headache, lethargy, and irritability, proceeding to seizures and ultimately coma. Mortality is 15%. Serious long-term sequelae include seizures, deafness, hemiplegia, and severe learning difficulties, affecting up to 40% of survivors.
- *SSPE* is a rare but devastating illness manifesting, on average, 7 years after measles infection in about 1 in 100 000 cases. Most children who develop SSPE had primary measles infection before 2 years of age. SSPE is caused by a variant of the measles virus, which persists in the CNS. The disorder presents with loss of neurological function, which progresses over several years to dementia and death. The diagnosis is essentially clinical, supported by finding high levels of measles antibody in both blood and CSF, and by characteristic electroencephalogram abnormalities. Since the introduction of immunization against measles, it has become extremely rare.

In low-income countries, where malnutrition and vitamin A deficiency lead to impaired cell-mediated immunity, measles often follows a protracted course with severe complications. Impaired cellular immune responses such as in HIV infection may result in a modified or absence of rash, with an increased risk of dissemination, including giant-cell pneumonia or encephalitis.

Treatment
Treatment for measles is supportive. Children who are admitted to hospital should be isolated. In immunocompromised patients, the antiviral drug ribavirin may be used. Vitamin A, which may modulate the immune response, should be given in low-income countries.

Prevention
Prevention by immunization is the most successful strategy for reducing the morbidity and mortality of measles.

> Measles remains a major cause of death in childhood in low-income countries

> **Summary**
>
> **Measles**
> - Incidence has declined dramatically since immunization was introduced; a recent small increase has resulted from the decline in immunization uptake.
> - Clinical features: fever, cough, runny nose, conjunctivitis, marked malaise, Koplik spots, and maculopapular rash.
> - Complications: common if malnourished or immunocompromised; major cause of death in low-income countries.

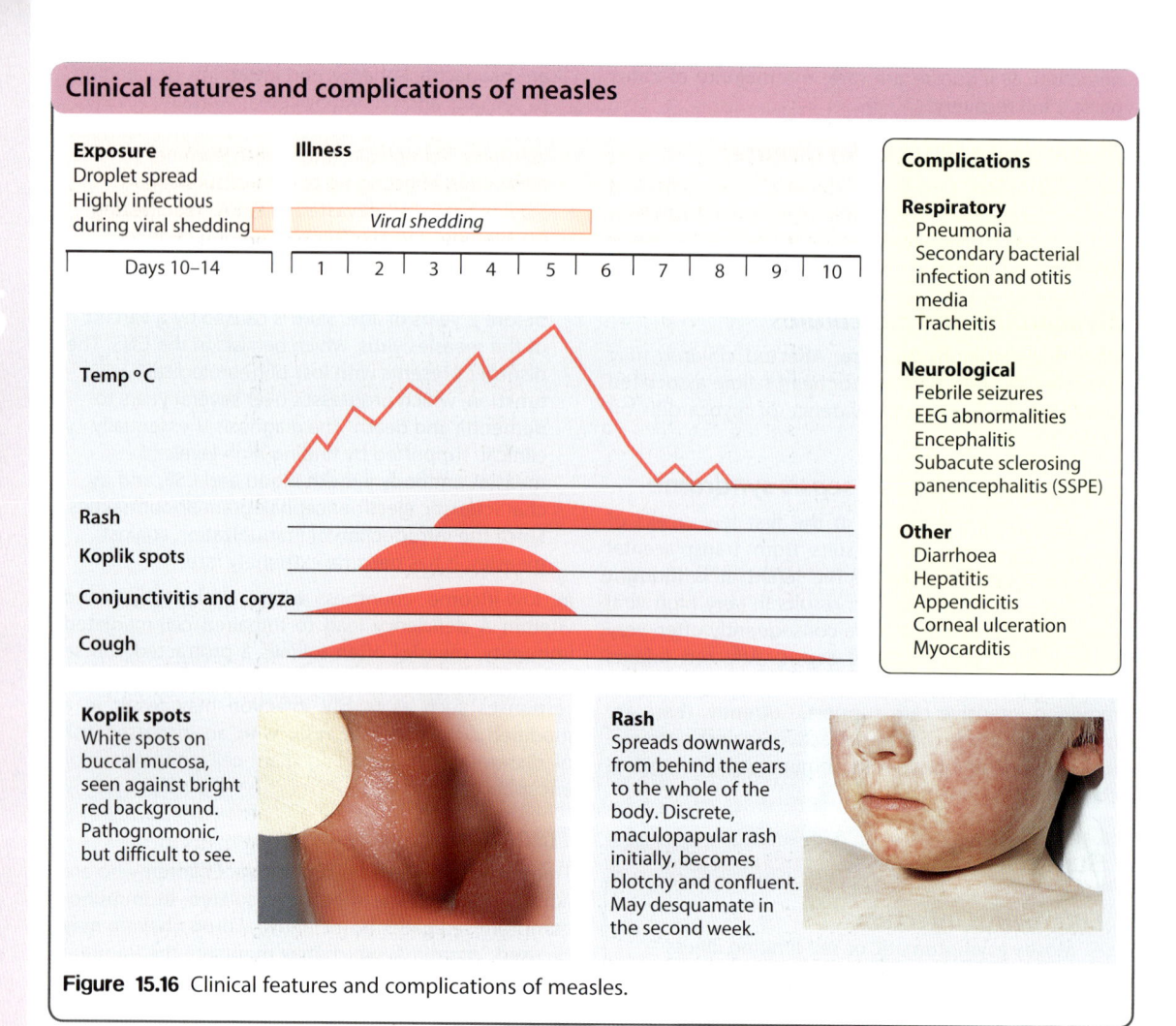

Clinical features and complications of measles

Exposure
Droplet spread
Highly infectious during viral shedding

Illness
Viral shedding

Complications

Respiratory
 Pneumonia
 Secondary bacterial infection and otitis media
 Tracheitis

Neurological
 Febrile seizures
 EEG abnormalities
 Encephalitis
 Subacute sclerosing panencephalitis (SSPE)

Other
 Diarrhoea
 Hepatitis
 Appendicitis
 Corneal ulceration
 Myocarditis

Koplik spots
White spots on buccal mucosa, seen against bright red background. Pathognomonic, but difficult to see.

Rash
Spreads downwards, from behind the ears to the whole of the body. Discrete, maculopapular rash initially, becomes blotchy and confluent. May desquamate in the second week.

Figure 15.16 Clinical features and complications of measles.

Mumps

Mumps occurs worldwide, but its incidence has declined dramatically because of the mumps component of the MMR vaccine. Following the decrease in the uptake of the MMR immunization in the late 1990s, there has been a rise in unimmunized children and young adults. Mumps usually occurs in the winter and spring months. It is spread by droplet infection to the respiratory tract where the virus replicates within epithelial cells. The virus gains access to the parotid glands before further dissemination to other tissues.

Clinical features

The incubation period is 15 days to 24 days. Onset of the illness is with fever, malaise, and parotitis, but in up to 30% of cases, the infection is subclinical. Only one side of the face may be swollen initially, but bilateral parotid involvement may occur over the next few days. The parotitis is uncomfortable and children may complain of earache or pain on eating or drinking. Examination of the parotid duct may show redness and swelling. Occasionally, parotid swelling may be absent. The fever usually disappears within 3 days to 4 days. Plasma amylase levels are often elevated due to parotid inflammation, and, when associated with abdominal pain, there may be evidence of pancreatic involvement. Infectivity is for up to 7 days after the onset of parotid swelling. The illness is generally mild and self-limiting. Although hearing loss can rarely follow mumps, it is usually unilateral and transient.

Viral meningitis and encephalitis

Lymphocytes are seen in the CSF in about 50%, meningeal signs are only seen in 10%, and encephalitis in about 1 in 5000 cases. The common clinical features are headache, photophobia, vomiting, and neck stiffness.

Orchitis

This is the most feared complication, although it is uncommon in prepubertal males. When it does occur, it is usually unilateral. Although there is some evidence of a reduction in sperm count, infertility is actually very unusual. Rarely, oophoritis, mastitis, and arthritis may occur.

Rubella (German measles)

Rubella is generally a mild disease in childhood. It typically occurs in the winter and spring. It is an important infection, as it can cause severe damage to the fetus (see Ch. 10). The incubation period is 15 days to 20 days. It is spread by the respiratory route, frequently from a known contact. The prodrome is usually mild with a low-grade fever or none at all. The maculopapular rash is often the first sign of infection, appearing initially on the face and then spreading centrifugally to cover the whole body. It fades in 3 days to 5 days. Lymphadenopathy, particularly the suboccipital and postauricular nodes, is prominent. Complications are rare in childhood but include arthritis, encephalitis, thrombocytopenia, and myocarditis. Clinical differentiation from other viral infections (including enteroviruses) is unreliable. The diagnosis should be confirmed serologically if there is any risk of exposure of a nonimmune pregnant woman. There is no effective antiviral treatment. Prevention therefore lies in immunization.

> **Summary**
>
> **Rubella**
> Generally, a mild illness, but can cause devastating congenital infection.

Prolonged fever

Most childhood infections are acute and resolve in a few days. If not, the child needs to be reassessed for complications of the original illness, e.g. a secondary bacterial infection, or the source of infection may not have been identified, e.g. urinary tract infection. Often, the child has developed another unrelated febrile illness. Assessment of prolonged fever is also required for prompt recognition of Kawasaki disease to avoid complications. Causes of prolonged fever are listed in Box 15.2.

Kawasaki disease

Kawasaki disease is a systemic vasculitis. Although uncommon, it is important to establish the diagnosis early, because aneurysms of the coronary arteries are a potentially devastating complication. Prompt treatment reduces their incidence.

Kawasaki disease mainly affects children of 6 months to 4 years of age, with a peak at the end of the 1st year of life. The disease is more common in children of Japanese and, to a lesser extent, Black-Caribbean ethnicity, than in Caucasians. Young infants are often very miserable and tend to be more severely affected than older children and are more likely to have 'incomplete' symptoms, in which not all the cardinal features are present. The aetiology of Kawasaki disease remains unknown.

There is no diagnostic test; instead, the diagnosis is made based on clinical findings alone (Fig. 15.17). In addition to the classic features, affected children are strikingly irritable, have a high fever that is difficult to control, and may also have inflammation of their BCG (bacillus Calmette–Guérin) vaccination scar. They have high inflammatory markers (C-reactive protein,

> **Box 15.2** Causes of prolonged fever
>
> ***Infective***
> - Localized infection: e.g. osteomyelitis
> - Bacterial infections: e.g. typhoid, *Bartonella henselae* (cat scratch disease), *Brucella* species
> - Deep abscesses: e.g. intra-abdominal, retroperitoneal, pelvic
> - Infective endocarditis
> - Tuberculosis
> - Nontuberculous mycobacterial infections: e.g. *Mycobacterium avium* complex
> - Viral infections: e.g. Epstein–Barr virus, cytomegalovirus, HIV (human immunodeficiency virus)
> - Parasitic infections: e.g. malaria, toxocariasis, *Entamoeba histolytica*
>
> ***Noninfective***
> - Systemic onset juvenile idiopathic arthritis
> - Systemic lupus erythematosus
> - Vasculitis (including Kawasaki disease)
> - Inflammatory bowel disease (Crohn's disease and ulcerative colitis)
> - Sarcoidosis
> - Malignancy: e.g. leukaemia, lymphoma, neuroblastoma, Ewing sarcoma
> - Macrophage activation syndromes: e.g. haemophagocytic lymphohistiocytosis
> - Drug fever
> - Fabricated or induced illness (including Munchausen syndrome by proxy).

erythrocyte sedimentation rate, white cell count), with a platelet count that rises typically in the 2nd week of the illness. The coronary arteries are affected in about one-third of affected children within the first 6 weeks of the illness. This can lead to aneurysms, which can be detected on echocardiography (see Case History 15.2). Subsequent narrowing of the vessels from scar formation can result in myocardial ischaemia and sudden death. Mortality is 1% to 2%.

Prompt treatment with intravenous immunoglobulin given within the first 10 days has been shown to lower the risk of coronary artery aneurysms. Aspirin is used to reduce the risk of thrombosis. It is given at a high anti-inflammatory dose until the fever subsides and inflammatory markers return to normal, and continued at a low antiplatelet dose until echocardiography at 6 weeks reveals the presence or absence of aneurysms. Children with giant coronary artery aneurysms may require long-term warfarin therapy and close follow-up. Children suspected of having the disease but who do not have all the clinical features should still be considered for treatment. Sometimes, fever recurs despite treatment and these children are given a second dose of intravenous immunoglobulin. Children with persistent inflammation and fever may require treatment with corticosteroids, infliximab (a monoclonal antibody against tumour necrosis factor-α), or cyclosporin.

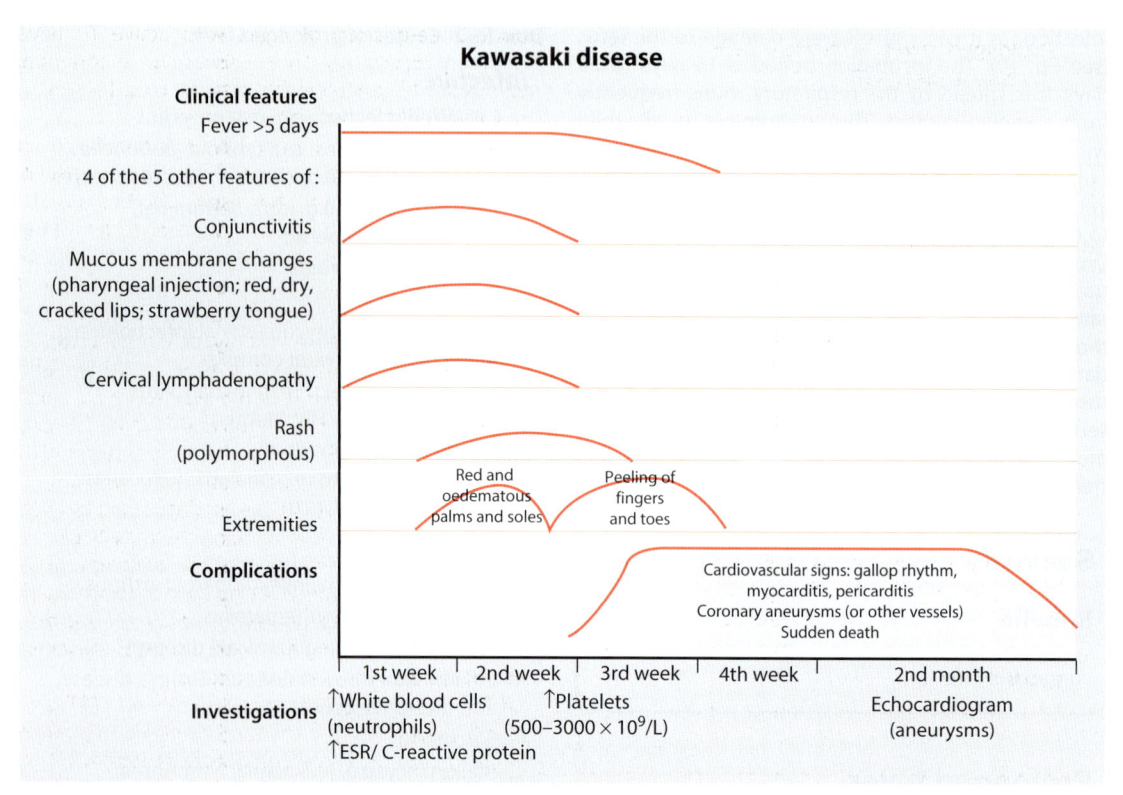

Figure 15.17 Evolution of clinical features and abnormal investigations in Kawasaki disease.

Case history 15.2

Kawasaki disease

This 2-year-old boy developed a high fever of 2 days' duration. Examination showed a miserable child with mild conjunctivitis, a rash, and cervical lymphadenopathy. A viral infection was diagnosed and his mother was reassured. When he presented to hospital 3 days later, he was noted to have cracked red lips (Fig. 15.18a). He was admitted and a full septic screen, including a lumbar puncture, was performed and antibiotics started. The following day, he was still febrile and irritable; his C-reactive protein and erythrocyte sedimentation rate were raised considerably above upper limit of normal. Kawasaki disease was suspected and he was treated with intravenous immunoglobulin and high-dose oral aspirin. His clinical condition improved and he became afebrile the following morning. An echocardiogram at this stage showed no aneurysms of the coronary arteries, which are the most serious complication associated with delayed diagnosis and treatment. On the 15th day of the illness there was peeling of the fingers and toes (Fig. 15.18b).

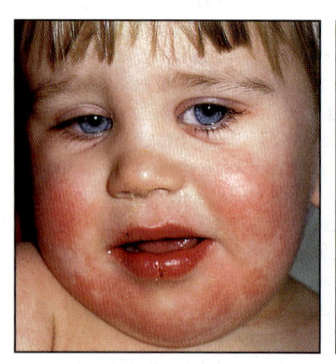

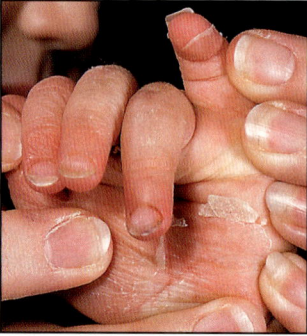

Figure 15.18 (a) Red, cracked lips and conjunctival inflammation; and (b) peeling of the fingers, which developed on the 15th day of the illness. (Courtesy of Professor Mike Levin.)

(a)   (b)

☀ Prolonged fever – check – is it Kawasaki disease?

> **Summary**
>
> **Kawasaki disease**
> - Mainly affects infants and young children.
> - The diagnosis is made on clinical features – fever over 5 days and four other features of nonpurulent conjunctivitis, red mucous membranes, cervical lymphadenopathy, rash, red and oedematous palms and soles, or peeling of fingers and toes. Children with Kawasaki disease are often strikingly miserable, which is not improved by oral antipyretic agents.
> - 'Incomplete' cases can occur, especially in infants, so a high index of suspicion should be maintained in a persistently febrile child.
> - Complications – coronary artery aneurysms and sudden death.
> - Treatment – intravenous immunoglobulin and aspirin.

Tuberculosis

The decline in the incidence and mortality from TB in developed countries was hailed as an example of how public health measures and antimicrobial therapy can dramatically modify a disease. However, TB is again becoming a public health problem, partly through its increased incidence in patients with HIV infection, and with the emergence of multidrug-resistant *Mycobacterium tuberculosis* strains (MDR-TB). Spread of TB is almost invariably by the respiratory route. Close proximity, a large infectious load in the index case (related to pulmonary cavitation and sputum smear positivity), and underlying immunodeficiency enhance the risk of transmission. There is an important distinction between latent TB (an asymptomatic infection state) and TB *disease* (active TB). Latent TB is more likely to progress to active TB in infants and young children compared with adults. In contrast to adults, children are generally not infectious, because their disease is typically paucibacillary. Children usually acquire TB from an infected adult in the same household.

Clinical features

These are outlined in Fig. 15.19.

Diagnosis

Diagnosis of TB in children is even more difficult than in adults. The clinical features of active TB are often nonspecific, such as prolonged fever, malaise, anorexia, weight loss, or focal signs of infection (e.g. lymph node swelling in TB lymphadenitis). The majority (about three-quarter) of cases with active TB have pulmonary TB; extrapulmonary disease is less common, and includes TB lymphadenitis, osteoarticular TB, genito-urinary TB, and TB meningitis.

Sputum samples are generally unobtainable from children under about 8 years of age, unless specialist induction techniques are used. Children usually swallow sputum, so gastric washings on three consecutive mornings can be used to identify *M. tuberculosis* originating from the lung, using special staining techniques for acid–fast bacilli (Ziehl–Neelsen stains or auramine stains) and mycobacterial cultures. To obtain these, a nasogastric tube is passed and secretions are washed out of the stomach with saline (before food intake). Urine, lymph node tissue, CSF, and radiological examinations should also be performed as appropriate. Although it is difficult to culture TB from children, the rise of MDR-TB makes it important to try to grow the organism so that antibiotic sensitivity can be assessed. PCR-based methods for the detection of *M. tuberculosis* are increasingly being used in parallel with mycobacterial cultures; however, these methods only provide limited information regarding drug resistance and therefore cannot replace cultures.

If TB is suspected, a tuberculin skin test (TST; also called Mantoux test) is performed by injecting purified protein derivative of tuberculin into the forearm (0.1 ml intradermal injection, read after 48 hours to 72 hours as induration measured in millimetres). Because purified protein derivative is a mixture of proteins, some of which are expressed by both *M. tuberculosis* and BCG, the TST may be positive because of past BCG vaccination rather than TB infection. Most international guidelines therefore suggest that a history of BCG immunization should be taken into account when interpreting the test result. This was also the case in previous TB guidelines in the UK, but recommendations were changed in 2016 (NICE). The new guideline states that an induration of 5 mm or more should be considered to be positive, regardless of prior BCG vaccination. Other countries use different cut-offs (typically 10 mm). Heaf tests are no longer used for screening for TB.

Interferon-gamma release assays (IGRAs) are newer, blood-based tests for TB. They assess the response of T cells to in vitro stimulation, with a small number of antigens expressed by *M. tuberculosis* but not by BCG. Positive results therefore indicate TB infection rather than BCG vaccination. However, a negative IGRA result does not reliably rule out TB infection. Also, there is increasing evidence that IGRAs perform worse in children compared with adults. Neither IGRA nor the TST can distinguish between latent TB and active TB, so correlation with clinical signs and symptoms is required.

Coinfection with HIV makes the diagnosis even more difficult. With advanced immunocompromise, both TST and IGRA can be false negative. Contact history, radiology, and possibly tissue diagnosis become even more important. One must avoid making an incorrect diagnosis of TB on chest X-ray appearances alone, as lymphoid interstitial pneumonitis can have a similar appearance and occurs in 20% of HIV-infected children. In view of the overlapping epidemiology, all individuals with TB should be tested for HIV, and vice versa.

Clinical features of TB

Primary infection

Asymptomatic

Nearly half of infants and 90% of older children have minimal or no symptoms or signs of infection. A local inflammatory reaction limits the progression of infection. However, the disease remains latent and may therefore develop into active disease at a later time. Asymptomatic children with a positive tuberculin skin test (TST) (Fig 18.19a) or interferon-gamma release assay result (i.e. latent TB) should be given chemoprophylaxis to prevent future conversion to active TB.

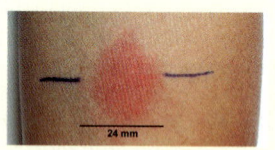

a) Example of a positive TST (24-mm induration). A TST (2 units PPD, Purified Protein Derivative) is positive if the palpable induration is 5 mm or more in diameter irrespective of whether or not had BCG immunization (NICE guidelines, 2016). Only the induration should be measured (not the surrounding erythema).

Symptomatic

In this case the local host response fails to contain inhaled *M. tuberculosis*, allowing spread via the lymphatic system to regional lymph nodes. The lung lesion plus the lymph node constitutes the 'Ghon (or primary) complex'. When the host's cellular immune system responds to the infection (3–6 weeks), mycobacterial replication diminishes but systemic symptoms develop:
- fever
- anorexia and weight loss
- cough
- chest X-ray changes (Fig. 18.19b).

The primary complex usually heals and may calcify. The inflammatory reaction may lead to local enlargement of peribronchial lymph nodes, which may cause bronchial obstruction, with collapse and consolidation of the affected lung. Pleural effusions may also be present. Further progression may be halted by the host's immunological response, or there may be local dissemination to other regions of the lung.

Although primary infection most commonly occurs in the lung, it may also involve other organs including lymph nodes, bones and joints, the genitourinary system, and the meninges.

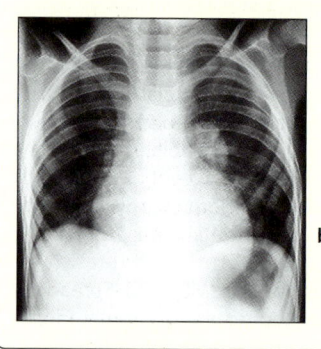

b) Chest X-ray of pulmonary TB. There is marked left hilar lymphadenopathy

Dormancy and dissemination

Both asymptomatic and symptomatic infections may become dormant but subsequently reactivate and spread by lymphohaematological routes.

Reactivation

Post-primary TB

This may present as localized disease or may be widely disseminated (called miliary TB), to sites such as bones, joints, kidneys, pericardium, and CNS. Infants and young children are particularly prone to tuberculous meningitis. This was always fatal before antimicrobial therapy was available, and is still associated with significant morbidity and mortality if treatment is not initiated early.

Figure 15.19 Clinical features of tuberculosis.

Treatment

Triple or quadruple therapy (rifampicin, isoniazid, pyrazinamide, ethambutol) is the recommended initial combination, unless MDR-TB is strongly suspected (e.g. when a household member has been recently diagnosed with MDR-TB). This is decreased to rifampicin and isoniazid alone after 2 months, by which time antibiotic sensitivities are often known. Treatment for uncomplicated pulmonary TB or TB lymphadenitis is usually for 6 months; longer treatment courses are required for osteoarticular TB, TB meningitis, or disseminated disease. In adolescents, pyridoxine is given weekly to prevent peripheral neuropathy associated with isoniazid therapy, a complication that does not occur in young children. In tuberculous meningitis, dexamethasone is given initially, to decrease the risk of long-term sequelae.

Asymptomatic children who are Mantoux or IGRA positive and therefore latently infected should also be treated (e.g. with rifampicin and isoniazid for 3 months or isoniazid alone for 6 months) as this will decrease the risk of reactivation (i.e. conversion to active TB) later in life.

Prevention and contact tracing

BCG immunization has been shown to reduce the incidence of TB, but its protective effect is incomplete (i.e. BCG-vaccinated children can still acquire TB infection). In the UK, BCG is recommended at birth for high-risk groups. The UK programme of routine BCG immunization for all tuberculin-negative children between 10 years and 14 years of age has been discontinued. BCG, which is a live vaccine, should not be given to HIV-positive or other immunocompromised children due to the risk of severe local reactions and dissemination.

As most children are infected by a household contact, it is essential to screen other family members for TB infection. Children who are exposed to individuals with pulmonary TB should be assessed for evidence of latent TB (by TST and IGRA). The latest NICE (National Institute for Health and Care Excellence) guidelines recommend that children under 2 years of age who had close contact with a sputum smear-positive pulmonary TB person should be started on prophylactic isoniazid; if the TST and the IGRA are negative at 6 weeks, isoniazid should be discontinued and the BCG vaccine should be given (unless previously immunized with BCG).

Nontuberculous mycobacterial infections

There are numerous nontuberculous mycobacteria found in the environment. Immunocompetent individuals rarely suffer from diseases caused by these organisms. They occasionally cause persistent lymphadenitis in young children, primarily affecting the cervicofacial region. Where technically possible without risk of damage to the facial nerve, the most commonly used treatment approach is complete lymph node excision, as biopsy or partial excision can result in formation of a chronic fistula and poor healing. Alternative treatment approaches are 'watchful waiting' (no intervention, as in the majority of cases spontaneous resolution occurs over several months), or treatment with antimycobacterial antibiotics. Unlike TB, these organisms are transmitted via soil and water, and therefore contact tracing is not required.

Nontuberculous mycobacteria may cause disseminated infection in immunocompromised individuals. *Mycobacterium avium-intracellulare* infections are particularly common in patients with advanced HIV disease. These infections do not respond to conventional TB treatment, and require a combination regimen of different antimycobacterial drugs. Recently, chronic pulmonary nontuberculous mycobacterial infections have become an increasing problem in adolescents and adults with cystic fibrosis. Treatment of these infections is often difficult, and only successful in some instances.

Summary

Tuberculosis

- TB affects millions of children worldwide; low but increasing incidence in many high-income countries.
- Clinical features follow a sequence – primary infection, then latency, which may be followed by conversion to active TB months to years later.
- Diagnosis is often difficult, so the decision to treat is then based on contact history, tuberculin skin test and interferon-gamma release assay results, X-ray findings, and clinical features.
- Adherence to drug therapy can be problematic but is essential for successful treatment.
- Contact tracing and identification of children with latent TB are important.
- TB is more difficult to diagnose and more likely to disseminate in immunocompromised individuals.

Tropical infections

Although tropical infections must be considered, most febrile children who have a recent travel history to a tropical region have a nontopical infection (e.g. a common viral infection). The most common or most serious imported infections are outlined in Fig. 15.20.

A febrile child returning from the tropics – most common causes are nontropical infections, but consider malaria, typhoid fever, and other tropical infections

An approach to the febrile child returning from the tropics

History
All places visited and duration of stay. immunization, malaria prophylaxis. History of food, drink (infected water), accommodation (exposure to insect vectors), infectious contacts e.g. TB, swimming (infested rivers and lakes).

Examination
Particular reference to: fever, jaundice, anaemia, enlarged liver or spleen.

Non-tropical causes of fever
Consider non-tropical causes of fever in childhood – upper and lower respiratory tract infections, gastroenteritis, urinary tract infection, septicaemia, meningitis, osteomyelitis, hepatitis, etc.

Tropical infections

Malaria

40% of the world's population live in an area where the female *Anopheles* mosquito transmits malaria. Causes over 300 000 child deaths in Africa each year, mainly from *Plasmodium falciparum* malaria. The clinical features include fever (often not cyclical), diarrhoea, vomiting, flulike symptoms, jaundice, anaemia, and thrombocytopenia. Whilst typically the onset is 7–10 days after inoculation, infections can present months later (depending on the *Plasmodium* species). Children are particularly susceptible to severe anaemia and cerebral malaria. Diagnosis is by examination of thick blood films. The species (*falciparum, vivax, ovale, malariae, or knowlesi*) is confirmed on a thin blood film. Repeated blood films may be necessary. Rapid diagnostic tests (RDTs) can also be used to establish the diagnosis.

Plasmodium falciparum is treated with quinine or artemisinin-based formulations. Travellers to endemic areas should seek up-to-date information on malaria prevention. Prophylaxis reduces but does not eliminate the risk of infection. Prevention of mosquito bites with repellants and bed nets is also important. In many countries there has been a marked reduction in the incidence of malaria in children from insecticide-treated bed nets, indoor residual spraying of houses with insecticides, destruction of mosquito larvae and breeding areas, and prompt treatment with artemisinin-based combination therapy.

Typhoid

A child with worsening fever, headaches, cough, abdominal pain, anorexia, malaise, and myalgia may be suffering from infection with *Salmonella typhi* or *paratyphi*. Gastrointestinal symptoms (diarrhoea or constipation) may not appear until the second week. Splenomegaly, bradycardia, and rose-coloured spots on the trunk may be present. The serious complications of this disease include gastrointestinal perforation, myocarditis, hepatitis, and nephritis. The recent increase in multi-drug resistant strains, particularly from the Indian subcontinent, means that treatment with cotrimoxazole, chloramphenicol or ampicillin is often inadequate. A third-generation cephalosporin or azithromycin is usually effective.

Viral infections transmitted by mosquitoes

Dengue fever is widespread in the tropics. The primary infection is characterized by a fine erythematous rash, myalgia, arthralgia, and high fever. After resolution of the fever, a secondary rash with desquamation may occur. Dengue haemorrhagic fever, (dengue shock syndrome), occurs when a previously infected child has a subsequent infection with a different strain of the virus. The partially effective host immune response augments the severity of infection causing severe capillary leak syndrome leading to hypotension as well as haemorrhagic manifestations. With fluid resuscitation, most children recover fully.

Chikungunya is endemic in parts of Africa, Asia, and India. In children, it can cause fever, arthralgia and arthritis.

Zika virus is usually transmitted by *Aedes* mosquitoes, mainly in Central and South America and the Caribbean. In children, it may cause fever, rash, conjunctivitis, and arthralgia. In pregnancy, it is associated with fetal microcephaly and other brain abnormalities.

Gastroenteritis and dysentery

Gastroenteritis frequently accompanies foreign travel. 'Traveller's diarrhoea' is commonly caused by a change in gut flora, viruses including rotavirus, and by *E. coli*. It rarely needs more than attention to rehydration. Fever accompanied by loose stools with blood or mucus suggests dysentery caused by *Shigella, Salmonella, Campylobacter,* or *Entamoeba histolytica*. Blood cultures and stool cultures should be taken and appropriate antibiotics started, if indicated.

Viral haemorrhagic fevers

Causes include the Lassa, Marburg, Ebola, and Crimean–Congo viruses. These rare infections are imported, are highly contagious, and have a high mortality. If suspected, strict isolation procedures should be initiated for any symptomatic patient who has returned from an endemic area within the 21-day incubation period of these infections. Specialist advice should be sought.

Figure 15.20 An approach to the febrile child returning from the tropics.

HIV infection

Globally, HIV infection affects over 3 million children, mostly in sub-Saharan Africa. There are still over 2 million adolescents living with HIV infection (Fig. 15.21). Though there has been a marked decline in the number of children becoming infected each year, there were still an estimated 150 000 in 2015 (Fig. 15.22). The major route of HIV infection in children is mother-to-child transmission, which occurs during pregnancy (intrauterine), at delivery (intrapartum), or through breastfeeding (postpartum). The virus may also be transmitted to children by infected blood products, contaminated needles, or through sexual abuse, but this is uncommon.

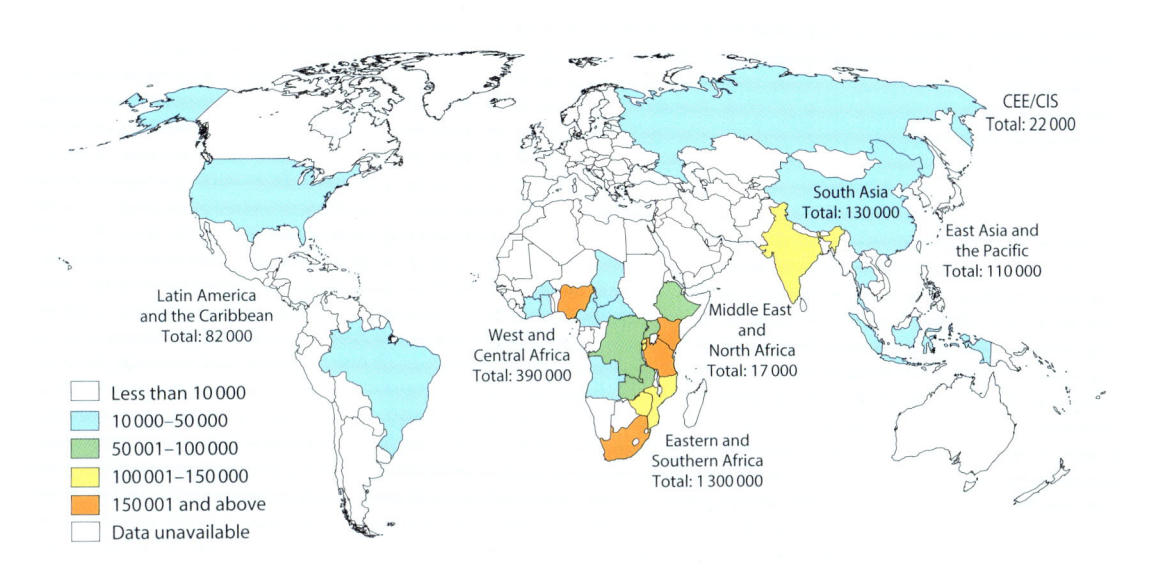

Figure 15.21 Adolescents (10–19 years) estimated to be living with human immunodeficiency virus (total estimated number: 2.1 million), 2012. (United Nations Children's Emergency Fund: *Towards an AIDS-Free Generation – Children and AIDS: Sixth Stocktaking Report, 2013*, New York, 2013, UNICEF. Reproduced with the permission of UNICEF.)

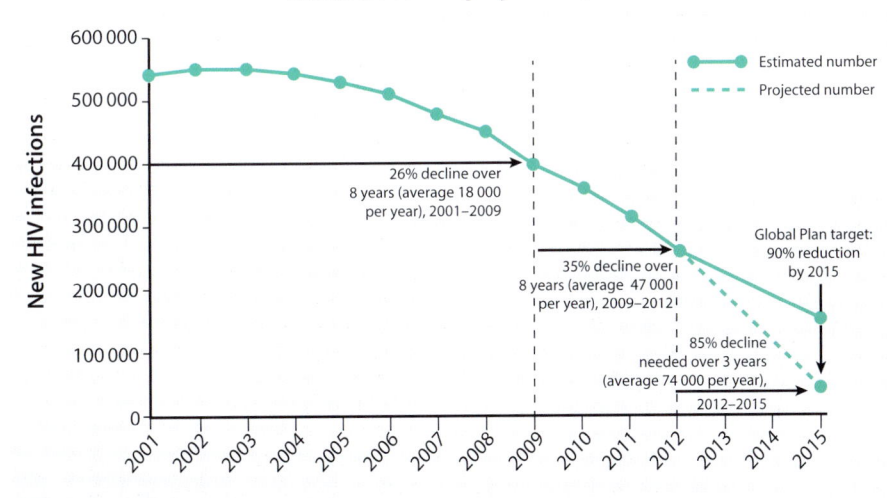

Figure 15.22 New human immunodeficiency virus (HIV) infections among children, 2001–2015 (with projected figures until 2015 of Global Plan target), showing a decline because HIV prevalence in mothers has stabilized and increasing prevention of mother-to-child transmission. (Data from United Nations Children's Emergency Fund: *Towards an AIDS-Free Generation – Children and AIDS: Sixth Stocktaking Report, 2013*, New York, 2016, UNICEF. Reproduced with the permission of UNICEF.)

Diagnosis

In children over 18 months of age, HIV infection is diagnosed by detecting antibodies against the virus. Children less than 18 months of age who are born to infected mothers will have transplacental maternal IgG HIV antibodies; therefore, at this age a positive antibody test confirms HIV exposure but not HIV infection. The most sensitive test for HIV diagnosis before 18 months of age is HIV DNA PCR. All infants born to HIV-infected mothers should be tested for HIV infection, whether or not they are symptomatic. Two negative HIV DNA PCRs within the first 3 months of life, at least 2 weeks after completion of postnatal antiretroviral therapy (ART), indicate the infant is not infected, although this is confirmed by the loss of maternal HIV antibodies from the infant's circulation after 18 months of age.

Clinical features

A proportion of HIV-infected infants progress rapidly to symptomatic disease and onset of acquired immune deficiency syndrome (AIDS) in the 1st year of life; however, other infected children remain asymptomatic for months or even years before progressing to clinical disease. Some asymptomatic children are only identified in adolescence at routine screening following diagnosis in another family member. Clinical presentation varies with the degree of immunocompromise. Children with mild immunocompromise may only have lymphadenopathy or parotid enlargement; if moderate, they may have recurrent bacterial infections, candidiasis, chronic diarrhoea, and lymphocytic interstitial pneumonitis (Fig. 15.23). This lymphocytic infiltration of the lungs may be caused by a response to the HIV infection itself, or it may be related to EBV infection. Severe AIDS diagnoses include opportunistic infections, e.g. *Pneumocystis jirovecii* (*carinii*) pneumonia (PCP), severe growth faltering, encephalopathy (Fig. 15.24), and malignancy, although the latter is rare in children. More than one clinical feature is often present. An unusual constellation of symptoms, especially if infectious, should alert one to the possibility of HIV infection.

> **Children with persistent lymphadenopathy, hepatosplenomegaly, recurrent fever, parotid swelling, thrombocytopenia, or any suggestion of serious, persistent, unusual, recurrent infections should be tested for HIV**

Treatment

A decision to start ART is based on a combination of clinical status, HIV viral load, and CD4 count, except in infants who should all start ART shortly after diagnosis, because they have a higher risk of disease progression. As in adults, combinations of three (or four) drugs are used. Prophylaxis against PCP with cotrimoxazole is prescribed for infants who are HIV-infected, and for older children with low CD4 counts.

Other aspects of management include

- Immunization, which is important because of the higher risk of infections, and should follow the routine vaccination schedule, with the exception that BCG should not be given as it is a live vaccine that can cause disseminated disease. Vaccination against influenza, hepatitis A and B, and VZV should be considered.
- Multidisciplinary management of children, if possible in a family clinic, where they can be seen together with other members of their family who may be HIV infected and where the team includes an adult specialist. The team will need to address issues such as adherence to medication, disclosure of HIV diagnosis, and planning for the future.
- Regular follow-up, with particular attention paid to weight, developmental progress, and clinical signs and symptoms of disease. Effective ART has transformed HIV infection into a chronic disease of childhood. Paediatric HIV clinics in the UK increasingly manage adolescents when there may be issues with ART adherence and need to address issues such as safe sex practices, fertility, and pregnancy.

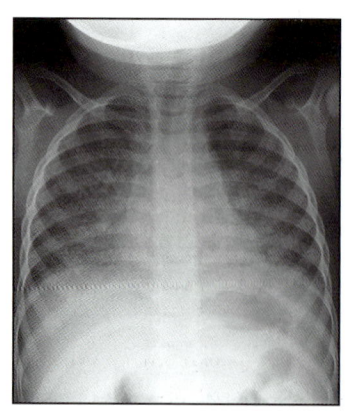

Figure 15.23 Lymphocytic interstitial pneumonitis in a child with human immunodeficiency virus infection. There is diffuse reticulonodular shadowing with hilar lymphadenopathy.

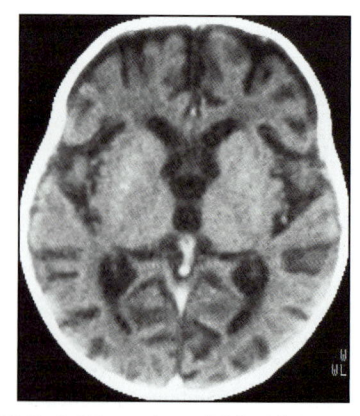

Figure 15.24 A CT scan in a child with HIV encephalopathy showing diffuse increase in cerebrospinal fluid spaces from cerebral atrophy and volume loss.

Reduction of vertical transmission

Mothers who are most likely to transmit HIV to their infants are those with a high HIV viral load and more advanced disease. Where mothers are not taking ART and breastfeed, 25% to 40% of infants become infected with HIV and it is known that avoidance of breastfeeding reduces the rate of transmission. In high-income countries, perinatal transmission of HIV has been reduced to less than 1% by using a combination of interventions:

- use of effective ART during pregnancy and intrapartum to achieve an undetectable maternal viral load at the time of delivery
- postexposure prophylaxis given to the infant after birth
- avoidance of breastfeeding
- active management of labour and delivery, to avoid prolonged rupture of the membranes and unnecessary instrumentation (e.g. forceps delivery)
- prelabour caesarean section if the mother's viral load is detectable close to the expected date of delivery.

This effective combination of interventions is not available to all women globally. Avoidance of breastfeeding is not practicable or safe in many parts of the world, where use of formula feeding increases the risk of gastroenteritis and malnutrition. It may be safer for babies in these environments to breastfeed, and ART may be given to the breastfeeding baby and/or mother to reduce the ongoing risk of mother-to-child transmission through this route.

> Antenatal antiretroviral treatment, active management of labour and delivery, and avoidance of breastfeeding can reduce the vertical transmission rate of HIV to less than 1%

Summary

HIV

- Affects over 3 million children (<15 years) worldwide.
- Treatment includes combination ART and prophylaxis against *Pneumocystis jirovecii* pneumonia.
- The majority of perinatally infected children are surviving into adulthood if ART is available and adhered to.
- Raises complex psychosocial issues for the family and healthcare providers, including when and what to tell the HIV-infected child (and the siblings), confidentiality, and adherence support.

Lyme disease

This disease, caused by the spirochaete *B. burgdorferi*, was first recognized in 1975 in a cluster of children with arthritis in Lyme, Connecticut. It also occurs in some regions in the UK and other European countries. *B. burgdorferi* is transmitted by hard ticks, which have a range of hosts but favour deer and moose. However, only in about half of the cases there is a history of a preceding tick bite. Infections occur most commonly in the summer months in rural settings.

Clinical features

Following an incubation period of 4 days to 20 days, an erythematous macule at the site of the tick bite enlarges to cause the classical skin lesion known as erythema migrans, a painless red expanding lesion with a bright red outer spreading edge. During early disease, the skin lesion is often accompanied by fever, headache, malaise, myalgia, arthralgia, and lymphadenopathy. Usually, these features fluctuate over several weeks and then resolve. Dissemination of infection in the early stages is rare, but may lead to cranial nerve palsies, meningitis, arthritis, or carditis.

The late stage of Lyme disease occurs after weeks to months with neurological, cardiac, and joint manifestations. Neurological disease includes meningoencephalitis and cranial (particularly facial nerve) and peripheral neuropathies. Cardiac disease includes myocarditis and heart block. Joint disease occurs in about 50% of cases and varies from brief migratory arthralgia to acute asymmetric monoarthritis and oligoarthritis of the large joints. Recurrent attacks of arthritis are common. In 10% of cases, chronic erosive joint disease occurs months to years after the initial attack.

Diagnosis

This is based on clinical and epidemiological features and serology. Serology may be negative in early disease, so repeat serological testing after 2 weeks to 4 weeks is advised. Isolation of the organism is difficult.

Treatment

The drug of choice for early uncomplicated cases over 12 years of age is doxycycline, and for younger children, amoxicillin. Intravenous treatment with ceftriaxone is required for carditis or neurological disease.

Immunization

Immunization is one of the most effective and economic public health measures to improve the health of both children and adults. The most notable success has been the worldwide eradication of smallpox achieved in 1979, and the prevalence of many other diseases, including polio, has been dramatically reduced.

Differences exist in the composition and scheduling of immunization programmes in different countries, and schedules change as new vaccines become available.

Immunization schedule in the UK (2016)

	Birth	1 month	2 months	3 months	4 months	1 year	2–7 years	3 years 4 months	12–13 years	14 years
BCG	BCG if at risk									
Hep B	Hep B if at risk	Hep B if at risk	Hep B if at risk			Hep B if at risk				
Diphtheria, tetanus, pertussis, polio, Haemophilus influenzae type B (DTaP/IPV/Hib)			5 in 1	5 in 1	5 in 1					
Pneumococcal conjugate vaccine (PCV)			PCV		PCV	PCV				
Rotavirus (oral)			Rotavirus	Rotavirus						
Meningococcal B vaccine (MenB)			MenB		MenB	MenB				
Meningococcal group C (MenC/MenACWY)										MenACWY
Hib/MenC						Hib/Men C				
MMR						MMR		MMR		
Intranasal influenza vaccine (annual from 2-6 years)							Flu vaccine			
Diphtheria, tetanus, pertussis, polio, (DTaP/IPV)								4 in 1		
Human papilloma-virus (HPV) Girls only, 2 doses 6 months apart									HPV	
Diphtheria tetanus, polio (Td/IPV)										3 in 1

Figure 15.25 Immunization schedule in the UK. (Available at: https://www.gov.uk/government/uploads/system/uploads/attachment_data/file/533863/PHE_2016_Routine_Childhood_Immunisation_Schedule_SUMMER2016.pdf Crown copyright)

The current UK schedule (Fig. 15.25) is available on the Department of Health website.
In summary:

- BCG is given to newborn infants at high risk of TB infection
- the '5 in 1' vaccine is given, against diphtheria, tetanus, pertussis, Hib and inactivated (killed) polio – at 2 months, 3 months, and 4 months of age. The oral, live polio vaccine has been replaced owing to the risk of vaccine-associated polio in the vaccinated person and unvaccinated family members or immunodeficient people following contact with gastrointestinal excretions of the vaccinated person
- pneumococcal conjugate vaccine (PCV13) is given at 2 months, 4 months, and 12 months of age
- meningococcal B vaccine is given at 2 months, 4 months, and 12 months of age
- rotavirus vaccine is given orally at 2 months and 3 months of age
- booster Hib and MenC, a conjugate vaccine against group C meningococcus is given at 1 year
- MMR against measles, mumps and rubella is given at 1 year and 3 years 4 months
- HPV, human papillomavirus vaccine, is given to girls at 12 years to 13 years of age.
- meningococcal ACWY conjugate vaccine is given at 14 years

Rationale behind the immunization programme

Diphtheria – infection causes local disease with membrane formation affecting the nose, pharynx, or larynx, or systemic disease with myocarditis and neurological manifestations. Immunization has practically eradicated the disease in the UK (Fig. 15.26a).

Pertussis – clinical features are described in Chapter 17. Marked decline in incidence with immunization, but epidemics recur when immunization rates fall (Fig. 15.26b). Following an increased number of infants less than 3 months with pertussis in the UK, pregnant women are now recommended to have pertussis immunization from 20 weeks gestation (booster dTaP/IPV)

Hib – causes invasive disease primarily in young children. The number of reports of infection dropped dramatically after the introduction of the Hib vaccine (Fig. 15.26c), but a gradual rise from 1988 occurred because protection was not maintained throughout childhood. This was addressed with a Hib catch-up programme, and to prevent a further resurgence, a Hib booster dose has been introduced at 12 months of age.

Poliovirus infection – although most infected children are asymptomatic or have a mild illness, some

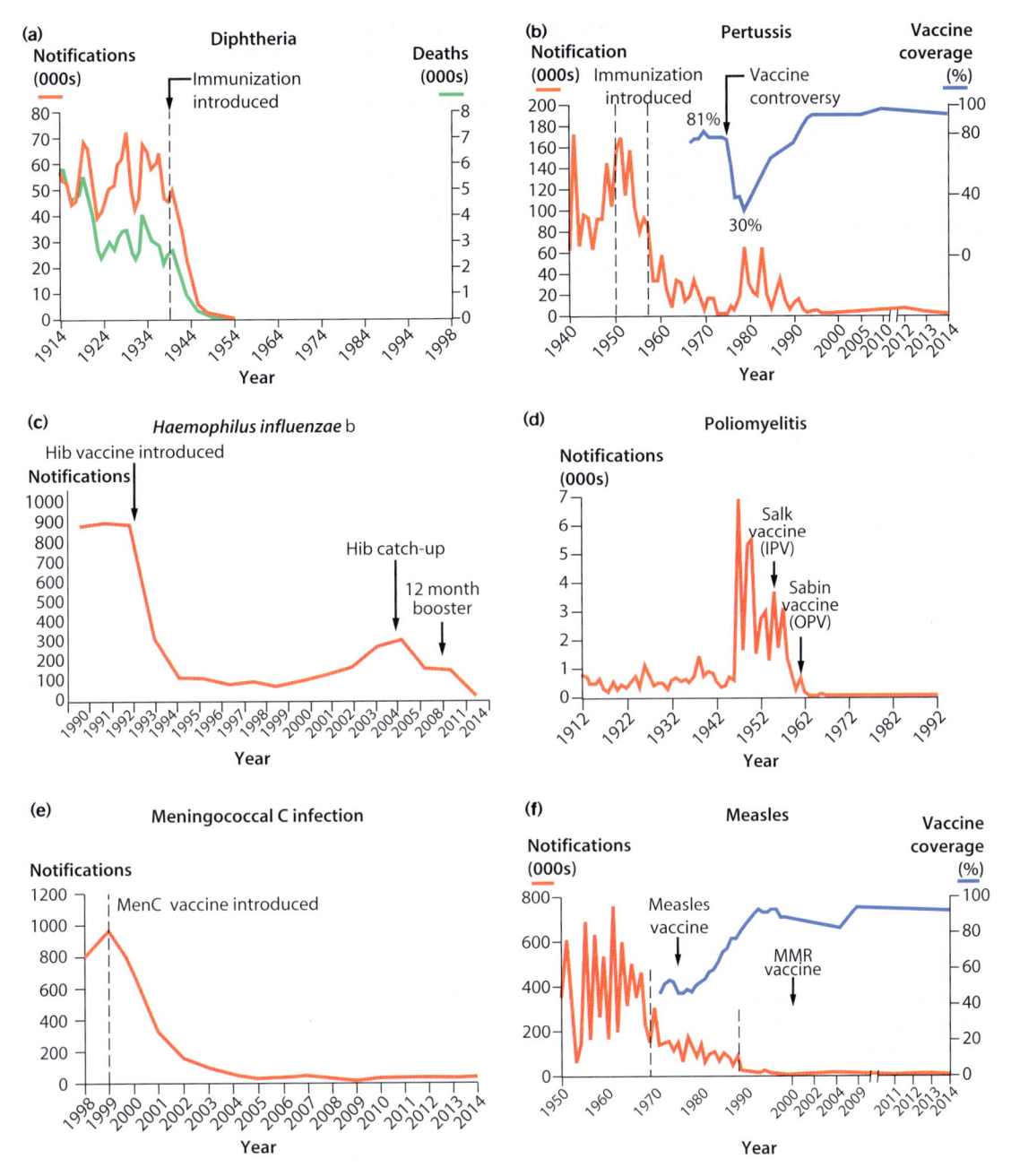

Figure 15.26 Effect of immunization on the number of notifications in England and Wales. (a) Diphtheria; (b) pertussis; (c) *Haemophilus influenzae* type b in children under 5 years of age; (d) poliomyelitis; (e) meningococcal disease; and (f) measles. (Data from Public Health England.)

develop aseptic meningitis and less than 1% develop paralytic poliomyelitis. Almost eradicated worldwide (Fig. 15.26d).

Meningococcal immunization – the marked fall in the number of reports of group C disease in all age groups is shown in Fig. 15.26e. The impact of the new meningococcal B vaccine programme has yet to be determined. Due to a rise in meningococcal Y and W disease in adolescents, ACWY conjugate vaccine has been introduced for this age group.

Pneumococcal vaccination – introduced into the UK immunization programme in 2006. Prior to this, more than 500 children under 2 years of age developed invasive pneumococcal disease in England and Wales each year. In 2010, a 13-valent conjugate vaccine (PCV, effective against 13 serotypes) was introduced, which protects against about 90% of the disease-causing pneumococcal serotypes.

Human papillomavirus vaccine – introduced in 2008. Provides protection against the two strains (human papillomavirus 16 and human papillomavirus 18) that cause 70% of cervical cancer. Two doses of vaccine are given over a 6-month period to girls aged 12–13 years of age.

BCG immunization – The number of notifications of TB in the UK has been declining slowly. TB is mainly confined to high-risk populations. BCG immunization in the neonatal period is therefore targeted to those at increased risk. The main value of BCG is in the prevention of disseminated disease (including meningitis) in younger children, hence the rationale for changing the timing of vaccination from early adolescence to the neonatal period.

Hepatitis B and *varicella vaccination* – these are included in the immunization programme in the USA and in many other countries. In the UK, hepatitis B immunization is given only to babies born to hepatitis B surface antigen (HBsAg)-positive mothers. It is given at 0 months, 1 month, 2 months, and 12 months of age. Babies born to highly infectious e-antigen (HBeAg)-positive mothers should additionally receive hepatitis B immunoglobulin at birth. Varicella vaccine is not routinely given in the UK, but may be given to the siblings of 'at-risk' children (e.g. those undergoing chemotherapy).

Low and middle-income countries – in 2012 all WHO member states endorsed the Global Vaccine Action Plan (GVAP) to provide immunization for all children. In 2015 about 85% of children received 3 doses of DTP immunization. Most countries, including low-income countries, have added hepatitis B and Hib to their routine immunizations, and many have added pneumococcal and rotavirus vaccines.

Complications and contraindications

Following vaccination, there may be swelling and discomfort at the injection site and a mild fever and malaise. Some vaccines, such as MMR vaccine, may be followed by a mild form of the disease 7 days to 10 days later. More serious reactions, including anaphylaxis, can occur but are very rare. Local guidelines about vaccination and its contraindications should be followed. Vaccination should be postponed if the child has an acute illness; however, a minor infection without fever or systemic features is not a contraindication. Live vaccines should not be given to immunocompromised children (except in children with HIV infection on ART in whom MMR vaccine can be given).

The controversy regarding a possible association between MMR vaccination and autism and inflammatory bowel disease has been discredited by a large number of well-conducted studies. However, public confidence in the immunization programme was damaged, and uptake rates consequently dropped (Fig. 15.26f). The MMR vaccine is only contraindicated in children with proven non-HIV-related immunodeficiency and those who are allergic to neomycin or kanamycin, which may be present in small quantities in the vaccine. There is a 10% vaccine failure rate from primary vaccination with MMR at 12 months of age, but the proportion of susceptible school-age children in the UK has been reduced by the introduction of a preschool booster of MMR. Detailed information on vaccines is available in the UK Department of Health Green Book.

Immunodeficiency

Immunodeficiency may be

- Primary (uncommon) – a genetically determined defect in the immune system
- Secondary (more common) – caused by another disease or treatment, such as malignancy/chemotherapy, malnutrition, HIV infection, immunosuppressive therapy, splenectomy, or nephrotic syndrome.

Primary immunodeficiencies

Many of the primary immunodeficiencies are inherited as X-linked or autosomal recessive disorders. There may be a family history of parental consanguinity and unexplained death, particularly in boys. Immunodeficiency should be considered in children who present with **S**evere, **P**rolonged, **U**nusual, or **R**ecurrent infections (Box 15.3). The clinical presentation of the different primary immune deficiencies is shown in Fig. 15.27.

Investigation

This is directed towards the most likely cause (Table 15.3). Investigations can quantify the essential components of the immune system and also provide a functional assessment of immunocompetence. Subsequent investigation can reveal known single-gene defects or novel diagnoses based on rapidly evolving exome and whole genome analytical technologies.

Box 15.3 Presentation of immunodeficiency

- Recurrent (proven) bacterial infections
- Severe infections (e.g. meningitis, osteomyelitis, pneumonia)
- Infections that present atypically, are unusually severe or chronic or fail to respond to regular treatment
- Infections caused by an unexpected or opportunistic pathogen or a pathogen the child has been immunized against
- Severe or long-lasting warts, generalized molluscum contagiosum
- Extensive candidiasis
- Complications following live vaccinations (e.g. disseminated BCG)
- Abscesses of internal organs; recurrent skin abscesses
- Prolonged or recurrent diarrhoea (often combined with faltering growth).

From de Vries E, Clinical Working Party of the European Society for Immunodeficiencies (ESID): Patient-centred screening for primary immunodeficiency: a multistage diagnostic protocol designed for nonimmunologists. *Clinical and Experimental Immunology* 145:204–215, 2006 with permission.

Clinical presentation of primary immune deficiency

Defect	Presentation	Examples
T-cell defects	Severe and/or unusual viral and fungal infections and faltering growth in first months of life, e.g. severe bronchiolitis, diarrhoea, oral thrush, *Pneumocystis jirovecii (carinii)* pneumonia (PCP), disseminated or severe cytomegalovirus infection.	**Severe combined immunodeficiency (SCID).** Heterogeneous group of inherited disorders of profoundly defective cellular and humoral immunity. Fatal without treatment. **HIV infection** **Wiskott–Aldrich syndrome** – triad of immunodeficiency, thrombocytopenia, and eczema (X-linked). **DiGeorge syndrome** – with abnormal development of the 5th branchial arch causing cardiac defects, palatal and facial defects, absence of thymus, and hypocalcaemia (deletion of section of chromosome 22; 22q11). **Duncan disease (X-linked lymphoproliferative disease)** – inability to generate a normal response to Epstein–Barr virus; either succumb to the initial infection or develop secondary lymphoma. **Ataxia telangiectasia** – defect in DNA repair, also increased risk of lymphoma. Cerebellar ataxia, developmental delay.
B-cell (antibody) defects	In first 2 years (beyond infancy because of passively acquired maternal antibodies) – severe bacterial infections, especially ear, sinus, pulmonary, and skin infections; recurrent diarrhoea and faltering growth. Recurrent pneumonias can lead to bronchiectasis; recurrent ear infections to impaired hearing.	**X-linked (Bruton) agammaglobulinaemia.** Abnormal tyrosine kinase gene; essential for B-cell maturation. **Common variable immune deficiency (CVID)** – B-cell deficiency. High risk of autoimmune disorders and malignancy. Later onset than Bruton agammaglobulinaemia. **Hyper IgM syndrome** – B-cells produce IgM but are prevented from switching to IgG and IgA. **Selective IgA deficiency** – most common primary immune defect. Usually asymptomatic, or recurrent ear, sinus, and pulmonary infections.
Neutrophil defects	Recurrent bacterial infections – abscesses (skin, lymph nodes, lung, liver, spleen, bone), poor wound healing, perianal disease and periodontal infections; invasive fungal infections, such as aspergillosis. Diarrhoea and faltering growth. Granulomas from chronic inflammation.	**Chronic granulomatous disease** – most are X-linked recessive, some autosomal recessive. Neutrophils fail to produce superoxide after phagocytosis of microorganisms.
Leucocyte function defects	Delayed separation of umbilical cord, delayed wound healing, chronic skin ulcers and deep-seated infections.	**Leucocyte adhesion deficiency (LAD)** – deficiency of neutrophil surface adhesion molecules, CD18, CD11b, leads to inability of neutrophils to migrate to sites of infection/inflammation.
Complement defects	Recurrent bacterial infections. SLE-like illness. Recurrent meningococcal, pneumococcal and Haemophilus influenzae infections – with deficiency of complement components.	**Early complement component deficiency** **Terminal complement component deficiency** **Mannose-binding lectin (MBL) deficiency.**

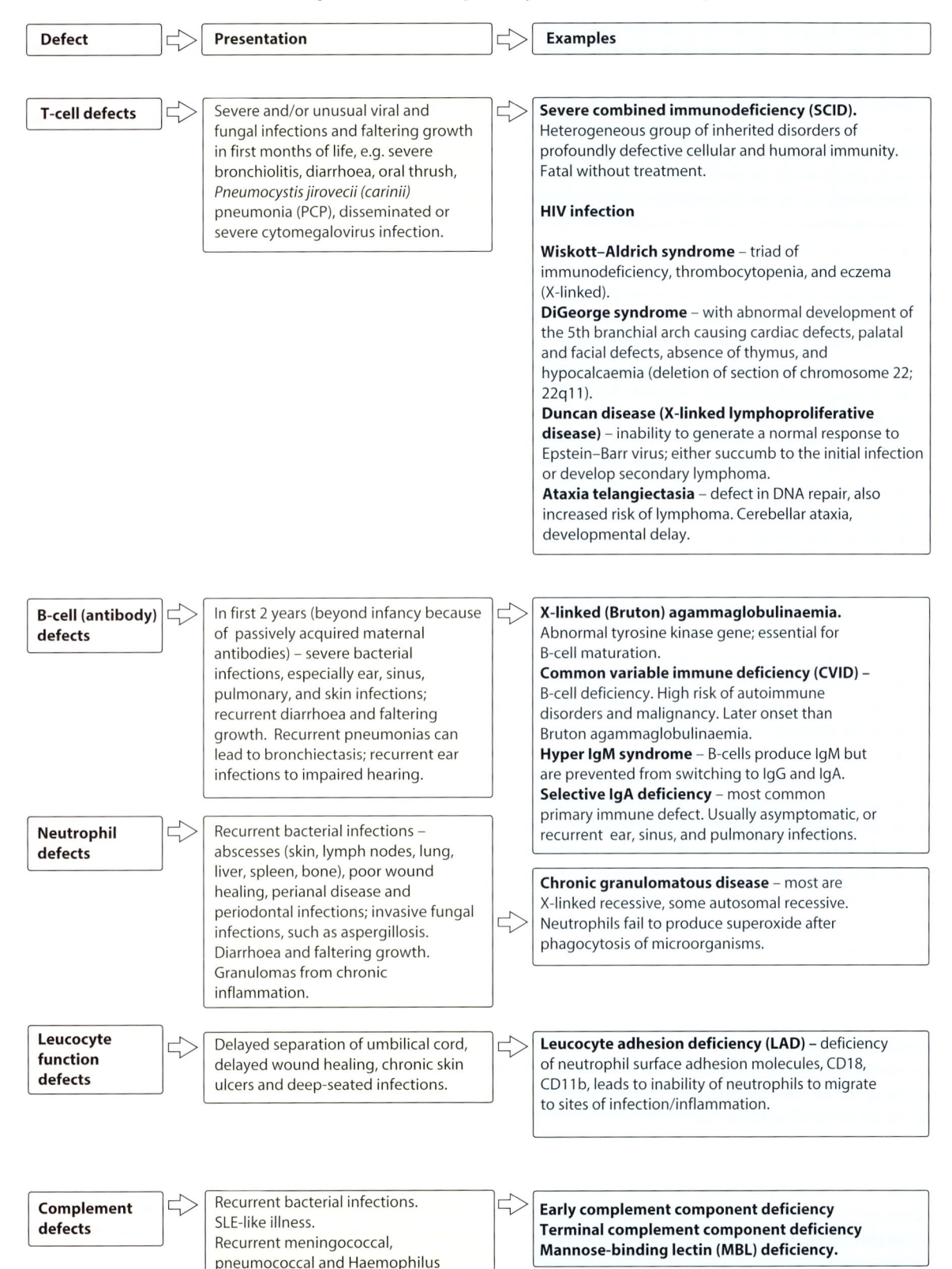

Figure 15.27 Clinical presentation of primary immunodeficiency.

Table 15.3 Investigation to identify primary immunodeficiency

Immune defect	Investigations
Cellular (T cells)	Full blood count (including lymphocyte count)
	Lymphocyte subsets [to assess $CD3^+$ (total T cell), $CD4^+$ (helper T cell), and $CD8^+$ (cytotoxic T cell) numbers]
	Ability of T cells to proliferate in response to mitogen
Antibody (humoral; B cells)	Immunoglobulin levels (IgG, IgM, IgA, and IgE)
	IgG subclasses (in children >2 years)
	Specific antibody responses (e.g. vaccine-induced antibodies to tetanus and pneumococci)
	Lymphocyte subsets (to assess B-cell numbers)
Combined (B and T cells)	Investigations as above
	Specific genetic/molecular tests for severe combined immunodeficiency
Neutrophils	Full blood count (to assess neutrophil numbers/neutropenia)
	Nitroblue tetrazolium test (NBT test) – abnormal in chronic granulomatous disease (most laboratories now use newer assays to determine superoxide production)
	Tests for leucocyte adhesion deficiency – CD11b/CD18 expression
	Tests of chemotaxis (neutrophil mobility)
Complement/ mannose-binding lectin	Tests of classical and alternative complement pathways (CH50, AP50)
	Assays for individual complement proteins
	Mannose-binding lectin levels

Management

Management options include
- Antimicrobial prophylaxis
  - For T-cell and neutrophil defects – cotrimoxazole to prevent PCP and itraconazole or fluconazole to prevent other fungal infections
  - For B-cell defects – antibiotic prophylaxis (e.g. azithromycin) to prevent recurrent bacterial (e.g. chest, ear, sinus) infections
- Antibiotic treatment
  - Prompt treatment of infections
  - Appropriate choice of antibiotics to cover likely organisms
  - Generally longer courses, with low threshold for intravenous therapy
- Screening for end-organ disease
  - E.g. CT scan in children with antibody deficiency to detect bronchiectasis
- Immunoglobulin replacement therapy
  - For children with antibody deficiency
  - Can be given intravenously, which may require central venous (Portacath or Hickman) line insertion, or subcutaneously
- Bone marrow transplantation
  - E.g. for severe combined immunodeficiency, chronic granulomatous disease
  - Can be matched sibling donor, matched unrelated donor, or haploidentical (parental) transplant
- Gene therapy
  - Currently an evolving area and not widely available

Acknowledgements

We would like to acknowledge contributors to this chapter in previous editions, whose work we have drawn on: Nigel Curtis (1st Edition), Nigel Klein (1st and 2nd Edition), Hermione Lyall (2nd and 3rd Edition), Saul Faust (3rd Edition), Gareth Tudor-Williams (4th Edition) and Andrew Prendergast (4th Edition).

Further reading

American Academy of Pediatrics: *Report of the Committee on Infectious Diseases. 'Red Book'*, ed 30, Illinois, 2015, American Academy of Pediatrics.
Useful manual on paediatric infection and immunization in the USA.

Feigin RD, Cherry JD, editors: *Textbook of Pediatric Infectious Diseases*, ed 7, Philadelphia, PA, 2013, Saunders.
Large comprehensive textbook.

Websites (Accessed November 2016)

Centers for Disease Control and Prevention, Atlanta, GA, USA: Available at: http://www.cdc.gov.

CHIVA (Children's HIV Association of UK and Ireland): Available at: http://www.chiva.org.uk.
Guidelines to reduce HIV vertical transmission and management of HIV-infected children.

Meningitis Research Foundation: Available at: http://www.meningitis.org.
Useful teaching material on meningitis.

Public Health England:
For incubation and exclusion periods, see www.gov.uk/health-protection/infectious-diseases.

UK Department of Health Green Book: Available at: https://www.gov.uk/government/collections/immunisation-against-infectious-disease-the-green-book.
Up-to-date information on vaccines and the immunization programme in the UK.

UK Department of Health Immunisation Schedule: Available at: https://www.gov.uk/government/uploads/system/uploads/attachment_data/file/533863/PHE_2016_Routine_Childhood_Immunisation_Schedule_SUMMER2016.pdf.
Up-to-date information on the immunization programme in the UK.

UNAIDS: Available at: http://www.unaids.org.
Worldwide information on HIV.

World Health Organization: Available at: http://www.who.int.

16 Allergy

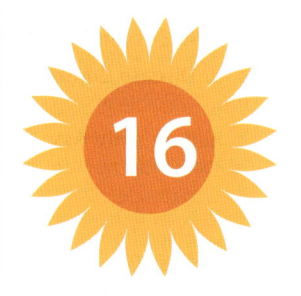

Mechanisms of allergic disease	288	Asthma	292
The hygiene hypothesis	289	Urticaria and angioedema	293
The allergic march	289	Drug allergy	293
Prevention of allergic diseases	289	Insect sting hypersensitivity	293
Food allergy and food intolerance	290	Anaphylaxis	293
Eczema	292		
Allergic rhinitis and conjunctivitis (rhinoconjunctivitis)	292		

Features of allergic disorders in children are:
- up to 40% of children in the UK have allergic rhinitis, eczema or asthma and 6% have food allergy
- they have increased in prevalence in the UK and in many other countries
- they are the most common chronic diseases of childhood and the most common cause of school absence and acute hospital admissions
- they cause significant morbidity and can be fatal, though this is rare, with about 20 children dying from asthma and two from food anaphylaxis in the UK each year.

An abnormal immune system may result in:
- allergic diseases
- immune deficiencies
- autoimmune disorders – either organ specific (e.g. type I diabetes mellitus) or systemic (e.g. systemic lupus erythematosus).

Explanations of some of the terms used in 'allergy' are listed in Box 16.1.

Mechanisms of allergic disease

Many genes have been linked to the development of allergic disease. Polymorphisms or mutations in these genes lead to a susceptibility to allergy.

Allergic diseases occur when individuals make an abnormal immune response to harmless environmental stimuli, usually proteins. The developing immune system must be 'sensitized' to an allergen before an allergic immune response develops. However, sensitization can be 'occult', e.g. sensitization to peanut from exposure to trace quantities of peanut in house dust.

Only a few stimuli account for most allergic disease:
- inhalant allergens, e.g. house-dust mite, plant pollens, pet dander and moulds
- ingestant allergens, e.g. cow's milk, nuts, soya, egg, wheat, seeds, legumes, seafood and fruits
- insect stings/bites, drugs, and natural rubber latex.

Box 16.1 Allergy definitions

- *Hypersensitivity* – objectively reproducible symptoms or signs following exposure to a defined stimulus (e.g. food, drug, pollen) at a dose that is usually tolerated by most people
- *Allergy* – a hypersensitivity reaction initiated by specific immunological mechanisms. This can be IgE mediated (e.g. peanut allergy) or non-IgE mediated (e.g. coeliac disease)
- *Atopy* – a personal and/or familial tendency to produce IgE antibodies in response to ordinary exposures to potential allergens, usually proteins. Strongly associated with asthma, allergic rhinitis and conjunctivitis, eczema and food allergy
- *Anaphylaxis* – a serious allergic reaction with bronchial, laryngeal, or cardiovascular involvement that is rapid in onset and may cause death

Proteins with an unstable tertiary structure may be rendered non-allergenic by heat degradation or other forms of processing. For example, some children are allergic to raw apples, but can tolerate eating cooked apples.

Allergic immune responses are classified as IgE mediated or non-IgE mediated. IgE-mediated allergic reactions have a characteristic clinical course:

- an early phase, occurring within minutes of exposure to the allergen, caused by release of histamine and other mediators from mast cells. Causes urticaria, angioedema, sneezing, vomiting, bronchospasm and/or cardiovascular shock
- a late phase response may also occur after 4–6 hours, especially in reactions to inhalant allergens. This causes nasal congestion in the upper airway, and cough and bronchospasm in the lower airway.

The majority of severe life-threatening allergic reactions are IgE mediated.

Non-IgE-mediated allergic immune responses usually have a delayed onset of symptoms and more varied clinical course.

The hygiene hypothesis

It is not clear why the prevalence of allergic diseases has increased in many countries and the speed of this change suggests an environmental cause. A consistent observation is that the risk is lower in younger children of large families and in children raised on farms. These findings have led to the hygiene hypothesis, which proposes that the increased prevalence is due to altered microbial exposure associated with modern living conditions (Fig. 16.1). Although the hypothesis remains the leading explanation for the increase in allergic disease, it is mainly supported by indirect evidence.

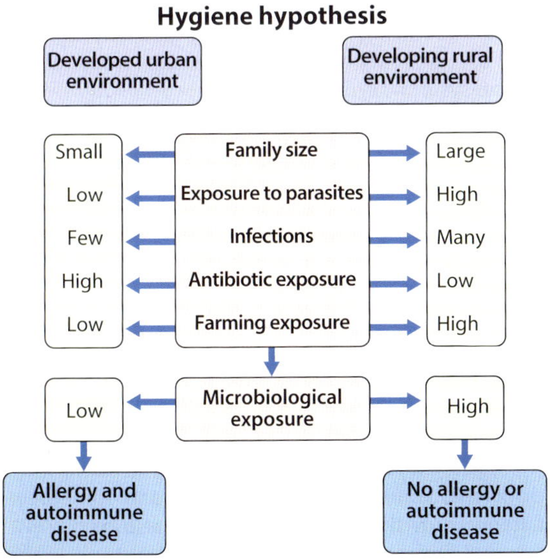

Figure 16.1 Hygiene hypothesis.

The allergic march

Allergic children develop individual allergic disorders at different ages:

- Eczema and food allergy usually develop in infancy.
- Allergic rhinitis, conjunctivitis and asthma begin most often in preschool and primary school years.
- Rhinitis and conjunctivitis may precede the development of asthma. Allergic disorders often overlap. Many children with food allergy have eczema and up to 80% of children with asthma have rhinitis.

The presence of eczema or food allergy in infancy is predictive of asthma and allergic rhinitis in later life. The progression is referred to as the 'allergic march'.

Prevention of allergic diseases

Many interventions have been tried to prevent allergic disease or interrupt the allergic march. Those with some evidence base include avoiding the use of formula milk from cow's milk to reduce the risk of eczema, using probiotics during late pregnancy and lactation for preventing eczema and early introduction of peanut or egg to the infant diet to prevent peanut or egg allergy (oral tolerance). Other approaches tried but not yet proven to work include prebiotics (nondigestible oligosaccharides naturally present in breast milk), nutritional supplements (e.g. omega-3 fatty acids, vitamin D, antioxidants, trace elements), and medications (e.g. antihistamines, immunotherapy).

History and examination

The child and family may not volunteer a history of allergic disease as they have come to consider the symptoms as normal, e.g. the child who coughs most nights or has a blocked nose most of the time may not perceive this as abnormal. As allergic diseases are multisystem, in addition to the signs of individual allergic diseases, examination may reveal:

- mouth breathing (Fig. 16.2a). Children who habitually breathe with their mouth open may have an obstructed nasal airway from rhinitis, and there may also be a history of snoring or obstructive sleep apnoea
- an allergic salute (Fig. 16.2b), from rubbing an itchy nose
- pale and swollen inferior nasal turbinates
- hyperinflated chest or Harrison sulci from chronic undertreated asthma
- atopic eczema affecting the limb flexures
- allergic conjunctivitis; may also be prominent creases (Dennie–Morgan folds) and blue-grey discoloration below the lower eyelids.

Growth needs to be checked, especially in those with food allergy, where dietary restrictions or malabsorption can lead to nutritional compromise, and in those treated with high-dose inhaled/nasal/topical corticosteroids.

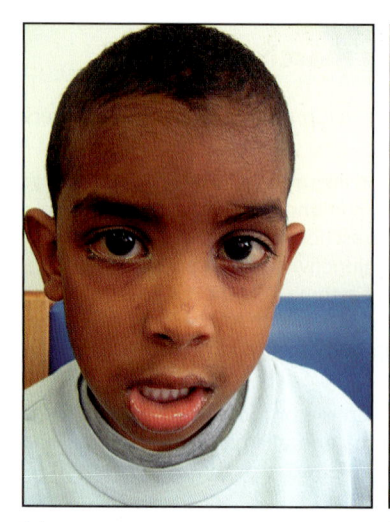

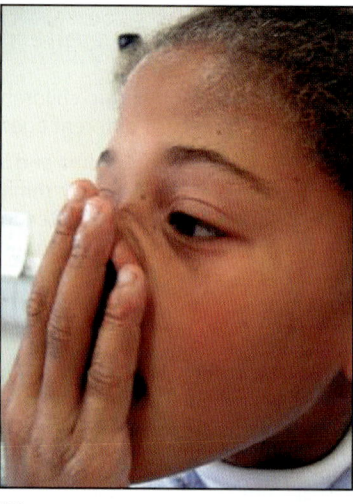

Figure 16.2 Allergic facies. (a) There is a habitually open mouth due to mouth breathing; and (b) an allergic salute, from rubbing an itchy nose. (Courtesy of Dr George Du Toit.)

Management

The individual diseases are managed by general practitioners, general paediatricians or organ-specific specialists, e.g. eczema by dermatologists, asthma by respiratory paediatricians. However, allergic diseases co-exist and it is therefore helpful to consider allergy as a systemic disease. The role of paediatric allergists is to identify triggers to avoid and to manage children with multisystem or severe disease.

Management of specific conditions is described in the following section. In addition, specific allergen immunotherapy can be used for treating allergic rhinitis and conjunctivitis, insect stings, anaphylaxis, and asthma. During immunotherapy, solutions of an allergen to which the patient is allergic are injected subcutaneously or administered sublingually on a regular basis for 3–5 years, with the aim of developing immune tolerance. It is highly effective in providing protection for many years. However, it must be carried out under specialist supervision due to the risk of inducing severe allergic reactions (anaphylaxis). Allergen immunotherapy is widely used in the United States and in some countries in Europe. Sublingual immunotherapy appears to be safer than subcutaneous injections and is used increasingly. Immunotherapy for food allergy is under investigation but has not yet been shown to be sufficiently safe for use in clinical practice.

Summary

Paediatric allergy
- Includes food allergy, eczema, allergic rhinitis and conjunctivitis, asthma, urticaria, insect sting hypersensitivity and anaphylaxis.
- Occurs when a genetically susceptible person reacts abnormally to an environmental antigen.
- There is an 'allergic march' of disorders.
- Different allergic diseases often co-exist – if a child has one, look for others.

Food allergy and food intolerance

A food allergy occurs when a pathological immune response is mounted against a specific food protein. It is usually IgE mediated, but may be non-IgE mediated. A non-immunological hypersensitivity reaction to a specific food is called food intolerance. An example of each in relation to cow's milk is shown in Fig. 16.3.

Food allergy is most commonly primary, where children usually react on first exposure. Presentation varies with the agent and the child's age:

- in infants – the most common causes are milk, egg and peanut
- in older children – peanut, tree nut, fish and shellfish.

Food allergy can also be secondary, which is usually due to cross-reactivity between proteins present in fresh fruits/vegetables/nuts and those present in pollens, e.g. a child who can eat apples may develop allergy to apples when older if they develop allergy to birch tree pollen, because the apple and birch pollen share a very similar protein. This common condition is termed the 'pollen food allergy syndrome' and generally leads to mild allergic reactions, often causing an itchy mouth but no systemic symptoms.

Non-IgE food allergy typically occurs hours after ingestion and usually involves the gastrointestinal tract. Food allergy and intolerance are different from food aversion, where the person refuses the food for psychological or behavioural reasons.

Clinical features

In IgE-mediated food allergy there is a history of allergic symptom varying from urticaria to facial swelling to anaphylaxis (Fig. 16.3), usually occurring 10–15 minutes (up to 2 hours) after ingestion of a food. Non-IgE mediated food allergy usually presents with diarrhoea, vomiting, abdominal pain and sometimes faltering growth. Colic or eczema may also be present. It sometimes presents with blood in the stools in the first few weeks of life from proctitis, or with severe

Examples of food allergy and hypersensitivity to milk

Condition	Clinical manifestation	
IgE mediated food allergy • Immediate cow's milk allergy	The clinical features of an acute allergic reaction are listed in (a). A 6-month-old breastfed infant developed widespread urticaria immediately after the first formula feed. Skin-prick test was strongly positive (8 mm weal) to cow's milk, confirming the diagnosis of IgE mediated cow's milk allergy. Widespread urticaria and lip swelling after milk ingestion are shown in **(b)** and **(c)**	**(a) Clinical features of an acute allergic reaction:** **Mild reaction** • Urticaria and itchy skin • Facial swelling **Severe reaction** • Wheeze • Stridor • Abdominal pain, vomiting, diarrhoea • Shock, collapse
Non-IgE mediated cow's milk allergy	A 4-month-old infant, formula fed since birth, has loose stools and faltering growth. Skin-prick test to cow's milk is negative (0 mm weal). Elimination of cow's milk results in resolution of symptoms, which return on trial re-introduction.	
Non-allergic food hypersensitivity • Temporary lactose intolerance	Previously well 12-month-old infant develops diarrhoea and vomiting. The vomiting settles but watery stools continue for several weeks. Stool sample – no pathogens but positive for reducing substances. Diagnosis – temporary lactose intolerance.	

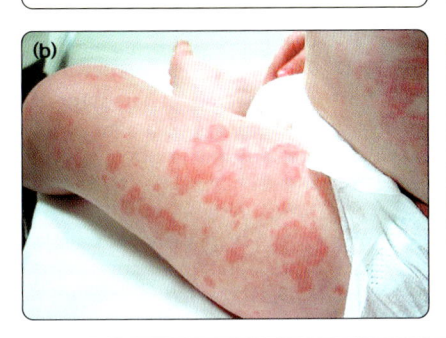

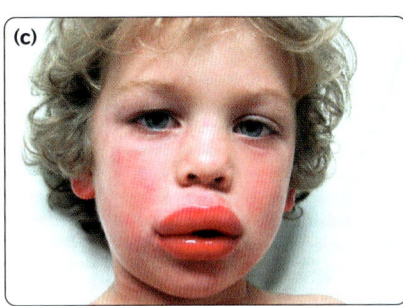

Figure 16.3 Examples of food allergy and hypersensitivity to milk. (**a**) Clinical features of an acute allergic reaction; and (**b**, **c**) Widespread urticaria and lip swelling after milk ingestion. (Courtesy of Dr Pete Smith.)

repetitive vomiting in an infant which can result in shock (food protein-induced enterocolitis syndrome).

Diagnosis

The clinical history is key in food allergy diagnosis. Food allergy should be suspected if typical symptoms occur following exposure to a particular food. For IgE-mediated food allergy, the most helpful confirmatory tests are skin-prick tests (Fig. 16.4) and measurement of specific IgE antibodies in blood. Both tests may yield false-positive results, but the greater the response, the more likely the child is to be allergic. Negative skin test results make IgE-mediated allergy unlikely.

Non-IgE-mediated food allergies are harder to diagnose. Diagnosis relies on clinical history and examination. If indicated, endoscopy and intestinal biopsy may be obtained; the diagnosis is supported by the presence of eosinophilic infiltrates.

For both IgE-mediated and non-IgE-mediated food allergies, the gold-standard investigation in cases of doubt is exclusion of the relevant food under a dietitian's supervision, followed by a double-blind placebo-controlled food challenge. This involves the child being given increasing amounts of the food or placebo, starting with a tiny quantity, until a full portion is reached. The test should be performed in hospital with full resuscitation facilities available, and close monitoring for signs of an allergic reaction.

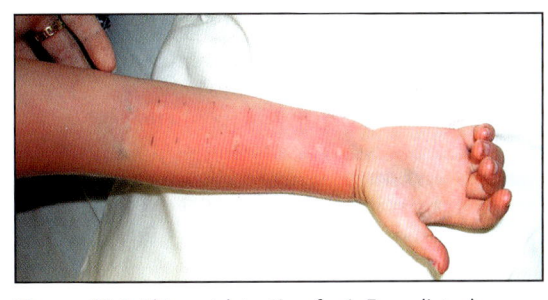

Figure 16.4 Skin-prick testing for IgE mediated allergy. A drop of the allergen is placed on the skin, the site is marked, and pricked with a needle, and any weals measured. Weals of 4 mm or greater are considered positive. Multiple positive results are present. (Courtesy of Dr Pete Smith.)

Management

The management of a food-allergic child involves avoidance of the relevant food(s). This can be very difficult as the most common food allergens are common ingredients in the human diet, and they may be present in small quantities in many foods. Food labelling in the European Union legally requires common food allergens to be clearly disclosed, including foods sold in catering outlets. The advice of a paediatric dietitian is essential to help patients avoid foods to which they are allergic, find appropriate alternatives, and avoid nutritional deficiencies.

In addition, the child and family must be able to manage an allergic attack. Written self-management plans and adequate training are essential. Drug management for mild reactions (no cardiorespiratory symptoms) is with non-sedating antihistamines. If the child has a severe reaction (i.e. with cardiovascular, laryngeal or bronchial involvement), treatment is with epinephrine (adrenaline) given intramuscularly by autoinjector (e.g. EpiPen), which the child or parent should carry with them at all times.

Food allergy to cow's milk and egg often resolves in early childhood, and gradual reintroduction under supervision of a paediatric dietician may be possible for these foods. However, food allergy to nuts and seafood usually persists through to adulthood.

> **The diagnosis of food allergy should not be made lightly – dietary restrictions and fear of accidental reactions make a major impact on family life**

Summary

Food allergy

- Affects up to 6% of children.
- The most common causes are milk, egg, nuts, seafood, wheat, legumes, seeds and fruits.
- Diagnosis of IgE-mediated food allergy is based on a suggestive history supported by skin-prick tests or specific IgE antibodies in blood.
- Supervised food challenge is sometimes necessary to clarify the diagnosis.
- Those at risk of a severe reaction, e.g. with previous anaphylaxis or coexistent asthma, should carry an epinephrine (adrenaline) autoinjector.

Eczema

Eczema can be either atopic (where there is evidence of IgE antibodies to common allergens) or non-atopic. Atopic eczema is classified as an allergic disease as many affected children have a family history of allergy, at least 50% develop other allergic diseases and IgE antibodies to common allergens are usually present. Filaggrin gene mutations have been identified as the key genetic risk factor for eczema development due to impairment of skin barrier function, which then leads to cutaneous sensitization to inhalant and food allergens. This means that filaggrin gene mutations predispose to food allergy, asthma and hay fever as well as eczema. Up to 40% of young infants with severe eczema have an IgE-mediated food allergy, in particular egg allergy. Screening by skin prick or IgE blood testing should be considered in these patients. Eczema is considered further in Chapter 25 (Dermatological disorders).

Allergic rhinitis and conjunctivitis (rhinoconjunctivitis)

This can also be atopic (associated with IgE antibodies to common inhalant allergens) or non-atopic. Rhinoconjunctivitis is classified according to the pattern and severity of symptoms experienced. Therefore it may be intermittent or persistent and mild, moderate or severe. In temperate climates it is often classified as seasonal (related to seasonal grass, weed or tree pollens) and perennial (related to perennial allergens such as house-dust mite or pets). It affects up to 20% of children and can severely disrupt their lives. In addition to its classic presentation of coryza and conjunctivitis, it can also present as 'cough-variant rhinitis' due to a post-nasal drip or as a chronically blocked nose causing sleep disturbance with impaired daytime behaviour and concentration, or with predominant eye symptoms. It is associated with eczema, sinusitis and adenoidal hypertrophy and is closely associated with asthma. Treatment of allergic rhinitis may improve the control of co-existent asthma. Treatment options are listed in Box 16.2.

Asthma

Allergy is an important component of asthma. Affected children often have IgE antibodies to aero-allergens (house-dust mite; tree, grass and weed pollens; moulds; animal danders). Allergen avoidance is difficult to achieve. Management of asthma is described in Chapter 17 (Respiratory disorders).

Box 16.2 Range of treatment for allergic rhinoconjunctivitis

- Second-generation non-sedating antihistamines (used topically or systemically)
- Topical corticosteroid nasal or eye preparations (the latter under specialist ophthalmology supervision)
- Cromoglycate eye drops
- Leukotriene receptor antagonists, e.g. montelukast
- Nasal decongestants (use for no more than 7–10 days due to risk of rebound effect)
- Allergen immunotherapy – sublingual or subcutaneous (limited by anaphylaxis risk)
- Systemic corticosteroids should not be used due to the risk of adverse effects

Urticaria and angioedema

Urticaria presents as hives or redness and results from local vasodilation and increased permeability of capillaries and venules. These changes are dependent on activation of skin mast cells, which release a range of mediators including histamine. It is itchy. A classification of urticaria is shown in Box 16.3. Acute urticaria usually results from either a viral infection (rash lasts for days) or allergen exposure (rash lasts for hours). Urticaria may involve deeper tissues to produce swelling (angioedema), especially of the lips and soft tissues around the eyes. When allergy (especially food allergy) is the cause of urticaria, there is a risk of anaphylaxis. Chronic urticaria (persisting >6 weeks) is usually non-allergic in origin. Treatment of urticaria is with second-generation non-sedating antihistamines, which may need to be increased up to four times the standard dose. In refractory cases, leukotriene receptor antagonists or anti-IgE antibody (omalizumab) are helpful.

Drug allergy

Drug allergies do occur in children, especially to antibiotics, but only a minority who are labelled 'drug allergic' are truly allergic. This is usually because viral illnesses, for which children are often prescribed antibiotics, themselves cause skin rashes. A detailed history is required of the nature and timing of the rash in relation to taking the antibiotics.

Allergy skin and blood tests can be used to support a diagnosis of drug allergy, but a drug challenge may be the only way to conclusively confirm or refute the diagnosis. This is contraindicated after a severe allergic reaction and an alternative drug should be sought.

Insect sting hypersensitivity

This arises mainly from bee and wasp stings, but also from ant species in the United States, Asia and Australia. The severity of the allergic reaction may be:

- mild – local swelling
- moderate – generalized urticaria
- severe – systemic symptoms with wheeze or shock.

Children with a previous mild or moderate reaction are unlikely to develop a severe reaction in the future and the family can be reassured. Those who had a severe reaction, or have significant anxiety about a further reaction, should be offered an epinephrine (adrenaline) autoinjector and allergen immunotherapy.

Box 16.3 Classification of urticaria/angioedema

- Acute – resolves within 6 weeks; infection, food allergy and drug reactions are common triggers
- Chronic idiopathic – intermittent for at least 6 weeks
- Physical urticarias
  - cold, delayed pressure, heat contact, solar, and vibratory urticaria
- Other causes
  - water (aquagenic), sweating (cholinergic), exercise induced
  - aspirin and other nonsteroidal anti-inflammatory agents
  - C1 esterase inhibitor deficiency (angioedema, but no urticaria or pruritus)

Summary

Insect sting hypersensitivity
- Mainly to bee and wasp stings.
- Following a severe reaction, an epinephrine (adrenaline) autoinjector should be carried.
- Immunotherapy is effective for preventing further reactions.

Anaphylaxis

This serious and potentially life-threatening allergic reaction is described in Chapter 6 (Paediatric emergencies).

Acknowledgements

We would like to acknowledge contributors to this chapter in previous editions, whose work we have drawn on: Gideon Lack and Tom Blyth (3rd Edition, Allergy and Immunity), Bob Boyle (4th Edition, Allergy).

Further reading

Burks AW: ICON: food allergy. Journal of Allergy and Clinical Immunology 2012;129:906–920.

Kay AB: Advances in immunology: allergy and allergic disease (first of two parts). New England Journal of Medicine 2001;344:30–37.

Strachan DP: Family size, infection and atopy: the first decade of the 'hygiene hypothesis'. Thorax 2000;55: S2–S10.

Websites (Accessed December 2016)

Allergy UK: Available at: http://www.allergyuk.org.
A charity for people with allergy problems.

Food Allergy and Anaphylaxis Network: Available at: http://www.foodallergy.org.
A nonprofit organisation for people with food allergy.

17

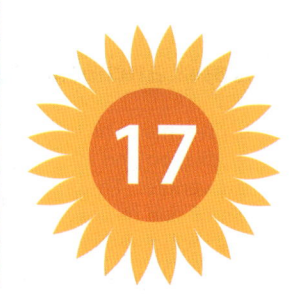

Respiratory disorders

Physiology of stridor and wheeze	295	Cystic fibrosis	313
Upper respiratory tract infection	295	Primary ciliary dyskinesia	317
Stridor	297	Immunodeficiency	317
Wheeze	300	Tuberculosis	317
Cough	310	Sleep-disordered breathing	317
Pneumonia	311	Tracheostomy	318
Chronic lung infection	313	Long-term ventilation	318

Features of respiratory disorders in children are:

- worldwide, they cause more than 750 000 deaths per year in children 1 month–5 years old
- in the UK, they account for half of consultations with general practitioners for acute illness in young children and a third of consultations in older children
- they are common and collectively responsible for about 25% of acute paediatric admissions to hospital in the UK
- asthma is the most common chronic illness of childhood in the UK; 1 in 11 children in the UK receives treatment for asthma
- modern management of cystic fibrosis has markedly extended life expectancy.

Presentation of respiratory disorders in children is with:

- upper respiratory tract symptoms of coryza, sore throat, earache, sinusitis or stridor
- lower respiratory tract symptoms of cough, wheeze and respiratory distress.

As children, especially infants, have compliant chest walls and poorly developed respiratory muscles, they are particularly susceptible to respiratory failure, and early detection and prevention are the cornerstone of management. Infants may develop signs of respiratory distress from most respiratory disorders. Its features are:

- moderate – tachypnoea, tachycardia, nasal flaring, use of accessory respiratory muscles, intercostal and subcostal recession, head retraction and inability to feed
- severe – cyanosis, tiring because of increased work of breathing, reduced conscious level, oxygen saturation < 92% despite oxygen therapy.

Oxygen saturation monitoring is helpful to detect hypoxaemia and to titrate the amount of additional oxygen required. Respiratory support, either non-invasive or occasionally invasive ventilation may be required [see Ch. 6 (Paediatric emergencies)]. However, signs of respiratory distress may become less marked when children become exhausted.

Children who are particularly susceptible to respiratory failure include ex-preterm infants with bronchopulmonary dysplasia, those with haemodynamically significant congenital heart disease or disorders causing muscle weakness, cystic fibrosis (CF) or immunodeficiency. Susceptibility to specific acute respiratory infections varies with age (Fig. 17.1).

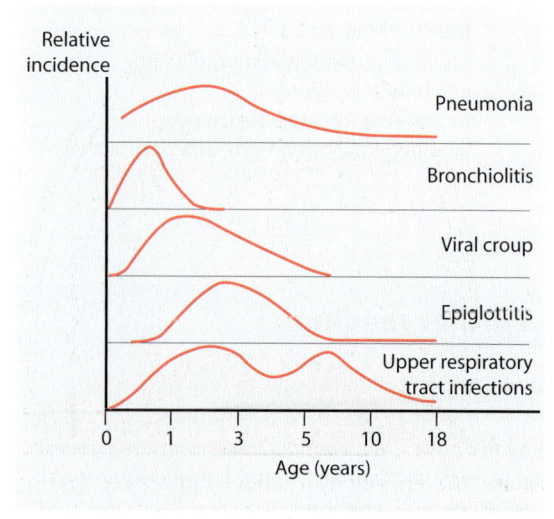

Figure 17.1 Age distribution of acute respiratory infections in children.

Physiology of stridor and wheeze

A review of the respiratory physiology explains why stridor, from extrathoracic airway obstruction in the trachea and larynx, is predominantly inspiratory, and wheeze, from intrathoracic airway narrowing, is predominantly expiratory. Inspiration is an active process in which the contraction and downward movement of the diaphragm combines with the upward and outward movement of the ribs to generate a negative pressure in the thoracic cavity, which sucks air into the lungs through the tube of the extrathoracic airways. A gradient of negative pressure is formed from the alveoli to the upper airway. Within the thoracic cavity the airway walls are pulled outwards by the negative intrathoracic pressure. Above the thoracic inlet, where the external pressure is atmospheric, the negative pressure within the airways leads to a degree of inward collapse during inspiration. The reverse happens during expiration, when the recoil pressure of the chest wall generates a positive intrathoracic pressure and pushes air out from the alveoli to the upper airway, compressing the intrathoracic airways but distending the extrathoracic airway. These changes are exaggerated during any form of airway obstruction, since the pressures generated to overcome the obstruction are even higher. As a result, obstruction to the extrathoracic airways is worse during inspiration, whereas obstruction to the intrathoracic airways is worse during expiration (Fig. 17.2). Snoring is also inspiratory, but because it is caused by variable partial upper airway obstruction, it is a rough inspiratory noise (stertor).

- Narrowing of the airway due to inflammation is a feature of many respiratory pathologies
- Upper airway narrowing results in increased effort and added respiratory noises during inspiration – stridor is harsh but musical whilst snoring (stertor) is rough and lacks a single note!
- Lower airway narrowing results in increased effort and added respiratory noises during expiration, such as crepitations and wheeze

Upper respiratory tract infection

Children have a median of five upper respiratory tract infections (URTIs) per year in the first few years of life, but some toddlers and primary school-aged children have as many as 10–12 per year. Approximately 80% of all respiratory infections involve only the nose, throat, ears or sinuses. The term URTI embraces a number of different conditions:

- common cold (coryza)
- sore throat (pharyngitis, including tonsillitis)
- acute otitis media
- sinusitis (relatively uncommon).

The most common presentation is a child with a combination of these conditions. Cough may be troublesome and in URTI may be secondary to postnasal drip or

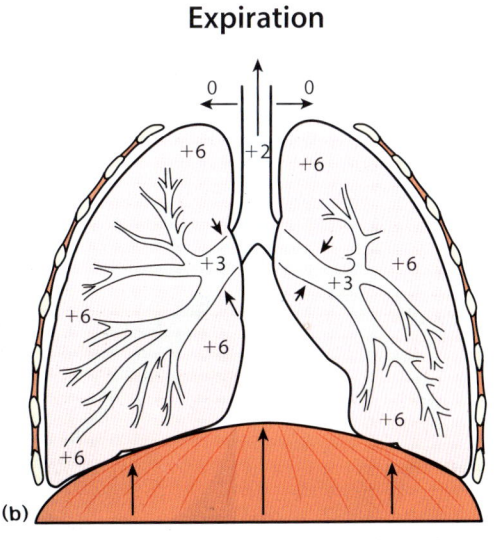

Figure 17.2 Physiology of stridor and wheeze. (a) Negative intrapleural pressure on inspiration dilates the intrathoracic airways but collapses the extrathoracic airway; and (b) positive intrapleural pressure on expiration does the opposite. This explains why extrathoracic obstruction causes difficulty in inspiration, whereas intrathoracic obstruction causes problems on expiration. Numbers represent pressures at different points.

attempts to clear upper airway secretions. URTIs may cause:

- difficulty in feeding in infants as their noses are blocked and this obstructs breathing
- febrile seizures
- acute exacerbations of asthma.

Hospital admission is rarely required but may be necessary if feeding and fluid intake is inadequate.

The common cold (coryza)

This is the most common infection of childhood. Classical features include a clear or mucopurulent nasal discharge and nasal blockage. The most common pathogens are viruses – rhinoviruses (of which there are >100 different serotypes), coronaviruses and respiratory syncytial virus (RSV). Health education to advise parents that colds are self-limiting and have no specific curative treatment may reduce anxiety and save unnecessary visits to doctors. Pain is best treated with paracetamol or ibuprofen. Antibiotics are of no benefit as the common cold is viral in origin and secondary bacterial infection is very uncommon. Cough may persist for up to 4 weeks after a common cold.

Sore throat (pharyngitis and tonsillitis)

In pharyngitis, the pharynx and soft palate are inflamed and local lymph nodes are enlarged and tender. It is usually due to viral infection (mostly adenoviruses, enteroviruses, as well as rhinoviruses). In the older child, group A β-haemolytic streptococcus is a common pathogen.

Tonsillitis is a form of pharyngitis where there is intense inflammation of the tonsils, often with a purulent exudate. Common pathogens are group A β-haemolytic streptococci and the Epstein–Barr virus (infectious mononucleosis). Group A β-haemolytic streptococcus can be cultured from many tonsils; however, it is uncertain why it causes recurrent tonsillitis in some children but not in others.

Although the surface exudates on the tonsils seen in infectious mononucleosis are reported to be more membranous in appearance compared with bacterial tonsillitis, in reality it is not possible to distinguish clinically between viral and bacterial causes. Marked constitutional disturbance, such as headache, apathy and abdominal pain, white tonsillar exudate and cervical lymphadenopathy, is more common with bacterial infection.

Antibiotics (e.g. penicillin V or erythromycin if there is penicillin allergy) are often prescribed for severe pharyngitis and tonsillitis even though only a third are caused by bacteria. They may hasten recovery from streptococcal infection. In order to eradicate the organism completely (and prevent rheumatic fever) 10 days of antibiotic treatment is required for pharyngitis or tonsillitis. Rarely, in severe cases, children may require hospital admission for intravenous fluid administration and analgesia if they are unable to swallow solids or liquids. Amoxicillin is best avoided as it may cause a widespread maculopapular rash if the tonsillitis is due to infectious mononucleosis.

Occasionally, group A streptococcal infection results in scarlet fever, which is most common in children aged 5–12 years. Fever usually precedes the presence of headache and tonsillitis by 2–3 days. The appearance of the rash is variable, although a typical appearance will include a 'sandpaper-like' maculopapular rash with flushed cheeks and perioral sparing. The tongue is often white and coated and may be sore or swollen. This is the only childhood exanthema caused by a bacterium, and requires treatment with antibiotics (penicillin V or erythromycin) to prevent complications including acute glomerulonephritis or, very rarely in high-income countries, rheumatic fever.

> ☀ **It is not possible to distinguish clinically between viral and bacterial tonsillitis**

Acute otitis media

Most children will have at least one episode of acute otitis media. This is most common at 6–12 months of age. Up to 20% will have three or more episodes. Infants and young children are prone to acute otitis media because their Eustachian tubes are short, horizontal, and function poorly. There is pain in the ear and fever. Every child with a fever must have his/her tympanic membranes examined (Fig. 17.3a–d). In acute otitis media, the tympanic membrane is seen to be bright red and bulging with loss of the normal light reflection (Fig. 17.3b). Occasionally, there is acute perforation of the eardrum with pus visible in the external canal. Pathogens include viruses, especially RSV and rhinovirus, and bacteria including pneumococcus,

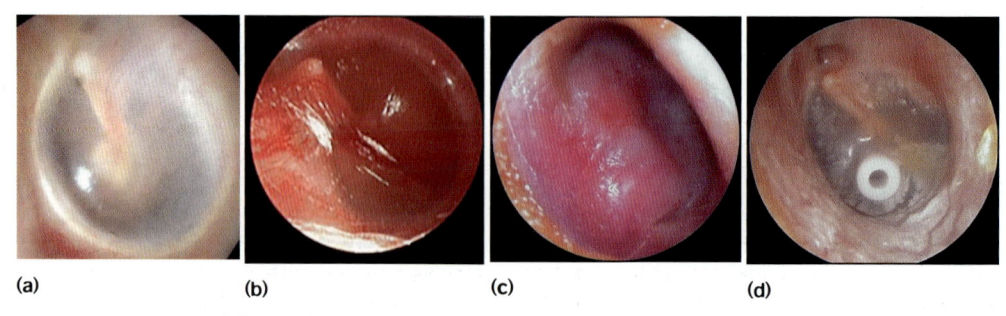

(a)   (b)   (c)   (d)

Figure 17.3 Appearance of the eardrum. (a) Normal; (b) acute otitis media; (c) otitis media with effusion; and (d) grommet. (Courtesy of Mr N Shah, Mr N Tolley, Mr Williamson, and Mr R Thevasagayam.)

nontypeable *Haemophilus influenzae* and *Moraxella catarrhalis*. Serious complications are mastoiditis and meningitis, but these are now uncommon. Pain should be treated with an analgesic such as paracetamol or ibuprofen. Regular analgesia is more effective than intermittent (as required) and may be needed for up to a week until the acute inflammation has resolved. Most cases of acute otitis media resolve spontaneously. Antibiotics marginally shorten the duration of pain but have not been shown to reduce the risk of hearing loss (see Evidence-based medicine Fig. 5.8, Ch. 5). A reasonable approach is to give the parents a prescription but ask them to use it only if the child remains unwell after 2–3 days. Amoxicillin is widely used. Neither decongestants nor antihistamines are beneficial.

Recurrent ear infections can lead to otitis media with effusion (also called glue ear, Fig. 17.3c). Children are usually asymptomatic apart from possible decreased hearing. The eardrum is seen to be dull and retracted, often with a fluid level visible. Otitis media with effusion is very common between the ages of 2–7 years, with peak incidence between 2.5–5 years of age. It usually resolves spontaneously, but may cause conductive hearing loss as shown on pure tone audiometry (possible if >4 years old) or a flat trace on tympanometry hearing testing in younger children. Cochrane reviews have shown no evidence of long-term benefit from the use of antibiotics, steroids, or decongestants. Otitis media with effusion is the most common cause of conductive hearing loss in children and can interfere with normal speech development and result in learning difficulties in school. In such children, insertion of ventilation tubes (grommets, Fig. 17.3d) is often performed, but benefits do not last more than 12 months. In practice, children with recurrent URTIs and chronic otitis media with effusion (glue ear) that does not resolve with conservative measures often also undergo grommet insertion. If problems recur after grommet extrusion, then reinsertion of grommets with adjuvant adenoidectomy is often advocated, as there is some evidence that adenoidectomy can offer more long-term benefit.

> **Summary**
>
> **Acute otitis media**
> - Is diagnosed by examining the tympanic membrane.
> - Antibiotics marginally shorten the duration of pain but do not reduce hearing loss.
> - If recurrent, may result in otitis media with effusion, which may cause speech and learning difficulties from hearing loss.

Sinusitis

Infection of the paranasal sinuses may occur with viral URTIs. Occasionally, there is secondary bacterial infection, with pain, swelling and tenderness over the cheek from infection of the maxillary sinus. As the frontal sinuses do not develop until late childhood, frontal sinusitis is uncommon in the first decade of life. Antibiotics and analgesia are used for acute sinusitis.

Tonsillectomy and adenoidectomy

Children with recurrent tonsillitis are often referred for removal of their tonsils, one of the most common operations performed in children. Many children have large tonsils, usually reaching a maximum size at about 8 years but this in itself is not an indication for tonsillectomy as they shrink spontaneously in late childhood.

The indications for tonsillectomy are controversial, and must be balanced against the risks of surgery, but include:

- recurrent severe tonsillitis (as opposed to recurrent URTIs) – tonsillectomy reduces the number of episodes of tonsillitis by a third, e.g. from three to two per year but is unlikely to benefit mild symptoms
- a peritonsillar abscess (quinsy)
- obstructive sleep apnoea (the adenoids will also often be removed).

Like the tonsils, adenoids increase in size until about the age of 8 years and then gradually regress. In young children, the adenoids grow proportionately faster than the airway, so that their effect of narrowing the airway lumen is greatest between ages 2–8 years. They may narrow the posterior nasal space sufficiently to justify adenoidectomy. Indications for the removal of both the tonsils and adenoids are controversial but include:

- recurrent otitis media with effusion with hearing loss, where it gives a significant long-term additional benefit
- obstructive sleep apnoea (an absolute indication).

Stridor

Stridor is a harsh, muscial sound due to partial obstruction of the lower portion of the upper airway including the upper trachea and the larynx. The causes of acute stridor are listed in Box 17.1. By far the most common cause is laryngeal and tracheal infection, where mucosal inflammation and swelling can rapidly cause life-threatening obstruction of the airway in young children.

The severity of upper airways obstruction is best assessed clinically by characteristics of the stridor (none, only on crying, at rest, or biphasic) and the degree of chest retraction (none, only on crying, at rest; Fig. 17.4).

Severe obstruction also leads to increasing respiratory rate, heart rate, and agitation. Central cyanosis, drooling or reduced level of consciousness suggest impending complete airway obstruction. The most reliable objective measure of hypoxaemia is by measuring the oxygen saturation by pulse oximetry, but, in contrast to lung disease, is a late feature of upper airways obstruction.

Total obstruction of the upper airway may be precipitated by examination of the throat using a spatula. One must avoid looking at the throat of a child with upper airways obstruction unless full resuscitation equipment and personnel are at hand.

Box 17.1 Differential diagnosis of acute stridor (upper airway obstruction)

Common causes

Viral laryngotracheobronchitis ('croup')

Rare causes

Epiglottitis
Bacterial tracheitis
Laryngeal or oesophageal foreign body
Allergic laryngeal angioedema (seen in anaphylaxis and recurrent croup)
Inhalation of smoke and hot fumes in fires
Trauma to the throat
Retropharyngeal abscess
Hypocalcaemia
Severe lymph node swelling (tuberculosis, infectious mononucleosis, malignancy)
Measles
Diphtheria
Psychological – vocal cord dysfunction

Table 17.1 Clinical features of croup (viral laryngotracheitis) and epiglottitis

	Croup	Epiglottitis
Onset	Over days	Over hours
Preceding coryza	Yes	No
Cough	Severe, barking	Absent or slight
Able to drink	Yes	No
Drooling saliva	No	Yes
Appearance	Unwell	Toxic, very ill
Fever	<38.5°C	>38.5°C
Stridor	Harsh, rasping	Soft, whispering
Voice, cry	Hoarse	Muffled, reluctant to speak

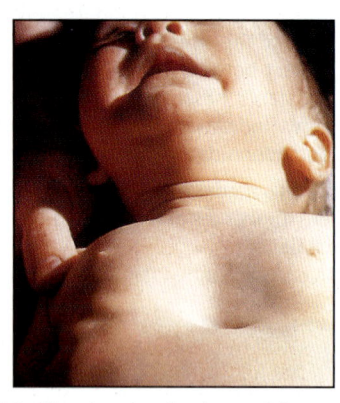

Figure 17.4. The degree of subcostal, intercostal, and sternal recession is a more useful indicator of severity of upper airways obstruction than the respiratory rate.

Croup

Viral croup accounts for over 95% of laryngotracheal infections. Parainfluenza viruses are the most common cause, but other viruses, such as rhinovirus, RSV and influenza, can produce a similar clinical picture. Croup typically occurs from 6 months to 6 years of age but the peak incidence is in the 2nd year of life. It is most common in the autumn. The typical features are coryza and fever followed by:

- hoarseness due to inflammation of the vocal cords
- a barking cough, like a sea lion, due to tracheal oedema and collapse
- harsh stridor
- variable degree of difficulty breathing with chest retraction
- the symptoms often start, and are worse, at night.

When the upper airway obstruction is mild, the stridor and chest recession disappear when the child is at rest and the child can usually be managed at home. The parents should observe the child closely for signs of increasing severity. The decision to manage the child at home or in hospital is influenced not only by the severity of the illness but also by the time of day, ease of access to hospital, the child's age (with a low threshold for admission for those <12 months old due to their narrow airway calibre) and parental understanding and confidence about the disorder.

Inhalation of warm moist air is a traditional and widely used therapy but it has not been shown to be beneficial. Oral dexamethasone, oral prednisolone, or nebulized steroids (budesonide) reduce the severity and duration of croup and are first-line therapy for croup causing chest recession at rest. They have been shown to reduce the need for hospitalization.

In severe upper airways obstruction, nebulized epinephrine (adrenaline) with oxygen by face mask provides rapid but transient improvement. The child must continue to be observed closely for 2–3 hours after administration as the effects wear off. Intubation for viral croup has become extremely unusual since the introduction of steroid therapy. Some children have a pattern of recurrent croup, which may be related to atopy.

Acute epiglottitis

In acute epiglottitis there is intense swelling of the epiglottis and surrounding tissues associated with septicaemia. It is a life-threatening emergency due to the high risk of respiratory obstruction. It is caused by *H. influenzae* type b (Hib). In the UK and many other countries, the introduction of universal Hib immunization in infancy has led to more than 99% reduction in the incidence of epiglottitis and other invasive Hib infections.

Epiglottitis is most common in children aged 1–6 years but affects all age groups. It is important to distinguish clinically between epiglottitis and croup (Table 17.1) as they require quite different treatment.

Case history 17.1

Acute epiglottitis

This 5-year-old girl developed a severe sore throat, drooling of saliva, a high fever, and increasing difficulty breathing over 8 hours (Fig. 17.5a). Epiglottitis was diagnosed and her airway was guaranteed with a nasotracheal tube. Antibiotics were started immediately (Fig. 17.5b, c). She made a full recovery.

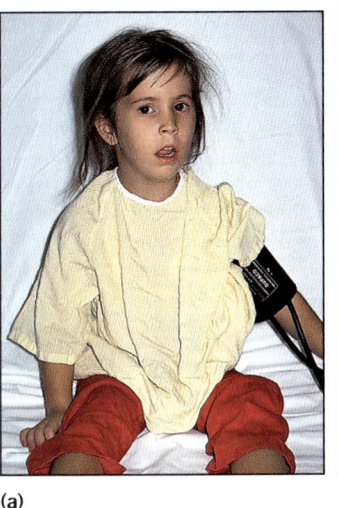

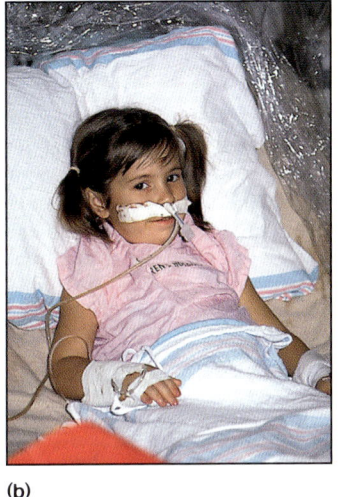

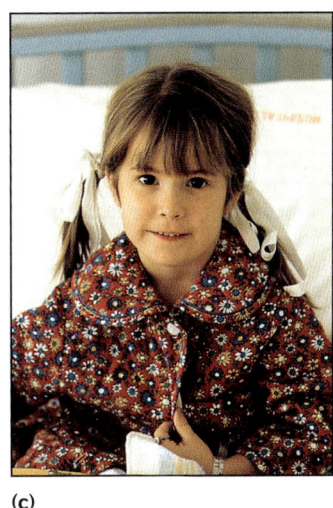

Figure 17.5 Acute epiglottitis. (a) At presentation; (b) at 16 hours, with nasotracheal and nasogastric tubes and an indwelling cannula for intravenous antibiotics; and (c) at 36 hours, following removal of the nasotracheal and nasogastric tubes.

The onset of epiglottitis is usually very acute (see Case History 17.1), with:

- high fever in a very ill, toxic-looking child
- an intensely painful throat that prevents the child from speaking or swallowing; saliva drools down the chin
- soft inspiratory stridor and rapidly increasing respiratory difficulty over hours
- the child sitting immobile, upright, with an open mouth to optimize the airway.

In contrast to viral croup, cough is minimal or absent. Attempts to lie the child down or examine the throat with a spatula or perform a lateral neck X-ray to identify a swollen epiglottis and surrounding tissues must not be undertaken as they can precipitate total airway obstruction and death.

If the diagnosis of epiglottitis is suspected, urgent hospital admission and treatment are required. A senior anaesthetist, paediatrician, and ear, nose, and throat (ENT) surgeon should be summoned and treatment initiated without delay. The child should be transferred directly to the intensive care unit or an anaesthetic room, and must be accompanied by senior medical staff in case respiratory obstruction occurs. The child should be intubated under controlled conditions with a general anaesthetic. Rarely, this is impossible and urgent tracheostomy is life-saving. Only after the airway is secured should blood be taken for culture and intravenous antibiotics such as cefuroxime started. The tracheal tube can usually be removed after 24 hours and antibiotics given for 3–5 days. With appropriate treatment, most children recover completely within 2–3 days. As with other serious *H. influenzae* infections, prophylaxis with rifampicin is offered to close household contacts.

Bacterial tracheitis (pseudomembranous croup)

This rare but dangerous condition is similar to severe epiglottitis in that the child has a high fever, appears very ill, and has rapidly progressive airways obstruction with copious thick airway secretions. It is typically caused by infection with *Staphylococcus aureus*. Management is by intravenous antibiotics and intubation and ventilation if required.

Other causes of stridor

When a child with acute stridor presents with atypical features or a poor response to treatment, other causes need to be considered (Box 17.1). If a child has an abrupt onset of stridor without apparent infection, consider anaphylaxis or inhaled foreign body.

Chronic stridor is usually due to a structural problem, either from intrinsic narrowing or collapse of the laryngotracheal airway, e.g. subglottic stenosis, laryngomalacia (floppy larynx), or external compression (e.g. vascular ring, lymph nodes, tumours). Investigations are required to determine the cause.

☀ **Basic management of acute upper airways obstruction is:**
- reduce anxiety by being calm, confident, and well organized
- observe carefully for signs of hypoxia or deterioration – agitation or fatigue or drowsiness or cyanosis. Provide oxygen if required and tolerated
- do not examine the throat with a spatula! It may precipitate upper airway obstruction
- oral, nebulized or intravenous steroids are beneficial in croup and have similar speed of onset (90–120 min)
- if severe, administer nebulized epinephrine (adrenaline) and contact an anaesthetist
- if respiratory failure develops from increasing airways obstruction, exhaustion or secretions blocking the airway, urgent tracheal intubation is required.

Wheeze

Acute wheeze is due to a partial obstruction of the intrathoracic airways. This is from mucosal inflammation and swelling as in bronchiolitis or bronchoconstriction as in asthma or mechanical obstruction (e.g. with foreign body or mucus). It may occur as a combination of all three.

Bronchiolitis

Bronchiolitis is the most common serious respiratory infection of infancy: 2–3% of all infants are admitted to hospital with the disease each year during annual winter epidemics; 90% are aged 1–9 months. RSV is the pathogen in 80%, the remainder are accounted for by parainfluenza virus, rhinovirus, adenovirus, influenza virus, and human metapneumovirus. There is evidence

---

Summary

The child with stridor

Clinical features to assess

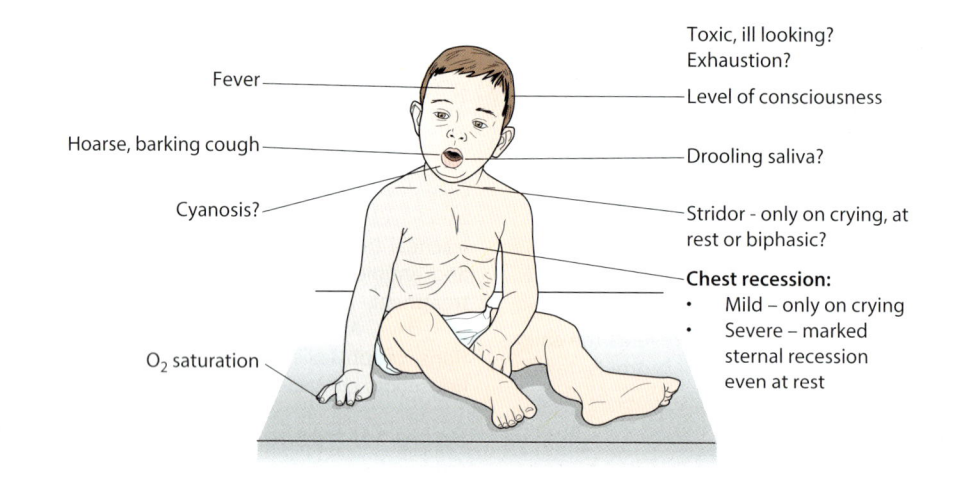

- Fever
- Hoarse, barking cough
- Cyanosis?
- O_2 saturation
- Toxic, ill looking? Exhaustion?
- Level of consciousness
- Drooling saliva?
- Stridor - only on crying, at rest or biphasic?
- Chest recession:
  - Mild – only on crying
  - Severe – marked sternal recession even at rest

Clinical conditions

Croup:
- Mostly viral
- 6 months to 6 years of age
- Harsh, loud stridor
- Coryza and mild fever, hoarse voice, barking cough

Epiglottitis:
- Caused by *H. influenzae* type b, rare since Hib immunization
- Mostly aged 1–6 years
- Acute, life-threatening illness
- High fever, ill, toxic-looking
- Painful throat, unable to swallow saliva, which drools down the chin

Bacterial tracheitis:
- High fever, toxic
- Loud, harsh stridor

Inhaled foreign body:
- Choking on peanut or toy or object in mouth
- Sudden onset of cough or respiratory distress

Chronic stridor:
- Recurrent or continuous stridor since birth or early infancy from laryngomalacia, congenital airway abnormality, or external compression, e.g. vascular ring

Other rare causes:
- See Box 17.1

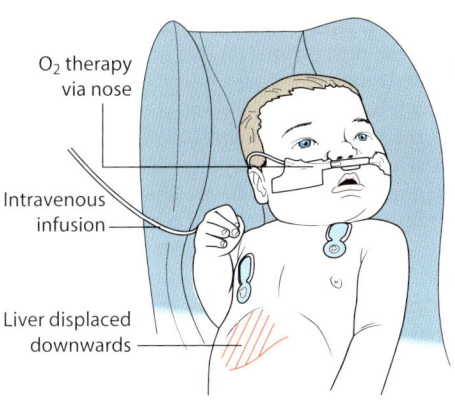

Bronchiolitis

Figure 17.6 Clinical features of severe bronchiolitis in an infant.

- O₂ therapy via nose
- Intravenous infusion
- Liver displaced downwards

- Dry, wheezy cough
- Cyanosis or pallor
- Hyperinflation of the chest:
  - sternum prominent
  - liver displaced downwards
- Subcostal and intercostal recession
- Auscultation:
  - fine end-inspiratory crackles (crepitations)
  - prolonged expiration/wheeze

Causes of acute respiratory distress in an infant:
- Bronchiolitis
- Viral episodic wheeze
- Pneumonia
- Heart failure
- Foreign body
- Anaphylaxis
- Pneumothorax or pleural effusion
- Metabolic acidosis
- Severe anaemia

that co-infection with more than one virus, particularly RSV and human metapneumovirus may lead to a more severe illness.

Coryzal symptoms precede a dry cough and increasing breathlessness. Feeding difficulty associated with increasing dyspnoea is often the reason for admission to hospital. Recurrent apnoea is a serious complication, especially in young infants. Infants born prematurely who develop bronchopulmonary dysplasia or with other underlying lung disease, such as cystic fibrosis, or have congenital heart disease are most at risk from severe bronchiolitis. The characteristic findings on examination (Fig. 17.6) are:

- dry wheezy cough
- tachypnoea and tachycardia
- subcostal and intercostal recession
- hyperinflation of the chest
- fine end-inspiratory crackles
- high-pitched wheezes – expiratory > inspiratory.

Investigations and decision to admit

Pulse oximetry should be performed on all children with suspected bronchiolitis. No other investigations are routinely recommended. In particular, chest X-ray or blood gases are only indicated if respiratory failure is suspected.

Hospital admission is indicated if any of the following are present:

- apnoea (observed or reported)
- persistent oxygen saturation of < 90% when breathing air
- inadequate oral fluid intake (50–75% of usual volume)
- severe respiratory distress – grunting, marked chest recession, or a respiratory rate over 70 breaths/minute.

Management

This is supportive. Humidified oxygen is either delivered via nasal cannulae or using a head box; the concentration required is determined by pulse oximetry. The infant is monitored for apnoea. No evidence for reducing severity or illness duration has been shown from use of mist, nebulized hypertonic saline, antibiotics, corticosteroids or nebulized bronchodilators, such as salbutamol or ipratropium. Fluids may need to be given by nasogastric tube or intravenously. Assisted ventilation in the form of non-invasive respiratory support with CPAP (continuous positive airway pressure) or else mechanical ventilation is required in a small percentage of infants admitted to hospital [see Case History 6.1 in Ch. 6 (Paediatric emergencies)]. RSV is highly infectious, and infection control measures, particularly good hand hygiene, cohort nursing, and gowns and gloves, have been shown to prevent cross-infection to other infants in hospital.

Most infants recover from the acute infection within 2 weeks. However, as many as half will have recurrent episodes of cough and wheeze (see the following section). Rarely, usually following adenovirus infection, the illness may result in permanent damage to the airways (*bronchiolitis obliterans*).

Prevention of bronchiolitis

A monoclonal antibody to RSV (palivizumab, given monthly by intramuscular injection) reduces the number of hospital admissions in high-risk preterm infants, although 17 babies need to be treated to avoid one admission. Its use is limited by cost and the need for multiple intramuscular injections.

Asthma

Asthma is the most common chronic respiratory disorder in childhood, affecting at least 1 in 11 children in the UK. Worldwide, there has been a significant increase in the incidence of asthma over the last 40 years, although this has now plateaued in many high-income countries. Although the symptoms of asthma are readily controlled in most children, it is an important cause of absence from school, restricted activity, and anxiety for the child and family. There are still about 20 deaths from asthma in children each year in the UK.

Diagnosing asthma in preschool children is often difficult. Approximately half of all children wheeze at some time during the first 3 years of life. In general, there are three patterns of wheezing (Fig. 17.7):

- viral episodic wheezing – wheeze only in response to viral infections

- multiple trigger wheeze – in response to multiple triggers and which is more likely to develop into asthma over time
- asthma.

Viral episodic wheeze

Most wheezy preschool children have *viral episodic wheeze*. This is thought to result from small airways being more likely to narrow and obstruct due to inflammation and aberrant immune responses to viral infection. This gives the condition its episodic nature, being triggered by viruses that cause the common cold. Studies have found that sufferers often have reduced small airway diameter from birth. Risk factors include maternal smoking during and/or after pregnancy and prematurity. A family history of asthma or allergy is not a risk factor, but a family history of early viral wheezing is common. Viral episodic wheezing is more common in males and usually resolves by 5 years of age, presumably from increase in airway size.

Multiple trigger wheeze and asthma

Some children, both preschool and school aged, have frequent wheeze triggered by many stimuli, not just viruses but also cold air, dust, animal dander and exercise. This has been called multiple-trigger wheeze. In the preschool age group, where a formal diagnosis of asthma may be unjustified, this distinction is helpful as many children in this group benefit from asthma preventer therapy and a significant proportion go on to have asthma. When recurrent wheezing is associated with symptoms between viral infections (interval symptoms) and evidence of allergy to one or more inhaled allergens such as house dust mite, pollens or pets, it is called 'atopic asthma'. Evidence of allergy may be accompanied by positive skin-prick testing or presence of IgE on blood testing. Atopic asthma is strongly associated with other atopic diseases such as eczema, rhinoconjunctivitis and food allergy, and is more common in those with a family history of such diseases.

A small number of persistent or recurrent wheezing children will have other causes, such as non-atopic asthma. Other causes of recurrent wheeze are listed in Box 17.2.

Pathophysiology of asthma

An outline of the pathophysiology of asthma is shown in Fig. 17.8.

Box 17.2 Causes of recurrent or persistent childhood wheeze

Viral episodic wheeze
Multiple trigger wheeze
Asthma
Recurrent anaphylaxis (e.g. in food allergy)
Chronic aspiration
Cystic fibrosis
Bronchopulmonary dysplasia
Bronchiolitis obliterans
Tracheo-bronchomalacia

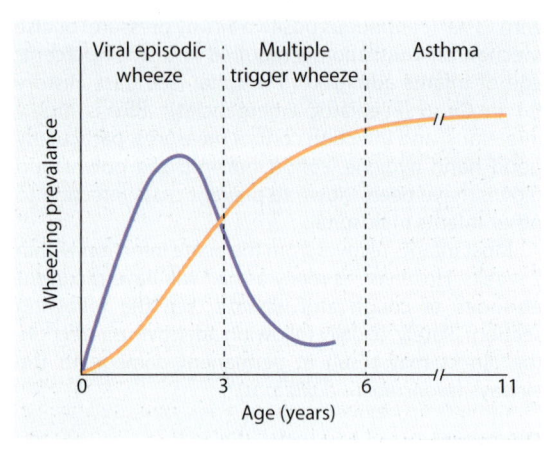

Figure 17.7 Prevalence of wheeze in children caused by the three major phenotypes by age.

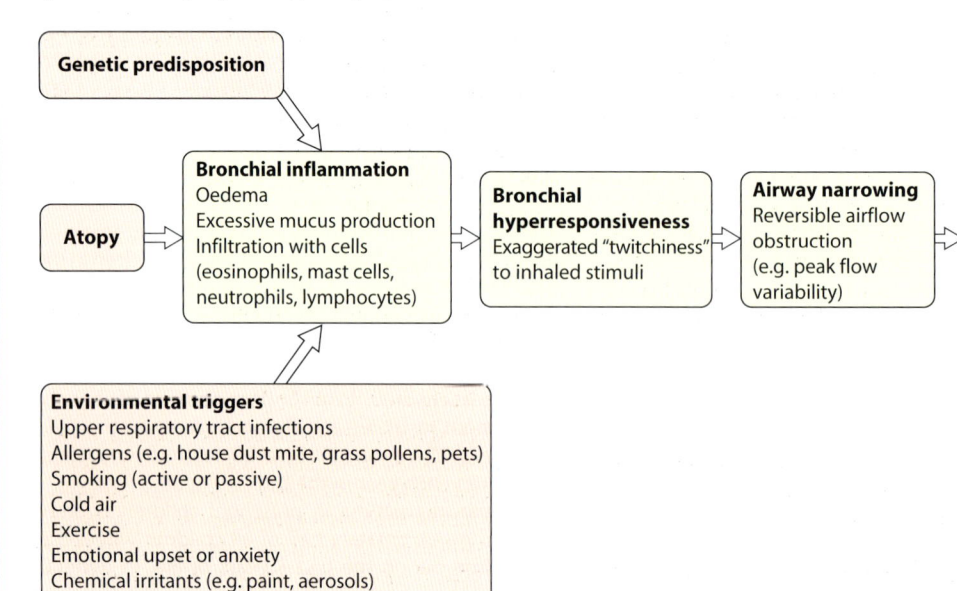

Figure 17.8 Pathophysiology of asthma.

Clinical features

Asthma should be suspected in any child with wheezing on more than one occasion, particularly if there are interval symptoms. It is more common in children with a personal or family history of atopy. Although it may be clear to most clinicians what 'wheezing' is, children and parents do not always mean the same thing. It is best to describe the sound (e.g. 'a whistling in the chest when your child breaths out') and ask if that fits with their child's symptoms. Ideally, the presence of wheeze is confirmed on auscultation by a health professional to distinguish it from transmitted upper respiratory noises, which are often loud and easy to hear in children. Asthmatic wheeze is a polyphonic (multiple pitch) noise coming from the airways. It is believed to represent many airways of different sizes vibrating from abnormal narrowing.

Key features associated with a high probability of a child having asthma include:

- Symptoms worse at night and in the early morning
- Symptoms that have nonviral triggers
- Interval symptoms, i.e. symptoms between acute exacerbations
- Personal or family history of an atopic disease
- Positive response to asthma therapy.

Once suspected, the pattern or phenotype should be further explored by asking

- How frequent are the symptoms?
- What triggers the symptoms? Specifically, are sport and general activities affected by the asthma?
- How often is sleep disturbed by asthma?
- How severe are the interval symptoms between exacerbations?
- How much school has been missed due to asthma?

Examination of the chest is usually normal between attacks. In long-standing asthma there may be hyperinflation of the chest, generalized polyphonic expiratory wheeze with a prolonged expiratory phase. Onset of the disease in early childhood may result in Harrison's sulci (Fig. 17.9). Evidence of eczema should be sought, as should examination of the nasal mucosa for allergic rhinitis. Growth should be plotted but is usually normal unless the asthma is extremely severe. The presence of a wet cough or sputum production, finger clubbing or poor growth suggests a condition characterized by chronic infection such as cystic fibrosis or bronchiectasis.

Investigations

In younger children, asthma is usually diagnosed from history and examination alone. Parental description of the symptoms and response to treatment is the cornerstone to diagnosis. Sometimes, specific investigations are required to confirm the diagnosis, or determine the severity and phenotype in more detail. Skin-prick testing for common allergens may be performed to aid the diagnosis of atopy and to identify allergens, which may be acting as triggers. A chest X-ray is usually normal and is not necessary unless other conditions need to be excluded.

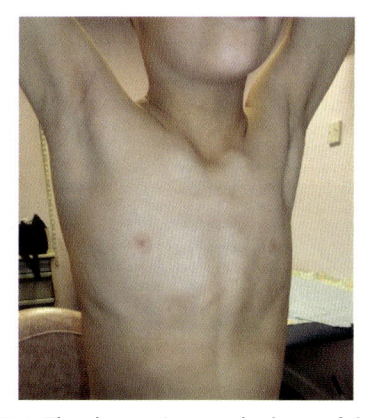

Figure 17.9 The depressions at the base of the thorax associated with the muscular insertion of the diaphragm are called Harrison's sulci, and are associated with chronic obstructive airways disease such as asthma during childhood from chronic increased work of breathing.

If there is uncertainty in the diagnosis or disease severity needs to be monitored, peak expiratory flow rate (PEFR) may be measured or spirometry performed [see Ch. 2 (History and examination) and Appendix A5 and A6]. Peak flow is less sensitive to changes in airway calibre than spirometry but is portable and therefore helpful for serial measurements. Most children over 5 years of age can use a peak flow meter or undertake spirometry. Poorly controlled asthma leads to increased variability in peak flow, with both diurnal variability (morning usually lower than evening peak flow) and day-to-day variability. Spirometry involves measurement of forced expiratory volume in 1 second blowing out as hard and as fast as possible (FEV_1). This provides a non-invasive measure of flow through the larger airways (to the bronchioles). Often, response to a bronchodilator is the most helpful investigation. This can be demonstrated as an improvement in peak flow rate or in FEV_1 before and after inhaling a bronchodilator (an improvement of 12% or more confirms bronchodilator reversibility and is characteristic of asthma). Following treatment, this reversibility often reduces or disappears completely.

Management

Medications used to treat children with asthma are shown in Table 17.2.

Bronchodilator therapy

Inhaled $β_2$-agonists are the most commonly used and most effective bronchodilators. *Short-acting $β_2$-agonists* (often called *relievers*) such as salbutamol or terbutaline have a rapid onset of action (maximum effects after 10–15 min), are effective for 2–4 hours and have few side-effects. They are used "as required" for increased symptoms and in high doses for acute asthma attacks.

Table 17.2 Drugs in chronic asthma

Type of drug	Drug
Bronchodilators	
β$_2$-agonists (relievers)	Salbutamol
	Terbutaline
Anticholinergic bronchodilator	Ipratropium bromide
Preventer therapy	
Inhaled steroids	Budesonide
	Beclometasone
	Fluticasone
	Mometasone
Long-acting β$_2$-agonists (LABA)	Salmeterol
	Formoterol
Methylxanthines	Theophylline
Leukotriene receptor antagonists (LTRA)	Montelukast
Oral steroids	Prednisolone
Anti-IgE monoclonal antibody	Omalizumab

All are given by inhalation, except prednisolone, leukotriene modulators and theophylline preparations, which are by mouth, and omalizumab, which is by subcutaneous injection.

By contrast, *long-acting β$_2$-agonists* (*LABAs*) such as salmeterol or formoterol are effective for 12 hours. They are not used in acute asthma and should not be used without an inhaled corticosteroid. LABAs are useful in exercise-induced asthma.

Ipratropium bromide, an anticholinergic bronchodilator, is sometimes given to young infants when other bronchodilators are found to be ineffective or in the treatment of severe acute asthma.

Preventer therapy
Inhaled corticosteroids

Prophylactic drugs are effective only if taken regularly. *Inhaled corticosteroids* (often called *preventers*) are the most effective inhaled prophylactic therapy. They decrease airway inflammation, resulting in decreased symptoms, asthma exacerbations and bronchial hyperactivity. They are often used in conjunction with an inhaled LABA or leukotriene receptor antagonist. They have no clinically significant side-effects when given in low dose, although they can cause mild reduction in height velocity, but this is usually followed by catch-up growth in late childhood. Systemic side-effects, including impaired growth, adrenal suppression and altered bone metabolism may be seen when high doses are used. To reduce the risk of unwanted side-effects, treatment with inhaled corticosteroids should always be at the lowest dose possible. Treatment for many children is effective at very low doses (see Fig. 17.10).

> Always monitor the growth of children with asthma, especially if taking regular inhaled or oral corticosteroids

Add-on therapy

The first choice of add-on therapy in a child over 5 years is a LABA, whereas in children under 5 years, an oral *leukotriene receptor antagonist* such as montelukast is recommended. The latter can also be used in older children when symptoms are not controlled by the addition of a LABA. *Slow-release oral theophylline* is an alternative; however, it has a high incidence of side-effects (vomiting, insomnia, headaches, poor concentration), so it is not often used in children.

Other therapies

Oral *prednisolone*, usually given on alternate days to minimize the adverse effect on growth, is required only in severe persistent asthma where other treatment has failed. All children on this therapy must be managed by a specialist in childhood asthma. *Anti-IgE therapy* (*omalizumab*) is an injectable monoclonal antibody that acts against IgE, the natural antibody that mediates allergy. It is used for the treatment of severe atopic asthma, and should also only be administered by a specialist in childhood asthma.

Most antibiotics are of no value in the absence of a bacterial infection and neither cough medicines nor decongestants are helpful. Antihistamines, e.g. loratadine and nasal steroids are useful in the treatment of allergic rhinitis.

The British Guideline on Asthma Management uses a stepwise approach, starting treatment with the step most appropriate to the severity of the asthma and aiming for optimal control of symptoms. Complete control is defined as the absence of daytime or night-time symptoms, no limit on activities (including exercise), no need for reliever use, normal lung function and no exacerbations (need for hospitalization or oral steroids) in the previous 6 months. Treatment increases from step 1 (mild intermittent asthma) to step 5 (chronic severe asthma requiring continuous or frequent use of oral steroids), stepping down when control is good (Fig. 17.10).

Allergen avoidance and other nonpharmacological measures

Although asthma in many children is precipitated or worsened by specific allergens, complete avoidance of the allergen is difficult to achieve. The value of identifying such triggers by history or allergy testing is controversial. Most studies of allergen avoidance have been disappointing, although dust mite-impermeable mattress covers may be beneficial in some children. Allergen immunotherapy is effective for treating atopic asthma due to a single allergen, but its use is limited by the risk of systemic allergic reactions associated with the treatment (see Ch. 16).

Parents should be advised about the harmful effects of cigarette smoking in the house. Although

A stepwise approach to the treatment of chronic asthma

Step 5: Continuous or frequent use of oral steroids
In **children 5–12 years:** maintain ICS at 800 µg/day.
Use lowest possible daily dose of oral steroids to maintain adequate control. Refer to respiratory paediatrician
In **adolescents and young adults:** maintain ICS at 1600 µg/day. Use lowest possible daily dose of oral steroids to maintain adequate control. Refer.

Step 4: Persistent poor control
In <5 years: refer to respiratory paediatrician
In 5–12 years: increase ICS to 800 µg/day
In adolescents and young adults: increase ICS to 1600 µg/day and consider LTRA, or SR theophylline
Issue steroid replacement warning card.

Step 3: Initial add-on therapy
In <5 years: add LTRA; if poor response, increase ICS to 400 µg/day.
>5 years and young adults: initially add inhaled long-acting β_2-agonist (LABA). Assess response:
• Good response—LABA
• Partial response—increase ICS to 400 µg/day [800 in adolescents and young adults].
• Poor response—stop LABA, increase ICS to 400 µg/day [800 µg in adolescents and young adults] and consider LTRA and/or slow release (SR) theophylline.

Step 2: Regular preventer therapy
In all ages: add inhaled corticosteroid 200 µg/day or in those <5 years consider leukotriene receptor antagonist (LTRA) if inhaled corticosteroid cannot be used. In adolescents and young adults doses of up to 400 µg/day may be used at this step.
Monitor height and weight of all children on asthma treatment.

Step 1: Mild intermittent asthma
In all ages: inhaled short-acting β_2-agonist as required

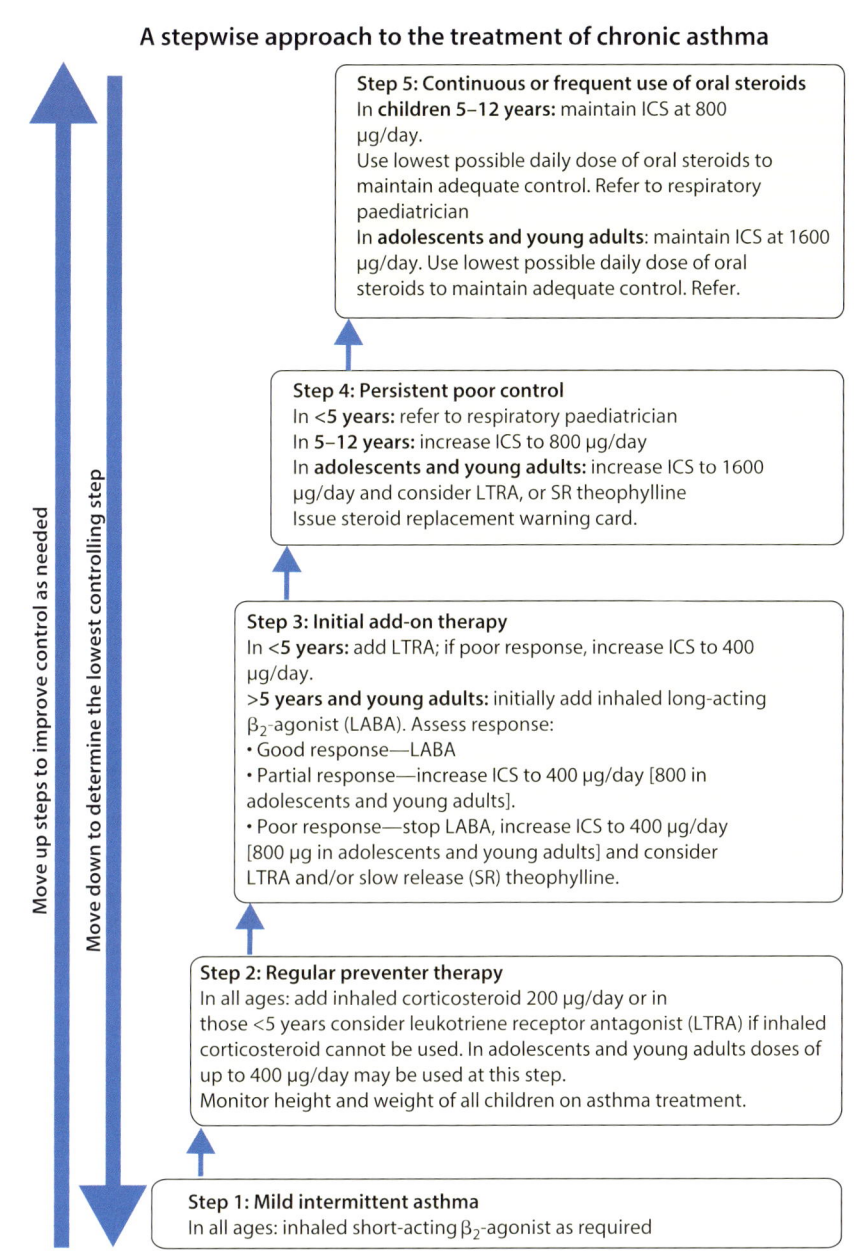

Move up steps to improve control as needed
Move down to determine the lowest controlling step

Figure 17.10 A stepwise approach to the treatment of asthma. All ICS doses expressed as beclometasone diproprionate (CFC-MDI) equivalent. The aim of treatment is to gain control of symptoms and to maintain this control at the lowest possible step of treatment. LTRA – leukotriene receptor antagonist; SR theophylline – slow release theophylline; LABA – long-acting β_2-agonist; ICS – inhaled corticosteroid. (From the Scottish Intercollegiate Guideline Network/British Thoracic Society: 2016 with permission (Accessed October 2016).)

exercise improves general fitness, there is no evidence that physical training improves asthma itself. Psychological intervention may be useful in chronic severe asthma.

Acute asthma

Assessment

With each acute attack, the duration of symptoms, the treatment already given, and the course of previous attacks should be noted. Clinical features which need to be determined are shown in Fig. 17.11.

Criteria for admission to hospital

Children require hospital admission if, after high-dose inhaled bronchodilator therapy, they:

- have not responded adequately clinically, i.e. there is persisting breathlessness or tachypnoea
- are becoming exhausted

Assessment of the child with acute asthma

Determine the severity of the attack (see Fig. 17.12):
- Mild
- Moderate
- Severe
- Life-threatening

This is determined by clinical features shown.

Too breathless to talk – severe

Increased work of breathing
Check respiratory rate:
- Tachypnoea – varies with age; poor guide to severity

Chest recession:
- Moderate – some intercostal recession
- Severe – use of accessory neck muscles
- Life-threatening – poor respiratory effort

Auscultation:
- Wheeze
- Silent chest – poor air entry from poor expiratory effort or exhaustion in life-threatening

Cardiovascular:
- Tachycardia – varies with age; better guide to severity than respiratory rate but affected by β_2-agonists
- Arrythmia, hypotension – life-threatening

Altered consciousness, agitation or confusion – in life-threatening
Exhaustion – life-threatening

Tongue:
- Cyanosis in life-threatening

Peak flow (% predicted or best or usual measurement):
- Moderate >50%
- Severe 33–50%
- Life-threatening <33%

O_2 saturation:
- Moderate ≥92%
- Severe or life-threatening <92%

Is there a trigger for the attack?:
- URTI or other viral illness
- Allergen, e.g. animal dander
- Exercise
- Cold air

Causes of acute breathlessness in the older child:
- **Asthma**
- Pneumonia or lower respiratory tract infection
- Foreign body
- Anaphylaxis
- Pneumothorax or pleural effusion
- Metabolic acidosis – diabetic ketoacidosis, inborn error of metabolism, lactic acidosis
- Severe anaemia
- Heart failure
- Panic attacks (hyperventilation)

Figure 17.11 Assessment of the child with acute asthma to determine severity of the attack.

- still have a marked reduction in their predicted (or usual best) peak flow rate or FEV_1 (<50%)
- have a reduced oxygen saturation (<92% in air).

A chest X-ray is indicated only if there are unusual features (e.g. asymmetry of chest signs suggesting pneumothorax, lobar collapse) or signs of severe infection. In children, blood gases are only indicated in life-threatening or refractory cases and often are normal until the child is *in extremis*.

Management

Acute breathlessness is frightening for both the child and the parents. Calm and skilful management is the key to their reassurance. High-dose inhaled bronchodilators, steroids, and oxygen form the foundation of therapy of severe acute asthma.

Management is summarized in Fig. 17.12. As soon as the diagnosis has been made, the child should be given oxygen if the oxygen saturation is <92%. All children should be given a β_2-bronchodilator, the dose and frequency increasing according to severity of the attack, the child's age and response to therapy.

It should be given via a spacer, as used by the child at home, unless the attack is severe to life-threatening when a nebulizer driven by high-flow oxygen may be indicated. The addition of nebulized ipratropium to the initial therapy in severe asthma is beneficial. A short course (3–7 days) of oral prednisolone expedites the recovery from moderate or severe acute asthma.

Inhaled therapies are not always be successful as the drugs may be delivered in suboptimal doses to areas of the lung that are poorly ventilated. Intravenous therapy therefore has a role in the minority of children who fail to respond adequately to inhaled bronchodilator therapy. Magnesium sulphate, aminophylline, or intravenous salbutamol are all potentially beneficial. Magnesium sulphate probably has the least side-effects and most evidence of benefit, and is increasingly being used as the first choice for intravenous therapy. For intravenous aminophylline, a loading dose is given over 20 minutes, followed by continuous infusion. Seizures, severe vomiting and fatal cardiac arrhythmias may follow a rapid infusion. If the child is already on oral theophylline, the loading dose should be omitted. With

Assessment and management of acute asthma

Assess severity

Moderate
- Able to talk
- Oxygen saturation >92%
- Peak flow >50% [best]
- Respiratory rate
  ≤40 breaths/min for 2–5 year
  ≤30 breaths/min for 5–12 year
  ≤25 breaths/min for 12–18 year
- Heart rate
  ≤140 beats/min for 2–5 year
  ≤125 beats/min for 5–12 year
  ≤110 beats/min for 12–18 year

Severe
- Too breathless to talk
- Oxygen saturation <92% for <12 year olds
- Peak flow 33%–50% [best]
- Respiratory rate
  >40 breaths/min for 2–5 year
  >30 breaths/min for 5–12 year
  >25 breaths/min for 12–18 year
- Heart rate
  >140 beats/min for 2–5 year
  >125 beats/min for 5–12 year
  >110 beats/min for 12–18 year

Life-threatening
- Silent chest, cyanosis
- Poor respiratory effort
- Exhaustion
- Arrhythmia, hypotension
- Altered consciousness
- Agitation, confusion
- Peak flow <33% [best]
- Oxygen saturation <92% (all ages)

Management

High flow oxygen (if available)

- Keep calm and reassure child and parents
- Short-acting β_2-agonist via spacer (with face mask for those under 3), 2–4 puffs, increasing by 2 puffs every 2 min to 10 puffs if required
- Oral prednisolone 1–2 mg/kg, maximum 40 mg
- Monitor response for 15–30 min

- Short-acting β_2-agonist via spacer, 10 puffs or nebulized (2.5 mg salbutamol in <8 years, 5 mg in >8 years), assess response and repeat as required
- Oral prednisolone or IV hydrocortisone
Consider:
- Inhaled ipratropium
- IV β_2-agonist (salbutamol) or aminophylline or magnesium

- Short-acting β_2-agonist nebulized (2.5 mg salbutamol in <8 years, 5 mg in >8 years), assess response continuously and repeat as required (back to back)
- Oral prednisolone or IV hydrocortisone
- Nebulized ipratropium
Consider:
- IV β_2-agonist (salbutamol) or aminophylline or magnesium
Discuss with PICU

Assess response to treatment

Responding:
- Continue bronchodilators 1–4 h prn
- Discharge when stable on 4-h treatment
- Continue oral prednisolone for 3–7 days

At discharge:
- Review medication and inhaler technique
- Provide personalized asthma action plan
- Arrange appropriate follow-up

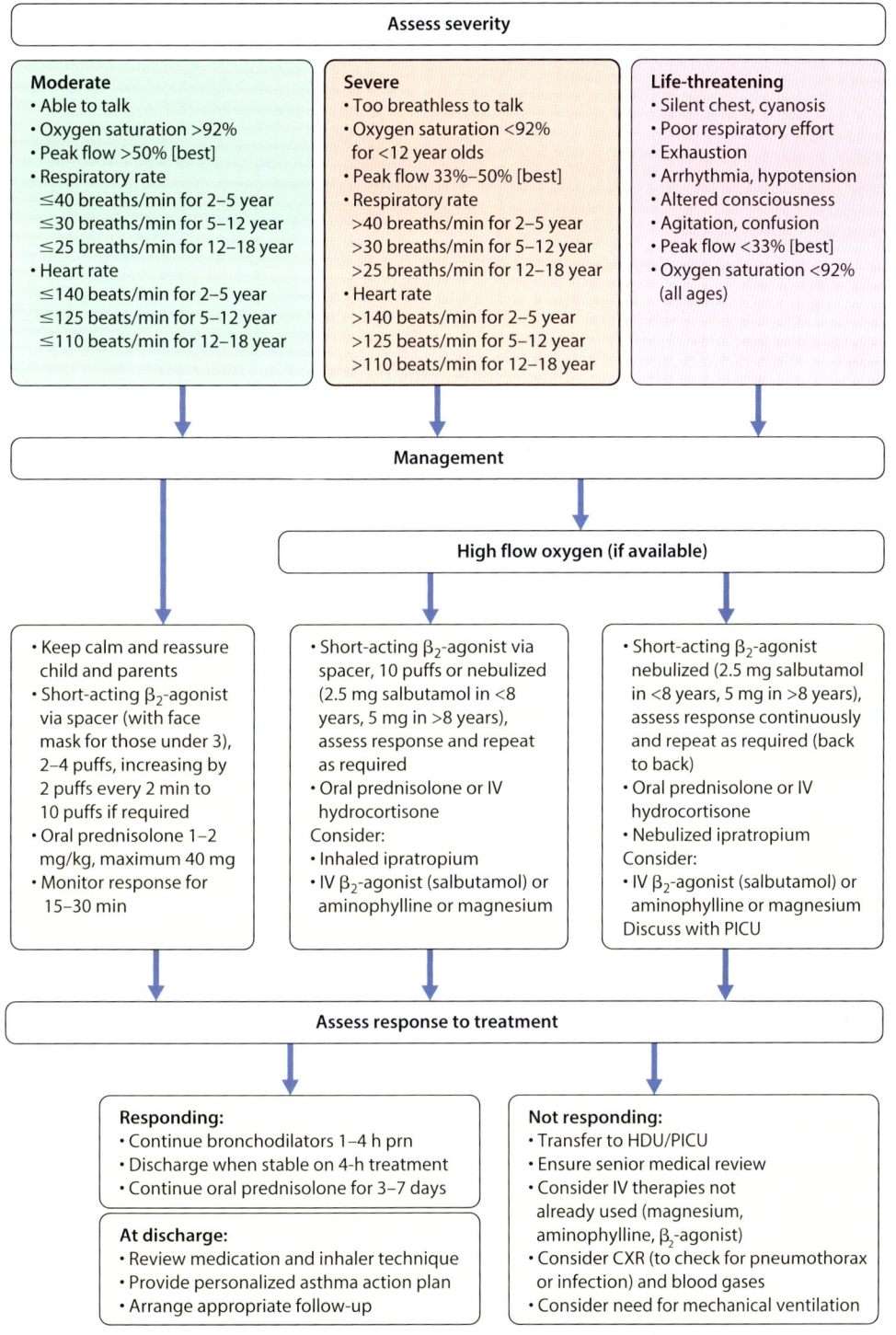

Not responding:
- Transfer to HDU/PICU
- Ensure senior medical review
- Consider IV therapies not already used (magnesium, aminophylline, β_2-agonist)
- Consider CXR (to check for pneumothorax or infection) and blood gases
- Consider need for mechanical ventilation

Figure 17.12 Assessment and management of acute asthma. (Adapted and modified from British Thoracic Society and Scottish Intercollegiate Guidelines Network (2016) with permission.)

Choosing the correct inhaler

Inhaled drugs may be administered via a variety of devices, chosen according to the child's age and preference
- *Pressurized metered dose inhaler and spacer* (Fig. 17.13).
  - Appropriate for all age groups: 0–2 years, spacer and face mask; >3 years, spacer alone.
  - A spacer is recommended for all children as it increases drug deposition to the lungs and reduces oropharyngeal deposition, reducing steroid side-effects.
  - Useful for acute asthma attacks when poor inspiratory effort may impair the use of inhalers direct to the mouth.
- *Breath-actuated metered dose inhalers* (e.g. *Autohaler*, *Easi-Breathe*): 6+ years. Less coordination needed than a pressurized metered dose inhaler without spacer. Useful for delivering β_2-agonists when 'out and about' in older children.
- *Dry powder inhaler*: 4+ years (Fig. 17.14). Needs a good inspiratory flow, therefore less good in severe asthma and during an asthma attack. Also easy to use when 'out and about' in older children.
- *Nebulizer*: any age (Fig. 17.15). Only used in acute asthma where oxygen is needed in addition to inhaled drugs; occasionally used at home as part of an acute management plan in those with rapid-onset severe asthma (brittle asthma).

Many children fail to gain the benefit of their treatment because they cannot use the inhaler correctly or the inhaler used is no longer appropriate for the child. They need to be shown and their ability to use it checked. In young children, parents need to be skilled in assisting their child to use the inhaler correctly. Assessing and reassessing inhaler technique is vital to good management and should be a routine part of any review.

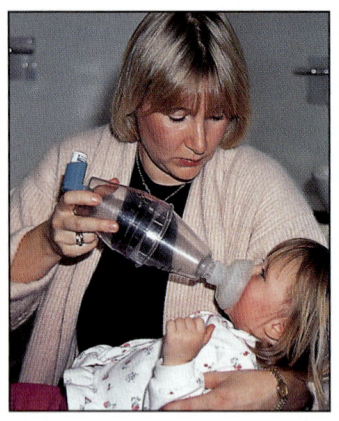

Figure 17.13 Pressurized metered dose inhaler and spacer. Suitable for all ages, with face mask if under 2 years of age.

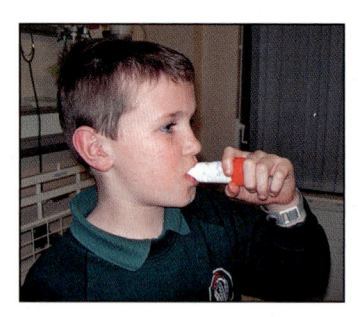

Figure 17.14 Dry powder inhaler, 4 years and older.

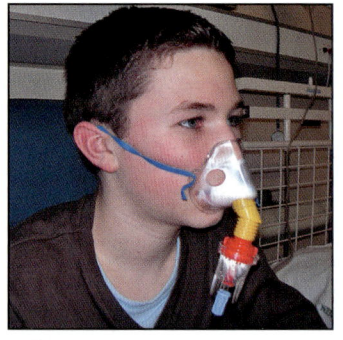

Figure 17.15 Nebulizer: all ages. Only used in acute asthma where oxygen is needed in addition to inhaled drugs.

both aminophylline and salbutamol, the ECG should be monitored and blood electrolytes checked. Antibiotics are only given if there are clinical features of bacterial infection. Occasionally, these measures are insufficient and mechanical ventilation is required.

Patient education

Prior to discharge from hospital after an acute admission, the following should be reviewed with the child and family:
- When drugs should be used (regularly or 'as required').
- How to use the drug (inhaler technique) (Figs 17.13–17.15).
- What each drug does (relief vs. prevention).
- How often and how much can be used (frequency and dosage).
- What to do if asthma worsens (a written personalized asthma management action plan should be compiled: see Appendix A3 for an example).

The child and parents need to be aware that increasing cough, wheeze, breathlessness and difficulty in walking, talking and sleeping, or decreasing relief from bronchodilators all indicate poorly controlled asthma. Some asthmatics find it difficult to identify gradual deterioration – measurement of peak flow rate at home allows earlier recognition. Patients with troublesome asthma are usually given a supply of oral steroids to keep at home, with details in the asthma action plan

Periodic assessment of the child with asthma

Clinical features to check

- Growth and nutrition
- Peak flow/spirometry
- Chest for:
  - Hyperinflation
  - Harrison's sulcus
  - Wheeze
- Are there other allergic disorders?
  - Allergic rhinitis
  - Eczema
  - Food allergy
- If atypical features present:
  - Sputum
  - Finger clubbing
  - Growth failure
  - then seek another diagnosis

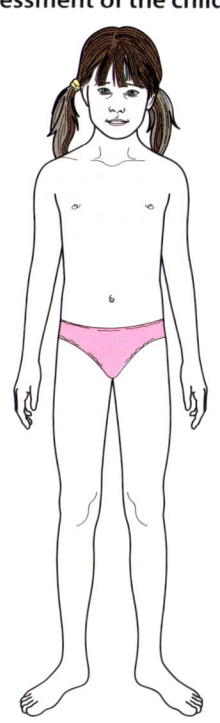

Monitor:
- Peak flow diary
- Severity and frequency of symptoms
- Exercise tolerance
- Interference with life, time off school
- Is sleep disturbed?
- Use of preventer and reliever medication – are they appropriate?
- Inhaler technique
- Lung function tests

Consider triggers:
- Untreated allergic rhinitis
- Allergens or cigarette smoke
- Stress

Check:
- Child has an up to date personalized asthma management action plan
- Family have necessary medication/equipment to manage an acute exacerbation

Figure 17.16 Outline of periodic assessment required for a child with asthma.

on when to start them. Outcomes are better for children with asthma who have a package of educational measures but no single component has been shown to be beneficial in isolation. Follow-up arrangements need to be made. The periodic assessment of the child with asthma is outlined in Fig. 17.16.

Other causes of acute wheezing

The most common cause of acute wheeze is an acute attack of asthma or viral episodic wheeze. In infants and toddlers it is also present in bronchiolitis. Other causes are:

- *Atypical pneumonia* – although pneumococcal pneumonia rarely causes wheezing, atypical pneumonia caused by *Mycoplasma*, *Chlamydia* or adenovirus can do so.
- *Foreign body inhalation* – abrupt onset of cough followed by wheeze in a previously well child. On passing below the glottis, a foreign body generally impacts in a main or lobar bronchus and may initially cause unilateral wheezing and air trapping. A chest X-ray performed during expiration will show persistent hyperinflation of the lung distal to the obstruction (see Case History 17.2). Eventually, airway swelling causes complete obstruction and lobar collapse is seen.
- *Anaphylaxis* – suspect if acute urticaria, facial swelling, stridor, or previous reaction to an allergen. The management of anaphylaxis is shown in Fig. 6.11.

Case history 17.2

Foreign body inhalation

A previously well 3-year-old boy presented with a 5-day history of severe cough and wheeze. His symptoms developed after choking on some peanuts. A chest X-ray revealed a hyperlucent right lung (Fig. 17.17). Bronchoscopy was performed and revealed a peanut wedged in the right main bronchus.

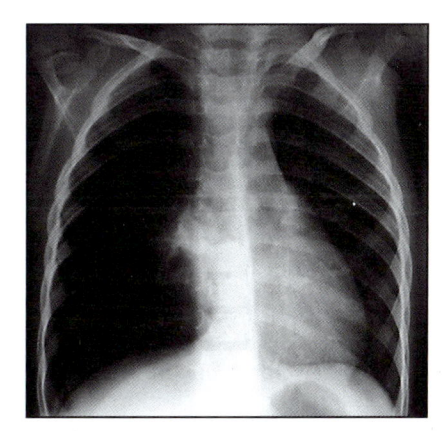

Figure 17.17 Hyperlucency of the right lung and mediastinal shift to the left. (Courtesy of Dr Abbas Khakoo.)

Cough

Acute cough

Cough is the most common symptom of respiratory disease. Identifying if the cough is dry or moist can be helpful diagnostically. A dry cough with a prolonged expiratory phase suggests that there is some narrowing of the small-sized to moderate-sized airways. A barking cough suggests a degree of tracheal inflammation, narrowing or collapse. A moist cough suggests that there is either increased mucus secretion or infection in the lower airway.

The cough reflex functions to expel unwanted material from the airway below the glottis. In most children, episodes of cough are due to tracheobronchial spread of URTIs caused by the common cold viruses and do not indicate the presence of long-term or serious underlying respiratory disease.

Whooping cough (pertussis)

This is a highly contagious respiratory infection caused by *Bordetella pertussis*. It is endemic, with epidemics every 3–4 years. After a week of coryza (catarrhal phase), the child develops a characteristic paroxysmal or spasmodic cough followed by a characteristic inspiratory whoop (paroxysmal phase). The spasms of cough are often worse at night and may culminate in vomiting. During a paroxysm, the child goes red or blue in the face, and mucus flows from the nose and mouth. The whoop may be absent in infants, but apnoea is common at this age. Epistaxis and subconjunctival haemorrhages can occur after vigorous coughing. The paroxysmal phase lasts up to 3 months. The symptoms gradually decrease (convalescent phase), but may persist for many months. Complications such as pneumonia, seizures and bronchiectasis are uncommon but there is still a significant mortality, particularly in infants who have not yet completed their primary vaccinations at 4 months. Infants and young children suffering severe spasms of cough or cyanotic attacks should be admitted to hospital and isolated from other children.

The organism can be identified early in the disease from culture of a pernasal swab, although PCR (polymerase chain reaction) is more sensitive. Characteristically, there is a marked lymphocytosis (>15 × 10^9/L) on a blood count. Although macrolide antibiotics eradicate the organism, they decrease symptoms only if started during the catarrhal phase. Siblings, parents and school contacts may develop a similar cough, and close contacts should receive macrolide prophylaxis. Unimmunized infant contacts should be vaccinated. Immunization reduces the risk of developing pertussis and the severity of disease in those affected but does not guarantee protection. The level of protection declines steadily during childhood. Reimmunization of mothers during pregnancy reduces the risk of pertussis in her infant during the first few months of life when it is particularly dangerous. It is currently recommended in the UK; this followed the re-emergence of pertussis in infants in the community.

Summary

Pertussis
- Caused by *Bordetella pertussis*.
- Paroxysmal cough followed by inspiratory whoop and vomiting; in infants, apnoea rather than whoop, which is potentially dangerous.
- Diagnosis: culture of organism on pernasal swab, marked lymphocytosis on blood film.

Persistent or recurrent cough

Children often have persistent or recurrent cough. By far the commonest reason for this is that the child has had a series of respiratory tract infections. However, some infections, such as pertussis and RSV and *Mycoplasma*, can cause a cough that persists for weeks or months. In about half of children with acute cough the symptoms will settle by 10 days, but in up to 10% it will persist for up to 25 days. A cough that lasts more than 8 weeks or one that has not improved after 3–4 weeks should be considered persistent in the absence of recurrent URTI.

Persistent cough after an acute infection may indicate unresolved lobar collapse (which will be demonstrable on a chest X-ray), persistent bacterial bronchitis (see the following section), or suppurative lung disease. Most children will swallow rather than expectorate sputum. If the cough is 'wet' (i.e. sounding like there is excess sputum in the airways) or if the cough is productive, further investigation is required. In any child with a severe, persistent cough, tuberculosis should be considered.

Asthma is another common cause of recurrent cough. Although there is usually associated wheeze and breathlessness, sometimes the wheezing is not recognized or not described accurately. Identifying wheeze on auscultation during an acute episode is helpful to make the diagnosis. However, many children with persistent cough without wheeze are treated incorrectly as having asthma. If the clinical features are not suggestive of asthma or if initial asthma treatment is not beneficial, other diagnoses should be considered or the child referred to a respiratory paediatrician.

Other, less common causes are listed in Box 17.3.

Aspiration of feeds may cause cough and wheeze. This may be caused by gastro-oesophageal reflux or as a result of swallowing disorders, e.g. in children with cerebral palsy. Inhaled foreign body needs to be considered when a cough has not resolved, especially if there is a persistent radiological abnormality. There may not be a clear history of choking; only in 50% of children with inhaled foreign body will a choking episode be recalled.

The significance of parental smoking on children is generally underestimated. If both parents smoke, young children are twice as likely to have recurrent cough and wheeze than in non-smoking households. In the older child, active smoking is an important factor: currently, 6% of 11–15 year olds and 19% of 16–19 year olds smoke regularly.

Box 17.3 Causes of persistent or recurrent cough

- Recurrent respiratory infections
- Following specific respiratory infections (e.g. pertussis, respiratory syncytial virus, *Mycoplasma*)
- Asthma
- Persistent lobar collapse following pneumonia
- Suppurative lung diseases (e.g. cystic fibrosis, ciliary dyskinesia or immune deficiency)
- Recurrent aspiration (±gastro-oesophageal reflux)
- Persistent bacterial bronchitis
- Inhaled foreign body
- Cigarette smoking (active or passive)
- Tuberculosis
- Habit cough
- Airway anomalies (e.g. tracheo-bronchomalacia, tracheo-oesophageal fistula)

Some older children and adolescents develop a barking, unproductive, habit cough following an infection or an asthma attack. The cough characteristically disappears during sleep and is dry in nature. Reassurance and explanation after a thorough examination are usually effective.

Pneumonia

The incidence of pneumonia peaks in infancy and old age, but is relatively high in childhood. It is a major cause of childhood mortality in low and middle-income countries. It is caused by a variety of viruses and bacteria, although in over 50% of cases no causative pathogen is identified. Viruses are the most common cause in younger children, whereas bacteria are more common in older children. In clinical practice, it is difficult to distinguish between viral and bacterial pneumonia.

The most common pathogens causing pneumonia vary according to the child's age:

- Newborn – organisms from the mother's genital tract, particularly group B streptococcus, but also Gram-negative enterococci and bacilli.
- Infants and young children – respiratory viruses, particularly RSV, are most common, but bacterial infections include *Streptococcus pneumoniae* or *H. influenzae*. *Bordetella pertussis* and *Chlamydia trachomatis* can also cause pneumonia at this age. An infrequent but serious cause is *Staphylococcus aureus*.
- Children over 5 years – *Mycoplasma pneumoniae*, *Streptococcus pneumoniae*, and *Chlamydia pneumoniae* are the main causes.
- At all ages *Mycobacterium tuberculosis* should be considered.

There has been a marked reduction in the incidence of pneumonia from *Haemophilus influenzae* since the introduction of Hib immunization. A polysaccharide conjugate vaccine (Prevenar 13), with immunogenicity against 13 of the most common serotypes of *Streptococcus pneumoniae* responsible for invasive disease, is now included in the routine immunization schedule in the UK and many countries. Initial resuults show, in young children, a decrease in septicaemia, meningitis and severe rhinosinusitis, but not in bacteraemic pneumonia.

Clinical features

Fever, cough and rapid breathing are the most common presenting symptoms. These are usually preceded by a URTI. Other symptoms include lethargy, poor feeding, and an 'unwell' child. Some children do not have a cough at presentation. Localized chest, abdominal, or neck pain is a feature of pleural irritation and suggests bacterial infection.

Examination reveals tachypnoea, nasal flaring and chest indrawing. In contrast to asthma, the most sensitive clinical sign of pneumonia in children is increased respiratory rate, and pneumonia can sometimes be missed if the respiratory rate is not measured in a febrile child (so-called silent pneumonia). There may be end-inspiratory coarse crackles over the affected area but the classic signs of consolidation with dullness on percussion, decreased breath sounds and bronchial breathing over the affected area are often absent in young children. Oxygen saturation may be decreased.

A chest X-ray may confirm the diagnosis (Fig. 17.18) but cannot reliably differentiate between bacterial and viral pneumonia. In younger children, a nasopharyngeal aspirate may identify viral causes, but blood tests, including full blood count and acute-phase reactants are generally unhelpful in differentiating between a viral and bacterial cause. In a small proportion of children the pneumonia is associated with a pleural effusion, where there may be blunting of the costophrenic angle on the chest X-ray (Fig. 17.19). Some of these effusions develop into empyema and fibrin strands may form, leading to septations.

Management

Evidence-based guidelines for the management of pneumonia in childhood have been published (British Thoracic Society). Most affected children can be managed at home but indications for admission include oxygen saturation <92%, recurrent apnoea, grunting and/or an inability to maintain adequate fluid/feed intake. General supportive care should include oxygen for hypoxia and analgesia if there is pain. Intravenous fluids should be given if necessary to correct dehydration and maintain adequate hydration and sodium balance. Physiotherapy has no proven role.

The choice of antibiotic is determined by the child's age and the severity of illness. Newborns require broad-spectrum intravenous antibiotics. Most older infants can be managed with oral amoxicillin, with broader-spectrum antibiotics such as co-amoxiclav reserved for complicated or unresponsive pneumonia. For children over 5 years of age, either amoxicillin or an oral macrolide such as erythromycin is the treatment of choice. There is no advantage in giving intravenous rather than oral treatment in mild/moderate pneumonia.

Chest X-ray interpretation in pneumonia

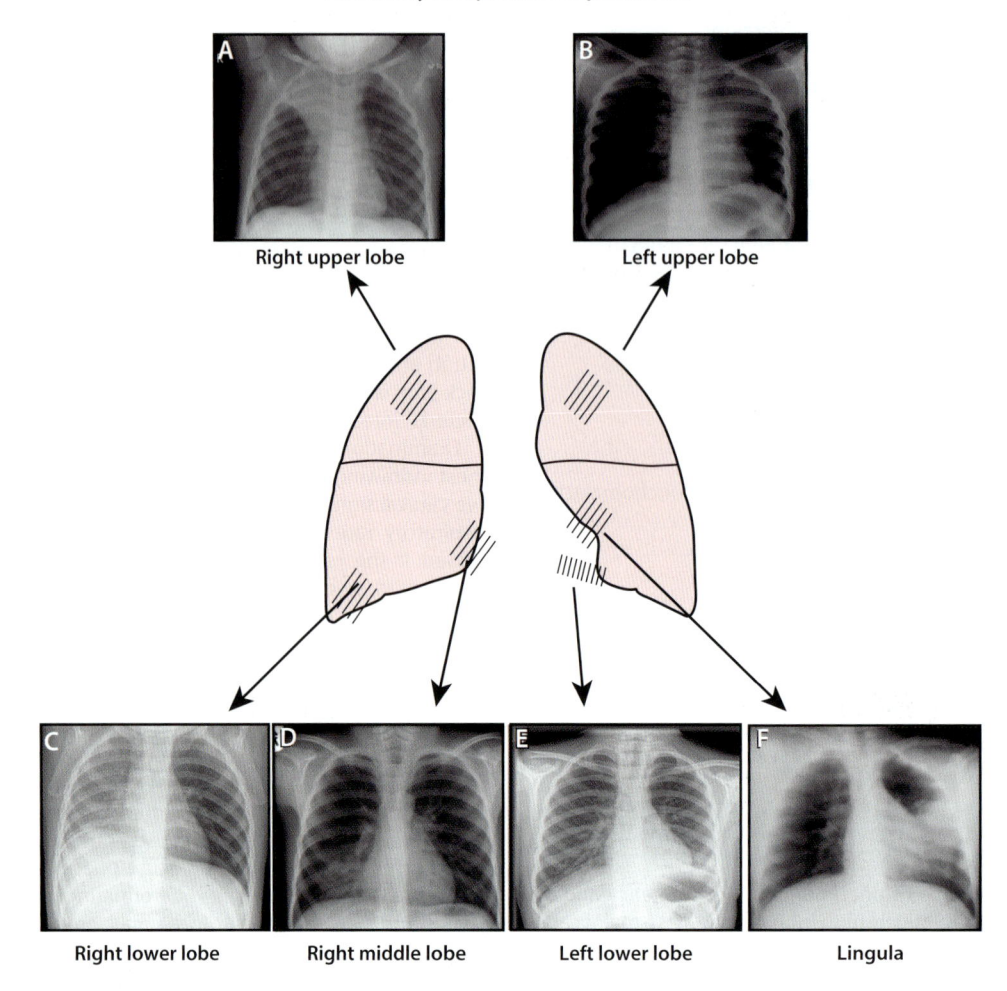

A. Consolidation of the right upper lobe with loss of volume of this lobe. The horizontal fissure has been shifted upwards.
B. Left upper lobe consolidation.
C. Right lower lobe consolidation with volume loss on the right. The heart silhouette is clearly seen but the right hemidiaphragm is raised and partially obscured.
D. A normal right hemidiaphragm but partial loss of the right heart border typical of right middle lobe consolidation.
E. Left lower lobe consolidation - the diaphragm is not clearly seen behind the cardiac silhouette.
F. Lingular consolidation with obvious loss of the left heart border.

Figure 17.18 A guide to the radiological appearances of pneumonia in different lobes of the lung. The diagram shows the horizontal fissures and shading illustrates the key finding in each lobar consolidation.

Small parapneumonic effusions occur in up to one-third of children with pneumonia and may resolve with appropriate antibiotics, but persistent fever despite 48 hours of antibiotics suggests a pleural collection which requires drainage (Fig. 17.19). This should be done with ultrasound guidance. The percutaneous placement of a small-bore chest drain and regular instillation of a fibrinolytic agent to break down the fibrin strands are usually effective, but more aggressive intervention such as video-assisted thoracoscopic surgery or even thoracotomy and decortication is sometimes necessary in refractory cases.

Prognosis and follow-up

Follow-up is not generally required for children with simple consolidation on chest X-ray and who recover clinically. Those with evidence of lobar collapse or atelectasis should have a repeat chest X-ray after 4–6 weeks to check that the lung fields look normal. Virtually all children with pneumonia, even those with empyema, make a full recovery.

Consider pneumonia in children with neck stiffness or acute abdominal pain

Chronic lung infection

Any child with a persistent cough that sounds 'wet' (i.e. sounds like there is excess sputum in the chest) or is productive requires further investigations. Persistent bacterial bronchitis, where there is persistent inflammation of the lower airways driven by chronic infection, is increasingly recognized as a cause of chronic wet cough in children. Common organisms are *Haemophilus influenzae* and *Moraxella catarrhalis*. It may be a precursor to bronchiectasis if investigations and treatment are not instituted. Referral to a specialist in paediatric respiratory disorders is indicated. Bacterial growth from sputum or bronchial lavage is consistent with the diagnosis. Treatment is with a high dose of antibiotic such as co-amoxiclav, coupled with physiotherapy.

Another cause is bronchiectasis (permanent dilatation of the bronchi). It may be generalized or restricted to a single lobe. Generalized bronchiectasis may be due to cystic fibrosis, primary ciliary dyskinesia, immunodeficiency, or chronic aspiration. Focal bronchiectasis is due to previous severe pneumonia, congenital lung abnormality, or obstruction by a foreign body. A plain chest X-ray may show gross bronchiectasis, but often it is not possible to identify it. It is best identified on a CT scan of the chest (Fig. 17.20a,b). To investigate focal disease, bronchoscopy is usually indicated to exclude a structural cause.

Cystic fibrosis

Epidemiology, genetics, and basic defect

CF is the most common life-limiting autosomal recessive condition in Caucasians, with an incidence of 1 in 2500 live births and carrier rate of 1 in 25. It is well recognized but less common in other ethnic groups. Average life expectancy has increased from a few years to the mid-30s, with a projected life expectancy for current newborns into the 40s.

The fundamental problem in CF is a defective protein called the CF transmembrane conductance regulator (CFTR). This is a cyclic AMP-dependent chloride channel found in the membrane of cells. The gene for CFTR is located on chromosome 7. Over 900 different gene mutations have been discovered that cause a number of distinct defects in CFTR, but by far the most frequent mutation (about 78%) in the UK is ΔF508 (Fig. 17.21).

Identification of the gene mutation involved within a family allows prenatal diagnosis and carrier detection in the wider family. Some genotypes are known to be associated with milder disease and pancreatic sufficiency. However, until recently, the precise genotype had little influence on treatment options. The discovery of CFTR potentiators (Ivacaftor) and CFTR correctors (Lumicaftor) have challenged this dogma. Potentiators are helpful in restoring function of CFTR in Class III and Class IV mutations (see Fig. 17.21) and correctors can partially restore CFTR number in Class II defects (ΔF508).

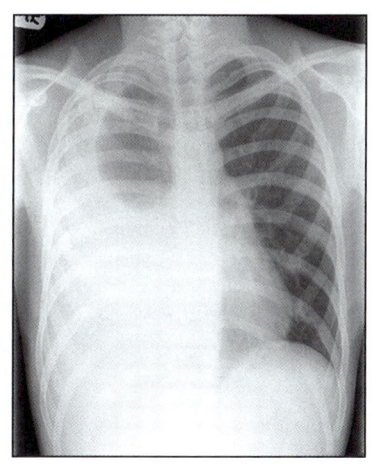

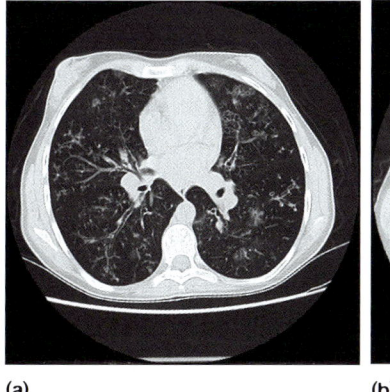

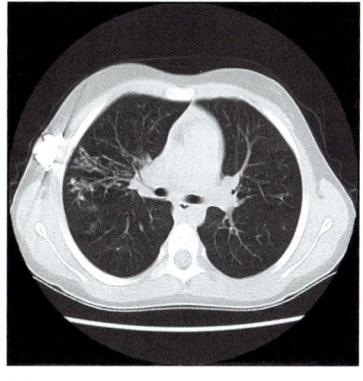

Figure 17.19 Right-sided empyema.

(a) (b)

Figure 17.20 Bronchiectasis on CT scan of the chest. (a) Generalized and (b) focal, in the right upper lobe.

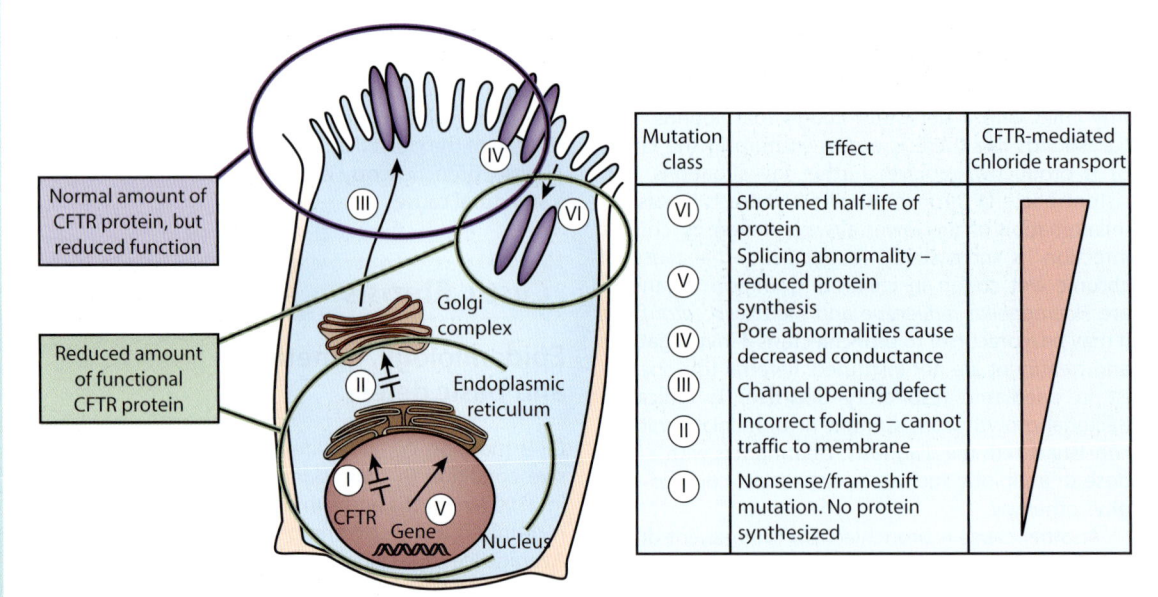

Figure 17.21 Effect of different classes of mutations on the function of the CFTR protein. ΔF508 is a class II mutation. G551D is a Class III mutation. Newer therapies are targeting specific classes of mutation and are potentially a major advance in treatment.

Mutation class	Effect	CFTR-mediated chloride transport
(VI)	Shortened half-life of protein	
(V)	Splicing abnormality – reduced protein synthesis	
(IV)	Pore abnormalities cause decreased conductance	
(III)	Channel opening defect	
(II)	Incorrect folding – cannot traffic to membrane	
(I)	Nonsense/frameshift mutation. No protein synthesized	

Pathophysiology

CF is a multisystem disorder, which results mainly from abnormal ion transport across epithelial cells. In the airways this leads to reduction in the airway surface liquid layer and consequent impaired ciliary function and retention of mucopurulent secretions. Chronic endobronchial infection with specific organisms such as *Pseudomonas aeruginosa* ensues. Defective CFTR also causes dysregulation of inflammation and defence against infection. In the intestine, thick viscid meconium is produced, leading to meconium ileus in 10–20% of infants. The pancreatic ducts also become blocked by thick secretions, leading to pancreatic enzyme deficiency and malabsorption. Abnormal function of the sweat glands results in excessive concentrations of sodium and chloride in the sweat.

Clinical features

All newborn infants born in the UK are screened for CF. Screening reduces diagnostic delay and lowers the risk of presenting with faltering growth or established chronic infection. Immunoreactive trypsinogen (IRT) is raised in newborn infants with CF and is measured in routine heel-prick blood taken for biochemical screening. Those samples with a raised immunoreactive trypsinogen are then screened for common CF gene mutations, and infants with two mutations have a sweat test to confirm the diagnosis.

The majority of children with CF are identified by screening; however, some may still present clinically with recurrent chest infections, faltering growth, or malabsorption (Box 17.4). Chronic infection with specific bacteria – initially *Staphylococcus aureus* and *Haemophilus influenzae* and subsequently with *Pseudomonas aeruginosa* or *Burkholderia* species results from viscid mucus in the smaller airways of the lungs. This leads

Box 17.4 Clinical features of cystic fibrosis

Newborn
- Diagnosed through newborn screening
- Meconium ileus

Infancy
- Prolonged neonatal jaundice
- Growth faltering
- Recurrent chest infections
- Malabsorption, steatorrhoea

Young child
- Bronchiectasis
- Rectal prolapse
- Nasal polyp
- Sinusitis

Older child and adolescent
- Allergic bronchopulmonary aspergillosis
- Diabetes mellitus
- Cirrhosis and portal hypertension
- Distal intestinal obstruction (meconium ileus equivalent)
- Pneumothorax or recurrent haemoptysis
- Sterility in males

to damage of the bronchial wall, bronchiectasis, and abscess formation (Fig. 17.22). The child has a persistent, 'wet' cough, productive of purulent sputum. On examination there is hyperinflation of the chest due to air trapping, coarse inspiratory crepitations, and/or expiratory wheeze. With established disease, there is finger clubbing. Ultimately, 95% die of respiratory failure.

Over 90% of children with CF have pancreatic exocrine insufficiency (lipase, amylase, and proteases),

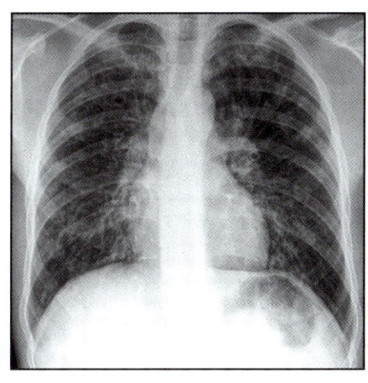

Figure 17.22 A chest X-ray in cystic fibrosis showing hyperinflation, marked peribronchial shadowing, bronchial wall thickening and ring shadows.

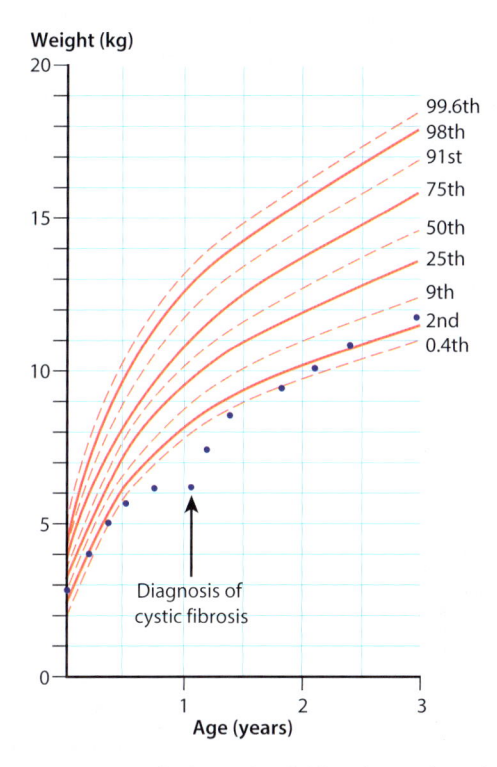

Figure 17.23 Growth chart of a child with cough and recurrent wheeze. Only when the diagnosis of cystic fibrosis was made and appropriate treatment started did he gain weight. (Adapted from growth chart © Child Growth Foundation. Further supplies and information from www.healthforallchildren.co.uk. Reproduced with permission.)

resulting in maldigestion and malabsorption. Untreated, this leads to faltering growth (Fig. 17.23) with frequent large, pale, and greasy stools (steatorrhoea). Pancreatic insufficiency can be diagnosed by demonstrating low faecal elastase.

About 10–20% of infants with CF present in the neonatal period with meconium ileus, in which inspissated meconium causes intestinal obstruction. Typically, there is vomiting, abdominal distension, and failure to pass meconium in the first few days of life. Surgery is usually required, but gastrografin enema may relieve the obstruction.

Diagnosis

The essential diagnostic procedure is the sweat test, to confirm that the concentration of chloride in sweat is markedly elevated (Cl 60–125 mmol/L in CF, 10–40 mmol/L in normal children). Sweating is stimulated by applying a low-voltage current to pilocarpine applied to the skin. The sweat is collected into a special capillary tube or absorbed onto a weighed piece of filter paper. Diagnostic errors are common if there is an inadequate volume of sweat collected. Confirmation of diagnosis can be made by testing for gene abnormalities in the CFTR protein.

Management

The effective management of CF requires a multidisciplinary team approach. All patients with CF should be reviewed at least annually in a specialist centre (Fig. 17.24). The aim of therapy is to prevent progression of the lung disease and to maintain adequate nutrition and growth.

Respiratory management

Recurrent and persistent bacterial chest infection is the major problem. In younger children, respiratory monitoring is based on symptoms; older children should have their lung function measured regularly by spirometry. The FEV_1 expressed as a percentage predicted for age, sex, and height, is an indicator of clinical severity and declines with disease progression.

With regular treatment, many infants and children with CF will have no respiratory symptoms, and often have no abnormal signs. From diagnosis, children should have physiotherapy at least twice a day, aiming to clear the airways of secretions. In younger children, parents are taught to perform airway clearance at home using chest percussion and postural drainage. Older patients perform controlled deep breathing exercises and use a variety of physiotherapy devices for airway clearance. Physical exercise is beneficial and is encouraged.

Many CF specialists recommend continuous prophylactic oral antibiotics (usually flucloxacillin), with additional rescue oral antibiotics for any increase in respiratory symptoms or decline in lung function. Persisting symptoms or signs require prompt and vigorous intravenous therapy to limit lung damage, usually administered for 14 days via a PIC (peripherally inserted central) line. Increasingly, parents are taught to administer courses of intravenous antibiotics at home, to decrease disruption of school and other activities. Chronic *Pseudomonas* infection is associated with a more rapid decline in lung function, which is slowed by the use of daily nebulized antipseudomonal antibiotics. Nebulized DNase or hypertonic saline may be helpful to decrease the viscosity of sputum and to increase its clearance. The macrolide antibiotic azithromycin, given regularly, decreases respiratory exacerbations, probably due to an immunomodulatory effect rather than

Periodic review of the child or adolescent with cystic fibrosis

Siblings may be affected – autosomal recessive condition

Sweat – salty, may lead to dehydration in hot weather

Central venous line, e.g. Portacath – for intravenous antibiotics to aggessively treat infection

Chest – determine if:
- Hyperexpansion due to air trapping
- Harrison's sulcus
- Coarse inspiratory crepitations and/or expiratory wheeze
- Chest infection

Clubbing of fingers?

Scar from operation for meconium ileus as neonate (10–20%)

Monitor for potential complications
- Nasal polyps, sinusitis, rectal prolapse
- Allergic bronchopulmonary aspergillosis (ABPA)
- Diabetes mellitus (often insulin-dependent)
- Cirrhosis and portal hypertension
- Distal intestinal obstruction syndrome (DIOS, meconium ileus equivalent)
- Pneumothorax or recurrent haemoptysis
- Concern about sterility in males

Sputum
– acute or chronic colonisation with *Pseudomonas aeruginosa* or *Burkholderia cepacia*

Growth
- Aim for normal growth

Nutrition
- Gastrostomy for overnight feeding for extra calories?
- Pancreatic exocrine insufficiency
– taking sufficient pancreatic replacement therapy?
– taking fat-soluble vitamins?

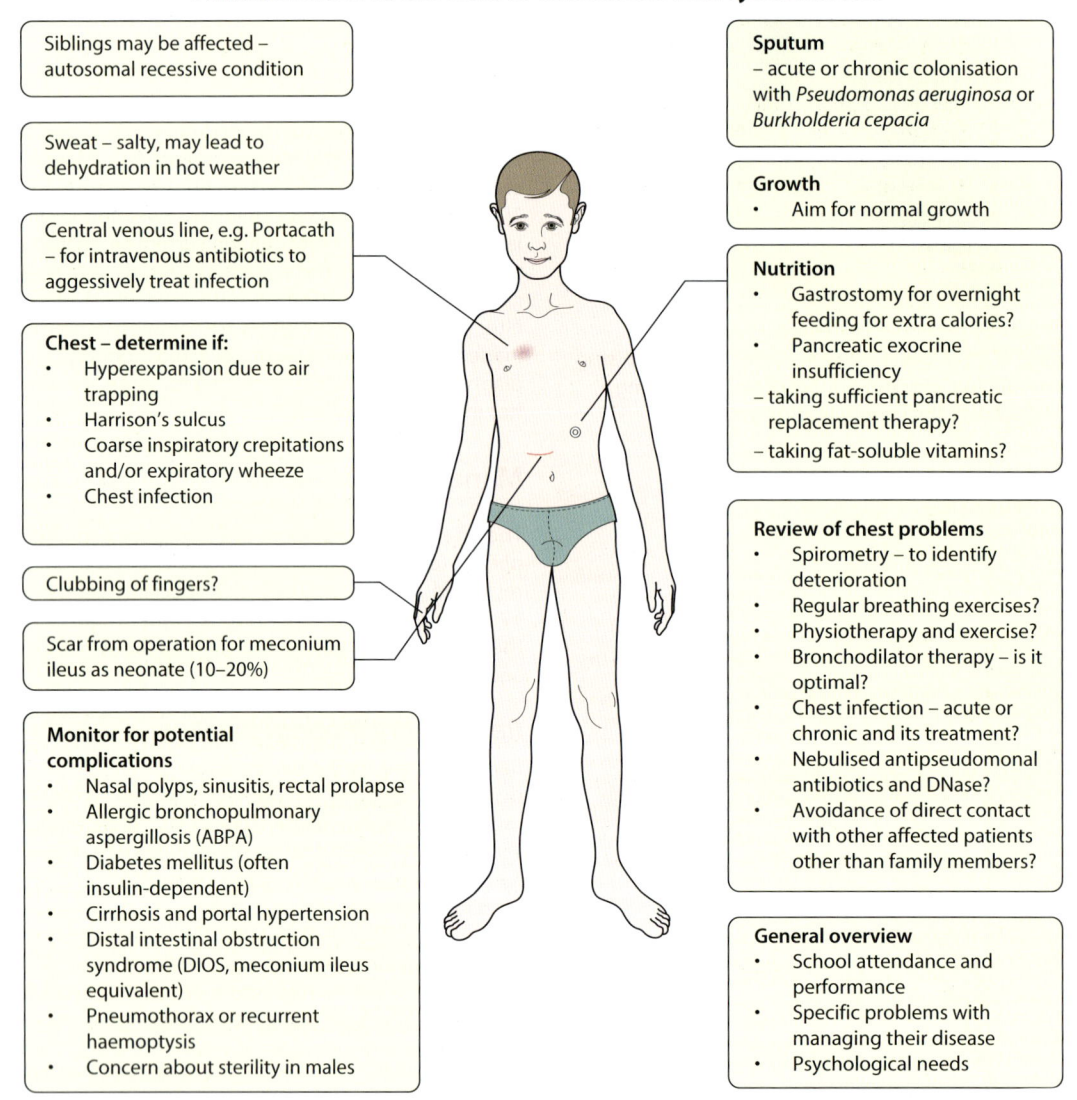

Review of chest problems
- Spirometry – to identify deterioration
- Regular breathing exercises?
- Physiotherapy and exercise?
- Bronchodilator therapy – is it optimal?
- Chest infection – acute or chronic and its treatment?
- Nebulised antipseudomonal antibiotics and DNase?
- Avoidance of direct contact with other affected patients other than family members?

General overview
- School attendance and performance
- Specific problems with managing their disease
- Psychological needs

Figure 17.24 Periodic review of the child or adolescent with cystic fibrosis.

antibiotic action. Regular, nebulized hypertonic saline may decrease the number of respiratory exacerbations.

More severe CF requires more regular intravenous antibiotic therapy. If venous access becomes troublesome, implantation of a central venous catheter with a subcutaneous access port (e.g. Portacath) simplifies venous access, although they require monthly flushing and complications may develop.

Bilateral sequential lung transplantation is the only therapeutic option for end-stage CF lung disease. Outcomes following lung transplantation continue to improve, with over 50% survival at 10 years. Meticulous assessment, for example, with regard to comorbidities and microbiology, psychological preparation, optimal timing of transplantation, and expert post-transplant care, are all essential parts of the multidisciplinary transplant process.

Nutritional management

Dietary status should be assessed regularly. Pancreatic insufficiency is treated with oral enteric-coated pancreatic replacement therapy taken with all meals and snacks. Dosage is adjusted according to clinical response. A high-calorie diet is essential, and dietary intake is recommended at 150% of normal. To achieve this, overnight feeding via a gastrostomy is increasingly used. Most patients require fat-soluble vitamin supplements.

Teenagers and adults

Most children with CF survive into adult life. With increasing age come increased complications, most commonly diabetes mellitus due to decreasing pancreatic endocrine function. Up to one-third of adolescent patients will have evidence of liver disease with hepatomegaly on liver palpation, abnormal liver function on blood tests, or an abnormal ultrasound. Regular ursodeoxycholic acid, to improve flow of bile, may be beneficial. Rarely, the liver disease progresses to cirrhosis, portal hypertension, and ultimately liver failure. Liver transplant is generally very successful in CF-related liver failure.

In distal intestinal obstruction syndrome (DIOS, meconium ileus equivalent), viscid mucofaeculent material obstructs the bowel. This is usually cleared by a combination of oral laxative agents.

As the disease progresses there may be increasing chest infections, as well as other late respiratory complications including pneumothorax and life-threatening haemoptysis. There is increasing concern over transmission of virulent strains of *Pseudomonas* and *Burkholderia cepacia* between patients, causing rapid decline in lung function. Consequently, patients are often segregated and advised not to socialise with other people with CF.

Females have normal fertility, and unless they have severe lung disease, tolerate pregnancy well. Males are virtually always infertile due to absence of the vas deferens, although they can father children through intracytoplasmic sperm injection.

The psychological repercussions on affected children and their families of a chronic and ultimately fatal illness that requires regular physiotherapy and drugs, frequent hospital admissions and absences from school are considerable. The CF team should provide psychological and emotional support. Adolescents have particular needs, which must receive special consideration. Older adolescents with CF should transfer to specialist adult CF care.

Despite early hopes, gene therapy has not yet proven to be a useful treatment in CF. However, there is considerable optimism that CFTR potentiators and CFTR correctors may significantly improve outcomes. The availability of these treatments is currently limited by their high cost.

> Cystic fibrosis should be considered in any child with recurrent infections, loose stools or faltering growth

Primary ciliary dyskinesia

In primary ciliary dyskinesia there is congenital abnormality in the structure or function of cilia lining the respiratory tract. This leads to impaired mucociliary clearance. Affected children have recurrent infection of the upper and lower respiratory tracts, which if untreated may lead to severe bronchiectasis. They characteristically have a recurrent productive cough, purulent nasal discharge, and chronic ear infections. Since ciliary action is responsible for normal organ situs, 50% have dextrocardia and situs inversus (Kartagener syndrome, where major organs are in mirror position of normal). The diagnosis is made by examination of the structure and function of the cilia of nasal epithelial cells brushed from the nose. The cornerstones of management are daily physiotherapy to clear secretions, proactive treatment of infections with antibiotics, and appropriate ENT follow-up.

Immunodeficiency

Children with immunodeficiency may develop severe, unusual, or recurrent chest infections. The immune deficiency may be secondary to an illness, e.g. malignant disease or its treatment with chemotherapy. Less commonly, it is due to HIV infection or a primary immune deficiency. Different types of immune deficiency predispose to different lung infections: IgG deficiency predisposes to infections with polysaccharide-capsulated bacteria such as *S. pneumoniae*; cell-mediated immunodeficiencies make one susceptible to opportunistic infections such as *Pneumocystis jirovecii* and fungi, and neutrophil-killing defects predispose to staphylococcal infection (See Chapter 15 Infection and Immunity).

Tuberculosis

Tuberculosis remains an important cause of chronic lung infection [see Ch. 15. (Infection and immunity)]. All children with a persistent productive cough should have a chest X-ray and either a tuberculin skin test or tuberculosis blood tests (IGRA, interferon-gamma release assays). Marked hilar or paratracheal lymphadenopathy is highly suggestive of tuberculosis.

Sleep-disordered breathing

During REM (rapid eye movement) sleep, the control of breathing becomes unstable and there is relaxation of voluntary muscles in the upper airway and chest. This makes upper airway collapse more likely.

Sleep-disordered breathing occurs either due to airway obstruction, central hypoventilation or a combination of these. Key aspects of the history include loud snoring, witnessed pauses in breathing (apnoeas), restlessness, and disturbed sleep. However, symptoms alone are neither a sensitive nor specific marker of actual difficulties. Up to 12% of prepubertal school children snore, but true estimates of the prevalence of obstructive sleep apnoea resulting in gas-exchange abnormalities range from 0.7–3%.

Obstructive sleep apnoea leads to excessive daytime sleepiness or hyperactivity, learning and behaviour problems, faltering growth, and in severe cases, pulmonary hypertension. In childhood, it is usually due to upper airway obstruction secondary to adenotonsillar hypertrophy. Predisposing causes of sleep-disordered breathing are neuromuscular disease (e.g. Duchenne muscular dystrophy), craniofacial abnormalities (e.g. Pierre Robin sequence, achondroplasia), dystonia of upper airway muscles (e.g. cerebral palsy), and severe obesity. Children with Down syndrome have anatomical upper airway restriction as well as hypotonia and are particularly at risk. These high-risk groups should be screened for sleep-disordered breathing.

The most basic assessment is overnight pulse oximetry, which can be performed in the child's home. The frequency and severity of periods of desaturation can be quantified. Normal oximetry does not exclude the condition, but means that severe physical consequences are unlikely. Polysomnography is required in more complex cases. This should include monitoring of heart rate, respiratory effort, airflow, CO_2 measurement and video recording. This provides more information about gas exchange and can distinguish between

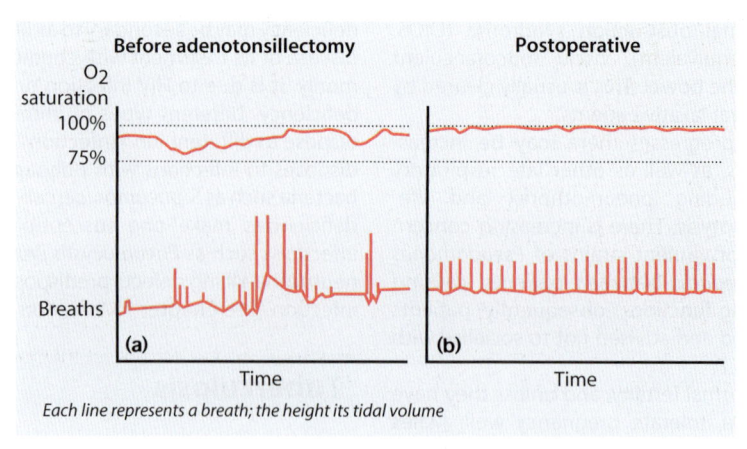

Figure 17.25 Extract from cardiorespiratory monitoring in a child with obstructive sleep apnoea. (a) Irregular breathing with periodic pauses associated with oxygen desaturation; and (b) post-adenotonsillectomy, the breathing is regular and the desaturation has resolved. (Courtesy of Dr Parviz Habibi.)

central and obstructive events. Sometimes more detailed electrophysiological assessment is needed to assess neurological arousals and sleep staging.

In children with adenotonsillar hypertrophy, adenotonsillectomy usually dramatically improves their condition (Fig. 17.25a,b). Before surgery for obstructive sleep apnoea, overnight oximetry should be performed to identify severe hypoxaemia, which may increase the risk of perioperative complications. For children with other sleep-related breathing disorders, nasal or face mask continuous positive pressure (CPAP) or BiPAP (bilevel positive airway pressure) to maintain their upper airway may be required at night.

Congenital central hypoventilation syndrome is a rare congenital condition resulting in disordered central control of breathing as well as other autonomic dysfunction. In severe cases, life-threatening hypoventilation occurs during sleep, which may result in death in infancy. Long-term ventilation, either continuous or only during sleep is the mainstay of treatment.

> **Summary**
>
> **Sleep disordered breathing**
> - The majority are due to adenotonsillar hypertrophy, and surgical removal usually dramatically improves symptoms.

Tracheostomy

The number of children of all ages with a tracheostomy is increasing. Indications are listed in Table 17.3.

If a child with a tracheostomy develops sudden and severe breathing difficulties, it may be that the tracheostomy tube is blocked with secretions and needs urgent suction or needs changing immediately. If this does not relieve the difficulty in breathing, respiratory support is given via the tracheostomy tube. All children with a tracheostomy should have a spare tracheostomy tube with them at all times, and a carer competent to change it.

Table 17.3 Some indications for tracheostomy in children

Narrow upper airways	Subglottic stenosis
	Laryngeal anomalies (e.g. atresia, haemangiomas, webs)
	Pierre Robin sequence (small jaw and cleft palate)
	Other craniofacial anomalies (e.g. Crouzon disease)
Lower airway anomalies	Severe tracheo-bronchomalacia
Long-term ventilation	Muscle weakness
	Head or spinal injury
Wean from ventilation	Any prolonged period of ventilation
Airway protection	To facilitate clearance of secretions

Long-term ventilation

An increasing number of children are receiving long-term respiratory support. Preterm infants with severe bronchopulmonary dysplasia may require additional oxygen for many months. Children with sleep-disordered breathing due to neuromuscular diseases such as Duchenne muscular dystrophy will benefit in both quality and duration of life from nocturnal respiratory support. This requires BiPAP (bilevel positive airway pressure), which can be delivered non-invasively by a nasal mask or full face mask (Fig. 17.26). Children who have more severe respiratory failure may need

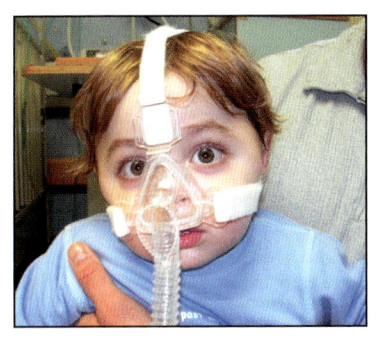

Figure 17.26 Long-term non-invasive respiratory support given overnight via nasal mask to a child with muscle weakness.

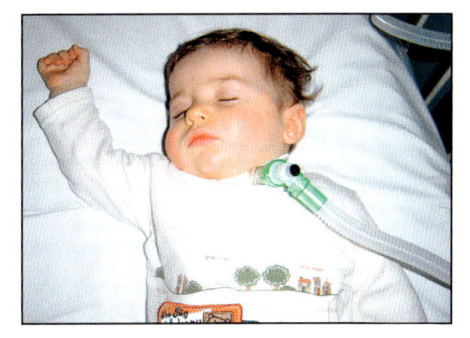

Figure 17.27 Long-term ventilation via a tracheostomy.

24-hour respiratory support via a tracheostomy (Fig. 17.27). In some severe and progressive conditions such as type 1 spinal muscular atrophy, difficult ethical decisions need to be made about admission for intensive care and whether to initiate long-term full ventilation.

Acknowledgements

We would like to acknowledge contributors to this chapter in previous editions, whose work we have drawn on: Jon Couriel (1st, 2nd Edition), Iolo Doull (3rd Edition), Michael McKean (4th Edition), Gerard Siou (4th Edition), Malcolm Brodie (4th Edition).

Further reading

Primhak R, O'Brien C: Best practice: sleep apnoea. *Archives of Disease in Childhood – Education and Practice Edition* 90:ep87–ep91, 2005.
Short review of obstructive sleep apnoea in children.

Taussig LM, Landau LI: *Pediatric Respiratory Medicine*, ed 2, St Louis, MO, 2008, Mosby.
Definitive textbook.

Websites (Accessed November 2016)

British Thoracic Society: *Guidelines for the Management of Community Acquired Pneumonia in Childhood.* London, 2011, British Thoracic Society. Available at: http://www.brit-thoracic.org.uk/clinical-information/pneumonia/pneumonia-guidelines.aspx. (Accessed November 2016).

Scottish Intercollegiate Guideline Network: *Management of Sore Throat and Indications for Tonsillectomy.* Edinburgh, 2010, Scottish Intercollegiate Guideline Network. Available at: http://www.sign.ac.uk/pdf/sign117.pdf. (Accessed November 2016).

Scottish Intercollegiate Guideline Network/British Thoracic Society: *The British Guideline on Asthma Management.* Edinburgh, 2016, Scottish Intercollegiate Guideline Network. Available at: http://www.sign.ac.uk/pdf/SIGN153.pdf (Updated September 2016).

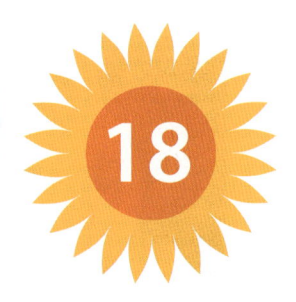

Cardiac disorders

Epidemiology	320	Outflow obstruction in the sick infant	337
Aetiology	321	Care following cardiac surgery	339
Circulatory changes at birth	321	Cardiac arrhythmias	339
Presentation	322	Syncope	340
Diagnosis	323	Chest pains	340
Nomenclature	325	Rheumatic fever	340
Left-to-right shunts	325	Infective endocarditis	342
Right-to-left shunts	329	Myocarditis/cardiomyopathy	342
Common mixing (blue and breathless)	333	Kawasaki disease	343
		Pulmonary hypertension	343
Outflow obstruction in the well child	335		

Recent developments in paediatric cardiac disease are:
- lesions are being increasingly identified on antenatal ultrasound screening
- most lesions are diagnosed by echocardiography, the mainstay of diagnostic imaging
- magnetic resonance imaging allows three-dimensional reconstruction of complex cardiac disorders, assessment of haemodynamics and flow patterns, and assists interventional cardiology, reducing the need for cardiac catheterization
- most defects can be corrected by definitive surgery at the initial operation
- an increasing number of defects (60%) are treated non-invasively, e.g. persistent ductus arteriosus
- new therapies are available to treat pulmonary hypertension and delay transplantation
- the overall infant cardiac surgical mortality has been reduced from approximately 20% in 1970 to 1.8% in 2016.

Epidemiology

Heart disease in children is mostly congenital. It is the most common single group of structural malformations in infants:

- 8 per 1000 liveborn infants have significant cardiac malformations, 30% of which require intervention in the 1st year of life
- some abnormality of the cardiovascular system, e.g. a bicuspid aortic valve, is present in 1–2% of live births
- about 1 in 10 stillborn infants have a cardiac anomaly.

The nine most common anomalies account for 80% of all lesions (Box 18.1), but:

- about 10–15% have complex lesions with more than one cardiac abnormality and
- about 10–15% also have a non-cardiac abnormality.

Box 18.1 The most common congenital heart lesions

Left-to-right shunts (breathless)
- Ventricular septal defect 30%
- Persistent arterial duct 12%
- Atrial septal defect 7%

Right-to-left shunts (blue)
- Tetralogy of Fallot 5%
- Transposition of the great arteries 5%

Common mixing (breathless and blue)
- Atrioventricular septal defect (complete) 2%

Outflow obstruction in a well child (asymptomatic with a murmur)
- Pulmonary stenosis 7%
- Aortic stenosis 5%

Outflow obstruction in a sick neonate (collapsed with shock)
- Coarctation of the aorta 5%.

Aetiology

Genetic causes are increasingly recognized in the aetiology of congenital heart disease, now in more than 10%. These might affect whole chromosomes, point mutations, or microdeletions (Table 18.1). Polygenic abnormalities probably explain why having a child with congenital heart disease doubles the risk for subsequent children and the risk is higher still if either parent has congenital heart disease. A small number are related to external teratogens.

Circulatory changes at birth

In the fetus, the left atrial pressure is low, as relatively little blood returns from the lungs. The pressure in the right atrium is higher than in the left, as it receives all the systemic venous return including blood from the placenta. The flap valve of the foramen ovale is held open, blood flows across the atrial septum into the left atrium, and then into the left ventricle, which in turn pumps it to the upper body (Figs 18.1 and 10.8).

With the first breaths, resistance to pulmonary blood flow falls and the volume of blood flowing through the lungs increases six-fold. This results in a rise in the left atrial pressure. Meanwhile, the volume of blood returning to the right atrium falls as the placenta is excluded from the circulation. The change in the pressure difference causes the flap valve of the foramen ovale to be closed. The ductus arteriosus, which connects the pulmonary artery to the aorta in fetal life, will normally close within the first few hours or days. Some babies with congenital heart lesions rely on blood flow through the duct (duct-dependent circulation). Their clinical condition will deteriorate dramatically when the duct closes, which is usually at 1–2 days of age but occasionally later.

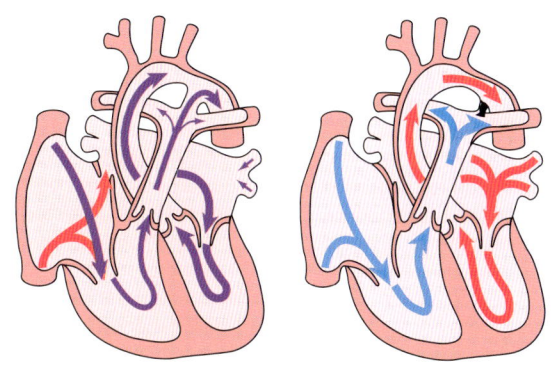

Antenatal circulation   Postnatal circulation

Figure 18.1 Changes in the circulation from the fetus to the newborn. When congenital heart lesions rely on blood flow through the duct (a duct-dependent circulation), there will be a dramatic deterioration in the clinical condition when the duct closes.

Table 18.1 Causes of congenital heart disease

	Cardiac abnormalities	**Frequency**
Maternal disorders		
Rubella infection	Peripheral pulmonary stenosis, PDA	30–35%
Systemic lupus erythematosus	Complete heart block (anti-Ro and anti-La antibody)	35%
Diabetes mellitus	Incidence increased overall	2%
Maternal drugs		
Warfarin therapy	Pulmonary valve stenosis, PDA	5%
Fetal alcohol syndrome	ASD, VSD, tetralogy of Fallot	25%
Chromosomal abnormality		
Down syndrome (trisomy 21)	Atrioventricular septal defect, VSD	30%
Edwards syndrome (trisomy 18)	Complex	60–80%
Patau syndrome (trisomy 13)	Complex	70%
Turner syndrome (45XO)	Aortic valve stenosis, coarctation of the aorta	15%
Chromosome 22q11.2 deletion	Aortic arch anomalies, tetralogy of Fallot, common arterial trunk	80%
Williams syndrome (7q11.23 microdeletion)	Supravalvular aortic stenosis, peripheral pulmonary artery stenosis	85%
Noonan syndrome (PTPN11 mutation and others)	Hypertrophic cardiomyopathy, atrial septal defect, pulmonary valve stenosis	50%

ASD, atrial septal defect; PDA, persistent ductus arteriosus; VSD, ventricular septal defect.

Presentation

Congenital heart disease presents with:
- antenatal cardiac ultrasound diagnosis
- detection of a heart murmur
- heart failure
- shock
- cyanosis.

Antenatal diagnosis

Checking the anatomy of the fetal heart has become a routine part of the fetal anomaly scan performed in developed countries between 18 weeks' and 20 weeks' gestation and can lead to 70% of those infants who require surgery in the first 6 months of life being diagnosed antenatally. If an abnormality is detected, detailed fetal echocardiography is performed by a paediatric cardiologist. Any fetus at increased risk, e.g. suspected Down syndrome, where the parents have had a previous child with heart disease or where the mother has congenital heart disease is also checked. Early diagnosis allows the parents to be counselled. Depending on the diagnosis, some choose termination of pregnancy; the majority continue with the pregnancy and can have their child's management planned antenatally. Mothers of infants with duct-dependent lesions likely to need treatment within the first 2 days of life may be offered delivery at or close to the cardiac centre.

Heart murmurs

The most common presentation of congenital heart disease is with a heart murmur. Even so, the vast majority of children with murmurs have a normal heart. They have an 'innocent murmur', which can be heard at some time in almost 30% of children. It is obviously important to be able to distinguish an innocent murmur from a pathological one.

Hallmarks of an innocent ejection murmur are (all have an 'S', 'innoSent'):
- aSymptomatic
- Soft blowing murmur
- Systolic murmur only, not diastolic
- left Sternal edge.

Also:
- normal heart sounds with no added sounds
- no parasternal thrill
- no radiation.

During a febrile illness or anaemia, innocent or flow murmurs are often heard because of increased cardiac output. Therefore it is important to examine the child when such other illnesses have been corrected.

Differentiating between innocent and pathological murmurs can be difficult. If a murmur is thought to be significant, or if there is uncertainty about whether it is innocent, the child should be seen by an experienced paediatrician to decide about referral to a paediatric cardiologist for echocardiography. A chest radiograph and electrocardiography (ECG) may help with the diagnosis beyond the neonatal period.

Many newborn infants with potential shunts have neither symptoms nor a murmur at birth, as the pulmonary vascular resistance is still high. Therefore conditions such as a ventricular septal defect (VSD) or ductus arteriosus may only become apparent at several weeks of age when the pulmonary vascular resistance falls.

> The features of an innocent murmur can be remembered as the five Ss:
> 'InnoSent' murmur = Soft, Systolic, aSymptomatic, left Sternal edge

Heart failure

Symptoms
- Breathlessness (particularly on feeding or exertion)
- Sweating
- Poor feeding
- Recurrent chest infections.

Signs
- Poor weight gain or faltering growth
- Tachypnoea
- Tachycardia
- Heart murmur, gallop rhythm
- Enlarged heart
- Hepatomegaly
- Cool peripheries.

Signs of right heart failure (ankle oedema, sacral oedema, and ascites) are rare in developed countries, but may be seen with long-standing rheumatic heart disease or pulmonary hypertension, with tricuspid regurgitation and right atrial dilatation.

In the first week of life, heart failure (Box 18.2) usually results from left heart obstruction, e.g. coarctation of the aorta. If the obstructive lesion is very severe, then

---

Box 18.2 Causes of heart failure

1 Neonates – obstructed (duct-dependent) systemic circulation
- Hypoplastic left heart syndrome
- Critical aortic valve stenosis
- Severe coarctation of the aorta
- Interruption of the aortic arch

2 Infants (high pulmonary blood flow)
- Ventricular septal defect
- Atrioventricular septal defect
- Large persistent ductus arteriosus

3 Older children and adolescents (right or left heart failure)
- Eisenmenger syndrome (right heart failure only)
- Rheumatic heart disease
- Cardiomyopathy.

Table 18.2 Types of presentation with congenital heart disease

Type of lesion	Left-to-right shunt	Right-to-left shunt	Common mixing	Well children with obstruction	Sick neonates with obstruction
Symptoms	Breathless or asymptomatic	Blue	Breathless and blue	Asymptomatic	Collapsed with shock
Examples	ASD VSD PDA	Tetralogy of Fallot TGA	AVSD Complex congenital heart disease	AS PS Adult-type CoA	Coarctation HLHS

AS, aortic stenosis; ASD, atrial septal defect; AVSD, atrioventricular; CoA, coarctation of the aorta; HLHS, hypoplastic left heart syndrome; PDA, patent ductus arteriosus; PS, pulmonary stenosis; TGA, transposition of the great arteries; VSD, ventricular septal defect.

arterial perfusion may be predominantly by right-to-left flow of blood via the arterial duct, so-called duct-dependent systemic circulation (Fig. 18.2). Closure of the duct under these circumstances rapidly leads to severe acidosis, collapse and death unless ductal patency is restored (Case History 18.1).

After the first week of life, progressive heart failure is most likely due to a left-to-right shunt (Case History 18.2). During the subsequent weeks, as the pulmonary vascular resistance falls, there is a progressive increase in left-to-right shunt and increasing pulmonary blood flow. This causes pulmonary oedema and breathlessness.

Such symptoms of heart failure will increase up to the age of about 3 months, but may subsequently improve as the pulmonary vascular resistance rises in response to the left-to-right shunt. If left untreated, these children will develop Eisenmenger syndrome, which is irreversibly raised pulmonary vascular resistance resulting from chronically raised pulmonary arterial pressure and flow. Now the shunt is from right to left and the teenager is blue. If this develops, the only surgical option is a heart–lung transplant, if available, although medication is now available to palliate the symptoms.

Cyanosis

- Peripheral cyanosis (blueness of the hands and feet) may occur when a child is cold or unwell from any cause or with polycythaemia.
- Central cyanosis, seen on the tongue as a slate blue colour, is associated with a fall in arterial blood oxygen tension. It can only be recognized clinically if the concentration of reduced haemoglobin in the blood exceeds 50 g/L, so it is less pronounced if the child is anaemic.
- Check with a pulse oximeter that an infant's oxygen saturation is normal (≥94%). Persistent cyanosis in an otherwise well infant is nearly always a sign of structural heart disease.

Cyanosis in a newborn infant with respiratory distress (respiratory rate >60 breaths/min) may be due to:

- cardiac disorders – cyanotic congenital heart disease
- respiratory disorders, e.g. respiratory distress syndrome (surfactant deficiency), meconium aspiration, pulmonary hypoplasia
- persistent pulmonary hypertension of the newborn – failure of the pulmonary vascular resistance to fall after birth
- infection – septicaemia from group B streptococcus and other organisms
- inborn error of metabolism – metabolic acidosis and shock.

Whether the presentation of congenital heart disease is with a heart murmur, heart failure, cyanosis or shock depends on the underlying anatomic lesion causing:

- left to right shunt
- right to left shunt
- common mixing
- outflow obstruction in the well or sick child.

This is summarized in Table 18.2.

Diagnosis

If congenital heart disease is suspected, a chest radiograph and ECG (Box 18.3) should be performed. Although rarely diagnostic, they may be helpful in establishing that there is an abnormality of the cardiovascular system and as a baseline for assessing future changes. Echocardiography, combined with Doppler ultrasound, enables almost all causes of congenital heart disease to be diagnosed. Even when a paediatric cardiologist is not available locally a specialist echocardiography opinion may be available via telemedicine, or else transfer to the cardiac centre will be necessary. A specialist opinion is required if the child is haemodynamically unstable, if there is heart failure, if there is cyanosis, when the oxygen saturations are less than 94% due to heart disease, and when there are reduced volume pulses.

Case history 18.1

Shock

A 2-day-old baby had been discharged home the day after delivery following a normal routine examination. He suddenly collapsed and was rushed to hospital. He was pale, with grey lips. The right brachial pulse could just be felt, the femoral pulses were impalpable and his liver was significantly enlarged. Blood gases showed a severe metabolic acidosis. The differential diagnosis was:

- congenital heart disease
- septicaemia
- inborn error of metabolism.

He was ventilated and treated with volume support. Blood cultures were taken and antibiotics started for possible sepsis. Blood and urine samples were taken for an amino acid screen and urine for organic acids. As the femoral pulses remained impalpable, a prostaglandin infusion was started. Within 2 hours, he was pink and well perfused and the acidosis was resolving. Severe coarctation of the aorta (Fig. 18.2) was diagnosed on echocardiography. He had developed shock from a left heart outflow tract obstruction once the arterial duct had closed.

☀ **Maintaining ductal patency is the key to early survival in neonates with a duct-dependent circulation**

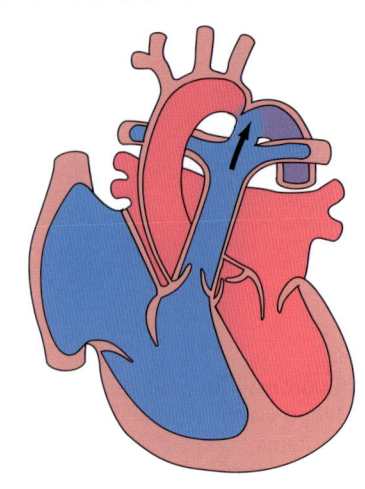

Duct-dependent coarctation

Figure 18.2 The systemic circulation is maintained by blood flowing right to left across the ductus arteriosus – a duct-dependent systemic circulation.

Case history 18.2

Heart failure

A 5-week-old female infant was referred to hospital because of wheezing, poor feeding and poor weight gain during the previous 2 weeks. Before this she had been well. Her routine neonatal examination had been normal. She was tachypnoeic (50–60 breaths/min) and there was some sternal and intercostal recession. The pulses were normal. There was a thrill, a pansystolic murmur at the lower left sternal edge and a slightly accentuated pulmonary component to the second heart sound. There were scattered wheezes. The liver was enlarged, palpable at two finger breadths below the costal margin. The ECG was unremarkable. The chest radiograph showed cardiomegaly and increased pulmonary vascular markings. An echocardiogram showed a moderate-sized ventricular septal defect (VSD; Fig. 18.3). Treatment was medical with diuretics and captopril. The VSD closed spontaneously at 18 months.

This infant developed heart failure from a moderate VSD presenting at several weeks of age when the pulmonary resistance fell, causing increased left-to-right shunting of blood. The defect closed spontaneously.

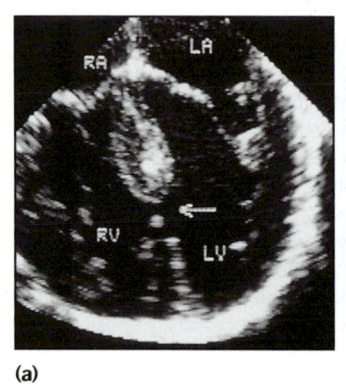

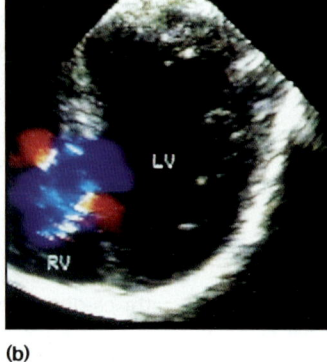

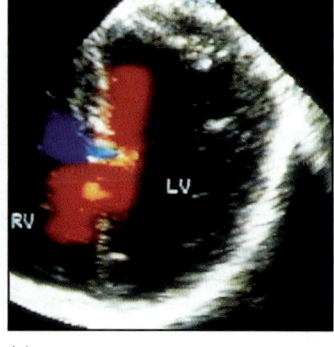

Figure 18.3 (a) Echocardiogram showing a medium-sized muscular ventricular septal defect (arrow); (b) the colour Doppler shows a left-to-right shunt (blue) during systole; and (c) there is also a small right-to-left shunt (red) during diastole. LA, left atrium; LV, left ventricle; RA, right atrium; RV, right ventricle.

Box 18.3 ECG in children

Important features
- Arrhythmias
- Superior QRS axis (negative deflection in AVF; see Fig. 18.4f)
- Right ventricular hypertrophy (upright T wave in V_1 over 1 month of age; see Fig. 18.5d)
- Left ventricular strain (inverted T wave in V_6; see Fig. 18.13d)

Pitfalls
- P-wave morphology is rarely helpful in children
- Partial right bundle branch block – most are normal children, although it is common in ASD
- Sinus arrhythmia is a normal finding.

ASD, atrial septal defect.

Nomenclature

The European (as opposed to American) system for naming congenital heart disease is referred to as sequential segmental arrangement. The advantage is that it is not necessary to remember the pattern of an eponymous syndrome, e.g. tetralogy of Fallot. The disadvantage is that it is long-winded. The idea is that each component is described in turn, naming the way the atria, then the ventricles, and then the great arteries are connected. Hence, a normal heart will be described as situs solitus (i.e. the atria are in the correct orientation), concordant atrioventricular connection and concordant ventriculo–arterial connection. Therefore a heart of any complexity can be described in a logical step-by-step process. This system is not described here, as it is beyond the scope of this book.

Summary

Presentation of congenital heart disease
- Antenatal ultrasound screening – increasing proportion detected antenatally.
- Detection of a heart murmur – need to differentiate innocent from pathological murmur.
- Cyanosis – if duct dependent, prostaglandin to maintain ductal patency is vital for initial survival.
- Heart failure – usually from left-to-right shunt when pulmonary vascular resistance falls.
- Shock – when duct closes in severe left heart obstruction.

Left-to-right shunts

These are:
- atrial septal defects (ASDs)
- VSDs
- persistent ductus arteriosus (PDA).

Atrial septal defect

There are two main types of ASD:
- secundum ASD (80% of ASDs; Fig. 18.4a)
- partial atrioventricular septal defect (AVSD or primum ASD; Fig. 18.4b).

Both present with similar symptoms and signs, but their anatomy is quite different. The secundum ASD is a defect in the centre of the atrial septum involving the foramen ovale.

Partial AVSD is a defect of the atrioventricular septum and is characterized by:
- an interatrial communication between the bottom end of the atrial septum and the atrioventricular valves (primum ASD)
- abnormal atrioventricular valves, with a left atrioventricular valve which has three leaflets and tends to leak (regurgitant valve).

Clinical features
Symptoms
- None (commonly)
- Recurrent chest infections/wheeze
- Arrhythmias (fourth decade onwards).

Physical signs
- An ejection systolic murmur best heard at the upper left sternal edge – due to increased flow across the pulmonary valve because of the left-to-right shunt (Fig. 18.4c).
- A fixed and widely split second heart sound (often difficult to hear) – due to the right ventricular stroke volume being equal in both inspiration and expiration.
- With a partial AVSD, an apical pansystolic murmur from atrioventricular valve regurgitation.

Investigations
Chest radiograph
The chest radiograph (Fig. 18.4d) shows cardiomegaly, enlarged pulmonary arteries and increased pulmonary vascular markings.

ECG
- Secundum ASD – partial right bundle branch block is common (but may occur in normal children), right axis deviation due to right ventricular enlargement (Fig. 18.4e).
- Partial AVSD – a 'superior' QRS axis (mainly negative in AVF; Fig. 18.4f). This occurs because there is a defect of the middle part of the heart where the atrioventricular node is. The displaced node then conducts to the ventricles superiorly, giving the abnormal axis.

Echocardiography
This will delineate the anatomy and is the mainstay of diagnostic investigations.

Management
Children with significant ASD (large enough to cause right ventricle dilation) will require treatment. For

secundum ASDs, this is by cardiac catheterization with insertion of an occlusion device (Fig. 18.4g), but for partial AVSD surgical correction is required. Treatment is usually undertaken at about 3 years to 5 years of age in order to prevent right heart failure and arrhythmias in later life.

Ventricular septal defects

VSDs are common, accounting for 30% of all cases of congenital heart disease. There is a defect anywhere in the ventricular septum, perimembranous (adjacent to the tricuspid valve) or muscular (completely surrounded by muscle). They can most conveniently be considered according to the size of the lesion.

Small VSDs

These are smaller than the aortic valve in diameter, perhaps up to 3 mm.

Clinical features

Symptoms
- Asymptomatic.

Physical signs
- Loud pansystolic murmur at lower left sternal edge (loud murmur implies smaller defect).
- Quiet pulmonary second sound (P_2).

Atrial septal defect

(a) Secundum atrial septal defect
(b) Partial AVSD
(c) A2 P2 Fixed
(d) Enlarged heart
Enlarged pulmonary arteries
Increased pulmonary vascular markings
(e) Secundum ASD
V_1
RSR^1 in V_1
Right axis deviation
Partial right bundle branch block
(f) Partial AVSD
AVF
Superior axis
(negative deflection in lead AVF)
(g)

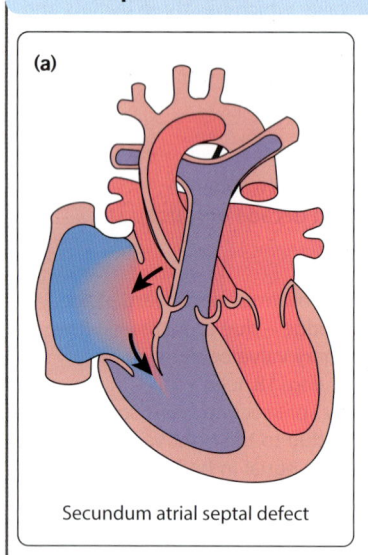

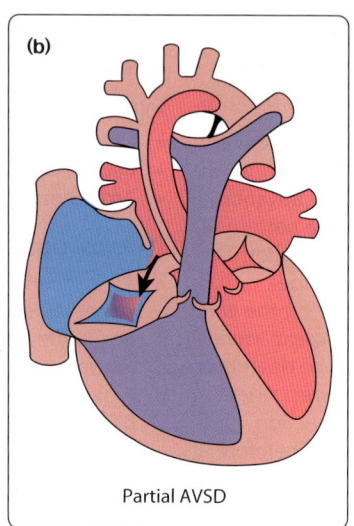

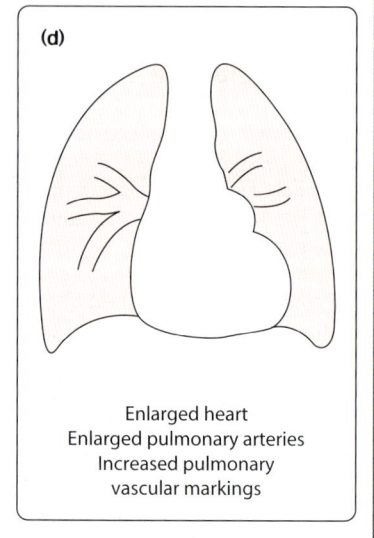

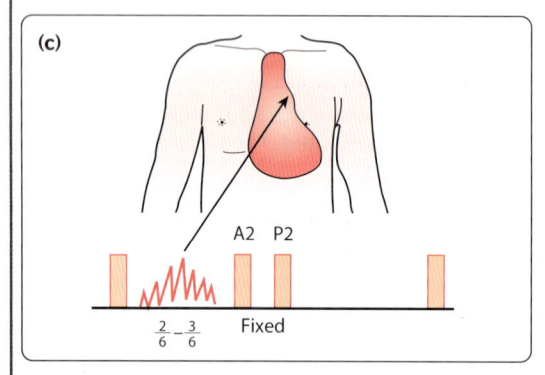

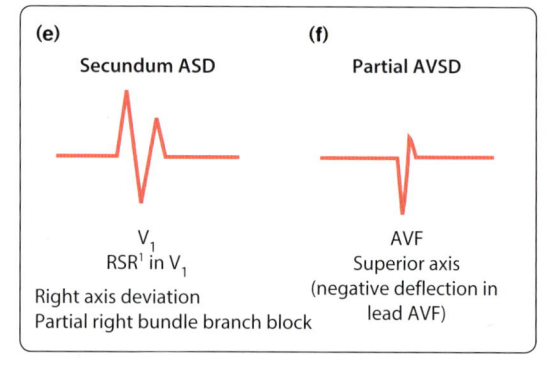

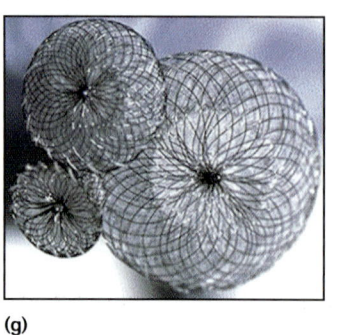

Figure 18.4 Atrial septal defect. (a) The ostium secundum atrial septal defect is a deficiency of the foramen ovale and surrounding atrial septum; (b) partial atrioventricular septal defect (AVSD) is a deficiency of the atrioventricular septum; (c) murmur; (d) chest radiograph; (e and f) ECG; and (g) examples of an occlusion device used to close secundum atrial septal defects.

Investigations

Chest radiograph
- Normal.

ECG
- Normal.

Echocardiography
- Demonstrates the precise anatomy of the defect. It is possible to assess its haemodynamic effects using Doppler echocardiography. There is no pulmonary hypertension.

Management

These lesions will close spontaneously. This is ascertained by the disappearance of the murmur with a normal ECG on follow-up by a paediatrician or paediatric cardiologist and by a normal echocardiogram. While the VSD is present, prevention of bacterial endocarditis is by maintaining good dental hygiene.

Large VSDs

These defects are the same size or bigger than the aortic valve (Fig. 18.5a).

Clinical features

Symptoms
- Heart failure with breathlessness and faltering growth after 1 week old.
- Recurrent chest infections.

Physical signs (Fig. 18.5b)
- Tachypnoea, tachycardia and enlarged liver from heart failure.
- Active precordium.
- Soft pansystolic murmur or no murmur (implying large defect).
- Apical mid-diastolic murmur (from increased flow across the mitral valve after the blood has circulated through the lungs).
- Loud pulmonary second sound (P_2) – from raised pulmonary arterial pressure.

Large ventricular septal defect

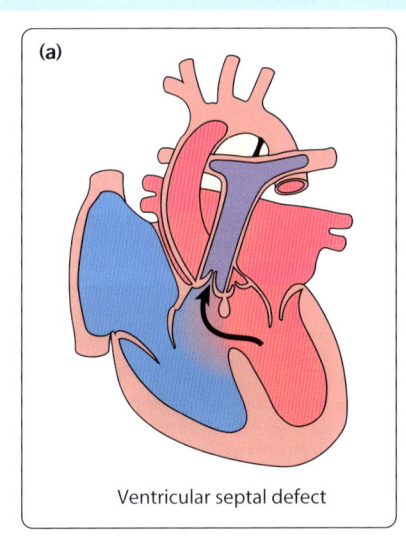

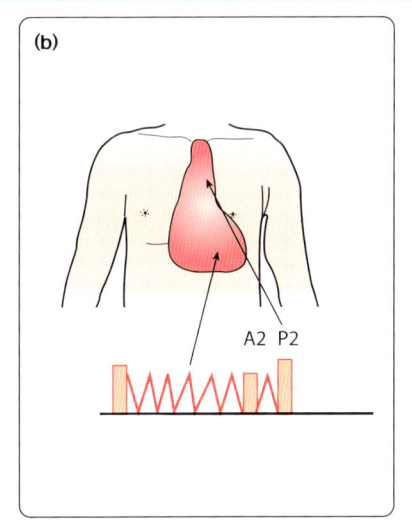

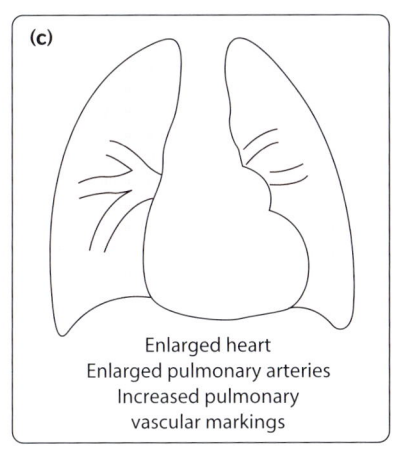

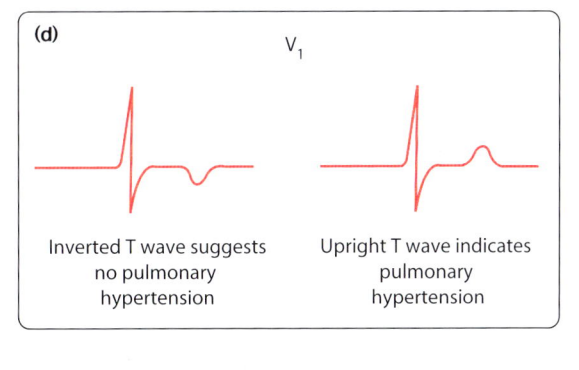

Figure 18.5 Ventricular septal defect. (a) Ventricular septal defect showing a left-to-right shunt; (b) murmur; (c) chest radiograph; and (d) ECG.

Investigations

Chest radiograph (Fig. 18.5c)
- Cardiomegaly
- Enlarged pulmonary arteries
- Increased pulmonary vascular markings
- Pulmonary oedema.

ECG (Fig. 18.5d)
- Biventricular hypertrophy by 2 months of age.

Echocardiography
- Demonstrates the anatomy of the defect, haemodynamic effects and pulmonary hypertension (due to high flow).

Management

Drug therapy for heart failure is with diuretics, often combined with captopril. Additional calorie input is required. There is always pulmonary hypertension in children with large VSD and left-to-right shunt. This will ultimately lead to irreversible damage of the pulmonary capillary vascular bed (see the 'Eisenmenger Syndrome' section). To prevent this, surgery is usually performed at 3 months to 6 months of age in order to:

- manage heart failure and faltering growth
- prevent permanent lung damage from pulmonary hypertension and high blood flow.

Persistent ductus arteriosus (persistent arterial duct)

The ductus arteriosus connects the pulmonary artery to the descending aorta. In term infants, it normally closes shortly after birth. In PDA it has failed to close by 1 month after the expected date of delivery due to a defect in the constrictor mechanism of the duct. The flow of blood across a PDA is then from the aorta to the pulmonary artery (i.e. left to right), following the fall in pulmonary vascular resistance after birth. In the preterm infant, the presence of a PDA is not from congenital heart disease but due to prematurity. This is described in Chapter 11.

Clinical features

Most children present with a continuous murmur beneath the left clavicle (Fig. 18.6a). The murmur continues into diastole because the pressure in the pulmonary artery is lower than that in the aorta throughout the cardiac cycle. The pulse pressure is increased, causing a collapsing or bounding pulse. Symptoms are unusual, but when the duct is large there will be increased pulmonary blood flow with heart failure and pulmonary hypertension.

Investigations

The chest radiograph and ECG are usually normal, but if the PDA is large and symptomatic the features on

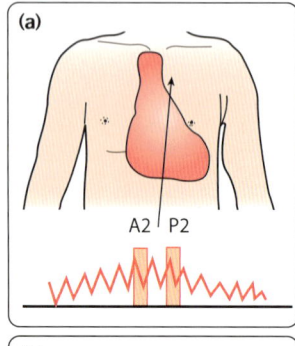

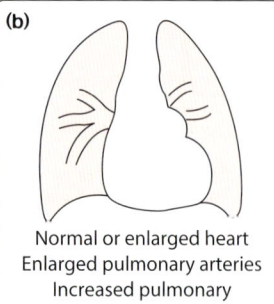

Persistent ductus arteriosus

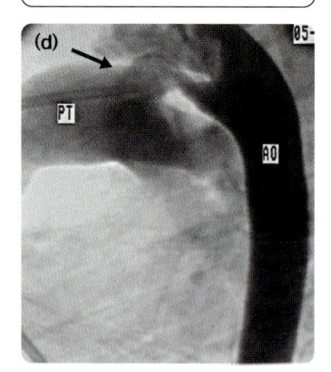

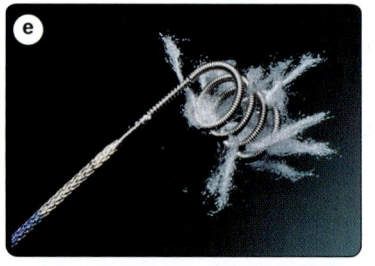

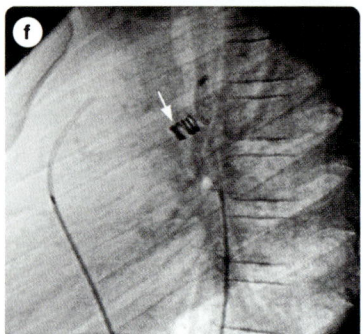

Figure 18.6 Persistent ductus arteriosus. (a) Murmur; (b) chest radiograph; (c) ECG; (d) a persistent ductus arteriosus visualized on angiography; (e) a coil used to close ducts. It is passed through a catheter via the femoral artery or vein; and (f) angiogram to show coil in the duct. AO, aorta; PT, pulmonary trunk.

Summary

Left-to-right shunts

Lesion	Symptoms	Signs	Management
ASD			
Secundum	None	ESM at ULSE Fixed split S$_2$	Catheter device closure at 3–5 years of age
Partial AVSD	None	ESM at ULSE Fixed split S$_2$ Pansystolic murmur at apex	Surgery at 3 years of age
VSD			
Small (80–90% of cases)	None	Pansystolic murmur at LLSE	None
Large (10–20% of cases)	Heart failure	Active precordium, loud P$_2$, soft murmur, tachypnoea, hepatomegaly	Diuretics, captopril, calories Surgery at 3–6 months of age
PDA	None	Continuous murmur at ULSE ± bounding pulses	Coil or device closure at cardiac catheter at 1 year of age, or ligation

ASD, atrial septal defect; AVSD, atrioventricular septal defect; ESM, ejection systolic murmur; LLSE, lower left sternal edge; PDA, persistent ductus arteriosus; ULSE, upper left sternal edge; VSD, ventricular septal defect.

---

chest radiograph (Fig. 18.6b) and ECG (Fig. 18.6c) are indistinguishable from those seen in a patient with a large VSD. However, the duct is readily identified on echocardiography.

Management

Closure is recommended to abolish the lifelong risk of bacterial endocarditis and of pulmonary vascular disease. Closure is with a coil or occlusion device introduced via a cardiac catheter at about 1 year of age (Fig. 18.6d–f). Occasionally, surgical ligation is required.

Right-to-left shunts

These are:
- tetralogy of Fallot
- transposition of the great arteries.

Presentation is with cyanosis (blue, oxygen saturations ≤94%, or collapsed), usually in the first week of life.

Hyperoxia (nitrogen washout) test

The test is used to help determine the presence of heart disease in a cyanosed neonate. The infant is placed in 100% oxygen (headbox or ventilator) for 10 minutes. If the right radial arterial partial pressure of oxygen (PaO$_2$) from a blood gas remains low (<15 kPa, 113 mmHg) after this time, a diagnosis of 'cyanotic' congenital heart disease can be made if lung disease and persistent pulmonary hypertension of the newborn have been excluded. If the PaO$_2$ is over 20 kPa, it is not cyanotic heart disease. Blood gas analysis must be performed as oxygen saturations are not reliable enough in this range of values.

Management of the cyanosed neonate

- Stabilize the airway, breathing, and circulation (ABC), with artificial ventilation if necessary.
- Start prostaglandin infusion (5 ng/kg per min). Most infants with cyanotic heart disease presenting in the first few days of life are duct dependent, i.e. there is reduced mixing between the pink oxygenated blood returning from the lungs and the blue deoxygenated blood from the body. Maintenance of ductal patency is the key to early survival of these children (Fig. 18.7). Observe for potential side-effects of prostaglandin – apnoea, jitteriness and seizures, flushing, vasodilatation and hypotension.

Tetralogy of Fallot

This is the most common cause of cyanotic congenital heart disease (Fig. 18.8a).

Clinical features

In tetralogy of Fallot, as implied by the name, there are four cardinal anatomical features:
- a large VSD
- overriding of the aorta with respect to the ventricular septum
- subpulmonary stenosis causing right ventricular outflow tract obstruction
- right ventricular hypertrophy as a result.

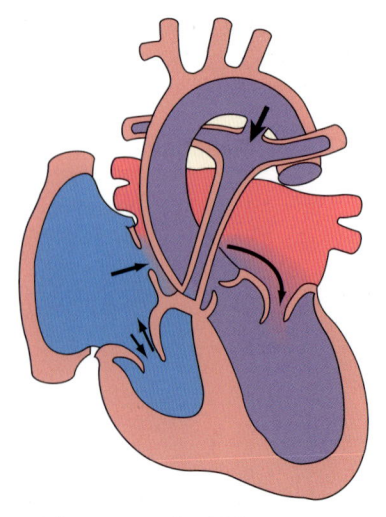

Pulmonary atresia with intact septum

Figure 18.7 An example of cyanotic congenital heart disease from duct-dependent pulmonary circulation – the pulmonary circulation is maintained by blood flowing left to right across the duct. Maintaining ductal patency with prostaglandin is crucial for early survival.

Symptoms

Most are diagnosed:

- antenatally *or*
- following the identification of a murmur in the first 2 months of life. Cyanosis at this stage may not be obvious, although a few present with severe cyanosis in the first few days of life.

The classical description of severe cyanosis, hypercyanotic spells and squatting on exercise developing in late infancy, is now rare in developed countries, but still common where access to the necessary paediatric cardiac services is not available. It is important to recognize hypercyanotic spells, as they may lead to myocardial infarction, cerebrovascular accidents and even death if left untreated. They are characterized by a rapid increase in cyanosis, usually associated with irritability or inconsolable crying because of severe hypoxia and breathlessness and pallor because of tissue acidosis. On auscultation, there is a very short murmur during a spell.

Signs

- Clubbing of the fingers and toes will develop in older children.
- A loud harsh ejection systolic murmur at the left sternal edge from day 1 of life (Fig. 18.8b). With increasing right ventricular outflow tract obstruction, which is predominantly muscular and below the pulmonary valve the murmur will shorten and cyanosis will increase.

Tetralogy of Fallot

(a) Tetralogy of Fallot

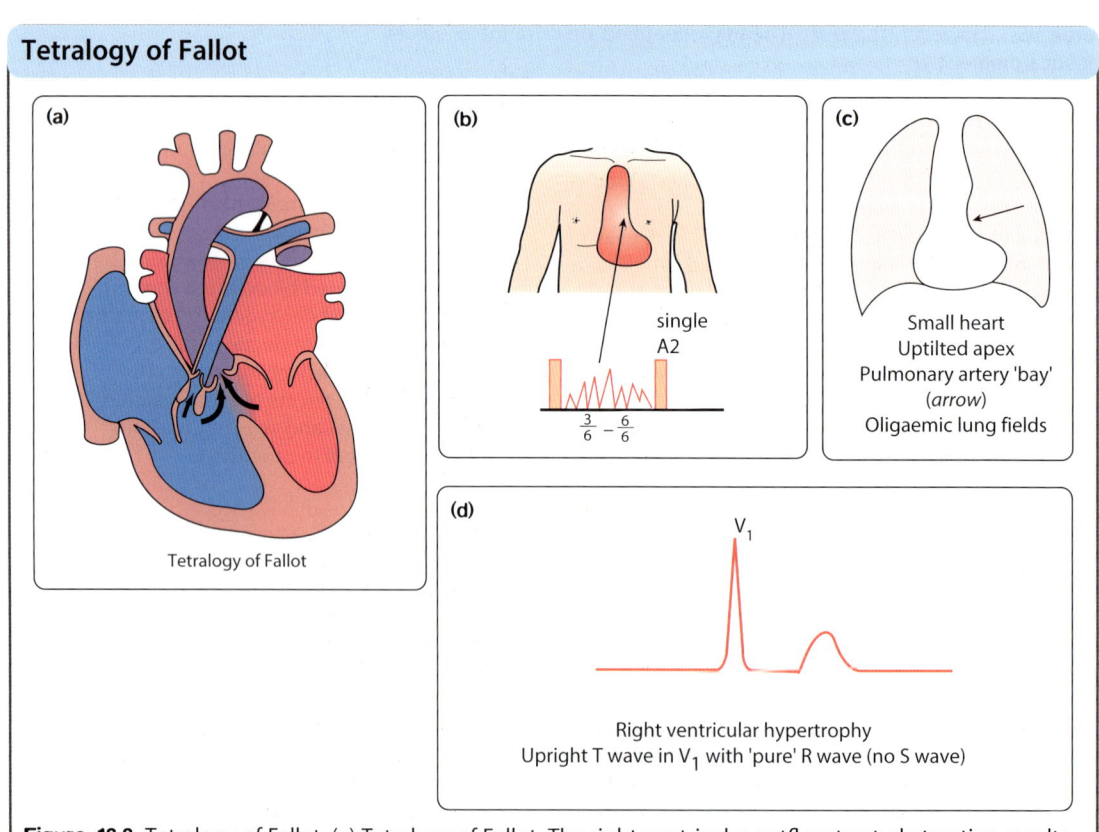

(b) single A2
$\frac{3}{6} - \frac{6}{6}$

(c) Small heart
Uptilted apex
Pulmonary artery 'bay' (*arrow*)
Oligaemic lung fields

(d) V_1
Right ventricular hypertrophy
Upright T wave in V_1 with 'pure' R wave (no S wave)

Figure 18.8 Tetralogy of Fallot. (a) Tetralogy of Fallot. The right ventricular outflow tract obstruction results in blood flowing from right to left across the ventricular septal defect; (b) murmur; (c) chest radiograph; and (d) ECG.

Investigations

Chest radiograph (Fig. 18.8c)

A radiograph will show a relatively small heart, possibly with an uptilted apex (boot shaped) due to right ventricular hypertrophy, more prominent in the older child. There may be a right-sided aortic arch, but characteristically there is a pulmonary artery 'bay', a concavity on the left heart border where the convex-shaped main pulmonary artery and right ventricular outflow tract would normally be profiled. There may also be decreased pulmonary vascular markings reflecting reduced pulmonary blood flow.

ECG (Fig. 18.8d)

Normal at birth. Right ventricular hypertrophy when older.

Echocardiography

This will demonstrate the cardinal features, but cardiac catheterization may be required to show the detailed anatomy of the coronary arteries.

Management

- Initial management is medical, with definitive surgery at around 6 months of age. It involves closing the VSD and relieving right ventricular outflow tract obstruction, sometimes with an artificial patch which extends across the pulmonary valve.
- Infants who are very cyanosed in the neonatal period require a shunt to increase pulmonary blood flow. This is usually done by surgical placement of an artificial tube between the subclavian artery and the pulmonary artery (a modified Blalock–Taussig shunt), or sometimes by balloon dilatation of the right ventricular outflow tract.
- Hypercyanotic spells are usually self-limiting and followed by a period of sleep. If prolonged (beyond about 15 min), they should be given prompt treatment, according to need, with:
  - sedation and pain relief (morphine is excellent)
  - intravenous propranolol (or an α adrenoceptor agonist), which probably works both as a peripheral vasoconstrictor and by relieving the subpulmonary muscular obstruction that is the cause of reduced pulmonary blood flow
  - intravenous volume administration
  - bicarbonate to correct acidosis
  - muscle paralysis and artificial ventilation in order to reduce metabolic oxygen demand.

Transposition of the great arteries

The aorta is connected to the right ventricle and the pulmonary artery is connected to the left ventricle (discordant ventriculo–arterial connection). The blue blood is therefore returned to the body and the pink blood is returned to the lungs (Fig. 18.9a). There are two parallel circulations – unless there is mixing of blood between them, this condition is incompatible with life. Fortunately, there are a number of naturally occurring associated anomalies, e.g. VSD, ASD and PDA as well as therapeutic interventions which can achieve this mixing in the short term.

Clinical features

Symptoms

Cyanosis is the predominant symptom. It may be profound and life-threatening. Presentation is usually on day 2 of life when ductal closure leads to a marked reduction in mixing of the desaturated and saturated blood. Cyanosis will be less severe and presentation delayed if there is more mixing of blood from associated anomalies, e.g. an ASD.

Physical signs (Fig. 18.9b)

- Cyanosis is always present.
- The second heart sound is often loud and single.
- Usually no murmur, but may be a systolic murmur from increased flow or stenosis within the left ventricular (pulmonary) outflow tract.

Investigations

Chest radiograph (Fig. 18.9c)

This may reveal the classic findings of a narrow upper mediastinum with an 'egg on side' appearance of the cardiac shadow (due to the anteroposterior relationship of the great vessels, narrow vascular pedicle, and hypertrophied right ventricle, respectively). Increased pulmonary vascular markings are common due to *increased* pulmonary blood flow.

ECG (Fig. 18.9d)

This is usually normal.

Echocardiography

This is essential to demonstrate the abnormal arterial connections and associated abnormalities.

Management

- In the sick cyanosed neonate, the key is to improve mixing.
- Maintaining the patency of the ductus arteriosus with a prostaglandin infusion is mandatory.
- A balloon atrial septostomy may be a life-saving procedure, which may need to be performed in 20% of those with transposition of the great arteries (Fig. 18.9e–g). A catheter with an inflatable balloon at its tip is passed through the umbilical or femoral vein and then on through the right atrium and foramen ovale. The balloon is inflated within the left atrium and then pulled back through the atrial septum. This tears the atrial septum, renders the flap valve of the foramen ovale incompetent and so allows mixing of the systemic and pulmonary venous blood within the atrium.
- All patients with transposition of the great arteries will require surgery, which is usually the arterial switch procedure in the neonatal period. In this operation, performed in the first few days of life, the pulmonary artery and aorta are transected

Transposition of the great arteries

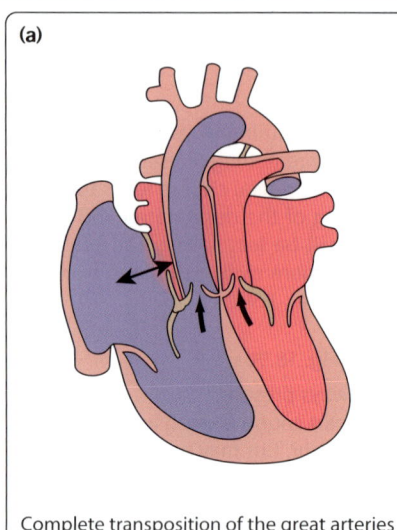

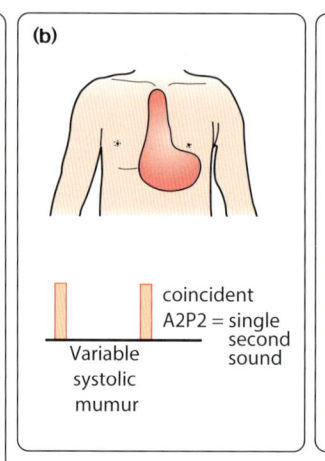

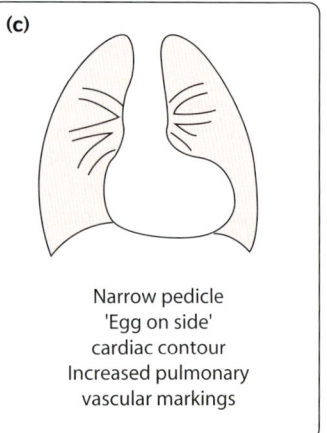

(a) Complete transposition of the great arteries

(b) Variable systolic mumur — coincident A2P2 = single second sound

(c) Narrow pedicle 'Egg on side' cardiac contour Increased pulmonary vascular markings

(d) ECG Usually normal neonatal pattern

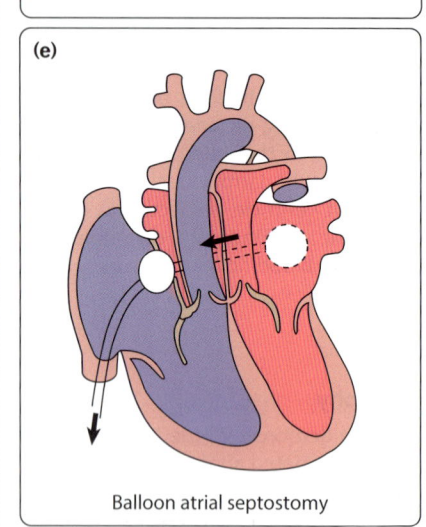

(e) Balloon atrial septostomy

In transposition of the great arteries:
- Establishing a prostaglandin infusion to maintain patency of the ductus arteriosis is essential
- Balloon atrial septostomy may be life-saving

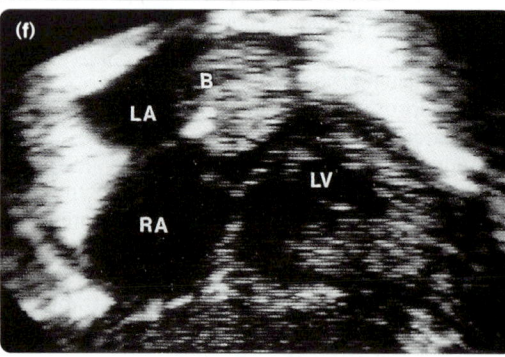

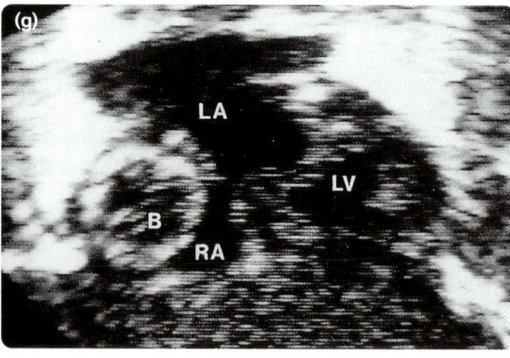

Figure 18.9 Transposition of the great arteries. (a) Transposition of the great arteries. There must be mixing of blood between the two circulations for this to be compatible with life; (b) heart sounds; (c) chest radiograph; (d) ECG; (e) balloon atrial septostomy. A balloon (about 2-ml) is pulled through the atrial septum from the left atrium to the right atrium in order to increase the size of the atrial defect. This is done with echocardiographic guidance; (f) echocardiogram showing balloon in the left atrium; and (g) balloon has been pulled through the atrial septum and is now in the right atrium. B, balloon; LA, left atrium; LV, left ventricle; RA, right atrium.

Summary

Cyanotic congenital heart disease

Lesion	Clinical features	Management
Tetralogy of Fallot	Loud murmur at upper left sternal edge	Surgery at 6–9 months of age
	Clubbing of fingers and toes (older)	
	Hypercyanotic spells	
Transposition of the great arteries	Neonatal cyanosis	Prostaglandin infusion
	No murmur	Balloon atrial septostomy
		Arterial switch operation in neonatal period
Eisenmenger syndrome	No murmur	Medication to delay transplantation
	Right heart failure (late)	

above the arterial valves and switched over. In addition, the coronary arteries have to be transferred across to the new aorta.

Eisenmenger syndrome

If high pulmonary blood flow due to a large left-to-right shunt or common mixing is not treated at an early stage, then the pulmonary arteries become thick walled and the resistance to flow increases (Fig. 18.10). Gradually, those children that survive become less symptomatic as the shunt decreases. Eventually, at about 10–15 years of age, the shunt reverses and the teenager becomes blue, which is Eisenmenger syndrome. This situation is progressive and the adult will die in right heart failure at a variable age, usually in the fourth or fifth decade of life. Treatment is aimed at prevention of this condition, with early intervention for high pulmonary blood flow. Transplantation is not easily available although there are now medicines to palliate such pulmonary vascular disease (see the 'Pulmonary hypertension' section).

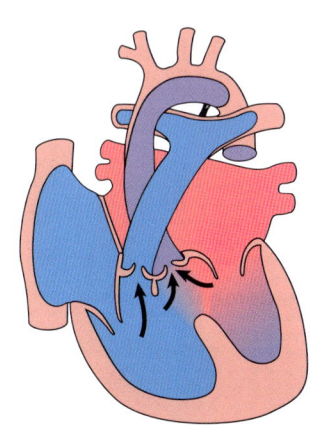

Common mixing (blue and breathless)

These include:

- AVSD (complete)
- complex congenital heart disease, e.g. tricuspid atresia.

Atrioventricular septal defect (complete)

This is most commonly seen in children with Down syndrome (Fig. 18.11). A complete AVSD is a defect in the middle of the heart with a single five-leaflet (common) valve between the atria and ventricles, which stretches across the entire atrioventricular junction and tends to leak. As there is a large defect there is pulmonary hypertension.

Features of a complete AVSD are:

- presentation on antenatal ultrasound screening
- cyanosis at birth or heart failure at 2 weeks to 3 weeks of life
- no murmur heard, the lesion being detected on routine echocardiography screening in a newborn baby with Down syndrome
- there is always a superior axis on the ECG
- management is to treat heart failure medically (as for large VSD) and surgical repair at 3 months to 6 months of age.

Eisenmenger syndrome

Figure 18.10 Eisenmenger syndrome with right-to-left shunting from pulmonary vascular disease following increased pulmonary blood flow and pulmonary hypertension with large ventricular septal defect.

Complex congenital heart disease

It is difficult to generalize about these conditions, (tricuspid atresia, mitral atresia, double inlet left ventricle,

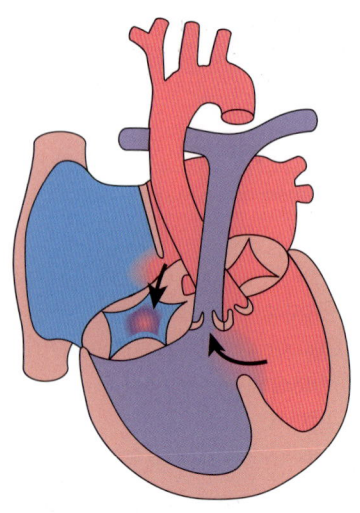

Atrioventricular septal defect

Figure 18.11 Complete atrioventricular septal defect, with a common atrioventricular valve between a large atrial and ventricular component to the atrioventricular septal defect.

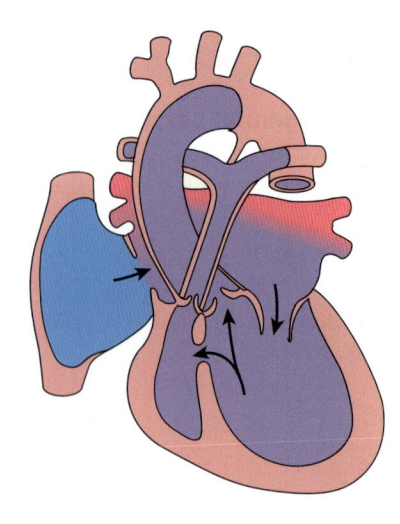

Tricuspid atresia

Figure 18.12 In tricuspid atresia, there is only one effective ventricle because of complete absence of the tricuspid valve.

common arterial trunk – truncus arteriosus) because their main presenting feature depends on whether cyanosis or heart failure is more predominant. Tricuspid atresia is the most common.

Tricuspid atresia

In tricuspid atresia (Fig. 18.12), only the left ventricle is effective, the right being small and nonfunctional.

Clinical features

There is 'common mixing' of systemic and pulmonary venous return in the left atrium. Presentation is with cyanosis in the newborn period if duct dependent, or the child may be well at birth and become cyanosed or breathless.

Management

Early palliation (as with all the common mixing complex diseases) is performed to maintain a secure supply of blood to the lungs at low pressure, by:

- a Blalock–Taussig shunt insertion (between the subclavian and pulmonary arteries) in children who are severely cyanosed
- pulmonary artery banding operation to reduce pulmonary blood flow if breathless.

Completely corrective surgery is not possible with most, as there is often only one effective functioning ventricle. Palliation is performed (Glenn or hemi-Fontan operation connecting the superior vena cava to the pulmonary artery after 6 months of age and a Fontan operation to also connect the inferior vena cava to the pulmonary artery at 3–5 years of age).

Thus the left ventricle drives blood around the body and systemic venous pressure supplies blood to the lungs. The Fontan operation results in a less than ideal functional outcome, but has the advantages of relieving cyanosis and removing the long-term volume load on the single functional ventricle.

Summary

Common mixing

Lesion	Clinical features	Management
Atrioventricular septal defect (complete)	Down syndrome (often) Cyanosis at birth Breathless at 2–3 weeks of life	Treat heart failure medically Surgical repair at 3 months
Complex diseases (e.g. tricuspid atresia)	Cyanosis Breathless	Shunt (Blalock–Taussig) or pulmonary artery banding, then surgery (Glenn and later Fontan operation)

Outflow obstruction in the well child

These lesions are:
- aortic stenosis
- pulmonary stenosis
- adult-type coarctation of the aorta.

Aortic stenosis

The aortic valve leaflets are partly fused together, giving a restrictive exit from the left ventricle (Fig. 18.13a). There may be one to three aortic leaflets. Aortic stenosis may not be an isolated lesion. It is often associated with mitral valve stenosis and coarctation of the aorta, and their presence should always be excluded.

Clinical features

Most present with an asymptomatic murmur. Those with severe stenosis may present with reduced exercise tolerance, chest pain on exertion, or syncope.

In the neonatal period, those with *critical* aortic stenosis and a duct-dependent systemic circulation may present with severe heart failure leading to shock.

Physical signs (Fig. 18.13b)
- Small volume, slow rising pulses.
- Carotid thrill (always).
- Ejection systolic murmur maximal at the upper right sternal edge radiating to the neck.
- Delayed and soft aortic second sound.
- Apical ejection click.

Investigations

Chest radiograph (Fig. 18.13c)
Normal or prominent left ventricle with poststenotic dilatation of the ascending aorta.

ECG (Fig. 18.13d)
There may be left ventricular hypertrophy.

Management

In children, regular clinical and echocardiographic assessment is required in order to assess when to intervene. Children with symptoms on exercise or who have a high resting pressure gradient (>64 mmHg) across the aortic valve will undergo balloon valvotomy. Balloon dilatation in older children is generally safe and uncomplicated, but in neonates this is much more difficult and dangerous.

Most neonates and children with significant aortic valve stenosis requiring treatment in the first few years of life will eventually require aortic valve replacement. Early treatment is therefore palliative and directed towards delaying this for as long as possible.

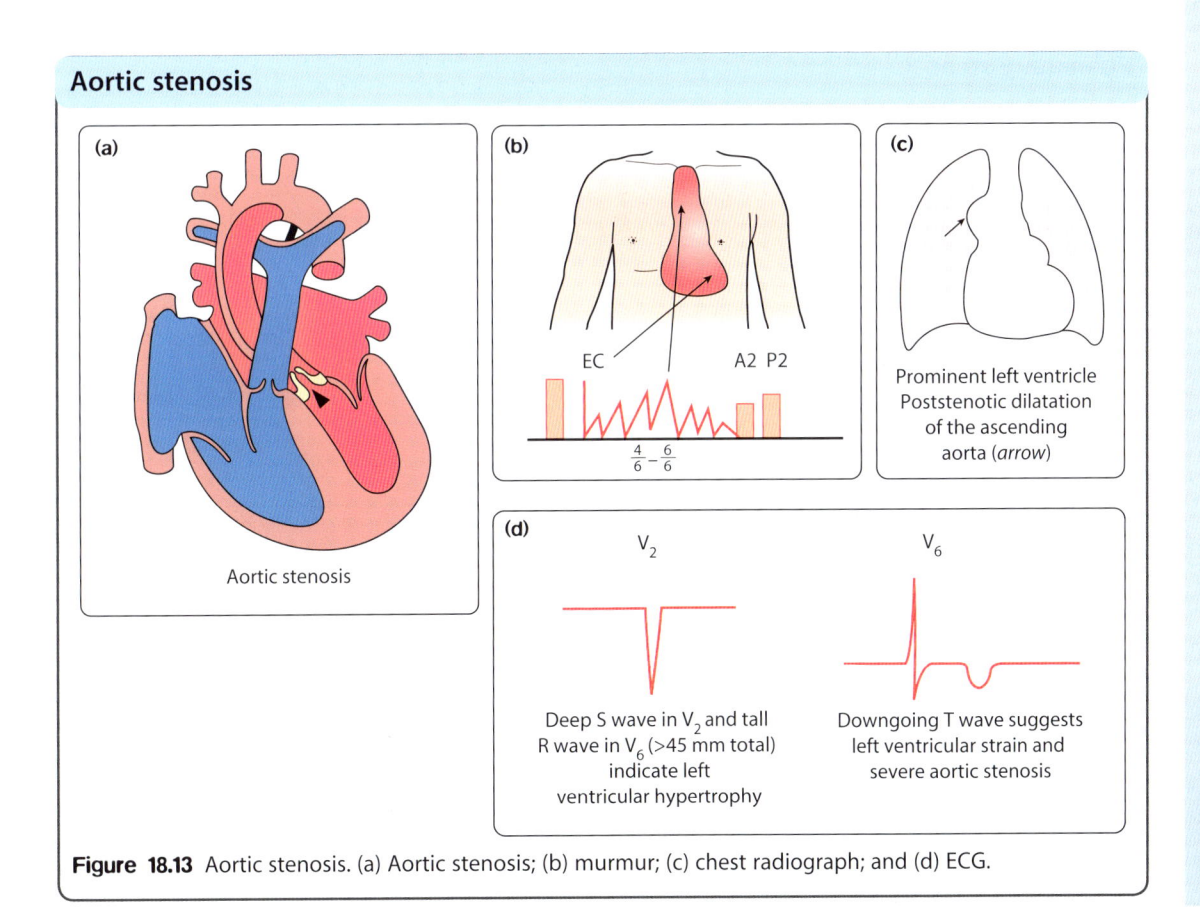

Aortic stenosis

(a) Aortic stenosis

(b) EC A2 P2 $\frac{4}{6} - \frac{6}{6}$

(c) Prominent left ventricle
Poststenotic dilatation of the ascending aorta (*arrow*)

(d) V_2 V_6
Deep S wave in V_2 and tall R wave in V_6 (>45 mm total) indicate left ventricular hypertrophy
Downgoing T wave suggests left ventricular strain and severe aortic stenosis

Figure 18.13 Aortic stenosis. (a) Aortic stenosis; (b) murmur; (c) chest radiograph; and (d) ECG.

Pulmonary stenosis

The pulmonary valve leaflets are partly fused together, giving a restrictive exit from the right ventricle.

Clinical features

Most are asymptomatic (Fig. 18.14a). It is diagnosed clinically. A small number of neonates with *critical* pulmonary stenosis have a duct-dependent pulmonary circulation and present in the first few days of life with cyanosis.

Physical signs (Fig. 18.14b)

- An ejection systolic murmur best heard at the upper left sternal edge; thrill may be present.
- An ejection click best heard at the upper left sternal edge.
- When severe, there is a prominent right ventricular impulse (heave).

Investigations

Chest radiograph (Fig. 18.14c)

Normal or poststenotic dilatation of the pulmonary artery.

ECG (Fig. 18.14d)

Shows evidence of right ventricular hypertrophy (upright T wave in V_1).

Management

Most children are asymptomatic and when the pressure gradient across the pulmonary valve becomes markedly increased (>about 64 mmHg), intervention will be required. Transcatheter balloon dilatation is the treatment of choice in most children.

Adult-type coarctation of the aorta

This uncommon lesion (Fig. 18.15a) is not duct dependent. It gradually becomes more severe over many years.

Clinical features (Fig. 18.15b)

- Asymptomatic.
- Systemic hypertension in the right arm.
- Ejection systolic murmur at upper sternal edge.
- Collaterals heard with continuous murmur at the back.
- Radio-femoral delay. This is due to blood bypassing the obstruction via collateral vessels in the chest wall and hence the pulse in the legs is delayed.

Investigations

Chest radiograph (Fig. 18.15c)

- 'Rib notching' due to the development of large collateral intercostal arteries running

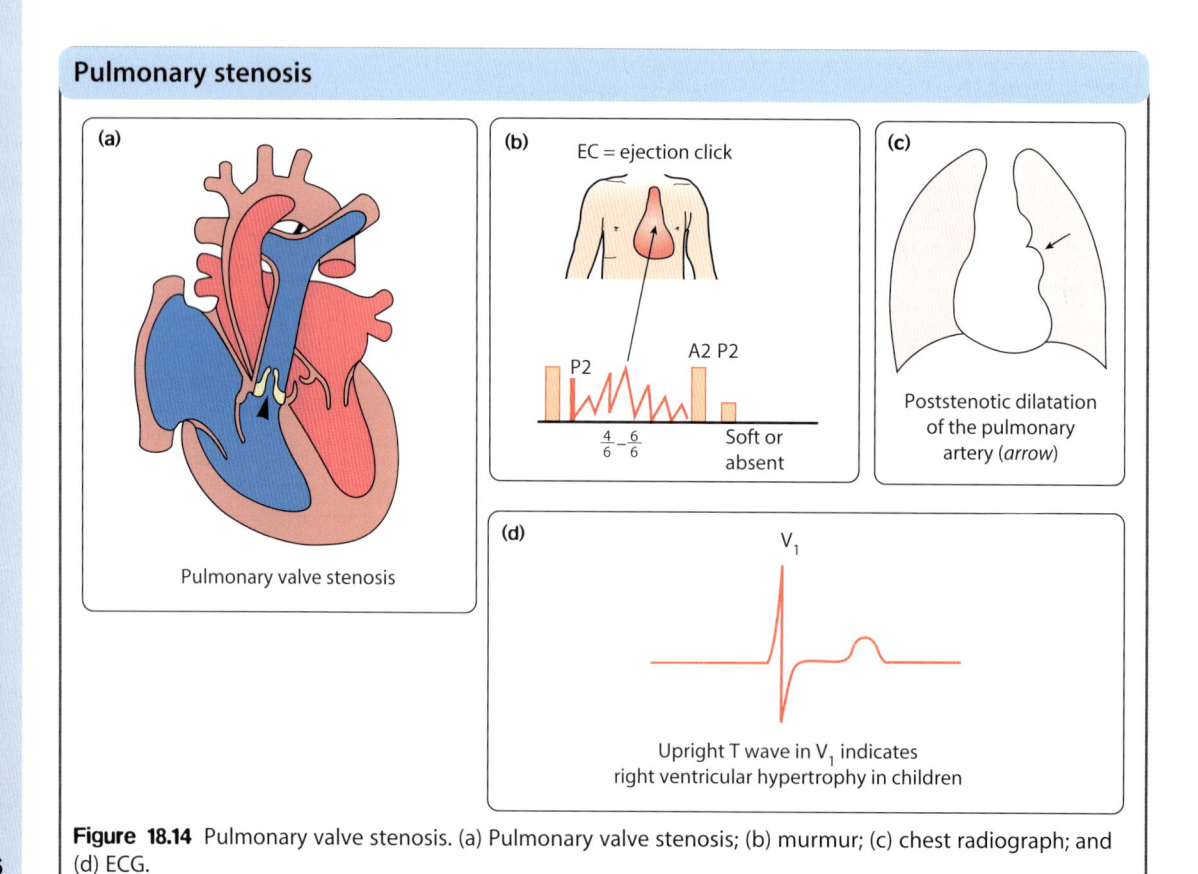

Pulmonary stenosis

(a) Pulmonary valve stenosis

(b) EC = ejection click; Soft or absent

(c) Poststenotic dilatation of the pulmonary artery (*arrow*)

(d) Upright T wave in V_1 indicates right ventricular hypertrophy in children

Figure 18.14 Pulmonary valve stenosis. (a) Pulmonary valve stenosis; (b) murmur; (c) chest radiograph; and (d) ECG.

under the ribs posteriorly to bypass the obstruction.
- '3' sign, with visible notch in the descending aorta at site of the coarctation.

ECG
- Left ventricular hypertrophy (Fig. 18.15d).

Management
When the condition becomes severe, as assessed by echocardiography, a stent may be inserted at cardiac catheter. Sometimes surgical repair is required.

Outflow obstruction in the sick infant

These lesions include:
- coarctation of the aorta
- interruption of the aortic arch
- hypoplastic left heart syndrome.

Clinical features are:
- in all of these children, they usually present sick with heart failure and shock in the neonatal period, unless diagnosed on antenatal ultrasound

Summary

Outflow obstruction in the well child

Lesion	Signs	Management
Aortic stenosis	Murmur, upper right sternal edge; carotid thrill	Balloon dilatation
Pulmonary stenosis	Murmur, upper left sternal edge; no carotid thrill	Balloon dilatation
Coarctation (adult type)	Systemic hypertension Radio-femoral delay	Stent insertion or surgery

Adult-type coarctation of the aorta

(a) Adult-type coarctation of the aorta

(b) Ejection systolic mumur between shoulder blades or normal

(c) Usually normal. Rib notching from aortic-to-aortic collateral arteries in teenagers and adults

(d) V_2 — Deep S wave in V_2 and tall R wave in V_6 (>45 mm total) and upright T wave indicate left ventricular hypertrophy

V_6 — Downgoing T wave suggests left ventricular strain and severe coarctation and/or hypertension

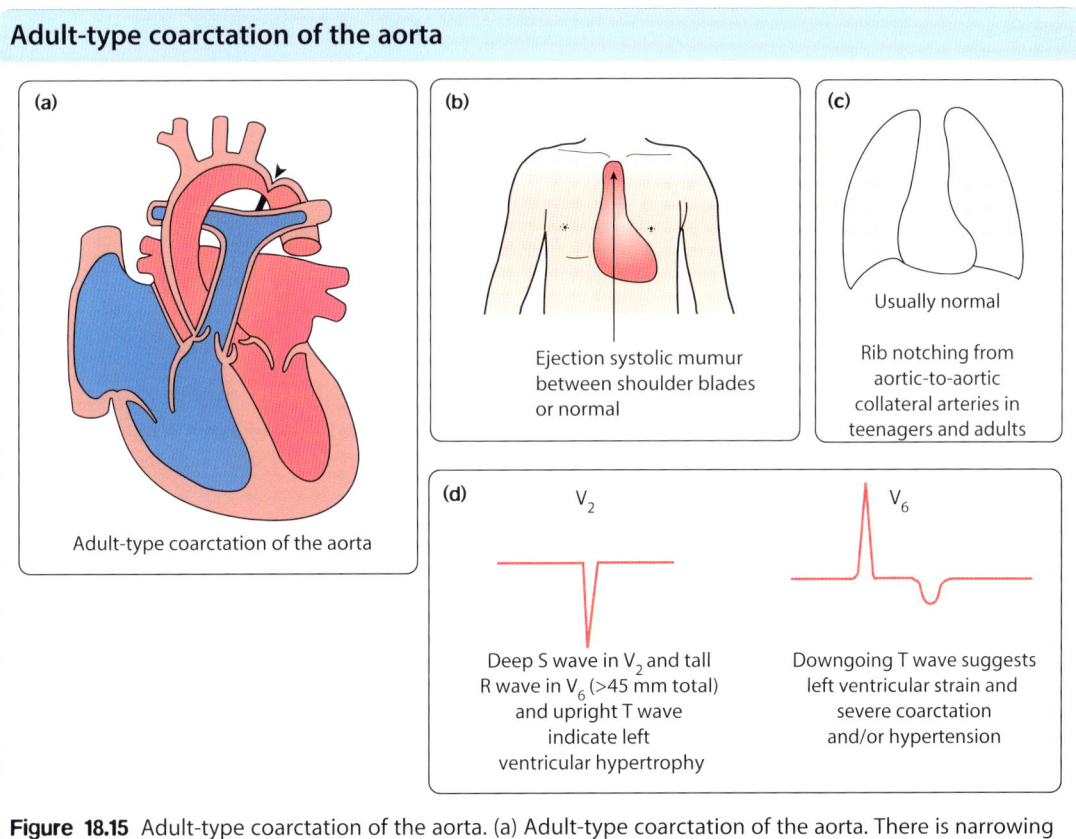

Figure 18.15 Adult-type coarctation of the aorta. (a) Adult-type coarctation of the aorta. There is narrowing of the aorta distal to the left subclavian artery adjacent to the insertion of the arterial duct; (b) murmur; (c) chest radiograph; and (d) ECG.

Management is:
- resuscitate (ABC)
- prostaglandin should be commenced at the earliest opportunity
- referral is made to a cardiac centre for early surgical intervention.

Coarctation of the aorta

This is due to arterial duct tissue encircling the aorta just at the point of insertion of the duct (Fig. 18.2). When the duct closes, the aorta also constricts, causing severe obstruction to the left ventricular outflow. This is the most common cause of collapse due to left outflow obstruction.

Clinical features

Examination on the first day of life is usually normal. The neonates usually present with acute circulatory collapse at 2-days of age when the duct closes.

Physical signs
- A sick baby, with severe heart failure.
- Absent femoral pulses.
- Severe metabolic acidosis.

Investigations

Chest radiograph
Cardiomegaly from heart failure and shock.

ECG
Normal.

Management

This is the same as for all the children in this section with outflow obstruction in the sick infant. Surgical repair is performed soon after diagnosis.

Interruption of the aortic arch

- Uncommon, with *no* connection between the proximal aorta and distal to the arterial duct, so that the cardiac output is dependent on right-to-left shunt via the duct (Fig. 18.16).
- A VSD is usually present.
- Presentation is with shock in the neonatal period as above.
- Complete correction with closure of the VSD and repair of the aortic arch is usually performed within the first few days of life.
- Association with other conditions (DiGeorge syndrome – absence of thymus, palatal defects, immunodeficiency and hypocalcaemia, and chromosome 22q11.2 microdeletion).

Hypoplastic left heart syndrome

In this condition there is underdevelopment of the entire left side of the heart (Fig. 18.17). The mitral valve is small or atretic, the left ventricle is diminutive, and there is usually aortic valve atresia. The ascending aorta

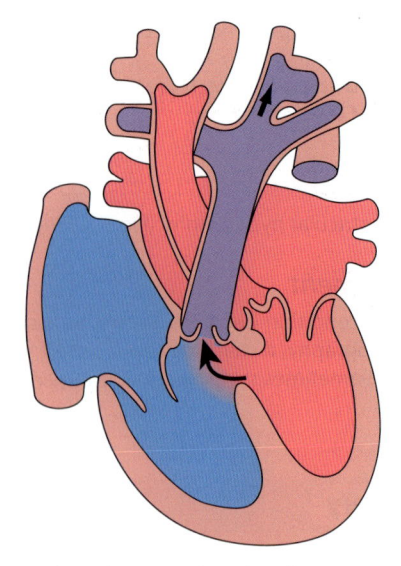

Interrupted aortic arch

Figure 18.16 Interruption of the aortic arch. The lower body circulation is maintained by right-to-left flow of blood across the duct.

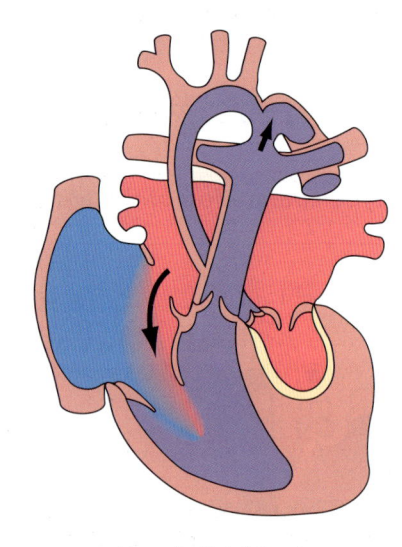

Hypoplastic left heart

Figure 18.17 Hypoplastic left heart syndrome. The entire left side of the heart is underdeveloped.

is very small, and there is almost invariably coarctation of the aorta.

Clinical features

These children may be detected antenatally at ultrasound screening. This allows for effective counselling and prevents the child from becoming sick after birth. If they do present after birth, they are the sickest of all neonates presenting with a duct-dependent systemic circulation. There is no flow through the left side of the heart, so ductal constriction leads to profound acidosis and rapid cardiovascular collapse. There is weakness or absence of all peripheral pulses, in contrast to weak femoral pulses in coarctation of the aorta.

Summary

Left heart outflow obstruction in the sick infant – duct-dependent lesions

Lesion	Clinical features	Management
Coarctation of the aorta	Circulatory collapse Absent femoral pulses	Maintain ABC Prostaglandin infusion
Interruption of the aortic arch	Circulatory collapse Absent femoral pulses and absent left brachial pulse	Maintain ABC Prostaglandin infusion
Hypoplastic left heart syndrome	Circulatory collapse All peripheral pulses absent	Maintain ABC Prostaglandin infusion

Management

The management of this condition consists of a difficult neonatal operation called the Norwood procedure. Children who have complex lesions or are small for gestational age undergo hybrid procedures that are a combination of cardiac catheter and surgical operation. This is followed by a further operation (Glenn or hemi-Fontan) at about 6 months of age and again (Fontan) at about 3 years of age.

Care following cardiac surgery

Most children recover rapidly following cardiac surgery and are back at nursery or school within a month. Exercise tolerance will be variable and most children can be allowed to find their own limits. Restricted exercise is advised only for children with severe residual aortic stenosis and for ventricular dysfunction.

Most of the children are followed up in specialist cardiac clinics. Most lead normal, unrestricted lives, but any change in symptoms, e.g. decreasing exercise tolerance or palpitations requires further investigation. An increasing number of adolescents and young adults require revision of surgery performed in early life. The most common reason for this is replacement of artificial valves and relief of postsurgical suture line stenosis, e.g. recoarctation or pulmonary artery stenosis.

Cardiac arrhythmias

Sinus arrhythmia is normal in children and is detectable as a cyclical change in heart rate with respiration. There is acceleration during inspiration and slowing on expiration (the heart rate changing by up to 30 beats/min).

Supraventricular tachycardia

This is the most common childhood arrhythmia. The heart rate is rapid, between 250–300 beats/min. It can cause poor cardiac output and pulmonary oedema. It typically presents with symptoms of heart failure in the neonate or young infant. It is a cause of *hydrops fetalis* and intrauterine death. The term re-entry tachycardia

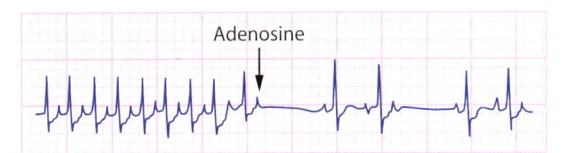

Figure 18.18 Rhythm strip showing supraventricular re-entry tachycardia, in which there is a narrow complex (<120 ms or three small squares) tachycardia of 250–300 beats/min, and response to treatment with adenosine.

is used because a circuit of conduction is set up, with premature activation of the atrium via an accessory pathway. There is rarely a structural heart problem, but an echocardiogram should be performed.

Investigation

The ECG will generally show a narrow complex tachycardia of 250–300 beats/min (Fig. 18.18). It may be possible to discern a P wave after the QRS complex due to retrograde activation of the atrium via the accessory pathway. If heart failure is severe, there may be changes suggestive of myocardial ischaemia, with T-wave inversion in the lateral precordial leads. When in sinus rhythm, a short P–R interval may be discernible. In the Wolff–Parkinson–White syndrome, the early antegrade activation of the ventricle via the pathway results in a short P–R interval and a delta wave.

Management

In the severely ill child, prompt restoration of sinus rhythm is the key to improvement. This is achieved by:

- circulatory and respiratory support – tissue acidosis is corrected, positive pressure ventilation if required
- vagal stimulating manoeuvres, e.g. carotid sinus massage or cold ice pack to face, successful in about 80%
- intravenous adenosine – the treatment of choice. This is safe and effective, inducing atrioventricular block after rapid bolus injection. It terminates the tachycardia by breaking the re-entry circuit that is set up between the atrioventricular node and

accessory pathway. It is given incrementally in increasing doses
- electrical cardioversion with a synchronized direct current shock (0.5–2 J/kg body weight) if adenosine fails.

Once sinus rhythm is restored, maintenance therapy will be required, e.g. with flecainide or sotalol. Digoxin can be used on its own when there is no overt pre-excitation wave (delta wave) on the resting ECG, but propranolol can be added in the presence of pre-excitation. Even though the resting ECG may remain abnormal, 90% of children will have no further attacks after infancy. Treatment is therefore stopped at 1 year of age. Those who have Wolff–Parkinson–White syndrome need to be assessed to ensure they cannot conduct quickly and this may be undertaken in teenage life, with atrial pacing. This will reduce the small chance of sudden death in such patients. Those who relapse or are at risk are usually treated with percutaneous radiofrequency ablation or cryoablation of the accessory pathway.

Congenital complete heart block

This is a rare condition (Fig. 18.19) that is usually related to the presence of anti-Ro or anti-La antibodies in maternal serum. These mothers will have either manifest or latent connective tissue disorders. Subsequent pregnancies are often affected. This antibody appears to prevent normal development of the electrical conduction system in the developing heart, with atrophy and fibrosis of the atrioventricular node. It may cause fetal hydrops, death in utero and heart failure in the neonatal period. However, most remain symptom free for many years, but a few become symptomatic with presyncope or syncope. All children with symptoms require insertion of an endocardial pacemaker. There are other rare causes of complete heart block.

Other arrhythmias

Long QT syndrome may be associated with sudden loss of consciousness during exercise, stress or emotion, usually in late childhood. It may be mistakenly diagnosed as epilepsy. If unrecognized, sudden death from ventricular tachycardia may occur. Inheritance is autosomal dominant; there are several phenotypes. It has been associated with erythromycin therapy, electrolyte disorders and head injury.

It is one of the group of channelopathies caused by specific gene mutations. Abnormalities of the sodium, potassium or calcium channels lead to gain or loss of function. Anyone with a family history of sudden unexplained death or a history of syncope on exertion should be assessed.

Atrial fibrillation, atrial flutter, ectopic atrial tachycardia, ventricular tachycardia and ventricular fibrillation occur in children, but all are rare. They are most often seen in children who have undergone surgery for complex congenital heart disease.

Syncope

Transient loss of consciousness is usually due to syncope, when it is associated with a loss of postural tone with spontaneous recovery. It is caused by a transient impairment of brain oxygen delivery, generally due to impaired cerebral perfusion [see also Ch. 29. Neurological disorders].

This is common in adolescents and is usually benign, but rarely it is due to cardiac disease, which may be life-threatening.

The causes are:

- neurally mediated syncope – is in response to a range of provocations and stressors. These may be from just standing up too quickly (a symptom of 'orthostatic intolerance'), to the sight of blood or needles or to a sudden unexpected pain. There is usually a prodrome of dizziness and light-headed feeling and abnormal vision often with nausea, sweating, or pallor. When associated with jerking movements, it can easily be misdiagnosed as epilepsy. In most episodes there is a maladaptive drop in blood pressure; in a significant minority there is a marked fall in heart rate and in a few there is asystole
- cardiac syncope – may be arrhythmic, from heart block, supraventricular tachycardia, ventricular tachycardia, e.g. associated with long QT syndrome or structural, associated with aortic stenosis, hypertrophic cardiomyopathy.

Features suggestive of a cardiac cause are:

- symptoms on exercise – potentially dangerous
- family history of sudden unexplained death
- palpitations.

Check blood pressure and for signs of cardiac disease (murmur, femoral pulses, signs of Marfan syndrome). Investigate all presenting with transient loss of consciousness with a standard 12-lead ECG, and check the corrected Q-T interval.

Chest pains

Rarely due to cardiac disease in children. Only those occurring with palpitations or on exertion suggest a possible cardiac origin.

Rheumatic fever

This is now rare in the developed world, but remains the most important cause of heart disease in children worldwide. Improvements in sanitation, reduction in

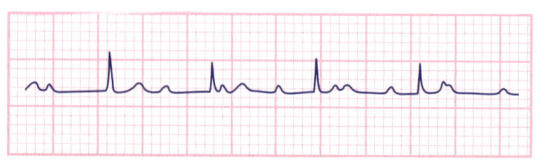

Figure 18.19 Electrocardiography of congenital complete heart block. The P waves and QRS complexes are dissociated.

overcrowded living conditions, treatment of streptococcal pharyngitis with 10-day course of antibiotics and changes in streptococcal virulence have led to its virtual disappearance in developed countries. The estimated prevalence of rheumatic heart disease among 5–15-year-olds in Sub-Saharan Africa is 6/1000 compared with 0.3/1000 in developed countries. Acute rheumatic fever is a short-lived, multisystem autoimmune response to a preceding infection with group A β-haemolytic streptococcus. The disease mainly affects children aged 5–15 years. It progresses to chronic rheumatic heart disease in up to 80% of cases.

Clinical features

After a latent interval of 2–6 weeks following a pharyngeal or skin infection, polyarthritis, mild fever and malaise develop. The clinical features and diagnostic criteria are shown in Fig. 18.20.

Chronic rheumatic heart disease

The most common form of long-term damage from scarring and fibrosis of the valve tissue of the heart is mitral stenosis. If there have been repeated attacks of rheumatic fever with carditis, this may occur as early as the second decade of life, but usually symptoms do not develop until early adult life. Although the mitral valve is the most frequently affected, aortic, tricuspid and rarely, pulmonary valve disease may occur.

Management

Acute rheumatic fever is usually treated with bed rest and anti-inflammatory agents. While there is evidence of active myocarditis (echocardiographic changes with a raised erythrocyte sedimentation rate), bed rest and limitation of exercise are essential. Aspirin is very effective at suppressing the inflammatory response of the joints and heart. It needs to be given in high dosage

---

Jones criteria for diagnosis of rheumatic fever

Required to make the diagnosis

Two major, or one major and two minor, criteria plus supportive evidence of preceding group A streptococcal infection (markedly raised or rising ASO titre or positive rapid streptococcal antigen test or positive group A streptococcus on throat culture)

Major manifestations

Carditis (50%)
Endocarditis
• significant murmur
• valvular dysfunction
Myocarditis
• may lead to heart failure and death
Pericarditis
• pericardial friction rub
• pericardial effusion
• tamponade

Migratory arthritis (80%)
Ankles, knees, and wrists
Exquisite tenderness, moderate rednes, and swelling
'Flitting', lasting <1 week in a joint, but migrating to other joints over 1–2 months

Sydenham chorea (10%)
2–6 months after the streptococcal infection
Involuntary movements and emotional lability for 3–6 months

Erythema marginatum (<5%)
Uncommon, early manifestation
Rash on trunk and limbs
Pink macules spread outwards, causing pink border with fading centre. Borders may unite to give a maplike outline

Subcutaneous nodules (rare)
Painless, pea-sized, hard
Mainly on extensor surfaces

Minor manifestations

| Fever | Raised acute-phase reactants: ESR, C-reactive protein, leucocytosis |
| Polyarthralgia | Prolonged P–R interval on ECG |

Figure 18.20 Jones criteria for diagnosis of rheumatic fever.

and serum levels monitored. If the fever and inflammation do not resolve rapidly, corticosteroids may be required. Symptomatic heart failure is treated with diuretics and angiotensin-converting enzyme inhibitors, and significant pericardial effusions will require pericardiocentesis. Anti-streptococcal antibiotics may be given if there is any evidence of persisting infection.

Following resolution of the acute episode, recurrence should be prevented. Monthly injections of benzathine penicillin is the most effective prophylaxis. Alternatively, penicillin can be given orally every day, but it is less effective and compliance may be a problem. Oral erythromycin can be substituted in those sensitive to penicillin. The length of prophylaxis is controversial. Most recommend prophylaxis for either 10 years after the last episode of acute rheumatic fever or until the age of 21 years, whichever is the longer, or lifelong prophylaxis if there is severe valvular disease. The severity of eventual rheumatic valvular disease relates to the number of childhood episodes of rheumatic fever. Symptomatic patients are given medical therapy to relieve symptoms and disease progression, but surgical intervention with valvular repair or replacement may be required, but carry significant risk.

Infective endocarditis

All children of any age with congenital heart disease (except secundum ASD), including neonates, are at risk of infective endocarditis. The risk is highest when there is a turbulent jet of blood, as with a VSD, coarctation of the aorta and PDA or if prosthetic material has been inserted at surgery. It may be difficult to diagnose, but should be suspected in any child or adult with a sustained fever, malaise, raised erythrocyte sedimentation rate, unexplained anaemia or haematuria. The presence of the classical peripheral stigmata of infective endocarditis should not be relied upon.

Clinical signs

- Fever
- Anaemia and pallor
- Splinter haemorrhages in nailbed
- Clubbing (late)
- Necrotic skin lesions (Fig. 18.21)
- Changing cardiac signs
- Splenomegaly
- Neurological signs from cerebral infarction
- Retinal infarcts
- Arthritis/arthralgia
- Haematuria (microscopic).

Diagnosis

Multiple blood cultures should be taken before antibiotics are started. Detailed cross-sectional echocardiography may confirm the diagnosis by identification of vegetations but can never exclude it. The vegetations consist of fibrin and platelets and contain infecting organisms. Acute-phase reactants are raised and can be useful to monitor response to treatment.

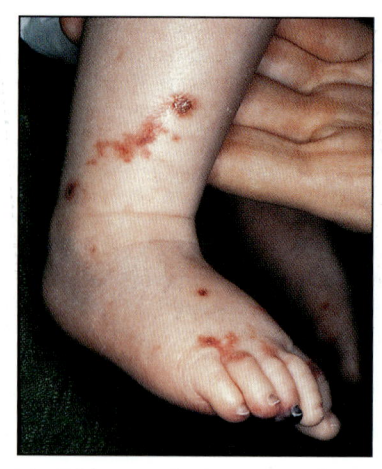

Figure 18.21 Widespread infected emboli and infarcts in a child with bacterial endocarditis. The tip of the third toe is gangrenous.

The most common causative organism is α-haemolytic streptococcus (*Streptococcus viridans*). Bacterial endocarditis is usually treated with high-dose penicillin in combination with an aminoglycoside, giving 6 weeks of intravenous therapy and checking that the serum level of the antibiotic will kill the organism. If there is infected prosthetic material, e.g. prosthetic valves, VSD patches or shunts, there is less chance of complete eradication and surgical removal may be required.

Prophylaxis

The most important factor in prophylaxis against endocarditis is good dental hygiene that should be strongly encouraged in all children with congenital heart disease along with avoidance of body piercing and tattoos.

Antibiotic prophylaxis is *no longer recommended in the UK*, but may be required in other countries for:

- dental treatment, however, trivial
- surgery which is likely to be associated with bacteraemia.

Myocarditis/cardiomyopathy

Dilated cardiomyopathy (a large, poorly contracting heart) may be inherited, secondary to metabolic disease or may result from a direct viral infection of the myocardium. It should be suspected in any child with an enlarged heart and heart failure who has previously been well. The diagnosis is readily made on echocardiography. Treatment is symptomatic with diuretics and angiotensin-converting enzyme inhibitors and carvedilol, a β-adrenoceptor blocking agent. The role of steroids and immunoglobulin infusion is controversial. Myocarditis usually improves spontaneously, but some children ultimately require heart transplantation. Other cardiomyopathies (hypertrophic/restrictive) are rare in childhood and are usually related to a systemic disease (e.g. Hurler, Pompe or Noonan syndromes).

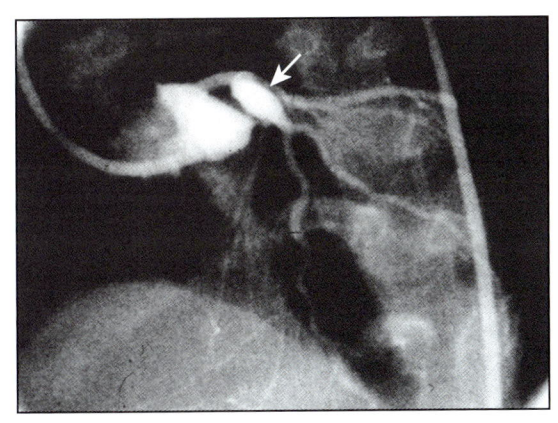

Figure 18.22 Kawasaki disease. Angiogram showing coronary artery aneurysm.

Kawasaki disease

This mainly affects children of 6 months to 5 years of age. Clinical features are described in Chapter 15. It is uncommon (9/100 000 children) but can cause significant cardiac disease. An echocardiogram is performed at diagnosis that may show a pericardial effusion, myocardial disease (poor contractility), endocardial disease (valve regurgitation) or coronary disease with aneurysm formation, which can be giant (>8 mm in diameter). If the coronary arteries are abnormal, angiography (Fig. 18.22) or magnetic resonance imaging will be required.

Pulmonary hypertension

This is of increasing importance in paediatric cardiology, as there is now effective medication for most causes. It can be caused by a number of different diseases (Box 18.4). From the cardiac perspective, most children with pulmonary hypertension (high pulmonary artery pressure, mean >25 mmHg) have a large post-tricuspid shunt with high pulmonary blood flow and low resistance, e.g. VSD, AVSD or PDA. The pressure falls to normal if the defect is corrected by surgery within 6 months of age. If these children are left untreated, however, the high flow and pressure cause irreversible damage to the pulmonary vascular bed

Box 18.4 Causes of pulmonary hypertension

- **Pulmonary arterial hypertension**
  Idiopathic: sporadic or familial
  Post-tricuspid shunts (e.g. VSD, AVSD, PDA)
  HIV infection
  Persistent pulmonary hypertension of the newborn
- **Pulmonary venous hypertension**
  Left-sided heart disease
  Pulmonary vein stenosis or compression
- **Pulmonary hypertension with respiratory disease**
  Chronic obstructive lung disease or bronchopulmonary dysplasia in preterm infants
  Interstitial lung disease
  Obstructive sleep apnoea or upper airway obstruction
- **Pulmonary thromboembolic disease**
- **Pulmonary inflammatory or capillary disease.**

AVSD, atrioventricular septal defect; HIV, human immunodeficiency virus; PDA, persistent ductus arteriosus; VSD, ventricular septal defect.

(pulmonary vascular disease), which is not correctable other than by heart/lung transplantation.

Many medical therapies are now available, which may act on the pulmonary vasculature on the cyclic guanosine monophosphate pathway (e.g. inhaled nitric oxide, intravenous magnesium sulphate and oral phosphodiesterase inhibitors including sildenafil) or on the cyclic adenosine monophosphate pathway (intravenous prostacyclin or inhaled iloprost). In addition, endothelin receptor antagonists are valuable but expensive therapy, e.g. oral bosentan. Anticoagulation is often given with heparin, aspirin or warfarin. These medications allow transplantation to be delayed for many years.

Acknowledgements

We would like to acknowledge contributors to this chapter in previous editions, whose work we have drawn on: Andrew Redington (1st and 2nd Editions), Robert Tulloh (3rd and 4th Editions).

Further reading

Anderson RH, Baker E, Penny D, et al: *Paediatric Cardiology*, ed 3, Edinburgh, 2009, Churchill Livingstone.

Website (Accessed November 2016)

Children's Heart Federation: Available at: http://www.chfed.org.uk.

Kidney and urinary tract disorders

Assessment of the kidneys and urinary tract	344	Hypertension	360
Congenital abnormalities	344	Renal masses	360
Urinary tract infection	349	Renal calculi	360
Enuresis	353	Renal tubular disorders	361
Proteinuria	355	Acute kidney injury	361
Haematuria	357	Haemolytic uraemic syndrome	363
		Chronic kidney disease	363

Features of kidney and urinary tract disorders in children are:

- many structural abnormalities of the kidneys and urinary tract are identified on antenatal ultrasound screening
- urinary tract infection, vesicoureteric reflux, and urinary obstruction have the potential to damage the growing kidney
- nephrotic syndrome is usually steroid sensitive and only rarely leads to chronic kidney disease
- chronic renal disorders may affect growth and development.

Assessment of the kidneys and urinary tract

The glomerular filtration rate (GFR) is low in the newborn infant and is especially low in premature infants; the GFR at 28 weeks' gestation is only 10% of the term infant. In term infants, the corrected GFR (15–20 ml/min per 1.73 m^2) rapidly rises from 1-year to 2-years of age when the adult rate of 80 ml/min to 120 ml/min per 1.73 m^2 is achieved (Fig. 19.1). The assessment of renal function in children is listed in Table 19.1. The radiological investigations of the kidneys and urinary tract are presented in Table 19.2.

Congenital abnormalities

Before antenatal ultrasound scanning became routine, few congenital abnormalities of the kidneys and urinary tract were diagnosed until they caused symptoms in infancy, childhood, or occasionally, adult life. Now the majority are identified in utero and can be managed prospectively. Abnormalities are identified in 1 in 200 to 1 in 400 births. They are potentially important because they may:

- be associated with abnormal renal development or function (chronic kidney disease)
- predispose to postnatal infection
- involve urinary obstruction which requires surgical treatment.

The antenatal detection and early treatment of urinary tract anomalies provide an opportunity to minimize or prevent progressive renal damage. A disadvantage is that minor abnormalities are also detected, most commonly mild unilateral pelvic dilatation, which do not require intervention but may lead to over-investigation, unnecessary treatment, and unwarranted parental anxiety.

Anomalies detectable on antenatal ultrasound screening

Absence of both kidneys (renal agenesis) – As amniotic fluid is mainly derived from fetal urine, there is severe

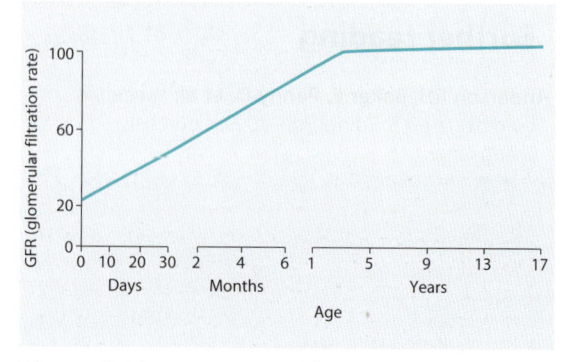

Figure 19.1 Increase in renal function (glomerular filtration rate, ml/min per 1.73 m^2) with age.

Table 19.1 Assessment of renal function in children

Plasma creatinine concentration	Main test of renal function. Rises progressively throughout childhood according to height and muscle bulk. May not be outside laboratory 'normal range' until renal function has fallen to less than half normal
Estimated glomerular filtration rate (eGFR)	The formula eGFR = k × height (cm) ÷ creatinine (μmol/L) provides estimate of GFR. Better measure of renal function than creatinine and useful to monitor renal function serially in children with renal impairment (k is 31 if measured enzymatically or 40 if creatinine measured using older Jaffe method)
Inulin or EDTA (ethylenediaminetetraacetic acid) glomerular filtration rate	More accurate as clearance from the plasma of substances freely filtered at the glomerulus, and is not secreted or reabsorbed by the tubules. Need for repeated blood sampling over several hours limits use in children
Creatinine clearance	Requires timed urine collection and blood tests. Rarely done in children as inconvenient and often becomes inaccurate
Plasma urea concentration	Increased in renal failure, often before creatinine starts rising, and raised levels may be symptomatic. Urea levels also increased by high protein diet, in catabolic states, or due to gastrointestinal bleeding

Table 19.2 Radiological investigation of the kidneys and urinary tract

Ultrasound	Standard imaging procedure of the kidneys and urinary tract provides anatomical assessment but not function. Excellent at visualizing urinary tract dilatation, stones, and nephrocalcinosis (small, multiple calcium deposits within renal parenchyma)
	Advantages: noninvasive, mobile
	Disadvantages: operator dependent, will not detect all renal scars
DMSA scan (^{99m}Tc dimercaptosuccinic acid)	*Static* scan of the renal cortex
	Detects functional defects, such as scars or areas of nonfunctioning renal tissue, but very sensitive, so need to wait at least 2 months after a urinary tract infection to avoid diagnosing false 'scars'
Micturating cystourethrogram (MCUG)	Contrast introduced into the bladder through urethral catheter
	Can visualize bladder and urethral anatomy. Detects vesicoureteric reflux (VUR) and urethral obstruction
	Disadvantages: invasive and unpleasant investigation especially beyond infancy, high radiation dose, and can introduce infection
MAG3 renogram (mercapto-acetyl-triglycine, labelled with ^{99m}Tc)	*Dynamic* scan, isotope-labelled substance MAG3 excreted from the blood into the urine. Measures drainage, best performed with a high urine flow so furosemide often given
	In children old enough to cooperate (usually >4 years of age), scan during micturition is used to identify VUR (indirect cystogram)
Plain abdominal X-ray	Identifies unsuspected spinal abnormalities
	May identify renal stones, but poor at showing nephrocalcinosis

oligohydramnios resulting in Potter syndrome (Fig. 19.2a,b), which is fatal.

Multicystic dysplastic kidney – Results from the failure of union of the ureteric bud (which forms the ureter, pelvis, calyces, and collecting ducts) with the nephrogenic mesenchyme. It is a non-functioning structure with large fluid-filled cysts with no renal tissue and no connection with the bladder (Fig. 19.3). Half will have involuted by 2 years of age, and nephrectomy is indicated only if it remains very large or hypertension develops, but this is rare. Because they produce no urine, Potter syndrome will result if the lesion is bilateral. Other causes of large cystic kidneys are *autosomal recessive polycystic kidney disease* (ARPKD; Fig. 19.4), *autosomal dominant polycystic kidney disease* (ADPKD; Fig. 19.5), and tuberous sclerosis. In contrast to a multicystic dysplastic kidney, in these disorders some or normal renal function is maintained but both

Some congenital abnormalities of the kidneys and urinary tract

Bilateral renal agenesis or bilateral multicystic dysplastic kidneys
↓
Reduced fetal urine excretion
↓
Oligohydramnios causing fetal compression

Potter facies:
Low-set ears
Beaked nose
Prominent epicanthic folds and downward slant to eyes

Pulmonary hypoplasia causing respiratory failure

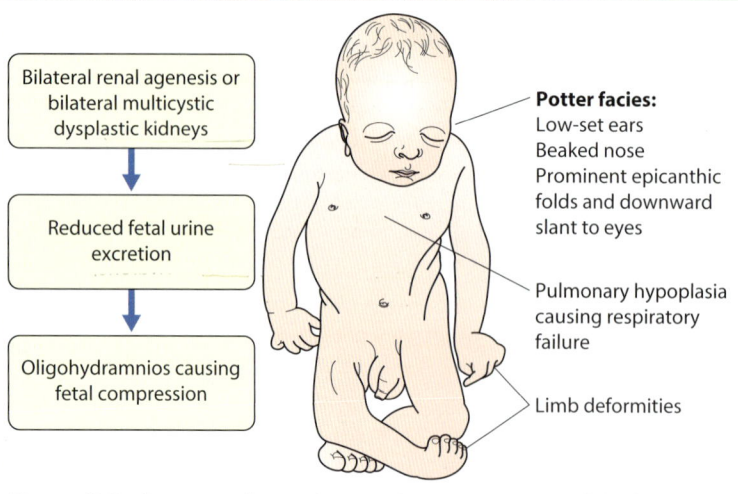

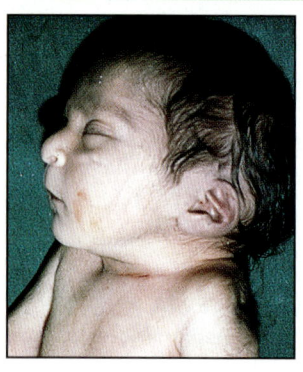

Limb deformities

Figure 19.2b Facies in Potter syndrome.

Figure 19.2a Potter syndrome. Intrauterine compression of the fetus from oligohydramnios caused by lack of fetal urine causes a characteristic facies, lung hypoplasia, and postural deformities including severe talipes. The infant may be stillborn or die soon after birth from respiratory failure.

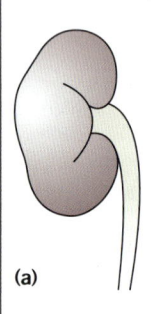

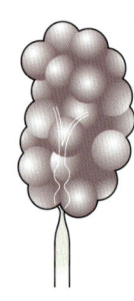

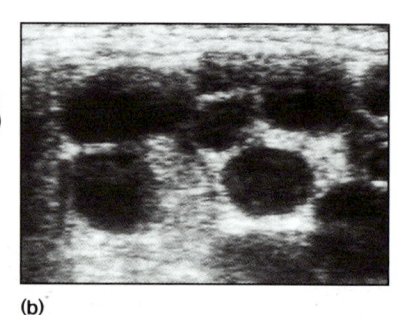

Figure 19.3 (a) Multicystic renal dysplasia. The kidney is replaced by cysts of variable size, with atresia of the ureter; and (b) renal ultrasound showing discrete cysts of variable size.

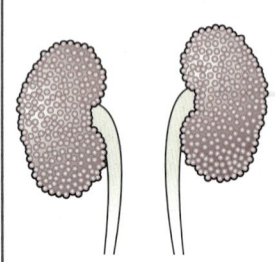

Figure 19.4 Autosomal recessive polycystic kidney disease (ARPKD). There is diffuse bilateral enlargement of both kidneys.

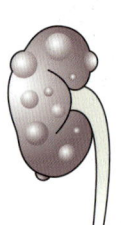

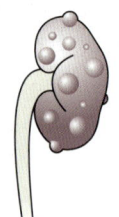

Figure 19.5 Autosomal dominant polycystic kidney disease (ADPKD). There are separate cysts of varying size between normal renal parenchyma. The kidneys are enlarged.

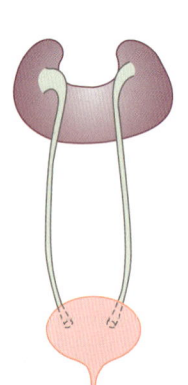

Figure 19.6 Horseshoe kidney.

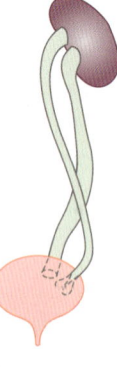

Figure 19.7 Duplex kidney showing ureterocele of upper moiety and reflux into lower pole moiety.

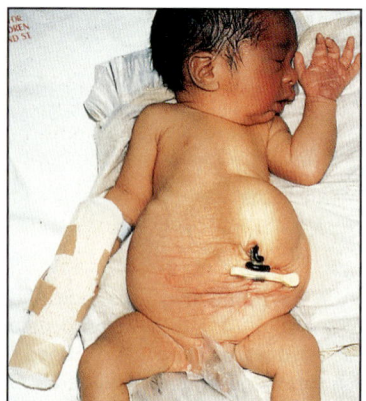

Figure 19.8 Prune-belly syndrome (absent musculature syndrome). The name arises from the wrinkled appearance of the abdomen. It is associated with a large bladder, dilated ureters, and cryptorchidism. (Courtesy of Jane Deal.)

Urinary tract obstruction

Unilateral hydronephrosis
– Pelviureteric junction obstruction
– Vesicoureteric junction obstruction

Bilateral hydronephrosis
– Bladder neck obstruction
– Posterior urethral valves

Figure 19.9a Obstruction to urine flow results in dilatation of the urinary tract proximal to the site of obstruction. Obstruction may be at the pelviureteric or vesicoureteric junction (left), the bladder neck, or urethra (right).

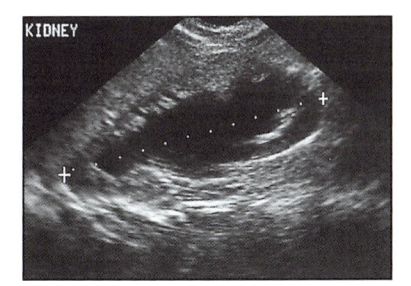

Figure 19.9b An ultrasound showing a dilated renal pelvis from pelviureteric junction obstruction.

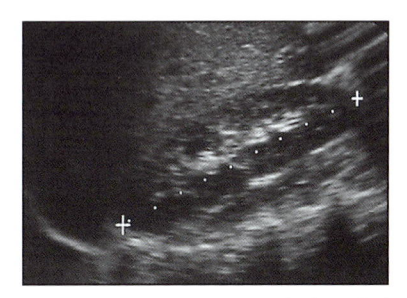

Figure 19.9c A normal ultrasound of the kidney is shown for comparison.

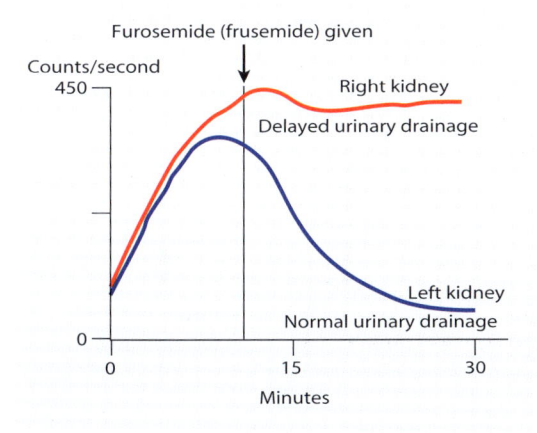

Figure 19.9d Graph from dynamic nuclear medicine scan MAG3 showing delayed excretion from a pelviureteric junction obstruction.

Kidney and urinary tract disorders

347

kidneys are always affected. ADPKD has an incidence of 1 in 1000; the main symptoms in childhood are hypertension and it causes renal failure in late adulthood. It is associated with several extrarenal features including cysts in the liver and pancreas, cerebral aneurysms, and mitral valve prolapse.

Abnormal caudal migration may result in a *pelvic kidney* or a *horseshoe kidney* (Fig. 19.6), when the lower poles are fused in the midline. The abnormal position may predispose to infection or obstruction of urinary drainage.

Premature division of the ureteric bud gives rise to a *duplex system*, which can vary from simply a *bifid renal pelvis* to complete division with two ureters. These ureters frequently have an abnormal drainage so that the ureter from the lower pole moiety often refluxes, whereas the upper pole ureter may drain ectopically into the urethra or vagina or may prolapse into the bladder (ureterocele) and urine flow may be obstructed (Fig. 19.7).

Failure of fusion of the infraumbilical midline structures results in exposed bladder mucosa (*bladder exstrophy*). Absence or severe deficiency of the anterior abdominal wall muscles is frequently associated with a large bladder and dilated ureters (megacystis-megaureter) and cryptorchidism, the *prune-belly syndrome* (*absent musculature syndrome*; Fig. 19.8).

Obstruction to urine flow may occur at the pelviureteric or vesicoureteric junction, at the *bladder neck* (e.g. due to disruption of the nerve supply, *neuropathic bladder*), or at the *posterior urethra* in a boy due to mucosal folds or a membrane, known as *posterior urethral valves*. The consequences of obstruction to urine flow are shown in Fig. 19.9a–d. At worst, this results in a *dysplastic kidney* which is small, poorly functioning, and may contain cysts. In the most severe and bilateral cases Potter syndrome is present. Renal dysplasia can also occur in association with severe intrauterine vesicoureteric reflux (VUR), in isolation, or in certain rare, inherited syndromes affecting multiple systems.

Antenatal treatment

The male fetus with posterior urethral valves may develop severe urinary outflow obstruction resulting in progressive bilateral hydronephrosis, poor renal growth, and declining liquor volume with the potential to lead to pulmonary hypoplasia. Intrauterine bladder drainage procedures to prevent severe renal damage have been attempted but results have been disappointing. Early delivery is rarely indicated.

Postnatal management

An example of a protocol for infants with antenatally diagnosed anomalies is shown in Fig. 19.10. Prophylactic antibiotics may be started at birth to try to prevent urinary tract infection (UTI), although practice varies between centres. As the newborn kidney has a low GFR, urine flow is low and mild outflow obstruction may not be evident in the first few days of life. The ultrasound scan should therefore be delayed for a few weeks. However, bilateral hydronephrosis in a male infant warrants investigations including an ultrasound and micturating cystourethrogram (MCUG) shortly after birth to exclude posterior urethral valves, which always requires urological intervention such as cystoscopic ablation (Case History 19.1).

Antenatally diagnosed urinary tract anomalies – a protocol

Antenatal diagnosis of urinary tract anomaly
↓
Start prophylactic antibiotics
↓
- Bilateral hydronephrosis and/or dilated lower urinary tract in a male
  - Ultrasound within 48 h of birth to exclude posterior urethral valves
    - Abnormal → MCUG → Surgery if required
    - Normal → Stop antibiotics, Repeat ultrasound after 2–3 months
- Unilateral hydronephrosis in a male / Any anomaly in female
  - Ultrasound at 4–6 weeks
    - Normal → Stop antibiotics, Repeat ultrasound after 2–3 months
    - Abnormal → Further investigations

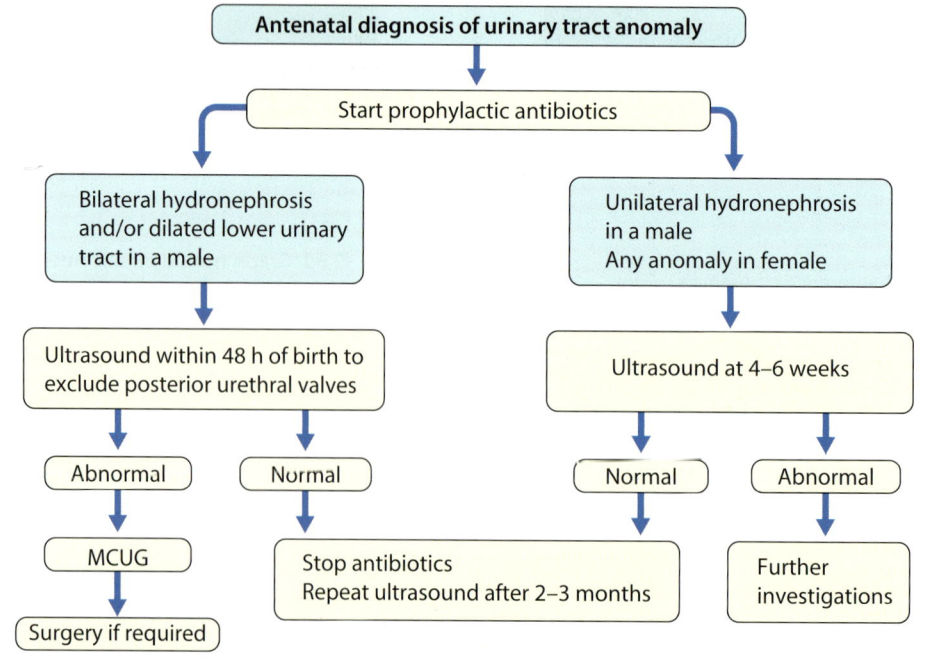

Figure 19.10 An example of a protocol for the management of infants with antenatally diagnosed urinary tract anomalies. MCUG, micturating cystourethrogram.

Case history 19.1

Posterior urethral valves

Bilateral hydronephrosis was noted on antenatal ultrasound at 20 weeks' gestation in a male fetus. There was progressive hydronephrosis, poor renal growth with reduced renal cortex, and decreasing volume of amniotic fluid on repeated scans (Fig. 19.11a). After birth, a urethral catheter was inserted and prophylactic antibiotics were started. An urgent ultrasound showed bilateral hydronephrosis with small dysplastic kidneys and cyst formation. A micturating cystourethrogram showed severe, bilateral vesicoureteric reflux, a small thickened bladder, and a dilated posterior urethra (Fig. 19.11b). Posterior urethral valves were confirmed on cystoscopy and ablated surgically. Caden's subsequent progress is described in Case history 19.4.

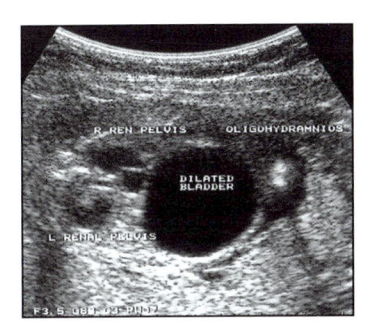

☼ **Bilateral hydronephrosis in a male infant requires urgent investigation to exclude posterior urethral valves**

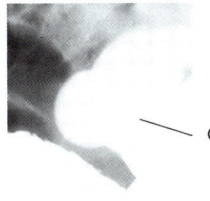

Figure 19.11a Antenatal ultrasound scan in an infant with urinary outflow obstruction from posterior urethral valve. (Courtesy of Karl Murphy.)

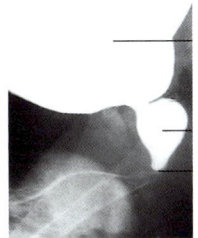

Figure 19.11b Micturating cystourethrogram (MCUG) in the same patient.

Urinary tract infection

About 3–7% of girls and 1–2% of boys have at least one symptomatic UTI before the age of 6 years, and 12–30% of them have a recurrence within a year. UTI may involve the kidneys (pyelonephritis), when it is usually associated with fever and systemic involvement, or may be due to cystitis, when there may be no fever. UTI in childhood is important because:

- up to half of patients have a structural abnormality of their urinary tract
- pyelonephritis may damage the growing kidney by forming a scar, predisposing to hypertension and to progressive chronic kidney disease if the scarring is bilateral.

The NICE (National Institute for Health and Care Excellence) guidelines on UTI in children were published in 2007, although they have proved to be controversial as they recommend fewer children being investigated and the investigations are less extensive.

Box 19.1 Presentation of urinary tract infection in infants and children

Infants	Children
• Fever	• Dysuria, frequency and urgency
• Vomiting	• Abdominal pain or loin tenderness
• Lethargy or irritability	• Fever with or without rigors (exaggerated shivering)
• Poor feeding/faltering growth	
• Jaundice	• Lethargy and anorexia
• Septicaemia	• Vomiting, diarrhoea
• Offensive urine	• Haematuria
• Febrile seizure (>6 months)	• Offensive/cloudy urine
	• Febrile seizure
	• Recurrence of enuresis

Clinical features

Presentation of UTI varies with age (Box 19.1). In infants, symptoms are nonspecific; fever is usually but not always present, and **septicaemia may develop rapidly**. The classical symptoms of dysuria, frequency, and loin pain become more common with increasing age. Serious illness from septicaemia is described in Chapter 6. Dysuria alone is usually due to cystitis, or vulvitis in girls or balanitis in uncircumcised boys. Symptoms suggestive of a UTI may also occur following sexual abuse.

Table 19.3 Methods and interpretation of dipstick testing in children

Methods of dipstick testing	
Nitrite stick testing	Positive result useful as very likely to indicate a true urinary tract infection (UTI)
	But some children with a UTI are nitrite negative
Leucocyte esterase stick testing (for white blood cells)	May be present in children with UTI but may also be negative
	Present in children with febrile illness without UTIs
	Positive in balanitis and vulvovaginitis
Interpretation of results	
Leucocyte esterase and nitrite positive	Regard as UTI
Leucocyte esterase negative and nitrite positive	Start antibiotic treatment if clinical evidence of UTI
	Diagnosis depends on urine culture
Leucocyte esterase positive and nitrite negative	Only start antibiotic treatment if clinical evidence of UTI
	Diagnosis depends on urine culture
Leucocyte esterase and nitrite negative	UTI unlikely. Repeat or send urine for culture if clinical history suggests UTI
Blood, protein, and glucose present on stick testing	Useful in any unwell child to identify other diseases, e.g. nephritis, diabetes mellitus, but will not discriminate between children with and without UTIs

Collection of samples

The most common error in the management of UTI in children, and especially in infants, is failure to establish the diagnosis properly in the first place. If the diagnosis of a UTI is not made, the opportunity to prevent renal damage may be missed, or, if incorrectly diagnosed, may lead to unnecessary invasive investigations.

For the child in nappies, urine can be collected by:

- a 'clean-catch' sample into a waiting clean pot when the nappy is removed. This is the recommended method
- an adhesive plastic bag applied to the perineum after careful washing, although there may be contamination from the skin
- a urethral catheter if there is urgency in obtaining a sample and no urine has been passed
- suprapubic aspiration, when a fine needle attached to a syringe is inserted directly into the bladder just above the symphysis pubis under ultrasound guidance; it may be used in severely ill infants requiring urgent diagnosis and treatment, but it is an invasive procedure, and is increasingly replaced by urethral catheter sampling.

In the older child, urine can be obtained by collecting a midstream sample. Careful cleaning and collection are necessary, as contamination with both white cells and bacteria can occur from under the foreskin in boys, and from reflux of urine into the vagina during voiding in girls.

Ideally, the urine sample should be observed under a microscope to identify organisms and cultured straight away. This is indicated in all infants and children under the age of 3 years with a suspected UTI. If this is not possible, the urine sample should be refrigerated to prevent the overgrowth of contaminating bacteria.

Urinary white cells are not a reliable feature of a UTI, as they may lyse during storage and may be present in febrile children without a UTI and in children with balanitis or vulvovaginitis. Dipsticks can be used as a screening test. Urine culture should still be performed unless both leucocyte esterase and nitrite are negative or if the clinical symptoms and dipstick tests do not correlate (Table 19.3).

A bacterial culture of more than 10^5 colony-forming units (CFU) of a single organism per millilitre in a properly collected specimen gives a 90% probability of infection. If the same result is found in a second sample, the probability rises to 95%. A growth of mixed organisms usually represents contamination, but if there is doubt, another sample should be collected. Any bacterial growth of a single organism per millilitre in a catheter sample or suprapubic aspirate is considered diagnostic of infection.

> A urine sample should be tested in all infants with an unexplained fever >38°C

Bacterial and host factors that predispose to infection

Infecting organism

UTI is usually the result of bowel flora entering the urinary tract via the urethra, although it can be haematogenous, e.g. in the newborn. The most common organism is *Escherichia coli*, followed by *Klebsiella*, *Proteus*, *Pseudomonas*, and *Streptococcus faecalis*. *Proteus* infection is more commonly diagnosed in boys than in girls, possibly because of its presence under the prepuce. *Proteus* infection predisposes to the formation of phosphate stones by splitting urea to ammonia, and thus alkalinizing the urine. *Pseudomonas* infection may indicate the presence of some structural abnormality in the urinary tract affecting drainage and it is also more common in children with plastic catheters.

Antenatally diagnosed renal or urinary tract abnormality

Increases risk of infection and investigation of a UTI may lead to urinary tract abnormality being detected if antenatal diagnosis was not made or missed to follow-up.

Incomplete bladder emptying

Contributing factors in some children are:

- infrequent voiding, resulting in bladder enlargement
- vulvitis
- incomplete micturition with residual postmicturition bladder volumes
- obstruction by a loaded rectum from constipation
- neuropathic bladder
- vesicoureteric reflux.

Vesicoureteric reflux

VUR is a developmental anomaly of the vesicoureteric junctions. The ureters are displaced laterally and enter directly into the bladder rather than at an angle, with a shortened or absent intramural course. Severe cases may be associated with renal dysplasia. It is familial, with a 30% to 50% chance of occurring in first-degree relatives. It may also occur with bladder pathology, e.g. a neuropathic bladder or urethral obstruction, or temporarily after a UTI. Its severity varies from reflux into the lower end of an undilated ureter during micturition to the severest form with reflux during bladder filling and voiding, with a distended ureter, renal pelvis, and clubbed calyces (Fig. 19.12). Mild reflux is unlikely to be of significance, but the more severe degrees of VUR may be associated with *intrarenal reflux*, which is the backflow of urine from the renal pelvis into the papillary collecting ducts and is associated with a particularly high risk of renal scarring if UTIs occur. The incidence of renal defects increases with increasing severity of reflux. There is considerable controversy as to whether renal scarring is a congenital abnormality already present in children with reflux and which predisposes to infection or if children with reflux have normal kidneys at birth which are damaged by UTIs and that preventing UTIs in these children prevents scars. VUR tends to resolve with age, especially lower grades of VUR.

VUR-associated ureteric dilatation is important as:

- urine returning to the bladder from the ureters after voiding results in incomplete bladder emptying which encourages infection
- the kidneys may become infected (pyelonephritis) especially if there is intrarenal reflux
- bladder voiding pressure is transmitted to the renal papillae which may contribute to renal damage if voiding pressures are high.

Infection may destroy renal tissue, leaving a scar, resulting in a shrunken, poorly functioning segment of kidney (reflux nephropathy). If scarring is bilateral and severe, progressive chronic kidney disease may

Mild reflux
Reflux into ureter only

Severe reflux
Gross dilatation of ureter, renal pelvis and calyces
Predisposes to intrarenal reflux and renal scarring with UTI

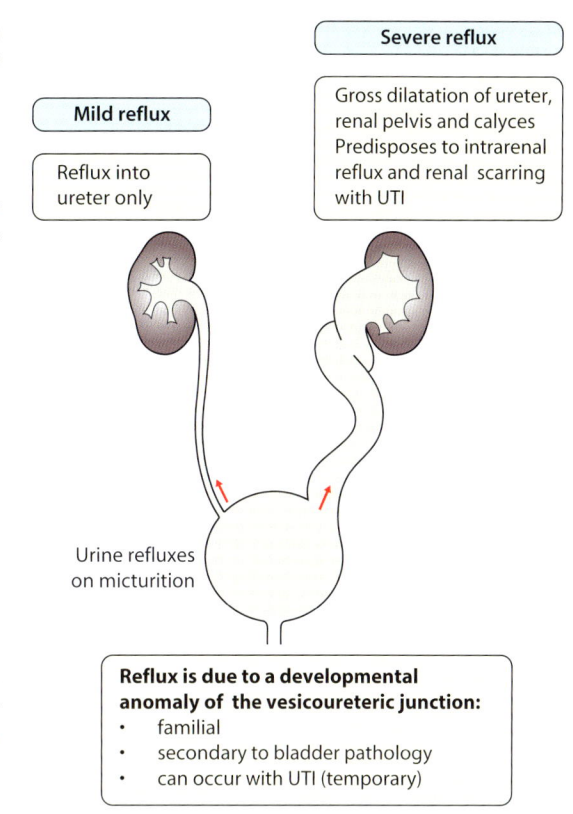

Urine refluxes on micturition

Reflux is due to a developmental anomaly of the vesicoureteric junction:
- familial
- secondary to bladder pathology
- can occur with UTI (temporary)

Figure 19.12 Vesicoureteric reflux.

develop. The risk of hypertension in childhood or early adult life is variously estimated to be up to 10%.

Investigation

The extent to which a child with a UTI should be investigated is controversial. This is not only because of the invasive nature and radiation burden of the tests but also because of the lack of an evidence base to show that outcome is improved (unless urinary obstruction is demonstrated). Mild VUR usually resolves spontaneously and operative intervention to stop mild VUR has not been shown to decrease renal damage. Furthermore, there is no evidence that antibiotic prophylaxis is any better than prompt treatment. There has, therefore, been a move away from extensive investigation of all children with UTIs to those who have had atypical or recurrent UTIs. Atypical UTI includes:

- seriously ill or septicaemia
- poor urine flow
- abdominal or bladder mass
- raised creatinine
- failure to respond to suitable antibiotics within 48 hours
- infection with atypical (non-*E. coli*) organisms.

An initial ultrasound will identify:

- serious structural abnormalities and urinary obstruction
- renal defects (although it is not the gold standard for detecting renal scars).

First urinary tract infection – a protocol for initial management and investigation

```
First proven urinary tract infection
              ⇓
      Antibiotic therapy
              ⇓
Ultrasound of kidneys and urinary tract
       ⇓         ⇓           ⇓
    <1 year   >1 year –    >3 years
              <3 years   ultrasound normal
       ⇓         ⇓           ⇓
    MCUG and   DMSA       No further
     DMSA                 investigations
```

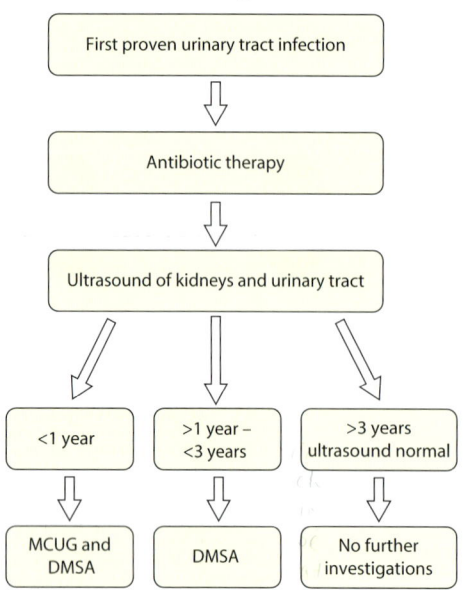

Figure 19.13 An example of a protocol for the initial management and investigation of a first urinary tract infection. This is controversial. The 2007 UK NICE (National Institute for Health and Care Excellence) guidelines do not recommend ultrasound examination for first urinary tract infection if there was response to antibiotic treatment within 48 hours, unless under 6 months of age or atypical or recurrent, but many paediatric nephrologists consider this approach too minimalistic and follow protocols like the one shown here.

Subsequent investigations will depend on the results of the ultrasound. The need for any investigations in a child with only bladder symptoms (lower UTI/cystitis) is also controversial. If urethral obstruction is suspected (abnormal bladder in a boy), MCUG should be performed promptly. Functional scans should be deferred for 3 months after a UTI, unless the ultrasound is suggestive of obstruction, to avoid missing a newly developed scar and because of false-positive results from transient inflammation. Medical measures for the prevention of UTI should be initiated.

A suggested schema for investigation of the first proven UTI is shown in Fig. 19.13, but there is significant variation of practice.

Management

All infants under 3 months of age with suspicion of a UTI or if seriously ill should be referred immediately to hospital. They require intravenous antibiotic therapy (e.g. co-amoxiclav) for at least 5–7 days at which point oral prophylaxis can then be commenced (see Case History 19.2).

Infants aged over 3 months and children with acute pyelonephritis/upper UTI (bacteriuria and fever ≥38°C or bacteriuria and loin pain/tenderness even if fever is <38°C) are usually treated with oral antibiotics (e.g. trimethoprim for 7 days); or else intravenous antibiotics, e.g. co-amoxiclav, are given for 2–4 days followed by oral antibiotics for a total of 7–10 days. The choice of antibiotic is adjusted according to sensitivity on urine culture.

Children with cystitis/lower UTI (dysuria but no systemic symptoms or signs) can be treated with oral antibiotics such as trimethoprim or nitrofurantoin for 3 days.

Medical measures for the prevention of UTI

The aim is to ensure washout of organisms that ascend into the bladder from the perineum; and to reduce the presence of aggressive organisms in the stool, perineum, and under the foreskin:

- high fluid intake to produce a high urine output
- regular voiding
- ensure complete bladder emptying by encouraging the child to try a second time to empty his bladder after a minute or two, commonly known as double voiding, which empties any urine residue or refluxed urine returning to the bladder
- treatment and/or prevention of constipation
- good perineal hygiene
- *Lactobacillus acidophilus*, a probiotic to encourage colonization of the gut by this organism and reduce the number of pathogenic organisms that might potentially cause invasive disease
- antibiotic prophylaxis, although this is controversial. It is often used in those under 2 years to 3 years of age with a congenital abnormality of the kidneys or urinary tract or who have had an upper UTI and those with severe reflux until out of nappies. Trimethoprim (2 mg/kg at night) is used most often, but nitrofurantoin or cephalexin may be given. Broad-spectrum, poorly absorbed antibiotics such as amoxicillin should be avoided.

Follow-up of children with recurrent UTIs, renal scarring, or reflux

In these children:

- urine should be dipsticked with any nonspecific illness in case it is caused by a UTI and urine sent for microscopy and culture if suggestive of UTI

Case history 19.2

Urinary tract infection

Jack, a 2-month-old infant, stopped feeding and had a high, intermittent fever. He was referred to hospital, where he had an infection screen. Urine microscopy showed more than 100 white blood cells and cultured more than 10^5 *E. coli* CFU/ml. He was treated with intravenous antibiotics. An ultrasound showed that the left kidney was smaller than the right kidney with dilated ureters. He was started on prophylactic antibiotics. A DMSA (dimercaptosuccinic acid) scan (Fig. 19.14) performed 3 months later confirmed bilateral renal scarring, with the left kidney contributing 33% of renal function. The MCUG (Fig. 19.15) showed bilateral vesicoureteric reflux. At 4 years of age, the reflux had resolved and antibiotic prophylaxis was stopped. His blood pressure, urine protein-to-creatinine ratio, and renal growth and function continue to be monitored in clinic.

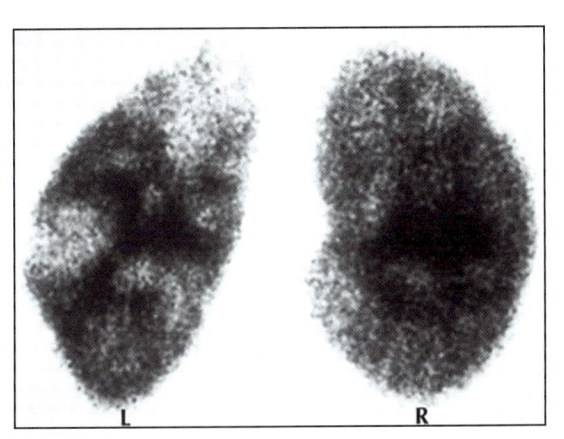

Figure 19.14 DMSA (Dimercaptosuccinic acid) scan showing bilateral renal scarring, more severe on left upper pole.

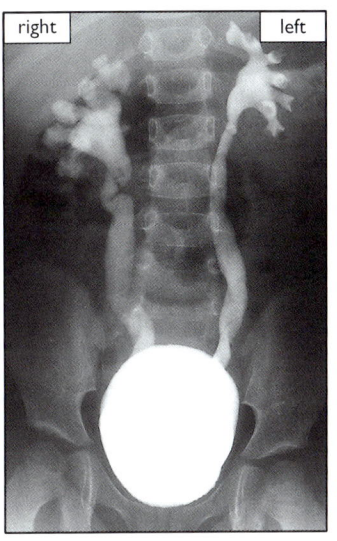

Figure 19.15 Micturating cystourethrogram (MCUG) showing bilateral vesicoureteric reflux with ureteric dilatation and dilated clubbed calyces on the right.

- long-term, low-dose antibiotic prophylaxis can be used. There is no evidence for when antibiotic prophylaxis should be stopped
- circumcision in boys may sometimes be considered as there is evidence that it reduces the incidence of UTI
- anti-VUR surgery may be indicated if there is progression of scarring with ongoing VUR but it has not been shown to improve outcome in mild VUR
- blood pressure should be checked annually if renal defects are present
- urinalysis to check for proteinuria which is indicative of progressive chronic kidney disease
- regular assessment of renal growth and function is necessary if there are bilateral defects because of the risk of progressive chronic kidney disease.

If there are further symptomatic UTIs in younger children, investigations may be required to determine whether there is new scar formation and if so whether there is ongoing VUR, which may require prophylactic antibiotic therapy or surgical anti-VUR treatment.

Enuresis

Primary nocturnal enuresis

This is considered in Chapter 24. Child and Adolescent Mental Health.

Daytime enuresis

This is a lack of bladder control during the day in a child old enough to be continent (over the age of 3–5 years). Nocturnal enuresis is also usually present. It may be caused by:

- lack of attention to bladder sensation: a manifestation of a developmental or psychogenic problem, although it may occur in otherwise normal children who are too preoccupied with what they are doing to respond to the sensation of a full bladder
- detrusor instability (sudden, urgent urge to void induced by sudden bladder contractions)
- bladder neck weakness
- a neuropathic bladder (bladder is enlarged and fails to empty properly, irregular thick wall, and is

Kidney and urinary tract disorders

19

Summary

A child with a first urinary tract infection

Why important?
Up to half have a structural abnormality of their urinary tract
Pyelonephritis may damage the growing kidney by forming a renal scar, which may result in hypertension and chronic renal failure

Predisposing factors?
Incomplete bladder emptying
Constipation
Vesicoureteric reflux

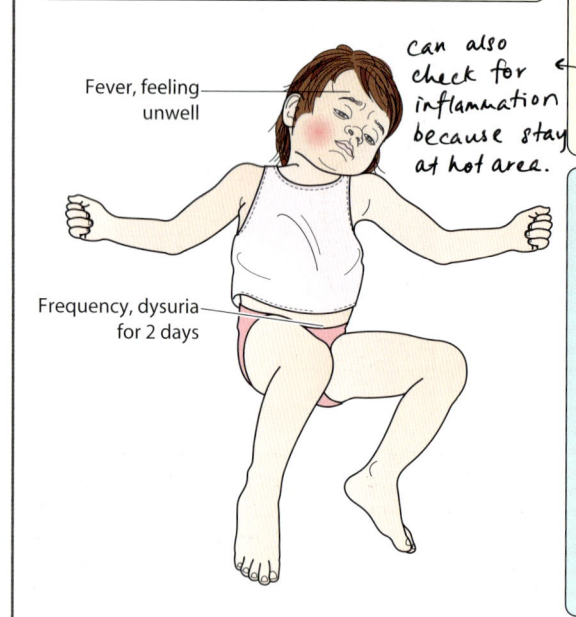

- Fever, feeling unwell
- Frequency, dysuria for 2 days

(handwritten note: can also check for inflammation because stay at hot area)

Diagnosis secure?
- Suggestive clinical features?
- Upper or lower urinary tract infection?
- Urine sample properly collected and processed?
- Culture of single organism >10^5/ml if clean catch or mid-stream urine or else any organisms on suprapubic aspirate or catheter sample?

Why investigate?
To identify serious structural abnormalities, urinary obstruction, renal scars, vesicoureteric reflux.

What investigation?
Consider:
- Ultrasound of kidneys and urinary tract
- DMSA to check for renal scars 3 months after UTI
- MAG3 or MCUG to detect obstruction and vesicouretic reflux.

Management
Treat infection with antibiotics
Advice about medical preventative measures to consider:
- High fluid intake
- Regular voiding, double micturition
- Prevent or treat constipation
- Good perineal hygiene
- *Lactobacillus acidophilus*

Advise to check urine culture if develops clinical features suggestive of non-specific illness

If renal scarring or reflux on investigation, or develops recurrent UTIs:
- Consider low-dose antibiotic prophylaxis
- Monitor blood pressure, renal growth and function

---

associated with spina bifida and other neurological conditions)
- a UTI (rarely in the absence of other symptoms)
- constipation
- an ectopic ureter, causes constant dribbling and child is always damp.

Examination may reveal evidence of a neuropathic bladder, i.e. the bladder may be distended, there may be abnormal perineal sensation and anal tone, or abnormal leg reflexes and gait. Sensory loss in the distribution of the S2, S3, and S4 dermatomes should be sought. A spinal lesion may be present. Girls who are dry at night but wet on getting up are likely to have pooling of urine from an ectopic ureter opening into the vagina.

A urine sample should be examined for microscopy, culture, and sensitivity. Other investigations are performed if indicated. An ultrasound may show bladder pathology, with incomplete bladder emptying or thickening of the bladder wall. Urodynamic studies may be required. An X-ray of the spine may reveal a vertebral anomaly. A MRI scan may be required to confirm or exclude a spinal defect such as tethering of the cord.

Affected children in whom a neurological cause has been excluded may benefit from star charts, bladder training, and pelvic floor exercises. Constipation should be treated. A small portable alarm with a pad in the pants, which is activated by urine, can be used when there is lack of attention to bladder sensation. Anticholinergic drugs, such as oxybutynin, to dampen down bladder contractions, may be helpful if other measures fail.

Secondary (onset) enuresis

The loss of previously achieved urinary continence may be due to:
- emotional upset, which is the most common cause
- UTI
- polyuria from an osmotic diuresis in diabetes mellitus or a renal concentrating disorder, e.g. sickle cell disease or chronic kidney disease or very rarely diabetes insipidus, which can be central or nephrogenic.

Investigation should include:
- testing a urine sample for infection, glycosuria, and proteinuria using a dipstick

- assessment of urinary concentrating ability by measuring the osmolality of an early morning urine sample. Rarely, a formal water deprivation test may be needed to exclude a urinary concentrating defect
- ultrasound of the renal tract.

> **Summary**
>
> **Enuresis**
> **Daytime enuresis**
> - Consider possible causes: developmental or psychogenic, bladder instability or neuropathy, UTI, constipation, ectopic ureter.
>
> **Secondary (onset) enuresis**
> - Consider – emotional upset, UTI, polyuria from an osmotic diuresis in diabetes mellitus or a renal concentrating disorder.

Proteinuria

Transient proteinuria may occur during febrile illnesses or after exercise and does not require investigation. Persistent proteinuria is significant and should be quantified by measuring the urine protein-to-creatinine ratio in an early morning sample (normal protein-to-creatinine ratio <20 mg/mmol).

A common cause is orthostatic (postural) proteinuria when proteinuria is only found when the child is upright during the day. It can be diagnosed by measuring the urine protein-to-creatinine ratio in a series of early morning urine specimens. The prognosis is excellent and further investigations are not necessary. Other causes of proteinuria, which need further evaluation, are listed in Box 19.2.

Nephrotic syndrome

In nephrotic syndrome, heavy proteinuria results in a low plasma albumin and oedema. The cause of the condition is unknown, but a few cases are secondary to systemic diseases such as Henoch–Schönlein purpura and other vasculitides, e.g. SLE (systemic lupus erythematosus), infections (e.g. malaria) or allergens (e.g. bee sting).

Clinical signs of the nephrotic syndrome are:

- periorbital oedema (particularly on waking) which is often the earliest sign
- scrotal or vulval, leg, and ankle oedema (Fig. 19.16)
- ascites
- breathlessness due to pleural effusions and abdominal distension
- infection such as peritonitis, septic arthritis, or sepsis due to loss of protective immunoglobulins in the urine.

Case history 19.3 shows typical presentation, and initial investigations are listed in Box 19.3.

Steroid-sensitive nephrotic syndrome

In 85–90% of children with nephrotic syndrome, the proteinuria resolves with corticosteroid therapy

Box 19.2 Causes of proteinuria

- Orthostatic proteinuria
- Glomerular abnormalities
  - Minimal change disease
  - Glomerulonephritis
  - Abnormal glomerular basement membrane (familial nephritides)
- Increased glomerular filtration pressure
- Reduced renal mass in chronic kidney disease
- Hypertension
- Tubular proteinuria

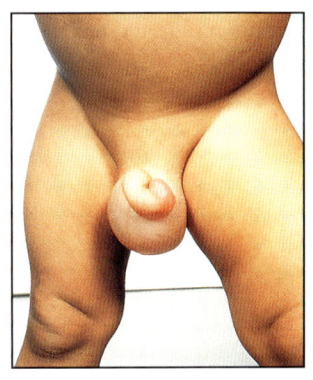

Figure 19.16 Gross oedema of the scrotum and legs as well as abdominal distension from ascites.

(steroid-sensitive nephrotic syndrome). These children do not progress to chronic kidney disease. It is more common in boys than in girls, in Asian children than in Caucasians, and there is an association with atopy. It is often precipitated by respiratory infections. Features suggesting steroid-sensitive nephrotic syndrome are:

- age between 1–10 years
- no macroscopic haematuria
- normal blood pressure
- normal complement levels
- normal renal function.

Management

The most widely used protocol is to initially give oral corticosteroids (60 mg/m^2 per day of prednisolone), unless there are atypical features. After 4 weeks, the dose is reduced to 40 mg/m^2 on alternate days for 4 weeks and then weaned or stopped. The median time for the urine to become free of protein is 11 days. However, there is now good evidence that extending the initial course of steroids by gradually tapering the alternate day part of the course leads to a marked reduction in the proportion of children who develop a frequently relapsing or steroid-dependent course, although there are increased side-effects from steroid treatment. Children who do not respond to 4–6 weeks of corticosteroid therapy or have atypical features may have a more complex diagnosis and require a renal biopsy. Renal histology in steroid-sensitive nephrotic syndrome is usually normal on light microscopy but

Case history 19.3

Nephrotic syndrome

Zakariya developed periorbital oedema (Fig. 19.17) which improved during day. He was seen by several doctors who diagnosed allergy, conjunctivitis, and hay fever. When he developed ascites and bilateral leg oedema his urine was dipsticked and showed 4+ protein and nephrotic syndrome was diagnosed. Periorbital oedema is often the initial sign of nephrotic syndrome but diagnosis is often delayed until other complications develop. Investigations performed are listed in Box 19.3. He is most likely to have steroid-responsive nephrotic syndrome, and the clinical course is outlined in Fig. 19.18.

Box 19.3 Investigations performed at presentation of nephrotic syndrome

- Urine protein – on test strips (dipstick)
- Full blood count and erythrocyte sedimentation rate
- Urea, electrolytes, creatinine, albumin
- Complement levels – C3, C4
- Antistreptolysin O or anti-DNAse B titres and throat swab
- Urine microscopy and culture
- Urinary sodium concentration
- Hepatitis B and hepatitis C screen
- Malaria screen if travel abroad

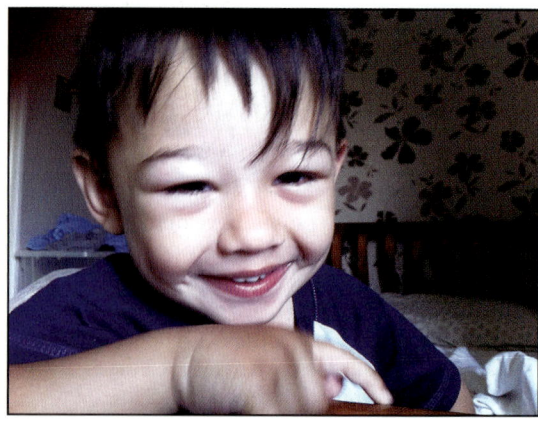

Figure 19.17 Facial oedema in nephrotic syndrome which improves during the day and is often misdiagnosed as an allergy.

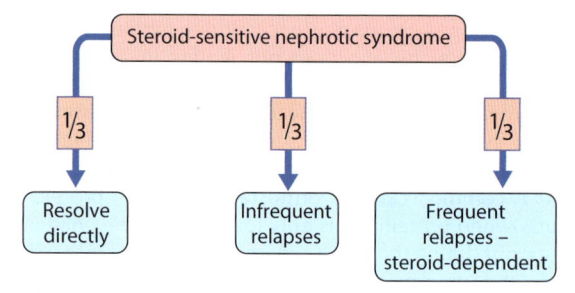

Figure 19.18 Clinical course in steroid-responsive nephrotic syndrome.

---

fusion of the specialized epithelial cells that invest the glomerular capillaries (podocytes) is seen on electron microscopy. For this reason, it is called minimal change disease.

The child with nephrotic syndrome is susceptible to several serious complications at presentation or relapse

- *Hypovolaemia* – during the initial phase of oedema formation, the intravascular compartment may become volume depleted. The child who becomes hypovolaemic characteristically complains of abdominal pain and may feel faint. There is peripheral vasoconstriction and urinary sodium retention. A low urinary sodium (<10 mmol/L) and a high packed cell volume of red blood cells are indications of hypovolaemia, which requires urgent treatment with intravenous fluid (0.9% saline or 4.5% albumin solution) as the child is at risk of vascular thrombosis and shock. Increasing peripheral oedema, assessed clinically and by daily weight, may cause discomfort and respiratory compromise. If severe, this may need treatment with intravenous 20% albumin infusion with furosemide. Care must be taken with the use of 20% albumin as it may precipitate pulmonary oedema and hypertension from fluid overload, and also with diuretics, which may cause or worsen hypovolaemia.
- *Thrombosis* – a hypercoagulable state, due to urinary losses of antithrombin III, thrombocytosis which may be exacerbated by steroid therapy, increased synthesis of clotting factors, and increased blood viscosity from the raised haematocrit, all predispose to thrombosis. This may affect the lungs, brain, limbs, and splanchnic circulation with potentially catastrophic results.
- *Infection* – children in relapse are at risk of infection with capsulated bacteria, especially *Pneumococcus*. Spontaneous peritonitis may occur. Pneumococcal and seasonal influenza vaccination is widely recommended. Chickenpox and shingles should be treated with aciclovir.
- *Hypercholesterolaemia* – this correlates inversely with the serum albumin, but the cause of the hyperlipidaemia is not fully understood.

Prognosis

This is summarized in Fig. 19.18. Relapses are identified by parents on urine testing. The side-effects

Table 19.4 Steroid-resistant nephrotic syndrome

Cause	Specific features	Prognosis
Focal segmental glomerulosclerosis	Most common Familial or idiopathic	30% progress to end-stage renal failure in 5 years; 20% respond to cyclophosphamide, cyclosporin, tacrolimus, or rituximab Recurrence post-transplant is common
Mesangiocapillary glomerulonephritis (membranoproliferative glomerulonephritis)	More common in older children Haematuria and low complement level present	Decline in renal function over many years
Membranous nephropathy	Associated with hepatitis B May precede SLE (systemic lupus erythematosus)	Most remit spontaneously within 5 years

of corticosteroid therapy may be reduced by an alternate-day regimen. If relapses are frequent, or if a high maintenance dose is required, involvement of a paediatric nephrologist is advisable as steroid-sparing agents may be considered to enable reduction in steroid use. Possible steroid-sparing agents include the immunomodulator levamisole, alkylating agents (e.g. cyclophosphamide), calcineurin inhibitors such as tacrolimus and cyclosporin A, the immunosuppressant mycophenolate mofetil, and for difficult cases the anti-B-cell monoclonal antibody rituximab.

Steroid-resistant nephrotic syndrome

These children should be referred to a paediatric nephrologist (Table 19.4). Management of the oedema is by diuretic therapy, salt restriction, angiotensin-converting enzyme inhibitors, and sometimes nonsteroidal anti-inflammatory drugs, which may reduce proteinuria. Genetic testing for steroid-resistant nephrotic syndrome is available and helps in the management of children, e.g. withdrawal of immunosuppression or supplementation of CoQ10 if there is a CoQ10 pathway defect.

Congenital nephrotic syndrome

Congenital nephrotic syndrome presents in the first 3 months of life. It is rare. The most common kind is recessively inherited and the gene frequency is particularly high in Finns. In the UK, it is more common in consanguineous families. It is associated with a high mortality, usually due to complications of hypoalbuminaemia rather than progressive chronic kidney disease. The albuminuria is so severe that unilateral nephrectomy may be necessary for its control, followed by dialysis for stage 5 (most severe) chronic kidney disease, which is continued until the child is no longer nephrotic and old enough for renal transplantation.

> An oedematous child – test for proteinuria to diagnose nephrotic syndrome

> **Summary**
>
> **Nephrotic syndrome**
> - Clinical signs: oedema (periorbital, scrotal or vulval, leg, and ankle oedema; ascites; pleural effusions).
> - Diagnosis: heavy proteinuria and low plasma albumin.
>
> **Steroid-sensitive nephrotic syndrome**
> - Characteristic features: 1–10-years-old; no macroscopic haematuria; and normal blood pressure, complement levels, and renal function.
> - Management: oral corticosteroids, renal biopsy if unresponsive or atypical features.
> - Complications: hypovolaemia, thrombosis, infection (pneumococcal), hypercholesterolaemia.
> - Prognosis: may resolve or else there may be infrequent or frequent relapses.

Haematuria

Urine that is red in colour or tests positive for haemoglobin on urine sticks should be examined under the microscope to confirm haematuria (>10 red blood cells per high-power field). Glomerular haematuria is suggested by brown urine, the presence of deformed red cells (which occurs as they pass through the basement membrane), and casts, and is often accompanied by proteinuria. Lower urinary tract haematuria is usually red, occurs at the beginning or end of the urinary stream, is not accompanied by proteinuria, and is unusual in children.

UTI is the most common cause of haematuria (Box 19.4), although seldom as the only symptom. The history and examination may suggest the diagnosis, e.g. a family history of stone formation or nephritis or a history of trauma. A plan of investigation is outlined in Box 19.5.

Haematuria

Box 19.4 Causes of haematuria

Nonglomerular
- Infection (bacterial, viral, tuberculosis, schistosomiasis)
- Trauma to genitalia, urinary tract, or kidneys
- Stones
- Tumours
- Sickle cell disease
- Bleeding disorders
- Renal vein thrombosis
- Hypercalciuria

Glomerular
- Acute glomerulonephritis (usually with proteinuria)
- Chronic glomerulonephritis (usually with proteinuria)
- IgA nephropathy
- Familial nephritis, e.g. Alport syndrome
- Thin basement membrane disease

Box 19.5 Investigation of haematuria

All patients
- Urine microscopy (with phase contrast) and culture
- Protein and calcium excretion
- Kidney and urinary tract ultrasound
- Plasma urea, electrolytes, creatinine, calcium, phosphate, albumin
- Full blood count, platelets, coagulation screen, sickle cell screen

If suggestive of glomerular haematuria
- ESR, complement levels, and anti-DNA antibodies
- Throat swab and antistreptolysin O/anti-DNAse B titres
- Hepatitis B and C screen
- Renal biopsy if indicated
- Test mother's urine for blood (if Alport syndrome suspected)
- Hearing test (if Alport syndrome suspected)

A renal biopsy may be indicated if:
- there is significant persistent proteinuria
- there is recurrent macroscopic haematuria
- renal function is abnormal
- the complement levels are persistently abnormal.

Acute nephritis

The causes of acute nephritis in childhood are listed in Box 19.6. Increased glomerular cellularity restricts glomerular blood flow, and therefore glomerular filtration is decreased. This leads to:

- decreased urine output and volume overload
- hypertension, which may cause seizures
- oedema, characteristically initially periorbital
- haematuria and proteinuria.

Management is by attention to both water and electrolyte balance and the use of diuretics when necessary. Rarely, there may be a rapid deterioration in renal function (rapidly progressive glomerulonephritis). This may occur with any cause of acute nephritis, but is uncommon when the cause is poststreptococcal. If left untreated, irreversible chronic kidney disease may occur over weeks or months, so renal biopsy and subsequent treatment with immunosuppression and plasma exchange may be necessary.

Post-streptococcal and post-infectious nephritis

Usually follows a streptococcal sore throat or skin infection and is diagnosed by evidence of a recent streptococcal infection (culture of the organism, raised ASO/anti-DNAse B titres), and low complement C3 levels that return to normal after 3 weeks to 4 weeks.

Box 19.6 Causes of acute nephritis

- Post-infectious (including streptococcus)
- Vasculitis (Henoch–Schönlein purpura or, rarely, SLE (systemic lupus erythematosus), Wegener granulomatosis, microscopic polyarteritis, polyarteritis nodosa)
- IgA nephropathy and mesangiocapillary glomerulonephritis
- Antiglomerular basement membrane disease (Goodpasture syndrome) – very rare

Streptococcal nephritis is a common condition in developing countries, but has become uncommon in developed countries. Long-term prognosis is good.

Henoch–Schönlein purpura

Henoch–Schönlein purpura is the combination of some of the following features:

- characteristic skin rash on extensor surfaces
- arthralgia
- periarticular oedema
- abdominal pain
- glomerulonephritis.

It usually occurs between the ages of 3–10 years, is twice as common in boys, peaks during the winter months, and is often preceded by an upper respiratory infection. Despite much research, the cause is unknown. It is postulated that genetic predisposition and antigen exposure increase circulating IgA levels and disrupt IgG synthesis. The IgA and IgG interact to produce complexes that activate complement and are deposited in affected organs, precipitating an inflammatory response with vasculitis.

Clinical findings

At presentation, affected children often have a fever. The *rash* is the most obvious feature (Fig. 19.19). It is symmetrically distributed over the buttocks, the extensor surfaces of the arms and legs, and the ankles. The trunk is usually spared. The rash may initially be urticarial, rapidly becoming maculopapular and purpuric, is characteristically palpable, and may recur over several weeks. The rash is the first clinical feature in about 50% and is the cornerstone of the diagnosis, which is clinical.

- *Joint pain* occurs in two-thirds of patients, particularly of the knees and ankles. There is *periarticular oedema*. Long-term damage to the joints does not occur, and symptoms usually resolve before the rash goes.
- *Colicky abdominal pain* occurs in many children and, if severe, can be treated with corticosteroids. Gastrointestinal involvement can cause haematemesis and melaena. Intussusception can occur and can be particularly difficult to diagnose under these circumstances. Ileus, protein-losing enteropathy, orchitis, and occasionally central nervous system involvement are other rare complications.
- *Renal involvement* is common, but is rarely the first symptom. Over 80% have microscopic or macroscopic haematuria or mild proteinuria. These children usually make a complete recovery. If proteinuria is more severe, nephrotic syndrome may result. Risk factors for progressive chronic kidney disease are heavy proteinuria, oedema, hypertension, and deteriorating renal function, when a renal biopsy will determine if treatment is necessary. All children with Henoch–Schönlein purpura should be followed for a year to detect those with persisting haematuria or proteinuria (5–10%). Children who have persistent renal involvement or required treatment for Henoch–Schönlein purpura nephritis require long-term follow-up. This is necessary as hypertension and progressive chronic kidney disease may develop after an interval of several years.

IgA nephropathy

This may present with episodes of macroscopic haematuria, commonly in association with upper respiratory tract infections. Histological findings and management are as for Henoch–Schönlein purpura, which may be a variant of the same pathological process but not restricted to the kidney. The prognosis in children is better than that in adults.

Familial nephritis

The most common familial nephritis is Alport syndrome. This is usually an X-linked recessive disorder that progresses to progressive end-stage chronic kidney disease by early adult life in males and is associated with nerve deafness and ocular defects. The mother may have haematuria. The differential diagnosis is thin basement membrane disease, which also required long-term follow-up to detect proteinuria and chronic kidney disease, which rarely develops in later life.

Vasculitis

The most common vasculitis to involve the kidney is Henoch–Schönlein purpura (see the 'Henoch–Schönlein Purpura' section). However, renal involvement may occur in rarer vasculitides such as polyarteritis nodosa, microscopic polyarteritis, and granulomatosis with polyangiitis (formerly known as Wegener granulomatosis). Characteristic symptoms are fever, malaise, weight loss, skin rash, and arthropathy with prominent involvement of the respiratory tract in granulomatosis with polyangiitis. ANCA (antineutrophil cytoplasm antibodies) are present and diagnostic in these diseases. Renal arteriography, to demonstrate the presence of aneurysms, will diagnose polyarteritis nodosa. Renal involvement may be severe and rapidly progressive. Treatment is with corticosteroids, plasma exchange, and intravenous cyclophosphamide, which may need to be continued for many months.

Systemic lupus erythematosus (SLE)

SLE is a disease that presents mainly in adolescent girls and young women. It is much more common in Asian and Black than White ethnic groups. It is characterized by the presence of multiple autoantibodies, including antibodies to double-stranded DNA. The C3 and C4 components of complement may be low, particularly during active phases of the disease. Haematuria and proteinuria are indications for renal biopsy, as immunosuppression is always necessary and its intensity will depend on the severity of renal involvement.

Henoch-Schönlein purpura

Rash (a)
Buttocks (a)
Extensor surfaces of legs and arms
Ankles (b)

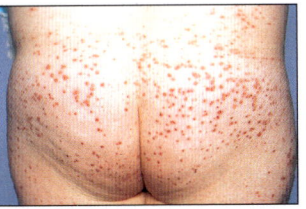

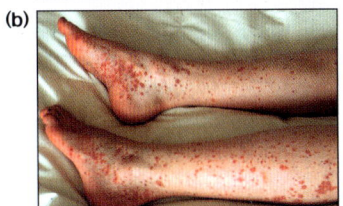

Joint pain and swelling
Knees and ankles (b)

Abdominal pain
Haematemesis and melaena
Intussusception

Renal
Microscopic/macroscopic haematuria (80%)
Nephrotic syndrome (rare)

Figure 19.19 Main clinical manifestations of Henoch–Schönlein purpura. (a) Rash on buttocks (Courtesy of Michael Markiewicz); and (b) rash around the extensor surfaces of the legs and slight joint swelling (Courtesy of Tauny Southwood).

> **Summary**
>
> **Acute nephritis**
> - Cause: usually post-infectious or follows a streptococcal infection, but also vasculitis (including Henoch–Schönlein purpura), IgA nephropathy, and familial nephritis.
> - Clinical features: oedema (around the eyes), hypertension, decreased urine output, haematuria and proteinuria.
> - Management: fluid and electrolyte balance, diuretics, monitor for rapid deterioration in renal function.

Hypertension

Blood pressure in children needs to be measured with a cuff over two-thirds the length of the upper arm (see Fig. 2.14). Blood pressure increases with age and height and readings should be plotted on a centile chart (see Appendix A4). Hypertension is blood pressure above 95th percentile for height, age, and sex. Children who are overweight or obese are at increased risk. Symptomatic hypertension in children is usually secondary to renal, cardiac, or endocrine causes (Box 19.7).

Presentation includes vomiting, headaches, facial palsy, hypertensive retinopathy, convulsions, or proteinuria. Faltering growth and cardiac failure are the most common features in infants. Pheochromocytoma may also cause paroxysmal palpitations and sweating.

Some causes are correctable, e.g. nephrectomy for unilateral scarring, angioplasty for renal artery stenosis, surgical repair of coarctation of the aorta, resection of a pheochromocytoma, but in most cases medical treatment is necessary with antihypertensive medications.

Early detection of hypertension is important. All children with a renal tract abnormality should have their blood pressure checked annually throughout life. Children with a family history of essential hypertension should be encouraged to restrict their salt intake, avoid obesity, and have their blood pressure checked regularly.

Renal masses

An abdominal mass identified on palpating the abdomen should be investigated promptly by ultrasound scan. The causes of palpable kidneys are shown in Box 19.8. Bilaterally enlarged kidneys in early life are most frequently due to autosomal recessive polycystic kidney disease (ARPKD), which is associated with hypertension, hepatic fibrosis, and progression to chronic kidney disease. This form of polycystic kidney disease must be distinguished from ADPKD (autosomal dominant adult-type polycystic kidney disease), which has a more benign prognosis in childhood with onset of progressive chronic kidney disease in adulthood, although hypertension is found in at least 10% of affected children.

Box 19.7 Causes of hypertension
- **Renal**
  - Renal parenchymal disease
  - Renovascular, e.g. renal artery stenosis
  - Polycystic kidney disease (autosomal recessive polycystic kidney disease and autosomal dominant polycystic kidney disease)
  - Renal tumours
- **Coarctation of the aorta**
- **Catecholamine excess**
  - Pheochromocytoma
  - Neuroblastoma
- **Endocrine**
  - Congenital adrenal hyperplasia
  - Cushing syndrome or corticosteroid therapy
  - Hyperthyroidism
- **Essential hypertension**
  - A diagnosis of exclusion.

Box 19.8 Causes of palpable kidneys

Unilateral
- Multicystic kidney
- Compensatory hypertrophy
- Obstructed hydronephrosis
- Renal tumour (Wilms tumour)
- Renal vein thrombosis

Bilateral
- Autosomal recessive polycystic kidneys
- Autosomal dominant polycystic kidneys
- Tuberous sclerosis
- Renal vein thrombosis

Renal calculi

Renal stones are uncommon in childhood (Fig. 19.20). When they occur, predisposing causes must be sought:
- UTI
- structural anomalies of the urinary tract
- metabolic abnormalities.

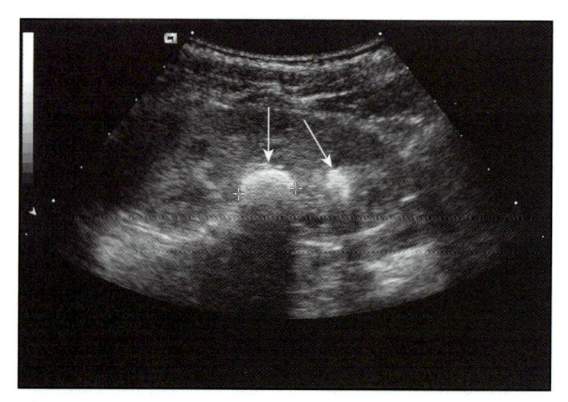

Figure 19.20 Renal ultrasound showing a staghorn calculus.

The most common are phosphate stones associated with infection, especially with *Proteus*. Calcium-containing stones occur in idiopathic hypercalciuria, the most common metabolic abnormality, and with increased urinary urate and oxalate excretion. Deposition of calcium in the parenchyma (nephrocalcinosis) may occur with hypercalciuria, hyperoxaluria, and distal renal tubular acidosis. Nephrocalcinosis may be a complication of furosemide therapy in the neonate. Cystine and xanthine stones are rare.

Presentation may be with haematuria, loin or abdominal pain, UTI, or passage of a stone. Stones that are not passed spontaneously should be removed, by either lithotripsy or surgery, and any predisposing structural anomaly repaired if possible. A high fluid intake is recommended in all affected children. If the cause is a metabolic abnormality, specific therapy may be possible.

Renal tubular disorders

Abnormalities of renal tubular function may occur at any point along the length of the nephron and affect any of the substances handled by it.

Generalized proximal tubular dysfunction (Fanconi syndrome)

Proximal tubule cells are among the most metabolically active in the body, so are especially vulnerable to cellular damage. The cardinal features are excessive urinary loss of amino acids, glucose, phosphate, bicarbonate, sodium, calcium, potassium, and magnesium. The causes are listed in Box 19.9. Fanconi syndrome should be considered in a child presenting with:

- polydipsia and polyuria
- salt depletion and dehydration
- hyperchloraemic metabolic acidosis
- rickets
- faltering or poor growth.

Box 19.9 Causes of Fanconi syndrome

Idiopathic
Secondary to inborn errors of metabolism
- Cystinosis (an autosomal recessive disorder causing intracellular accumulation of cystine)
- Glycogen storage disorders
- Lowe syndrome (oculocerebrorenal dystrophy)
- Galactosaemia
- Fructose intolerance
- Tyrosinaemia
- Wilson disease

Acquired
- Heavy metals
- Drugs and toxins
- Vitamin D deficiency

Specific transport defects

See Fig. 19.21.

Acute kidney injury

Acute kidney injury has acute renal failure at the most severe end of the spectrum where there is a sudden, potentially reversible, reduction in renal function. Oliguria (<0.5 ml/kg per hour) is usually present. It can be classified as (see Box 19.10):

- prerenal: the most common cause in children
- renal: there is salt and water retention; blood, protein, and casts are often present in the urine; and there may be symptoms specific to an accompanying disease [e.g. haemolytic uraemic syndrome (HUS)]
- postrenal: from urinary obstruction.

Acute-on-chronic renal failure is suggested by the child having growth failure, anaemia, and disordered bone mineralization (renal osteodystrophy).

Management

Children with acute renal failure should have their circulation and fluid balance meticulously monitored. Investigation by ultrasound scan will identify obstruction of the urinary tract, the small kidneys of chronic kidney disease, or large, bright kidneys with loss of cortical medullary differentiation typical of an acute process.

Prerenal failure

This is suggested by hypovolaemia. The fractional excretion of sodium is very low as the body tries to retain volume. The hypovolaemia needs to be urgently corrected with fluid replacement and circulatory support if acute tubular injury and necrosis are to be avoided.

Renal failure

If there is circulatory overload, restriction of fluid intake and challenge with a diuretic may increase urine output sufficiently to allow gradual correction of sodium and water balance. A high-calorie, normal protein feed will decrease catabolism, uraemia, and hyperkalaemia. Emergency management of metabolic acidosis, hyperkalaemia, and hyperphosphataemia is shown in Table 19.5. If the cause of renal failure is not obvious, a renal biopsy should be performed to identify rapidly progressive glomerulonephritis, as this may need immediate treatment with immunosuppression. The two most common renal causes of acute renal failure in children in the UK are haemolytic uraemic syndrome and acute tubular necrosis, the latter usually in the setting of multisystem failure in the intensive care unit or following cardiac surgery.

Postrenal failure

This requires assessment of the site of obstruction and relief by nephrostomy or bladder catheterization.

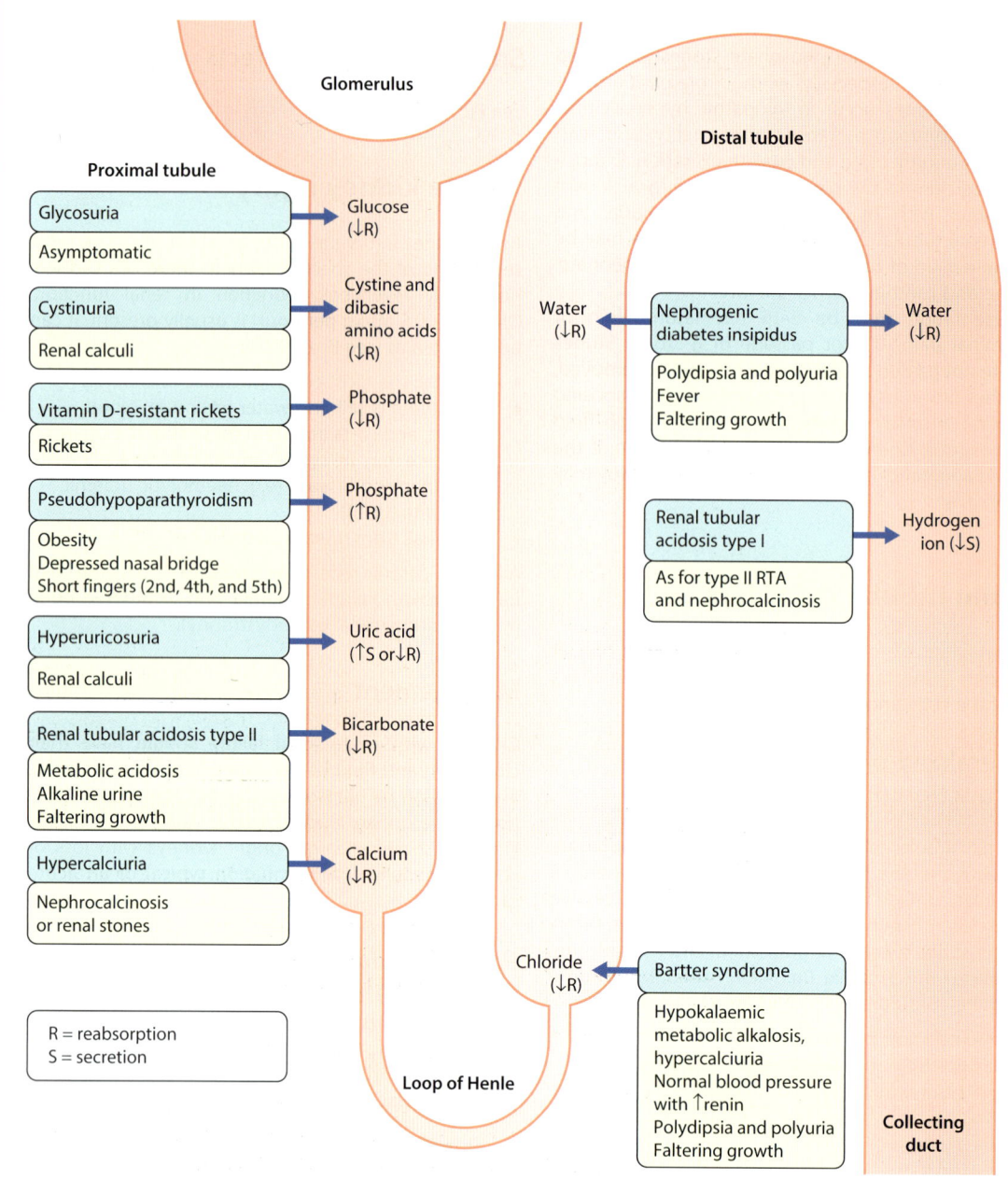

Figure 19.21

Schematic diagram of specific transport defects in some renal tubular disorders.

Proximal tubule:

- **Glycosuria** → Glucose (↓R)
  - Asymptomatic
- **Cystinuria** → Cystine and dibasic amino acids (↓R)
  - Renal calculi
- **Vitamin D-resistant rickets** → Phosphate (↓R)
  - Rickets
- **Pseudohypoparathyroidism** → Phosphate (↑R)
  - Obesity
  - Depressed nasal bridge
  - Short fingers (2nd, 4th, and 5th)
- **Hyperuricosuria** → Uric acid (↑S or ↓R)
  - Renal calculi
- **Renal tubular acidosis type II** → Bicarbonate (↓R)
  - Metabolic acidosis
  - Alkaline urine
  - Faltering growth
- **Hypercalciuria** → Calcium (↓R)
  - Nephrocalcinosis or renal stones

Distal tubule:

- **Nephrogenic diabetes insipidus** → Water (↓R)
  - Polydipsia and polyuria
  - Fever
  - Faltering growth
- **Renal tubular acidosis type I** → Hydrogen ion (↓S)
  - As for type II RTA and nephrocalcinosis

Loop of Henle: Water (↓R), Chloride (↓R)

- **Bartter syndrome** (Collecting duct)
  - Hypokalaemic metabolic alkalosis, hypercalciuria
  - Normal blood pressure with ↑renin
  - Polydipsia and polyuria
  - Faltering growth

R = reabsorption
S = secretion

Box 19.10 Causes of acute kidney injury

Prerenal
- Hypovolaemia:
  - gastroenteritis
  - burns
  - sepsis
  - haemorrhage
  - nephrotic syndrome
- Circulatory failure

Renal
- Vascular:
  - haemolytic uraemic syndrome
  - vasculitis
  - embolus
  - renal vein thrombosis
- Tubular:
  - acute tubular necrosis
  - ischaemic
  - toxic
  - obstructive
- Glomerular:
  - glomerulonephritis
- Interstitial:
  - interstitial nephritis
  - pyelonephritis

Postrenal
- Obstruction:
  - congenital, e.g. posterior urethral valves
  - acquired, e.g. blocked urinary catheter

Surgery can be performed once fluid volume and electrolyte abnormalities have been corrected.

Dialysis

Dialysis in acute kidney injury is indicated when there is:

- failure of conservative management
- hyperkalaemia
- severe hyponatraemia or hypernatraemia
- pulmonary oedema or severe hypertension due to volume overload
- severe metabolic acidosis
- multisystem failure.

Peritoneal dialysis or haemodialysis can be undertaken for acute kidney injury. If plasma exchange is part of the treatment (e.g. in vasculitis), haemodialysis is used. If there is cardiac decompensation or hypercatabolism, continuous arteriovenous or venovenous haemofiltration provides gentle, continuous dialysis and fluid removal. Acute kidney injury in childhood generally carries a good prognosis for renal recovery unless complicating a life-threatening condition, e.g. severe infection, following cardiac surgery or multisystem failure.

> **Summary**
>
> **Acute kidney injury**
> - Prerenal: most common cause in children, from hypovolaemia and circulatory failure.
> - Renal: most often haemolytic uraemic syndrome or multisystem failure.
> - Postrenal: from urinary obstruction.
> - Management: treat underlying cause, metabolic abnormalities, dialysis if necessary.

Haemolytic uraemic syndrome

HUS is a triad of acute renal failure, microangiopathic haemolytic anaemia, and thrombocytopenia. Typical HUS is secondary to gastrointestinal infection with verocytotoxin-producing *E. coli* O157:H7, acquired through contact with farm animals or eating uncooked beef, or, less often, *Shigella*. It follows a prodrome of bloody diarrhoea. The toxin from these organisms enters the gastrointestinal mucosa and preferentially localizes to the endothelial cells of the kidney where it causes intravascular thrombogenesis. Coagulation cascade is activated and clotting is normal (unlike in disseminated intravascular coagulation). Platelets are consumed in this process and microangiopathic haemolytic anaemia results from damage to red blood cells as they circulate through the microcirculation, which is occluded. Other organs such as the brain, pancreas, and heart may also be involved.

With early supportive therapy, including dialysis, the typical diarrhoea-associated HUS usually has a good prognosis, although long-term follow-up is necessary as there may be persistent proteinuria and the development of hypertension and progressive chronic kidney disease in subsequent years. By contrast, atypical HUS has no diarrhoeal prodrome, may be familial, and frequently relapses. It has a high risk of hypertension and progressive chronic kidney disease with a high mortality. A new treatment, the monoclonal anti-terminal complement antibody eculizumab, has greatly improved the prognosis of this condition although it is very expensive, and therefore plasma exchange is still used in many cases, especially in cerebral atypical HUS.

Table 19.5 Some metabolic abnormalities in acute renal failure and their therapy

Metabolic abnormality	Treatment
Metabolic acidosis	Sodium bicarbonate
Hyperphosphataemia	Calcium carbonate
	Dietary restriction
Hyperkalaemia	Calcium gluconate if ECG changes
	Salbutamol (nebulized or intravenous)
	Calcium exchange resin
	Glucose and insulin
	Dietary restriction
	Dialysis

> **Haemolytic uraemic syndrome – the triad of:**
> - acute kidney injury
> - haemolytic anaemia
> - thrombocytopenia

Chronic kidney disease

Chronic kidney disease is progressive loss of renal function due to numerous conditions and has five stages as shown in Table 19.6. Stage 5 chronic kidney disease, with GFR less than 15 ml/min per 1.73 m^2, is much less common in children than in adults, with an incidence of only 10 per million of the child population each year. Congenital and familial causes are more common in childhood than are acquired diseases (Table 19.7).

Clinical features

Stage 4 and stage 5 chronic kidney disease presents with:

- anorexia and lethargy
- polydipsia and polyuria
- faltering growth/growth failure
- bony deformities from renal osteodystrophy (renal rickets)
- hypertension
- acute-on-chronic renal failure (precipitated by infection or dehydration)
- incidental finding of proteinuria
- unexplained normochromic, normocytic anaemia.

Table 19.6 Grading of severity of chronic kidney disease

Stage	Estimated glomerular filtration rate	Description
1	>90 ml/min per 1.73 m^2	Normal renal function but structural abnormality or persistent haematuria or proteinuria
2	60–89 ml/min per 1.73 m^2	Mildly reduced function, asymptomatic
3	30–59 ml/min per 1.73 m^2	Moderately reduced renal function, renal osteodystrophy
4	15–29 ml/min per 1.73 m^2	Severely reduced renal function with metabolic derangements and anaemia. Need to make plans for renal replacement therapy
5	<15 ml/min per 1.73 m^2	End stage renal failure, renal replacement therapy required

Many children with chronic kidney disease have had their renal disease detected before birth by antenatal ultrasound or have previously identified renal disease. Symptoms rarely develop before renal function falls to less than one-third of normal or chronic kidney disease stage 4.

Management

The aims of management are to prevent the symptoms and metabolic abnormalities of chronic kidney disease, to allow normal growth and development, and to preserve residual renal function. The management of these children should be conducted in a specialist paediatric nephrology centre.

Diet

Anorexia and vomiting are common. Improving nutrition using calorie supplements and nasogastric or gastrostomy feeding is often necessary to optimize growth. Protein intake should be sufficient to maintain growth and a normal albumin, whilst preventing the accumulation of toxic metabolic by-products.

Prevention of renal osteodystrophy

Phosphate retention and hypocalcaemia due to decreased activation of vitamin D lead to secondary hyperparathyroidism, which results in osteitis fibrosa and osteomalacia of the bones. Phosphate restriction by decreasing the dietary intake of milk products, calcium carbonate as a phosphate binder, and activated vitamin D supplements help to prevent renal osteodystrophy.

Control of salt and water balance and acidosis

Many children with chronic kidney disease caused by congenital structural malformations and renal dysplasia have an obligatory loss of salt and water. They need salt supplements and free access to water. Treatment with bicarbonate supplements is necessary to prevent acidosis.

Anaemia

Reduced production of erythropoietin and circulation of metabolites that are toxic to the bone marrow result in anaemia. This responds well to the administration of recombinant human erythropoietin which is administered subcutaneously.

Hormonal abnormalities

Many hormonal abnormalities occur in progressive chronic kidney disease. Most importantly, there is growth hormone resistance with high growth hormone levels but poor growth. Recombinant human growth hormone has been shown to be effective in improving growth for up to 5 years of treatment, but whether it improves final height remains unknown. Many children with stage 4 and stage 5 chronic kidney disease have delayed puberty and a subnormal pubertal growth spurt.

Dialysis and transplantation

It is now possible for all children to enter renal replacement therapy programmes when stage 5 chronic kidney disease is reached. The optimum management is by renal transplantation (Case History 19.4).

Table 19.7 Causes of chronic kidney disease

Cause	%
Renal dysplasia ± reflux	34
Obstructive uropathy	18
Glomerular disease	10
Congenital nephrotic syndrome	10
Tubulointerstitial diseases	7
Renovascular disease	5
Polycystic kidney disease	4
Metabolic	4

Data from UK Renal Registry 2014.

Case history 19.4

Renal transplantation

Caden was born with a severe form of posterior urethral valves and had chronic kidney disease from birth (see Fig. 19.11a, b). He was managed for the first 3 years with intensive nutritional input. He underwent treatment for UTIs and received medications including salt supplements and erythropoietin. He needed to have his bladder augmented and went on to dialysis briefly (Fig. 19.22) before he had a live related transplant from his father at the age of 4 years. He is now growing and developing well although he continues to need immunosuppressants and occasionally suffers from UTIs.

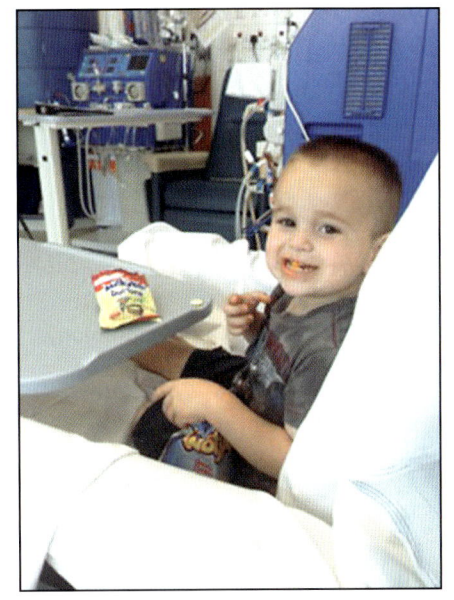

Figure 19.22 Caden enjoying treats whilst on dialysis. Children with chronic kidney disease have a diet restricted in potassium and phosphate, which means no chocolate, crisps, or pizza – unless on the dialysis machine!

Technically, this is difficult in very small children and a minimum weight, e.g. 10 kg, needs to be reached before transplantation to avoid renal vein thrombosis. Kidneys obtained from living related donors have a higher success rate than deceased donor kidneys, which are matched as far as possible to the recipient's HLA (human leukocyte antigen) type. Patient survival is high and first-year graft survival is around 95% for living related and 96% for deceased kidneys in the UK. Graft losses from both acute and chronic rejection or recurrent disease mean that the 5-year graft survival is reduced to 94% for living related kidneys and 84% for deceased donor kidney transplants and some children need retransplantation. Current immunosuppression is mainly with combinations of tacrolimus and mycophenolate mofetil and prednisolone and there is increasing use of minimal steroid regimens which improve growth.

Ideally, a child is transplanted before dialysis is required, but if this is not possible, a period of dialysis may be necessary. Peritoneal dialysis, either by cycling overnight using a machine (continuous cycling peritoneal dialysis) or by manual exchanges over 24 hours (continuous ambulatory peritoneal dialysis), can be done by the parents at home and is therefore less disruptive to family life and the child's schooling. Haemodialysis is an alternative and is usually done in hospital three to four times a week.

Summary

Chronic kidney disease
- Causes: congenital (structural malformations and hereditary nephropathies) most common.
- Presentation: abnormal antenatal ultrasound, anorexia and lethargy, polydipsia and polyuria, faltering growth/growth failure, renal rickets (osteodystrophy), hypertension, proteinuria, anaemia.
- Management: diet and nasogastric or gastrostomy feeding, phosphate restriction and activated vitamin D to prevent renal osteodystrophy, salt supplements and free access to water to control salt and water balance, bicarbonate supplements to prevent acidosis, erythropoietin to prevent anaemia, growth hormone, and dialysis and transplantation.

Acknowledgements

We would like to acknowledge contributors to this chapter in previous editions, whose work we have drawn on: Lesley Rees (1st, 2nd, 3rd Edition), George Haycock (3rd Edition), Larissa Kerecuk (4th Edition).

Further reading

Avner ED, Harmon WE, Niaudet P, et al: *Pediatric Nephrology*, ed 7, Philadelphia, PA, 2016, Lippincott Williams & Wilkins.
A comprehensive textbook.

Rees L, Brogan P, Bockenhauer D, et al: *Handbook of Paediatric Nephrology*, ed 2, Oxford, 2012, Oxford University Press.

Websites (Accessed November 2016)

American Society of Pediatric Nephrology: Available at: http://www.aspneph.com.

British Association of Paediatric Nephrology: Available at: http://www.renal.org/BAPN#sthash.jZQVJSKo.dpbs

Emedicine: Available at: http://emedicine.medscape.com/pediatrics_general
Details about a range of paediatric nephrology conditions.

Royal College of Paediatrics and Child Health/British Kidney Patient Association and British Association for Paediatric Nephrology InfoKid: Available at: http://www.infokid.org.uk.
Information for parents and carers about children's kidney conditions.

The Renal Association Rarerenal.org: Available at: http://rarerenal.org.
Provides up to date information for clinicians and patients on rare renal diseases which are relatively common in paediatric nephrology.

20

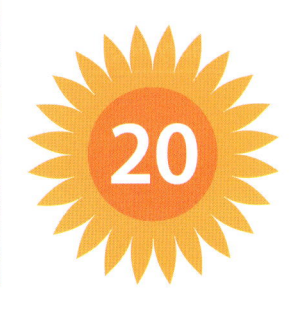

Genital disorders

| Inguinoscrotal conditions | 367 | Genital disorders in girls | 374 |
| Abnormalities of the penis | 371 | | |

Features of genital disorders in children are:
- hydroceles, inguinal hernias and undescended testes usually arise from abnormal embryological development
- the acute scrotum is a surgical emergency
- foreskin conditions and hypospadias are common in boys
- vulvovaginitis and labial adhesions are common in girls.

Inguinoscrotal conditions

Embryology

Development of a testis from an early indeterminate gonad is determined by genes associated with a Y chromosome. For a testis to descend from its origin on the posterior abdominal wall, it must produce testosterone which acts on peripheral tissues. The testis, guided by the mesenchymal gubernaculum, migrates down into the inguinal canal (Fig. 20.1a). The structures that are found in the scrotum in a boy (testis, vas and blood vessels) or labium in a girl (attachment of the round ligament of the uterus) pass through the abdominal wall and pick up layers corresponding to those of the abdominal wall. In a boy these make up the coverings of the spermatic cord. In boys and girls there is a remnant of peritoneal invagination, the processus vaginalis (Fig. 20.1b), which, if it remains patent and in continuity with the abdomen, explains why fluid or abdominal contents can become a hydrocele or hernia, respectively (Fig. 20.1c–e).

Inguinal hernia

Inguinal hernias are common, occurring in up to 5% of boys, and are even more common in premature babies. As explained by the embryology, a hernia is usually caused by a persistently patent processus vaginalis and emerges from the deep inguinal ring through the inguinal canal. It is therefore usually indirect, although in premature babies where the tissues are weak and friable, direct hernias are more likely than in older children.

A hernia presents as a lump in the groin which may extend into the scrotum (Fig. 20.2) or labium. They are usually asymptomatic but may be intermittent, visible during straining. On examination, sometimes a lump or thickened cord structures can be palpated in the groin.

The contents of the hernia may become irreducible (incarcerated), causing pain and sometimes intestinal obstruction or damage to the testis (strangulation). In these circumstances the lump is tender and the infant may be irritable and may vomit. The risk of incarceration is much higher in infants than in older children.

Most hernias can be successfully reduced by 'taxis' (gentle compression in the line of the inguinal canal) with good analgesia. Surgery can then be planned for a suitable time when any oedema has settled and the child is well. If reduction is impossible, emergency surgery is required because of the risk of compromise of the bowel or testis. In girls, sometimes the ovary can become incarcerated within a hernia.

Surgery (see Fig. 20.1d) involves ligation and division of the processus vaginalis, which has become the hernial sac (herniotomy, removal of the hernia sac – as opposed to herniorrhaphy in adults, when the inguinal abdominal wall is also reinforced, usually with a mesh). Beyond the first three months of age, this can be safely performed as a day case.

> **Prompt surgical repair is indicated for inguinal hernias in infants to lower the risk of incarceration**

Hydrocele

A hydrocele has the same underlying anatomy as a hernia, but the processus vaginalis, although patent, is not sufficiently wide to form an inguinal hernia.

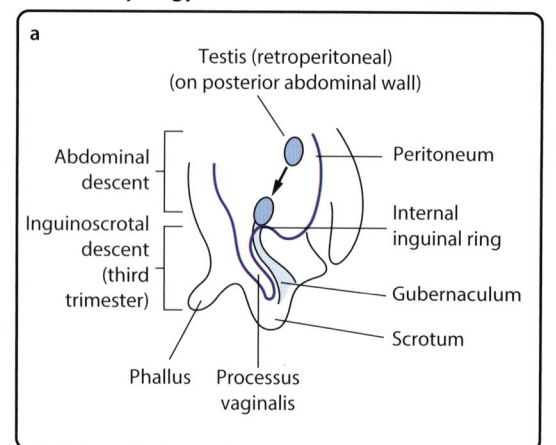

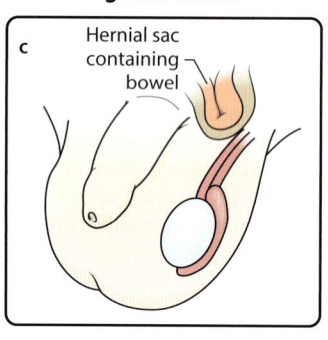

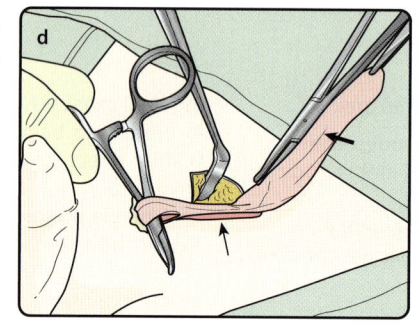

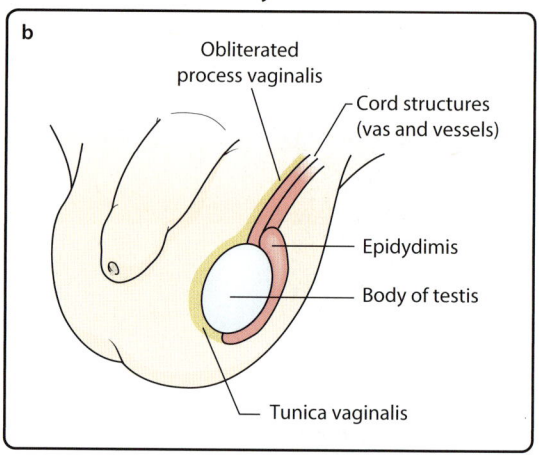

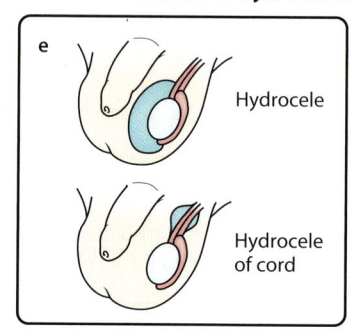

Figure 20.1 (a) Normal embryology of testicular descent; (b) normal groin structures showing remnant of processus vaginalis above and medial to cord structures; (c) relationship of inguinal hernia sac to cord; (d) surgical repair showing hernia sac (thick arrow) separated from cord structures (thin arrow); and (e) variants of hydrocele from patent processus vaginalis.

Hydroceles are usually asymptomatic and sometimes appear blue. It is usually possible to feel the testis, however tense the hydrocele. Sometimes the hydrocele is separate from the testis (see Fig. 20.1e) in the cord. The key to differentiating a hernia from a hydrocele is the ability to 'get above' a hydrocele. Hydroceles usually transilluminate (Fig. 20.3).

Although the processus vaginalis is often patent at birth it usually closes within months. Hydroceles therefore usually resolve spontaneously, and can be managed expectantly. Surgery may be considered if it persists beyond the first two years of life, but resolution may take longer than this. In a girl, a hydrocele (of the 'canal of Nuck') is much less common than in boys.

Varicocele

This is a scrotal swelling comprising dilated (varicose) testicular veins and occurs in up to 15% of boys, usually at puberty (Fig. 20.4). Its cause is multifactorial; valvular incompetence plays a role. It is commoner on the left side because of drainage of the gonadal vein into the left renal vein, which also receives blood containing catecholamines from the left adrenal vein. It is usually asymptomatic, but may cause a dull ache. On examination it may have a bluish colour and feel like a 'bag of worms'. Sometimes the testis is smaller or softer than normal. Management is conservative if asymptomatic. Occlusion of the gonadal veins can be achieved by surgical ligation – through the groin laparoscopically or by radiological embolization.

Undescended testis

Most undescended testes become arrested along their normal pathway of descent (see Fig. 20.1a). Undescended testes are present in up to 5% of newborn term infants but are more common in premature infants. By three months of age, only 1% are still undescended. The diagnosis should ideally be made at the routine examination of the newborn (Ch. 10. Perinatal medicine) but since there is still a small spontaneous rate of descent after this time the decision to operate for undescended testis should be delayed.

Examination of the testes in babies must be made in a warm environment and with warm hands. The testes may be felt in the scrotum or may need to be delivered by gentle pressure along the line of the inguinal canal to the scrotum.

An undescended testis may be palpable or impalpable. A palpable undescended testis is usually seen or felt in the groin, but cannot be manipulated into the scrotum. Occasionally it can be palpated below the

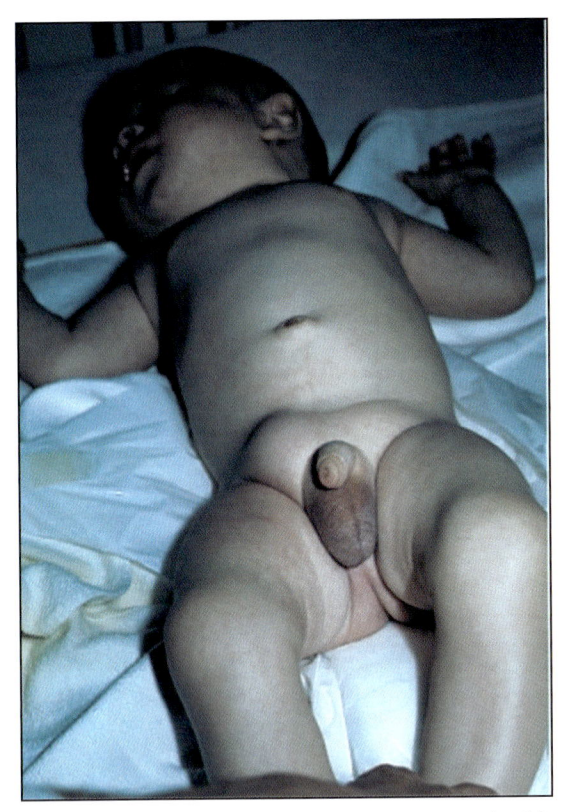

Figure 20.2 Bilateral inguinal hernias in 2-month-old boy. (Courtesy of Mike Coren).

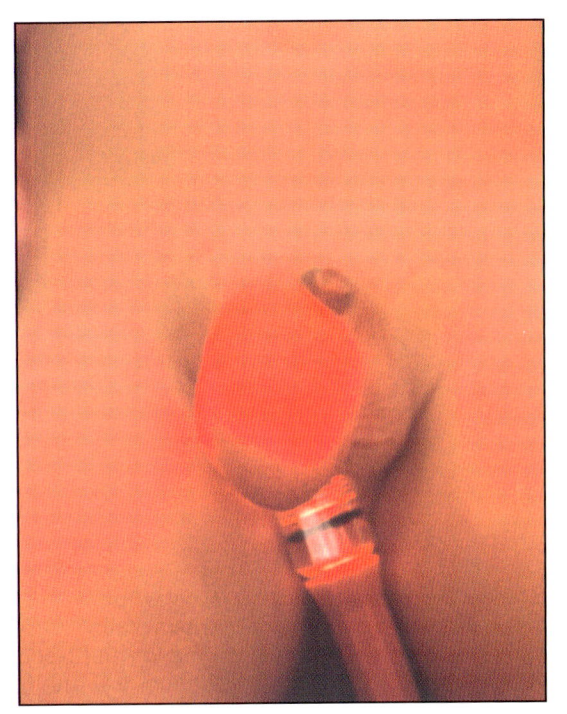

Figure 20.3 Transilluminated right hydrocele. (Courtesy of Anette Jacobsen).

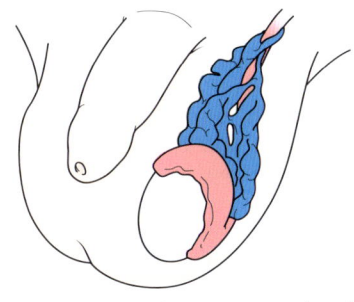

Figure 20.4 Varicocele showing convoluted vessels occupying much of the left hemiscrotum.

external inguinal ring but outside the scrotum – the so-called 'ectopic' testis.

If the testis is impalpable, it may be in the inguinal canal but cannot be identified or it may be intra-abdominal or absent. If there are bilateral impalpable testes, the karyotype must be established to exclude disorders of sex development. This should be regarded as a medical emergency.

A testis may also be retractile. The crucial difference between a retractile and undescended testis is that a retractile testis can be manipulated into the scrotum with ease and without tension. Action of the cremaster muscle (as seen in eliciting the cremasteric reflex by light touch on the abdominal wall) pulls up the testis. Parents of boys with a retractile testis often report that the testis is sometimes obvious, particularly when the boy is warm and relaxed, and sometimes not. This is why a boy with a suspected undescended testis should be examined in a warm environment and when warm and relaxed.

Investigations and management

Imaging is not helpful in the assessment of an undescended testis.

Orchidopexy, the surgical placement of the testis in the scrotum, is performed for the following reasons:

- Cosmetic – to achieve the same, symmetrical appearance as other boys. This may be of psychological benefit. If the testis is absent, a prosthesis can be inserted when older.
- Reduced risk of torsion and trauma compared to groin location
- Fertility – the testis needs to be in the scrotum, below body temperature, in order to allow spermatogenesis. The effect is probably marginal in unilateral undescended testis but is more important if bilateral. There is some evidence that delaying orchidopexy beyond the first two years of life adversely affects testicular development.
- Malignancy – increased risk in an undescended testis, which is greater if bilateral or intra-abdominal. Placing the testis in the scrotum facilitates self-examination but may not influence the risk of malignancy.

The timing of orchidopexy depends on local surgical and anaesthetic facilities, but should be performed before or around one year of age. Thereafter, spontaneous descent is unlikely, and there is evidence that testicular growth, hormonal function and spermatogenesis is improved by operating at this early age rather than waiting until older.

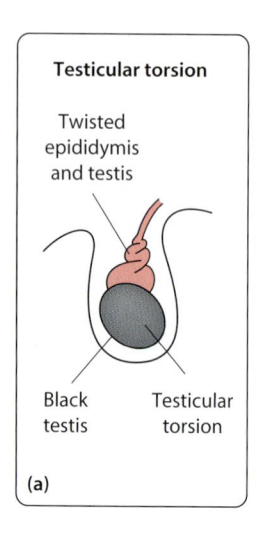

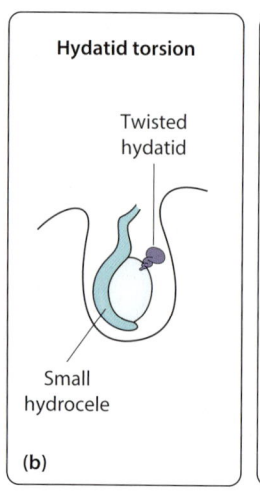

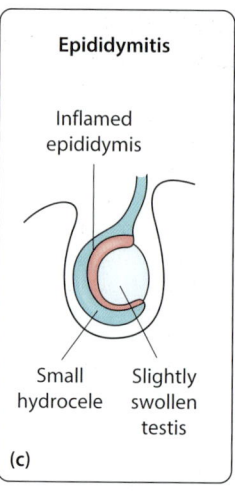

Figure 20.5 **(a)** Testicular torsion; **(b)** hydatid torsion; and **(c)** epididymitis.

Groin approach orchidopexy involves opening the inguinal canal in a similar manner to herniotomy, mobilizing the testis whilst preserving the vas and blood vessels and placing it within the scrotum. It is usually performed as a day case. An *intra-abdominal testis* is usually managed laparoscopically; it may be amenable to placement in the scrotum in a single operation or may require a staged approach.

Regarding *impalpable testes*, about 10% have regressed in development and are, in fact, absent. Laparoscopy allows both diagnosis and treatment.

For a *retractile testis*, follow up is recommended because some high testes require surgery to place them in the scrotum. Whether or not this is true ascent of the testis is controversial.

> Undescended testes should be referred to a paediatric surgeon when detected. If surgery is required, the optimum time is within the first year of life.

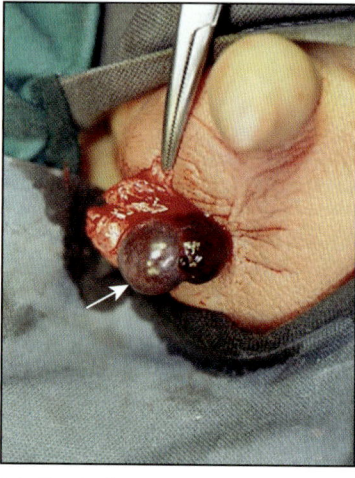

Figure 20.6 Testicular torsion on the right side showing nonviable testis (arrow). (Courtesy of Anette Jacobsen, Singapore).

Acute inguinoscrotal conditions ('the acute scrotum')

Torsion of the testis

This is commonest in post-pubertal boys (Fig. 20.5a), but may occur at any age, including the newborn when it usually presents at birth and is believed to be perinatal. It is usually very painful, with redness and oedema of the scrotal skin. However, the pain may be localised to the groin or lower abdomen, highlighting the need to always examine the testes in a boy presenting with sudden-onset pain in the groin, abdomen or scrotum. It must be distinguished from an incarcerated hernia. An undescended testis is at increased risk of torsion, as is a testis lying transversely on its attachment to the spermatic cord (the so-called 'clapper bell' testis).

Torsion of the testis must be treated within hours of the onset of symptoms to lower the risk of testicular loss. In fact, surgical exploration in any acute scrotal presentation is mandatory (Fig. 20.6) unless torsion can be excluded with certainty (see below). Fixation of the contralateral testis is essential because of the increased risk of a contralateral torsion, especially if an anatomical abnormality is present in the torted testis. Outcome is variable, depending on time to correction. If delayed, testicular loss is likely. In perinatal testicular torsion, testicular loss is almost inevitable.

Torsion of appendix testis

A testicular appendage (Hydatid of Morgagni) is a Mullerian (paramesonephric) remnant usually located on the upper pole of the testis. Torsion of the appendix testis (Fig. 20.5b) tends to affect prepubertal boys and is more common than torsion of the testis. Pain evolves over days, but is not as dramatic as in testicular torsion. Scrotal exploration and excision of the appendage is often necessary because it cannot be differentiated reliably from torsion of the testis. If a 'blue dot' can be seen through the scrotal skin and pain is controlled with analgesia, surgery may not be necessary.

Other acute inguinoscrotal conditions

Infection may cause an acute scrotum. *Epididymo-orchitis* (Fig. 20.5c) is commoner in infants and small children, and more likely with a pre-existing urological or anorectal malformation. As it may be indistinguishable from torsion, scrotal exploration may be necessary. Doppler ultrasound of flow pattern in the testicular blood vessels may allow differentiation of epididymitis from torsion of the testis, but must not delay surgical exploration if torsion remains a possibility. A urine sample should be obtained to identify an associated urinary tract infection. Pus should be sent at operation for microbiology to characterize the nature of the infection, but infection may be bacterial or viral. Antibiotics are started empirically.

In *idiopathic scrotal oedema* there is redness and swelling extending beyond the scrotum into the thigh, perineum and suprapubic area, but the testis is normal and non-tender. It requires analgesia and review. It may recur. An *incarcerated hernia* may also cause an acute scrotum, although symptoms usually affect the groin.

Trauma to the scrotum is an uncommon cause of testicular damage, but may need exploration, debridement and surgical repair. Sexual abuse needs to be considered in all genital injuries.

Recurrent scrotal pain in boys can be difficult to manage. Any associated symptoms or signs such as swelling or redness should be regarded as intermittent testicular torsion and the testes fixed. Sometimes prophylactic fixation is required to exclude intermittent torsion as a cause for recurrent pain. In adulthood, chronic scrotal pain can follow scrotal surgery.

> Torsion of the testis must be excluded (by emergency exploration if necessary) in boys with an 'acute scrotum'. Delay leads to testicular loss

Abnormalities of the penis

The foreskin

A normal foreskin does not retract in infancy, and retraction should not be attempted. At 1 year of age, about half of uncircumcised boys have a non-retractile (normal) foreskin. Only 1% of boys over 16 years old have a non-retractile foreskin. The prepuce develops adherent to the underlying glans, and acts as protection to the non-keratinised glanular and meatal squamous epithelium in an environment where astringent urine can cause inflammation or even ulceration. This can be manifest as ammoniacal dermatitis (napkin rash) in infants and young children, where the preputial opening can be reddened and sore. It usually only needs reassurance and attention to routine hygiene. This needs to be differentiated from infection, or balanoposthitis, where the redness is more extensive, and, crucially, there is a purulent discharge. It occurs in about 3% of boys, reaches a peak incidence around the third year of life, and recurs in about a third. The infection is usually bacterial and needs antibiotic treatment, either topical or systemic. As it is rarely fungal, antifungal agents are not indicated. Topical corticosteroids may sometimes be beneficial.

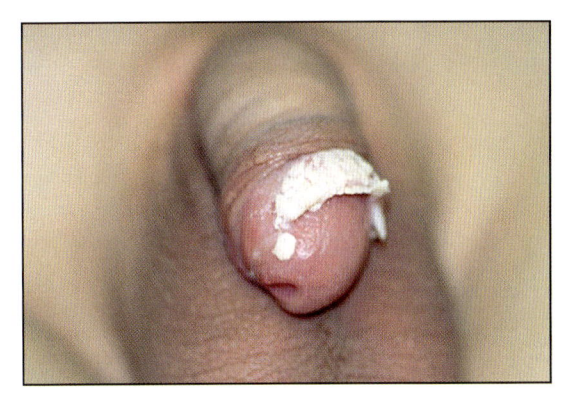

Figure 20.7 Smegma. (Courtesy of Anette Jacobsen, Singapore).

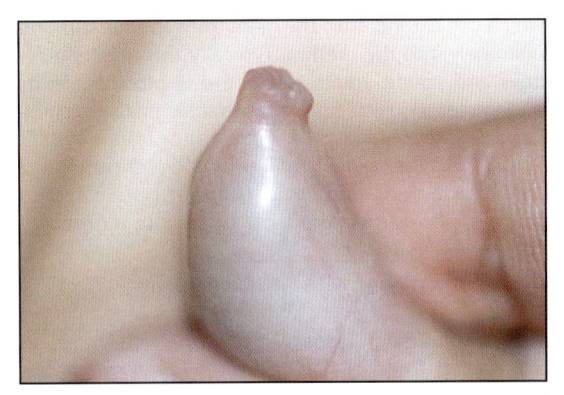

Figure 20.8 Normal foreskin in an infant. (Courtesy of Anette Jacobsen, Singapore).

Ballooning of the foreskin on urination is a common cause of parental concern. It can look dramatic but seldom causes any trouble. It results from lysis of preputial adhesions around the glans before those at the preputial opening. Ballooning may also occur on the shaft of the penis, arising from the attachment of shaft skin below the coronal sulcus of the glans. Ballooning stops when preputial adhesions have lysed completely. It has no functional consequence, does not represent obstruction, and does not need intervention.

Another cause of parental concern is sub-preputial smegma. It appears as a lump which grows briefly, seemingly under the non-retractile or partially retractile foreskin. It is yellowish and malleable, and simply comprises desquamated skin and secretions. There is no need to intervene – it will discharge in due course (with typical appearance of smegma – 'cottage cheese'; Fig. 20.7) when the preputial adhesions break down.

Non-retractile foreskin and phimosis

When traction is applied (gently) to a normal foreskin, the skin at the preputial opening is seen to evert, even if it does not necessarily open up (Fig. 20.8). A foreskin that is pathologically non-retractile will not do this, and will truly render the glans 'muzzled', (Greek word 'phimos'). This differentiates a foreskin that is simply non-retractile (i.e. normal, physiological) from one which is problematic. The commonest condition that gives rise to a true phimosis is balanitis xerotica obliterans, or BXO, which gives rise to progressive scarring

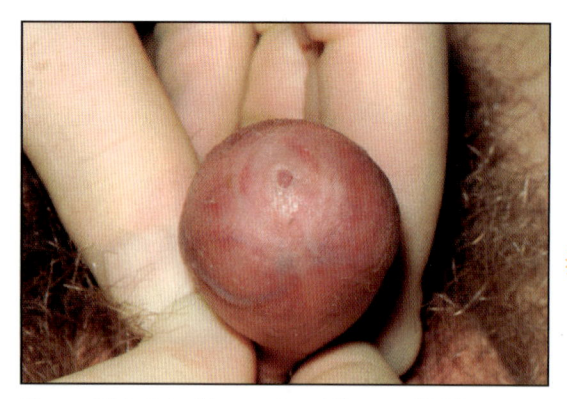

Figure 20.9 Balanitis xerotica obliterans (BXO) causing a true phimosis. (Courtesy of Alun Williams).

which can extend onto the glans, into the meatus and ultimately into the urethra. Typically this affects older boys and young adults, and there is often a history that the foreskin was normally retractile in earlier childhood. Figure 20.9 shows the typical appearance of BXO.

BXO is the index indication for circumcision, although there is some evidence that potent topical steroids, closely monitored, can cause it to regress.

Paraphimosis

This is a condition, usually in post-pubertal boys, of a retracted foreskin that cannot be reduced easily. There is a ring of narrower skin. The glans swells, and if the prepuce is not reduced it may result in compromise of the blood supply to the glans. Treatment (by reduction) is an emergency, which may require general anaesthesia. Paraphimosis has been regarded as an indication for circumcision, but this is no longer considered to be the case unless the foreskin is abnormal (as with BXO).

Circumcision

Circumcision remains a tradition in Jewish and Muslim religions.

Medical reasons for circumcision include:

- BXO causing a true phimosis
- recurrent balanoposthitis causing refractory symptoms
- prophylaxis of recurrent urinary infection, especially in the presence of a congenital uropathy (such as posterior urethral valves or vesicoureteric reflux) or if renal reserve is limited
- if access to the urethra is required reliably for intermittent catheterization, e.g. spina bifida.

There are inevitably other indications for circumcision, some of which are highly dependent on the individual family and surgeon. There is some evidence that circumcision affords protection against transmission of HIV and HPV (human papillomavirus), and there are programmes promoting circumcision in newborn infants and young adult males in some countries with high prevalence of HIV infection.

There have been many techniques described for circumcision, and complications are uncommon. Up to one boy in fifty has post-operative bleeding requiring a return to the operating theatre. Infection in the skin margin or ulceration of exposed granular skin may occur. Meatal stenosis can also occur, more often after circumcisions done for BXO, and this may require subsequent surgery. Rarer complications include urethral fistula.

> **A non-retractile foreskin is normal in preschool children**

Hypospadias

This is a common condition, with an incidence of up to 1 in 200 boys. It is thought to arise from failure of development of ventral tissues of the penis – in particular failure of ventral urethral closure. For that reason it is really a constellation of 'ventral hypoplasia' of the penis.

Typically there are three features, although their occurrence is variable:

- a ventral urethral meatus – the urethral meatus is variable in position (Fig. 20.10), but in most (80%) is on the distal shaft or glans penis (Fig. 20.11a)
- ventral curvature of the shaft of the penis (formerly called 'chordee') (Fig. 20.11b), more apparent on erection
- hooded appearance of the foreskin – characteristic in appearance because of ventral foreskin deficiency but of no functional significance.

There is rarely an associated or underlying disorder of sex development, and only very rarely another congenital urinary tract abnormality. Investigation of the urinary tract with imaging is not routinely indicated.

Management

Surgery is not mandatory, especially in a distal hypospadias when the penis and urinary stream are straight. However, it may be performed on functional or cosmetic grounds. The ultimate functional aim of hypospadias surgery is to allow a boy to pass urine in a straight line whilst standing, and to have a straight erection. Surgery, if needed, is usually performed in the first two to three years of life. The commonest surgical complications are breakdown of the repair or meatal narrowing. The prepuce may be preserved and reconstructed, although for more proximal hypospadias it is sometimes required for the repair itself. For this reason it is important that a boy with hypospadias is not circumcised before the repair.

> **Infants with hypospadias must not be circumcised, to preserve tissue for reconstruction.**

Other conditions of the penis

Variations in penoscrotal skin attachment and in the infant or child's body habitus may make the penis look buried. This is common with obesity, when the only treatment is weight loss, but improves with growth of the penis after puberty. However, it may persist if there is marked obesity.

Hypospadias

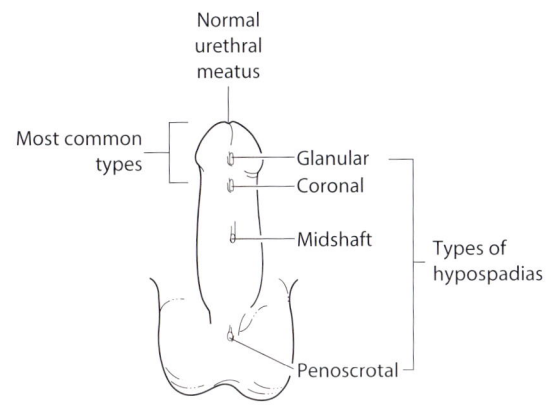

Figure 20.10 Varieties of hypospadias.

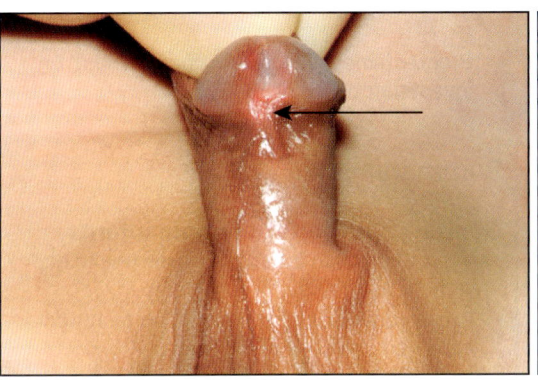

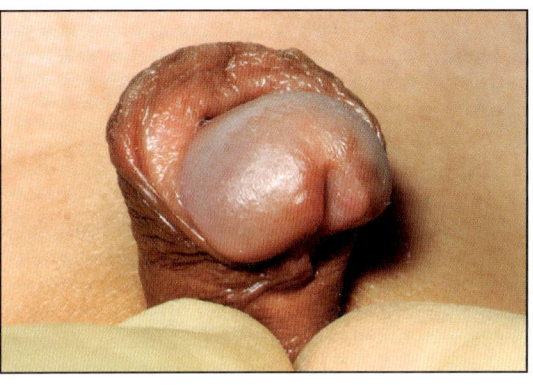

Figure 20.11 (a) Penile shaft in hypospadias showing the urethral meatus (arrow). (b) In oblique view, the dorsal hooded prepuce and ventral curvature of the penis (chordee) can be seen. (Courtesy of Alun Williams).

Summary

Genital conditions in male infants
Inguinal hernia/hydrocele
- Cause inguinoscrotal swellings: clinically one can get above a hydrocele
- Expedient surgical repair of inguinal hernias is required in infants to prevent bowel strangulation or after reduction of an irreducible hernia

Undescended testis
- Common – up to 5% of term boys
- If testis palpable, requires orchidopexy
- If impalpable, may require laparoscopy to establish presence of a testis
- If bilateral impalpable, urgent karyotype is essential
- Retractile testes usually do not require surgery

Acute scrotal conditions
- May occur at any age but torsion of testis must be considered not only for acute pain of the scrotum but also for acute abdominal and groin pain
- scrotal surgical exploration is required unless torsion of the testis can be reliably excluded

Non-retractile foreskin
- Is normal in preschool children
- Is pathological if associated with BXO
- Circumcision is not recommended routinely but is still traditional in some communities worldwide

Hypospadias
- Common – 1 in 200 boys
- Variable ventral urethral meatus and penile curvature
- Surgery may be required in first two years of life
- Infants with hypospadias must not be circumcised

Genital disorders in girls

Normal anatomy

Recognition of the normal female anatomy and its variations is crucial (Fig. 6.1a), in order to avoid incorrectly diagnosing them as pathological conditions or the result of abuse.

Vulvovaginitis/vaginal discharge

The commonest problem is redness of the vulva. In infants, this is often due to a nappy rash due to ammoniacal dermatitis. Less often, the vulvovaginitis is infective, occasionally with Candida infection. Vaginal discharge is common, and is usually innocuous unless it is green or offensive when it may indicate infection. Foreign bodies are more often suspected than found; they are actually rare. The 'red flag' symptom is a bloody vaginal discharge, and needs referral to a specialist as vaginal rhabdomyosarcoma is a rare but important cause in preschool girls.

Labial adhesions

Fusion of the labia minora can be a cause of local irritation in the prepubertal girl. There is usually an adequate orifice for the passage of urine. The characteristic appearance is of superficial fusion of the labia minora with a translucent (or even slightly bluish) area of flimsy tissue between the labia. The appearance sometimes raises parental concern about abnormal vaginal development, although these conditions are rare. Unless the labial adhesion causes significant symptoms, no specific treatment is required. Topical corticosteroids or oestrogens can be helpful to lyse the adhesions, especially if it allows the underlying introital anatomy to be seen, but readhesion is common. Examination under anaesthesia, or formal 'division of adhesions' should be undertaken only exceptionally because of the high rate of recurrence.

Other conditions

True obstruction or atresia of the vagina is rare. It may present with primary amenorrhoea in adolescence. This might co-exist with cyclical abdominal or pelvic pain representing obstruction to the flow of menses. Clinical examination usually reveals the cause. If there is a bulging introitus that appears blue, the diagnosis is imperforate hymen – and the treatment is hymenotomy under anaesthesia. Absence of an imperforate hymen represents a problem of vaginal septation, canalization or more complex abnormality with paramesonephric (Mullerian) duct development, and needs further imaging (often with MRI) to plan appropriate management.

In contrast to problems of the testes in boys, ovarian problems tend to be more difficult to diagnose because they are intra-abdominal. An ovarian cause for symptoms should be considered in a girl who presents with acute abdominal pain (from ovarian cyst or torsion) or a mass (cyst or tumour). Disorders of sex differentiation are considered in Chapter 26. Diabetes and endocrinology.

> Blood-stained vaginal discharge must be investigated

Summary

Genital conditions in female infants
- Vulvovaginitis in infants is usually due to nappy rash
- Labial adhesions tend to recur; no treatment is indicated unless symptomatic

Acknowledgements

We would like to acknowledge contributors to this chapter in previous editions, whose work we have drawn on. The chapter was originally written by Nick Madden (1st Edition), and was extensively rewritten by Mark Stringer and David Thomas (2nd, 3rd and 4th Editions). Additional contributions by Aruna Abhyankar (4th edition). We are grateful to Prof Annette Jacobsen and Mr Alun Williams for providing some of the clinical photographs.

Further reading

Balen AH, Creighton SM, Davies MC, MacDougall J, Stanhope R: *Paediatric and Adolescent Gynaecology*, 2011, Cambridge University Press.

Edmonds DK: *Dewhurst's Paediatric and Adolescent Gynaecology*, 2013, Butterworth-Heinemann.

Thomas DFM, Duffy PG, Rickwood AMK: *Essentials of Paediatric Urology*, ed 2, 2008, CRC Press.

21 Liver disorders

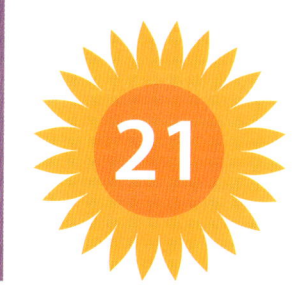

Neonatal cholestasis	375	Liver disease in older children	380
Neonatal metabolic liver disease	378	Complications of chronic liver disease	382
Viral hepatitis	378	Liver transplantation	384
Acute liver failure (fulminant hepatitis)	380		

Features of liver disorders in children are
- Prolonged neonatal jaundice (>14 days of age if term, >3 weeks if preterm) requires investigation to identify liver disease (conjugated jaundice).
- The earlier in life biliary atresia is diagnosed and treated surgically, the better the prognosis.
- Chronic hepatitis B virus (HBV) infection in children can be prevented.
- Hepatitis C is now curable with oral antiviral drugs, supporting the need to screen children at risk.
- Liver transplantation is an effective therapy for acute or chronic liver failure, with a greater than 80% 20-year survival rate.

Many of the clinical features and complications of liver disease are shown in Fig. 21.1.

> Liver disease in children is uncommon and should be managed by, or in conjunction with national centres

Neonatal cholestasis

Physiological jaundice in newborns is common but 90% will have resolved by 2 weeks (3 weeks if preterm). Prolonged (or persistent) neonatal jaundice requires prompt investigation to distinguish unconjugated (resolves spontaneously) from conjugated which indicates liver disease. Early diagnosis and management of neonatal liver disease improves prognosis.

The differential diagnosis of prolonged jaundice in infancy is shown in Box 21.1.

> In prolonged (persistent) jaundice, always look to see if the stools are pale, which suggests bile duct obstruction

Biliary atresia

This occurs in 1 in 15 000 live births. There is progressive fibrosis and obliteration of the extrahepatic and intrahepatic biliary tree. Without intervention, chronic liver failure develops and death occurs within 2 years. The exact aetiology is unknown. Clinical presentation is with mild jaundice and pale stools (the colour may fluctuate but becomes increasingly pale as the disease

Hepatic dysfunction

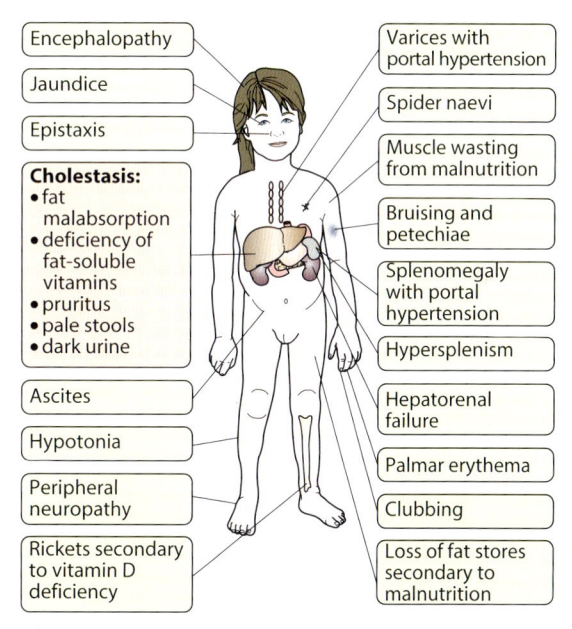

- Encephalopathy
- Jaundice
- Epistaxis
- Cholestasis:
  - fat malabsorption
  - deficiency of fat-soluble vitamins
  - pruritus
  - pale stools
  - dark urine
- Ascites
- Hypotonia
- Peripheral neuropathy
- Rickets secondary to vitamin D deficiency
- Varices with portal hypertension
- Spider naevi
- Muscle wasting from malnutrition
- Bruising and petechiae
- Splenomegaly with portal hypertension
- Hypersplenism
- Hepatorenal failure
- Palmar erythema
- Clubbing
- Loss of fat stores secondary to malnutrition

Figure 21.1 The symptoms and signs of hepatic dysfunction. In addition, faltering growth and malnutrition may occur.

Box 21.1 Causes of prolonged (persistent) neonatal jaundice

Unconjugated
- Breastmilk jaundice
- Infection (particularly urinary tract)
- Haemolytic anaemia, e.g. G6PD deficiency
- Hypothyroidism
- High gastrointestinal obstruction
- Crigler–Najjar syndrome

Conjugated (>25 μmol/L)
Bile duct obstruction
- Biliary atresia
- Choledochal cyst

Neonatal hepatitis syndrome
- Congenital infection
- Inborn errors of metabolism
- α_1-Antitrypsin deficiency
- Galactosaemia
- Tyrosinaemia (type 1)
- Errors of bile acid synthesis
- Progressive familial intrahepatic cholestasis
- Cystic fibrosis
- Intestinal failure-associated liver disease – associated with long-term parenteral nutrition

Intrahepatic biliary hypoplasia
- Alagille syndrome

---

progresses). (See Case History 21.1) They have normal birthweight followed by faltering growth. Hepatomegaly is often present initially. Splenomegaly develops due to portal hypertension.

Investigations

There is a raised conjugated bilirubin and abnormal liver function test. A fasting abdominal ultrasound may demonstrate a contracted or absent gallbladder, though it may be normal. The diagnosis is confirmed by a cholangiogram (ERCP (endoscopic retrograde cholangiopancreatography), or operative), which fails to outline a normal biliary tree. Liver biopsy initially demonstrates neonatal hepatitis with features of extrahepatic biliary obstruction developing with time.

Treatment

Palliative surgery with a Kasai hepatoportoenterostomy (a loop of jejunum is anastomosed to the cut surface of the porta hepatis) bypasses the fibrotic ducts and facilitates drainage of bile from any remaining patent ductules. Early surgery increases the success rate, with 80% clearing the jaundice if performed before 60 days. Even with successful clearance of jaundice, the disease progresses in most children who may develop cholangitis and cirrhosis with portal hypertension. Nutrition and fat-soluble vitamin supplementation is essential. If the Kasai is unsuccessful, liver transplantation is considered. Biliary atresia is the single most common indication for liver transplantation in the paediatric age group.

Choledochal cysts

These are cystic dilatations of the extrahepatic biliary system. They may be detected on antenatal ultrasound scan, present with neonatal jaundice or, in older children, presentation is with abdominal pain, a palpable mass, jaundice, or cholangitis. The diagnosis is established by ultrasound or magnetic resonance cholangiopancreatography. Treatment is by surgical excision of the cyst with the formation of a Roux-en-Y anastomosis to the biliary duct. Future complications include cholangitis and a 2% risk of malignancy, which may develop in any part of the biliary tree.

Neonatal hepatitis syndrome

In neonatal hepatitis syndrome, there is prolonged neonatal jaundice and hepatic inflammation. It is termed idiopathic if no specific cause can be found (Box 21.1). Babies may have a low birthweight and faltering growth. Other clinical features depend on the diagnosis. Jaundice may be severe and differentiation from biliary atresia is essential. Liver biopsy is often nonspecific but shows giant cell hepatitis.

Alagille syndrome

This is a rare autosomal dominant condition with widely varying penetrance even within families. Clinical presentation is with a characteristic triangular facies (Fig. 21.4), skeletal abnormalities (including butterfly vertebrae), congenital heart disease (classically peripheral pulmonary stenosis), renal tubular disorders, and defects in the eye. Infants may be profoundly cholestatic with severe pruritus and faltering growth. Identifying the gene mutations confirms the diagnosis. Treatment is to provide nutrition and fat-soluble vitamins. Pruritus is profound and difficult to manage. A small number will require liver transplant, but most survive into adult life. Mortality is most likely secondary to the cardiac disease.

Progressive familial intrahepatic cholestasis

These autosomal recessive disorders all affect bile salt transport. Clinical presentation is with jaundice, intense pruritus, faltering growth, rickets, and in some

Case history 21.1

Biliary atresia

A term infant, birthweight 3.4 kg, was initially breastfed and developed mild jaundice on the 3rd day of life. At 5 weeks she was still jaundiced. She was constantly hungry on an infant formula. On questioning, her stools were pale (Fig. 21.2) but showed no other features of liver disease.

Investigations revealed:

- Serum bilirubin 160 micromol/L, with 140 micromol/L conjugated.

She was referred to a national paediatric liver centre, where further investigations revealed:

- Alanine transferase elevated – 120 IU/L,
- Gamma glutamyl transferase elevated – 430 IU/L.

Ultrasound – absent gallbladder despite 4 hours of fasting.

Treatment with fat-soluble vitamins and ursodeoxycholic acid were commenced.

Feeds were changed to a high MCT (medium chain triglyceride) feed and she settled on to a 3-hour feeding pattern. No other causes of conjugated jaundice were identified.

A cholangiogram confirmed biliary atresia and she underwent a Kasai portoenterostomy at 6 weeks of age. Fig. 21.3 shows her a few months after her operation.

At 4 years of age she had developed increasing splenomegaly. Endoscopy identified oesophageal varices. She remains stable at age 6-years.

> In prolonged (persistent) neonatal jaundice, early diagnosis of biliary atresia improves the prognosis

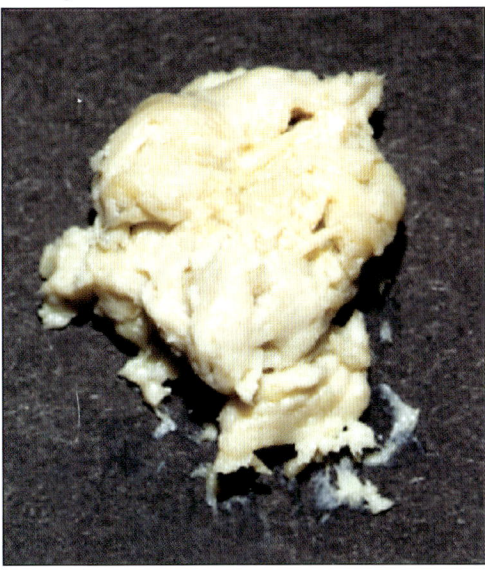

Figure 21.2 Pale stool secondary to biliary atresia.

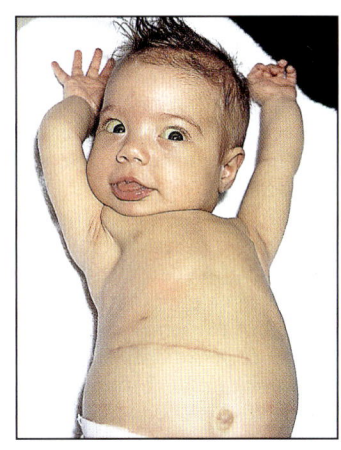

Figure 21.3 Several months after successful bile drainage by hepatoportoenterostomy (Kasai procedure) for biliary atresia. The scar is from her surgery.

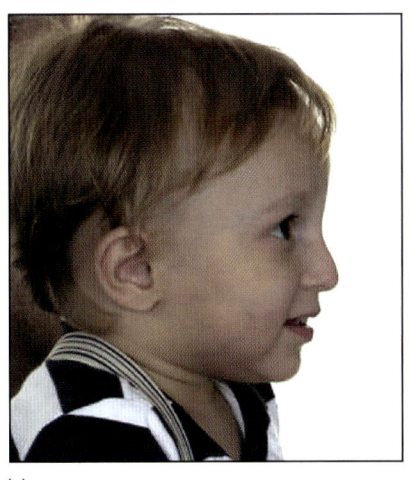

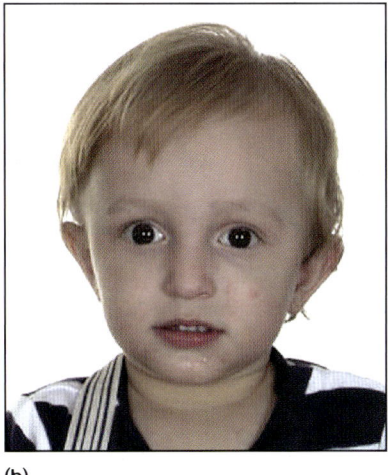

(a) (b)

Figure 21.4 The typical facial features of a child with Alagille syndrome with (a) pointed chin and (b) wide spaced eyes and prominent forehead.

cases diarrhoea and hearing loss. Older children may present with gallstones.

The diagnosis is confirmed by identifying mutations in bile salt transport genes. Treatment is with nutritional support and fat-soluble vitamins. Pruritus can be severe. Progression of fibrosis is usual with most requiring liver transplantation.

Neonatal metabolic liver disease

α₁-Antitrypsin deficiency

It is inherited as an autosomal recessive disorder with an incidence of 1 in 2000 to 1 in 4000 in the UK. There are many phenotypes of the protease inhibitor (Pi) which are coded on chromosome 14, with liver disease primarily associated with the protein phenotype PiZZ. Abnormal folding of the protease α₁-antitrypsin is associated with accumulation of the protein within the hepatocytes and hence liver disease in infancy and childhood. The lack of circulating α₁-antitrypsin results in emphysema in adults.

The majority of children who present with α₁-antitrysin deficiency will either have prolonged neonatal jaundice or, less commonly, bleeding due to vitamin K deficiency (haemorrhagic disease of the newborn). Hepatomegaly is present. Splenomegaly develops with cirrhosis and portal hypertension. The diagnosis is confirmed by estimating the level of α₁-antitrypsin in the plasma and identifying the protein phenotype. Approximately 50% of children have a good prognosis, but the remainder will develop liver disease and may require transplantation. Pulmonary disease is not significant in childhood, but is likely to develop in adult life. Advice to avoid smoking (both active and passive) should be given. The disorder can be diagnosed antenatally.

Galactosaemia

This very rare disorder has an incidence of 1 in 23 000 to 1 in 44 000. The infants develop poor feeding, vomiting, jaundice, and hepatomegaly when fed milk. Liver failure, cataracts, and developmental delay are inevitable if it is untreated. A rapidly fatal course with shock, haemorrhage, and disseminated intravascular coagulation, often due to Gram-negative sepsis, may occur.

On investigating prolonged (persistent) jaundice, it can be identified by detecting galactose, a reducing substance, in the urine. The diagnosis is made by measuring the enzyme galactose-1-phosphate-uridyl transferase in red cells. A recent blood transfusion may mask the diagnosis. A galactose-free diet prevents progression of liver disease, but ovarian failure and learning difficulties may occur later.

Other causes

Neonatal hepatitis may occur following prolonged parenteral nutrition. Rare causes include tyrosinaemia type 1, cystic fibrosis, lipid and glycogen storage disorders, peroxisomal disorders, and inborn errors of bile acid synthesis.

Viral hepatitis

The clinical features of acute viral hepatitis include nausea, vomiting, abdominal pain, lethargy, and jaundice; however, 30% to 50% of children do not develop jaundice. A large tender liver is common and 30% will have splenomegaly. The liver transaminases are usually markedly elevated. Coagulation is usually normal.

Hepatitis A

Hepatitis A virus is an RNA virus which is spread by faecal–oral transmission. The incidence of hepatitis A in childhood has fallen as socioeconomic conditions have improved. Many adults are now not immune. Vaccination is required for travellers to endemic areas.

The disease may be asymptomatic, but the majority of children have a mild illness and recover both clinically and biochemically within 2 weeks to 4 weeks. Some may develop prolonged cholestatic hepatitis (which is self-limiting), or fulminant hepatitis. Chronic liver disease does not occur.

Diagnosis can be confirmed by detecting IgM antibody to the virus. There is no treatment and no evidence that bed rest or change of diet is effective. Close contacts should be vaccinated within 2 weeks of the onset of the illness. In those at increased risk e.g. chronic liver disease, HNIG (human normal immunoglobulin) should be considered.

Hepatitis B

Hepatitis B virus (HBV) is a DNA virus that is an important cause of acute and chronic liver disease worldwide, with high prevalence and carrier rates in sub-Saharan Africa and the Far East (Fig. 21.5). HBV is transmitted by:

- perinatal transmission from carrier mothers or horizontal spread within families
- inoculation with infected blood via blood transfusion, needlestick injuries, or renal dialysis
- among adults it can also be transmitted sexually.

Infants who contract HBV perinatally are asymptomatic, but at least 90% become chronic carriers. Older children who contract HBV may be asymptomatic or have classical features of acute hepatitis. The majority will resolve spontaneously, but 1% to 2% develop fulminant hepatic failure, while 5% to 10% become chronic carriers.

The diagnosis is made by detecting HBV antigens and antibodies. IgM antibodies to the core antigen (anti-HBc) are positive in acute infection. Hepatitis B surface antigen (HBsAg) denotes ongoing infectivity. There is no treatment for acute HBV infection.

Chronic hepatitis B

Approximately 30% to 50% of asymptomatic carrier children will develop chronic HBV liver disease, which may progress to cirrhosis in 10%. There is a long-term

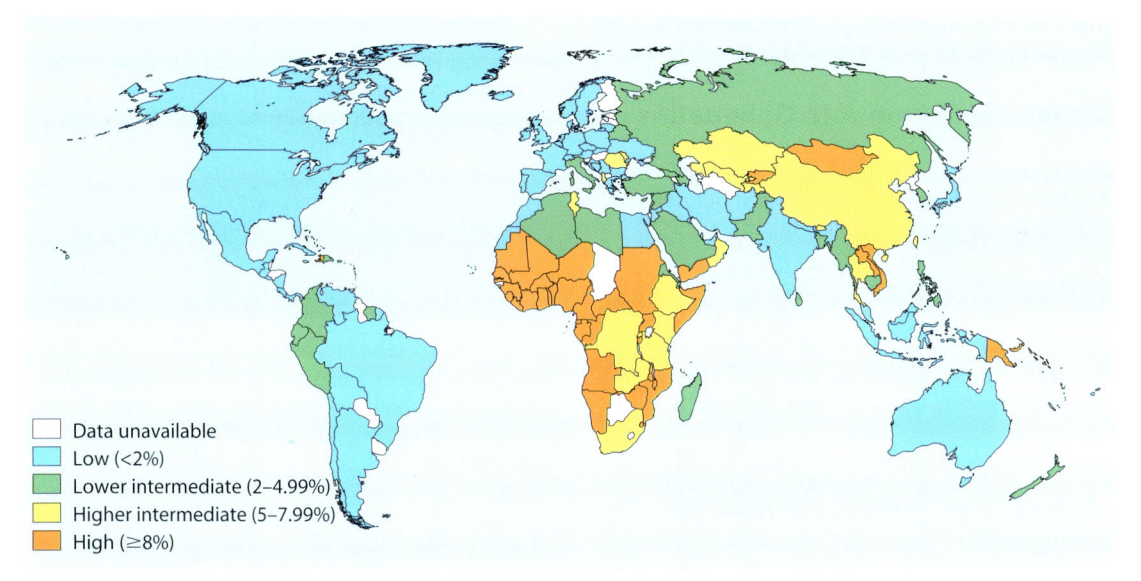

Figure 21.5 Global HBsAg prevalence. (From Schweitzer A, Horn J, Mikolajczyk RT, Krause G, Ott JJ: Estimations of worldwide prevalence of chronic hepatitis B virus infection: a systematic review of data published between 1965 and 2013, *Lancet* 386:1546–1555, 2015 with permission.)

risk of hepatocellular carcinoma. Current treatment regimens for chronic HBV have poor efficacy. Interferon or pegylated interferon (a long acting formulation) treatment for chronic hepatitis B is successful in 50% of children infected horizontally and 30% of children infected perinatally. Oral antiviral therapy such as lamivudine and adefovir is effective in 25% but may be limited by the development of resistance. Newer drugs (such as entecavir, tenofovir, and telbivudine) may be more effective.

Prevention

Prevention of HBV infection is important. All pregnant women should have antenatal screening for HBsAg. Babies of all HBsAg-positive mothers should receive a course of hepatitis B vaccination (given routinely to all infants in many countries), with hepatitis B immunoglobulin also being given if the mother is also hepatitis B e antigen (HBeAg)-positive. Antibody response to the vaccination course should be checked in high-risk infants at 12 months as 5% require further vaccination. Other members of the family should also be vaccinated. There is evidence that effective neonatal vaccination reduces the incidence of HBV-related cancer.

> **Summary**
>
> **Hepatitis B virus (HBV)**
> - Perinatal transmission from carrier mothers should be prevented in the UK by maternal screening and giving the infant a course of hepatitis B vaccine with hepatitis B immunoglobulin if indicated. Universal hepatitis B immunization is given in many countries.
> - Infection may result in chronic HBV liver disease, which may progress to cirrhosis and hepatocellular carcinoma.

Hepatitis C

Hepatitis C virus (HCV) is an RNA virus that was responsible for 90% of post-transfusion hepatitis until the screening of donor blood was introduced in 1991. In the UK, about 1 in 2000 donors have HCV antibodies. The prevalence is high among intravenous drug users. Vertical transmission is now the most common cause of HCV transmission in children. Six percent of transmission occurs from infected mothers, but is twice as common if there is coinfection with HIV. It seldom causes an acute infection, but the majority become chronic carriers, with a 20% to 25% lifetime risk of progression to cirrhosis or hepatocellular carcinoma. Standard treatment with a combination of pegylated interferon and ribavirin is successful. Recent developments with oral antiviral drugs such as sofosbuvir are likely to be 100% curative, thus increasing the need to screen high risk children, such as the children of drug abusers. Treatment is not undertaken before 3 years of age, as HCV may resolve spontaneously following vertically acquired infections.

Hepatitis D virus

Hepatitis D virus (HDV) is a defective RNA virus that depends on hepatitis B virus for replication. It occurs as a coinfection with hepatitis B virus or as a superinfection causing an acute exacerbation of chronic hepatitis B virus infection. Cirrhosis develops in 50% to 70% of those who develop chronic HDV infection.

Hepatitis E virus

This is an RNA virus that is enterally transmitted, usually by contaminated water. It is found worldwide but is more prevalent in low-income countries. Hepatitis E virus causes a mild self-limiting illness in most people and is known to be transmitted by blood transfusion or eating infected pork. In pregnant women it causes fulminant hepatic failure with a high mortality rate.

Seronegative (non-A to G) hepatitis

Clinical presentation is similar to hepatitis A. When a viral aetiology of hepatitis is suspected but not identified, it is known as seronegative hepatitis.

Epstein–Barr virus

Children with Epstein–Barr virus infection are usually asymptomatic. Some 40% have hepatitis with marked hepatosplenomegaly, which may become fulminant. Less than 5% are jaundiced.

Acute liver failure (fulminant hepatitis)

Acute liver failure in children is the development of massive hepatic necrosis with subsequent loss of liver function, with or without hepatic encephalopathy. The disease is uncommon, but has a high mortality. Most are caused by infection and metabolic conditions (Table 21.1). The child may present within hours or weeks with jaundice, encephalopathy, coagulopathy, hypoglycaemia, and electrolyte disturbance. Early signs of encephalopathy include alternate periods of irritability and confusion with drowsiness. Older children may be aggressive and unusually difficult. Complications include cerebral oedema, haemorrhage from gastritis or coagulopathy, sepsis and pancreatitis.

Diagnosis

Bilirubin may be normal in the early stages, particularly with metabolic disease. Transaminases are greatly elevated (10–100 times normal), alkaline phosphatase is increased, coagulation is very abnormal and plasma ammonia is elevated. It is essential to monitor the acid–base balance, blood glucose and coagulation times. An EEG will show acute hepatic encephalopathy and a CT scan may demonstrate cerebral oedema.

Management

Early referral to a national paediatric liver centre is essential.

Steps to stabilize the child prior to transfer include:
- maintaining the blood glucose (>4 mmol/L) with intravenous dextrose
- preventing sepsis with broad-spectrum antibiotics and antifungal agents
- preventing haemorrhage, particularly from the gastrointestinal tract, with intravenous vitamin K and H_2-blocking drugs or proton pump inhibitors
- prevent cerebral oedema by fluid restriction and mannitol diuresis if oedema develops.

Features suggestive of a poor prognosis are a shrinking liver, rising bilirubin with falling transaminases, a worsening coagulopathy, or progression to coma. Without liver transplantation, 70% of children who progress to coma will die.

Liver disease in older children

The causes of chronic liver disease are listed in Box 21.2. The clinical presentation varies from an apparent acute hepatitis to the insidious development of hepatosplenomegaly, cirrhosis, and portal hypertension with lethargy and malnutrition. The most common causes are hepatitis viruses (B or C) and autoimmune hepatitis and non-alcholic fatty liver disease, but Wilson disease should always be excluded.

Autoimmune hepatitis and sclerosing cholangitis

The mean age of presentation is 7 years to 10 years. It is more common in girls. It may present as an acute hepatitis, as fulminant hepatic failure or chronic liver disease with autoimmune features such as skin rash, arthritis, haemolytic anaemia, or nephritis. Diagnosis is based on elevated total protein, hypergammaglobulinaemia (IgG >20 g/L); positive autoantibodies, a low serum complement (C4); and typical histology. Autoimmune hepatitis may occur in isolation or in association with inflammatory bowel disease, coeliac disease, or other autoimmune diseases. Some 90% of children with autoimmune hepatitis will respond to prednisolone and azathioprine. Scerosing cholangitis is treated with ursodeoxycholic acid.

Table 21.1 Causes of acute liver failure

Children <2 years old	Children >2 years
Infection (most common is herpes simplex)	Seronegative hepatitis
	Paracetamol overdose
Metabolic disease	Mitochondrial disease
Seronegative hepatitis	Wilson disease
Drug induced	Autoimmune hepatitis
Neonatal haemochromatosis	

Box 21.2 Causes of chronic liver disease in older children

Postviral hepatitis B, C
Autoimmune hepatitis and sclerosing cholangitis
Drug-induced liver disease (NSAIDs)
Cystic fibrosis
Wilson disease
Fibropolycystic liver disease
Non-alcoholic fatty liver disease
α_1-Antitrypsin deficiency

Cystic fibrosis

Liver disease is the second most common cause of death after respiratory disease in cystic fibrosis. The most common liver abnormality is hepatic steatosis (fatty liver). It may be associated with protein energy malnutrition or micronutrient deficiencies. Steatosis does not generally progress and treatment involves ensuring optimal nutritional support. More significant liver disease arises from thick tenacious bile with abnormal bile acid concentration leading to progressive biliary fibrosis. Cirrhosis and portal hypertension develop in 20% of children by mid-adolescence. Early liver disease is difficult to detect by biochemistry, ultrasound or radioisotope scanning. Liver histology includes fatty liver, focal biliary fibrosis, or focal nodular cirrhosis. Supportive therapy includes endoscopic treatment of varices and nutritional therapy and treatment with ursodeoxycholic acid. Liver transplantation may be considered for those with end-stage liver disease, either alone or in combination with a heart–lung transplant.

Wilson disease

Wilson disease is an autosomal recessive disorder with an incidence of 1 in 200 000. Many mutations have now been identified. The basic genetic defect is a combination of reduced synthesis of caeruloplasmin (the copper-binding protein) and defective excretion of copper in the bile, which leads to an accumulation of copper in the liver, brain, kidney, and cornea. Wilson disease rarely presents in children under the age of 3 years. In those presenting in childhood, a hepatic presentation is more likely. They may present with almost any form of liver disease, including acute hepatitis, fulminant hepatitis, cirrhosis, and portal hypertension. Neuropsychiatric features are more common in those presenting from the second decade onwards and include deterioration in school performance, mood and behaviour change, and extrapyramidal signs such as incoordination, tremor, and dysarthria. Renal tubular dysfunction, with vitamin D-resistant rickets, and haemolytic anaemia also occur. Copper accumulation in the cornea (Kayser–Fleischer rings) (Fig. 21.6) is not seen before 7 years of age.

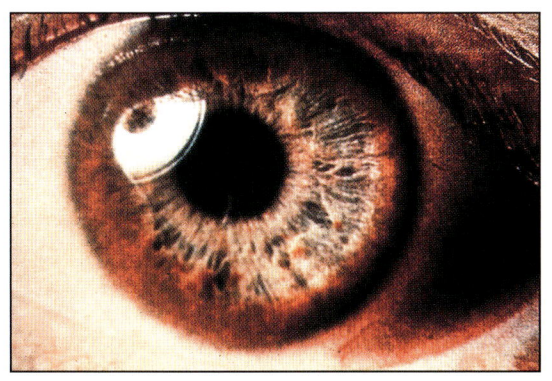

Figure 21.6 Kayser–Fleischer rings from copper in the cornea in a child with Wilson disease.

A low serum caeruloplasmin and copper is characteristic, but not universal. Urinary copper excretion is increased and this further increases after administering the chelating agent penicillamine. However, the diagnosis is confirmed by the finding of elevated hepatic copper on liver biopsy or identification of the gene mutation.

Treatment is with penicillamine or trientine. Both promote urinary copper excretion, reducing hepatic and central nervous system copper. Zinc is given to reduce copper absorption. Pyridoxine is given to prevent peripheral neuropathy. Zinc is used in asymptomatic children identified by screening families with an index case. Neurological improvement may take up to 12 months of therapy. About 30% of children with Wilson disease will die from hepatic complications if untreated. Liver transplantation is considered for children with acute liver failure or severe end-stage liver disease.

Fibropolycystic liver disease (ciliopathies)

This is a range of inherited conditions affecting the development of the intrahepatic biliary tree. Presentation is with liver cystic disease or fibrosis and renal disease.

Congenital hepatic fibrosis presents in children over 2 years old with hepatosplenomegaly, abdominal distension, and portal hypertension. It differs from cirrhosis in that liver function tests are normal in the early stage. Liver histology shows large bands of hepatic fibrosis containing abnormal bile ductules. Complications include portal hypertension with varices and recurrent cholangitis. Cystic renal disease may coexist and may cause hypertension or renal dysfunction. Indications for liver transplant include severe recurrent cholangitis or deterioration of renal function requiring renal transplant, in which case a combined transplant would be offered.

Non-alcoholic fatty liver disease

Non-alcoholic fatty liver disease is the single most common cause of chronic liver disease in the high-income world. It is a spectrum of disease, ranging from simple fatty deposition (steatosis) through to inflammation (steatohepatitis), fibrosis, cirrhosis, and end-stage liver failure. In childhood, it may be associated with a metabolic syndrome or with obesity. The prognosis in childhood is uncertain; few develop cirrhosis in childhood in contrast to 8% to 17% of adults. They are usually asymptomatic, although some complain of vague right upper quadrant abdominal pain or lethargy. The diagnosis is often suspected following the incidental finding of an echogenic liver on ultrasound or mildly elevated transaminases carried out for some other reason. Liver biopsy demonstrates marked steatosis with or without inflammation or fibrosis. The pathogenesis is not fully understood but may be linked to insulin resistance. Treatment targets weight loss through diet and exercise, which may lead to liver function tests returning to normal.

Complications of chronic liver disease

Nutrition

Effective nutrition is essential. It may improve and stabilize patients with liver disease. Barriers to effective nutrition include:

fat malabsorption – long chain fat is not effectively absorbed without bile. Therefore, medium chain triglyceride containing milk (specialist formula) is required if children are persistently cholestatic, as it does not require bile micelles for absorption. Up to 40% of fat needs to be long chain fat to prevent essential fatty acid deficiency. Fat-soluble vitamins are carried on the long chain fats and hence deficiency is common unless these vitamins are supplemented

protein malnutrition – poor intake combined with high catabolic rate of the diseased liver makes protein malnutrition common at presentation of liver disease. Protein intake should not be restricted unless the child is encephalopathic

anorexia – when unwell children cannot take the required amount of nutrition and many will require nasogastric tube feeding or occasionally parenteral nutrition.

Fat-soluble vitamins

All fat-soluble vitamins (Table 21.2) can be given orally. Monitoring of the levels and adjustment of dose is required to prevent deficiency. In severe deficiency, intramuscular administration may be required.

Pruritus

Severe pruritus is associated with cholestasis, although the aetiology is not clear. Pruritis is difficult to manage and may lead to excoriation of the skin. Treatment includes:

- Loose cotton clothing, avoiding overheating, keep nails short.
- Moisturising the skin with emollients.
- Medication: phenobarbital to stimulate bile flow; cholestyramine, a bile salt resin to absorb bile salts; ursodeoxycholic acid, an oral bile acid to solubilise the bile; rifampicin, an enzyme inducer.

Encephalopathy

This occurs in end-stage liver disease and may be precipitated by gastrointestinal haemorrhage, sepsis, sedatives, renal failure, or electrolyte imbalance. It is difficult to diagnose in children as the level of consciousness may vary throughout the day. Infants present with irritability and sleepiness, while older children present with abnormalities in mood, sleep rhythm, intellectual performance, and behaviour. Plasma ammonia may be elevated and an EEG is always abnormal. Oral lactulose and a nonabsorbable oral antibiotic (e.g. rifaximin) will help reduce the ammonia by lowering the colonic pH and increasing gut transit time.

Cirrhosis and portal hypertension

Cirrhosis is the end result of many forms of liver disease. It is defined pathologically as extensive fibrosis with regenerative nodules. It may be secondary to hepatocellular disease or to chronic bile duct obstruction (biliary cirrhosis). The main pathophysiological effects of cirrhosis are diminished hepatic function and portal hypertension with splenomegaly, varices, and ascites (Fig. 21.7). Hepatocellular carcinoma may develop.

Table 21.2 The effects of fat-soluble vitamin deficiency

Fat-soluble vitamin	Effect of deficiency
Vitamin K	Bleeding diathesis including intracranial bleeding
Vitamin A	Retinal changes in infants and night blindness in older children
Vitamin E	Peripheral neuropathy, haemolysis, and ataxia
Vitamin D	Rickets and fractures

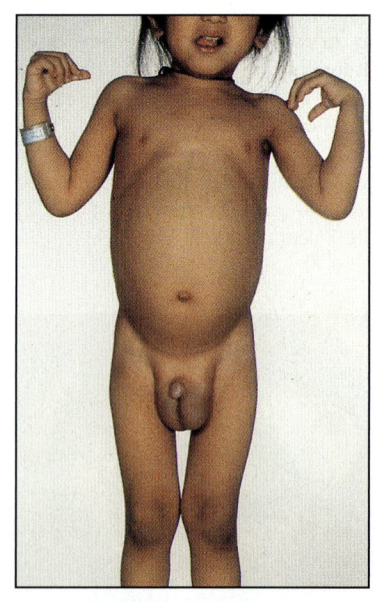

Figure 21.7 Cirrhosis and portal hypertension. (i) Malnutrition with loss of fat and muscle bulk; (ii) distended abdomen from hepatosplenomegaly and ascites; (iii) scrotal swelling from ascites; and (iv) no jaundice, despite advanced liver disease.

Children with compensated cirrhosis may be asymptomatic if liver function is adequate. They will not be jaundiced and may have normal liver function tests. As the cirrhosis increases, however, the results of deteriorating liver function and portal hypertension become obvious. Physical signs include jaundice, palmar (Fig. 21.8) and plantar erythema, telangiectasia and spider naevi (Fig. 21.9), malnutrition, and hypotonia. Dilated abdominal veins and splenomegaly suggest portal hypertension, although the liver may be shrunken and impalpable.

Investigations include:

- screening for the known causes of chronic liver disease
- upper gastrointestinal endoscopy to detect the presence of oesophageal varices and/or erosive gastritis
- abdominal ultrasound – may show a shrunken liver and splenomegaly with gastric and oesophageal varices
- liver biopsy – may be difficult because of increased fibrosis but may indicate the aetiology (e.g. typical changes in congenital hepatic fibrosis, copper storage).

As cirrhosis decompensates, biochemical tests may demonstrate an elevation of aminotransferases and alkaline phosphatase. The plasma albumin falls and the prothrombin time becomes increasingly prolonged.

Oesophageal varices

These are an inevitable consequence of portal hypertension and may develop rapidly in children. They are best diagnosed by upper gastrointestinal endoscopy. Acute bleeding is treated conservatively with blood transfusions and H_2-blockers (e.g. ranitidine) or omeprazole. If bleeding persists, octreotide infusion, vasopressin analogues, endoscopic band ligation, or sclerotherapy may be effective. Portacaval shunts may preclude liver transplantation, but radiological placement of a stent between the hepatic and portal veins can be used as a temporary measure if transplantation is being considered.

Ascites

Ascites is a major problem (Fig. 21.10). The pathophysiology of ascites is uncertain, but contributory factors include hypoalbuminaemia, sodium retention, renal impairment and fluid redistribution. It is treated by sodium and fluid restriction and diuretics. Additional therapy for refractory ascites includes albumin infusions or paracentesis.

Spontaneous bacterial peritonitis

This should always be considered if there is undiagnosed fever, abdominal pain, tenderness, or an

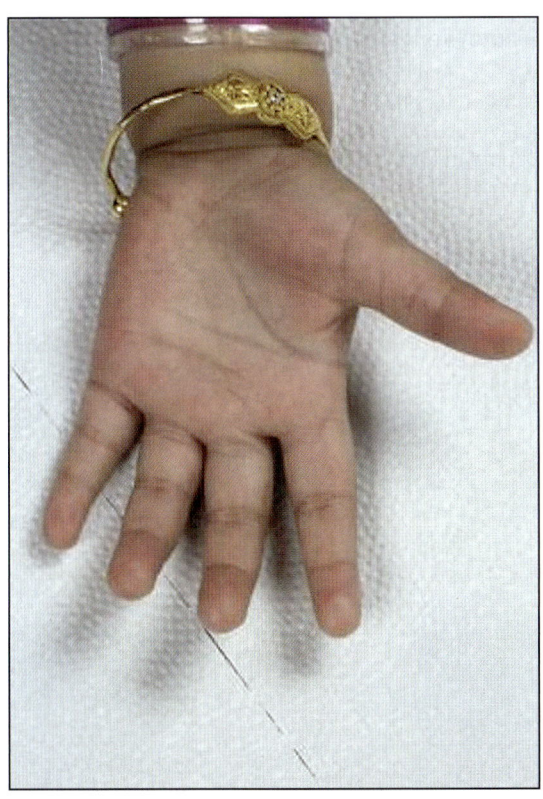

Figure 21.8 Palmar erythema in a child with biliary atresia.

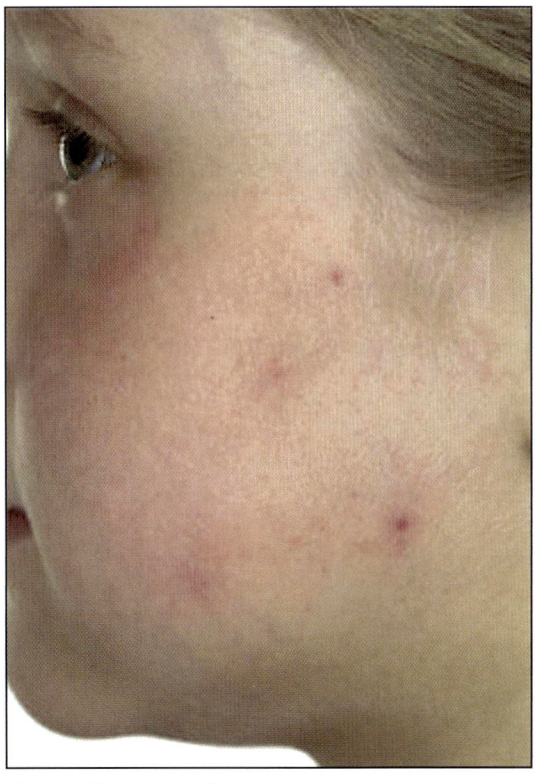

Figure 21.9 Facial telangiectasia, spider naevi, and mild jaundice in a child with progressive familial intrahepatic cholestasis type 2.

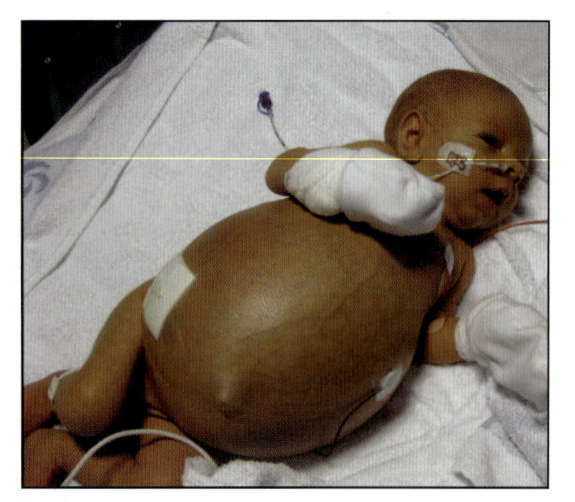

Figure 21.10 Tense ascites in a baby with end stage liver disease.

unexplained deterioration in hepatic or renal function. A diagnostic paracentesis should be performed and the fluid sent for white cell count and differential and culture. Treatment is with broad-spectrum antibiotics.

Renal failure

This may be secondary to renal tubular acidosis, acute tubular necrosis, or functional renal failure (hepatorenal syndrome).

Liver transplantation

Liver transplantation is an accepted therapy for acute or chronic end-stage liver failure and has revolutionized the prognosis for these children. Transplantation is also considered for some hepatic malignancy (hepatoblastoma or hepatocellular carcinoma).

The indications for transplantation in chronic liver failure are:
- severe malnutrition unresponsive to intensive nutritional therapy
- complications refractory to medical management (bleeding varices, resistant ascites)
- failure of growth and development
- poor quality of life.

Liver transplant evaluation includes assessment of the vascular anatomy of the liver and exclusion of irreversible disease in other systems. Absolute contraindications include sepsis, untreatable cardiopulmonary disease or cerebrovascular disease.

There is considerable difficulty in obtaining small organs for children. Most children receive part of an adult's liver, either a cadaveric graft or more recently from a living related donor. A cadaveric organ may either be reduced to fit the child's abdomen (reduction hepatectomy) or split (shared between an adult and child).

Complications post-transplantation include:
- primary non-function of the liver (5%)
- hepatic artery thrombosis (10–20%)
- biliary leaks and strictures (20%)
- rejection (30–60%)
- sepsis, the main cause of death.

In large national centres, the overall 1-year survival is approximately 90%, and the overall 20-year survival is greater than 80%. Most deaths occur in the first 3 months. Children who survive the initial postoperative period usually do well. Long-term studies indicate normal psychosocial development and quality of life in survivors.

Acknowledgements

We would like to acknowledge contributors to this chapter in previous editions, whose work we have drawn on: Deirdre Kelly (1st, 2nd, 3rd Edition), Ulrich Baumann (3rd Edition), Stephen Hodges (4th Edition), Jonathan Bishop (4th Edition).

Further reading

Kelly DA, Bremner R, Hartley JL, Flynn D: *Practical Approach to Pediatric Gastroenterology, Hepatology and Nutrition*, ed 1, 2014, Wiley-Blackwell. *Comprehensive textbook.*

Kelly DA: *Diseases of the Liver and Biliary System in Childhood*, ed 4, Oxford, 2017, Blackwell Science. *A practical handbook*

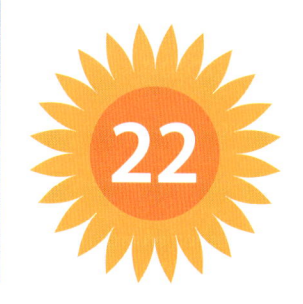

Malignant disease

Aetiology	386	Neuroblastoma	394
Clinical presentation	386	Wilms tumour (nephroblastoma)	395
Investigations	386	Soft tissue sarcomas	396
Treatment	387	Bone tumours	396
Supportive care and side-effects of treatment	388	Retinoblastoma	397
		Kaposi sarcoma	398
Leukaemia	390	Rare tumours	398
Brain tumours	391	Long-term survivors	398
Lymphomas	393	Palliative and end-of-life care	399

Features of malignant disease in children are:

- the pattern of malignant disease varies with age and between continents
- awareness of clinical presentation is important as early diagnosis often optimises outcome
- management is conducted by specialist centres, but in the UK shared care arrangements usually allow supportive care to be provided by hospitals nearer home
- prognosis for many types of malignant disease has improved markedly, but often involves intensive therapy with short and long-term complications.

Cancer in children is not common:

- Around 1 child in 500 develops cancer by 15 years of age.
- Each year, in Western countries, there are 120 to 140 new cases per million children aged under 15 years, equivalent to about 1500 new cases each year in the UK.

The types of disease seen (Fig. 22.1) are very different from those in adults, where carcinomas of the lung, breast, gut, and prostate predominate. The age at presentation varies with the different types of disease:

- leukaemia affects children at all ages (although there is an early childhood peak)
- neuroblastoma and Wilms tumour are almost always seen in the first 6 years of life
- Hodgkin lymphoma and bone tumours have their peak incidence in adolescence and early adult life.

Despite significant improvements in survival over the last four decades (Fig. 22.2), cancer is the most common disease causing death in childhood (beyond the neonatal period). Overall, the 5-year survival of children with all forms of cancer is about 75%, most of whom can be considered cured, although cure rates vary considerably for different diagnoses. This improved life expectancy can be attributed mainly to the introduction of multiagent chemotherapy, supportive care, and specialist multidisciplinary management. However, for some children, the price of survival is long-term medical or psychosocial difficulties.

> For children in the developed world, leukaemia is the most common malignancy followed by brain tumours

% of all childhood cancers in the UK

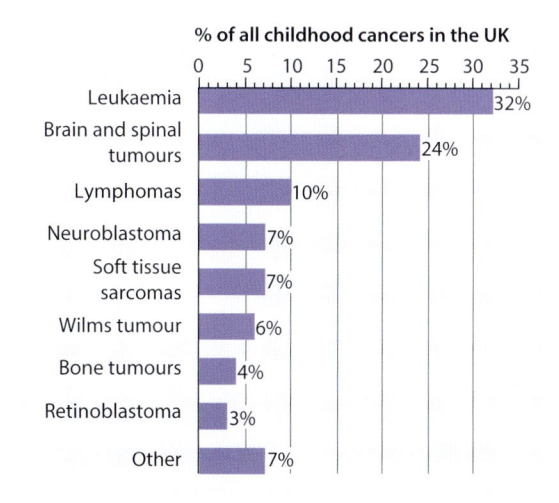

Type	%
Leukaemia	32%
Brain and spinal tumours	24%
Lymphomas	10%
Neuroblastoma	7%
Soft tissue sarcomas	7%
Wilms tumour	6%
Bone tumours	4%
Retinoblastoma	3%
Other	7%

Figure 22.1 Relative frequency of different types of cancer in children in the UK.

Aetiology

In most cases, the aetiology of childhood cancer is unclear, but it is likely to involve an interaction between environmental factors (e.g. viral infection) and host genetic susceptibility. In fact, there are very few established environmental risk factors. Cancer is usually sporadic but may be inherited, although in most cases a specific gene mutation is unknown. One example of an inherited cancer is bilateral retinoblastoma, which is associated with a mutation within the RB gene located on chromosome 13. There are also syndromes associated with an increased risk of cancer in childhood, e.g. associations exist between Down syndrome and leukaemia, and neurofibromatosis and glioma. In time, the further identification of biological characteristics of specific tumour cells may also help elucidate the basic pathogenetic mechanisms behind their origin.

Examples of infection-related childhood cancers are Burkitt lymphoma, Hodgkin lymphoma and nasopharyngeal carcinoma (all associated with Epstein-Barr virus), liver carcinoma (hepatitis B), and Kaposi sarcoma (HIV and human herpes virus 8). Burkitt lymphoma and Kaposi sarcoma are the most common childhood cancers in Africa, but account for a very small proportion of childhood cancer in Western countries (Fig. 22.3).

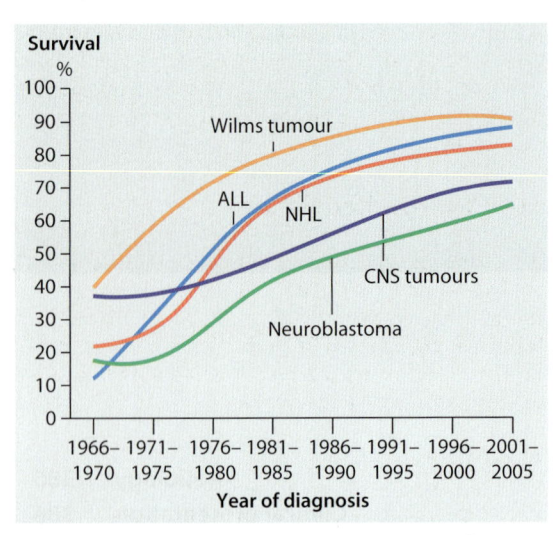

Figure 22.2 Five-year survival rates showing the considerable improvement over the last 50 years. ALL, acute lymphoblastic leukaemia; CNS, central nervous system; NHL, non-Hodgkin lymphoma. (From National Registry of Childhood Tumours, Childhood Cancer Research Group with permission.)

Clinical presentation

Cancer in children can present with:
- a localized mass
- the consequences of disseminated disease, e.g. bone marrow infiltration, causing systemic ill-health
- the consequences of pressure from a mass on local structures or tissue, e.g. airway obstruction secondary to enlarged lymph nodes in the mediastinum.

Investigations

Initial symptoms can be very nonspecific and this can often lead to significant delays in diagnosis. Once a diagnosis of malignancy is suspected, the child should be referred to a specialist centre for further investigation.

Radiology

The location of solid tumours and evidence of any metastases are identified and localised, using a combination of ultrasound, plain X-rays, CT and MRI

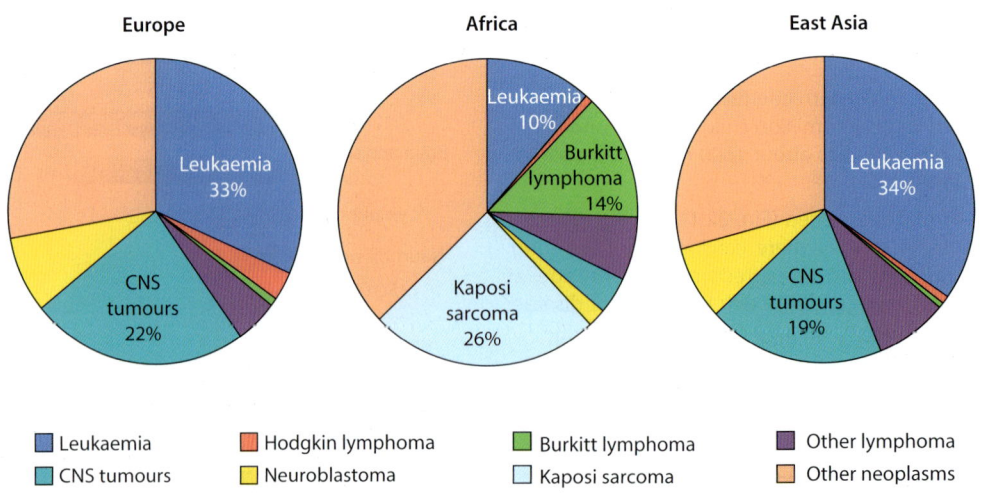

Figure 22.3 International distributions of cancer in children highlighting much higher frequency of Burkitt lymphoma and Kaposi sarcoma in Africa than in Europe or East Asia populations. (Data from Global Cancer Facts and Figures. ed 2, 2011, American Cancer Society.)

scans. Nuclear medicine imaging (e.g. radiolabelled technetium bone scan) may be useful to identify bone or bone marrow disease or, using special markers MIBG scan localise tumours of neural crest origin, e.g. neuroblastoma.

Tumour marker studies

Increased urinary catecholamine excretion (e.g VMA, vanillylmandelic acid, and HVA, homovanillic acid) is useful in confirming the diagnosis of neuroblastoma. High α-fetoprotein (αFP) production is often observed in germ cell tumours and liver tumours and can be used to monitor treatment response.

Pathology

Typically, diagnoses are confirmed histologically, either by bone marrow aspiration for cases of leukaemia or by biopsy for most solid tumours, although this may not always be possible for brain tumours. Histological techniques such as immunohistochemistry are routinely used to differentiate tumour types. Molecular and genetic techniques are also used to confirm diagnosis (e.g. translocation of chromosomes 11 and 22 in Ewing sarcoma) and to predict prognosis (e.g. amplification of the oncogene associated with a poor prognosis in neuroblastoma).

Management

Once malignancy has been diagnosed, the parents and child need to be seen and the diagnosis explained to them in a realistic, yet positive way. Detailed investigation to define the extent of the disease (staging) is paramount to planning treatment. Children are usually treated as part of national and international collaborative studies that offer consistency in care and have contributed to improvements in outcome.

In the UK, children with cancer are initially investigated and treated in specialist centres where experienced multidisciplinary teams can provide the intensive medical and psychosocial support required. Subsequent management is often shared between the specialist centre, referral hospital, and local services within the community, to provide the optimum care with the least disruption to the family.

Teenagers and young adults

Survival statistics suggest that teenagers and young adults have poorer outcomes than children and constitute a distinct population. This relates both to the specific types and biological behaviour of their tumours and to their particular social/psychological needs. This has prompted the development of age-appropriate treatment protocols, facilities, and support networks.

Treatment

Treatment may involve chemotherapy, surgery, or radiotherapy, alone or in combination.

Chemotherapy

Cytotoxic chemotherapy agents target cells that are rapidly proliferating and typically cause cell death by interfering with DNA replication/repair mechanisms, cell division, or metabolic pathways.

Chemotherapy is used:

- as primary curative treatment, e.g. in acute lymphoblastic leukaemia
- to control primary or metastatic disease before definitive local treatment with surgery and/or radiotherapy (neoadjuvant treatment), e.g. in sarcoma or neuroblastoma
- as adjuvant treatment to deal with residual disease and to eliminate presumed micrometastases, e.g. after initial local treatment with surgery in Wilms tumour.

High-dose therapy with stem cell rescue

The limitation of chemotherapy (and radiotherapy) is the risk of irreversible damage to normal tissues, particularly bone marrow. Transplantation of bone marrow stem cells can be used as a strategy to intensify the treatment of patients with the administration of potentially lethal doses of chemotherapy and/or radiation. The source of stem cells may be allogeneic (from a compatible donor) or autologous (from the patient him/herself, harvested beforehand, while the marrow is uninvolved or in remission). Allogeneic transplantation is principally used in the management of high-risk or relapsed leukaemia and autologous stem cell support is used most commonly in the treatment of children with solid tumours whose prognosis is poor using conventional chemotherapy, e.g. high-risk neuroblastoma.

Targeted therapies

A growing understanding of the molecular biology of cancer has led to the increasing development and use of targeted therapies. Examples include:

- tyrosine kinase inhibitors, such as imatinib that targets the BCR-ABL fusion gene that causes Philadelphia chromosome positive (Ph+) acute lymphatic leukaemia and chronic myeloid leukaemia
- monoclonal antibodies, such as rituximab (anti-CD20) for lymphoma and anti-GD2 for treatment of high-risk neuroblastoma.

Radiotherapy

Radiotherapy uses high-energy radiation to kill cancer cells. It is most commonly administered as 'external beam' electron radiotherapy, although there is growing interest in the use of proton beam radiotherapy that may allow the radiation dose to be delivered in a more controlled fashion, reducing the dose to normal adjacent structures. In addition, radiotherapy can be administered as an intravenous medicine (e.g.

radioactive iodine for thyroid cancer or MIBG therapy for high-risk neuroblastoma). Radiotherapy has an important role in the treatment of some tumours, but the risk of damage to growth and function of normal tissue is greater in a child than in an adult. The need for adequate protection of normal tissues and for careful positioning and immobilisation of the patient during treatment raises practical difficulties, particularly in young children. Cranial radiotherapy in children under the age of 3 years is particularly problematic because of the significant risk of severe damage to neurocognitive development.

Surgery

Initial surgery is frequently restricted to biopsy to establish the diagnosis, and more extensive operations are usually undertaken to remove residual tumour after chemotherapy and/or radiotherapy.

Supportive care and side-effects of treatment

Cancer treatment produces frequent, predictable, and often severe multisystem side-effects (Fig. 22.4). Supportive care is an important part of management and improvements in this aspect of cancer care have contributed to the increasing survival rates.

Infection from immunosuppression

Due to both treatment (chemotherapy or wide-field radiation) and underlying disease, children with cancer are immunocompromised and at risk of serious infection. Children with fever and neutropenia must be admitted promptly to hospital for cultures and treatment with broad-spectrum antibiotics. Some important opportunistic infections associated with therapy for cancer include *Pneumocystis jiroveci* (*carinii*) pneumonia (especially in children with leukaemia), disseminated fungal infection (e.g. aspergillosis and candidiasis) and coagulase-negative staphylococcal infections of central venous catheters.

Most common viral infections are no worse in children with cancer than in other children, but measles and varicella zoster (chickenpox) may have atypical presentation and can be life-threatening. If non-immune, immunocompromised children are at risk from contact with measles or varicella, some protection can be afforded by prompt administration of immunoglobulin or zoster immune globulin. Aciclovir is used to treat established varicella infection, but no treatment is available for measles. During chemotherapy and from 6 months to a year subsequently, the use of live vaccines is contraindicated due to depressed immunity. After this period, reimmunisation against common childhood infections is recommended.

> **Fever with neutropenia requires hospital admission, investigation and treatment**

Bone marrow suppression

Anaemia may require blood transfusions. Thrombocytopaenia presents the hazard of bleeding, and considerable blood product support may be required, particularly for children with leukaemia, those undergoing intensive therapy requiring bone marrow transplantation, and in the more intensive solid tumour protocols.

Gastrointestinal damage, nausea and vomiting, and nutritional compromise

Mouth ulcers are common, painful and, when severe, can prevent a child eating adequately. Many chemotherapy agents are nauseating and induce vomiting, which may be only partially prevented by the routine use of antiemetic drugs. These two complications can result in significant nutritional compromise. Chemotherapy-induced gut mucosal damage also causes diarrhoea and may predispose to Gram-negative infection.

Drug-specific side-effects

Many individual drugs have specific side-effects: e.g. cardiotoxicity with doxorubicin; renal failure and deafness with cisplatin; haemorrhagic cystitis with cyclophosphamide; and neuropathy with vincristine. The extent of these side-effects is not always predictable and patients require careful monitoring during, and in some cases, after treatment is complete.

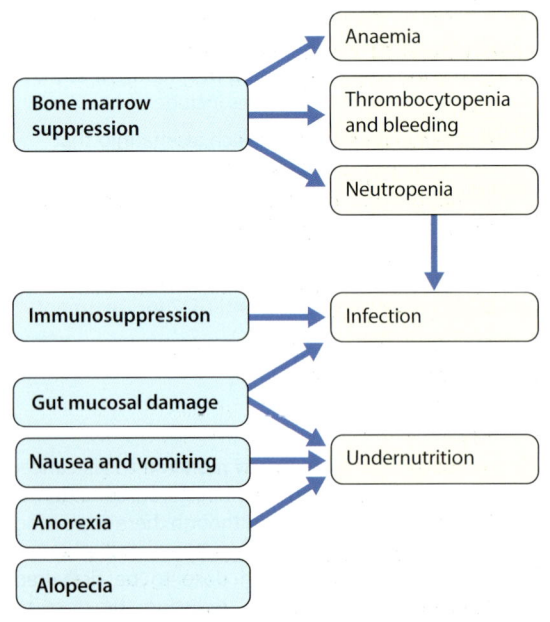

Figure 22.4 Short-term side-effects of chemotherapy.

Other supportive care issues

Fertility preservation
Some patients may be at risk of infertility as a result of their cancer treatment. Appropriate fertility preservation techniques may involve surgically moving a testis or ovary out of the radiotherapy field; sperm banking (which should be offered to boys mature enough to achieve this); and consideration of newer techniques such as cryopreservation of ovarian cortical tissue, although the long-term efficacy of this is still uncertain.

Venous access
The discomfort of multiple venepunctures for blood sampling and intravenous infusions can be avoided with central venous catheters. Different types of catheters are used including tunnelled venous catheters (Hickman lines) and implantable ports. A port is similar to a tunnelled catheter but is left entirely under the skin (Fig. 22.5a and b). Central venous catheters can remain in situ for many months if not years, i.e. the duration of chemotherapy treatment but they carry a risk of infection and can get blocked or split.

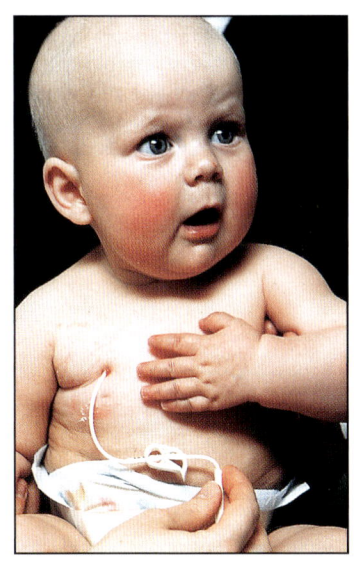

Psychosocial support
The diagnosis of a potentially fatal illness has an enormous and long-lasting impact on the whole family. They need the opportunity to discuss the implications of the diagnosis and its treatment and their anxiety, fear, guilt, and sadness. Most will benefit from the counselling and practical support provided by health professionals. Help with practical issues, including transport, finances, accommodation, and care of siblings, is an early priority. The provision of detailed written material for parents will help them understand their child's disease and treatment. The children themselves, and their siblings, need an age-appropriate explanation of the disease. Once treatment is established and the disease appears to be under control, families should be encouraged to return to as normal a lifestyle as possible. Early return to school is important and children with cancer should not be allowed to under-achieve the expectations previously held for them. It is easy to underestimate the severe stress that persists within families in relation to the uncertainty of the long-term outcome. This often manifests itself as marital problems in parents and behavioural difficulties in both the child and siblings.

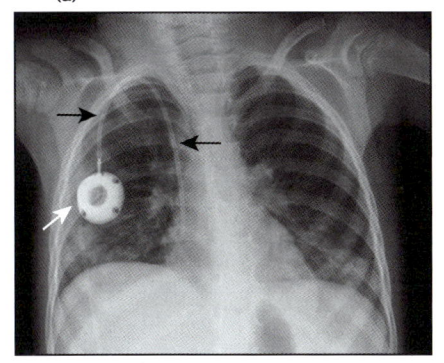

Figure 22.5 (a) A central venous catheter allows pain-free blood tests and injections for this child on chemotherapy, which has caused the alopecia; and (b) a port device visualised on a chest X-ray.

Summary

Malignant disease in children
- Uncommon, but affects 1 in 500 by 15 years of age.
- Can present with a localised mass or its pressure effects or disseminated disease.
- Treatment may involve chemotherapy, surgery, radiotherapy, or high-dose therapy with stem cell rescue.
- Fever with neutropenia must be investigated and treated urgently.
- Measles and varicella zoster infection are potentially life-threatening.
- A multidisciplinary team is required to provide supportive care and psychosocial support.
- Supportive care includes not only management of side-effects but also pain management and fertility preservation.
- Psychosocial support – includes not only the patient and parents but also siblings and other family and community members.

Leukaemia

Acute lymphoblastic leukaemia (ALL) accounts for 80% of leukaemia in children. Most of the remainder is acute myeloid leukaemia/acute nonlymphocytic leukaemia (AML/ANLL). Chronic myeloid leukaemia and other myeloproliferative disorders are rare.

Clinical presentation

Presentation of ALL peaks at 2–5 years of age. Clinical symptoms and signs result from disseminated disease and systemic ill-health from infiltration of the bone marrow or other organs with leukemic blast cells (Fig. 22.6). In most children, leukaemia presents insidiously over several weeks (see Case History 22.1) but in some children the illness presents and progresses very rapidly.

Investigations

In most but not all children, the full blood count is abnormal, with low haemoglobin, thrombocytopenia, and evidence of circulating leukemic blast cells. Bone marrow examination is essential to confirm the diagnosis and to identify immunological and cytogenetic characteristics which give useful prognostic information. A clotting screen should be performed as approximately 10% of patients with acute leukaemia have disseminated intravascular coagulation (DIC) at the time of diagnosis. These patients may present with haemorrhagic or thrombotic complications. A lumbar puncture is performed to identify disease in the CSF. Chest X-ray is required to identify a mediastinal mass characteristic of T-cell disease.

Both ALL and AML are classified by morphology. Immunological phenotyping further subclassifies ALL; the common (75%) and T-cell (15%) subtypes are the most common. Prognosis and some aspects of clinical presentation vary according to different subtypes, and treatment intensity is adjusted accordingly.

Management of acute lymphoblastic leukaemia

A number of factors contribute to prognosis in ALL including patient age, white cell count at presentation, cytogenetics of the leukemic cells, and response to treatment. The intensity of therapy is adapted according to risk (Table 22.1).

Remission induction

Before starting treatment of the disease, anaemia may require correction with blood transfusion, the risk of bleeding minimised by transfusion of platelets, and infection must be treated. Additional hydration and allopurinol (or urate oxidase when the white cell count is high and the risk is greater) are given to protect renal function against the effects of rapid cell lysis. Remission implies eradication of the leukemic blasts and restoration of normal marrow function. Combination chemotherapy including steroids is given and current induction treatment schedules achieve remission rates of 95%.

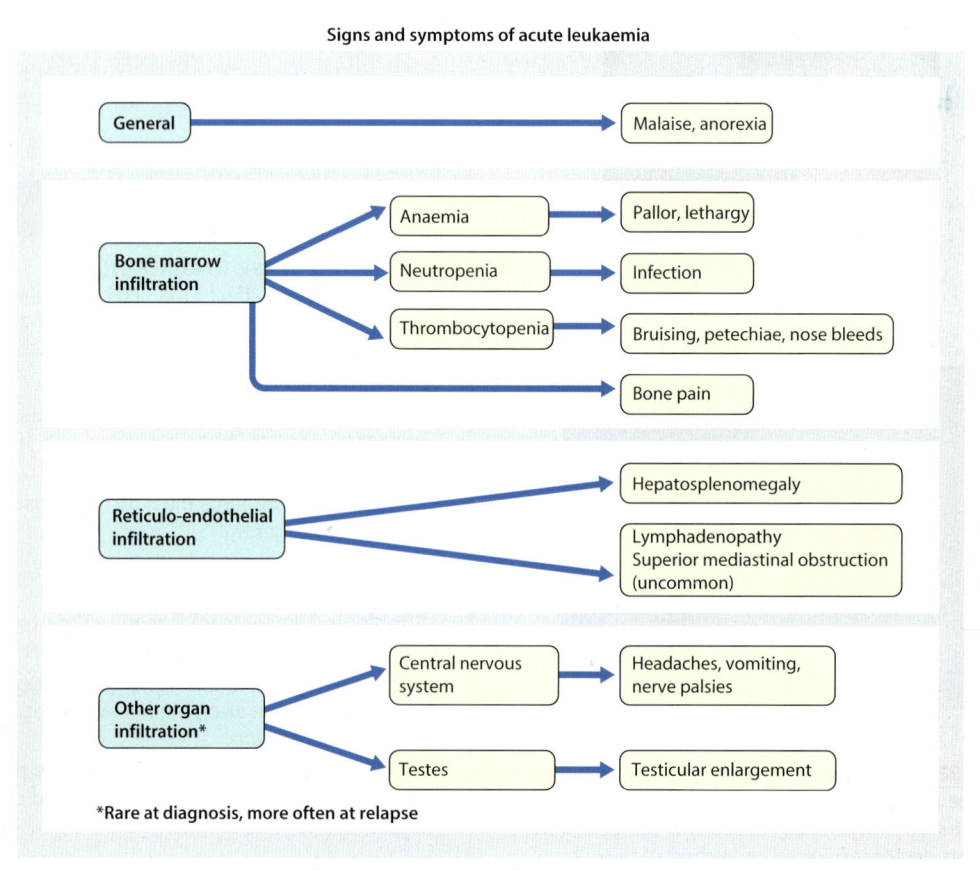

Signs and symptoms of acute leukaemia

- General → Malaise, anorexia
- Bone marrow infiltration
  - Anaemia → Pallor, lethargy
  - Neutropenia → Infection
  - Thrombocytopenia → Bruising, petechiae, nose bleeds
  - Bone pain
- Reticulo-endothelial infiltration
  - Hepatosplenomegaly
  - Lymphadenopathy / Superior mediastinal obstruction (uncommon)
- Other organ infiltration*
  - Central nervous system → Headaches, vomiting, nerve palsies
  - Testes → Testicular enlargement

*Rare at diagnosis, more often at relapse

Figure 22.6 Signs and symptoms of acute leukaemia.

Case history 22.1

Disseminated disease, e.g. bone marrow infiltration, causing systemic ill-health

A 4-year-old girl was generally unwell, lethargic, looking pale, and occasionally febrile over a period of 9 weeks. Two courses of antibiotics for recurrent sore throat failed to result in any benefit. Her parents returned to their general practitioner when she developed a rash. Examination showed pallor, petechiae, modest generalised lymphadenopathy, and mild hepatosplenomegaly. A full blood count showed:

- Haemoglobin 83 g/L
- White blood cells 15.6×10^9/L
- Platelets 44×10^9/L.

Blast cells were seen on the peripheral blood film. CSF examination was normal. Bone marrow examination confirmed acute lymphoblastic leukaemia (Fig. 22.7).

Diagnosis: Acute lymphoblastic leukaemia.

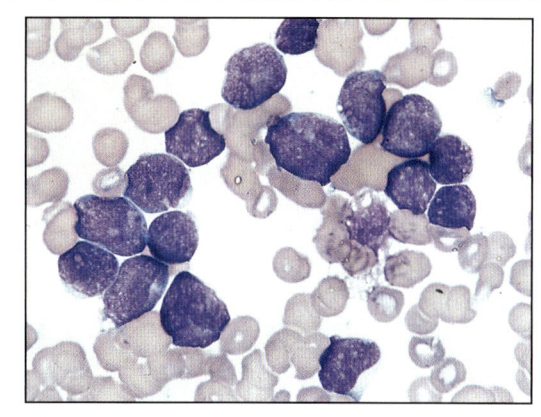

Figure 22.7 Leukemic blast cells on a bone marrow smear.

Table 22.1 Prognostic factors in acute lymphatic leukaemia

Prognostic factor	High-risk features
Age	<1 year or >10 years
Tumour load (measured by the white cell count)	$>50 \times 10^9$/L
Cytogenetic/molecular genetic abnormalities in tumour cells	e.g. MLL rearrangement, t(4;11) hypodiploidy (<44 chromosomes)
Speed of response to initial chemotherapy	Persistence of leukemic blasts in the bone marrow
Minimal residual disease (MRD) assessment (submicroscopic levels of leukaemia detected by PCR)	Detectable MRD after induction therapy

Intensification
A block of intensive chemotherapy is given to consolidate remission. This improves cure rates but at the expense of increased toxicity.

Central nervous system
Cytotoxic drugs penetrate poorly into the central nervous system (CNS). As leukemic cells in this site may survive effective systemic treatment, treatment with intrathecal chemotherapy is used to prevent CNS relapse. Patients with evidence of CNS disease at diagnosis receive additional doses of intrathecal chemotherapy during induction.

Continuing therapy
Chemotherapy of modest intensity is continued over a relatively long period of time, up to 3 years from diagnosis. Cotrimoxazole prophylaxis is given routinely to prevent *Pneumocystis* pneumonia.

Treatment of relapse
High-dose chemotherapy, with or without total body irradiation followed by bone marrow transplantation, is used as an alternative to conventional chemotherapy after a relapse.

Brain tumours

In contrast to adults, brain tumours in children are almost always primary rather than metastatic and 60% are infratentorial (located below the tentorium cerebelli). They are the most common solid tumour in children and are the leading cause of childhood cancer deaths in the UK. Types of brain tumour in children (Fig. 22.8) include

- Astrocytoma (~40%) – varies from benign to highly malignant (*glioblastoma multiforme*).
- Medulloblastoma (~20%) – arises in the midline of the posterior fossa. May seed through the CNS via the CSF and up to 20% have spinal metastases at diagnosis.
- Ependymoma (~8%) – mostly in posterior fossa where it behaves like medulloblastoma.
- Brainstem glioma (6%) – malignant tumours associated with a very poor prognosis.
- Craniopharyngioma (4%) – a developmental tumour arising from the squamous remnant of Rathke pouch. It is not truly malignant but is locally invasive and grows slowly in the suprasellar region.
- Atypical teratoid/rhabdoid tumour – a rare type of aggressive tumour that most commonly occurs in young children.

Brain tumours – sites, presentation and typical case histories

Supratentorial:
- Cortex – astrocytoma

Midline:
- Craniopharyngioma

Infratentorial:
- Cerebellar – medulloblastoma, astrocytoma, ependymoma
- Brainstem – brainstem glioma

Spinal cord:
- Astrocytoma, ependymoma

(a)

Clinical presentation

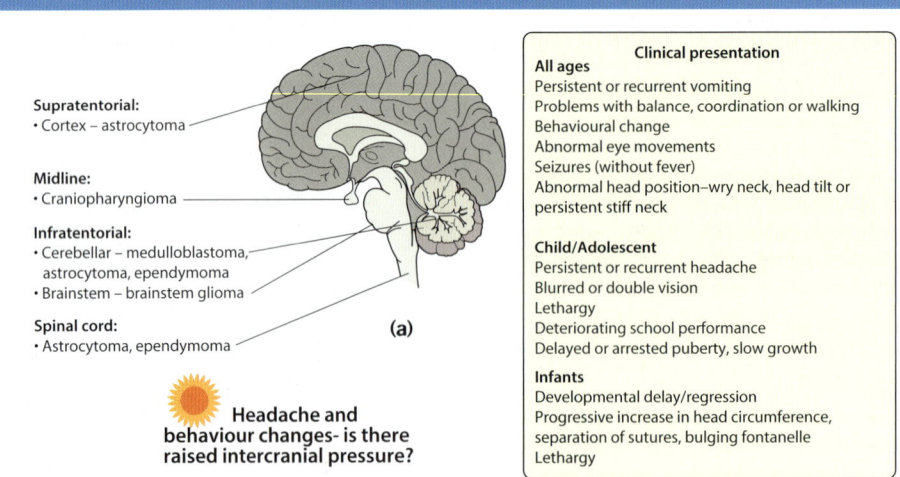

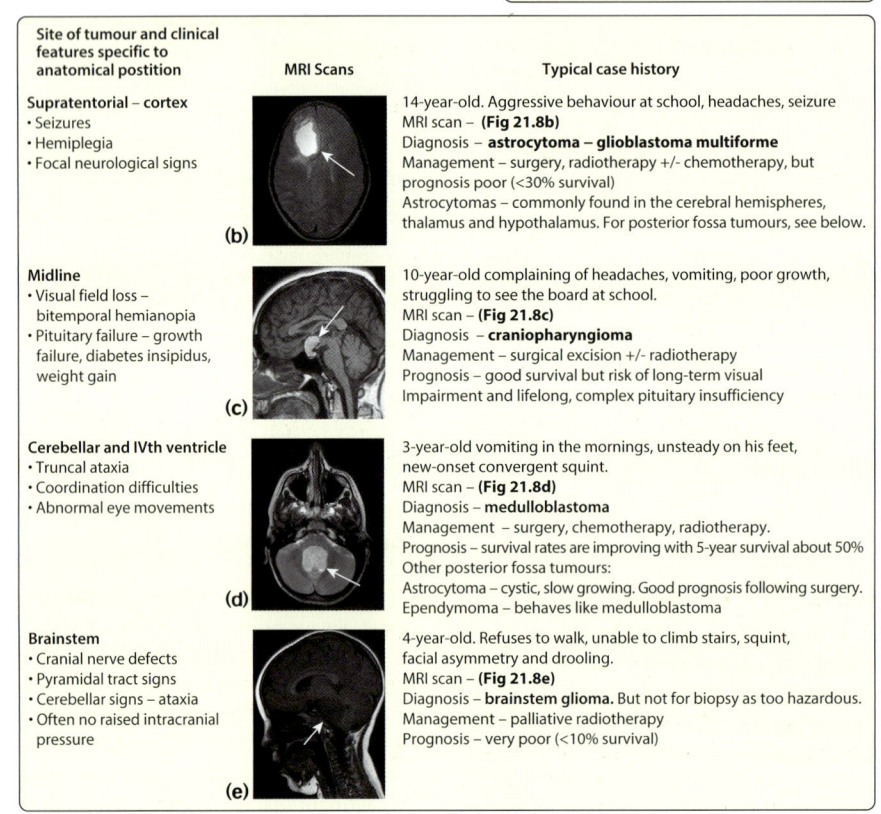

All ages
Persistent or recurrent vomiting
Problems with balance, coordination or walking
Behavioural change
Abnormal eye movements
Seizures (without fever)
Abnormal head position–wry neck, head tilt or persistent stiff neck

Child/Adolescent
Persistent or recurrent headache
Blurred or double vision
Lethargy
Deteriorating school performance
Delayed or arrested puberty, slow growth

Infants
Developmental delay/regression
Progressive increase in head circumference, separation of sutures, bulging fontanelle
Lethargy

☀ Headache and behaviour changes- is there raised intercranial pressure?

Site of tumour and clinical features specific to anatomical position	MRI Scans	Typical case history
Supratentorial – cortex • Seizures • Hemiplegia • Focal neurological signs	(b)	14-year-old. Aggressive behaviour at school, headaches, seizure MRI scan – **(Fig 21.8b)** Diagnosis – **astrocytoma – glioblastoma multiforme** Management – surgery, radiotherapy +/- chemotherapy, but prognosis poor (<30% survival) Astrocytomas – commonly found in the cerebral hemispheres, thalamus and hypothalamus. For posterior fossa tumours, see below.
Midline • Visual field loss – bitemporal hemianopia • Pituitary failure – growth failure, diabetes insipidus, weight gain	(c)	10-year-old complaining of headaches, vomiting, poor growth, struggling to see the board at school. MRI scan – **(Fig 21.8c)** Diagnosis – **craniopharyngioma** Management – surgical excision +/- radiotherapy Prognosis – good survival but risk of long-term visual Impairment and lifelong, complex pituitary insufficiency
Cerebellar and IVth ventricle • Truncal ataxia • Coordination difficulties • Abnormal eye movements	(d)	3-year-old vomiting in the mornings, unsteady on his feet, new-onset convergent squint. MRI scan – **(Fig 21.8d)** Diagnosis – **medulloblastoma** Management – surgery, chemotherapy, radiotherapy. Prognosis – survival rates are improving with 5-year survival about 50% Other posterior fossa tumours: Astrocytoma – cystic, slow growing. Good prognosis following surgery. Ependymoma – behaves like medulloblastoma
Brainstem • Cranial nerve defects • Pyramidal tract signs • Cerebellar signs – ataxia • Often no raised intracranial pressure	(e)	4-year-old. Refuses to walk, unable to climb stairs, squint, facial asymmetry and drooling. MRI scan – **(Fig 21.8e)** Diagnosis – **brainstem glioma.** But not for biopsy as too hazardous. Management – palliative radiotherapy Prognosis – very poor (<10% survival)

Figure 22.8 (a) Location of brain tumours. Clinical features of brain tumours. MRI scans showing **(b)** fronto-parietal mass; **(c)** large midline suprasellar mass; **(d)** cerebellar mass; and **(e)** brainstem mass.

Clinical features

The developmental age of the child is important as presentation varies according to age and their ability to report symptoms (see 'Brain tumours – clinical presentation'). Signs and symptoms are often related to evidence of raised intracranial pressure but focal neurological signs may be detected depending on the site of the tumour. Papilloedema may be present, but can be a late sign and difficult to detect.

Spinal tumours, primary or metastatic, can present with back pain, peripheral weakness of arms or legs, or bladder/bowel dysfunction, depending on the level of the lesion.

☀ **Persistent back pain in children warrants investigation with MRI scan**

Investigations

Brain tumours are best characterised on MRI scan. Magnetic resonance spectroscopy can be used to examine the biological activity of a tumour. Some tumour types can metastasize within the CSF and a lumbar puncture is therefore required for complete staging of the disease. Lumbar puncture must not be performed without neurosurgical advice if there is any suspicion of raised intracranial pressure.

Management
Surgery is usually the first treatment and is aimed at treating hydrocephalus, providing a tissue diagnosis and attempting maximum resection. In some cases the anatomical position of the tumour means biopsy is not safe, e.g. tumours in the brainstem and optic pathway. Even tumours which are histologically 'benign' can threaten survival. The use of radiotherapy and/or chemotherapy varies with tumour type and the age of the patient.

Late effects
The functional implications of the site of the tumour, the potential hazards of surgery and the importance of radiotherapy in treatment all combine to place children with brain tumours at particular risk of neurological disability and of growth, endocrine, neuropsychological, and educational problems. Survivors may present complex combinations of these problems.

Lymphomas

Lymphomas are malignancies of the cells of the immune system and can be divided into Hodgkin and non-Hodgkin lymphoma (NHL). NHL is more common in childhood, while Hodgkin lymphoma is seen more frequently in adolescence.

Hodgkin lymphoma

Clinical features
Classically presents with painless lymphadenopathy, most frequently in the neck. Lymph nodes are much larger and firmer than the benign lymphadenopathy commonly seen in young children. The lymph nodes may cause airways obstruction (see Case History 22.2). The clinical history is often long (several months) and systemic symptoms (sweating, pruritus, weight loss and fever – the so-called 'B' symptoms) are uncommon, even in more advanced disease.

Investigations
Lymph node biopsy, radiological assessment of all nodal sites and bone marrow biopsy is used to stage disease and determine treatment.

Management
Combination chemotherapy with or without radiotherapy. Positron emission tomography (PET) scanning is used in the UK to monitor treatment response and guide further management (Fig. 22.9).

Overall, about 80% of all patients can be cured. Even with disseminated disease, about 60% can be cured.

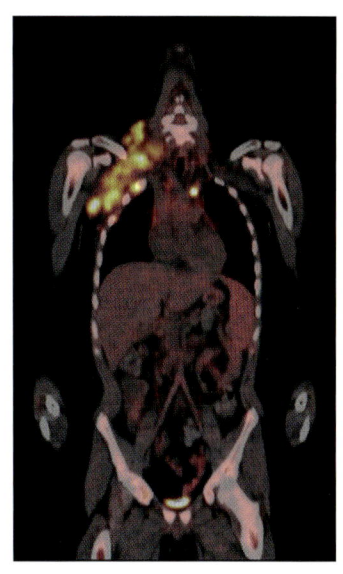

Figure 22.9 PET scan showing active disease in Hodgkin lymphoma in the right cervical and axillary nodes.

Non-Hodgkin lymphoma

T-cell malignancies may present as acute lymphoblastic leukaemia or non-Hodgkin lymphoma, with both being characterised by a mediastinal mass with varying degrees of bone marrow infiltration. The mediastinal mass may cause superior vena cava obstruction presenting with dyspnoea, facial swelling and flushing, venous distention in the neck, and distended veins in the upper chest and arms. B-cell malignancies present more commonly as non-Hodgkin lymphoma, with localised lymph node disease usually in the head and neck or abdomen. Abdominal disease presents with pain from intestinal obstruction, a palpable mass or even intussusception in cases with involvement of the ileum.

Investigations
Biopsy, radiological assessment of all nodal sites (CT or MRI), and examination of the bone marrow and CSF.

Management
Multiagent chemotherapy. The majority of patients now do well and survival rates of over 80% are expected for both T-cell and B-cell disease.

Burkitt lymphoma

Burkitt lymphoma is a type of B-cell non-Hodgkin lymphoma and has three variants. The **endemic variant** most commonly occurs in children living in malaria endemic regions of the world and is the most common childhood cancer in Africa. Epstein–Barr virus (EBV) infection is found in nearly all patients as chronic malaria is believed to reduce resistance to EBV, allowing it to take hold. The disease characteristically involves the jaw or other facial bone (Fig. 22.11) and it is not uncommon for patients to present with advanced stage disease. In the Western world cases

Case history 22.2

Pressure from a mass on local structures or tissue, e.g. airway obstruction secondary to enlarged lymph nodes

A 14-year-old girl complained of a cough for 2 weeks which was non-productive and worse at night. She had seen her general practitioner and her chest was clear. She returned 2 weeks later, as she had noticed a swelling in her neck. On examination, she had a large anterior cervical lymph node which was non-tender. On referral to hospital, she had a chest X-ray, which showed a large mediastinal mass (Fig. 22.10).

Differential diagnosis
- T-cell non-Hodgkin lymphoma/acute leukaemia
- Hodgkin lymphoma

Her full blood count was normal. A biopsy of the mass was consistent with a diagnosis of Hodgkin lymphoma.

Diagnosis: Hodgkin lymphoma.

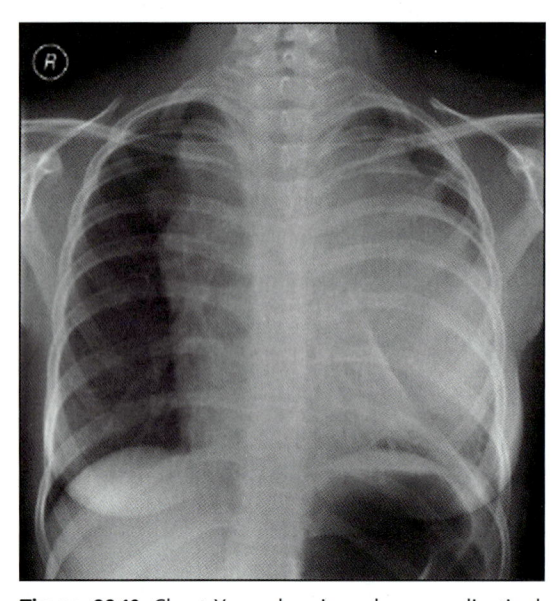

Figure 22.10 Chest X-ray showing a large mediastinal mass.

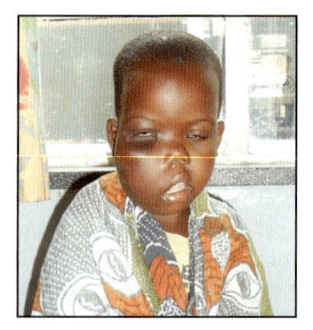

Figure 22.11 Burkitt lymphoma involving facial bones. (Courtesy of Liz Molyneux.)

are **sporadic** and can be associated with EBV infection. **Immunodeficiency-associated** Burkitt lymphoma is usually associated with HIV infection or occurs in patients on immunosuppression post-transplant. Treatment is with multiagent chemotherapy.

Neuroblastoma

Neuroblastoma and related tumours arise from neural crest tissue in the adrenal medulla and sympathetic nervous system. It is a biologically unusual tumour in that spontaneous regression sometimes occurs in very young infants. There is a spectrum of disease from the benign (ganglioneuroma) to the highly malignant (neuroblastoma). Neuroblastoma is most common before the age of 5 years.

Clinical features

At presentation (Box 22.1), most children have an abdominal mass, but the primary tumour can lie anywhere along the sympathetic chain from the neck to the pelvis. Classically, the abdominal primary is of adrenal origin, but at presentation the tumour mass is often large and complex, crossing the midline and enveloping major blood vessels and lymph nodes. Paravertebral tumours may invade through the adjacent intervertebral foramen and cause spinal cord compression requiring emergency intervention to prevent devastating long-term neurological damage. Over the age of 2 years, clinical symptoms are mostly from metastatic disease, particularly bone pain, bone marrow suppression causing weight loss, and malaise (see Case History 22.3).

Investigations

Characteristic clinical and radiological features with raised urinary catecholamine metabolite levels (VMA/HVA) suggest neuroblastoma. Confirmatory biopsy is usually obtained and evidence of metastatic disease detected with bone marrow sampling and MIBG scan (as in Fig. 22.13).

Age and stage of disease at diagnosis are the major factors which influence prognosis. Unfortunately, the majority of children over 1 year present with advanced disease and have a poor prognosis. Increasingly,

Box 22.1 Presentation of neuroblastoma

Common	Less common
Pallor	Paraplegia
Weight loss	Cervical lymphadenopathy
Abdominal mass	Proptosis
Hepatomegaly	Periorbital bruising
Bone pain	Skin nodules
Limp	

Case history 22.3

Neuroblastoma

Jack, a 3-year-old boy, was taken to his general practitioner by his mother because he was not eating as well as usual and had a distended abdomen. Recently, he appeared reluctant to walk and sometimes cried when he was picked up. His grandmother thought he had lost weight. On examination, the general practitioner confirmed that he seemed generally miserable and pale. He was concerned to note a large abdominal mass. Urgent referral to his local hospital was made and, on arrival, he was also noted to be hypertensive.

Differential diagnosis and specific investigations

An initial ultrasound examination confirmed the abdominal mass and an MRI scan characterised a very large upper abdominal mass in complex relationship with the left kidney and the major vessels but extending towards the midline, suggestive of neuroblastoma (Fig. 22.12). Subsequent investigations confirmed bone marrow infiltration by tumour cells and a positive MIBG scan showing uptake at the primary and distant sites consistent with metastatic disease (Fig. 22.13).

Diagnosis: Metastatic neuroblastoma.

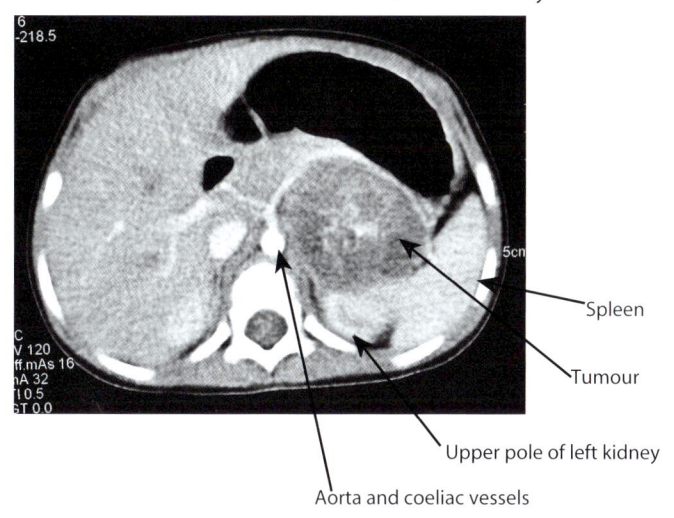

Figure 22.12 Transverse MRI image showing a large left-sided primary neuroblastoma arising from the adrenal region and distorting coeliac and mesenteric blood vessels.

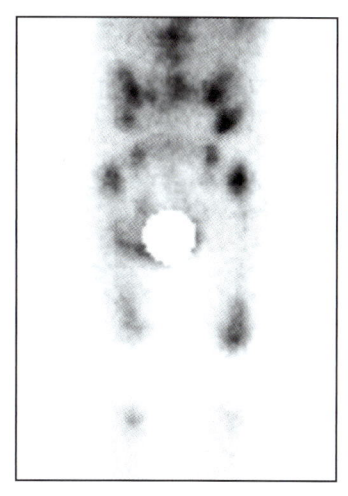

Figure 22.13 The MIBG scan 'maps' metastatic tumour marrow. This image shows the lower half of the abdomen, pelvis, and legs. The dark areas are evidence of high isotope uptake and the pattern is consistent with widespread metastatic disease. (Normal uptake from excretion of isotope into urine in the bladder has been blocked in this exposure.)

---

information about the biological characteristics of neuroblastoma is being used to guide therapy and prognosis. Amplification of the *MYCN* oncogene predicts aggressive behaviour of the tumour and evidence of deletion or gain of genetic material on part of one or more chromosomes (as compared with a change in the number of copies of whole chromosomes) is also associated with a poorer prognosis.

Management

Localised primaries without metastatic disease can often be cured with surgery alone and in some infants neuroblastoma (including when metastatic) may resolve spontaneously.

Metastatic disease in older children is treated with chemotherapy, including high-dose therapy with autologous stem cell rescue, surgery, and radiotherapy. Risk of relapse is high and the prospect of cure for children with metastatic disease is still little better than 40%. Immunotherapy and the use of 'maintenance' treatment with differentiating agents (retinoic acid) are now establishing a role in those with high-risk disease.

Wilms tumour (nephroblastoma)

Wilms tumour originates from embryonal renal tissue and is the most common renal tumour of childhood. Over 80% of patients present before 5 years of age and it is very rarely seen after 10 years of age.

Clinical features

Most children present with a large abdominal mass, often found incidentally in an otherwise well child. Other clinical features are listed in Box 22.2.

Box 22.2 Presentation of Wilms tumour

Common	Less common
Abdominal mass	Abdominal pain
Haematuria	Anorexia
	Anaemia (haemorrhage into mass)
	Hypertension

Investigations

Ultrasound and/or CT/MRI (Fig. 22.14) is usually characteristic, showing an intrinsic renal mass distorting the normal structure. Staging is to assess for distant metastases (usually in the lung), initial tumour resectability and function of the contralateral kidney.

Management

In the UK, children receive initial chemotherapy followed by delayed nephrectomy, after which the tumour is staged histologically and subsequent treatment is planned according to the surgical and pathological findings. Radiotherapy is restricted to those with more advanced disease. Around 5% of patients have bilateral disease at diagnosis and require particularly careful management in order to preserve as much renal function as possible.

Prognosis is good, with more than 80% of all patients cured. Cure rate for patients with metastatic disease at presentation (~15%) is over 60%, but relapse carries a poor prognosis.

Soft tissue sarcomas

Sarcomas are cancers of connective tissue such as muscle or bone. Rhabdomyosarcoma is the most common form of soft tissue sarcoma in childhood. The tumour is thought to originate from primitive mesenchymal tissue and there are a wide variety of primary sites, resulting in varying presentations and prognosis.

Clinical features

Head and neck are the most common sites of disease (40%), causing, e.g. proptosis, nasal obstruction, or bloodstained nasal discharge.

Genitourinary tumours may involve the bladder, paratesticular structures, or the female genitourinary tract. Symptoms include dysuria and urinary obstruction, scrotal mass, or bloodstained vaginal discharge.

Metastatic disease (lung, liver, bone, or bone marrow) is present in approximately 15% of patients at diagnosis and is associated with a particularly poor prognosis.

Investigations

Biopsy and full radiological assessment of primary disease and any evidence of metastasis (Fig. 22.15).

Management

Multimodality treatment (chemotherapy, surgery, and radiotherapy) is used, dependent on the age of the patient and the site, size, and extent of disease. The tumour margins are deceptively ill-defined, and attempts at primary surgical excision are often unsuccessful and are not attempted unless this can be achieved without mutilation or irreversible organ damage. Overall cure rates are about 65%.

Bone tumours

Malignant bone tumours are uncommon before puberty. Osteosarcoma is more common than Ewing sarcoma, but Ewing sarcoma is seen more often in younger children. Both have a male predominance.

Clinical features

The limbs are the most common site. Persistent localised bone pain is the characteristic symptom, usually preceding the detection of a mass, and is an indication for early X-ray. At diagnosis, most patients are otherwise well.

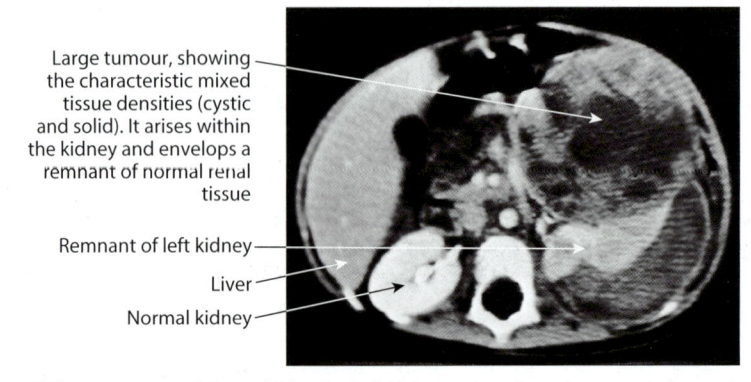

Figure 22.14 Large Wilms tumour arising within the left kidney, showing characteristic cystic and solid tissue densities.

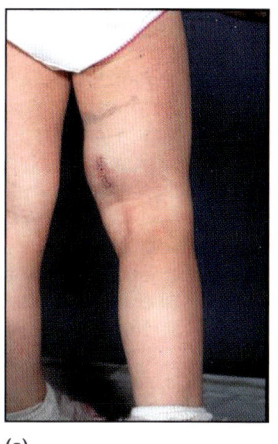

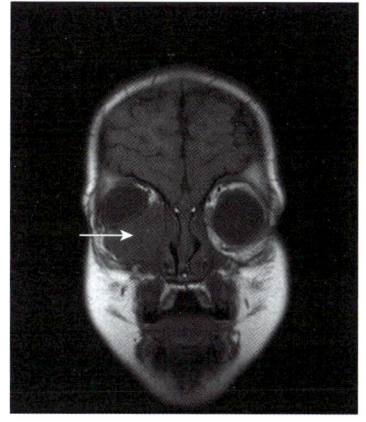

Figure 22.15 Rhabdomyosarcoma. (a) Soft tissue mass of lower limb. The scar is from a biopsy. (b) MRI scan of a child presenting with proptosis of the right eye. It shows a right periorbital soft tissue mass displacing the globe and compressing other orbital structures. Histology confirmed the diagnosis of rhabdomyosarcoma.

Investigations

Plain X-ray is followed by MRI and bone scan (Fig. 22.16a–c). A bone X-ray shows destruction and variable periosteal new bone formation. In Ewing sarcoma, there is often a substantial soft tissue mass. Chest CT is used to assess for lung metastases and bone marrow sampling to exclude marrow involvement.

Management

In both tumours, treatment involves the use of combination chemotherapy given before surgery. Whenever possible, amputation is avoided by using *en bloc* resection of tumours with endoprosthetic resection (Fig. 22.16d). In Ewing sarcoma, radiotherapy is also used in the management of local disease, especially when surgical resection is impossible or incomplete, e.g. in the pelvis or axial skeleton.

Retinoblastoma

Retinoblastoma is a malignant tumour of retinal cells and, although rare, it accounts for about 5% of severe visual impairment in children. It may affect one or both eyes. All bilateral tumours are hereditary, as are about 20% of unilateral cases. The retinoblastoma susceptibility gene is on chromosome 13, and the pattern of inheritance is dominant, but with incomplete penetrance. Most children present within the first 3 years of life. Children from families with the hereditary form of the disease should be screened regularly from birth.

Clinical features

The most common presentation of unsuspected disease is when a white pupillary reflex is noted to replace the normal red one (Fig. 22.17) or with a squint.

Investigations

MRI and examination under anaesthetic. Tumours are frequently multifocal.

Treatment

The aim is to cure, yet preserve vision. Biopsy is not undertaken and treatment is based on the

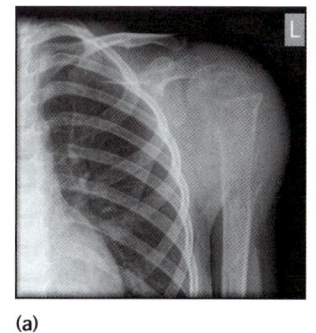

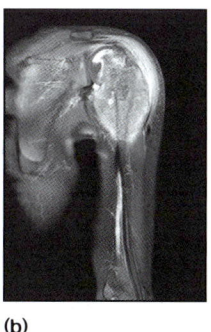

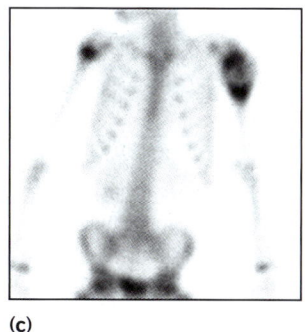

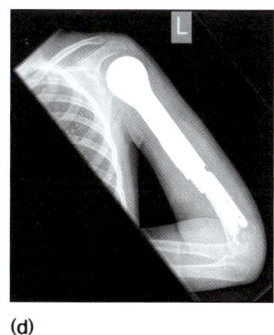

Figure 22.16 Ewing sarcoma of the humerus. (a) Plain X-ray shows a destructive bone lesion within the proximal humeral metaphysis; (b) MRI shows a large destructive soft tissue mass arising from the proximal metadiaphysis of the left humerus; (c) bone scan shows prominent abnormal tracer uptake in the proximal left humerus; and (d) postsurgery, most of the humerus has been resected and replaced by a metallic prosthesis.

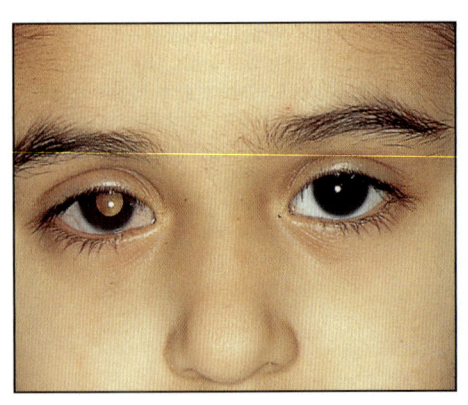

Figure 22.17 White pupillary reflex in retinoblastoma.

ophthalmological findings. Enucleation of the eye may be necessary for more advanced disease. Chemotherapy is used, particularly in bilateral disease, to shrink the tumour(s), followed by local laser treatment to the retina. Radiotherapy may be used in advanced disease, but it is more often reserved for the treatment of recurrence. Most patients are cured, although many are visually impaired. There is a significant risk of second malignancy (especially sarcoma) among survivors of hereditary retinoblastoma.

Kaposi sarcoma

Kaposi sarcoma is a low-grade cancer that arises from the cells of the blood or lymph vessels and is triggered by human herpes virus-8. Although very rare in children in the UK, the prevalence of HIV infection in sub-Saharan Africa means that it is one of the most common paediatric malignancies in this region. Whilst adults typically present with a purple/brown skin rash, these appearances are less common in children who may have only generalised lymphadenopathy suggestive of lymphoma. Diagnosis requires biopsy confirmation. Treatment involves a combination of chemotherapy and antiretroviral therapy.

Rare tumours

Liver tumours

Primary malignant liver tumours are mostly hepatoblastoma (65%) or hepatocellular carcinoma (25%). Presentation is usually with abdominal distension or with a mass. Pain and jaundice are rare. Elevated serum αFP is detected in nearly all cases of hepatoblastoma and in some cases of hepatocellular carcinoma. Management includes chemotherapy, surgery and, in inoperable cases, liver transplantation is required. The majority of children with hepatoblastoma can now be cured, but the prognosis for children with hepatocellular carcinoma is less satisfactory.

Germ cell tumours

Germ cell tumours (GCTs) may be benign or malignant. They arise from the primitive germ cells which migrate from yolk sac endoderm to form gonads in the embryo. Benign tumours are most common in the sacrococcygeal region, and most malignant germ cell tumours are found in the gonads. Serum markers (αFP and β-HCG) are invaluable in confirming the diagnosis and in monitoring response to treatment. Malignant germ cell tumours are very sensitive to chemotherapy, and a very good outcome can be expected for disease at most sites, including the brain.

Langerhans cell histiocytosis

Langerhans cell histiocytosis (LCH) is a rare disorder characterised by an abnormal proliferation of histiocytes (a type of dendritic antigen presenting cells). Whether it truly represents a malignancy remains uncertain, however its sometimes aggressive behaviour and its response to chemotherapy place it within the practice of oncologists. Clinically, its manifestations include:

- bone lesions – present at any age with pain, swelling, or even fracture. X-ray reveals a characteristic lytic lesion with a well-defined border, often involving the skull (Fig. 22.18)
- diabetes insipidus – may be associated with skull disease with proptosis and hypothalamic infiltration
- systemic LCH – the most aggressive form which tends to present in infancy with a seborrhoeic rash (Fig. 22.19) and soft tissue involvement of the gums, ears, lungs, liver, spleen, lymph nodes, and bone marrow. This form of LCH is usually progressive and requires chemotherapy, although spontaneous regression may occur.

The prognosis is variable, but most patients are cured.

Long-term survivors

Improved survival rates means an ever-increasing population of adult survivors of childhood cancer. Over half have at least one residual problem as a consequence of either the disease or its treatment (Table 22.2).

All survivors need regular long-term follow-up to provide appropriate treatment or advice. This need for specialist multidisciplinary follow-up continues into adulthood, and its provision presents a challenge within adult healthcare services. Until recently, the majority of survivors have remained under the care of paediatric oncologists, although specialist adult clinics are being established. Some survivors will require specific counselling for problems such as poor or asymmetric growth, infertility and sexual dysfunction, and advances in the use of adult growth hormone. Assisted reproductive technology has enhanced the lives of many patients. The risk of second cancer is small, but nevertheless survivors are at increased risk and this may rise with increasing survival rates. When new treatment protocols

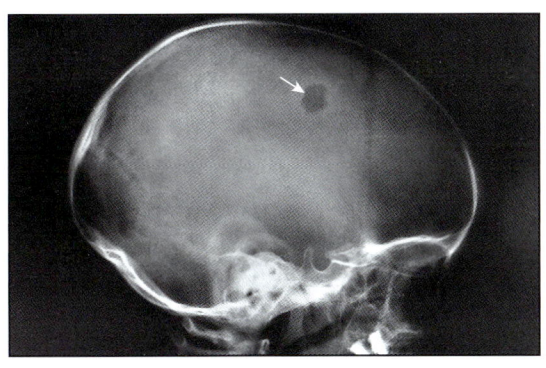

Figure 22.18 Lytic bone lesions on a skull X-ray in Langerhans cell histiocytosis.

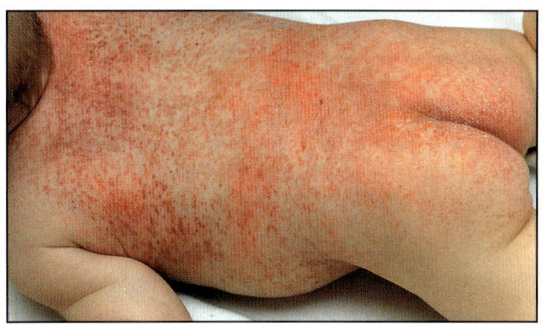

Figure 22.19 Rash in systemic Langerhans cell histiocytosis. It is often mistaken for seborrhoeic dermatitis or eczema.

Table 22.2 Some problems that may occur following cure of childhood cancer

Problem	Cause
Specific organ dysfunction	Nephrectomy for Wilms tumour
	Toxicity from chemotherapy, e.g. renal from cisplatin or ifosfamide, cardiac from doxorubicin or mediastinal radiotherapy
Growth/endocrine problems	Growth hormone deficiency from pituitary irradiation
	Bone growth retardation at sites of irradiation
Infertility	Gonadal irradiation
	Alkylating agent chemotherapy (cyclophosphamide, ifosfamide)
Neuropsychological problems	Cranial irradiation (particularly at age <5 years)
	Brain surgery
Second malignancy	Irradiation
	Alkylating agent chemotherapy
Social/educational disadvantage	Chronic ill health
	Absence from school

for childhood cancers are developed, there is a need to reduce, whenever possible, the toxicity of treatment to spare adverse short-term and long-term effects.

Palliative and end-of-life care

Palliative care assists with symptom management, psychosocial support for the child and family, attention to practical needs and spiritual care throughout the child's illness. If a child relapses, further treatment may be considered. A reasonable number can still be cured and others may have a further significant remission with good-quality life. However, for some children, a time comes when death is inevitable and the staff and family must make the decision to concentrate on end-of-life care (see Ch. 5. Care of the sick child and young person).

Most parents prefer to care for their terminally ill child at home, but will need practical help and emotional support. Pain control and symptom relief are a serious source of anxiety for parents, but they can often be achieved successfully at home. Health professionals with experience in palliative and end-of-life care for children work together with the family and local healthcare workers. Some families may choose for the child's care to be provided in conjunction with a children's hospice. After the child's death, families should be offered continuing contact with an appropriate member of the team who looked after their child, and be given support through their bereavement.

☀ **With adequate support from health professionals, end-of-life care for children can often be provided at home**

Summary

Presentation of malignant disease in children

Brain tumours:
- Raised intracranial pressure
- Neurological signs – depends on anatomical position

Retinoblastoma:
- Screening if positive family history
- White pupillary reflex or squint

Lymphomas:
- Enlarged lymph nodes in the neck or abdomen
- Mediastinal mass – may cause superior vena caval obstruction.

Wilms tumour:
- Large abdominal mass in a well child
- Occasionally anorexia, abdominal pain, haematuria

Langerhans cell histiocytosis:
- Seborrhoeic rash
- Widespread soft tissue infiltration
- Bone pain, swelling or fracture
- Diabetes insipidus

Soft tissue sarcomas:
- Mass any site

Neuroblastoma:
- Abdominal mass
- Spinal cord compression
- Weight loss and malaise
- Pallor, bruising
- Bone pain

Acute lymphoblastic leukaemia (ALL):
- Malaise, anorexia
- Pallor, lethargy
- Infections
- Bruising, petechiae, nose bleeds
- Lymphadenopathy
- Hepatosplenomegaly
- Bone pain

Malignant bone tumours:
- Localised bone pain

Pre-school (<5 years old)	School-aged	Adolescence
Acute lymphoblastic leukaemia (ALL) – peak incidence Non-Hodgkin lymphoma	Acute lymphoblastic leukaemia (ALL)	Acute lymphoblastic leukaemia (ALL) Hodgkin lymphoma
Neuroblastoma	Brain tumours	Malignant bone tumours
Wilm tumour		Soft tissue sarcomas
Retinoblastoma		

Acknowledgements

We would like to acknowledge contributors to this chapter in previous editions, whose work we have drawn on: Michael Stevens (1st, 2nd, 3rd, 4th Edition), Helen Jenkinson (2nd, 3rd Edition), Rachel Dommett (4th Edition).

Further reading

Bailey S, Skinner R, editors: 2009 *Paediatric Haematology and Oncology.* Oxford Specialist Handbooks in Paediatrics. Oxford, Oxford University Press.
Short textbook

Goldman A, Hains R, Lieben S, editors: Oxford Textbook of Palliative Care in Children, ed 2, Oxford, 2012, Oxford University Press.

Pizzo PA, Poplack DG, editors: *Principles and Practice of Pediatric Oncology,* ed 7, 2015, Lippincott, Williams and Wilkins.
Comprehensive textbook

Stevens MCG, Caron HN, Biondi A, editors: *Cancer in Children: Clinical Management,* ed 6, Oxford, 2011, Oxford University Press.
Short textbook

Websites (Accessed November 2016)

CCLG (Children Cancer and Leukaemia Group): Available at: http://www.cclg.org.uk
Association of healthcare professionals involved in the treatment and care of children and younger teenagers with cancer, underpins all the activity in paediatric oncology in the UK.

Cure4Kids. Available at: http://www.cure4kids.org
Dedicated to improving healthcare for children with cancer and other catastrophic diseases around the globe. Provides continuing medical education and communication tools to healthcare professionals and scientists worldwide.

23

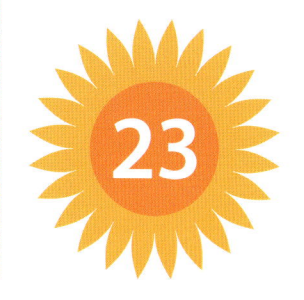

Haematological disorders

Anaemia	402	Bleeding disorders	413
Bone marrow failure syndromes	413	Thrombosis in children	421

Features of haematological disorders in children are:
- the composition and concentration of haemoglobin changes during childhood
- iron deficient anaemia is common
- causes of haemolytic anaemia include sickle cell disease, thalassaemia, G6PD deficiency, and hereditary spherocytosis
- the most common inherited causes of abnormal bleeding are haemophilia A and B and von Willebrand disease (vWD)
- petechiae or purpura may be nonthrombocytopenic (Henoch-Schonlein purpura, sepsis, trauma) or thrombocytopenic (immune thrombocytopenia, leukaemia, disseminated intravascular coagulation).

Haemopoiesis is the process which maintains lifelong production of haemopoietic (blood) cells. The main site of haemopoiesis in fetal life is the liver, whereas throughout postnatal life it is the bone marrow. All haemopoietic cells are derived from *pluripotent haemopoietic stem cells*, which are crucial for normal blood production; deficiency causes bone marrow failure because stem cells are required for the ongoing replacement of dying cells. Haemopoietic stem cells can also be used for treatment, e.g. cells from healthy donors can be transplanted into children with bone marrow failure (*stem cell transplantation*).

Haemoglobin production in the fetus and newborn

The most important difference between haemopoiesis in the fetus compared with postnatal life is the changing pattern of haemoglobin (Hb) production at each stage of development. The composition and names of these haemoglobins are shown in Table 23.1. Understanding the developmental changes in haemoglobin helps to explain the patterns of abnormal haemoglobin production in some inherited childhood anaemias. Fetal haemoglobin (HbF) is made up of 2 α chains and 2 γ chains ($\alpha_2\gamma_2$) and is the main Hb during fetal life. HbF has a higher affinity for oxygen than adult Hb (HbA), and is therefore better able to hold on to oxygen, an advantage in the relatively hypoxic environment of the fetus (Fig. 23.1). At birth, the types of Hb are: HbF, HbA and HbA$_2$. HbF is gradually replaced by HbA and HbA$_2$ during the first year of life. By 1 year of age, the percentage of HbF is very low in healthy children. The higher HbF in the first few months of life is protective in some types of inherited anaemia, such as sickle cell disease, which explains why neonates are asymptomatic and signs of the disease only develop later in the first year of life. An increased proportion of HbF can also be a sensitive indicator of thalassaemia and some types of bone marrow failure.

Table 23.1 Embryonic, fetal, and adult haemoglobins

	Globin chains	
Haemoglobin type	α-gene cluster	β-gene cluster
Embryonic		
Hb Gower 1	ξ_2	ε_2
Hb Gower 2	α_2	ε_2
Hb Portland	ξ_2	γ_2
Fetal		
HbF	α_2	γ_2
Adult		
HbA	α_2	β_2
HbA$_2$	α_2	δ_2
Haemoglobin types in newborns and adults		
Newborn	HbF 74%, HbA 25%, HbA$_2$ 1%	
Children >1 year old and adults	HbA 97%, HbA$_2$ 2%	

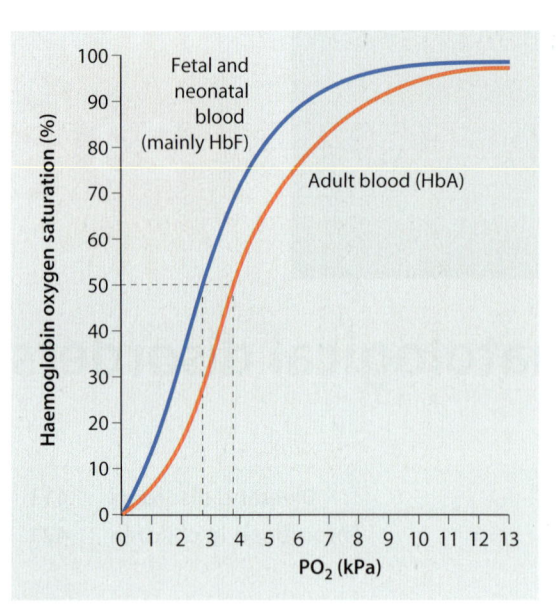

Figure 23.1 Oxygen dissociation curve showing the left shift of HbF compared with HbA. HbF-containing red cells have a higher affinity for oxygen and hold on to oxygen, delivering less to the tissues.

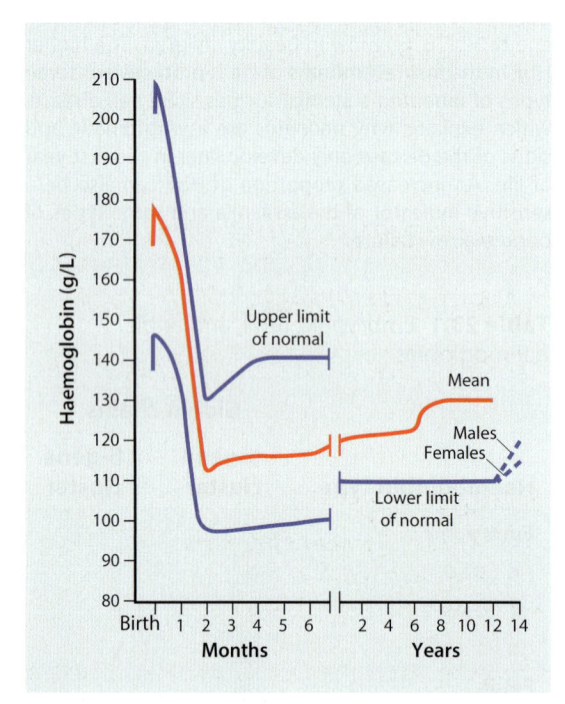

Figure 23.2 Changes in haemoglobin concentration with age, showing that the haemoglobin is high at birth, falling to its lowest concentration at 2 months to 3 months of age.

Haematological values at birth and the first few weeks of life

Features are

- At birth, the Hb in term infants is high, 140 g/L to 215 g/L, to compensate for the low oxygen concentration in the fetus. The Hb falls over the first few weeks due to reduced red cell production, reaching a nadir of around 100 g/L at 2 months of age (Fig. 23.2). Normal haematological values at birth and during childhood are shown in the Appendix (Table A.3).
- Preterm babies have a steeper fall in Hb to a mean of 65 g/L to 90 g/L at 4 weeks to 8 weeks chronological age.
- Normal blood volume at birth varies with gestational age. In healthy term infants the average blood volume is 80 ml/kg; in preterm infants the average blood volume is 100 ml/kg.
- Stores of iron, folic acid, and vitamin B_{12} in term and preterm babies are adequate at birth. However, in preterm infants, stores of iron and folic acid are lower and are depleted more quickly, leading to deficiency after 2 months to 4 months if the recommended daily intakes are not maintained by supplements.
- White blood cell counts in neonates are higher than in older children (10–25 × 10^9/L).
- Platelet counts at birth are within the normal adult range (150–400 × 10^9/L).

Summary

Haemoglobin at birth
- The Hb concentration is high at birth (>140 g/L) but falls to its lowest level at 2 months of age.
- HbF is gradually replaced by HbA (HbA + HbA_2) during infancy.

Anaemia

Anaemia is defined as an Hb level below the normal range. The normal range varies with age, so anaemia can be defined as:

- neonate: Hb less than 140 g/L
- 1 month to 12 months of age: Hb less than 100 g/L
- 1 year to 12 years of age: Hb less than 110 g/L

Anaemia results from one or more of the following mechanisms:

- reduced red cell production – either due to ineffective erythropoiesis (e.g. iron deficiency, the most common cause of anaemia) or due to red cell aplasia
- increased red cell destruction (*haemolysis*)
- blood loss – relatively uncommon cause in children.

There may be a combination of these three mechanisms, e.g. *anaemia of prematurity*.

Using this approach, the principal causes of anaemia are shown in Fig. 23.3 and a diagnostic approach to identifying their causes is shown in Fig. 23.4.

> The definition of anaemia varies with age: Hb <100 g/L in infants (postneonatal), Hb <110 g/L from 1 year old to 12 years old

Causes of anaemia in infants & children

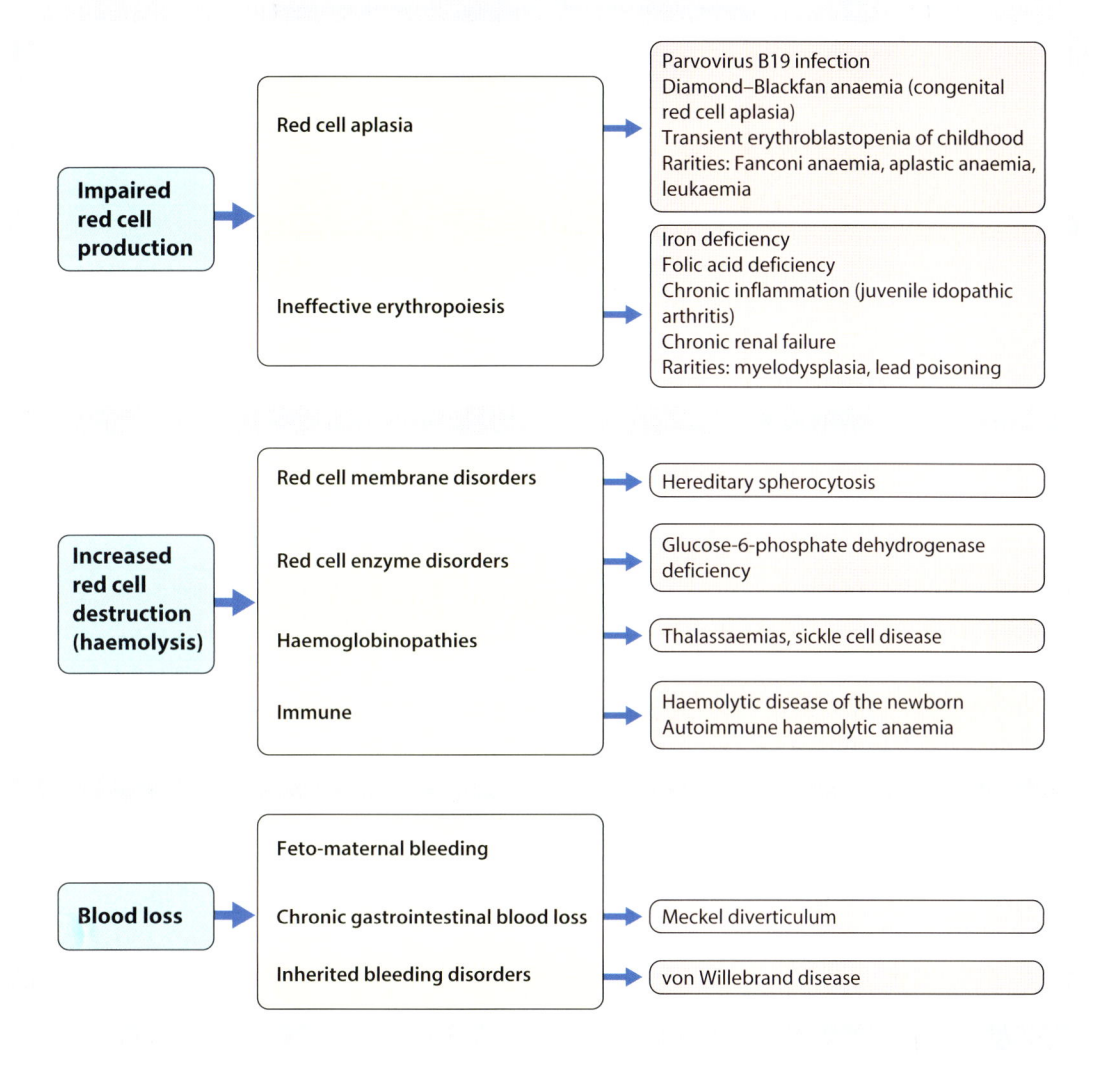

Impaired red cell production
- Red cell aplasia
  - Parvovirus B19 infection
  - Diamond–Blackfan anaemia (congenital red cell aplasia)
  - Transient erythroblastopenia of childhood
  - Rarities: Fanconi anaemia, aplastic anaemia, leukaemia
- Ineffective erythropoiesis
  - Iron deficiency
  - Folic acid deficiency
  - Chronic inflammation (juvenile idopathic arthritis)
  - Chronic renal failure
  - Rarities: myelodysplasia, lead poisoning

Increased red cell destruction (haemolysis)
- Red cell membrane disorders → Hereditary spherocytosis
- Red cell enzyme disorders → Glucose-6-phosphate dehydrogenase deficiency
- Haemoglobinopathies → Thalassaemias, sickle cell disease
- Immune → Haemolytic disease of the newborn / Autoimmune haemolytic anaemia

Blood loss
- Feto-maternal bleeding
- Chronic gastrointestinal blood loss → Meckel diverticulum
- Inherited bleeding disorders → von Willebrand disease

Figure 23.3 Causes of anaemia in infants and children.

Anaemia due to impaired red cell production

Reduced red cell production may be due to:
- 'ineffective erythropoiesis': here red cell production occurs at a normal or increased rate but differentiation and survival of the red cells is defective (e.g. iron deficiency)
- complete absence of red cell production (red cell aplasia).

Diagnosis of ineffective erythropoiesis

Diagnostic clues to ineffective erythropoiesis are:
- normal reticulocyte count
- abnormal mean cell volume (MCV) of the red cells: low in iron deficiency and raised in folic acid deficiency.

Iron deficiency

The main causes of iron deficiency are:
- inadequate intake
- malabsorption
- blood loss.

Inadequate intake of iron is common in infants because additional iron is required for the increase in blood volume accompanying growth and to build up the child's iron stores (Fig. 23.5). A 1-year-old infant requires an intake of iron of about 8 mg/day, which is about the same as his father (9 mg/day) but only half that of his mother (15 mg/day).

Iron may come from:
- breastmilk (low iron content but 50% of the iron is absorbed)
- infant formula (supplemented with adequate amounts of iron)
- cow's milk (higher iron content than breastmilk but only 10% is absorbed)

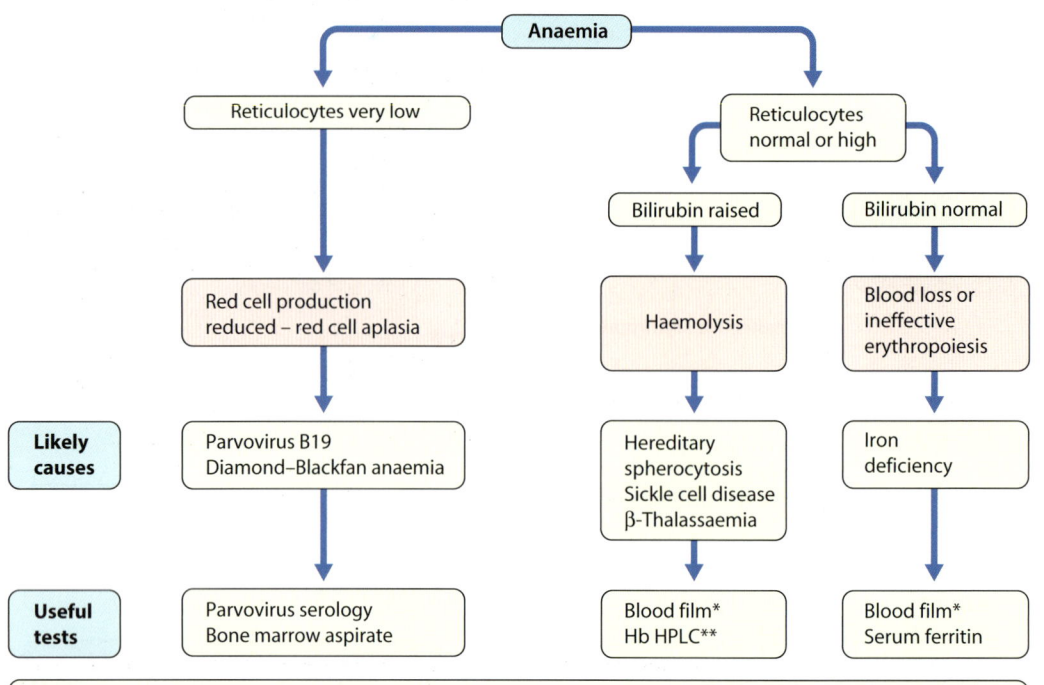

Simple diagnostic approach to anaemia in children

```
                        Anaemia
                   ┌──────┴──────┐
         Reticulocytes         Reticulocytes
         very low              normal or high
              │               ┌──────┴──────┐
              │         Bilirubin raised   Bilirubin normal
              ▼               ▼               ▼
         Red cell        Haemolysis     Blood loss or
         production                     ineffective
         reduced –                      erythropoiesis
         red cell aplasia
```

Likely causes
- Parvovirus B19 / Diamond–Blackfan anaemia
- Hereditary spherocytosis / Sickle cell disease / β-Thalassaemia
- Iron deficiency

Useful tests
- Parvovirus serology / Bone marrow aspirate
- Blood film* / Hb HPLC**
- Blood film* / Serum ferritin

*Blood film shows spherocytes in hereditary spherocytosis, sickle cells and target cells in sickle cell disease, hypochromic/microcytic red cells in thalassaemia and in iron deficiency.

** Hb HPLC, high performance liquid chromatography (in some laboratories Hb electrophoresis is used instead) shows:
- in sickle cell disease – HbS and no HbA is present
- in β-thalassaemia major – only HbF is present
- in β-thalassaemia trait – the main abnormality is an increased level of HbA_2
- in α-thalassaemia trait – Hb HPLC is normal

Figure 23.4 Diagnostic approach to anaemia.

- solids introduced at weaning, e.g. cereals (cereals are supplemented with iron but only 1% is absorbed).

Iron deficiency may develop because of a delay in the introduction of mixed feeding beyond 6 months of age or to a diet with insufficient iron-rich foods, especially if it contains a large amount of cow's milk (Box 23.1). Iron absorption is markedly increased when eaten with food rich in vitamin C (fresh fruit and vegetables) and is inhibited by tannin in tea

> Infants should not be fed unmodified cow's milk as its iron content is low and poorly absorbed

Clinical features

Most infants and children are asymptomatic until the Hb drops below 60 g/L to 70 g/L. As the anaemia worsens, children tire easily and young infants feed more slowly than usual. The history should include asking about blood loss and symptoms or signs suggesting malabsorption. They may appear pale but pallor is an unreliable sign unless confirmed by pallor of the conjunctivae, tongue or palmar creases. Some

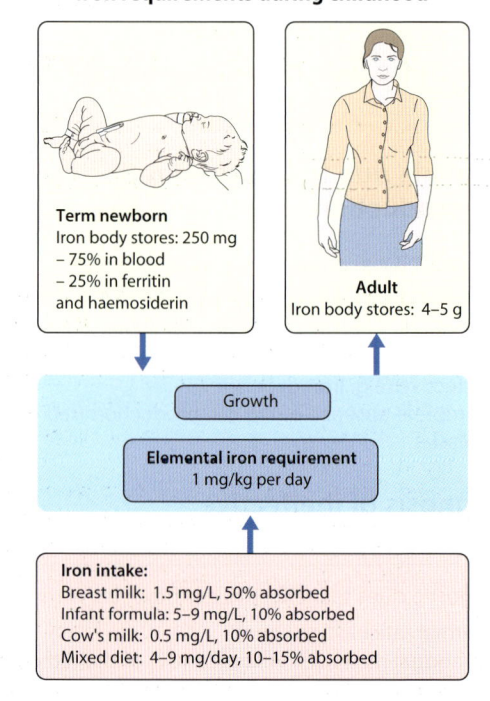

Iron requirements during childhood

Term newborn
Iron body stores: 250 mg
– 75% in blood
– 25% in ferritin and haemosiderin

Adult
Iron body stores: 4–5 g

Growth

Elemental iron requirement
1 mg/kg per day

Iron intake:
Breast milk: 1.5 mg/L, 50% absorbed
Infant formula: 5–9 mg/L, 10% absorbed
Cow's milk: 0.5 mg/L, 10% absorbed
Mixed diet: 4–9 mg/day, 10–15% absorbed

Figure 23.5 Iron requirements during childhood.

Box 23.1 Dietary sources of iron

High in iron
- Red meat – beef, lamb
- Liver, kidney
- Oily fish – pilchards, sardines, etc.

Average iron
- Pulses, beans, and peas
- Fortified breakfast cereals with added vitamin C
- Wholemeal products
- Dark green vegetables – broccoli, spinach, etc.
- Dried fruit – raisins, sultanas
- Nuts and seeds – cashews, peanut butter, etc.

Foods to avoid in excess in toddlers
- Cow's milk
- Tea: tannin inhibits iron uptake
- High-fibre foods: phytates inhibit iron absorption.

Case history 23.1

Iron deficiency anaemia

Ayesha, aged 2 years, was noted to look pale when she attended her general practitioner for an upper respiratory tract infection. A blood count showed Hb 50.0 g/L, MCV 54 fl (normal 72–85 fl) and MCH 16 pg (normal 24–39 pg). She was drinking three pints of cow's milk per day and was a very fussy eater, refusing meat. She had started eating soil when playing in the garden.

Because of the inappropriately large volume of milk she was drinking, she was not sufficiently hungry to eat solid food. Replacing some of the milk with iron-rich food and treatment with oral iron produced a rise in the Hb to 75 g/L within 4 weeks. Her pica (eating non-food materials) stopped. Oral iron was continued until her Hb had been normal for 3 months.

---

children have 'pica', a term which describes the inappropriate eating of non-food materials such as soil, chalk, gravel, or foam rubber (see Case History 23.1). There is evidence that iron deficiency anaemia may be detrimental to behaviour and intellectual function.

Diagnosis

The diagnostic clues are:

- microcytic, hypochromic anaemia (low MCV and MCH; Mean Cell Haemoglobin)
- low serum ferritin.

The other main causes of microcytic anaemia are:

- β-thalassaemia trait (usually children of Asian, Arabic, or Mediterranean origin)
- anaemia of chronic disease (e.g. due to chronic kidney disease).

Children with α-thalassaemia trait (usually children of African or Far Eastern origin) also have a microcytic/hypochromic blood picture but most of these children are not anaemic.

Management

For most children, management involves *dietary advice* and supplementation with *oral iron*. The best tolerated preparations are Sytron (sodium iron edetate) or Niferex (polysaccharide iron complex) – unlike some other preparations these do not stain the teeth. Iron supplementation should be continued until the Hb is normal and then for a minimum of a further 3 months to replenish the iron stores. With good compliance, the Hb will rise by about 10 g/L per week. Failure to respond to oral iron usually means the child is not getting the treatment. However, investigation for other causes, in particular malabsorption (e.g. due to coeliac disease) or chronic blood loss (e.g. due to Meckel diverticulum) is advisable if the history or examination suggests a non-dietary cause or if there is failure to respond to therapy in compliant patients. Blood transfusion should never be necessary for dietary iron deficiency. Even children with an Hb as low as 20 g/L to 30 g/L due to iron deficiency have arrived at this low level over a prolonged period and can tolerate it.

Treatment of iron deficiency with normal Hb

Some children have biochemical evidence of iron deficiency (e.g. low serum ferritin) but have not yet developed anaemia. Whether these children should be treated with oral iron is controversial. In favour of treatment is the knowledge that iron is required for normal brain development and there is evidence that iron deficiency anaemia is associated with behavioural and intellectual deficiencies, which may be reversible with iron therapy. However, it is not yet clear whether treatment of subclinical iron deficiency confers significant benefit. Treatment also carries a risk of accidental poisoning with oral iron, which is very toxic. A simple strategy is to provide dietary advice to increase oral iron and its absorption in all children with subclinical deficiency and to offer parents the option of additional treatment with oral iron supplements.

> **Treatment of iron deficiency anaemia is with dietary advice and oral iron therapy for several months**

Red cell aplasia

There are three main causes of red cell aplasia in children:

- congenital red cell aplasia ('Diamond–Blackfan anaemia')
- transient erythroblastopenia of childhood
- parvovirus B19 infection (this infection only causes red cell aplasia in children with inherited haemolytic anaemias and not in healthy children).

(a) (b) (c)

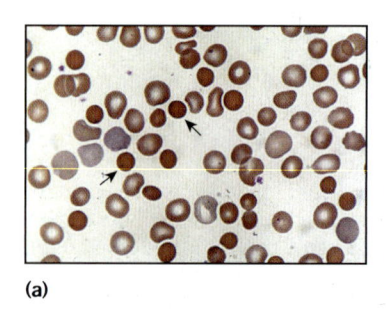

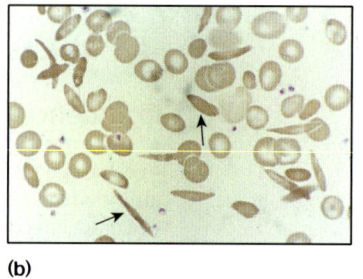

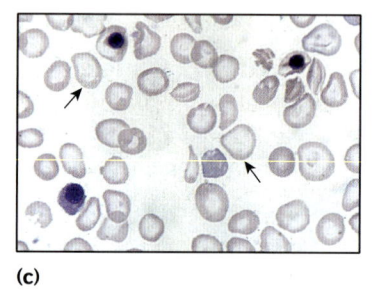

Figure 23.6 Abnormally shaped red blood cells help make the diagnosis in haemolytic anaemias. **(a)** Spherocytes (arrows) in hereditary spherocytosis; **(b)** sickle cells (arrows) in sickle cell disease; and **(c)** hypochromic cells (arrows) in thalassaemia.

The diagnostic clues to red cell aplasia are:

- low reticulocyte count despite low Hb
- normal bilirubin
- negative direct antiglobulin test (Coombs test)
- absent red cell precursors on bone marrow examination.

Diamond–Blackfan anaemia (DBA) is a rare disease (5–7 cases/million live births). There is a family history in 20% of cases; the remaining 80% are sporadic. Specific gene mutations in ribosomal protein (RPS) genes are implicated in some cases. Most cases present at 2 months to 3 months of age, but 25% present at birth. Affected infants have symptoms of anaemia; some have other congenital anomalies, such as short stature or abnormal thumbs. Treatment is by oral steroids; monthly red blood cell transfusions are given to children who are steroid unresponsive and some may also be offered stem cell transplantation.

Transient erythroblastopenia of childhood (TEC) is usually triggered by viral infections and has the same haematological features as Diamond–Blackfan anaemia. The main differences between them is that, unlike Diamond–Blackfan anaemia, transient erythroblastopenia of childhood always recovers, usually within several weeks, there is no family history or RPS gene mutations and there are no congenital anomalies.

Increased red cell destruction (haemolytic anaemia)

Haemolytic anaemia is characterised by reduced red cell lifespan. It is caused by increased red cell destruction in the circulation (intravascular haemolysis) or liver or spleen (extravascular haemolysis). The lifespan of a normal red cell is 120 days and the bone marrow produces 173 000 million red cells per day. In haemolysis, red cell survival may be reduced to a few days but bone marrow production can increase about eightfold, so haemolysis only leads to anaemia when the bone marrow is no longer able to compensate for the premature destruction of red cells.

In children, unlike neonates, immune haemolytic anaemias are uncommon. The main cause of haemolysis in children is *intrinsic* abnormalities of the red blood cells:

- red cell membrane disorders (e.g. hereditary spherocytosis)
- red cell enzyme disorders (e.g. glucose-6-phosphate dehydrogenase deficiency)
- haemoglobinopathies (abnormal haemoglobins, e.g. β-thalassaemia major, sickle cell disease).

Haemolysis from increased red cell breakdown leads to:

- anaemia
- hepatomegaly and splenomegaly
- increased blood levels of unconjugated bilirubin
- excess urinary urobilinogen.

The diagnostic clues to haemolysis are:

- raised reticulocyte count (on the blood film this is called 'polychromasia' as the reticulocytes have a characteristic lilac colour on a stained blood film)
- unconjugated bilirubinaemia and increased urinary urobilinogen
- abnormal appearance of the red cells on a blood film (e.g. spherocytes, sickle shaped or very hypochromic) (Fig. 23.6)
- positive direct antiglobulin test (only if an immune cause, as this test identifies antibody-coated red blood cells)
- increased red blood cell precursors in the bone marrow.

Hereditary spherocytosis

Hereditary spherocytosis (HS) occurs in 1 in 5000 births in Caucasians. It usually has an autosomal dominant inheritance, but in 25% there is no family history and it is caused by new mutations. The disease is caused by mutations in genes for proteins of the red cell membrane (mainly spectrin, ankyrin, or band 3). This results in the red cell losing part of its membrane when it passes through the spleen. This reduction in its surface-to-volume ratio causes the cells to become spheroidal, making them less deformable than normal red blood cells and leads to their destruction in the microvasculature of the spleen.

Clinical features

The disorder is often suspected because of the family history. The clinical manifestations are highly variable. Although affected individuals may be completely asymptomatic, the clinical features include:

- Jaundice – usually develops during childhood but may be intermittent; may cause severe haemolytic jaundice in the first few days of life.

- Anaemia – presents in childhood with mild anaemia (Hb 90–110 g/L), but the Hb level may transiently fall during infections.
- Mild to moderate splenomegaly – depends on the rate of haemolysis.
- Aplastic crisis – uncommon, transient (2–4 weeks), caused by parvovirus B19 infection.
- Gallstones – due to increased bilirubin excretion.

Diagnosis

The blood film is usually diagnostic but more specific tests are available (e.g. dye binding assay or osmotic fragility), although seldom required. Autoimmune haemolytic anaemia is also associated with spherocytes but this can be excluded by a positive direct antibody test and the absence of a family history of hereditary spherocytosis.

Management

Most children have mild chronic haemolytic anaemia and the only treatment they require is oral folic acid as they have a raised folic acid requirement secondary to their increased red blood cell production. Splenectomy is beneficial but is only indicated for poor growth or troublesome symptoms of anaemia (e.g. severe tiredness, loss of vigour) and is usually deferred until after 7 years of age because of the risks of postsplenectomy sepsis. Prior to splenectomy all patients should be checked that they have been vaccinated against *Haemophilus influenzae* (Hib), meningitis C and *Streptococcus pneumoniae* and lifelong daily oral penicillin prophylaxis is advised. Aplastic crisis from parvovirus B19 infection usually requires one or two blood transfusions over the 3-week to 4-week period when no red blood cells are produced. If gallstones are symptomatic, cholecystectomy may be necessary.

Glucose-6-phosphate dehydrogenase deficiency

Glucose-6-phosphate dehydrogenase (G6PD) deficiency is the most common red cell enzymopathy affecting over 100 million people worldwide. It has a high prevalence (10–20%) in individuals originating from central Africa, the Mediterranean, the Middle East, and the Far East. Many different mutations of the gene have been described, leading to different clinical features in different populations.

G6PD is the rate-limiting enzyme in the pentose phosphate pathway and is essential for preventing oxidative damage to red cells. Red cells lacking G6PD are susceptible to oxidant-induced haemolysis (usually caused by certain drugs – see Box 23.2). G6PD deficiency is X-linked and therefore predominantly causes symptoms in males. Females who are heterozygotes are usually clinically normal as they have about half the normal G6PD activity. Females may be affected either if they are homozygous or, more commonly, when by chance more of the normal than the abnormal X chromosomes have been inactivated (extreme Lyonisation – the Lyon hypothesis is that, in every XX cell, one of the X chromosomes is inactivated and that this is random). In Mediterranean, Middle Eastern, and Oriental populations, affected males have very low or absent enzyme activity in their red cells. Affected African Americans have 10–15% normal enzyme activity.

Box 23.2 Drugs and chemicals which can cause haemolysis in children with G6PD deficiency

Antimalarials
- Primaquine
- Quinine
- Chloroquine

Antibiotics
- Sulphonamides (including co-trimoxazole)
- Quinolones (ciprofloxacin, nalidixic acid)
- Nitrofurantoin

Analgesics
- Aspirin (in high doses)

Chemicals
- Naphthalene (mothballs)
- Divicine (fava beans – also called broad beans)

Adapted from: *British National Formulary for Children 2015*.

Clinical manifestations

Children usually present clinically with

- *Neonatal jaundice* – onset is usually in the first 3 days of life. Worldwide it is the most common cause of severe neonatal jaundice requiring exchange transfusion.
- *Acute haemolysis* – precipitated by:
  – infection, the most common precipitating factor
  – certain drugs (see Box 23.2)
  – fava beans (broad beans; other types of beans do not cause haemolysis)
  – naphthalene in mothballs.

Haemolysis due to G6PD deficiency is predominantly intravascular. This is associated with fever, malaise, abdominal pain, and the passage of dark urine, as it contains haemoglobin as well as urobilinogen. The haemoglobin level falls rapidly and may drop below 50 g/L over 24 hours to 48 hours.

Diagnosis

Between episodes, almost all patients have a completely normal blood picture and no jaundice or anaemia. The diagnosis is made by measuring G6PD activity in red blood cells. During a haemolytic crisis, G6PD levels may be misleadingly elevated due to the higher enzyme concentration in reticulocytes, which are produced in increased numbers in response to the destruction of mature red cells. A repeat assay is then required once the haemolytic episode is over to confirm the diagnosis.

Management

The parents should be given advice about the signs of acute haemolysis (jaundice, pallor, and dark urine) and provided with a list of drugs, chemicals, and food to avoid (Box 23.2). Transfusions are rarely required, even for acute episodes.

Haematological disorders

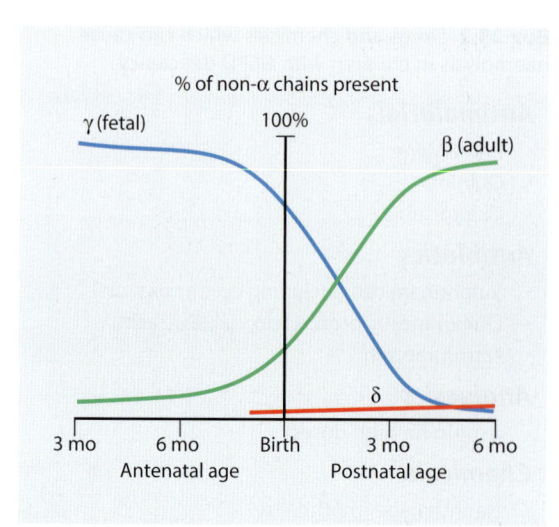

Figure 23.7 Changes in haemoglobin chains in the fetus and infancy.

Table 23.2 Haemoglobins in haemoglobinopathies

	HbA	HbA$_2$	HbF	HbS
Newborn	25%	1%	74%	–
Adult	97%	2%	–	–
β-Thalassaemia trait	>90%	↑	+ ↑	–
β-Thalassaemia major	–	↑	↑	–
Sickle cell trait	✓	✓	+ ↑	✓
Sickle cell disease	–	✓	+ ↑	✓

Haemoglobinopathies

These are red blood cell disorders which cause haemolytic anaemia because of reduced or absent production of HbA (α-thalassaemias and β-thalassaemias) or because of the production of an abnormal Hb (e.g. sickle cell disease). α-Thalassaemias are caused by deletions (occasionally mutations) in the α-globin gene. β-Thalassaemia and sickle cell disease are caused by mutations in the β-globin gene. Clinical manifestations of the haemoglobinopathies affecting the β-chain are delayed until after 6 months of age when most of the HbF present at birth has been replaced by HbA (Fig. 23.7, Table 23.2).

Sickle cell disease

This is now the most common inherited disorder in children in many European countries, including the UK (prevalence 1 in 2000 live births). The inheritance is autosomal recessive. Sickle cell disease is the collective name given to haemoglobinopathies in which HbS is inherited. HbS forms as a result of a point mutation in codon 6 of the β-globin gene, which causes a change in the amino acid encoded from glutamine to valine. Sickle cell disease is most common in patients whose parents are black and originate from tropical Africa or the Caribbean but it is also found in the Middle East and in low prevalence in most other parts of the world except for northern Europeans.

There are three main forms of sickle cell disease

- *Sickle cell anaemia* (*HbSS*) – patients are homozygous for HbS, i.e. virtually all their Hb is HbS; they have small amounts of HbF and *no* HbA because they have the sickle mutation in both β-globin genes.
- *HbSC disease* (*HbSC*) – affected children inherit HbS from one parent and HbC from the other parent (HbC is formed as a result of a different point mutation in β-globin), so they also have *no* HbA because they have no normal β-globin genes.
- *Sickle β-thalassaemia* – affected children inherit HbS from one parent and β-thalassaemia trait from the other. They have no normal β-globin genes and most patients can make no HbA and therefore have similar symptoms to those with sickle cell anaemia.
- *Carriers* (*Sickle trait*) – where there is inheritance of HbS from one parent and a normal β-globin gene from the other parent, patients are carriers and approximately 40% of their haemoglobin is HbS. As carriers, these individuals do not have sickle cell disease and are asymptomatic. However, they can transmit HbS to their offspring. Sickle trait can only be identified as a result of blood tests.

Pathogenesis

In all forms of sickle cell disease, HbS polymerises within red blood cells forming rigid tubular spiral bodies which deform the red cells into a sickle shape. Irreversibly sickled red cells have a reduced lifespan and may be trapped in the microcirculation, resulting in blood vessel occlusion (vaso-occlusion) and therefore ischaemia in an organ or bone. This is exacerbated by low oxygen tension, dehydration, and cold.

The clinical manifestations of sickle cell disease vary widely between different individuals. Disease severity also varies with different forms of sickle cell disease; in general, HbSS is the most severe form of the disease. One of the most important factors which modifies severity of sickle cell disease is the amount of HbF. While most patients with sickle cell disease have HbF levels of 1%, genetic variation means that some patients naturally produce more HbF (e.g. 10–15% of their Hb may be HbF) and this results in a marked reduction in disease severity. As a result, considerable research is being carried out into drugs which increase HbF.

Clinical features

These are listed in Fig. 23.8.

Management

Prophylaxis – Because of increased susceptibility to infection, especially encapsulated organisms, e.g. *Streptococcus pneumoniae* and *Haemophilus influenzae* type B because of functional asplenia, children should be fully immunized, including

Clinical manifestations of sickle cell disease

Anaemia → All have moderate anaemia (usually Hb 60–100 g/L) with clinically detectable jaundice from chronic haemolysis

Infection → All have marked increase in susceptibility to infection from encapsulated organisms such as pneumococci and *Haemophilus influenzae*. There is also an increased incidence of osteomyelitis caused by *Salmonella* and other organisms. This susceptibility to infection is due to **hyposplenism** secondary to chronic sickling and **microinfarction** in the spleen in infancy. The risk of overwhelming sepsis is greatest in early childhood

Painful crises → **Vaso-occlusive crises** causing pain affect many organs of the body with varying frequency and severity. A common mode of presentation in late infancy is the hand-foot syndrome, in which there is dactylitis with swelling and pain of the fingers and/or feet from vaso-occlusion (Fig. 23.9).
The bones of the limbs and spine are the most common sites. The most serious type of painful crisis is acute chest syndrome, which can lead to severe hypoxia and the need for mechanical ventilation and emergency transfusion. Avascular necrosis of the femoral heads may also occur. Acute vaso-occlusive crises may be precipitated by exposure to cold, dehydration, excessive exercise or stress, hypoxia or infection

Acute anaemia → Sudden drop in haemoglobin from
Haemolytic crises – sometimes associated with infection
Aplastic crises – haemoglobin may fall precipitously. Parvovirus infection causes complete, though temporary, cessation of red blood cell production
Sequestration crises – sudden splenic or hepatic enlargement, abdominal pain and circulatory collapse from accumulation of sickled cells in spleen

Priapism → Needs to be treated promptly with exchange transfusion as it may lead to fibrosis of the corpora cavernosa and subsequent erectile impotence

Splenomegaly → Common in young children, but becomes much less frequent in older children

Long-term problems → Short stature and delayed puberty
Stroke and cognitive problems – although 1 in 10 children with sickle cell disease have a stroke, twice that number develop more subtle neurological damage (Fig. 23.10), often manifest with poor concentration and school performance
Adenotonsillar hypertrophy – causing sleep apnoea syndrome leading to nocturnal hypoxaemia, which can cause vaso-occlusive crises and/or stroke
Cardiac enlargement – from chronic anaemia
Heart failure – from uncorrected anaemia
Renal dysfunction – may exacerbate enuresis because of inability to concentrate urine
Pigment gallstones – due to increased bile pigment production
Leg ulcers – uncommon in children
Psychosocial problems – difficulties with education and behaviour exacerbated by time off school may occur

Figure 23.8 Clinical manifestations of sickle cell disease.

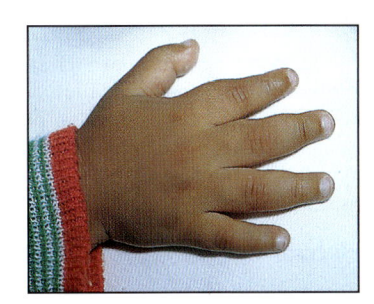

Figure 23.9 Dactylitis in sickle cell disease.

against pneumococcal, *Haemophilus influenzae* type B and meningococcus infection. To ensure full coverage of all pneumococcal subgroups, daily oral penicillin throughout childhood should be given. Patients should receive once-daily oral folic acid because of the increased demand for folic acid caused by the chronic haemolytic anaemia. Vaso-occlusive crises should be minimized by avoiding exposure to cold, dehydration, excessive exercise, undue stress, or hypoxia. This requires practical measures such as dressing children warmly, giving drinks especially before exercise,

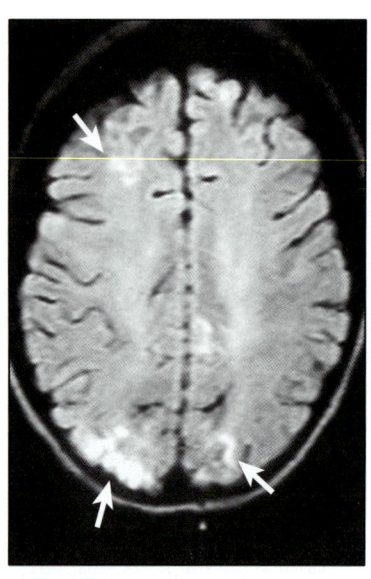

Figure 23.10 Magnetic resonance image of the brain in sickle cell disease showing multiple cerebral infarcts.

and taking extra care to keep children warm after swimming or when playing outside in the winter.

Treatment of acute crises – Painful crises should be treated with oral or intravenous analgesia according to need (may require opiates) and good hydration (oral or intravenous as required); infection should be treated with antibiotics; oxygen should be given if the oxygen saturation is reduced. Exchange transfusion is indicated for acute chest syndrome, stroke and priapism.

Treatment of chronic problems – Children who have recurrent hospital admissions for painful vaso-occlusive crises or acute chest syndrome (see Case History 23.2) may benefit from hydroxycarbamide, a drug which increases their HbF production and helps protect against further crises. It requires monitoring for side-effects, especially white blood cell suppression. The most severely affected children (1–5%) who have had a stroke or who do not respond to hydroxycarbamide may be offered a bone marrow transplant. This is the only cure for sickle cell disease but is usually only possible if the child has an HLA-identical sibling who can donate their bone marrow – the cure rate is 90% but there is a 5% risk of fatal transplant-related complications.

Prognosis

Sickle cell disease is a cause of premature death due to one or more of these severe complications; around 50% of patients with the most severe form of sickle cell disease die before the age of 40 years. However, the mortality rate during childhood is around 3%, usually from bacterial infection.

Prenatal diagnosis and screening

Many countries with a high prevalence of haemoglobinopathies, including the UK, perform neonatal screening using the dried blood spots (Guthrie test) collected in the first week of life for neonatal

Case history 23.2

Acute sickle chest syndrome

Princess, a 9-year-old girl with known sickle cell anaemia (HbSS), presented with increasing chest pain for 6 hours. She had a nonproductive cough. On examination, she had a fever of 39.7°C. Her breathing was laboured, respiratory rate increased and there was reduced air entry at both bases.

Investigations

- Haemoglobin 60 g/L, white blood cells (WBC) 14 × 10^9/L, platelets 350 × 10^9/L
- Chest X-ray (see Fig. 23.11)
- Oxygen saturation – 89% in air
- Arterial PO_2 – 9.3 kPa (70 mmHg) breathing face-mask oxygen
- Blood cultures were taken and viral titres performed

A diagnosis of acute sickle chest syndrome was made, a potentially fatal condition. She was given oxygen by continuous positive airways pressure (CPAP). An exchange transfusion was performed. Broad-spectrum antibiotics were commenced. She responded well to treatment.

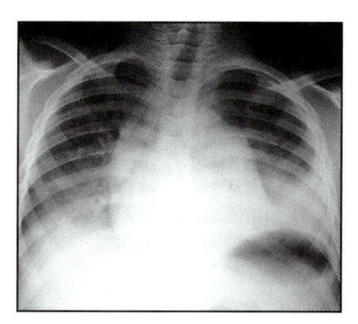

Figure 23.11 Chest X-ray in acute sickle chest syndrome showing bilateral lower zone consolidation. (Courtesy of Parviz Habibi.)

biochemical screening. Early diagnosis of sickle cell disease allows penicillin prophylaxis to be started in early infancy instead of awaiting clinical presentation, possibly due to a severe infection. Prenatal diagnosis can be carried out by chorionic villus sampling at the end of the first trimester if parents wish to choose this option to prevent the birth of an affected child.

Haemoglobin SC disease

Children with SC disease usually have a nearly normal haemoglobin level and fewer painful crises than those with HbSS, but they may develop proliferative retinopathy in adolescence. Their eyes should be checked periodically. They are also prone to develop osteonecrosis of the hips and shoulders.

Sickle cell trait

This is asymptomatic and is not considered as a disease. Potential carriers should be screened prior to general anaesthesia to make sure that additional effort to prevent hypoxia is made since sickling is theoretically possible if carriers are exposed to low oxygen tension.

β-Thalassaemias

The β-thalassaemias occur most often in people from the Indian subcontinent, Mediterranean, and Middle East (Fig. 23.12). In the UK, most affected children are born to parents from the Indian subcontinent; in the past, many were born to Greek Cypriots, but this has become uncommon through active genetic counselling within their community.

There are two main types of β-thalassaemia (β-thalassaemia major and β-thalassaemia intermedia) both of which are characterised by a severe reduction in the production of β-globin (and thereby reduction in HbA production). All affected individuals have a severe reduction in β-globin and disease severity depends on the amount of residual HbA and HbF production.

- *β-Thalassaemia major* – This is the most severe form of the disease. HbA ($\alpha_2\beta_2$) cannot be produced because of the abnormal β-globin gene.
- *β-Thalassaemia intermedia* – This form of the disease is milder and of variable severity. The β-globin mutations allow a small amount of HbA and/or a large amount of HbF to be produced.

Clinical features (Fig. 23.13)

These are

- Severe anaemia, which is transfusion dependent, from 3 months to 6 months of age and jaundice.
- Faltering growth/growth failure.
- Extramedullary haemopoiesis, prevented by regular blood transfusions. In the absence of regular blood transfusion, develop hepatosplenomegaly and bone marrow expansion; the latter leads to the classical facies with maxillary overgrowth and skull bossing (very rare in the UK and developed countries).

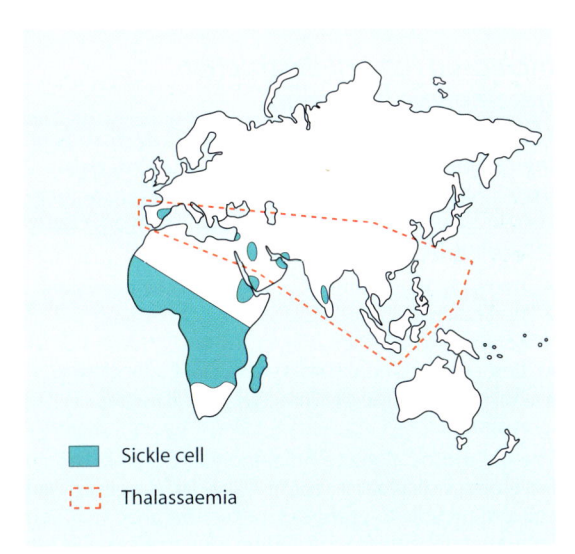

Figure 23.12 Ethnic origin of most families with sickle cell disease and thalassaemia.

Management

β-Thalassaemia major is uniformly fatal without regular blood transfusions, so all patients are given lifelong monthly transfusions of red blood cells. The aim is to maintain the haemoglobin concentration above 100 g/L in order to reduce growth failure and prevent bone deformation. Repeated blood transfusion causes chronic iron overload, which if untreated causes cardiac failure, liver cirrhosis, diabetes, infertility, and growth failure. For this reason, all patients are treated with iron chelation with subcutaneous desferrioxamine, or with an oral iron chelator drug, such as deferasirox, starting from 2 years to 3 years of age. Patients who comply well with transfusion and chelation have a greater than 90% chance of living into their forties and beyond. However, compliance is difficult. Those who cannot comply have a high mortality in early adulthood from iron overload. The complications of multiple transfusions are shown in Box 23.3. An alternative treatment for β-thalassaemia major is bone marrow transplantation, which is currently the only cure. It is generally reserved for children with an HLA-identical sibling as there is then a 90% to 95% chance of success (i.e. transfusion independence and long-term cure) but a 5% chance of transplant-related mortality.

Prenatal diagnosis

For parents who are both heterozygous for β-thalassaemia trait, there is a 1 in 4 risk of having an affected child. Prenatal diagnosis of β-thalassaemia (DNA analysis of a chorionic villus sample) should be offered together with genetic counselling to help parents to make informed decisions about whether or not to continue the pregnancy.

β-Thalassaemia trait

Heterozygotes are usually asymptomatic. The red cells are hypochromic and microcytic. Anaemia is mild or absent, with a disproportionate reduction in MCH (18–22 fl) and MCV (60–70 fl). The red blood cell count is therefore usually increased (>5.5 × 10^{12}/L). The most important diagnostic feature is a raised HbA_2, usually about 5%, and in about half there is a mild elevation of HbF level of 1% to 3%. β-Thalassaemia trait can cause confusion with mild iron deficiency because of the hypochromic/microcytic red cells but can be distinguished by measuring serum ferritin, which is low in iron deficiency but not β-thalassaemia trait.

To avoid unnecessary iron therapy, serum ferritin levels should be measured in patients with mild anaemia and microcytosis prior to starting iron supplements.

α-Thalassaemias

Healthy individuals have four α-globin genes. The manifestation of α-thalassaemia syndromes depends on the number of functional α-globin genes.

The most severe α-thalassaemia, *α-thalassaemia major* (also known as Hb Barts hydrops fetalis) is caused by deletion of all four α-globin genes, so no HbA ($\alpha_2\beta_2$) can be produced. It occurs mainly in families of South-East Asian origin and presents in midtrimester with fetal hydrops (oedema and ascites) from fetal anaemia, which is always fatal in utero or within hours of delivery. The only long-term survivors of α-thalassaemia major

Clinical features and complications of β-thalassaemia major

- Pallor
- Jaundice
- Bossing of the skull / Maxillary overgrowth
- Splenomegaly and hepatomegaly
- Need for repeated blood transfusions — Complications shown in Box 22.3

Figure 23.13 Facies in β-thalassaemia showing maxillary overgrowth and skull bossing in a child who has not been adequately transfused. This is now very rare in the UK and developed countries.

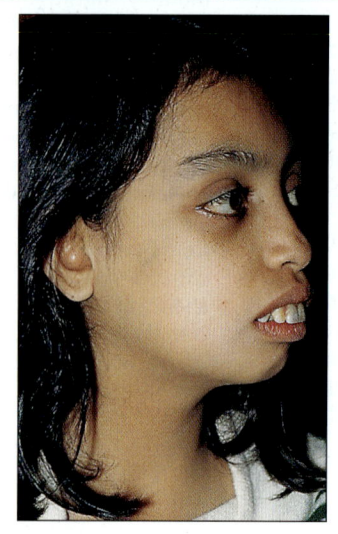

Box 23.3 Complications of long-term blood transfusion in children

Iron deposition – the most important (all patients)
- Heart – cardiomyopathy
- Liver – cirrhosis
- Pancreas – diabetes
- Pituitary gland – impaired growth and sexual maturation
- Skin – hyperpigmentation

Antibody formation (10% of children)
- Allo-antibodies to transfused red cells in the patient make finding compatible blood very difficult

Infection – now uncommon (<10% of children)
- Hepatitis A, B, C
- HIV
- Malaria
- Prions (e.g. new variant Creutzfeldt-Jakob disease)

Venous access (common problem)
- Often traumatic in young children
- Central venous access device (e.g. Portacath) may be required; these predispose to infection

---

are those who have received monthly intrauterine transfusions until delivery followed by lifelong monthly transfusions after birth. The diagnosis is made by Hb high-performance liquid chromatography (HPLC) or Hb electrophoresis, which shows only, or mainly, Hb Barts.

When only three of the α-globin genes are deleted (*HbH disease*), affected children have mild–moderate anaemia but occasional patients are transfusion-dependent.

Deletion of one or two α-globin genes (known as α-thalassaemia trait) is usually asymptomatic and anaemia is mild or absent. The red cells may be hypochromic and microcytic, which may cause confusion with iron deficiency.

Anaemia in the newborn

Reduced red blood cell production

There are two main but rare causes in the newborn and both cause red cell aplasia:

- Congenital infection with parvovirus B19.
- Congenital red cell aplasia (Diamond–Blackfan anaemia).

In this situation, the Hb is low and the red blood cells look normal. The diagnostic clue is that the reticulocyte count is low and the bilirubin is normal.

Increased red cell destruction (haemolytic anaemia)

This occurs either because of an antibody destroying the red blood cells (i.e. an extrinsic cause) or because there is an intrinsic abnormality of the surface or intracellular contents of the red blood cell. The main causes of haemolytic anaemia in neonates are:

- Immune (e.g. haemolytic disease of the newborn).
- Red cell membrane disorders (e.g. hereditary spherocytosis).
- Red cell enzyme disorders (e.g. G6PD deficiency).
- Abnormal haemoglobins (e.g. α-thalassaemia major).

The diagnostic clues to a haemolytic anaemia are an increased reticulocyte count (due to increased red cell production to compensate for the anaemia) and increased unconjugated bilirubin (due to increased red cell destruction with release of this bile pigment into the plasma).

Haemolytic disease of the newborn (immune haemolytic anaemia of the newborn) is due to antibodies against blood group antigens. The most important are: anti-D (a 'rhesus' antigen), anti-A or anti-B (ABO blood group antigens), and anti-Kell. The mother is always negative for the relevant antigen (e.g. rhesus D-negative) and the baby is always positive; the mother then makes antibodies against the baby's blood group antigen and these antibodies cross the placenta into the baby's circulation causing fetal or neonatal haemolytic anaemia. The diagnostic clue to this type of haemolytic anaemia is a positive direct anti-globulin test (Coombs test). This test is only positive in antibody-mediated anaemias and so is negative in all the other types of haemolytic anaemia. (These conditions are considered further in Ch. 11.)

The most common causes of nonimmune haemolytic anaemia in neonates are: G6PD deficiency and hereditary spherocytosis. Haemoglobinopathies, apart from α-thalassaemia, rarely present with clinical features in the neonatal period but are detected on neonatal haemoglobinopathy screening (Guthrie test).

Blood loss

The main causes are

- Feto-maternal haemorrhage (occult bleeding into the mother).
- Twin-to-twin transfusion (bleeding from one twin into the other one).
- Blood loss around the time of delivery (e.g. placental abruption).

The main diagnostic clue is severe anaemia with a raised reticulocyte count and normal bilirubin.

Anaemia of prematurity

The main causes are

- Inadequate erythropoietin production.
- Reduced red cell lifespan.
- Frequent blood sampling whilst in hospital.
- Iron and folic acid deficiency (after 2–3 months).

Bone marrow failure syndromes

Bone marrow failure (also known as aplastic anaemia) is a rare condition characterised by a reduction or absence of all three main lineages in the bone marrow leading to peripheral blood pancytopenia. It may be inherited or acquired. The acquired cases may be due to viruses (especially hepatitis viruses), drugs (such as sulphonamides, chemotherapy), or toxins (such as benzene, glue); however, many cases are labelled as 'idiopathic' because a specific cause cannot be identified.

The condition may be partial or complete. It may start as failure of a single lineage but progress to involve all three cell lines.

The clinical presentation is with:

- anaemia due to reduced red cell numbers
- infection due to reduced white cell numbers (especially neutrophils)
- bruising and bleeding due to thrombocytopenia.

Inherited aplastic anaemia

These disorders are all rare.

Fanconi anaemia

This is the most common inherited form of aplastic anaemia. It is an autosomal recessive condition caused by mutations in one of the many FANC genes, most commonly FANCA. The majority of children have congenital anomalies, including short stature, abnormal radii and thumbs, renal malformations, microphthalmia, and pigmented skin lesions. Children may present with one or more of these anomalies or with signs of bone marrow failure which do not usually become apparent until the age of 5 years or 6 years. Neonates with Fanconi anaemia nearly always have a normal blood count but it can be diagnosed by demonstrating increased chromosomal breakage of peripheral blood lymphocytes. This test can be used to identify affected family members or for prenatal diagnosis. Affected children are at high risk of death from bone marrow failure or transformation to acute leukaemia. The recommended treatment is bone marrow transplantation using normal donor marrow from an unaffected sibling or matched unrelated marrow donor.

Shwachman–Diamond syndrome

This rare autosomal recessive disorder is characterised by bone marrow failure, together with signs of pancreatic exocrine failure and skeletal abnormalities. Most are caused by mutations in the SBDS gene, which can be used for identifying unusual cases or prenatal diagnosis. The most common haematological problem is an isolated neutropenia or mild pancytopenia. Like Fanconi anaemia, there is an increased risk of transforming to acute leukaemia.

Bleeding disorders

Normal haemostasis

Haemostasis describes the normal process of blood clotting. It takes place via a series of tightly regulated interactions involving cellular and plasma factors.

There are five main components

1. *Coagulation factors* – are produced (mainly by the liver) in an inactive form and are activated when coagulation is initiated (usually by tissue factor (TF), which is released by vessel injury; see Fig. 23.14).
2. *Coagulation inhibitors* – these either circulate in plasma or are bound to endothelium and are necessary to prevent widespread coagulation throughout the body once coagulation has been initiated.
3. *Fibrinolysis* – this process limits fibrin deposition at the site of injury due to activity of the key enzyme plasmin.
4. *Platelets* – are vital for haemostasis as they aggregate at sites of vessel injury to form the

Summary

Anaemia

Causes of anaemia:
- Reduced red cell production
- Increased red cell destruction (haemolysis)
- Combination of causes, e.g. anaemia of prematurity
- Blood loss (uncommon)

Reduced red cell production

Iron deficiency anaemia
- Common in infants and toddlers, especially if of Indian subcontinent origin
- Usually dietary in origin
- Occurs because of high iron requirement (1 mg/kg/day) for growth and body stores
- Will not occur if infants are weaned at 6 months of age on to a mixed diet including iron-rich food
- Is diagnosed from a hypochromic microcytic anaemia and low serum ferritin
- Is treated with dietary advice and oral iron therapy for at least 3 months

Red cell aplasia
- Congenital red cell aplasia ('Diamond–Blackfan anaemia')
- Transient erythroblastopenia of childhood (TEC)
- Parvovirus B19 infection

Increased red cell production (haemolysis)

Hereditary spherocytosis
- Inheritance is autosomal dominant, but in 25% of cases there is no family history
- May cause early, severe jaundice in newborn infants
- Is often asymptomatic, but it may cause anaemia, jaundice, splenomegaly, aplastic crisis and gallstones
- Can usually be diagnosed from the blood film
- Treatment is with folic acid, splenectomy if symptomatic

β-Thalassaemia major
- Mutation of the β-globin gene results in an inability to produce HbA ($\alpha_2\beta_2$)
- Clinical features: severe anaemia, faltering growth and hepatosplenomegaly
- Condition is fatal without regular blood transfusions, but blood transfusions cause iron overload
- Iron chelation therapy with desferrioxamine or oral iron chelation is essential in all patients to minimise iron overload

β-Thalassaemia trait and α-thalassaemia trait
- Can cause diagnostic confusion with mild iron deficiency

α-Thalassaemia major
- Deletion of all 4 α-globin genes, α-thalassaemia major is fatal in utero (Hb Barts) or within hours of birth

Isoimmune
- Haemolytic disease of the newborn

Immune haemolytic anaemia

G6PD deficiency
- Affects over 100 million people worldwide, usually of Mediterranean, Middle East, Far East and Central African ethnicity
- Is X-linked and therefore predominantly affects males, but females may be affected
- May present with neonatal jaundice
- Causes acute intermittent haemolysis precipitated by infection, certain drugs, fava beans (broad beans) and naphthalene in mothballs
- Parents should be given a list of drugs, chemicals and food to avoid

Sickle cell disease
- Family usually originates from tropical Africa or the Caribbean
- Autosomal recessive
- Sickled red cells result in ischaemia in organs or bones
- Main clinical features are: anaemia, infection, painful crises, sequestration crises, splenomegaly in some young children, growth failure, gallstones, behaviour and learning problems
- The most serious clinical complications are bacterial infection, acute chest syndrome, strokes and priapism
- Management: prophylactic penicillin and immunisation; folic acid; maintain good hydration Treat crises: analgesia, hydration, antibiotics, exchange or blood transfusion as indicated Long-term: hydroxycarbamide *Chemo drug* or occasionally bone marrow transplant

---

primary haemostatic plug, which is then stabilized by fibrin.

5. *Blood vessels* – both initiate and limit coagulation. Intact vascular endothelium secretes prostaglandin I$_2$ and nitric oxide (which promote vasodilatation and inhibit platelet aggregation). Damaged endothelium releases TF and procoagulants (e.g. collagen and von Willebrand factor, vWF) and there are inhibitors of coagulation on the endothelial surface (thrombomodulin,

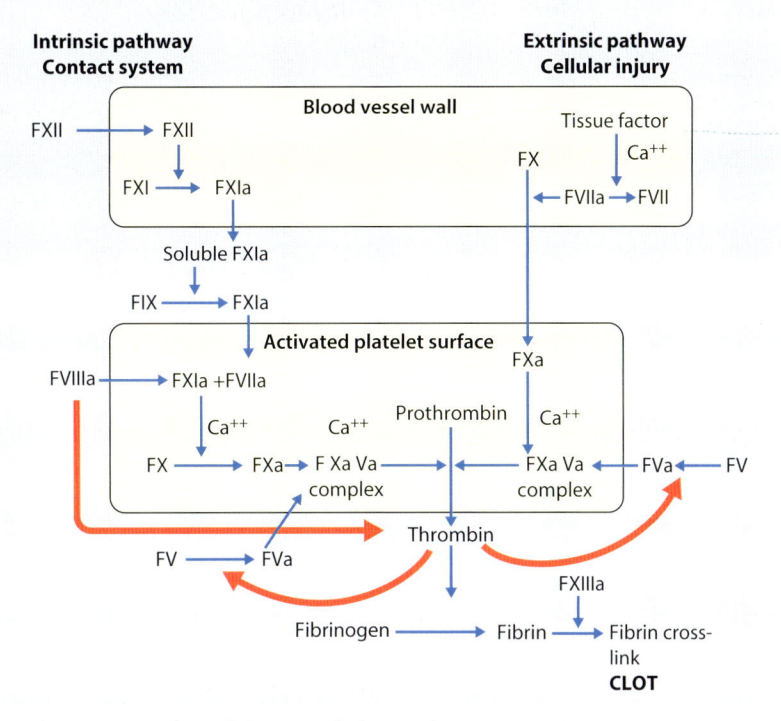

Figure 23.14 Schematic representation of the coagulation pathway.

antithrombin and protein S) to modulate coagulation.

The endpoint of the coagulation cascade is generation of thrombin. A simplified model is shown in Fig. 23.14. The two main pathways for thrombin generation were identified many years ago as the intrinsic and extrinsic pathways. Important components of these pathways are still being discovered. In recent years, the crucial role of TF in haemostasis has been recognized and it is now thought that the extrinsic pathway is the one primarily responsible for initiating both normal haemostasis and thrombotic disease.

Diagnostic approach

Defects in the coagulation factors, in platelet number or function, or in the fibrinolytic pathway are associated with an increased risk of bleeding. In contrast, defects in the naturally occurring inhibitors of coagulation (e.g. antithrombin) or in the vessel wall (e.g. damage from vascular catheters) are associated with thrombosis. In some cases, both procoagulant and anticoagulant abnormalities can occur at the same time, as seen in disseminated intravascular coagulation (DIC).

The diagnostic evaluation of an infant or child for a possible bleeding disorder includes

- Identifying features in the clinical presentation that suggest the underlying diagnosis, as indicated in Box 23.4.
- Initial laboratory screening tests to determine the most likely diagnosis (Table 23.3).
- Specialist investigation to characterize a deficiency or exclude important conditions that can present with normal initial investigations, e.g. mild vWD, factor XIII deficiency and platelet function disorders.

The most useful initial screening tests are

- Full blood count and blood film.
- Prothrombin time (PT) – measures the activity of factors II, V, VII and X.
- Activated partial thromboplastin time (APTT) – measures the activity of factors II, V, VIII, IX, X, XI and XII.
- If PT or APTT is prolonged, a 50:50 mix with normal plasma will distinguish between possible factor deficiency or presence of inhibitor.
- Thrombin time – tests for deficiency or dysfunction of fibrinogen.
- Quantitative fibrinogen assay.
- D-dimers – to test for fibrin degradation products.
- Biochemical screen, including renal and liver function tests.

The 'bleeding time' is no longer used to investigate platelet disorders, as it is unreliable. It has been replaced by in vitro tests of platelet function on a platelet function analyzer, which can be performed on a peripheral blood sample.

In the neonate, the levels of all clotting factors except factor VIII (FVIII) and fibrinogen are lower; preterm infants have even lower levels. Therefore the results have to be compared with normal values in infants of a similar gestational and postnatal age. In view of this, and because it is often difficult to obtain good-quality neonatal samples, it is sometimes necessary to exclude an inherited coagulation factor deficiency by testing the coagulation of both parents.

Box 23.4 Helpful clinical features in evaluating bleeding disorders

Age of onset
- Neonate – in 20% of haemophilias, bleeding occurs in the neonatal period, usually with intracranial haemorrhage or bleeding after circumcision
- Toddler – haemophilias may present when starting to walk
- Adolescent – von Willebrand disease may present with menorrhagia

Family history
- Family tree – detailed family tree required
- Gender of affected relatives (if all boys, suggests haemophilia)

Bleeding history
- Previous surgical procedures and dental extractions – if uncomplicated, suggests bleeding tendency is acquired rather than inherited
- Presence of systemic disorders
- Drug history, e.g. anticoagulants
- Unusual pattern or inconsistent history – consider nonaccidental injury

Pattern of bleeding
- Mucous membrane bleeding and skin haemorrhage – characteristic of platelet disorders or von Willebrand disease
- Bleeding into muscles or into joints – characteristic of haemophilia
- Scarring and delayed haemorrhage – suggestive of disorders of connective tissue, e.g. Marfan syndrome, osteogenesis imperfecta or factor XIII deficiency

Table 23.3 Investigations in haemophilia A and von Willebrand disease

	Haemophilia A	von Willebrand disease
PT	Normal	Normal
APTT	↑↑	↑ or normal
Factor VIII:C	↓↓	↓ or normal
vWF Antigen	Normal	↓
RiCoF (activity)	Normal	↓
Ristocetin-induced platelet aggregation	Normal	Abnormal
vWF multimers	Normal	Variable

APTT, activated partial thromboplastin time; PT, prothrombin time; RiCoF, ristocetin cofactor, measures vWD activity; vWF, von Willebrand factor.

Haemophilia

The most common severe inherited coagulation disorders are haemophilia A and haemophilia B. Both have X-linked recessive inheritance. In haemophilia A, there is FVIII deficiency (Fig. 23.15); it has a frequency of 1 in 5000 male births. Haemophilia B (FIX deficiency) has a frequency of 1 in 30 000 male births. Two-thirds of newly diagnosed infants have a family history of haemophilia, whereas one-third are sporadic. Identifying female carriers requires a detailed family history, analysis of coagulation factors and DNA analysis. Prenatal diagnosis is available using DNA analysis.

Clinical features

The disorder is graded as severe, moderate, or mild, depending on the FVIII (or IX in haemophilia B) level (Table 23.4). The hallmark of severe disease is recurrent spontaneous bleeding into joints and muscles, which can lead to crippling arthritis if not properly treated (Fig. 23.16). Most children present towards the end of the first year of life, when they start to crawl or walk

Table 23.4 Severity of haemophilia

Factor VIII	Severity	Bleeding tendency
<1%	Severe	Spontaneous joint/muscle bleeds
1–5%	Moderate	Bleed after minor trauma
>5–40%	Mild	Bleed after surgery

(and fall over). Bleeding episodes are most frequent in joints and muscles. Where there is no family history, nonaccidental injury may initially be suspected. Almost 40% of cases present in the neonatal period, particularly with intracranial haemorrhage, bleeding postcircumcision or prolonged oozing from heel stick and venepuncture sites. The severity usually remains constant within a family.

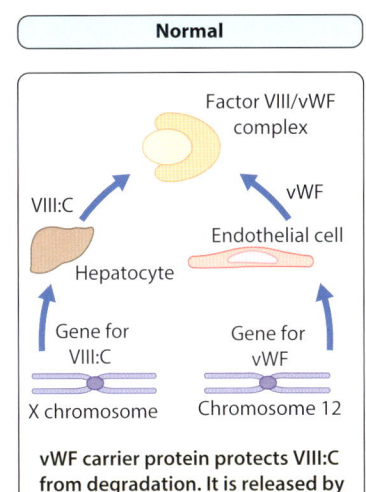

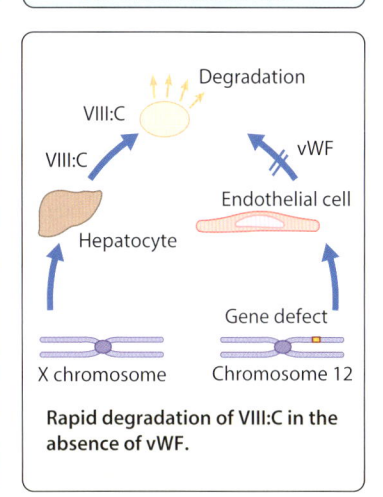

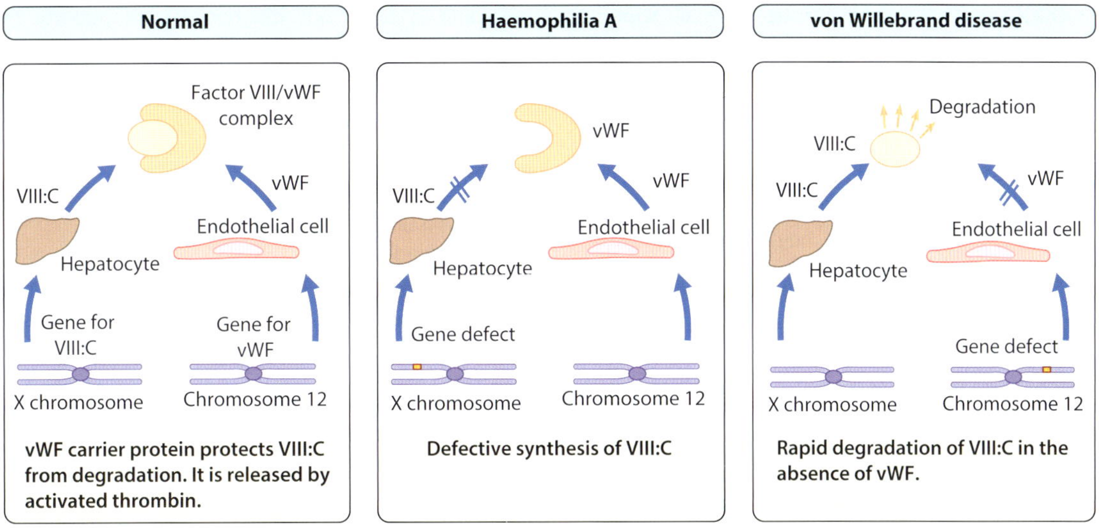

Figure 23.15 Factor VIII synthesis: normal, haemophilia A and von Willebrand disease.

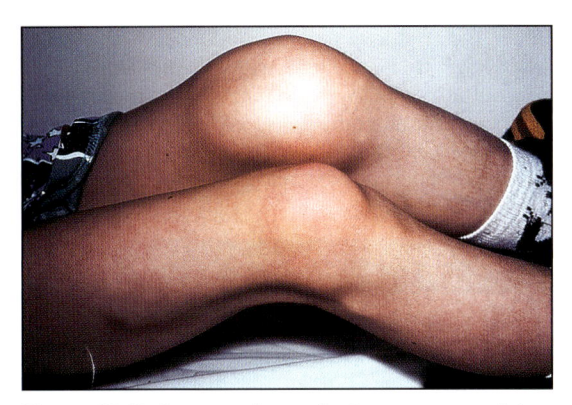

Figure 23.16 Severe arthropathy from recurrent joint bleeds in haemophilia. The aim of modern management is to prevent this from occurring.

Management

Recombinant FVIII concentrate for haemophilia A or recombinant FIX concentrate for haemophilia B is given by prompt intravenous infusion whenever there is any bleeding. If recombinant products are unavailable, highly purified, virally inactivated plasma-derived products should be used. The quantity required depends on the site and nature of the bleed. In general, raising the circulating level to 30% of normal is sufficient to treat minor bleeds and simple joint bleeds. Major surgery or life-threatening bleeds require the level to be raised to 100% and then maintained at 30% to 50% for up to 2 weeks to prevent secondary haemorrhage. This can only be achieved by regular infusion of factor concentrate (usually 8–12-hourly for FVIII, 12–24-hourly for FIX, or by continuous infusion) and by closely monitoring plasma levels. *Intramuscular injections, aspirin, and nonsteroidal anti-inflammatory drugs should be avoided in all patients with haemophilia.*

Complications are listed in Box 23.5.

Home treatment is encouraged to avoid delay in treatment, which increases the risk of permanent damage, e.g. progressive arthropathy. Parents are usually taught to give replacement therapy at home when the child is 2 years to 3 years of age and many children are able to administer their own treatment from 7 years to 8 years of age.

Prophylactic FVIII is given to all children with severe haemophilia A to further reduce the risk of chronic joint damage by raising the baseline level above 2%. Primary prophylaxis usually begins at age 2 years to 3 years, and is given two to three times per week. If peripheral venous access is poor, a central venous access device (e.g. Portacath) may be required. Prophylaxis has been shown to result in better joint function in adult life. Similarly, patients with severe haemophilia B are usually given prophylactic FIX.

Desmopressin (DDAVP) may allow mild haemophilia A to be managed without the use of blood products. It is given by infusion and stimulates endogenous release of FVIII:C and vWF. Adequate levels can be achieved to enable minor surgery and dental extraction to be undertaken. DDAVP is ineffective in haemophilia B.

Box 23.5 Complications of treatment of haemophilia

Inhibitors, i.e. antibodies to FVIII or FIX
- Develop in 5% to 20%
- Reduce or completely inhibit the effect of treatment
- Require the use of very high doses of factor VIII or bypassing agents (e.g. FVIIa) for treating bleeding
- May be amenable to immune tolerance induction

Transfusion-transmitted infections
- Hepatitis A, B, and C
- HIV
- Other, e.g. Prions, parvovirus B19

Vascular access
- Peripheral veins – may be difficult to cannulate
- Central venous access devices may become infected or thrombosed

Designated haemophilia centres normally supervise the management of children with bleeding disorders. They provide a multidisciplinary approach with expert medical, nursing, and laboratory input. Specialised physiotherapy is needed to preserve muscle strength and avoid damage from immobilization. Psychosocial support is an integral part of maintaining compliance.

Self-help groups such as the Haemophilia Society may provide families with helpful information and support.

von Willebrand disease

vWF has two major roles

- It facilitates platelet adhesion to damaged endothelium.
- It acts as the carrier protein for FVIII, protecting it from inactivation and clearance.

vWD results from either a quantitative or qualitative deficiency of vWF. This causes defective platelet plug formation and, since vWF is a carrier protein for FVIII, patients with vWD also are deficient in FVIII (see Fig. 23.15).

There are many different mutations in the vWF gene resulting in many different types of vWD. The inheritance is usually autosomal dominant. The most common subtype, type 1 (60–80%), is usually fairly mild and is often not diagnosed until puberty or adulthood.

Clinical features

These are:
- bruising
- excessive, prolonged bleeding after surgery
- mucosal bleeding such as epistaxis and menorrhagia.

In contrast to haemophilia, spontaneous soft tissue bleeding such as large haematomas and haemarthroses are uncommon.

Management

Treatment depends on the type and severity of the disorder. Type 1 vWD can usually be treated with DDAVP, which causes secretion of both FVIII and vWF into plasma. DDAVP should be used with caution in children less than 1 year of age as it can cause hyponatraemia due to water retention and may cause seizures, particularly after repeated doses, and if fluid intake is not strictly regulated. More severe types of vWD have to be treated with *plasma-derived* FVIII concentrate, as DDAVP is ineffective and recombinant FVIII concentrate contains no vWF. Cryoprecipitate is no longer used to treat vWD as it has not undergone viral inactivation. *Intramuscular injections, aspirin, and*

Summary

The child with abnormal bleeding – into soft tissues, mucocutaneous or following surgery

Acquired disorders

Vitamin K deficiency:
- mainly neonates or early infancy

Liver disease

Thrombocytopenia:
- immune, DIC, etc.

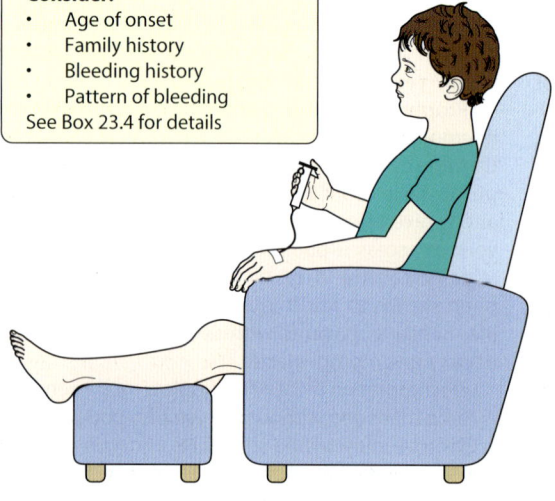

Consider:
- Age of onset
- Family history
- Bleeding history
- Pattern of bleeding

See Box 23.4 for details

Inherited disorders

Haemophilia A (factor VIII deficiency) and haemophilia B (factor IX deficiency):
- Are X-linked recessive disorders affecting males
- Presentation of severe disease – usually with recurrent spontaneous bleeding into joints and muscles at about 1 year of age
- Treatment – recombinant FVIII concentrate for haemophilia A or recombinant FIX concentrate for haemophilia B. Desmopressin (DDAVP) to treat mild haemophilia A
- Treatment complications – inhibitors and intravenous access

von Willebrand disease (vWD):
- Results from either a quantitative or qualitative deficiency of von Willebrand factor (vWF)
- Autosomal dominant
- Presentation – mucosal bleeding, e.g. epistaxis or menorrhagia in adolescence or excessive, prolonged bleeding after surgery
- Treatment – mild disease with DDAVP, severe disease with plasma-derived FVIII concentrate

nonsteroidal anti-inflammatory drugs should be avoided in all patients with vWD.

Acquired disorders of coagulation

The main acquired disorders of coagulation affecting children are those secondary to

- Haemorrhagic disease of the newborn due to vitamin K deficiency (see Ch. 10).
- Liver disease.
- Immune thrombocytopenia (ITP).
- Disseminated intravascular coagulation (DIC).

Vitamin K is essential for the production of active forms of factors II, VII, IX, X, and for the production of naturally occurring anticoagulants such as protein C and protein S. Vitamin K deficiency therefore causes reduced levels of all of these factors. The main clinical consequence of this is a prolonged prothrombin time and an increased risk of bleeding. Children may become deficient in vitamin K due to:

- inadequate intake (e.g. neonates, long-term chronic illness with poor intake)
- malabsorption (e.g. coeliac disease, cystic fibrosis, obstructive jaundice)
- vitamin K antagonists (e.g. warfarin).

Thrombocytopenia

Thrombocytopenia is a platelet count less than 150×10^9/L. The risk of bleeding depends on the level of the platelet count.

- Severe thrombocytopenia (platelets $<20 \times 10^9$/L) – risk of spontaneous bleeding.
- Moderate thrombocytopenia (platelets $20–50 \times 10^9$/L) – at risk of excess bleeding during operations or trauma but low risk of spontaneous bleeding.
- Mild thrombocytopenia (platelets $50–150 \times 10^9$/L) – low risk of bleeding unless there is a major operation or severe trauma.

Thrombocytopenia may result in bruising, petechiae, purpura and mucosal bleeding (e.g. epistaxis, bleeding from gums when brushing teeth). Major haemorrhage in the form of severe gastrointestinal haemorrhage, haematuria, and intracranial bleeding is much less common. The causes of easy bruising and purpura are listed in Table 23.5. While purpura may signify thrombocytopenia, it also occurs with a normal platelet count from platelet dysfunction and vascular disorders.

Immune thrombocytopenia

ITP is the most common cause of thrombocytopenia in childhood. It has an incidence of around 4 per 100 000 children per year. It is usually caused by destruction of circulating platelets by antiplatelet IgG autoantibodies. The reduced platelet count may be accompanied by a compensatory increase of megakaryocytes in the bone marrow.

Clinical features

Most children present between the ages of 2 years and 10 years, with onset often 1 week to 2 weeks after a viral infection. In the majority of children, there is a short history of days or weeks. Affected children develop petechiae, purpura, and/or superficial bruising (see Case History 23.3). It can cause epistaxis and other mucosal bleeding but profuse bleeding is uncommon, despite the fact that the platelet count often falls to less than 10×10^9/L. Intracranial bleeding is a serious but rare complication, occurring in 0.1% to 0.5%, mainly in those with a long period of severe thrombocytopenia.

Diagnosis

ITP is a diagnosis of exclusion, so careful attention must be paid to the history, clinical features, and blood film to ensure that another more sinister diagnosis is not missed. In the younger child, a congenital cause (such as Wiskott–Aldrich or Bernard–Soulier syndromes) should be considered. Any atypical clinical features, such as the presence of anaemia, neutropenia, hepatosplenomegaly, or marked lymphadenopathy, should prompt a bone marrow examination to exclude acute leukaemia or aplastic anaemia. A bone marrow examination should also be performed if the child is going to be treated with steroids, since this treatment may temporarily mask the diagnosis of acute lymphoblastic leukaemia (ALL). Inadvertent steroid therapy in undiagnosed ALL mimicking ITP is likely to delay effective treatment of the leukaemia and reduce the chance of cure of such patients. Systemic lupus erythematosus (SLE) should also be considered. However, if the clinical features are characteristic, with no abnormality in the blood other than a low platelet count and no intention to treat, there is no need to examine the bone marrow.

Management

In about 80% of children, the disease is acute, benign, and self-limiting, usually remitting spontaneously within 6 weeks to 8 weeks. Most children can be managed at home and do not require hospital admission. Treatment is controversial. Most children do not need any therapy even if their platelet count is less than 10×10^9/L but treatment should be given if there is evidence of major bleeding (e.g. intracranial or gastrointestinal haemorrhage) or persistent minor bleeding that affects daily life such as excessive epistaxis or menstrual bleeding. The treatment options include oral prednisolone, intravenous anti-D or intravenous immunoglobulin and all have significant side-effects. Platelet transfusions are reserved for life-threatening haemorrhage as they raise the platelet count only for a few hours. The parents need immediate 24-hour access to hospital treatment, and the child should avoid trauma, as far as possible, and contact sports while the platelet count is very low.

Chronic ITP

In 20% of children, the platelet count remains low 6 months after diagnosis; this is known as chronic ITP. In the majority of children, treatment is mainly supportive; drug treatment is only offered to children with chronic persistent bleeding that affects daily activities or impairs quality of life. Children with significant bleeding are rare and require specialist care. A variety of treatment modalities are available, including rituximab, a monoclonal antibody directed against B

Table 23.5 Causes of purpura or easy bruising

Platelet count reduced, i.e. thrombocytopenia	
Increased platelet destruction or consumption	
Immune	Immune thrombocytopenic purpura (ITP)
	Systemic lupus erythematosus (SLE)
	Alloimmune neonatal thrombocytopenia
Nonimmune	Haemolytic uraemic syndrome
	Thrombotic thrombocytopenic purpura
	DIC
	Congenital heart disease
	Giant haemangiomas (Kasabach–Merritt syndrome)
	Hypersplenism
Impaired platelet production	
Congenital	Fanconi anaemia
	Wiskott–Aldrich syndrome
	Bernard–Soulier syndrome
Acquired	Aplastic anaemia
	Marrow infiltration (e.g. leukaemia)
	Drug-induced
Platelet count normal	
Platelet dysfunction	
Congenital	Rare disorders, e.g. Glanzmann thrombasthenia, Hermansky Pudlak Syndrome Type 2
Acquired	Uraemia, cardiopulmonary bypass
Vascular disorders	
Congenital	Rare disorders, e.g. Ehlers–Danlos, Marfan syndrome, hereditary haemorrhagic telangiectasia
Acquired	Meningococcal and other severe infections
	Vasculitis, e.g. Henoch–Schönlein purpura, SLE
	Scurvy

lymphocytes. Newer agents such as thrombopoietic growth factors have shown clinical response in adults and may be used in children with severe nonresponsive disease. Splenectomy can be effective for this group but is mainly reserved for children who fail drug therapy as it significantly increases the risk of infection and patients require lifelong antibiotic prophylaxis. If ITP in a child becomes chronic, regular screening for SLE should be performed, as the thrombocytopenia may predate the development of autoantibodies.

Disseminated intravascular coagulation

DIC describes a disorder characterised by coagulation pathway activation leading to diffuse fibrin deposition in the microvasculature and consumption of coagulation factors and platelets.

The most common causes of activation of coagulation are severe sepsis or shock due to circulatory collapse, e.g. in meningococcal septicaemia, or extensive tissue damage from trauma or burns. DIC may be acute or chronic and is likely to be initiated through the tissue factor pathway. The predominant clinical feature is bruising, purpura, and haemorrhage. However, the pathophysiological process is characterised by microvascular thrombosis and purpura fulminans may occur.

No single test reliably diagnoses DIC. However, DIC should be suspected when the following abnormalities coexist – thrombocytopenia, prolonged PT, prolonged APTT, low fibrinogen, raised fibrinogen degradation products, and D-dimers and microangiopathic haemolytic anaemia. There is also usually a marked reduction in the naturally occurring anticoagulants, protein C and protein S and antithrombin.

The most important aspect of management is to treat the underlying cause of the DIC (usually sepsis) while providing intensive care. Supportive care may be provided with fresh frozen plasma (to replace clotting factors), cryoprecipitate and platelets. Antithrombin and protein C concentrates have been used, particularly

Case history 23.3

Immune thrombocytopenic purpura (ITP)

Sian, aged 5 years, developed bruising and a skin rash over 24 hours. She had had an upper respiratory tract infection the previous week. On examination she appeared well but had a purpuric skin rash with some bruises on the trunk and legs (Fig. 23.17). There were three blood blisters on her tongue and buccal mucosa, but no fundal haemorrhages, lymphadenopathy, or hepatosplenomegaly. Urine was normal on dipsticks testing. A full blood count showed Hb 115 g/L with normal indices, WBC and differential normal, platelet count 17×10^9/L. The platelets on the blood film were large; the film was otherwise normal. A diagnosis of ITP was made and she was discharged home. Her parents were counselled and given emergency contact names and telephone numbers. They were also given literature on the condition and advised that she should avoid contact sports but should continue to attend school. Over the next 2 weeks she continued to develop bruising and purpura but was asymptomatic. By the third week, she had no new bruises, and her platelet count was 25×10^9/L; the blood count and film showed no new abnormalities. The following week, the platelet count was 74×10^9/L and a week later it was 200×10^9/L. She was discharged from follow-up.

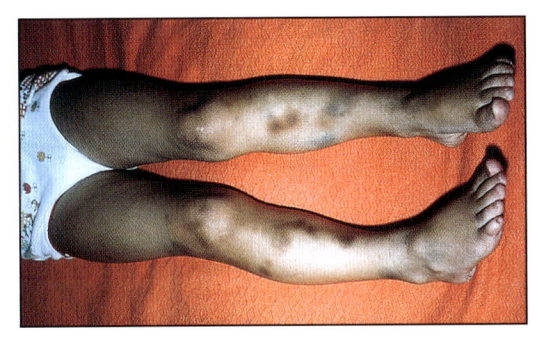

Figure 23.17 Bruising and purpura from immune thrombocytopenic purpura.

> In children with immune thrombocytopenic purpura, in spite of impressive cutaneous manifestations and extremely low platelet count, the outlook is good and most will remit quickly without any intervention

---

in severe meningococcal septicaemia with purpura fulminans. The use of heparin remains controversial.

Thrombosis in children

Thrombosis is uncommon in children and about 95% of venous thromboembolic events are secondary to underlying disorders associated with hypercoagulable states. Thrombosis of cerebral vessels usually presents with signs of a stroke. (The condition is considered further in Ch. 11 and 29.) Rarely, children may inherit abnormalities in the coagulation and fibrinolytic pathway that increase their risk of developing clots even in the absence of underlying predisposing factors. These conditions are termed congenital prothrombotic disorders (thrombophilias). They are

- Protein C deficiency
- Protein S deficiency
- Antithrombin deficiency
- Factor V Leiden
- Prothrombin gene G20210A mutation.

Proteins C and S and antithrombin are natural anticoagulants and their deficiencies are inherited in an autosomal dominant manner. Heterozygotes are also predisposed to thrombosis, usually venous, during the second or third decade of life and only rarely in childhood. Homozygous deficiency of protein C and protein S are very uncommon and present with life-threatening thrombosis with widespread haemorrhage and purpura into the skin (known as 'purpura fulminans') in the neonatal period. Homozygous antithrombin deficiency is not seen, probably because it is lethal in the fetus.

Factor V Leiden is an inherited abnormality in the structure of the coagulation protein factor V, which makes it resistant to degradation by activated protein C as part of the body's normal anticoagulant mechanism. The prothrombin gene mutation is associated with high levels of plasma prothrombin.

Acquired disorders are:

- catheter-related thrombosis
- DIC
- hypernatraemia
- polycythaemia (e.g. due to congenital heart disease)
- malignancy
- SLE and persistent antiphospholipid antibody syndrome.

Diagnosis

Although inherited thrombophilia is very uncommon, these disorders predispose to life-threatening thrombosis and so it is important not to miss the diagnosis in any child presenting with an unexplained thrombotic event. Therefore, screening tests for the presence of an inherited thrombophilia should be carried out in the following situations:

- any child with unanticipated or extensive venous thrombosis, ischaemic skin lesions, or neonatal purpura fulminans

Summary

The child with petechiae or purpura

Non-thrombocytopenic

Henoch–Schönlein purpura
- Lesions confined to buttocks, extensor surfaces of legs and arms
- Swollen painful knees and ankles
- Abdominal pain
- Haematuria

Sepsis
- Meningococcal or viral
- Clinical features – fever, septicaemia, meningitis
- Rash in meningococcal sepsis – positive glass test
- If suspected, give parenteral penicillin immediately

Trauma
- Accidental or non-accidental

Other causes (rare)

Positive glass test – rash does not blanch when pressed

Thrombocytopenia

Immune thrombocytopenia (ITP)
- 2–10 years
- Widespread petechiae and purpura and superficial bruising
- Distinguish from acute leukaemia and aplastic anaemia – clinical features, full blood count and blood film
- Bone marrow examination not required if only the platelet count is low, characteristic clinical features and no steroid treatment given
- Is acute, benign and self-limiting in about 80% of children
- Treatment – controversial, usually not required unless there is bleeding

Leukaemia
- Clinical features – malaise, infection, pallor, hepatosplenomegaly, lymphadenopathy
- Blood count – also low Hb, blasts on film, confirmed on bone marrow

Disseminated intravascular coagulation (DIC)
- Critically ill – severe sepsis or shock or extensive tissue damage

Other causes (uncommon)

- any child with a positive family history of neonatal purpura fulminans.

The screening tests are assays for protein C and protein S, antithrombin assay, polymerase chain reaction (PCR) for factor V Leiden, and for the prothrombin gene mutation.

Mutations in factor V (factor V Leiden) and the prothrombin gene, respectively, are present in 5% and 2% of the northern European population. Children with protein C deficiency or factor V Leiden have 4-times to 6-times higher risk of developing recurrent thromboses. The risk increases significantly if these conditions are inherited together. Therefore it is reasonable to screen children who develop thrombosis for all of these factors in order to plan the best management to prevent thrombosis. In the UK, current practice is not to screen asymptomatic children for genetic defects, which are not going to affect their medical management, e.g. on the basis of family history alone, until they are old enough to receive appropriate counselling and make decisions for themselves.

Summary

Thrombosis

All children with thrombosis should be screened for inherited or acquired predisposing disorders.

Acknowledgements

We would like to acknowledge contributors to this chapter in previous editions, whose work we have drawn on: Lynne Ball (1st Edition), Paula Bolton-Maggs (2nd Edition), Irene Roberts (3rd, 4th Edition), Michele Cummins 3rd Edition), Subarna Chakravorty (4th Edition).

Further reading

Bailey S, Skinner R: *Paediatric Haematology and Oncology. Oxford Specialist Handbooks in Paediatrics.* Oxford, 2009, Oxford University Press.

Lanzkowsky P, Lipton JM, Fish JD, editors: *Lanzkowsky's Manual of Pediatric Hematology and Oncology,* ed 6, 2016, Academic Press.

Lilleyman JS, Hann IM, Blanchette VS, editors: *Pediatric Haematology,* ed 3, Edinburgh, 2005, Churchill Livingstone.
A two-volume, comprehensive textbook

Orkin SH, Nathan DG, Ginsburg D, et al: *Nathan and Oski's Hematology and Oncology of Infancy and Childhood, 2-Volume Set, 8e (Nathan and Oskis Hematology of Infancy and Childhood),* 2014, Elsevier Saunders.

Websites (Accessed November 2016)

British Committee for Standards in Haematology guidelines: Available at: http://www.bcshguidelines.com.

Diamond–Blackfan syndrome: *UK Diamond Blackfan Anaemia Support Group.* Available at: http://www.diamondblackfan.org.uk.

Haemophilia: *World Federation of Haemophilia.* Available at: http://www.wfh.org or The Haemophilia Society. Available at: http://www.haemophilia.org.uk.

Sickle Cell Society: Available at: http://www.sicklecellsociety.org.

UK Thalassaemia Society: Available at: http://www.ukts.org.

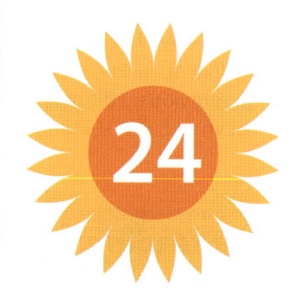

24 Child and adolescent mental health

How to ask about emotional and behavioural problems	424	Specific paediatric mental health problems	428
Adversities in the family	427	Management of emotional and behavioural problems	439

Features of child mental health are:
- good emotional health in childhood is a stronger predictor of high satisfaction in adult life than any other factor, including wealth, education and physical health
- suicide is the second most common cause of death in adolescents, both male and female
- more than 50% of adult mental illness is apparent by age 15 years
- mental illness is the single biggest cause of morbidity in adults.

Mental health has many confusing definitions. We will use the term to denote the emotional and behavioural aspects of children and young people. Therefore, the terms 'mental health' and 'emotional and behavioural' are used interchangeably in this chapter.

Also, when we refer to 'mental health problems' we mean any emotional and behavioural difficulty that adversely affects the child's life. Mental health disorders are diagnosed in a subset of children with emotional and behavioural problems, according to diagnostic criteria; these are often, but not always, applied to the more severely affected individuals. When we refer to 'child', 'children', or 'childhood', we include adolescence.

Mental health problems are common in paediatric populations (Table 24.1).

They are also complex. There is seldom, if ever, a single cause for a mental health problem, and factors in their evolution span biological, psychological and social domains, and can occur at any age. The key implications are:
- mental health assessments take time
- assessment needs to be undertaken in a flexible way
- no one agency can span the complexity of factors involved, so child mental health is 'everyone's business'.

How to ask about emotional and behavioural problems

Effective history taking must be open, explorative, non-judgemental and empathic. A technique of Socratic Questioning, with disciplined questioning to get the person or family to answer their own questions. Allowing complex issues to be explored, is advised.

It is best to interview both parents if possible. While doing so, consider the quality of their relationship and the parents' mental state. Ask open questions where possible and feel able to ask directly about feelings. Assess the attitudes of the parents to the child. Obtain examples of the problem and estimate its frequency, severity, duration and the impact it has on both the child and family.

Interview the child and ask to see the older child alone as part of the assessment. Explain to the parents that you always like to have a few words with children

Table 24.1 Prevalence of diagnosable mental health disorders and mental health problems

Population	Diagnosable mental health disorder	Total mental health problems
General population	10%	20%
Paediatric outpatients	20–30%	50%
Epilepsy	40%	up to 70% in complicated epilepsy

on their own as they may have things they may feel too embarrassed to discuss with parents present. Assess the extent of the child's suffering (they may be somewhat brazen and minimize this). Keep your questions very simple and specific, making sure the child understands what it is you want to know. This also applies to adolescents, who you need to ask about use of drugs and alcohol, experience of abuse, thoughts of self-harm and suicide. Consider whether reports from school or other involved agencies might help.

When taking a history from parents about the problem, the following questions may be useful:

- How does the problem affect the child and family?
- Who is in the family? Are there other problems in the family?
- Has the child themselves suffered any adversity?
- How did the current difficulties start?
- What else was happening at the time?

This is standard medical history, of course. However, the next set of questions will reveal more:

- How do people respond to the problem?
- What do you think about the problem? What does the child think?
- What worries everyone most?
- What are you doing about it already?
- Are there any times when it gets better?

When talking to adolescents, the following techniques may be helpful:

- *Clarifying their thinking,* e.g. 'Could you explain that further?'
- *Challenging their assumptions,* e.g. 'Is this always the case?'
- *Requesting evidence,* e.g. 'Why do you say that?'
- *Exploring implications and consequences,* e.g. 'How does…affect…?'
- *Questioning the question,* e.g. 'Why do you think that I asked that?'

Also, asking them to rate their mood (in the last fortnight) on a scale of 1–10 gives a useful baseline.

How mental health problems evolve in childhood

The process by which mental health problems evolve is closely related to the process of child development (see Ch. 3), and many of the same factors are in play. We will describe biological, psychological and social factors in turn, then bring these together in a 'biopsychosocial formulation'.

Biological/developmental factors

Genetic factors are important in the aetiology of many mental health problems. For developmental problems in which emotion and behaviour are integral to the presentation, such as autism spectrum disorder (ASD) and attention deficit hyperactivity disorder (ADHD), genetic factors are predominant in determining the neurobiology that underpins them. For instance, the heritability of autism spectrum disorder is usually estimated as being in excess of 80%. For disorders of a less

Box 24.1 Effect of chronic illness on mental health

Biological: direct effect on neurobiology, either from condition itself (e.g. epilepsy) or treatment (e.g. steroids for asthma).

Psychological: often marked by a similar psychological process to bereavement, with both denial and over-acceptance possible adverse results.

Social: effect on family wide-ranging and complex. Difference from peers becomes increasingly important and difficult in adolescence.

clearly developmental nature (e.g. anxiety), genetics and family history are still of great importance, although less is known and heritability is invariably lower.

Early biological adversity is an important risk factor both for developmental conditions and mental health problems. These include:

- prematurity
- exposure to toxins in utero, most commonly alcohol
- serious illness in infancy (e.g. meningitis).

In addition, later illness and chronic conditions (e.g. epilepsy) can represent a biological psychological and social challenge all in one (Box 24.1).

Developmental status is important to ascertain when assessing mental health, whether or not the child has a known specific developmental diagnosis. It may be that a behaviour that is thought to be abnormal is, in a child with developmental delay, normal for the developmental age. Specific problems with communication, interaction, and behavioural inhibition will affect the child's ability to respond in a constructive way to frustration and other challenges (Box 24.2).

Psychological factors

Self-esteem

Children develop views and make attributions about themselves. Most children experience praise and success in enough areas of their lives to develop a sense of inner self-confidence and self-worth. Those who do not are at increased risk of developing emotional and behavioural disorders which in turn may breed further

Box 24.2 Developmental problems and behavioural responses

Language impairment: child unable to verbalize feelings, so expresses them in behaviour problem – if this is not appreciated early on, this will escalate

Autism spectrum disorder (ASD): difficulty by the child understanding and accepting even quite subtle changes can lead to avoidant and often extreme behaviours

Attention deficit hyperactivity disorder (ADHD): child 'acts before thinking' and so frequently lashes out or shouts when frustrated

shame and failure. A child who does not consider himself/herself worthwhile and valued by others will play safe and not attempt new activities or explore new situations because of a fear of failure. This restricts the development of coping skills and knowledge of the world generally. It may also be a vulnerability factor for depression and anxiety disorders. Children who lack a belief in their own worth may adopt extraordinary and problematic behaviours in order to attract the attention and acclaim of others. For instance, one child took to openly eating dog faeces because it attracted a crowd of amazed children around her. Repeated failure, academically or socially, will undermine self-esteem, as will some disorders themselves (dyspraxia, enuresis and faecal soiling in particular). An important source of low self-esteem, however, is the child's parents, either because of their own low self-esteem or because of abuse (emotional, sexual or physical, and neglect).

Cognitive style

As children grow older, their thinking style evolves from one that is concrete to one that is able to cope with abstract thought. Below the age of about 5 years, thought is fundamentally egocentric, with the child being at the centre of his world (Box 24.3). During middle childhood, the dominant mode of thought is practical and orderly but tied to immediate circumstances and specific experiences rather than hypothetical possibilities or metaphors. Not until the mid-teens does the adult style of abstract thought begin to appear.

☼ **Adjust the way you talk to children to be compatible with their thinking style**

Social factors

Early relationships and attachment

In the first 2 months of a baby's life, infants are not fussy about who responds to their needs. From 3–6 months of age they become more selective, demanding comfort from one or two caregivers. By age 6–8 months they are particular about who responds to their needs or holds them, especially when distressed, and show tearful

Box 24.3 The quality of preschool thought

- The child is at the centre of his world ('I'm tired so it's getting dark')
- Everything has a purpose ('The sea is there for us to swim in')
- Inanimate objects are alive ('Naughty table hurt me') and have feelings and motives
- Poor categorization (all men are Daddies)
- Use of magical thinking ('If I close my eyes, she'll go away')
- Use of sequences or routines rather than a sense of time
- The use of toys and other aspects of imaginative play as aids to thought (particularly in making sense of experience and social relationships)

separation anxiety if their main caregiver, usually the mother, is not there. If tired, fearful, unhappy, or in pain, they will cling to her and be comforted by her presence as an *attachment figure*. At this time, the child learns to crawl, and so is able to leave a primary caregiver and possibly encounter danger. The development of attachment behaviour allows the infant to keep track of their parent's whereabouts and resist separation. This close attachment relationship derives from social interaction and the mother's sensitive responsiveness to the baby's needs, not from any blood tie. It need not be with the biological mother, although it usually is. Its importance lies in it being:

- a particularly close relationship within which the child's development of trust, empathy, conscience and ideals is promoted, forming a prototype for future close relationships
- the child's primary source of comfort, providing the principal method of coping with stress (fear, anxiety, pain, etc.).

Children who have never had the opportunity for a close, secure attachment relationship in their early years are at risk of growing up as self-centred individuals who seek the affection and attention of others but have difficulty with close personal relationships and with learning to conform with social rules of conduct.

The selective clinging of early attachment behaviour diminishes over time, so that in the second year of life children extend their emotional attachments to other family members and carers. By school age, they can tolerate separations from their parents for several hours. Children vary in their ability to do this depending on their temperament and social circumstances. For example, a child who is constitutionally apprehensive, who has an exceptionally anxious mother, or who has parents who threaten abandonment is likely to continue to cling to his/her mother for protection and comfort. A series of frightening events will tend to perpetuate clinging, which may persist well into middle childhood (age 5–12 years). This interferes with children's capacity to learn how to cope with anxiety on their own (Fig. 24.1).

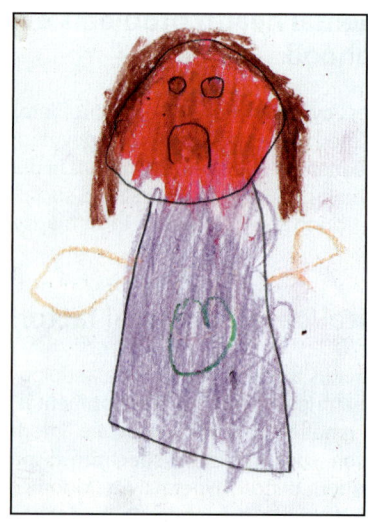

Figure 24.1 A 6-year-old with separation anxiety, showing what it feels like to leave her mother to go to school.

With entry into school, the importance of teachers and other children in shaping psychosocial development increases and their influence must be taken into account in understanding any schoolchild's development.

> **Summary**
>
> **Early relationships**
> Young children:
> - develop a close attachment relationship with their mother (or main caregiver)
> - if separated from their mother, may develop separation anxiety
> - if admitted to hospital, should be able to have their parents stay with them.

Adversities in the family

Family relationships are, for most children, the source of their most powerful emotions. Similarly, parents have more effect than anyone else on children's social learning and behaviour. The ecological model of child development indicates that families are generally the most potent environmental influence on a child's mental health. They are not all-powerful, since a predisposition to particular childhood emotional and behavioural problems can be inherited, but family influences interact with this so that overt disorder may or may not emerge. As mentioned above, not all disorders have their origin in family adversities; some (e.g. ASD and ADHD) arise independently of them. Nevertheless, the non-genetic contribution of family interactions to emotional and behavioural disorders is often substantial and the mechanisms whereby they produce disorder are various. The following are some of the known risk factors:

- angry discord between family members
- parental mental ill health, especially maternal depression
- bereavement
- divorce and subsequent loss of a parent figure (in some cases)
- intrusive overprotection
- lack of parental authority
- physical and sexual abuse
- emotional rejection or excessive criticism
- inconsistent, unpredictable discipline
- using the child to fulfil the unreasonable personal emotional needs of a parent
- inappropriate responsibilities or expectations for the child's level of maturity.

While parents need to be made aware of changes required to improve the situation, it is unwise to blame them for causing their child's problem as it makes them less likely to engage in treatment. It is more constructive and accurate to place the difficulties at home in the context of a biopsychosocial formulation.

Adversities outside the family

Experiences with other children are increasingly recognized as highly significant in psychosocial development. Bullying is a known adversity, and other forms of peer-mediated persecution. Conversely, having a number of steady, good-quality peer relationships is a marker for good prognosis in an emotional or behavioural problem which has resulted from environmental influences.

The majority of older children and adolescents in the developed world have internet access and utilize social media websites regularly, often using smartphone devices. Social media platforms are transforming the way young people communicate with one another. Whilst there are benefits in the form of online support groups and fora, and promising tools for education and mental health awareness, there is increasing evidence that vulnerable adolescents can be harmed by exposure to websites which may promote eating disordered or addictive behaviour. There are many online fora where discussions about self-harm and suicide can have a toxic effect on the adolescent. Cyberbullying over the internet is usually carried out by the same people as conventional bullying, but appears to be more damaging.

Excessive use of electronic devices can impact on sleep and reduce interpersonal interactions.

> **Summary**
>
> **Regarding adversities**
> - The child's family is the most potent influence on the child's mental health.
> - Adversities outside the family, e.g. bullying, may aggravate the situation.

Resilience

Given all the possible adversities that children could suffer, it may seem amazing that mental health problems are not universal! The reason for this is that for every adverse factor there is a corresponding factor that may increase the child's resilience and compensate for any adversity encountered.

Most are simply the converse of the factors listed above (for instance, good social interactions skills), but there are some specific resilience factors that should be enquired about:

- time spent together as a family
- meals eaten as a family
- regular exercise
- regular and sufficient sleep
- absence of bullying.

Putting it together: the biopsychosocial formulation

Once you have a wide-ranging history, the following structure can be used. It is useful to split factors into:

- predisposing – which usually can't be helped
- precipitating – which are useful in explaining the situation

Table 24.2 The 4p format to assist to develop a biopsychosocial formulation

	Biological/developmental	Psychological	Social
Predisposing factors			
Precipitating factors			
Perpetuating factors			
Protective factors (resilience)			

Case history 24.1

Ahmed, 2 years old, refuses to go to bed at bedtime, and screams loudly instead of going to sleep. His health visitor has advised his mother to shut the bedroom door and ignore him, but it's not working and is upsetting her. Table 24.3 shows her 4p framework.

This leads to some simple, hopefully helpful interventions:

- Stop screen time before bedtime.
- Mother to seek counselling/treatment for depression.
- Grandparents asked to help with domestic tasks so mother can spend time with Ahmed.
- Gradual withdrawal of mother from bedroom at bedtime, following good 'wind-down' with bath followed by reading stories.

Table 24.3 Use of 4p framework for Ahmed

	Biological/developmental	Psychological	Social
Predisposing	Preterm birth	Maternal anxiety	
Precipitating		Break-up of parents' relationship	Domestic violence
Perpetuating	Screen use (TV) in bedroom up till bedtime	Anxiety of mother	Mother unavailable due to depression

- perpetuating factors – which are ongoing and usually the easiest to target, along with encouraging identified resilience factors.

You can then use the information (Table 24.2) to agree a story with the family about what is happening. This will be far more useful than any single explanation of the child's predicament, and it can lead to wide-ranging, helpful intervention. An example is shown in Case history 24.1.

Specific paediatric mental health problems

Problems of the preschool years

Meal refusal

A common scenario is a mother complaining that her child refuses to eat any or much of what she provides; mealtimes have become a battleground. Examination reveals a healthy, well-nourished child whose height and weight are securely within normal limits on a centile growth chart.

An account of what goes on at a typical mealtime may reveal:

- A past history of force-feeding
- Irregular meals so that the child is not predictably hungry
- Unsuitable meals
- Unreasonably large portions
- Multiple opportunities for distraction, e.g. TV.

Most importantly, how much does the child eat between meals? A well-nourished child is getting food from somewhere. Not all parents regard sweets and crisps as being food. Some mothers, while concerned about their child's apparently poor food intake, provide little variety in the child's diet. For strategies for dealing with meal refusal, see Box 24.4.

Box 24.4 Strategy for meal refusal

Mealtime history
What is the parent most concerned about?
- Nutrition?
  - Refer to growth chart
- Discipline and parenting?
  - Family history of eating problems
  - Parenting style
  - What do others say?
  - Is it part of a broader behavioural problem?

How much food is eaten between meals?
- Food diary to record child's intake over a number of days

Advice
- As long as offered wholesome food with adequate range, children are remarkably good at eating an appropriate quantity of food when allowed a reasonable choice
- As it is impossible to force a child to eat, avoid confrontation at mealtimes
- Develop a relaxed atmosphere
- Use favourite foods as a reward. Introduce other rewards for compliance at mealtimes (e.g. additional privileges such as extra TV time)
- Reduce eating between meals if necessary, although many young children prefer small, frequent snacks

---

Box 24.5 Reasons for a child not settling at night

- Too much sleep in the late afternoon
- Displaced sleep/wake cycle – not waking child in morning because did not settle until late on the previous night
- Separation anxiety
- Overstimulated or overwrought in the evening
- Kept awake by siblings or noisy neighbours or TV in the bedroom
- Erratic parental practices: no bedtime or routine to cue child into sleep readiness, sudden removal from play to go to bed without prior warning to wind down
- Use of bedroom as punishment
- Dislike of darkness and silence – night light and playing story tapes can be helpful
- Some chronic physical conditions may be associated with sleep problems, e.g. painful crisis in sickle cell disease

---

Sleep-related problems
Difficulty in settling to sleep at bedtime

This is a common problem in the toddler years. The child will not go to sleep unless the parent is present. Most instances are normal expressions of separation anxiety, but there may be other obvious reasons for it which can be explored in taking a history (Box 24.5), supplemented if necessary by the parents keeping a prospective sleep diary. Many cases will respond to simple advice:

- creating a bedtime routine which cues the child to what is required
- telling the child to lie quietly in bed until he/she falls asleep, recognizing that children cannot fall asleep to order (although that is what everyone tells them to do)
- having a period of an hour before sleep time when the child is not involved with screens.

If that advice does not resolve the problem, a more active intervention may be required. This involves parents imposing a graded pattern of lengthening periods between tucking their child up in bed and coming back after a few minutes to visit, but leaving the room before the child falls asleep, even if they are protesting. The object is to provide the opportunity for the child to learn how to fall sleep alone, a skill not yet developed. More refractory cases may require specialist referral.

Waking at night

This is normal, but some children cry because they cannot settle themselves back to sleep without their parent's presence. This is often associated with difficulty settling in the evenings, which should be treated first. Some children who can settle in the evening may be unable to settle when they wake in the night because the circumstances are different – it is quieter, darker, etc. The graded approach described above for evening settling can also be used in the middle of the night. Parents will find it helpful to take alternate nights on duty to share the burden.

Nightmares

These are bad dreams which can be recalled by the child. They are common, rarely requiring professional attention unless they occur frequently or are stereotyped in content, indicating a morbid preoccupation or symptomatic of a psychiatric disorder such as posttraumatic stress disorder. Unless a disorder is suspected, reassuring the child and his family will usually suffice.

Night (sleep) terrors

These are different from nightmares, occurring about 1.5 hours after settling. The parents find the child sitting up in bed, eyes open, seemingly awake but obviously disorientated, confused and distressed, and unresponsive to their questions and reassurances. The child settles back to sleep after a few minutes and has no recollection of the episode in the morning. A night terror is a *parasomnia*, a disturbance of the structure of sleep wherein a very rapid emergence from the first period of deep slow-wave sleep produces a state of high arousal and confusion. Sleepwalking has similar origins and the two may be combined. Most night terrors need little more than reassurance directed towards the parents. The most important intervention for sleepwalking is to make the environment safe to prevent injury to the child (e.g. not sleeping on the

> **Box 24.6** Managing toddler disobedience
>
> - Ensure your demand is reasonable for the developmental stage of the child
> - Tell the child what you want him/her to do rather than nagging about what you do not want him/her to do
> - Praise for compliance, especially when it is spontaneous (catch doing the right thing)
> - Use simple incentives to reward good behaviour
> - Use instructions like 'If you (do this or that) … then we/I can do such and such' (not the other way round)
> - Avoid threats that cannot be carried out
> - Follow through with any consequences you indicated for noncompliance
> - Ignore some episodes of defiance if they are not significant

upper bunk of a double-bunk bed, putting gates before the staircase, locking the kitchen, etc.). Given that a common cause of night terrors and sleepwalking is a poor and erratic sleep schedule, a sleep routine can be helpful in preventing recurrence. Once parents have implemented the safety suggestions highlighted above, they can be reassured, as the natural course of these disorders is to decrease over time.

Disobedience, defiance, and tantrums

Normal toddlers often go through a phase of refusing to comply with parents' demands, sometimes angrily ('the terrible twos'). This is an understandable reaction to the discovery that the world is not organized around them. They also become confused and angered by the fact that the parent who provides them with comfort when they are distressed is also the person who is making them do things they do not wish to do. This seems exceptionally unfair to them. That is one reason why children play their parents up but may be fine with others. All this can exhaust and demoralize parents, not least because many people offer advice or criticism (everyone thinks themselves an expert in the area of children's development and behaviour). The points listed in Box 24.6 can be made.

Temper tantrums are ordinary responses to frustration, especially at not being allowed to have or do something. They are common and normal in young preschool children. If asked for advice, a sensible first move is to take a history, analyzing a couple of tantrums according to the ABC paradigm (Box 24.7).

> **Box 24.7** Analyzing a tantrum
>
> - **A**ntecedents – what happened in the minutes before the episode
> - **B**ehaviour – exactly what did the episode consist of
> - **C**onsequences – what happened as a result, including what you did and the outcome

Next, examine the child to identify potential medical or psychological factors. Medical factors include global or language delay, hearing impairment (e.g. glue ear), and medication with bronchodilators or anticonvulsants. If none are present, there are management strategies that can be adopted, some of which are shown in Box 24.8.

The easiest course of action is to distract the child or, if this cannot be done, to let the tantrum burn itself out while the parent leaves the room, returning a few minutes later when things quieten down (provided it is safe to leave the child alone). Obviously this should be done in a calm, neutral manner and certainly not accompanied by threats of abandonment. Tantrums which are essentially coercive (when a child is demanding something from a parent) must be met by a refusal to give in. They can often be forestalled by the simple expedient of making rules which the child can be reminded of before the situation presents itself. An alternative course is to use 'time out', which is a form of structured ignoring. The child in a tantrum is placed somewhere such as the hallway, where no-one will talk to him for a short time, e.g. 1 min per year of age. During this period they are ignored. Parents often expect this manoeuvre to produce a contrite child, complaining if it does not do so immediately. In fact, when used for tantrums, time out works according to different principles (not as a response to punishment but to the withdrawal of attention) and often takes several weeks to effect a gradual improvement. It may help to ask the mother to keep records to document this.

Disobedience can be dealt with by using a star chart to reward the child for complying with parental requests. The chart needs to be where the child can see it and it must be the case that the child knows what to do in order to get a star. It is wisest not to 'fine' the child by taking stars away once they have been earned. If the parent who is rewarding compliance by the child praises at the same time as giving the star, there may not be the need to tie stars with a material reward. However, if a tangible reward had been promised for a certain number of stars, it is important to follow through with this.

> **Box 24.8** Tantrums: management strategies
>
> - Affection and attention before the tantrum
> - Distraction
> - Avoiding antecedents
> - Ignoring:
>   - effective but can be difficult
>   - no surrender (when parents give in, tantrums become harder to deal with over time)
> - Time out from positive reinforcement:
>   - walk away, returning when quietens down
>   - separate from siblings
> - Holding firmly if the child is putting themselves or others in danger
> - Star chart to prevent future episodes.

The 1–2–3 principle for tantrums or aggressive behaviour

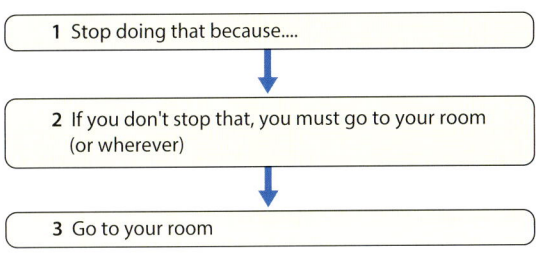

1. Stop doing that because....

2. If you don't stop that, you must go to your room (or wherever)

3. Go to your room

Figure 24.2 The 1–2–3 principle for tantrums or aggressive behaviour.

☀ For temper tantrums
- Analyse according to antecedents, behaviour and consequences
- Consider distraction, avoiding antecedents, ignoring and time out

Aggressive behaviour

Small children can be aggressive for a host of reasons, ranging from spite to exuberance. Much aggressive behaviour is learned, either by being rewarded (often inadvertently) or by copying parents, siblings or peers. For example, many instances of aggressive, demanding behaviour are provoked or intensified by a parent shouting at or smacking their child. In such cases, it is the parent's behaviour which needs to change. In most instances, the same principles as apply to tantrums are valid: make rules clear, stick to them, keep cool, do not give in and use time out if necessary. The latter can often be used on a 1–2–3 principle (Fig. 24.2). A tired or stressed child will be irritable and prone to angry outbursts, as will children whose communication skills are compromised by deafness or a developmental language disorder so that they are frustrated and exasperated. Optimistic reassurance that the child will spontaneously grow out of a pattern of aggressive behaviour is mistaken; once established, an aggressive behavioural style is remarkably persistent over a period of years. Thus, aggressive behaviour in children needs to be proactively managed. There are several evidence-based parenting programmes that are effective for teaching parents to manage aggression in their children. Parents should be encouraged to attend such programmes.

Autism spectrum disorder and attention deficit hyperactivity disorder

These are considered in Chapter 4.

Problems of middle childhood

Nocturnal enuresis

Children can wet themselves by day or night, but in colloquial speech, 'enuresis' is synonymous with bed-wetting. Infrequent bedwetting is common in children; nocturnal enuresis with bedwetting greater than 2 nights/week is present in about 6% of 5 year olds and 1.5% of 10 year olds. Boys outnumber girls by nearly 2 to 1. There is a genetically determined delay in acquiring sphincter competence, with two-thirds of children with enuresis having an affected first-degree relative. There may also be interference in learning to become dry at night. Small children need reasonable freedom from stress and a measure of parental approval in order to learn night-time continence. It is well recognized that emotional stress can interfere and cause secondary enuresis (relapse after a period of dryness). Most children with enuresis are psychologically normal and the treatment of nocturnal enuresis still relies mainly on the symptomatic approach described below, although any underlying stress, emotional or physical disorder must be addressed.

Organic causes of enuresis are uncommon but include:
- urinary tract infection
- faecal retention severe enough to reduce bladder volume and cause bladder neck dysfunction
- polyuria from osmotic diuresis, e.g. diabetes mellitus or renal concentrating disorders, e.g. chronic kidney disease.

It may also be associated with developmental, attention or learning difficulties.

Investigation with urinalysis is only indicated if the bed wetting is of recent onset, if it occurs during the day, if there are features of urinary tract infection, diabetes mellitus or ill health.

Daytime and secondary enuresis are considered in Chapter 19.

The management of nocturnal enuresis is straightforward but needs to be painstaking to succeed. After the age of 4 years, enuresis resolves spontaneously in only 5% of affected children each year. In practice, treatment is rarely undertaken before 5 years of age.

Explanation

The first step is to explain to both child and parent that the problem is common and beyond conscious control. The parents should stop punitive procedures, as these are counterproductive. Excessive or insufficient fluid intake and abnormal toileting patterns should be addressed. Waking or lifting during the night does not promote long-term dryness.

Star chart

The child earns praise and a star can be awarded for agreed behaviour helping to change the sheets rather than dry nights. Wet beds are treated in a matter-of-fact way and the child is not blamed for them.

Enuresis alarm

If a child does not respond to a star chart, it may be supplemented with an enuresis alarm. This is a sensor, usually placed in the child's pants or under the child, which sounds an alarm when it becomes wet. In order to be effective, the alarm must wake the child, who gets out of bed, goes to pass urine, returns and helps to remake a wet bed before going back to sleep. It is not necessary to reset the alarm that night. Parental help can be enlisted in the night using a baby alarm to transmit the noise of the alarm to the parents' bedroom.

The alarm method takes several weeks to achieve dryness but is effective in most cases so long as the child is motivated and the procedure is followed fully. About one-third relapse after a few months, in which case repeat treatment with the alarm usually produces lasting dryness.

Desmopressin

Desmopressin, a synthetic analogue of antidiuretic hormone, may be used in children over 7 years of age if treatment with the alarm is unsuccessful or unacceptable, or short-term relief is required, e.g. for holidays or sleep overs. It can be taken as tablets or sublingually. Fluid intake should be restricted after use. It may need to be continued for 3–6 months.

Self-help groups

These provide advice and assistance to parents and health professionals, e.g. ERIC, The Children's Bowel and Bladder Charity.

Summary

Nocturnal enuresis
- Common, males more than females.
- Most affected children are psychologically and physically normal.
- Treatment usually considered only at >5 years of age.
- Management – explanation, star charts, enuresis alarm, sometimes desmopressin.

Faecal soiling

It is abnormal for a child to soil after the age of 4 years. Thereafter, children who soil fall into two broad groups: those with and those without a rectum loaded with faeces. Because of this, it is important to ascertain whether there is faecal retention by abdominal palpation. The reasons why a child's rectum becomes loaded are various, and commonly involve an interplay between constitutional factors and experience. Some children have a rectum that only empties occasionally, perhaps because of poor coordination with anal sphincter relaxation, and are thus more prone to developing retention. Superimposed upon this are a number of other factors:

- constipation, possibly following dehydration during an illness
- inhibition of defecation because of pain from a fissure
- inhibition because of fear of punishment for incontinence
- anxieties about using the toilet.

Once established, a huge bolus of hard faeces may be beyond the capacity of the child to shift. Furthermore, a rectum loaded with hard or soft faeces (both are found) dilates and habituates to distension so that the child becomes unaware of the need to empty it. The loaded rectum inhibits the anus via the rectoanal reflex and stool may seep out with spontaneous rectal contractions beyond the child's control. Soiling occurs in the child's pants, which may then be removed and hidden out of shame.

Any reasons for faecal retention, such as an anal fissure, should be identified and treated, but the most important thing is to empty the rectum as soon as possible. The child and parents need to understand that retention is present and how it leads to incontinence.

A stool softener (macrogol) is given for a couple of weeks, followed, if necessary, by a stimulant laxative. Rarely, an enema is required. Once the rectum is disimpacted, maintenance laxative therapy is maintained (see Fig. 14.15 for details). The child can be encouraged to defecate regularly in the toilet, which earns stars on a star chart. Such retraining may take a number of weeks while the distended rectum shrinks to a normal size. Throughout this period a regular laxative is usually needed.

In some cases, repeated soiling will have been such a humiliating experience for the child that they psychologically deny there is a problem and cooperation is doubtful. Other children find that their involuntary soiling allows them a measure of control over parents and they are reluctant to surrender an apparently useful weapon. Such cases may need psychiatric referral.

Soiling may occur in conjunction with an empty rectum for various other uncommon reasons. Some children have an urgency of defecation for apparently constitutional reasons and can only postpone defecation for a few minutes; they can be taken by surprise. Some children have neuropathic bowel secondary to occult spinal abnormality, usually associated with urinary incontinence. Similarly, diarrhoea can overwhelm bowel control. The child may have a general learning disability with a mental age below 4 years, so that expectations of social bowel control need to be revised accordingly. Lastly, the child may defecate intentionally as a hostile act. Such children may be entrenched in distorted relationships with their parents and may have other behavioural problems requiring psychiatric referral.

Summary

Faecal retention
- Present in most children who soil.
- May be due to constipation or reluctance to open the bowels because of pain or reluctance to use the toilet.
- When present, the rectum needs to be emptied, initially with a stool softener and laxative, followed by retraining.

Recurrent unexplained somatic symptoms/somatisation

Recurrent medically unexplained (functional somatic) symptoms are common in childhood and adolescence. In many cases, they are aggravated by stress but they can also be the expression of an anxiety or depressive disorder. Somatisation is the term used for the communication of emotional distress, troubled relationships, and personal predicaments through bodily symptoms. The prepubertal child may experience affective distress as recurrent abdominal pain (this symptom peaking at age 9 years) and headaches (peaking at age 12 years). With increasing age, limb pain, aching muscles, fatigue, and neurological symptoms become more prominent.

Recurrent central abdominal pain, often sharp and colicky, affects about 10% of school-age children. The causes are considered in Chapter 14. In the majority of cases, no organic cause can be objectively demonstrated, yet the child is obviously in pain. Some of these children have clinically significant anxiety; whether this came before the onset of the pain or afterwards, it is an important perpetuating factor.

The history must attend to possible sources of stress and the child should be interviewed about school, friends and family, noting the general level of anxiety and ability to communicate. This should be an integral part of the interview and not done as an afterthought when organic causes have been excluded. A thorough physical examination is important to reassure the child and family that there is no underlying organic cause. It also provides an opportunity to gain further information about the nature of the pain and the child's reaction to it. When examining the child, it is sensible to ask the child to point to where the pain is. In general, the further the pain is from the umbilicus, the more likely it is being caused by organic pathology (Apley's rule).

The pain may be limited to school days or coincide with upsetting events in the home, such as parental conflict, or other specific situations. A short interview with the child on their own can reveal sources of stress which may be otherwise unrecognized by parents or which the child is wary of mentioning in front of them. Problems at school, particularly bullying and teasing, or difficulties with a teacher or class work may only be known by the child. A report from the school may be helpful. Completing a 4p framework is often helpful. A joint interview with both parents and the child is a good arena for explaining to the child and family how organic disease has been ruled out and, if appropriate, how tension can give rise to pain using familiar examples such as headache. It is often necessary to promote communication between family members to avoid any tendency for somatic symptoms to replace verbal communication of distress. Learning pain-coping skills, such as relaxation, may be helpful, especially for headaches. Referral to child and adolescent mental health services is indicated if any identified stressors cannot be relieved by straightforward means, if there is serious family dysfunction, or if the pain impairs the child's general functioning at home or school.

Tics

A tic is a quick, sudden, coordinated movement, which is apparently purposeful and recurs in the same part of the child's body. It is not entirely involuntary in that it can be purposefully suppressed to some extent. About 1 in 10 children develop a tic at some stage, typically around the face and head – blinking, frowning, head-flicking, sniffing, throat clearing and grunting being the most common. Boys are more commonly affected. The average age of onset is 8 years old: the tics tend to peak in intensity aged 11 years, then improve thereafter. Tics are most likely to occur when the child is inactive (watching TV or on long car journeys) and often disappear when actively concentrating. They may worsen with anxiety but they are not themselves an emotional reaction. In many cases, there is a family history. Most children do not need treatment. *Transient tic disorder* clear up over the next few months, although they may recur from time to time. They should be treated with reassurance in the first place.

Less commonly, the child has tics from which he/she is hardly ever free. They may be multiple, although there is fluctuation in the predominance of any particular tic and in overall severity. If the tics continue for more than 12 months they are considered chronic in nature, although most cases still resolve in adulthood. If there is both multiple motor tics and vocal tics such as grunting, coughing, humming, squeaking, the condition is known as *Gilles de la Tourette* syndrome, or more simply, Tourette's. Swearing as a verbal tic (coprolalia) is uncommon. These conditions tend to be persistent in the medium term. The first line of treatment is cognitive behavioural therapy with habit reversal techniques. More serious cases may require medication (such as clonidine or risperidone) under specialist supervision.

Antisocial behaviour

Children steal, lie, disobey, light fires, destroy things and pick fights for various reasons:

- failure to learn when to exercise social restraint
- lack of social skills, such as the ability to negotiate a disagreement
- they may be responding to the challenges of their peers in spite of their parents' prohibitions
- they may be chronically angry and resentful
- they may find their own notions of good behaviour overwhelmed by emotion such as sadness or temptation.

When serious antisocial behaviour which infringes the rights of others is the dominant feature of the clinical picture and is so severe as to represent a handicap to general functioning, a diagnosis of *conduct disorder* is made. Children with conduct disorder may not have necessarily broken the law, although their behaviour excites strong social disapproval. They typically come from homes in which there are considerable discord,

---

Summary

Somatic symptoms
- May be a means of communicating emotional distress.
- Sources of stress should be identified and ameliorated if possible.
- In many children with unexplained recurrent abdominal pain or headaches, no significant sources of stress are identified.

coercive relationships, limited boundaries that are inconsistently enforced and poor supervision by adults. A milder form, characterized by angry, defiant behaviour to authority figures such as parents and teachers, is known as *oppositional-defiant disorder*.

Treating conduct disorder can be difficult. Parent management training programmes (such as Webster–Stratton and Triple P) have an excellent evidence base and are highly recommended as primary interventions. However, poor parental cooperation and motivation can result in minimal benefit. Where parents are unwilling or unable to take up parenting programmes, affected children can be offered individual or group-based interventions focusing on problem-solving skills and anger management. Although these interventions show benefit in research settings, affected children often do not have the level of motivation required to benefit in routine clinic settings. In the absence of a coexisting psychiatric condition responsive to medication, it is not considered standard clinical practice to use medication for conduct disorder in the UK.

> **Summary**
>
> **Antisocial behaviour**
> - It is important to exclude any coexisting psychiatric condition and treat this directly, e.g. ADHD or depression.
> - Parenting groups are an evidence-based treatment for these disorders, but require motivation.

Anxiety

Pathological anxiety exists in two forms: specific and general. In phobias there is fear of a specific object or situation that is excessive and handicapping and cannot be dealt with by reassurance. Most children have a number of irrational fears (the dark, ghosts, kidnappers, dogs, spiders, bats, snakes) which are common and do not usually handicap the child's ordinary life. Some of these persist into adulthood. If they are so severe that the child's ability to lead an ordinary life is affected, then treatment by cognitive behavioural therapy with graded exposure to the feared event may be indicated and is usually successful.

More diffuse general anxiety presents indirectly in childhood and it is uncommon for a child to complain directly about anxiety. Often, it is first manifest as physical complaints: nausea, headache or pain. It may take the form of health worries and the child repeatedly asks for reassurance that he is not going to die. Some children with generalized anxiety may develop unusual coping strategies that appear manipulative, in an attempt to gain control over their parents and the world in general. It may be a justifiable reaction to an event or situation, or be disproportionate. If the condition follows a recognizable precipitant such as a parental illness and the parents can be directed to provide comfort and support, prognosis is good. If it arises insidiously, specialist mental health referral is indicated.

> Children rarely say spontaneously that they are anxious – instead they tend to complain of aches and pains or behave in apparently manipulative ways to cope with or avoid the feared situation

School refusal

During the years of compulsory school attendance, a child may be absent from school because of illness, because parents keep the child off school, or because of truancy in which the child chooses to do something else rather than attend school. In truancy, a child leaves to go to school but never arrives or leaves early. It is often accompanied by other behavioural difficulties. A few non-attendees at school suffer from *school refusal*, an inability to attend school on account of overwhelming anxiety. Such children may not complain of anxiety but of its physical concomitants or the consequences of hyperventilation. Anxiety may present as complaints of nausea, headache or otherwise not being well, which are confined to weekday, term-time mornings, clearing up by midday. It may be rational, as when the child is being bullied or there is educational underachievement. If it is disproportionate to stresses at school, it is termed school refusal, an anxiety problem with two common causes – separation anxiety persisting beyond the toddler years and anxiety provoked by some aspect of school, true school phobia. These can coexist.

School refusal based on separation anxiety is typical of children under the age of about 11 years. It may be provoked by an adverse life event such as illness, a death in the family or a move of house. The child is unable to tolerate separation from their attachment figure without whom the child cannot go anywhere, including school. Treatment is aimed at gently promoting increasing separations from the parents (e.g. staying overnight with relatives or friends), while arranging an early return to school. Some adolescents with school refusal have a depressive disorder, but more usually there is an interaction between an anxiety disorder and long-standing personality issues such as intolerance of uncertainty.

True school phobia is seen in slightly older, anxious children who are frequently uncommunicative and stubborn.

The management of school refusal is shown in Box 24.9.

> **Box 24.9** Treatment of school refusal
>
> - Advise and support parents and school about the condition
> - Treat any underlying emotional disorder
> - Plan and facilitate an early and graded return to school at a pace tolerable for the child with all involved (child, family, teachers, educational psychologist and educational welfare officers)
> - Help the parents make it more rewarding for the child to return to school than stay at home
> - Address bullying or educational difficulties if present

Box 24.10 Causes of underachievement at school

Long-standing problem
- Visual problems
- Hearing problems
- Dyslexia
- Generalized or specific learning problems
- Hyperactivity
- Antieducation family background
- Chaotic family background

Recent onset of problem
- Preoccupations (parental divorce, bullying, etc.)
- Fatigue
- Depression
- Rebellion against teacher, parents, or 'swot' label
- Unsuspected poor attendance at school
- Sexual abuse
- Drug abuse
- Prodromal period of a psychotic illness (rare)
- Degenerative brain condition, rare but important

Box 24.11 Formal operational thought
- The ability to form abstract thoughts
- Comparing implications of hypotheses
- Thinking about one's own thinking
- Testing the logic that links propositions
- Manipulating interactive abstract concepts

Educational underachievement

Children who achieve less well in school than expected are sometimes brought to doctors. It is important to evaluate parents' and teachers' expectations and ensure the child is actually able to rise to them. The services of an educational psychologist are indispensable. Core medical responsibilities include checking sight and hearing and attempting to elicit the cause of underachievement according to the list in Box 24.10. The topic is considered further in Chapter 4.

Problems of adolescence

Although a popular image of adolescence is one of angry, rebellious teenagers, alienated from their parents and embroiled in emotional turmoil, studies show that most adolescents maintain good relationships with their parents. They do, however, tend to bicker with them about minor domestic matters and what they are allowed to do. This is a healthy process involving boundary testing, which precedes the separation phase of leaving home. Minor psychological symptoms such as moodiness or social sensitivity are quite common (as they are in adults), but serious psychiatric problems are no more prevalent than in adult life. Family relationships are often influenced by teenagers' negotiation of their own autonomy, the emergence of their own sense of themselves and the first moves towards a personal identity. At the same time, their parents may be experiencing midlife crises of confidence in career, physical appearance or sexuality, so that parental and teenage preoccupations coincide, not always helpfully.

Cognitive style

The style of thought specifically associated with adolescence is formal operational (abstract) thought (Box 24.11), but this is acquired at various ages by different individuals during the teenage years, and a substantial minority do not develop it at all. Doctors are at a disadvantage here, as they have been selected by a series of examinations for excellence of their ability to manipulate abstractions and compare hypothetical predictions; they have often forgotten what it is like to think otherwise and communicate poorly with patients who still think concretely and practically (school-age children, about half of all teenagers, and perhaps 1 in 5 adults). When interviewing adolescents, the skill is to avoid being patronising, while being sensitive as to whether abstract and reflective thought is solidly achieved. Using practical examples (not metaphors) and checking whether you have been understood will help to avoid the common problem of being faced with an adolescent who responds to questions with a sullen 'don't know'. This is considered further in Chapter 30. Adolescent medicine.

Anorexia nervosa and other eating disorders

Dieting to slim is endemic among teenage girls. Part of the reason for this is the contemporary equation between thinness and attractiveness, an assumption prevalent in advertising and fashion. Resonant with this is the finding that most teenage girls (but very few boys) overestimate their body width and depth, perceiving and judging themselves as fatter than they actually are.

Slimming through self-imposed calorie restriction is usually self-limiting because the goal is achieved or because the girl gives up; hunger wins through. In some girls, however, the slimming process takes over and there supervenes what has been called a 'relentless pursuit of thinness', typically with a phobic horror of normal body weight and shape. This is *anorexia nervosa*, and the features are:

- self-induced weight loss resulting in a low body mass index (BMI); in children this needs to be plotted on a BMI centile chart, in older adolescents it is ≤17.5 kg/m^2
- a distorted perception of her body, which increases with weight loss
- a determined attempt to lose weight or avoid weight gain, by either restricting food intake, self-induced vomiting, laxative abuse, excessive exercising or using a combination of these methods

- when body weight falls below a critical point, pubertal development is halted and reversed so that menstruation ceases and the girl effectively becomes a prepubertal child. This may spare her some of the challenges of adolescence, particularly those related to sexuality
- the discovery by a girl who has felt powerless that through self-starvation she can control her shape and development and thus increase her sense of self-worth and self-effectiveness
- pre-occupations and dreams of food and cooking which come to dominate mental life as a response to starvation. There ensues a tremendous mental struggle not to give in and eat, which assumes prime importance in the girl's mental life
- the dramatic and visible effects of self-starvation on the girl, which can unite some parents in caring for their daughter and save a discordant marriage from divorce, something which she may fear is imminent.

An affected person will often deny hunger, reassure everyone that she is in the peak of health, exercise to lose weight and disagree fervently that she is too thin. She will be careless of her own emaciation and seem unconcerned that she is starving herself to death. To the bewilderment of her parents, she may cook for others and read cookery books avidly. She may well be deceitful to anyone she perceives as thwarting her in her quest. Thus, she will conceal her poor eating by secretly disposing of her meals or lying about her weight. Both before and during her illness she will show obsessional, perfectionist character traits; without these she would not have the capacity to establish herself as a persistent dieter. Indeed, she is likely to be described as having been quiet, compliant and hard-working, 'the last person to develop anorexia nervosa'. Her parents will often present as nice people who avoid conflict.

As a result of starvation, her body develops a low metabolic rate with slow-to-relax tendon reflexes, reduced peripheral circulation, bradycardia and amenorrhea. Fine lanugo hair appears over her trunk and limbs. She does not lose pubic or axillary hair, although incompletely established puberty is delayed. Serum T_3 (triiodothyronine) may be low, giving rise to a false suspicion of hypothyroidism. Plasma proteins are sometimes low and ankle oedema not uncommon. Blood and urine levels of luteinising hormone and follicle-stimulating hormone are low and non-cyclical.

Some discover that self-restraint in carbohydrate intake can be bypassed by self-induced vomiting following repeated bouts of overeating. And that further weight loss can be achieved by diuretics and laxatives (in the belief that these will expedite food transit time and reduce absorption). This can cause wide fluctuations in weight and metabolic abnormalities such as hypokalaemia and alkalosis. This condition is *bulimia* which can occur at normal body weight or in association with low body weight as an ominous complication of anorexia nervosa. It tends to affect older rather than younger teenagers. Bulimia at normal body weight can be managed by encouraging a regular diet, monitoring this by a diary and providing individual or group cognitive behavioural therapy.

It has recently become clear that a variety of children fit with a new, wider classification of avoidant/restrictive food intake disorder, which does not require abnormal weight loss and includes, for instance, food restriction in autism spectrum disorders.

The prevalence rate among teenagers of anorexia nervosa was previously estimated at less than 1%, but recent estimates (using broader criteria) have been closer to 5% in adolescent girls, although it is not yet clear how much of this rise is genuine. The peak age of onset is 14 years and girls outnumber boys by about 10:1. Bulimia is more common, although prevalence rates vary widely, depending on the degree of severity. It also shows a markedly female preponderance and may also be becoming more frequent.

Management

Management is two-fold: medical and psychological. The initial management of anorexia nervosa is to restore near-normal body weight by refeeding. The emergence of physical complications may necessitate admission to hospital for refeeding, which may even involve nasogastric tube feeding in some instances. The cornerstone of treatment is family therapy. Individual psychological treatment is introduced to help the young person challenge the cognitions that drive anorexia and to acquire more constructive ways of confronting developmental demands, including handling conflict, maintaining self-esteem, personal autonomy and relationships.

Medical aspects

Anorexia has a high mortality rate compared with other psychiatric disorders. Some of the excess mortality arise from medical complications such as malnutrition, electrolyte imbalance and infection. This emphasizes the importance of thorough physical examination, investigations and medical management. "Refeeding syndrome", the metabolic abnormalities on reinstituting nutrition, can be life threatening, but is manageable if standard guidelines are followed, such as Junior MARSIPAN (Management of Really Sick Patients with Anorexia Nervosa under 18 years). In the UK, the National Institute for Health and Clinical Excellence (NICE) has produced a guideline for treatment of eating disorders including the physical management of anorexia nervosa.

Prognosis

The prognosis for children and adolescents is variable, with as many as 50% failing to make a full recovery. Factors predicting a poorer outcome include a low BMI and physical complications prior to treatment, bulimic symptoms, especially self-induced vomiting, as well as family disturbance and interpersonal difficulties. Anorexia has the highest mortality of all psychiatric disorders. In addition to medical complications, the next important cause of mortality is suicide.

Eating disorders have become a major problem in adolescent girls

> **Summary**
>
> **In anorexia nervosa**
> - Female:male ratio is 10:1.
> - Peak age of onset – 14 years.
> - Affected girls have a distorted body image, so seldom agree that they are too thin and may deceive everyone by pretending to eat.
> - Features include: determined efforts to lose weight, arrest of puberty, cessation of periods.
> - May be accompanied by bulimia – overeating followed by self-induced vomiting.
> - Management is family therapy and individual therapy to restore body weight.
> - Some require hospitalization; prognosis is variable, but has a mortality from suicide, malnutrition and infection.

Chronic fatigue syndrome

Chronic fatigue syndrome refers to persisting high levels of subjective fatigue, leading to rapid exhaustion on minimal physical or mental exertion. The term is broader and more neutral than the specific pathology or aetiology implied by myalgic encephalomyelitis or postviral fatigue syndrome, which follows an apparently viral febrile illness. There is sometimes serological evidence of recent infection with coxsackie B or Epstein–Barr virus or a hepatitis virus. Some cases have no history or evidence of a precipitating infection and there are no specific diagnostic tests. The clinical picture is somewhat diffuse and there are no pathognomonic symptoms. Myalgia, migratory arthralgia, headache, difficulty getting off to sleep, poor concentration and irritability are virtually universal. Stomach pains, scalp tenderness, eye pain and photophobia, and tender cervical lymphadenopathy are frequently encountered. Depressive symptoms are common and there is continuing debate as to how much of the clinical picture is physical and how much psychological. Usually parents insist on there being a physical cause and there is a risk that the doctor will carry out excessive unnecessary investigations. Most experienced doctors now regard the final clinical picture as resulting from both physical and psychological factors.

The majority of cases will remit spontaneously with time, but this takes months or sometimes years. Earlier recommendations of continuous rest have been shown to be unhelpful and can lead to secondary complications. The recommended treatment involves graded exercise therapy and/or cognitive behavioural therapy. Graded exercise therapy is usually provided by physiotherapists and aims to achieve gradual increase in exercise tolerance. If too much pressure is put upon the child, tantrums or mute withdrawal can occur. Argument about how much of the condition is physical and how much psychological is unhelpful. The parents and the child need continuing support to maintain as much of a normal life as possible, including school attendance. The mood of children with depressive symptoms may respond to antidepressant medication, but this is a treatment only for depressive symptoms and it is unlikely to result in alleviation of the fatigability. NICE guidelines are available.

> **Summary**
>
> **In chronic fatigue syndrome**
> - There is exhaustion on minimal exertion.
> - There is thought to be a combination of physical and psychological factors.
> - Management is with graded exercise and/or cognitive behavioural therapy, but recovery may take months or years.

Depression

Low mood can arise secondary to adverse circumstances or sometimes spontaneously. Depression as a clinical condition is more than sadness and misery; it extends to affect motivation, judgement, the ability to experience pleasure and provokes emotions of guilt and despair. It may disturb sleep, appetite and weight. It leads to social withdrawal, an important sign. Such a state is well recognized among adolescents, particularly girls, but occasionally affects prepubertal children. The general picture is comparable to depression in adults but there are differences (Box 24.12).

A diagnosis of depression depends crucially upon interviewing the adolescent on their own, as well as taking a history from the parents. Teenagers will, out of loyalty, often pretend to their parents that things are all right if interviewed in their presence. It is necessary to ask about feelings directly and to ask specifically about suicidal ideas and plans.

Treatment depends upon severity. Children with mild depression are managed initially in primary care and other non-specialist mental health settings. Many will recover spontaneously; hence a period of watchful waiting for up to 4 weeks may be appropriate. Alternatively, the child could be offered non-directive

Box 24.12 Features of depression in adolescents

More common than adults
- Apathy, boredom and an inability to enjoy oneself rather than depressed mood
- Separation anxiety which reappears, having resolved in earlier life
- Decline in school performance
- Social withdrawal
- Hypochondriacal ideas and complaints of pain in chest, abdomen, and head
- Irritable mood or frankly antisocial behaviour

Less common than adults
- Loss of appetite and weight
- Loss of sleep
- Loss of libido
- Slowing of thought and movement
- Delusional ideas

supportive therapy or guided self-help. However, if mild depression does not respond to these measures in 2–3 months, the child should be referred to specialist mental health services. Similarly, children with moderate and severe depression should be referred to specialist mental health services for more specific psychological intervention such as cognitive behavioural therapy, family therapy, or interpersonal therapy. In all cases, any identified contributing factor such as bullying needs to be addressed. If psychological therapy for moderate or severe depression is insufficient after 6 weeks, then a SSRI (selective serotonin reuptake inhibitor antidepressant), fluoxetine, should be considered. Depressed young people who are suicidal may need admission to an adolescent psychiatric in-patient unit. A NICE guidline has been published.

Deliberate self-harm

Young people deliberately cause themselves harm for multiple reasons and in multiple ways. Explanations range from a coping technique for dealing with negative feelings (such as low self-esteem) to an expressed wish to punish themselves. Often the young person will describe the positive feeling of control they experience when harming themselves. The physical pain acts as a distraction from emotional distress.

Self-harm is common and is increasing. Estimates of prevalence find that approximately 15% of adolescents harm themselves deliberately during this developmental phase. Many do not present to healthcare professions actively, therefore no assessment of an adolescent with emotional or behavioural difficulties is complete without screening for self-harm.

Common methods of self-harm include cutting, burning, biting, bruising or scratching the skin, or tying ligatures around the neck. Punching of walls should also be considered self-harm (the presentation of a boxers fracture should raise suspicion).

A full physical examination is an ideal time to look for signs of deliberate self-harm. Cutting to the thighs, for example, can often be missed. The patient wearing long sleeves, reluctant to show their skin, should raise concern.

How to ask about self-harm

This involves:

- a history taken with the young person alone. Often a history taken with parents present will result in non-disclosure
- creating a safe environment
- allowing sufficient time to conduct the consultation sensitively, without interruptions
- setting rules about confidentiality clearly
- validating the young person's distress
- giving assurance that they will be supported
- asking questions directly, but sensitively.

There is no single way to ask about self-harm and suicide. Normalization of the problem is key. All clinicians will find a style of asking these questions which suits them e.g. "sometimes if people are feeling particularly stressed, worried or low, they can have thoughts about harming themselves, or ending their lives. Has this ever happened to you?"

Box 24.13 PATHOS instrument to assess suicide risk after adolescent overdose

- **P:** Have you had **P**roblems for longer than a month?
- **A:** Were you **A**lone in the house at the time?
- **T:** Did you plan the overdose for longer than **T**hree hours?
- **HO:** Are you feeling **Ho**peless about the future?
- **S:** Were you feeling **S**ad for most of the time before the overdose?

Score 1 for Yes; 0 for No and add together. Child at high risk if score >2. However, the final judgement of suicide risk is a clinical and qualitative decision, not one based on a cut-off score.

From Kingsbury S: PATHOS: a screening instrument for adolescent overdose: a research note. *Journal of Child Psychology and Psychiatry* 37:609–611, 1996.

A screening tool such as PATHOS (Box 24.13) can be useful alongside a holistic assessment.

Drug misuse

Most teenagers are exposed to illicit drugs at some stage. A number will then experiment with them, some becoming habitual users. Usually, this is for recreational purposes, but a few use them to avoid unpleasant feelings or memories. A very small number become dependent, psychologically or physically. What is taken varies with culture and opportunity, but alcohol and cannabis are common; solvents, LSD, ecstasy and amphetamine derivatives somewhat less so; and cocaine or heroin currently least prevalent, though their use is increasing. The addictive potential of the last two is the greatest and their dangers are well known.

Abuse implies heavy misuse. The signs vary with the agent but may include:

- intoxication
- unexplained absences from home or school
- mixing with known users
- high rates of spending or stealing money
- possession of the equipment required for drug use
- medical complications associated with use.

Doctors may be approached by parents worried that their adolescent child may be abusing drugs. An assessment will involve interviewing the adolescent, possibly combined with taking a urine sample for drug screening. Most geographical areas have specific services for adolescents with drug and/or alcohol problems. These services usually take self-referrals, so that young people with these difficulties can access them directly. Medical involvement is predominantly focused on users who have other psychopathology including depression or with the physical consequences of intoxication or injection when these threaten health. Solvent abuse (mainly glue and aerosol sniffing) is quite widespread as a group activity of young adolescents in some areas. It can occasionally give rise to cardiac dysrhythmias, bone marrow suppression or renal failure, and any of these can cause death, as may a fall or road traffic accident when intoxicated. Cannabis and LSD use may trigger anxiety or psychotic disorders. Ecstasy taken at dances or raves can cause dangerous hyperthermia, dehydration and death.

Doctors need to ensure that any adolescent known to them who is thought to be using drugs knows the specific risks to health. Dependence is rare among teenagers and most likely to involve alcohol. The few who are using illicit drugs for respite from psychological distress need referral to a psychiatrist.

"Legal Highs" are of increasing concern to clinicians. These include chemical substances which produce similar effects to illegal drugs (e.g. cocaine, cannabis, ecstasy). They can have depressant or simulant, including hallucinogenic, properties. They are easily purchased online, unregulated, often labelled as incense or salts. They have been associated with a number of deaths, although the association may not be causative. Their long term effects are uncertain.

Psychosis

Psychosis is a breakdown in the perception and understanding of reality and a lack of awareness that the person is unwell. This can affect ideas and beliefs, resulting in delusional thinking where abnormal beliefs are held with an unshakeable quality and lead to odd behaviour. The connectedness and coherence of thoughts may break down, so that speech is hard to follow, leading to thought disorder. Perceptual abnormalities lead to hallucinations, where a perception is experienced in the absence of a stimulus.

Psychotic disorders include:

- Schizophrenia, where no specific medical cause is identified and there is generally no major disturbance of mood other than blunting or flattening of affect.
- Bipolar affective disorder, where the psychosis is associated with lowered mood as in depression or elevation in mood as in mania.
- Organic psychosis occurs in delirium, substance-induced disorders and dementia.

Both schizophrenia and bipolar affective disorder are rare before puberty, but increase in frequency of presentation during adolescence. In these disorders the psychotic symptoms occur in clear consciousness.

Investigations should include a urine drug screen, exclusion of medication-induced psychosis (e.g. high-dose stimulants or anticholinergic drugs), exclusion of medical causes (i.e. infection, seizures, thyroid abnormalities and sleep disorders) and dementia.

Where schizophrenia and bipolar disorder is suspected, urgent referral to a psychiatrist is needed for comprehensive assessment and treatment with antipsychotic medication, psycho-education, family therapy, and where appropriate, individual therapy. In the case of an organic psychosis the underlying cause needs to be treated promptly by the paediatric team, with help from mental health professionals as appropriate.

Psychosis
- May present during adolescence
- May be precipitated by or be a consequence of substance abuse

Management of emotional and behavioural problems

The first thing is to construct, with the family and young person, a story that you all 'own' about how the problem has come about and what is perpetuating it as a biopsychosocial formulation. Many simple but important intervention opportunities will simply 'fall out' of this formulation, as with the young child Ahmed in Case History 24.1. An example of the process in an adolescent is shown in Case History 24.2.

Cultural considerations

Many developed countries are increasingly ethnically diverse in relation to language, religion and culture. This diversity has many important clinical implications for child mental health. The first implication relates to the need to recognise the subgroup of young people who are refugees or asylum seekers. These children and their families have often experienced major traumatic events before arriving in their host country. They remain highly vulnerable to mental and socio-economic adversities due to past and ongoing stressful experiences.

Another implication of culture relates to the presentation of psychiatric symptoms. It is well recognized that the content of obsessions in children with obsessive compulsive disorder is sometimes shaped by the child's cultural and religious beliefs. This is also true of some delusions in young people with psychotic disorders, e.g. possession by "Jinn's" in Islamic traditions. In these examples, understanding the child's religious and cultural background is essential for making an accurate diagnosis.

There are also important cultural differences about normative behaviour in children and thresholds for help-seeking. Differences in the level of stigma attached to mental illness across cultures also influence parent's help-seeking behaviour and access to child and adolescent mental health services. Finally, it is important to understand that culture and race are not the same thing; education, religion and class all deeply affect the parenting 'culture' of a family.

It is therefore essential to avoid making assumptions about the significance of clinical information with cultural or religious meaning but instead to contextualize the information to the patient's culture, e.g. through the use of trained interpreters.

Treatment

Many doctors, general practitioners, and paediatricians in particular, are good generalists in child mental health issues and the mental health specialist should be seen as a specialist extension of their expertise, rather than a completely different sort of person. The main treatment interventions employed are shown in Box 24.14 and an approach to managing a child displaying an emotional or behavioural problem is shown in Fig. 24.3.

In general, the management of children's emotional and behavioural problems:

- should be psychological rather than pharmacological

Case history 24.2

Eating disorder

Ellie, 16 years old, has come to the attention of social services when Youth Offending services noticed that she is unusually thin after an arrest for shoplifting.

The 4p framework (Table 24.4) provides useful potential avenues for further intervention:

- Assessment for eating disorder and possible ADHD.
- Frank discussion, hopefully including her mother, of risks.
- Negotiation around how to retain positive aspects of peer group while mitigating risks.
- Possible use of cognitive behaviour therapy to exploit her good intellectual function.

Table 24.4 4p framework relating to Ellie's eating disorder

	Biological/developmental	Psychological	Social
Predisposing factors	Possible ADHD	Blames self for father leaving	Chronic conflict with mother
Precipitating factors		Relationship with new boyfriend who uses drugs	Exposure to delinquent peer group
Perpetuating factors	Impulsive, emotionally labile	Identification with 'alternative' lifestyle, distorted body image	Estrangement from family
Protective factors (resilience)	Very bright	Self of self-worth fairly strong	Many of her peers genuinely supportive

---

Box 24.14 Main psychological treatment interventions employed for emotional and behavioural problems

Explanation and formulation

Suitable for mild problems with a good prognosis arising in children from supportive families who can work out for themselves a sensible way of managing the problem until it subsides.

Counselling of child or parents

Used to provide non-directive, unstructured supportive therapy for children and families to aid coping with difficulties that are not severe enough to require specialist psychological interventions (e.g. bereavement counselling).

In parental counselling, the aim is to enhance parental coping not by telling the parent what to do but by helping them to find their own solutions, so increasing their confidence and effectiveness.

Parenting groups

Recently, parenting groups have become popular, where a number of parents are seen together and given techniques on how to play with their children and respond effectively to their challenging behaviour. Various approaches are rehearsed using role play and the facilitation of a therapist.

Behavioural therapy

A pragmatic approach to problems, which alters the environmental factors that trigger or maintain behaviours. It is particularly effective in the management of behavioural problems in young children.

Family therapy

Widely used by child mental health professionals. It uses a series of interviews with the entire household to alter dysfunctional patterns of relationships between family members on the basis that many children's problems are perpetuated by the ways in which family members live with and deal with each other.

Cognitive therapy

Used by specialists to explore the way thinking affects feelings and behaviour. It helps the young person to identify and challenge unhelpful thinking styles that perpetuate negative feelings and behaviour. Good evidence for efficacy in a range of disorders including depression.

Individual or group dynamic psychotherapy

More structured and intense extension of counselling, which can help children who, for example, have unconscious conflicts which are manifest as relationship difficulties with a parent. Once the mainstay of child psychiatry, it is now less commonly used.

- does not need the child to be admitted to hospital (unless required as a place of safety for suicidal children or for child protection)
- involves parents as key participants
- may involve a variety of health and social service professionals.

Often more than one intervention is required and treatments are combined and several professionals become involved.

Medication plays a comparatively small role, although particular instances for which there is evidence for their efficacy are the use of stimulant and non-stimulant drugs in hyperkinetic disorder (ADHD), neuroleptics in psychosis, and antidepressants for severely depressed adolescents. There is sometimes a temptation to sedate a child who is causing a problem but this is rarely effective and ethically questionable.

Acknowledgements

We would like to acknowledge contributors to this chapter in previous editions, whose work we have drawn on: Peter Hill (1st, 2nd Editions), Elena Garralda (3rd Edition), Sharon Taylor (3rd, 4th Editions), Cornelius Ani (4th Edition).

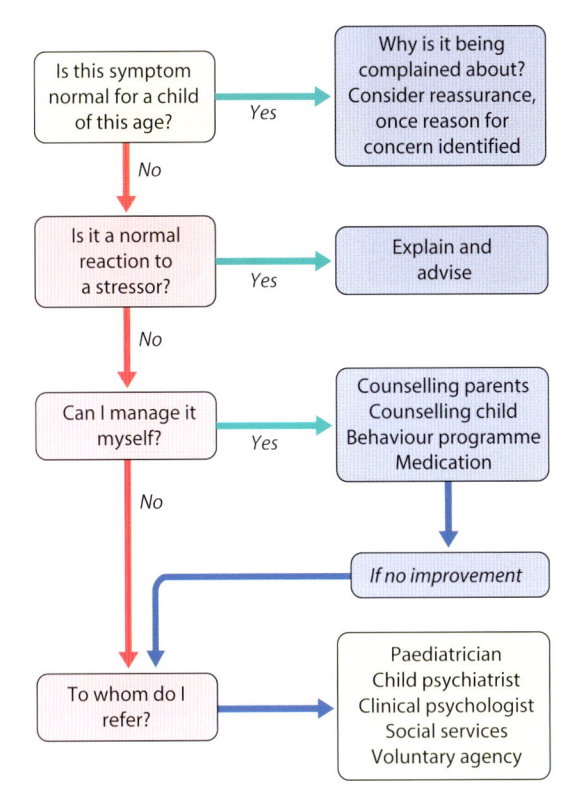

Figure 24.3 An approach to children's psychological problems.

Further reading

Coghill D, Bonnar S, Duke S, et al: *Child and Adolescent Psychiatry*, Oxford Specialist Handbooks in Psychiatry, Oxford, 2009, Oxford University Press.

Goodman R, Scott S: *Child and Adolescent Psychiatry*, ed 3, 2012, Wiley-Blackwell.

Huline-Dickens S: *Clinical Topics in Child Psychiatry*, 2014, RCPsych Publications.

Thapar A, Pine DS, Leckman JF et al: *Rutter's Child and Adolescent Psychiatry*, ed 6, 2015, Wiley-Blackwell.

Websites (Accessed November 2016)

e-learning for Child Mental Health: Available at: www.MindEd.org.uk

ERIC, The Children's Bowel and Bladder Charity: http://www.eric.org.uk/#
Advice about bowel and bladder continence problems in children

Junior Marsipan Guideline: Available at: http://www.rcpsych.ac.uk/usefulresources/publications/collegereports/cr/cr168.aspx
NICE (National Institute of Clinical Excellence) guidelines: *NICE on depression, anxiety, conduct disorder, eating disorders, nocturnal enuresis*

Paediatric mental health association (UK): Available at: http://pmha-uk.org/

Royal College of Psychiatrists: Available at: www.rcpsych.ac.uk

Young Minds: Available at: www.youngminds.org.uk
Charity for young people's mental health

25

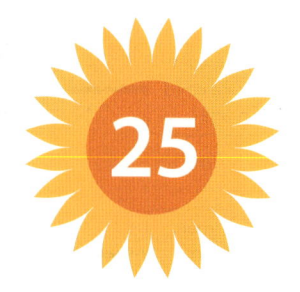

Dermatological disorders

The newborn	442	Other childhood skin disorders	450
Rashes of infancy	444	Rashes and systemic disease	451
Infections and infestations	448		

Features of dermatological disorders in children are:

- in the newborn, transient skin disorders are common but need to be distinguished from serious or permanent conditions
- atopic eczema affects up to 20% of children
- skin infections and infestations, especially viral warts and head lice, are common in school-aged children
- acne is troublesome for many during adolescence.

Skin complaints are common in children of all ages. The history gives important clues about the possible origin of any lesion. The child's age will often determine the most likely causes. Is it acute or chronic? A recent or ongoing febrile illness suggests that the rash may be one of the exanthema of childhood [see Ch. 15 (Infection and immunity)]. Rashes shared by family members or contacts are frequently infectious or represent infestations (e.g. scabies). Is the child otherwise well or is this part of a systemic illness? Is it itchy or otherwise causing upset? Examination will reveal the distribution and nature of the lesions (Table 25.1).

The newborn

The skin at birth is covered with a chalky-white greasy coat – the vernix caseosa. In the preterm infant, the skin is thin, poorly keratinized, and transepidermal water loss is markedly increased when compared with a term infant. Thermoregulation is also impaired as the preterm infant lacks subcutaneous fat and is unable to sweat until a few weeks old, whereas the term infant can sweat from birth.

Common naevi and rashes in the newborn period are described under the examination of the newborn infant [see Ch. 10 (Perinatal medicine)]. Some less common skin conditions presenting in the newborn period are described in this chapter.

Bullous impetigo

This is an uncommon but potentially serious blistering form of impetigo, the most superficial form of bacterial infection, seen particularly in the newborn (Fig. 25.1). It is most often caused by *Staphylococcus aureus*. Treatment is with systemic antibiotics, e.g. flucloxacillin (see also Ch. 15).

Melanocytic naevi (moles)

Congenital moles occur in up to 3% of neonates and any that are present are usually small. Congenital pigmented naevi involving extensive areas of skin (i.e. naevi >9 cm in diameter) are rare but disfiguring (Fig. 25.2) and carry a 4–6% lifetime risk of subsequent malignant melanoma. They require prompt referral to a paediatric dermatologist and plastic surgeon to assess the necessity for further investigation and/or feasibility of removal.

Melanocytic naevi become increasingly common as children get older and the presence of large numbers in an adult may be indicative of childhood sun exposure.

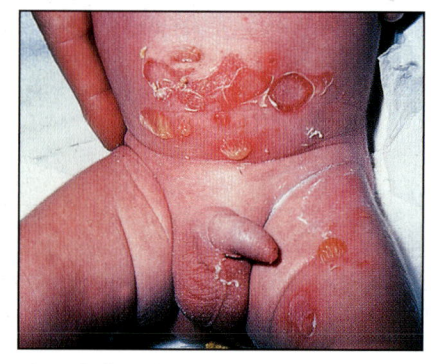

Figure 25.1 Bullous impetigo in a 2-week-old baby.

Table 25.1 Morphology of skin lesions

Primary skin lesions (arise de novo in the skin)

Lesion	Description	Example
Macule	A small flat area of altered colour or texture	Freckles, measles, rubella, roseola, café-au-lait macule of tuberous sclerosis
Patch	Larger flat area of altered colour or texture	Depigmented patch of vitiligo
Papule	A small raised lesion	Allergic, inflammatory papules of acne
Maculopapular	Combination of macules and papules	Measles, scarlet fever, parvovirus B19 (erythema infectiosum, fifth disease)
Plaque	A larger raised lesion	Scaly plaque of psoriasis
Nodule	A larger raised lesion with a deeper component (involvement of the dermis or subcutaneous fat)	Nodular lesion of erythema nodosum
Vesicle	A small clear blister	Varicella
Bulla	A large clear blister	Skin trauma, bullous impetigo
Wheal/weal	A transient raised lesion due to dermal oedema	Urticaria (hives)
Pustule	A pus-containing blister	Acute paronychia
Purpura	Bleeding into skin or mucosa. Small areas are petechiae, whereas large areas are ecchymoses. Do not blanch on pressure	Meningococcal septicaemia, Henoch–Schönlein purpura, immune thrombocytopenia, disseminated intravascular coagulation (DIC)

Secondary skin lesions (evolve from primary lesions or from scratching of primary lesions by the patient)

Excoriation	Scratch mark, loss of epidermis following trauma	Atopic dermatitis (from acute rubbing)
Lichenification	Roughening of skin with accentuation of skin markings	Atopic dermatitis (chronic rubbing)
Scales	Flakes of dead skin	Cradle cap in seborrhoeic dermatitis
Crust	Dry mass of exudates consisting of serum, dried blood, scales, and pus	Impetigo
Scar	Formation of new fibrous tissue postwound healing	Acne
Erosion	Loss of epidermis and dermis (heals with scarring)	Epidermolysis bullosa
Ulcer	Loss of epidermis and dermis (heals with scarring)	Ulcerating haemangioma

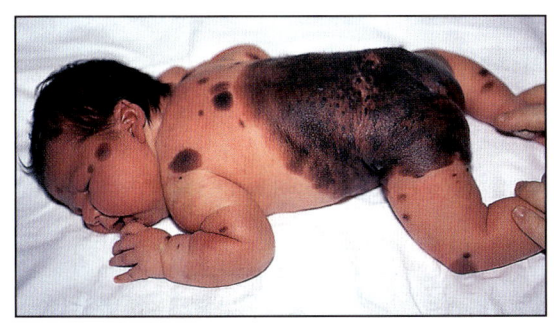

Figure 25.2 A large (giant) congenital pigmented hairy naevus. Other smaller naevi are also visible.

Prolonged exposure to sunlight should be avoided and sunscreen preparations with a sun protection factor of 30 or higher should be applied liberally to exposed skin in bright weather and reapplied every few hours.

Malignant melanoma is rare before puberty, except in giant naevi. However, in adults, the incidence of malignant melanoma has been increasing for many years. Risk factors for melanoma include a positive family history, having a large number of melanocytic naevi, fair skin, repeated episodes of sunburn, and living in a hot climate with chronic skin exposure to the sun.

☀ **Parents should prevent their children becoming sunburnt**

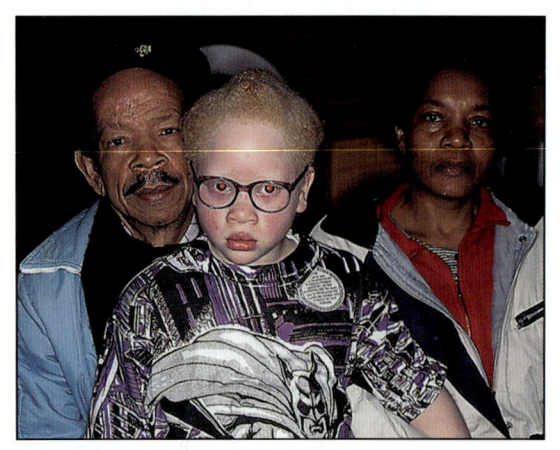

Figure 25.3 A child with oculocutaneous albinism, with her parents. The hair is silvery white.

Albinism

This is due to a defect in biosynthesis and distribution of melanin. The albinism may be oculocutaneous, ocular, or partial, depending on the distribution of depigmentation in the skin and eye (Fig. 25.3). The lack of pigment in the iris, retina, eyelids, and eyebrows results in failure to develop a fixation reflex. There is pendular nystagmus and photophobia, which causes constant frowning. Correction of refractive errors and tinted lenses may be helpful. In a few children, the fitting of tinted contact lenses from early infancy allows the development of normal fixation. The disorder is an important cause of severe visual impairment. The pale skin is prone to sunburn and skin cancer. In sunlight, a hat should be worn and high-factor barrier cream applied to the skin.

Epidermolysis bullosa

This is a rare group of genetic conditions with many types, characterized by blistering of the skin and mucous membranes. Autosomal dominant variants tend to be milder; autosomal recessive variants may be severe and even fatal. Blisters occur spontaneously or follow minor trauma (Fig. 25.4). Management is directed at avoiding injury from even minor skin trauma and treating secondary infection. In the severe forms, the fingers and toes may become fused, and contractures of the limbs develop from repeated blistering and healing. Mucous membrane involvement may result in oral ulceration and stenosis from oesophageal erosions. Management, including maintenance of adequate nutrition and analgesia when dressings are changed, should be by a multidisciplinary team including a paediatric dermatologist, paediatrician, plastic surgeon, and dietician.

Collodion baby

This is a rare manifestation of the inherited ichthyoses, a group of conditions in which the skin is dry and scaly. Infants are born with a taut, shiny parchment-like or collodion-like membrane (Fig. 25.5). There is a risk of dehydration. Emollients are applied to moisturize and soften the skin. The membrane becomes fissured and separates within a few weeks, usually leaving either ichthyotic or far less commonly, normal skin.

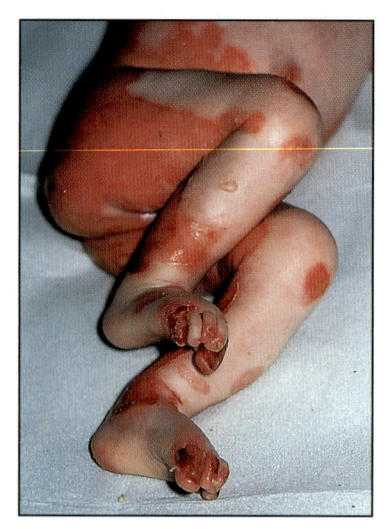

Figure 25.4 Severe, autosomal recessive form of epidermolysis bullosa. There is scarring following recurrent blistering.

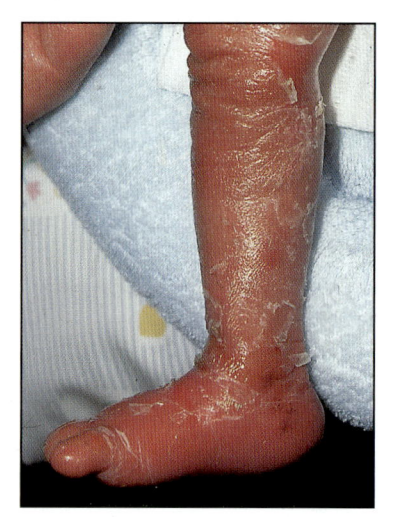

Figure 25.5 Collodion baby.

Rashes of infancy

Nappy rashes

Nappy rashes are common. Some causes are listed in Box 25.1.

Irritant dermatitis, the most common nappy rash, may occur if nappies are not changed frequently enough or if the infant has diarrhoea. However, irritant dermatitis can occur even when the nappy area is cleaned regularly. The rash is due to the irritant effect of urine on the skin of susceptible infants. Urea-splitting organisms in faeces increase the alkalinity and likelihood of a rash.

Box 25.1 Causes of nappy rashes

Common
- Irritant (contact) dermatitis
- Infantile seborrhoeic dermatitis
- *Candida* infection
- Atopic eczema

Rare
- Acrodermatitis enteropathica (see Fig. 14.13)
- Langerhans cell histiocytosis (see Fig. 22.19)
- Wiskott–Aldrich syndrome (see Fig. 15.27).

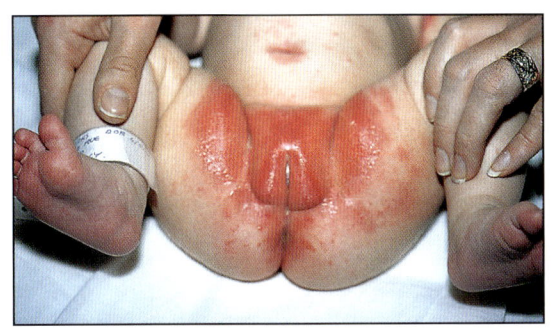

Figure 25.6 Napkin rash due to *Candida* infection. The skin flexures are involved and there are satellite pustules visible.

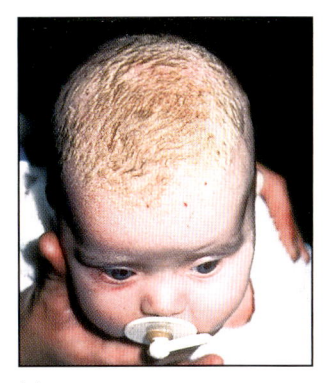

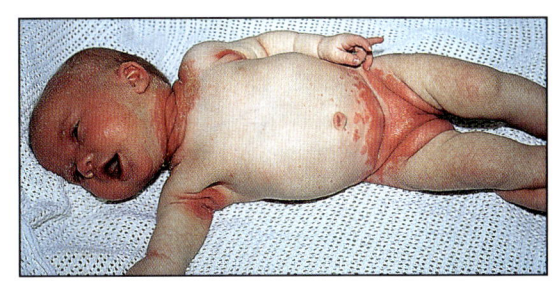

Figure 25.7 Infantile seborrhoeic dermatitis. (**a**) Cradle cap; and (**b**) involvement of face, axillae, and napkin area.

The irritant eruption affects the convex surfaces of the buttocks, perineal region, lower abdomen, and top of the thighs. Characteristically, the flexures are spared, which differentiates it from other causes of nappy rash. The rash is erythematous and may have a scalded appearance. More severe forms are associated with erosions and ulcer formation. Mild cases respond to the use of a protective emollient, whereas more severe cases may require mild topical corticosteroids. While leaving the child without a napkin will accelerate resolution, it is rarely practical at home.

Candida infection may cause and often complicates nappy rashes. The rash is erythematous, includes the skin flexures, and there may be satellite lesions (Fig. 25.6). Treatment is with a topical antifungal agent.

Infantile seborrhoeic dermatitis

This eruption of unknown cause presents in the first 3 months of life. It starts on the scalp as an erythematous scaly eruption. The scales form a thick yellow adherent layer, commonly called cradle cap (Fig. 25.7a). The scaly rash may spread to the face, behind the ears, and then extend to the flexures and napkin area (Fig. 25.7b). In contrast to atopic eczema, it is not itchy and the child is unperturbed by it. However, it is associated with an increased risk of subsequently developing atopic eczema. Mild cases will resolve with emollients. The scales on the scalp can be cleared with an ointment containing low-concentration sulphur and salicylic acid applied to the scalp daily for a few hours and then washed off. Widespread body eruption will clear with a mild topical corticosteroid, either alone or mixed with an antibacterial and antifungal agent.

Atopic eczema (atopic dermatitis)

The prevalence of atopic eczema in children in the UK is about 20%. A genetic deficiency of skin barrier function is important in the pathogenesis of atopic eczema. Onset of atopic eczema is usually in the first year of life. It is, however, uncommon in the first 2 months, unlike infantile seborrhoeic dermatitis, which is relatively common at this age. There is often a family history of atopic disorders: eczema, asthma, allergic rhinitis (hay fever). Around one-third of children with atopic eczema will develop asthma. Exclusive breast-feeding may delay the onset of eczema in predisposed children but does not appear to have a significant impact on the prevalence of eczema during later childhood. Atopic eczema is mainly a disease of childhood, being most severe and troublesome in the first year of life and resolving in 50% by 12 years of age, and in 75% by age 16 years.

Diagnosis

The diagnosis is made clinically. If the disease is unusually severe, atypical, or associated with unusual infections or faltering growth, an immune deficiency disorder should be excluded. Immunological changes in atopic disease are probably secondary to enhanced antigen penetration through a deficient epidermal barrier.

Itching

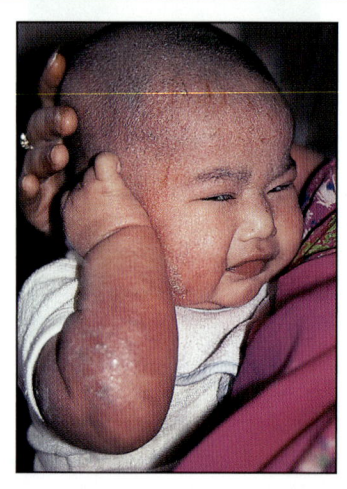

Figure 25.8 Atopic dermatitis. Inflamed skin worsened by rubbing/scratching. Itch is the key clinical feature in eczema at all ages, leading to an 'itch–scratch–itch' cycle.

Box 25.2 Some itchy rashes

- Atopic eczema
- Chickenpox
- Urticaria/allergic reactions
- Contact dermatitis
- Insect bites
- Scabies
- Fungal infections
- Pityriasis rosea

☀ No itch? – Then it is not eczema

Clinical features

Rashes may itch in many conditions (Box 25.2), but in atopic eczema, itching (pruritus) is the main symptom at all ages and this results in scratching and exacerbation of the rash (Fig. 25.8). The excoriated areas become erythematous, weeping, and crusted. Distribution of the eruption tends to change with age, as indicated in Fig. 25.9.

Atopic skin is usually dry and prolonged scratching and rubbing of the skin may lead to lichenification, in which there is accentuation of the normal skin markings (Fig. 25.10).

Complications

Causes of exacerbations of eczema are listed in Box 25.3. However, flare-ups are common, often for no obvious reason. Eczematous skin can readily become infected, usually with *Staphylococcus* or *Streptococcus* (Fig. 25.11). Inflammation increases the avidity of skin for *S. aureus* and reduces the expression of antimicrobial peptides, which are needed to control microbial infections. *S. aureus* thrives on atopic skin and releases superantigens, which seem to maintain and worsen eczema. Herpes simplex virus infection, although less frequent, is potentially very serious as it can spread rapidly on atopic skin, causing an extensive vesicular reaction, eczema herpeticum (see Fig. 15.13). Regional lymphadenopathy is common and often marked in active eczema; it usually resolves when the skin improves.

Management

A number of treatment modalities are available.

Avoiding irritants and precipitants

It is advisable to avoid soap and biological detergents. Clothing next to the skin should be of pure cotton where possible, avoiding nylon and pure woollen garments. Nails need to be cut short to reduce skin damage from scratching, and mittens at night may be helpful in the very young. When an allergen such as cow's milk has been proven to be a precipitant, it should be avoided.

Emollients

These are the mainstay of management, moisturizing, and softening the skin. They should be applied liberally two or more times a day and after a bath. They include ointments such as one containing equal parts of white soft paraffin and liquid paraffin. Ointments are preferable to creams when the skin is very dry. A daily or alternate day bath using emollient oil as a soap substitute is also beneficial.

Topical corticosteroids

These are an effective treatment for eczema, but must be used with care. Mildly potent corticosteroids, such as 1% hydrocortisone ointment, can be applied to the eczematous areas once or twice daily. Moderately potent topical steroids play a pivotal role in the management of acute exacerbations, but their use must be kept to a minimum. They should be applied thinly and their use on the face should be generally avoided. Excessive use of topical steroids may cause thinning of the skin as well as systemic side-effects. However, fear of these side-effects should not deter their use in controlling exacerbations.

Immunomodulators

In children over 2 years of age, short-term topical use of tacrolimus ointment or pimecrolimus cream may be indicated for eczema not controlled by topical corticosteroids and where there is a risk of important adverse effects from further topical steroid use.

Eczema

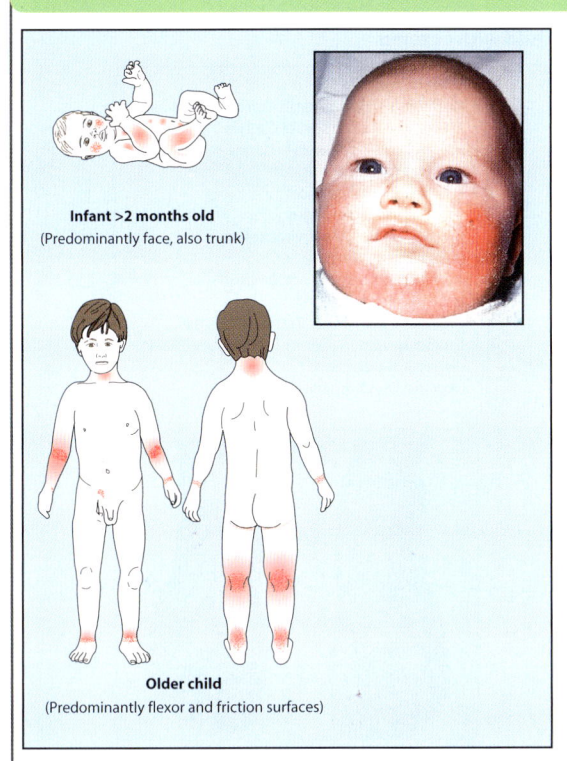

Figure 25.9 Distribution of atopic eczema. The distribution of eczema tends to change with age. In infants, the face and scalp are prominently affected, although the trunk may be involved. In older children, the skin flexures (cubital and popliteal fossae) and frictional areas, such as the neck, wrists, and ankles, are characteristically involved.

Box 25.3 Causes of exacerbation of eczema

- Bacterial infection, e.g. *Staphylococcus*, *Streptococcus* spp.
- Viral infection, e.g. herpes simplex virus
- Ingestion of an allergen, e.g. egg
- Contact with an irritant or allergen
- Environment: heat, humidity
- Change or reduction in medication
- Psychological stress
- Unexplained

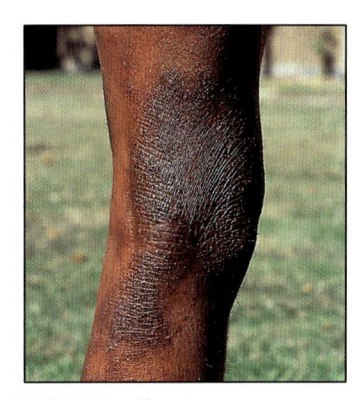

Figure 25.10 Lichenification.

Occlusive bandages

These are helpful over limbs when scratching and lichenification are a problem. They may be impregnated with zinc paste or zinc and tar paste. The bandages are worn overnight or for 2–3 days at a time until the skin has improved. For widespread itching in young children, short-term use of wet stockinette wraps may be helpful; diluted topical steroids mixed with emollient are applied to the skin and damp wraps fashioned for trunk and limbs are then applied with overlying dry wraps or clothes.

Antibiotics, antiviral agents, and antihistamines

Antibiotics with hydrocortisone can be applied topically for mildly infected eczema. Systemic antibiotics are indicated for more widespread or severe bacterial infection. Eczema herpeticum is acute and often widespread and is treated with systemic aciclovir.

Itch suppression in eczema is with an oral antihistamine. The second-generation antihistamines are not sedative. Antihistamines can be useful in raising the itching threshold so that scratching is reduced.

Dietary elimination

Food allergy may be suspected if the child reacts consistently to a food, or in infants and young children with moderate or severe atopic eczema, particularly if associated with gut dysmotility (colic, vomiting, altered bowel habit) or faltering growth. The most common food allergens resulting in eczema are egg and cow's milk. Allergen specific IgE antibodies in blood and skin prick testing may be helpful but must be interpreted with caution. Dietary elimination for 4–6 weeks may be required to detect a response.

A trial of an extensively hydrolyzed protein formula or amino acid formula in place of cow's milk formula may be undertaken in formula-fed infants under 6-months of age with severe atopic eczema that cannot be controlled by optimal treatment with emollients and moderately potent topical corticosteroids. Dietary elimination should be carried out with the advice of a dietician to ensure complete avoidance of specific food constituents and that the diet remains nutritionally adequate. A food challenge is required to be fully objective.

Psychosocial support

Eczema can be sufficiently severe to be disrupting both to the child and to the whole family. The parents and the child need considerable advice, help, and support from health professionals, other affected families, or fellow sufferers. In the UK, the National Eczema Society provides support and education about the disorder.

Summary

Assessment of the child with eczema

Condition of the skin
Distribution of the eczema: is the skin excoriated, weeping, crusted, lichenified?
How troublesome is the itching?
Worse or better than usual?
What causes exacerbation – food or other allergens, irritants, medications, stress?
Does it disturb sleep?
Does it interfere with life?
Family knowledgeable about condition and its management?

Check
- Any evidence of infection – bacterial or herpes simplex virus?
- Problems from other allergic disorders?
- Is growth normal?

Management
Avoiding soap, frequently using emollients?
Avoiding nylon and wool clothes?
Is there a need to give or change medications:
- Topical corticosteroids
- Immunomodulators
- Occlusive bandages
- Antibiotics or antiviral agents
- Antihistamines

Allergy test to egg +/- other foods – is it indicated to identify coexistent IgE – mediated food allergy?
On dietary elimination or is it indicated? If so, dietician supervision?
Need for psychosocial support?

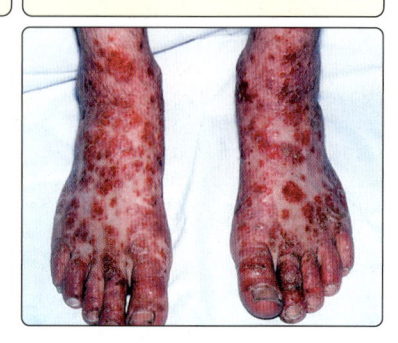

Figure 25.11 Infected, excoriated atopic eczema.

Infections and infestations

Bullous impetigo has been considered earlier in this chapter and acute bacterial and viral infections of the skin are considered in Chapter 15.

Viral infections

Viral warts
These are caused by the human papillomavirus, of which there are well over 150 types. Warts are common in children, usually on the fingers and soles (verrucae). Most disappear spontaneously over a few months or years and treatment is only indicated if the lesions are painful or are a cosmetic problem. They can be difficult to treat, but daily application of a proprietary salicylic acid and lactic acid paint or glutaraldehyde (10%) lotion can be used. Cryotherapy with liquid nitrogen is an effective treatment but can be painful and often needs repeated application, and its use should be reserved for older children.

Molluscum contagiosum
This is caused by a poxvirus. The lesions are small, skin-coloured, pearly papules with central umbilication (Fig. 25.12). They may be single but are usually multiple. Lesions are often widespread but tend to disappear spontaneously within a year. If necessary, a topical anti-bacterial can be applied to prevent or treat secondary bacterial infection, and cryotherapy for a few seconds

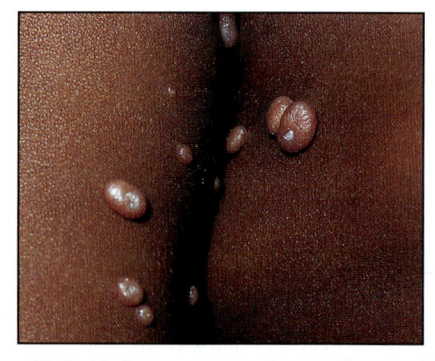

Figure 25.12 Molluscum contagiosum. Some of the pearly lesions show characteristic umbilication.

only can be used in older children, away from the face, to hasten the disappearance of more chronic lesions.

Fungal infections

Ringworm
Dermatophyte fungi invade dead keratinous structures, such as the horny layer of skin, nails, and hair. The term 'ringworm' is used because of the often ringed (annular) appearance of skin lesions. A severe inflammatory pustular ringworm patch is called a kerion (Fig. 25.13).

Tinea capitis (scalp ringworm), sometimes acquired from dogs and cats, causes scaling and patchy alopecia with broken hairs. Examination under filtered ultraviolet (Wood's) light may show bright greenish/

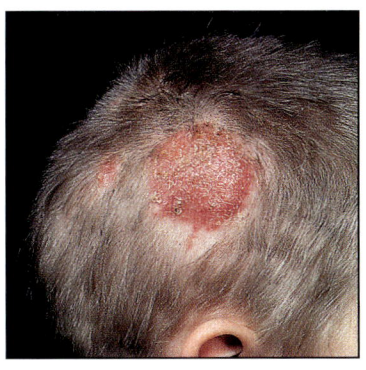

Figure 25.13 Ringworm of the scalp showing hair loss and kerion.

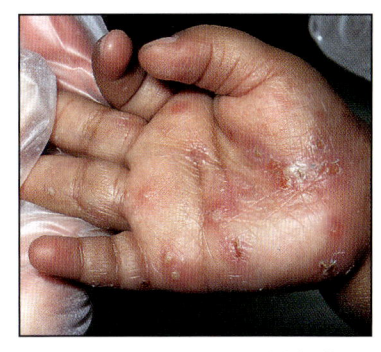

Figure 25.14 Scabies in a young child affecting the palm.

yellow fluorescence of the infected hairs with some fungal species.

Rapid diagnosis can be made by microscopic examination of skin scrapings for fungal hyphae. Definitive identification of the fungus is by culture. Treatment of mild infections is with topical antifungal preparations, but more severe infections require systemic antifungal treatment for several weeks. Any animal source of infection also needs to be treated.

> **Summary**
>
> **Tinea capitis (scalp ringworm)**
> - Annular scaling scalp lesion with patchy alopecia with broken hairs.
> - Fungal hyphae on skin scrapings.
> - Treated with topical or systemic antifungal.
> - Treat the dog or cat, if infected.

Parasitic infestations

Scabies

Scabies is caused by an infestation with the eight-legged mite *Sarcoptes scabiei*, which burrows down the epidermis along the stratum corneum. Severe itching occurs 2–6 weeks after infestation and is worse in warm conditions and at night.

In older children, burrows, papules, and vesicles involve the skin between the fingers and toes, axillae, flexor aspects of the wrists, belt line, and around the nipples, penis, and buttocks. In infants and young children, the distribution often includes the palms (Fig. 25.14), soles, and trunk. The presence of lesions on the soles can be helpful in making the diagnosis. The head, neck, and face can be involved in babies but is uncommon.

Diagnosis is made on clinical grounds with the history of itching and characteristic lesions. Although burrows are considered pathognomonic, they may be hard to identify because of secondary infection due to scratching. Itching in other family members is a helpful clinical indicator. Confirmation can be made by microscopic examination of skin scrapings from the lesions to identify mite, eggs, and mite faeces.

Complications

The skin becomes excoriated due to scratching and there may be a secondary eczematous or urticarial reaction masking the true diagnosis. Secondary bacterial infection is common, giving crusted, pustular lesions. Sometimes slowly resolving nodular lesions are visible.

Treatment

As it is spread by close bodily contact, the child and whole family should be treated, whether or not they have evidence of infestation. Permethrin cream (5%) should be applied below the neck to all areas and washed off after 8–12 hours. In babies, the face and scalp should be included, avoiding the eyes. Benzyl benzoate emulsion (25%) applied below the neck only, in diluted form according to age, and left on for 12 hours, is also effective but smells and has an irritant action. Malathion lotion (0.5% aqueous) is another effective preparation applied below the neck and left on for 12 hours.

> ☼ **If a child and other members of the family are itching, suspect scabies**

> **Summary**
>
> **Scabies**
> - Very itchy burrows, papules, and vesicles – distribution varies with age.
> - Scratching leads to excoriation, secondary eczematous, or urticarial reaction often with secondary bacterial infection.
> - Not only the child but also the whole family will need treatment.

Pediculosis

Pediculosis capitis (head lice infestation) is the most common form of lice infestation in children. It is widespread and troublesome among primary-school children. Presentation may be itching of the scalp and nape or from identifying live lice on the scalp or nits (empty egg cases) on hairs (Fig. 25.15). Louse eggs are cemented to hair close to the scalp and the nits

Dermatological disorders

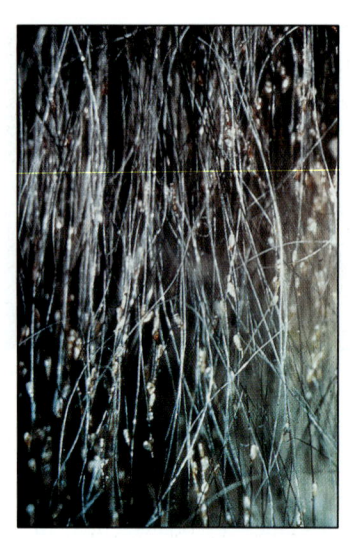

Figure 25.15 Head lice. Profuse nits (egg capsules) are visible on scalp hairs. Live lice were visible on the scalp.

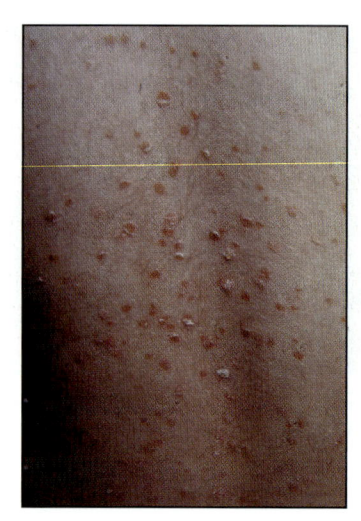

Figure 25.16 Guttate psoriasis over the back in a 5-year-old.

(small whitish oval capsules) remain attached to the hair shaft as the hair grows. There may be secondary bacterial infection, often over the nape of the neck, leading to a misdiagnosis of impetigo. Suboccipital lymphadenopathy is common. Once infestation is confirmed by finding live lice, dimeticone 4% lotion or an aqueous solution of malathion 0.5% is rubbed into the hair and scalp and left on overnight and the hair shampooed the following morning. Treatment should be repeated a week later. Flammability of an alcohol-based lotion should be noted. Wet combing with a fine-tooth comb to remove live lice (bug-busting) every 3–4 days for at least 2 weeks is a useful and safe physical treatment, particularly when parents treat with enthusiasm.

Other childhood skin disorders

Psoriasis

This familial disorder rarely presents before the age of 2 years. The guttate type (Fig. 25.16) is common in children and often follows a streptococcal or viral sore throat or ear infection. Lesions are small, raindrop-like, round or oval erythematous scaly patches on the trunk and upper limbs, and an attack usually resolves over 3 months to 4 months. However, most get a recurrence of psoriasis within the next 3–5 years. Chronic psoriasis with plaques or annular lesions is less common. Fine pitting of the nails may be seen in chronic disease but is unusual in children. Treatment for guttate psoriasis is with bland ointments. Coal tar preparations are useful for plaque psoriasis and scalp involvement. Calcipotriol, a vitamin D analogue, which does not stain the skin, is useful for plaque psoriasis in those over 6 years of age. Dithranol preparations are very effective in resistant plaque psoriasis. Occasionally, children with chronic psoriasis develop psoriatic arthritis. Chronic psoriasis may have a considerable effect on quality of life. The Psoriasis Association can be helpful in offering support and advice.

Pityriasis rosea

This acute, benign self-limiting condition is thought to be of viral origin. It usually begins with a single round or oval scaly macule, the herald patch, 2–5 cm in diameter, on the trunk, upper arm, neck, or thigh. After a few days, numerous smaller dull pink macules develop on the trunk, upper arms, and thighs. The rash tends to follow the line of the ribs posteriorly, described as the 'fir tree pattern'. Sometimes the lesions are itchy. No treatment is required and the rash resolves within 4–6 weeks.

Alopecia areata

This is a common form of hair loss in children and, understandably, a cause of much family distress. Hairless, single or multiple non-inflamed smooth areas of skin, usually over the scalp, are present (Fig. 25.17); remnants of broken-off hairs, visible as 'exclamation mark' hairs may be seen at the edge of active patches of hair fall. The more extensive the hair loss, the poorer the prognosis, but regrowth often occurs within 6 months to 12 months in localized hair loss. Prognosis should be more guarded in children with atopic disorders.

Granuloma annulare

Lesions are typically ringed (annular) with a raised flesh-coloured nonscaling edge (unlike ringworm; Fig. 25.18). They may occur anywhere but usually over bony prominences, especially over hands and feet. Lesions may be single or multiple, are usually 1–3 cm in diameter, and tend to disappear spontaneously but may take years to do so. There is also a subcutaneous form.

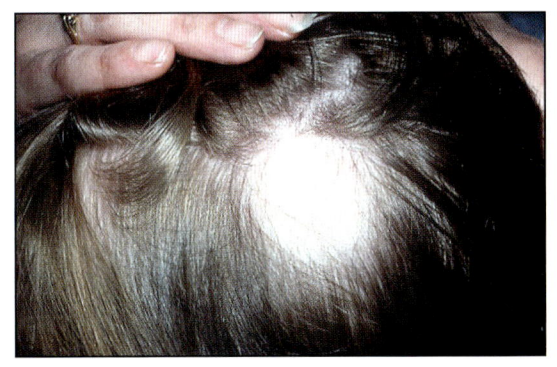

Figure 25.17 Alopecia areata. Smooth well-defined patch of noninflamed hair fall.

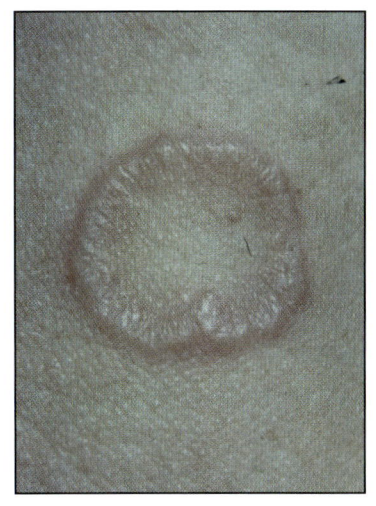

Figure 25.18 Granuloma annulare. Ringed lesion with a noninflamed, nonscaling raised edge.

Acne vulgaris

Acne may begin 1–2 years before the onset of puberty following androgenic stimulation of the sebaceous glands and an increased sebum excretion rate. Obstruction to the flow of sebum in the sebaceous follicle initiates the process of acne. Inflammation is also present. There are a variety of lesions, initially open comedones (blackheads) or closed comedones (whiteheads) progressing to papules, pustules, nodules, and cysts. Lesions occur mainly on the face, back, chest, and shoulders. The more severe cystic and nodular lesions often produce scarring. Menstruation and emotional stress may be associated with exacerbations. The condition usually resolves in the late teens, although it may persist.

Topical treatment is directed at encouraging the skin to peel using a keratolytic agent, such as benzoyl peroxide, applied once or twice daily after washing. Sunshine, in moderation, topical antibiotics, or topical retinoids may be helpful. For more severe acne, oral antibiotic therapy with tetracyclines (only when >12 years old, because they may discolour the teeth in younger children) or erythromycin is indicated. The oral retinoid isotretinoin is reserved for severe acne in teenagers unresponsive to other treatments.

Rashes and systemic disease

Skin rashes may be a sign of systemic disease. Examples are:

- facial rash in systemic lupus erythematosus or dermatomyositis
- purpura over the buttocks, lower limbs, and elbows in Henoch–Schönlein purpura
- erythema nodosum (Fig. 25.19, Box 25.4) and erythema multiforme (Fig. 25.20, Box 25.5); both can be associated with a systemic disorder, but often no cause is identified
- Stevens–Johnson syndrome, a severe bullous form of erythema multiforme also involving the mucous membranes (Fig. 25.21). It often starts with an

---

Erythema nodosum

Box 25.4 Causes of erythema nodosum

- Streptococcal infection
- Primary tuberculosis
- Inflammatory bowel disease
- Drug reaction
- Idiopathic
  (Sarcoidosis, a common association in adults, is rare in children)

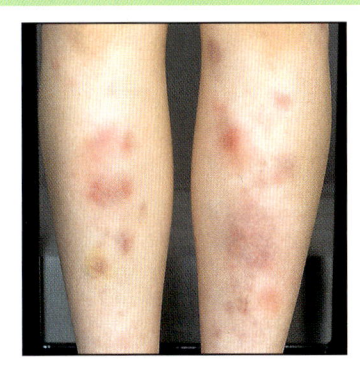

Figure 25.19 Erythema nodosum. There are tender nodules over the legs. She also had fever and arthralgia.

Erythema multiforme

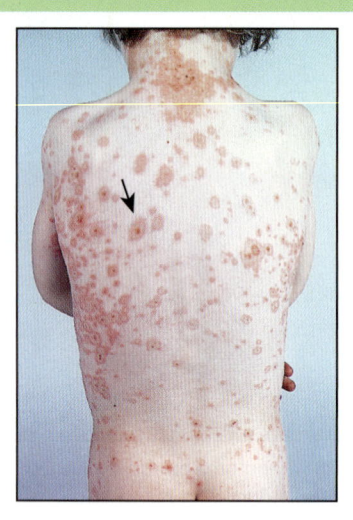

Figure 25.20 Erythema multiforme. There are target lesions with a central papule surrounded by an erythematous ring. Lesions may also be vesicular or bullous.

Box 25.5 Causes of erythema multiforme
- Herpes simplex infection
- *Mycoplasma pneumoniae* infection
- Other infections
- Drug reaction
- Idiopathic

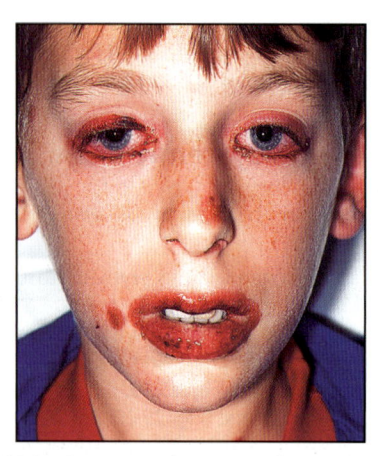

Figure 25.21 Stevens–Johnson syndrome showing severe conjunctivitis and ulceration of the mouth. (Courtesy of Rob Primhak.)

upper respiratory tract infection. Eye involvement may include conjunctivitis, corneal ulceration, and uveitis, and ophthalmological assessment is required. It may be caused by drug sensitivity, infection, or both with morbidity and sometimes even mortality from sepsis or electrolyte imbalance.

Urticaria

Urticaria (hives), characterized by flesh-coloured wheals, is described in Chapter 16 and the management of anaphylaxis in Chapter 6.

Papular urticaria is a delayed hypersensitivity reaction most commonly seen on the legs, following a bite from a flea, bedbug, animal or bird mite. Irritation, vesicles, papules and wheals appear and secondary infection due to scratching is common. It may last for weeks or months and may be recurrent.

Hereditary angioedema is a rare autosomal dominant disorder caused by a deficiency or dysfunction of C1-esterase inhibitor. There is no urticaria, but subcutaneous swellings occur, often accompanied by abdominal pain. The trigger is usually physical trauma or psychological stress. Most episodes develop over a few hours and subside over a few days. Angioedema may cause respiratory obstruction. Specific treatment of a severe acute attack is with a purified preparation of the inhibitor.

Acknowledgements

We would like to acknowledge contributors to this chapter in previous editions, whose work we have drawn on: Gill Du Mont (1st Edition), Julian Verbov (2nd, 3rd, 4th Edition).

Further reading

Website (Accessed November 2016)

Chiang NY, Verbov J: *Dermatology – A Handbook for Medical Students and Junior Doctors*, ed 2, London, 2014, British Association of Dermatologists. Available at: http://www.bad.org.uk/library-media/documents/Dermatology%20Handbook%20for%20medical%20students%202nd%20Edition%202014%20Final2%282%29.pdf.
A copy of the book can be obtained from the British Association of Dermatologists, London.

26

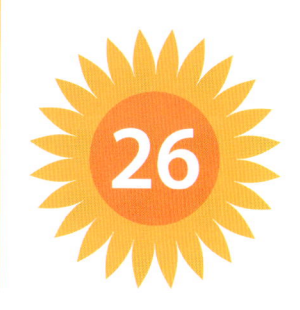

Diabetes and endocrinology

Diabetes mellitus	453	Pituitary disorders	466
Hypoglycaemia	462	Adrenal disorders	466
Thyroid disorders	464	Disorders of sex development	469
Parathyroid disorders	466		

Features of diabetes and endocrine disorders in children are:

- the UK has the 5th highest prevalence of type 1 diabetes in children in the world, and it's incidence is increasing
- tight glycaemic control has been shown to reduce the risk of long-term complications, which is particularly important in children given the length of time they will live with the disease
- the complications associated with diabetic ketoacidosis can be minimised by following national guidelines
- congenital hypothyroidism is identified on neonatal biochemical screening
- congenital adrenal hyperplasia may present with a salt-losing adrenal crisis in infancy
- the management of disorders of sex differentiation is complex and should be referred to specialist multidisciplinary teams.

Diabetes mellitus

There are about 30 500 children and young people under the age of 19 years with diabetes in the UK; a prevalence of almost 2 per 1000. Its incidence has increased steadily over the last 25 years, most likely from changes in environmental risk factors, but this is poorly understood. There is considerable ethnic and geographical variation – the condition is more common in northern countries, with a high incidence in Scotland and Finland. Almost all (96%) children have type 1 diabetes requiring insulin from the outset, although Type 2 diabetes due to insulin resistance is increasing in childhood, as obesity becomes more common and with a higher incidence in some ethnic groups, particularly Asian children. The other causes of diabetes are listed in Box 26.1.

Most children have type 1 diabetes (98%), although the number with type 2 diabetes is increasing

Box 26.1 Classification of diabetes according to aetiology

- **Type 1. Most childhood diabetes**
  - Destruction of pancreatic β-cells by an autoimmune process
- **Type 2. Insulin resistance followed later by β-cell failure**
  - Usually older children, obesity-related, positive family history, not as prone to ketosis, more common in some ethnic groups (e.g. Black and Asian children)
- **Other types**
  - Maturity onset diabetes of the young – various types caused by genetic defects in β-cell function. Strong family history.
  - Drugs, e.g. corticosteroids
  - Pancreatic insufficiency, e.g. cystic fibrosis, iron overload in thalassaemia
  - Endocrine disorders, e.g. Cushing syndrome
  - Genetic/chromosomal syndromes, e.g. Down and Turner
  - Neonatal diabetes: transient and permanent secondary to defective B cell function.
  - Gestational diabetes

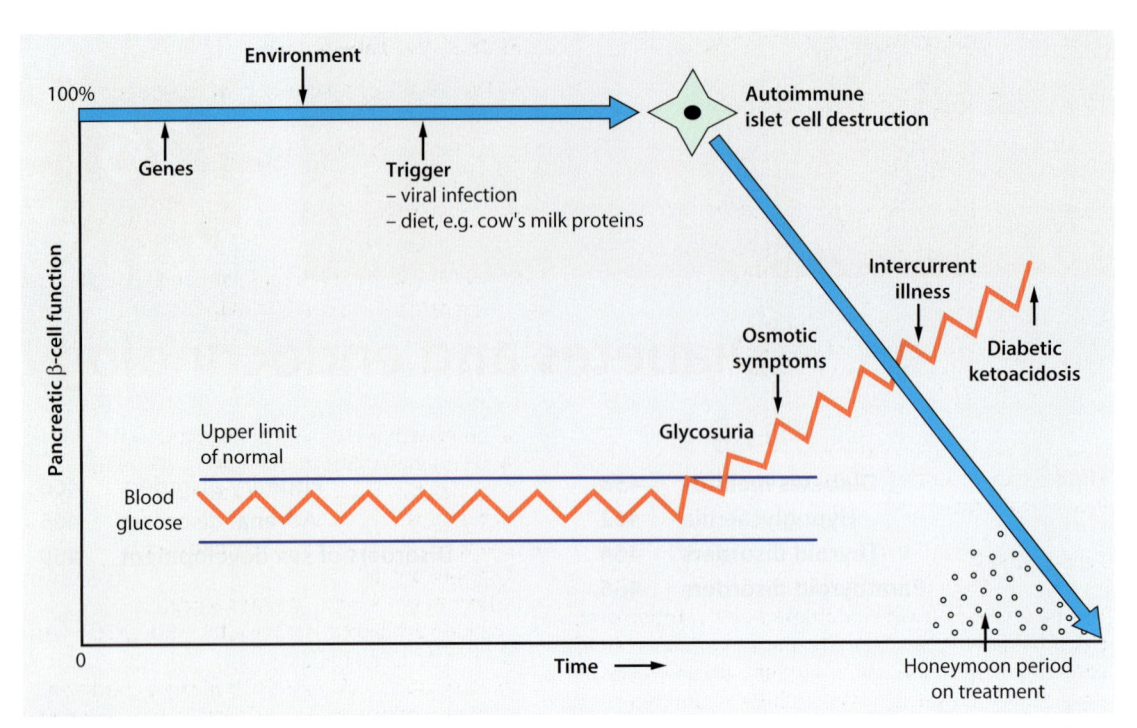

Figure 26.1 Stages in the development of diabetes.

Aetiology of type 1 diabetes

Both genetic predisposition and environmental precipitants play a role. Inherited susceptibility is demonstrated by:

- a 6% risk of developing diabetes by 20 years of age for each sibling if a child develops the disease, rising to 10–20% for a non-identical twin and 30–70% for an identical twin
- the increased risk of a child developing diabetes if a parent has insulin-dependent diabetes (6–9% if the father is affected, 2–4% if it is the mother).

Molecular mimicry probably occurs between an environmental trigger and an antigen on the surface of β-cells of the pancreas. Triggers which may contribute are enteroviral infections, accounting for the more frequent presentation in spring and autumn, and diet, possibly cow's milk proteins (Fig. 26.1) and overnutrition. In genetically predisposed individuals, this results in an autoimmune process which damages the pancreatic β-cells and leads to increasing insulin deficiency. Markers of β-cell destruction include antibodies to glutamic acid decarboxylase, the islet cells and insulin. There is an association with other autoimmune disorders such as hypothyroidism, Addison disease, coeliac disease, and rheumatoid arthritis in the patient or family.

Clinical features

There are peaks of presentation of type 1 diabetes in spring and autumn months. In contrast to adults, children usually present with only a few weeks of polyuria, excessive thirst (polydipsia) and weight loss; young children may also develop secondary nocturnal

Box 26.2 Symptoms and signs of diabetes

Early
Most common – the 'classical triad':
- excessive drinking (polydipsia)
- polyuria
- weight loss

Less common:
- enuresis (secondary)
- skin sepsis
- *candida* and other infections

Late – diabetic ketoacidosis
- Smell of acetone on breath
- Vomiting
- Dehydration
- Abdominal pain
- Hyperventilation due to acidosis (Kussmaul breathing)
- Hypovolaemic shock
- Drowsiness
- Coma and death

enuresis (Box 26.2). Diagnosis at an early stage of the illness is important in order to prevent development of diabetic ketoacidosis, so referral to a specialist team must be done immediately the diagnosis is suspected. Diabetic ketoacidosis requires urgent recognition and treatment as it carries a significant risk of mortality in children and young people. It can be misdiagnosed if hyperventilation is mistaken for pneumonia or abdominal pain for appendicitis or constipation.

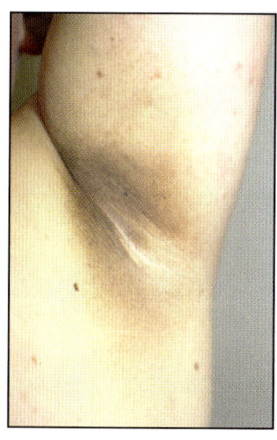

Figure 26.2 Acanthosis nigricans in axilla. A sign of insulin resistance.

Diagnosis

The diagnosis is usually confirmed in a symptomatic child by finding a markedly raised random blood glucose (>11.1 mmol/L by the current WHO definition), glycosuria, and ketosis. Where there is any doubt, a fasting blood glucose (>7 mmol/L) or a raised glycosylated haemoglobin (HbA$_{1c}$) are helpful. A diagnostic glucose tolerance test is rarely required to diagnose type 1 diabetes in children.

Type 2 diabetes should be suspected if there is a family history and in severely obese children with signs of insulin resistance (acanthosis nigricans – velvety dark skin on the neck or armpits (Fig. 26.2), skin tags or the polycystic ovary phenotype in teenage girls).

Initial management of type 1 diabetes

As type 1 diabetes in childhood is uncommon (1–2 children per large secondary school), much of the initial and routine care is delivered by specialist teams (Box 26.3).

The initial management will depend on the child's clinical condition. Those in diabetic ketoacidosis require urgent hospital admission and treatment. Most newly presenting children are alert and able to eat and drink and can be managed with subcutaneous insulin alone. Children newly presenting with diabetes who do not require intravenous therapy may be managed entirely at home if the necessary home-based care with support from the paediatric diabetes team can be provided.

An intensive educational programme is needed for the parents and child, which covers:

- a basic understanding of the pathophysiology of diabetes
- injection of insulin: technique and sites
- blood glucose (finger prick) monitoring to allow insulin adjustment and blood ketones when unwell
- healthy diet: same as for a child without diabetes, aiming for a minimum of five portions of fruit and vegetables per day. Patients should be taught 'carbohydrate counting' – estimating the amount of carbohydrate in food to allow calculation of the insulin required for each meal or snack

Box 26.3 The diabetes team

- Consultant paediatrician(s) with a special interest in diabetes
- Paediatric diabetes specialist nurse(s)
- Paediatric dietician
- Clinical psychologist
- Social worker
- Adult diabetes team for joint adolescent clinics
- Parent/patient support groups

- encouragement to exercise regularly with adjustments of diet and insulin for exercise
- 'sick-day rules' during illness to prevent ketoacidosis
- the recognition and staged treatment of hypoglycaemia
- where to get advice 24 hours a day
- the help available from voluntary groups, e.g. local groups or 'Diabetes UK'
- the psychological impact of a lifelong condition with potentially serious short-term and long-term complications.

A considerable period of time needs to be spent with the family to provide this information and psychological support. The information provided for the child must be appropriate for age, and updated regularly. The specialist nurse should liaise with the school (teachers, those who prepare school meals, physical education supervisors) and the primary care team.

Insulin

Insulin is made chemically identical to human insulin by recombinant DNA technology or by chemical modification of pork insulin. All insulin that is used in the UK in children is human and in concentrations of 100 units/ml (U-100). The types of insulin include:

- human insulin analogues. Rapid-acting insulin analogues, e.g. insulin lispro, insulin glulisine or insulin aspart (trade names Humalog, Apidra, and NovoRapid, respectively) – with a much faster onset and shorter duration of action than soluble regular insulin. There are also very long-acting insulin analogues, e.g. insulin detemir (Levemir) or glargine (Lantus)
- 'short-acting' soluble human regular insulin. Onset of action (30–60 min), peak 2–4 hours, duration up to 8 hours. Given 15–30 minutes before meals. Trade named examples are Actrapid and Humulin S
- intermediate-acting insulin. Onset 1–2 hours, peak 4–12 hours. Isophane insulin is insulin with protamine, e.g. Insulatard and Humulin I
- predetermined preparations of mixed rapid or short-acting and intermediate-acting insulins with 25% or 30% short-acting components.

Insulin can be given by continuous infusion of rapid-acting insulin from a pump or by injections using a variety of syringe and needle sizes or pen-like devices with insulin-containing cartridges.

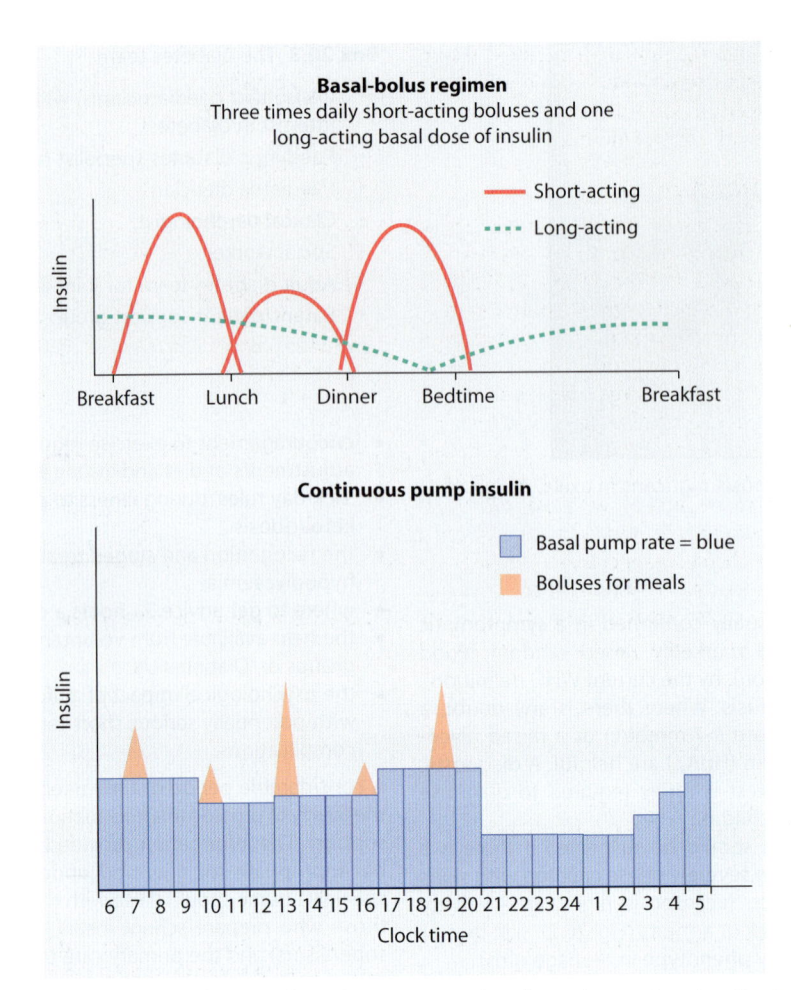

Figure 26.3 Basal-bolus insulin regimen and continuous pump insulin regimen, showing the basal levels of insulin programmed into the pump (blue bars) and the bolus insulin (red pulses) given before each meal/snack according to carbohydrate intake.

Insulin may be injected into the subcutaneous tissue of the anterior and lateral aspects of the thigh, the buttocks, and the abdomen. Rotation of the injection sites is essential to prevent lipohypertrophy or, more rarely, lipoatrophy. The skin should be gently pinched up and the insulin injected at a 45° angle. Using a long needle or an injection technique that is 'too vertical' causes a painful, bruised intramuscular injection. Shallow intradermal injections can also cause scarring and should be avoided.

Most children are started on a continuous subcutaneous insulin pump or a multiple daily injection regimen ('basal-bolus') with rapid-acting insulin (e.g. Lispro, Glulisine, or Insulin Aspart) being given (bolus) before each meal plus long-acting insulin (e.g. Glargine or Detemir) in the late evening and/or before breakfast to provide insulin background (basal). These treatments both allow greater flexibility by relating the insulin more closely to food intake and exercise (Fig. 26.3). Patients and families are taught to aim for blood glucose levels between 4 mmol/L and 7 mmol/L before meals and to give extra rapid acting insulin to 'correct' glucose down to target range at mealtimes. The input required by the child and family and team to start these intensive regimes is high, but they have been shown to achieve the best glycaemic control and reduce risks of long-term complications. Some patients and families still rely on twice-daily treatment with premixed insulin for simplicity.

Shortly after presentation, when some pancreatic function is preserved, insulin requirements often become minimal, the so-called 'honeymoon period'. Requirements subsequently increase to 0.5 units/kg to 1 unit/kg or even up to 2 units/kg per day during puberty.

Diet

Children and young people with diabetes mellitus are encouraged to eat a healthy diet and insulin doses need to match carbohydrate intake whichever regime is chosen. The aim is to optimise metabolic control while maintaining normal growth. The recommended diet has a high complex carbohydrate and modest fat content (<30% of total calories). The diet should be high in fibre, which will provide a sustained release of glucose, rather than refined carbohydrate, which causes rapid swings in glucose levels. 'Carbohydrate counting' allows patients to calculate their likely insulin requirements once their food choice for a meal is known, and taking into account their premeal sugar level and postmeal exercise pattern. Learning this balancing act requires a lot of educational input followed by refinement in the light of experience.

Blood glucose monitoring

Regular blood glucose measurements are required to adjust the insulin regimen and learn how changes in lifestyle, food, and exercise affect control (Fig. 26.4). A record should be kept in a diary or transferred from the memory of the blood glucose meter (see Case history 26.1). The aim is to maintain blood glucose as near to normal as possible, with a target of 4 mmol/L to 7 mmol/L before meals. During changes in routine (e.g. holidays) or illness, this means more than five tests per day. This can be a challenge without hypoglycaemia; realistic goals need to be agreed, with compromises reached about the frequency of monitoring and accommodation of lifestyle choices, especially in teenagers.

Continuous glucose monitoring sensors, using subcutaneous or transcutaneous sensors to provide a continuous reading of blood glucose, are available

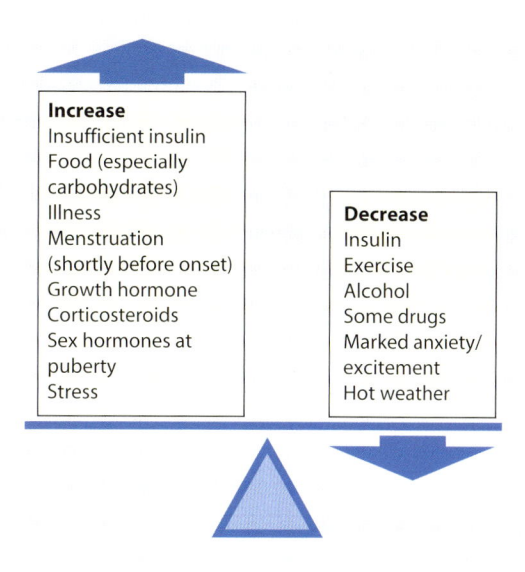

Increase
Insufficient insulin
Food (especially carbohydrates)
Illness
Menstruation (shortly before onset)
Growth hormone
Corticosteroids
Sex hormones at puberty
Stress

Decrease
Insulin
Exercise
Alcohol
Some drugs
Marked anxiety/excitement
Hot weather

Figure 26.4 Factors affecting blood glucose levels.

Case history 26.1

Blood glucose diary

This is the diary of an 8-year-old boy with Type 1 diabetes (Fig. 26.5).

It shows:

- his parents use carbohydrate counting for all meals, but this can be difficult when eating unfamiliar foods (August 3, blood glucose rises to 11.8 mmol/L)
- he uses correction doses if his blood glucose is high before meals, using 1 unit of Novorapid to bring his blood glucose down by approximately 4 mmol/L (July 29, from 9.3 before breakfast to 6.9 mmol/L before lunch)
- he reduces his rapid acting insulin before predictable sport to reduce the risk of hypoglycaemia (prelunch on August 2)
- he has good recognition of symptoms of hypoglycaemia and treats it with glucose tablets, then a snack. His blood glucose level sometimes 'overshoots' after treatment of hypoglycaemia (blood glucose low after physical exercise, high after treatment on August 6)
- when he is unwell or his blood glucose is unexpectedly high, he checks for blood ketones and gives extra Novorapid.

Date	Novorapid 1 unit:10 g (prebreakfast)	Novorapid 1 unit:10 g (prelunch)	Novorapid 1 unit:15 g (pretea)	Glargine units (before bed)	Before breakfast	2 hours post	Before lunch	2 hours post	Before tea	2 hours post	Before bed	During night	Comments
29/7	5 (+0.5)	6	5 (+0.5)	7	9.3		6.9		8.7		5.4	6.7 2 am	
30/7	4.5	6	5	7	7.2		5.9		6.7		7.1		
31/7	5	6.5	5.5	7	6.2	5.8 10.15 am	4.3		3.8/4.7		10.1		Hungry after hypo
1/8	5	7.0 (+0.5)	5	7	7.3		8.8		6.4		6.9		
2/8	4	5 (-2)	4.5	7	5.4		7.2		8.9		5.5		Football match
3/8	4.5	5.5 (+0.5)	5	7	5.0		9.0		6.8		11.8		Out for tea
4/8	4.5	5	5	7	3.5/5.6		5.4		7.3		7.0		
5/8	5	5	7 (+2)	7	6.6		7.1		14.2 Ketones mildly raised	13.3	8.2	7.2 2 am	Unwell after school
6/8	5	5.5	4	7	6.3		6.9		5.0		3.4/9.0	4.8 1 am	PE afternoon
7/8	4.5	4.5	4	7	4.6		5.4		7.0		7.9		

Figure 26.5 Blood glucose diary of an 8-year-old boy with type 1 diabetes

Case history 26.2

Continuous glucose monitoring in a child with an insulin infusion pump

A 5-year-old girl has recurrent hypoglycaemia affecting her behaviour and concentration at school. She is put on an insulin infusion pump with continuous glucose monitoring. The pump upload is shown in Fig. 26.6.

This shows her blood glucose profile on 2 days. On the first day, she has hypoglycaemia between 6 am and 8 am before waking, then a large peak in blood glucose after breakfast followed by further hypoglycaemia from 4 pm to 6 pm. The hourly basal rate of insulin was reduced from 4 am and again at 2 pm. The amount of insulin given per gram carbohydrate at breakfast was also increased. The second upload, some days later, shows steady blood glucose overnight, with smaller peaks after meals. The improvement in blood glucose levels improves her attention at school and she achieves an improved HbA1c.

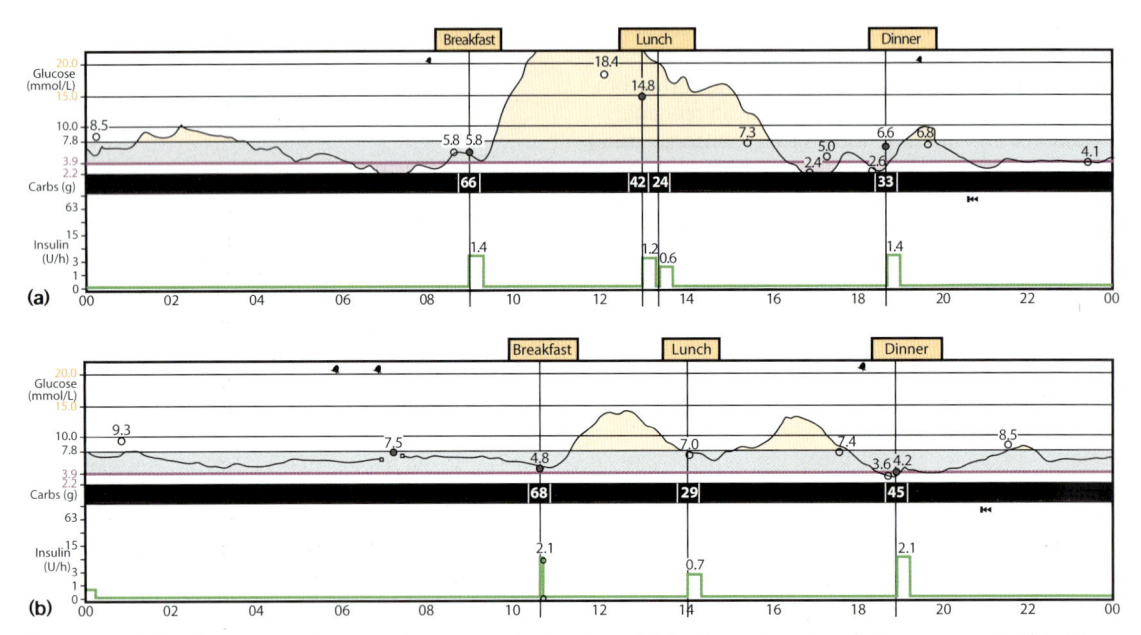

Figure 26.6 Read-out of continuous glucose monitoring in a child with an insulin infusion pump. **(a)** This 24 hour trace shows hypoglycaemia followed by a marked rise in glucose followed by further hypoglycaemia.; and **(b)** 24 hour trace following change in insulin regimen and elimination of both hypoglycaemia and marked rise in blood glucose

---

and help control the insulin delivered from a pump, e.g. suspending insulin delivery when anticipating hypoglycaemia. Continuous glucose monitoring sensors also allow the detection of unexpected asymptomatic episodes of nocturnal hypoglycaemia or times of poor control during the day (see Case History 26.2). Blood ketone testing (often using the same meter as for blood glucose) is mandatory during illness or when control is poor to try to avoid severe ketoacidosis.

The measurement of HbA_{1c} is particularly helpful as a guide of overall diabetes control over the previous 6–12 weeks and should be checked at least four times per year. The level is related to the risk of later complications in a nonlinear fashion, such that the risk of complications increases more rapidly with higher levels. However, it may be misleading if the red blood cell lifespan is reduced, such as in sickle cell trait or if the HbA molecule is abnormal, as in thalassaemia.

A HbA_{1c} level of less than 48 mmol/mol (6.5%) is the recommended target.

Acute complications

Hypoglycaemia

It is inevitable that children and young people who manage their diabetes well will experience hypoglycaemia. Most develop well-defined symptoms when their blood glucose falls below 4 mmol/L. The symptoms are highly individual and change with age, but most complain of hunger, tummy ache, sweatiness, feeling faint or dizzy or of a 'wobbly feeling' in their legs. If unrecognised or untreated, hypoglycaemia may progress to seizures and coma. Parents can often detect hypoglycaemia in young children by their pallor and irritability, sometimes presenting as unreasonable behaviour. If there is any doubt, the blood glucose concentration should be checked. Frequent episodes of hypoglycaemia can be associated with losing awareness of the symptoms.

Treating a 'hypo' at an early stage requires the administration of easily absorbed glucose in the form of glucose tablets or a sugary drink (e.g. Lucozade). Children should always have easy access to their hypo remedy, although young children quickly learn to complain of hypo-symptoms in order to leave class or obtain a sweet drink! Oral glucose gels (e.g. Glucogel) are quickly absorbed from the buccal mucosa and so are helpful if the child is unable to cooperate. It can be administered by teachers or other helpers. Parents and school should be provided with a glucagon injection kit for the treatment of severe hypoglycaemia, when the child has a reduced level of consciousness, and taught how to administer it intramuscularly to terminate severe hypos. After treatment of 'hypos', parents or carers should give the child some food (usually a biscuit or sandwich) to prevent the blood glucose dropping again.

Severe hypoglycaemia can usually be predicted (or explained in retrospect – missed meal, heavy exercise). The aim is anticipation and prevention. Hypoglycaemia in an unconscious child brought to hospital is treated with intravenous glucose.

Diabetic ketoacidosis

Presentation is described in Box 26.2, essential investigations in Box 26.4 and management in Fig. 26.7.

Long-term management

The aims of long-term management are:

- normal growth and development
- maintaining as normal a home and school life as possible
- good diabetes control through knowledge and good technique
- encouraging children to become self-reliant, but with adult supervision until they are able to take responsibility
- anticipating and minimising hypoglycaemia
- to maintain a HbA_{1c} of less than 48 mmol/mol (6.5%).

The long-term complications of diabetes are:

- macrovascular – hypertension, coronary heart disease, cerebrovascular disease
- microvascular – retinopathy, nephropathy, neuropathy.

It has been shown that meticulous diabetes control delays or prevents diabetic retinopathy and nephropathy and, if retinopathy occurs, it can slow its progression. There is also evidence that good early control reduces the risk of later complications even if control deteriorates later in life. Levels of HbA_{1c} above 48 mmol/mol (6.5%) are related to the risk of later complications in an almost exponential fashion, and so the ideal is to aim for a level as close to someone without diabetes as possible.

As these aims are difficult to achieve in all patients at all stages of their condition, children and their families should be reviewed regularly to assess their diabetes control, to monitor the development of complications, to ensure that have age-appropriate information, and that psychosocial aspects are addressed (Fig. 26.8).

Problems in diabetes control

Good blood glucose control is particularly difficult in the following circumstances:

- eating too many sugary foods, such as sweets or snacks taken without insulin, at parties or on the way home from school
- infrequent or unreliable blood glucose testing. 'Perfect' results are often invented and written down just before clinic to please the diabetes team. This is apparent if the blood glucose levels recorded are inconsistent with the HbA1c
- illness – viral illnesses are common in the young and although it is usually stated that infections cause insulin requirements to increase, in practice the insulin dose required is variable, partly because of reduced food intake. The dose of insulin should be adjusted according to regular blood glucose monitoring. Insulin *must* be continued during times of illness and blood tested for ketones. If ketosis is increasing along with a rising blood glucose, the family should know how to increase the rapid-acting insulin dose appropriately or seek medical help for advice or possible intravenous therapy
- exercise – vigorous or prolonged planned exercise (cross-country running, long-distance hiking, skiing) requires reduction of the insulin dose and increase in carbohydrate intake. Late hypoglycaemia may occur during the night or even the next day, but may be avoided by taking a bedtime snack, including slow-acting carbohydrate and fat such as cereal with milk. Less vigorous exercise such as sports lessons in school and spontaneous outdoor play can be managed with a reduction in short-acting insulin before the exercise
- eating disorders
- family disruption such as divorce or separation
- inadequate family motivation, support, or understanding. As children can never have a 'holiday' from their diabetes, they need a great deal of encouragement to continuously maintain good control. Educational programmes for children and families need to be arranged regularly and matched to their current level of education. Special courses and holiday camps are available; in the UK they are organised by Diabetes UK and local groups.

Management at school

An individualized care plan should be developed by the parents, diabetes team, and the school to address the specific needs of the child. This will include the child's dietary needs and what to do if the child becomes hypoglycaemic or loses consciousness. For younger children, support is needed to help test blood glucose, calculate and give the prelunch insulin injection or bolus from the pump.

Diabetic ketoacidosis

Box 26.4 Essential early investigations in diabetic ketoacidosis

- Blood glucose (>11.1 mmol/L)
- Blood ketones (>3.0 mmol/L)
- Urea and electrolytes, creatinine (dehydration)
- Blood gas analysis (severe metabolic acidosis)
- Evidence of a precipitating cause, e.g. infection (blood and urine cultures performed)
- Cardiac monitor for T-wave changes of hypokalaemia
- Weight (compare with recent clinic weight to ascertain level of dehydration)

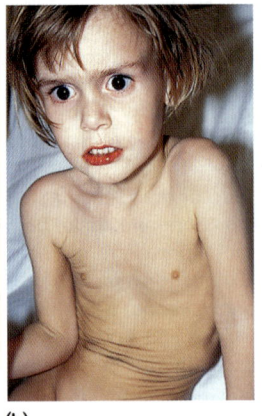

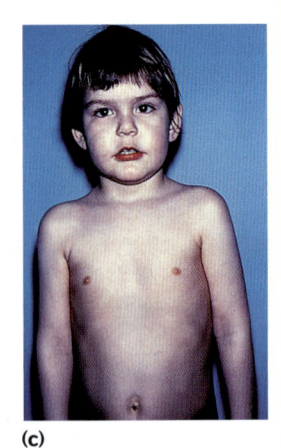

(b) **(c)**

(a) Diabetic ketoacidosis management

Follow this regimen if: hyperglycaemia (blood glucose >11 mmol/L, acidosis (pH <7.3 and/or bicarbonate <15 mmol/L), blood ketone usually >3 mmol/L and clinical dehydration and/or vomiting, drowsy or clinically acidotic.
(Follow guidelines from the British Society of Paediatric Endocrinology and Diabetes to reduce the risk from hypokalaemia, aspiration and cerebral oedema).

1. Fluids → If in shock, initial resuscitation is with 0.9% saline (10 ml/kg). Dehydration should then be corrected gradually over 48 hours (see Fig. 26.7b and c). Rapid rehydration should be avoided as it may lead to cerebral oedema. Initial rehydration fluids need to be taken into account in calculating fluid requirements. 0.9% saline with 40 mmol/L KCl is recommended for first 12 hours, adding 5% glucose when blood glucose <14 mmol/L. After 12 hours, if plasma sodium level is stable, 0.45% saline/5% glucose with 40 mmol/L KCl is recommended. Monitor:
- fluid input and output
- blood glucose (hourly), blood ketones (1-2 hourly), electrolytes, creatinine and acid–base status 2–4 hourly
- neurological state.

Consider transfer to PICU and central venous line (CVP) and urinary catheter if shocked or in coma. A nasogastric tube is passed for acute gastric dilatation if there is vomiting or depressed consciousness.

2. Insulin → Insulin infusion (0.1 units/kg per h) is started after intravenous fluids running for 1 hour. Do not give a bolus. Monitor the blood glucose hourly. Aim for gradual reduction of blood glucose. Change to a solution containing 5% glucose when the blood glucose has fallen to 14 mmol/L to avoid hypoglycaemia.

3. Potassium → Although the initial plasma potassium may be high, due to displacement from cells in exchange for hydrogen ions, it will fall following treatment with insulin and rehydration. Potassium replacement must be instituted as soon as maintenance fluids are started (unlike adults, it can be assumed that the child will have normal renal function and the greatest risk is from total body potassium depletion). Continuous cardiac monitoring and 2–4 hourly plasma potassium measurements are indicated until the plasma potassium is stable.

4. Acidosis → Although a metabolic acidosis is present, bicarbonate should be avoided unless the child is shocked. The acidosis will correct with fluid and insulin therapy.

5. Re-establish oral fluids, subcutaneous insulin and diet → Do not stop the intravenous insulin infusion until 1 hour after subcutaneous insulin has been given.

6. Identification and treatment of an underlying cause → Ketoacidosis may be precipitated by an intercurrent infection. Diabetic ketoacidosis causes neutrophilia but not a fever. Antibiotics may be indicated. If the child was known to have diabetes, consider the reason for the ketoacidosis.

Figure 26.7 (a) Diabetic ketoacidosis management; **(b)** boy with severe dehydration and weight loss from diabetic ketoacidosis; and **(c)** 4 months later. (Photos b and c courtesy of Jill Challener.)

Summary

Regular assessment of the child with diabetes

Assessment of diabetes:
- Any episodes of hypoglycaemia, diabetic ketoacidosis, hospital admission?
- Is there still awareness of hypoglycaemia?
- Absence from school? School supportive of diabetes care?
- Interference with normal life?
- HbA$_{1c}$ results – less than 48 mmol/mol (6.5%)?
- Diary of blood glucose results or blood glucose read-out– are appropriate actions to results being taken?
- Insulin regimen – appropriate?
- Lipohypertrophy or lipoatrophy (Fig. 26.8 a and b) at injection sites?
- Diet – healthy diet, manipulating food intake and insulin to maintain good control?

General overview (periodic):
- Normal growth and pubertal development, avoiding obesity – measure height and weight and BMI and plot on growth chart at each visit
- Blood pressure check for hypertension yearly (age-specific centiles)
- Renal disease – screening for microalbuminuria, an early sign of nephropathy, annually from 12 years
- Circulation: - check pulses and sensation
- Eyes – retinopathy or cataracts are rare in children, but should be monitored annually from 12 years, preferably with retinal photography
- Feet – maintain good care, avoid tight shoes and obtain prompt treatment of infections - annually
- Screening for coeliac and thyroid disease at diagnosis, thyroid screening annually, coeliac again if symptomatic.
- Annual reminder to have flu vaccination

Knowledge and psychosocial aspects:
- Good understanding of diabetes, would participation/holidays with other diabetic children be beneficial? Member of Diabetes UK?
- Becoming self-reliant, but appropriate supervision at home, school, diabetic team?
- Taking exercise, sport? Diabetes not interfering with it?
- Leading as normal life as possible?
- Smoking, alcohol?
- Is 'hypo' treatment readily available? Is stepped approach known?
- What are the main issues for the patient? Are there short-term goals to allow engagement with improving control?

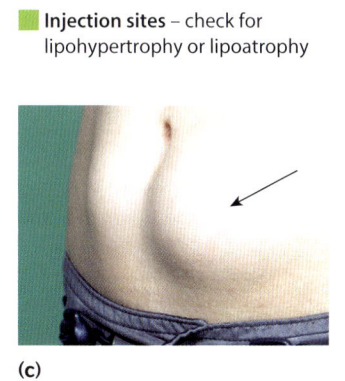

(a)

(b)

Injection sites – check for lipohypertrophy or lipoatrophy

(c)

Figure 26.8 (a) The regular assessment of the child or young person with diabetes; (b) injection sites; and (c) lipohypertrophy (arrow) of abdomen from insulin injections.

Puberty and adolescence

Diabetes in young people is influenced by biological, psychological, and social factors (see Table 26.1). The rapid growth spurt in early puberty is governed by a complex interaction of hormonal changes, some of which involve insulin and insulin-like growth factors. Growth hormone, oestrogen and testosterone all antagonise insulin action and there is an increase in the insulin requirement from the usual 0.5 unit/kg per day to 1.0 unit/kg per day of early childhood up to 2 units/kg per day. The increase may be especially marked first thing in the morning due to the peak of growth hormone secretion overnight.

In early adolescence, young people have concrete thinking and learn that they are not immediately ill if they eat less healthily or miss an injection. This is in contrast to what they are taught by adults and may discourage them from meticulous self-care. In later adolescence, their thinking is increasingly abstract but they may feel indestructible. Some test the degree to which the 'rules' can be broken as they 'feel OK'.

Table 26.1 The impact of diabetes in normal adolescence

Normal adolescence	How diabetes interferes
Biological factors	Insulin resistance secondary to growth and sex hormone secretion
	Growth and pubertal delay if diabetes control poor
Psychological factors	Reduced self-esteem e.g. related to impaired body image, difference from peers
Social factors	Different from peer group e.g. need for blood tests and injections
	Hypoglycaemic events – can be frightening and emphasise difference from friends
	Increased risk from alcohol, smoking, use of recreational drugs
	Vocational plans e.g. some restriction in choices such as heavy goods vehicle licence, pilot
	Separation from parents more complex

It is then important to focus on immediate benefits to good diabetes control and work with the young person to identify the challenges and support them to find solutions (see Ch. 30. Adolescent Medicine). One needs to keep track of the young person's social changes undertaken to keep abreast with their peers. With increasing independence, the young person may explore behaviours such as smoking, use of alcohol, and sexual relationships; the diabetes team need to ensure that the young person understands how to manage these safely alongside their diabetes. Conflict with parents (and sometimes professionals) is common during adolescence and may focus on diabetes management. Many parents are very protective and find it difficult to encourage their child, though now an adolescent, to take more responsibility for their diabetes. Support from a psychologist may be useful.

Some teenagers with diabetes, especially girls, have excessive weight gain and become obese if their insulin dose is not reduced towards the end of puberty. Intensive insulin regimens increase the risk of obesity and height and weight and body mass index should be plotted at each clinic visit. The weight gain not only affects their diabetes control, but may have a major impact on their body image. Eating disorders are more common in young people with diabetes, but do not always fit the typical pattern of anorexia nervosa or bulimia; for example, some learn that glycosuria can be used as an 'aid' to losing weight when they omit insulin.

It is generally unhelpful to give lectures about the long-term risks to health, as these are likely to be seen as irrelevant by many teenagers. However, they may be helped if:

- there are clear short-term goals, especially if suggested by themselves
- their efforts to improve their diabetes control, e.g. an improving or satisfactory HbA_{1c} level, are communicated promptly and enthusiastically
- there is a united team approach, with unambiguous guidelines for health and diabetes management
- peer group support is used to promote health. Activities that allow groups of teenagers to participate while learning about their diabetes management are encouraged.

Successful long-term diabetes management depends on education to understand their condition, increasing self-reliance and responsibility.

After many years in a children's clinic, it can be difficult for the patient and family to move to the adult care environment. This transition is helped by discussing and planning the move well ahead of time, and by the provision of joint clinics with the adult team through to the early twenties or end of tertiary education. Specialist periconceptional clinics have been established in some centres to help achieve tight control before conception in planned pregnancies. Conception of a fetus when the mother has a high HbA_{1c} increases the risks for the pregnancy, including the risk of congenital abnormalities in the offspring.

> **Summary**
>
> **Diabetes mellitus**
> - Type 1 diabetes is usually managed by an intensive insulin regime, matching insulin to the carbohydrate eaten in a balanced diet. Exercise is encouraged.
> - Diabetic ketoacidosis is associated with a significant morbidity and mortality rate in children and needs meticulous management.
> - Long-term complications are reduced if the HbA1c can be maintained at less than 48 mmol/mol (6.5%).

Hypoglycaemia

Hypoglycaemia is a common problem in neonates during the first few days of life (see Ch. 11). Thereafter, it is uncommon without diabetes. It is often defined as a plasma glucose less than 2.6 mmol/L, although the development of clinical features will depend on

Box 26.5 Tests to perform when hypoglycaemia is present

Blood
- Confirm hypoglycaemia with laboratory blood glucose
- Growth hormone, IGF-1, cortisol, insulin, C-peptide, fatty acids, ketones (acetoacetate, 3-hydroxybutyrate), glycerol, branched-chain amino acids, acylcarnitine profile, lactate, pyruvate

First urine after hypoglycaemia
- Organic acids
- Consider saving blood and urine for toxicology, e.g. salicylate, sulphonylurea

Box 26.6 Causes of hypoglycaemia beyond the immediate neonatal period

Fasting
- *Insulin excess*
  - Excess exogenous insulin, e.g. in diabetes mellitus/insulin given surreptitiously
  - β-cell tumours/disorders – persistent hypoglycaemic hyperinsulinism of infancy, insulinoma
  - Drug-induced (sulphonylurea)
  - Autoimmune (insulin receptor antibodies)
  - Beckwith syndrome
- *Without hyperinsulinaemia*
  - Liver disease
  - Ketotic hypoglycaemia of childhood
  - Inborn errors of metabolism, e.g. glycogen storage disorders
  - Hormonal deficiency: GH↓, ACTH↓, Addison disease, congenital adrenal hyperplasia

Reactive/nonfasting
- Galactosaemia
- Leucine sensitivity
- Fructose intolerance
- Maternal diabetes
- Hormonal deficiency
- Aspirin/alcohol poisoning

---

whether other energy substrates can be utilised. Clinical features include:

- sweating
- pallor
- central nervous system signs of irritability, headache, seizures, and coma.

The neurological sequelae may be permanent if hypoglycaemia persists and include epilepsy, severe learning difficulties and microcephaly. This risk is greatest in early childhood during the period of most rapid brain growth.

Infants have high energy requirements and relatively poor reserves of glucose from gluconeogenesis and glycogenesis. They are at risk of hypoglycaemia with fasting. Infants should never be starved for more than 4 hours, e.g. preoperatively. A blood glucose should be checked in any child who:

- becomes septicaemic or appears seriously ill. **ABC** then **DEFG** – '**D**on't **E**ver **F**orget **G**lucose'
- has a prolonged seizure
- develops an altered state of consciousness.

This is often done at the bedside, using glucose-sensitive strips with a meter. However, the strips only indicate that the glucose is within a low range of values and any low reading must always be confirmed by laboratory measurement.

If the cause of the hypoglycaemia is unknown, *it is vital that blood is collected at the time of the hypoglycaemia* and the first available urine sent for analysis, so that a valuable opportunity for making the diagnosis is not missed (Box 26.5).

Causes

These are listed in Box 26.6.

Ketotic hypoglycaemia is a poorly-defined entity in which young children readily become hypoglycaemic following a short period of starvation, probably due to limited reserves for gluconeogenesis. The child is often thin and the insulin levels are low. Regular snacks and extra glucose drinks when ill will usually prevent hypoglycaemia. The condition resolves spontaneously in later life. A number of rare endocrine and metabolic disorders may present with hypoglycaemia at almost any age in childhood. Hepatomegaly would suggest the possibility of an inherited glycogen storage disorder, in which hypoglycaemia can be profound.

Transient neonatal hypoglycaemia in neonates may be due to exposure to high levels of insulin in utero in mothers with diabetes or glucose intolerance. In contrast, recurrent, severe neonatal hypoglycaemia may be caused by persistent hypoglycaemic hyperinsulinism of infancy. This is a rare disorder of infancy where there are gene mutations of various pathways leading to dysregulation of insulin release by the islet cells of the pancreas leading to profound nonketotic hypoglycaemia. Treatment with high-concentration glucose solutions and diazoxide (plus other medications) may be required to maintain safe blood glucose levels pending investigation. Positron emission tomography scans reveal that up to 40% are caused by localised lesions in the pancreas amenable to partial resection, although the majority either require long-term medication or total pancreatectomy with the attendant risk of diabetes and exocrine pancreatic insufficiency.

Treatment

Hypoglycaemia can be corrected with an intravenous infusion of glucose (maximum of 5 ml/kg of 10% glucose bolus followed by 10% glucose infusion) or orally (see hypoglycaemia management in diabetes section). Care must be taken to avoid giving an excess volume as the intravenous solution is hypertonic and could cause cerebral oedema. If there is delay in establishing an infusion or failure to respond, glucagon is given intramuscularly. If a higher concentration than a

10% solution is required in a neonate, the low glucose is highly likely to be secondary to hyperinsulinism.

Corticosteroids may also be required if there is a possibility of pituitary or adrenal dysfunction. The correction of hypoglycaemia must always be documented with satisfactory laboratory glucose measurements.

> **Summary**
>
> **Hypoglycaemia**
> - Should be excluded in any child with septicaemia, who is seriously ill, has a prolonged seizure or altered state of consciousness ('**D**on't **E**ver **F**orget **G**lucose').
> - Low blood glucose on bedside testing must be confirmed by laboratory measurement.
> - If the cause is unknown, diagnostic blood and urine samples should, if possible, be taken at the time.

Thyroid disorders

Only a small amount of thyroxine is transferred from the mother to the fetus, although severe maternal hypothyroidism can affect the developing brain. The fetal thyroid predominantly produces 'reverse T_3', a derivative of T_3 which is largely inactive. After birth, there is a surge in the level of thyroid-stimulating hormone (TSH) which is accompanied by a marked rise in T_4 and T_3 levels. The TSH declines to the normal adult range within a week. Preterm infants may have very low levels of T_4 for the first few weeks of life, while the TSH is within the normal range; under these circumstances, additional thyroxine is not required.

Congenital hypothyroidism

Detection of congenital hypothyroidism is important in neonatal screening, as it is:

- relatively common, occurring in 1 in 4000 births
- a preventable cause of severe learning difficulties.

Causes of congenital hypothyroidism are:

- *maldescent of the thyroid and athyrosis* – the most common cause of sporadic congenital hypothyroidism. In early fetal life, the thyroid migrates from a position at the base of the tongue (sublingual) to its normal site below the larynx. The thyroid may fail to develop completely or partially. In maldescent, the thyroid remains as a lingual mass or a unilobular small gland. The reason for this failure of formation or migration is not well understood
- *dyshormonogenesis* – an inborn error of thyroid hormone synthesis, in about 5% to 10% of cases, although more common in some ethnic groups with consanguineous marriage
- *iodine deficiency* – the most common cause of congenital hypothyroidism worldwide but rare in the UK. It can be prevented by iodination of salt in the diet
- hypothyroidism due to *TSH deficiency* – isolated TSH deficiency is rare (<1% of cases) and is usually associated with pituitary dysfunction, which usually manifests with growth hormone, gonadotrophin and adrenocorticotrophic hormone (ACTH) deficiency leading to hypoglycaemia or micropenis and undescended testes in affected boys before the hypothyroidism becomes evident.

The clinical features (Box 26.7 and Fig. 26.9) are difficult to differentiate from normal in the first month of life, but become more prominent with age. There is a slight excess of other congenital abnormalities, especially heart defects.

Box 26.7 Clinical features of hypothyroidism

Congenital	Acquired
Usually asymptomatic and picked up on screening.	Females > males
	Short stature/poor growth
Clinical features:	Cold intolerance
• faltering growth	Dry skin
• feeding problems	Cold peripheries
• prolonged jaundice	Bradycardia
• constipation	Thin, dry hair
• pale, cold, mottled dry skin	Pale, puffy eyes with loss of eyebrows
• coarse facies	Goitre
• large tongue	Slow-relaxing reflexes
• hoarse cry	Constipation
• goitre (occasionally)	Delayed puberty/amenorrhoea
• umbilical hernia	Obesity
• delayed development	Slipped upper femoral epiphysis
	Poor concentration
	Deterioration in school work
	Learning difficulties

Figure 26.9 Untreated congenital hypothyroidism.

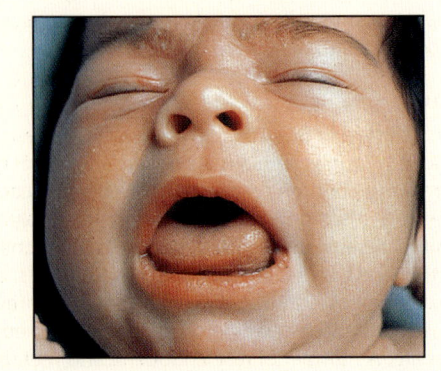

Most infants with congenital hypothyroidism are detected on routine neonatal biochemical screening (Guthrie test) performed on all newborn infants, by identifying a raised TSH in the blood. However, thyroid dysfunction secondary to pituitary abnormalities will not be picked up at neonatal screening as they have a low TSH. In some countries T_4 is also measured.

Treatment with thyroxine should be started before 2 weeks to 3 weeks of age to reduce the risk of impaired neurodevelopment. With neonatal screening, the results of long-term intellectual development have been satisfactory and intelligence should be in the normal range for the majority of children. Treatment is lifelong with oral replacement of thyroxine, titrating the dose to maintain normal growth, TSH and T_4 levels.

> **Summary**
>
> **Congenital hypothyroidism**
> - Is identified on routine neonatal biochemical screening (Guthrie test).
> - Although present antenatally, treatment started soon after birth results in satisfactory intellectual development.

Acquired hypothyroidism

This is usually caused by autoimmune thyroiditis. There is an increased risk in children with Down syndrome or Turner syndrome and of developing other autoimmune disorders, e.g. vitiligo, rheumatoid arthritis, diabetes mellitus. In some families, Addison disease may also occur.

The clinical features are listed in Box 26.7. It is more common in females. There is growth failure accompanied by delayed bone age. Goitre is often present but this may also be physiological in pubertal girls. Treatment is with thyroxine.

Hyperthyroidism

This usually results from autoimmune thyroiditis (Graves disease) secondary to the production of thyroid-stimulating immunoglobulins (TSIs). The clinical features are similar to those in adults, although eye signs are less common (Box 26.8 and Fig. 26.10). It is most often seen in teenage girls. The levels of thyroxine (T_4) and/or tri-iodothyronine (T_3) are elevated and TSH levels are suppressed to very low levels. Antithyroid peroxisomal antibodies may also be present which may eventually result in spontaneous resolution of the thyrotoxicosis but subsequently cause hypothyroidism.

The first-line of treatment is medical, with drugs such as carbimazole or propylthiouracil that interfere with thyroid hormone synthesis. There is a risk of neutropenia from antithyroid medication and all families should be warned to seek urgent help and a blood count if sore throat and high fever occur while

Box 26.8 Clinical features of hyperthyroidism

Systemic
Anxiety, restlessness
Increased appetite
Sweating
Diarrhoea
Weight loss
Rapid growth in height
Advanced bone maturity
Tremor
Tachycardia, wide pulse pressure
Warm, vasodilated peripheries
Goitre (bruit)
Learning difficulties/behaviour problems
Psychosis

Eye signs (uncommon in children)
Exophthalmos
Ophthalmoplegia
Lid retraction
Lid lag

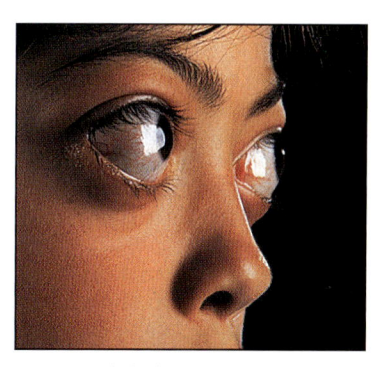

Figure 26.10 Exophthalmos in autoimmune thyroiditis (Graves disease).

on treatment. Initially, β-blockers can be added for symptomatic relief of anxiety, tremor, and tachycardia. Medical treatment is given for about 2 years, which should control the thyrotoxicosis, but the eye signs may not resolve. When medical treatment is stopped, 40% to 75% of patients relapse. A second course of drugs may then be given or an option for permanent remission considered such as radioiodine treatment or surgery in the form of subtotal thyroidectomy. Follow-up is always required as thyroxine replacement is often needed for subsequent hypothyroidism.

Neonatal hyperthyroidism may occur in infants of mothers with thyrotoxicosis from the transplacental transfer of TSIs. Treatment is required as it is potentially fatal, but it resolves with the regression of maternal antibodies.

> **Hyperthyroidism is less common in children than adults and can present with nonspecific symptoms**

Parathyroid disorders

Parathyroid hormone (PTH) promotes bone formation via bone-forming cells (osteoblasts). However, when calcium levels are low, PTH promotes bone resorption via osteoclasts, increases renal uptake of calcium, and activates metabolism of vitamin D to promote gut absorption of calcium. In hypoparathyroidism, which is rare in childhood, in addition to a low serum calcium, there is a raised serum phosphate and a normal alkaline phosphatase. The parathyroid hormone level is very low. Severe hypocalcaemia leads to muscle spasm, fits, stridor, and diarrhoea. Hypocalcaemia may also result in rickets (see Ch. 13). Other causes are rare in childhood.

Hypoparathyroidism in infants is usually due to a congenital deficiency (DiGeorge syndrome), associated with thymic aplasia, defective immunity, cardiac defects, and facial abnormalities. In older children, hypoparathyroidism is usually an autoimmune disorder and can be associated with Addison disease.

In *pseudohypoparathyroidism* there is end-organ resistance to the action of parathyroid hormone caused by a mutation in a signalling molecule. Serum calcium and phosphate levels are abnormal but the parathyroid hormone levels are normal or high. Associated abnormalities are short stature, obesity, subcutaneous nodules, short fourth metacarpals, and learning difficulties. There may be teeth enamel hypoplasia and calcification of the basal ganglia. A related state, in which there are the physical characteristics of pseudohypoparathyroidism but the calcium, phosphate and PTH are all normal, is called *pseudopseudohypoparathyroidism*. There may be a positive family history of both disorders in the same family.

Treatment of acute symptomatic hypocalcaemia is with an intravenous infusion of calcium gluconate. The 10% solution of calcium gluconate must be diluted as extravasation of the infusion will result in severe skin damage. Chronic hypocalcaemia is treated with oral calcium and high doses of vitamin D analogues, adjusting the dose to maintain the plasma calcium concentration just below the normal range. Hypercalcuria should be avoided as it may cause nephrocalcinosis, so urinary calcium excretion should be monitored.

Hyperparathyroidism results in a high calcium level, causing constipation, anorexia, lethargy and behavioural effects, polyuria, and polydipsia. Bony erosions of the phalanges may be seen on a hand radiograph. In neonates and young children, it is associated with some rare genetic abnormalities (e.g. William syndrome), but in later childhood can be secondary to adenomas occurring spontaneously or as part of the multiple endocrine neoplasia syndromes. Severe hypercalcaemia is treated with rehydration, diuretics, and bisphosphonates.

Pituitary disorders

Pituitary disorders (Box 26.9) are uncommon in childhood and can affect hormones in isolation e.g. growth hormone deficiency or a wider pattern of deficiencies across anterior and posterior segments of the pituitary gland. Excess hormone production from an adenoma e.g. prolactinoma or acromegaly is much less common than in adulthood.

Diabetes insipidus secondary to antidiuretic hormone insufficiency presents with polyuria although some children are unable to recognize thirst and will present with hypernatraemia. The syndrome of inappropriate antidiuretic hormone can be provoked by severe illness or neurosurgery and presents with hyponatraemia.

Box 26.9 Causes of pituitary disorders

Congenital	Acquired
Structural e.g. midline defects including septo-optic dysplasia	Brain tumours affecting hypothalamus or pituitary gland e.g. craniopharyngioma
Pituitary hypoplasia or aplasia	Cranial irradiation
	Trauma e.g. affecting pituitary stalk
	Infection e.g. post meningitis
	Infiltration e.g. histiocytosis
	Structural e.g. associated with cerebral malformation, hydrocephalus

Adrenal disorders

Congenital adrenal hyperplasia

Congenital adrenal hyperplasia (CAH) is the most common non-iatrogenic cause of insufficient cortisol and mineralocorticoid secretion. A number of autosomal recessive disorders of adrenal steroid biosynthesis result in congenital adrenal hyperplasia, with an incidence of about 1 in 17 000 births. Over 90% have a deficiency of the enzyme 21-hydroxylase, which is needed for cortisol biosynthesis. About 70% to 80% are also unable to produce aldosterone, leading to salt loss (low sodium and high potassium) (Fig. 26.11). In the fetus, the resulting cortisol deficiency stimulates the pituitary to produce ACTH, which drives overproduction of adrenal androgens.

Presentation is with:

- virilisation of the external genitalia in female infants, with clitoral hypertrophy and variable fusion of the labia (see Case History 26.3)
- in the infant male, the penis may be enlarged and the scrotum pigmented, but these changes are often only noted once the diagnosis has been made

Congenital adrenal hyperplasia

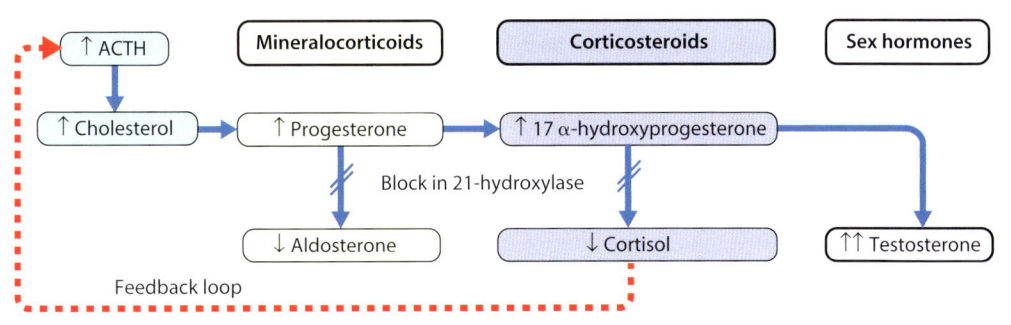

Figure 26.11 Abnormal adrenal steroid biosynthesis from 21-hydroxylase deficiency is the most common form of congenital adrenal hyperplasia. ACTH, adrenocorticotrophic hormone.

Case history 26.3

Abnormal genitalia at birth

The appearance of this newborn infant's genitalia is shown in Fig. 26.12
Investigation revealed:

- a normal female karyotype, 46XX
- the presence of a uterus on ultrasound examination
- a markedly raised plasma 17α-hydroxy-progesterone concentration, confirming congenital adrenal hyperplasia
- a low sodium and a high potassium level
- a low bicarbonate (metabolic acidosis), high urea (dehydration), and low blood glucose (cortisol deficiency).

The low sodium and high potassium indicate that the infant had the salt-losing form of CAH. After detailed explanation with her parents, she was started on oral hydrocortisone and fludrocortisone replacement therapy. Her growth, biochemistry, and bone age were monitored frequently and she attained normal adult height. Psychological counselling and support were offered around puberty and genital surgery was needed before she became sexually active.

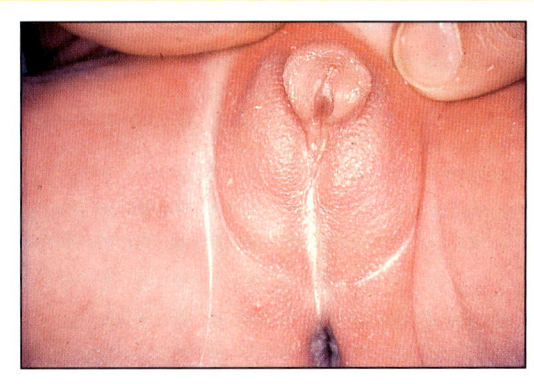

Figure 26.12 Abnormal genitalia at birth. Investigation established that this was a female infant with congenital adrenal hyperplasia causing clitoral hypertrophy with fusion of the labia.

> Severe hypospadias and bilateral undescended testes – a male or virilised female? The karyotype and a pelvic ultrasound are required

- a salt-losing adrenal crisis in the 80% of males who are salt losers; this occurs at 1 week to 3 weeks of age, presenting with vomiting and weight loss, hypotonia and circulatory collapse. A salt-losing crisis is less common in girls as the virilization is noted early and treatment started before salt loss is significant
- tall stature in the 20% of non-salt losers; both male and female non-salt losers also develop a muscular build, adult body odour, pubic hair, and acne from excess androgen production, leading to precocious pubarche.

There may be a family history of neonatal death if a salt-losing crisis had not been recognized and treated.

Diagnosis

This is made by finding markedly raised levels of the metabolic precursor 17α-hydroxy-progesterone in the blood. In salt losers, the biochemical abnormalities are:

- low plasma sodium
- high plasma potassium
- metabolic acidosis
- hypoglycaemia.

Management

Affected females will sometimes require corrective surgery to their external genitalia within the first year but as they have a uterus and ovaries they are reared as girls and are able to have children. Definitive surgical reconstruction is usually delayed until late puberty when females may require surgery to reduce clitoromegaly and a vaginoplasty before sexual intercourse is attempted. Infants with a salt-losing crisis require sodium chloride, glucose, and hydrocortisone intravenously.

The long-term management of both sexes is with:

- lifelong glucocorticoids (e.g. hydrocortisone) to suppress ACTH levels (and hence testosterone) to allow normal growth and maturation
- mineralocorticoids (fludrocortisone) if there is salt loss; before weaning, infants may need added sodium chloride
- monitoring of growth, skeletal maturity, and plasma androgens and 17α-hydroxy-progesterone – insufficient hormone replacement results in increased ACTH secretion and androgen excess, which will cause rapid initial growth and skeletal maturation at the expense of final height; excessive hormonal replacement will result in skeletal delay and slow growth
- additional hormone replacement to cover illness or surgery, as they are unable to mount a cortisol response.

Death can occur from adrenal crisis at the time of illness or injury. Some females experience psychosexual problems, which may relate to the high androgen levels experienced in utero prior to diagnosis.

Prenatal diagnosis is possible when a couple have had a previously affected child.

Primary adrenal insufficiency (Addison disease)

This is rare in childhood and may result from:

- an autoimmune process, sometimes in association with other autoimmune endocrine disorders, e.g. diabetes mellitus, hypothyroidism, hypoparathyroidism
- haemorrhage/infarction – neonatal, meningococcal septicaemia
- X-linked adrenoleucodystrophy, a rare neurodegenerative metabolic disorder
- tuberculosis, now rare.

Adrenal insufficiency may also be secondary to pituitary dysfunction from hypothalamic–pituitary disease or from hypothalamic–pituitary–adrenal suppression following long-term corticosteroid therapy.

Presentation

Infants present acutely (Box 26.10) with a salt-losing crisis, hypotension and/or hypoglycaemia. Dehydration may follow a gastroenteritis-like illness, from which the child recovers until the next episode. In older children, presentation is usually with nonspecific symptoms, such as fatigue, and pigmentation (Fig. 26.13). Postural hypotension can be a clue: check lying and standing blood pressure.

Box 26.10 Features of adrenal insufficiency

Acute	Chronic
Hyponatraemia	Vomiting
Hyperkalaemia	Lethargy
Hypoglycaemia	Brown pigmentation (gums, scars, skin creases)
Dehydration	
Hypotension	
Growth failure	
Circulatory collapse	

Summary

Congenital adrenal hyperplasia

- Autosomal recessive disorder of adrenal steroid biosynthesis.
- Females present with virilisation of the external genitalia.
- Males present with salt loss (80%) or tall stature and precocious puberty (20%).
- Long-term medical management with lifelong glucocorticoids, and mineralocorticoids/sodium chloride if salt loss.
- Additional corticosteroids must be given to cover illness or surgery.
- Salt-losing adrenal crisis needs urgent treatment with hydrocortisone, saline, and glucose given intravenously.
- Monitor growth, skeletal maturity, plasma androgens and 17α-hydroxyprogesterone.
- Surgery for females.

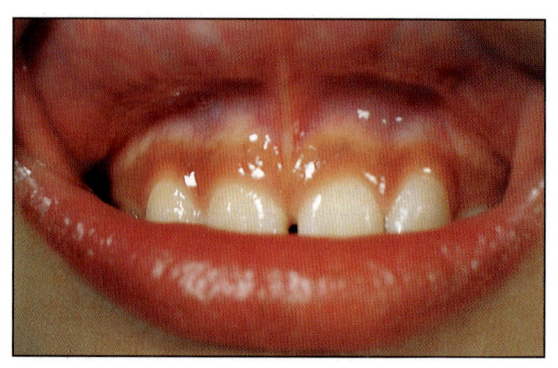

Figure 26.13 Buccal pigmentation in adrenal insufficiency (Addison disease). This 9-year-old boy presented with salt craving and pigmentation. (Courtesy of Steven Robinson.)

Diagnosis

This is made by finding hyponatraemia and hyperkalaemia, often associated with a metabolic acidosis and hypoglycaemia. The plasma cortisol is low and the plasma ACTH concentration high (except in pituitary dysfunction). With an ACTH (Synacthen) test, plasma cortisol concentrations remain low in both primary adrenal dysfunction and in long-standing pituitary/hypothalamic dysfunction. A normal response excludes adrenal insufficiency.

Management

An adrenal crisis requires urgent treatment with intravenous saline, glucose and hydrocortisone. Long-term treatment is with glucocorticoid and mineralocorticoid replacement. The dose of glucocorticoid needs to be increased by three times at times of illness or for an operation. Parents are taught how to inject intramuscular hydrocortisone in an emergency. All children at risk of an adrenal crisis should wear a MedicAlert bracelet or necklace and carry a steroid card.

> **Summary**
>
> **Adrenal insufficiency**
> - Usually due to withdrawal from long-term corticosteroid therapy, congenital adrenal hyperplasia or, rarely, Addison disease.
> - May result in an adrenal crisis requiring urgent treatment.

Cushing syndrome

Glucocorticoid excess in children is usually a side-effect of long-term glucocorticoid treatment (intravenous, oral or, more rarely, inhaled, nasal, or topical) for conditions such as nephrotic syndrome or asthma (Box 26.11 and Fig. 26.14). Corticosteroids are potent growth suppressors and prolonged use in high dosage will lead to reduced adult height and osteopenia. This unwanted side-effect of systemic corticosteroids is reduced by taking corticosteroid medication in the morning on alternate days.

Other causes of glucocorticoid excess are rare. It may be ACTH-driven, from a pituitary adenoma, usually in older children, or from ectopic ACTH-producing tumours, but these almost never occur in children. ACTH-independent disease is usually from corticosteroid therapy, but may be from adrenocortical tumours (benign or malignant), when there may also be virilisation; these usually occur in young children. A diagnosis of Cushing syndrome is often questioned in obese children. Most obese children from dietary excess are tall compared with their midparental height, in contrast to children with Cushing syndrome, who are short and have growth failure.

If Cushing syndrome is a possibility, then the normal diurnal variation of cortisol (high in the morning, low at midnight) may be shown to be lost – in Cushing syndrome the midnight concentration is also high. The 24-hour urine free cortisol is also high. After the administration of dexamethasone at night time, there is failure to suppress the plasma 09.00 hour cortisol levels the following morning. Adrenal tumours are identified on computed tomography or magnetic resonance imaging (MRI) scan of the abdomen and a pituitary adenoma on MRI brain scan. Adrenal tumours are usually unilateral and are treated by adrenalectomy and radiotherapy if indicated. Pituitary adenomas releasing ACTH (Cushing disease) are best treated by transsphenoidal resection, but radiotherapy can be used.

Box 26.11 Clinical features of Cushing syndrome

- Growth failure/short stature
- Face and trunk obesity
- Red cheeks
- Hirsutism
- Striae
- Hypertension
- Bruising
- Carbohydrate intolerance
- Muscle wasting and weakness
- Osteopenia
- Psychological problems.

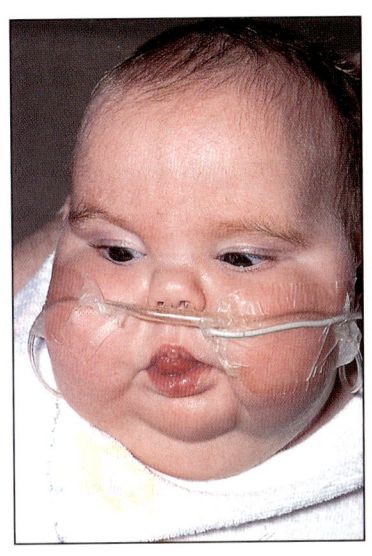

Figure 26.14 Facial obesity following prolonged course of high-dose corticosteroids in a preterm infant. Additional oxygen therapy is being given via nasal cannulae.

Disorders of sex development

The fetal gonad is initially bipotential (Fig. 26.15). In the male, a testis-determining gene on the Y chromosome (*SRY*) is responsible for the differentiation of the gonad into a testis. The production of testosterone and its metabolite, dihydrotestosterone, results in the development of male genitalia. In the absence of *SRY*, the gonads become ovaries and the genitalia female.

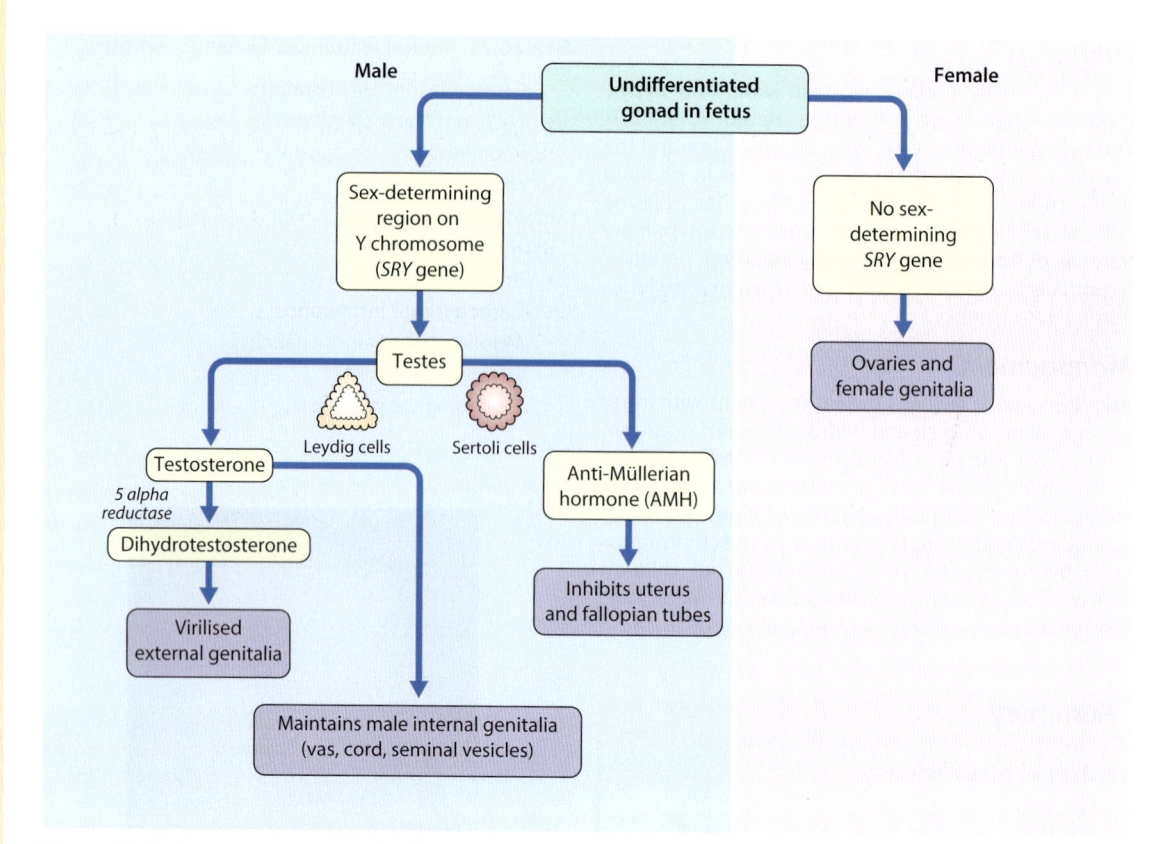

Figure 26.15 Sex development in the fetus.

Rarely, newborn infants may be born with a disorder of sex development (DSD) and there may be uncertainty about the infant's sex. A DSD may be secondary to:

- *excessive androgens producing virilisation in a female* – the most common cause of this is congenital adrenal hyperplasia
- *inadequate androgen action, producing under-virilisation in a male* – this can result from inability to respond to androgens (a receptor problem – androgen insensitivity syndrome, which may be complete or partial) or to convert testosterone to dihydrotestosterone (5α-reductase deficiency) or abnormalities of the synthesis of androgens from cholesterol
- *gonadotrophin insufficiency* – seen in several syndromes such as Prader–Willi syndrome and congenital pituitary dysfunction, which results in a small penis and cryptorchidism
- *ovotesticular DSD* (previously known as true hermaphroditism) – caused by both XX-containing cells and Y-containing cells being present in the fetus leading to both testicular and ovarian tissue being present and a complex external phenotype; this is rare.

All parents and their relatives are keen to know the sex of their newborn baby. However, if the genitalia are abnormal, the infant's sex must not be assigned until detailed assessment by medical, surgical, and psychological specialists has been performed followed by full discussion with the parents. Birth registration must be delayed until this has been completed.

Before the most appropriate sex of rearing is decided upon, the karyotype needs to be determined, adrenal and sex hormone levels measured, and ultrasound of the internal structures and gonads performed. Sometimes laparoscopic imaging and biopsy of internal structures are necessary. In many disorders of sex development, it has been usual to raise the child as a female, as it is easier to fashion female external genitalia, whereas it is not possible surgically to create an adequately functioning penis. However, it may be impossible to predict the sexual identity of the child in eventual adult life and further support or gender reassignment may be required. For this reason, there is a move toward delaying definitive surgery to allow the affected individual to give informed consent to any reconstructive procedures. This is a complex area and is best managed by experienced multidisciplinary teams.

If there is abnormal sexual differentiation at birth:

- do not guess the infant's gender
- the most common cause of a disorder of sexual development is female virilisation from congenital adrenal hyperplasia

Acknowledgements

We would like to acknowledge contributors to this chapter in previous editions, whose work we have drawn on: Tony Hulse (1st Edition), Jerry Wales (2nd, 3rd, 4th Edition), Paul Dimitri (4th Edition).

Further reading

Brook C, Clayton P, Brown R: *Brook's Paediatric Endocrinology*, ed 6, Oxford, 2009, Blackwell.

Sperling MA: *Pediatric Endocrinology*, ed 4, Amsterdam, 2014, Elsevier.

Websites (Accessed November 2016)

International Society for Pediatric and Adolescent Diabetes: Available at: http://www.ispad.org.

European Society for Paediatric Endocrinology: Available at: http://www.eurospe.org.

British Society of Paediatric Endocrinology and Diabetes, BSPED, guidelines: Available at: www.bsped.org.uk

NICE guidance on diagnosis and management of diabetes mellitus: Available at: https://www.nice.org.uk/guidance/NG18

Endotext.com Endocrine Source: Available at: http://www.endotext.org

27

Inborn errors of metabolism

Overview	472	Hypoglycaemia	476
Newborn screening	474	Lysosomal storage disorders	477
Metabolic disease and acid-base disturbance	475	Mitochondrial disease	477
		Lipid storage disorders	477
Hyperammonaemia	476	Disorders of lipid metabolism	479

Features of inborn errors of metabolism are:
- individually rare but collectively numerous
- some are diagnosed on neonatal biochemical screening
- wide range of presentations
- unlikely to be diagnosed unless specific investigations are performed
- genetic diagnosis is essential for confirmation and allow counselling
- with some conditions, delay in diagnosis may result in neurological damage or death.

Overview

Classification

Inborn errors of metabolism (IEM) represent disorders of the enzymatic reactions that degrade, synthesise, or interconvert molecules within cells. There are three broad pathophysiological groups – disorders of intoxication, energy metabolism, and complex organelles (Table 27.1).

Frequency

They are individually rare (Table 27.2), however, collectively they are not uncommon. Even when we exclude familial hypercholesterolaemia, they affect between 1 in 800 and 1 in 2500 children.

Presentation

Can present in a multitude of ways and at any age, although many present in early childhood. They should be considered in all children with:
- an unexpectedly severe presentation of an otherwise common illness
- significant metabolic acidosis
- an unexplained respiratory alkalosis

- hypoglycaemia
- cardiac failure or cardiomyopathy
- hepatomegaly or hepatosplenomegaly or liver dysfunction
- unexpected drowsiness, coma or irritability
- early onset seizures
- dysmorphic features
- developmental regression or loss of skills
- sudden unexplained death.

Table 27.1 Pathophysiological classification

Group	Examples of inborn errors of metabolism
Disorders leading to toxicity due to accumulated metabolite	Aminoacidopathies, e.g. homocystinuria
	Urea cycle disorders, e.g. citrullinaemia
	Organic acidaemias, e.g. isovaleric acidaemia
	Carbohydrate disorders, e.g. galactosaemia
	Neurotransmitter disorders, e.g. pyridoxine-dependent seizures
Disorders of energy metabolism	Mitochondrial diseases, e.g. MELAS, MERRF
	Fatty acid oxidation disorders, e.g. carnitine transporter deficiency
	Glycogen storage disorders, e.g. McArdle disease
Disorders of complex organelles	Lysosomal storage disorders, e.g. mucopolysaccharidoses
	Peroxisomal disorders, e.g. Zellweger syndrome

Table 27.2 Frequency

Disorder	Type of IEM	Incidence (live births)
Galactosaemia	Carbohydrate disorder	1 in 23 000 to 1 in 44 000
Ornithine transcarbamylase deficiency	Urea cycle disorder	1 in 14 000
Methylmalonic acidaemia	Organic acidaemia	1 in 50 000
Glycogen storage disorder type 1	Carbohydrate metabolism	1 in 100 000
Familial hypercholesterolaemia	Lipid disorder	1 in 500

In the history, specific questions are:
- a family history of inborn error of metabolism; draw a family tree
- a family history of sudden unexplained death(s), particularly in childhood, epilepsy, or learning difficulties
- consanguinity detailing if first, second, or third cousins.

On examination, there may not be any specific clinical findings. However, examination including the skin, musculoskeletal, and ophthalmological systems is required.

If an inborn error of metabolism is suspected, contact a specialist metabolic centre for advice

Genetics

Inborn errors of metabolism are inherited disorders and display specific inheritance patterns. Although mitochondrial and de novo occurrence are seen, the most common mode of inheritance is autosomal recessive, where consanguineous parentage increases the risk.

Investigations

If metabolic disease is not considered within the differential diagnosis, it is unlikely to be identified through standard blood, urine, or cerebral spinal fluid investigations. Early discussion with a specialist centre is vital. If a diagnosis is clear, then specific diagnostic investigations can be performed, including genetic testing. Often the diagnosis is uncertain, as many present with chronic, non-specific signs such as developmental delay, faltering growth, dysmorphism or seizures. Even those presenting acutely with metabolic acidosis or hyperammonaemia will need multiple investigations to elucidate the aetiology. Investigations are often staged. First line investigations are shown in Table 27.3. These are often followed by more specialist testing, such as muscle, skin or liver biopsy, genetic analyses, and specific cerebrospinal fluid testing, e.g. for glutamate or glycine. These should be guided by specialist advice.

Table 27.3 Typical first line investigations (guided by clinical picture)

Sample	Test	Indication
Blood	Amino acids and acyl-carnitines	Suspected urea cycle disorders, organic acidaemia or aminoacidopathy – presenting with developmental delay, seizures, faltering growth, dysmorphism
	Ammonia	Suspected urea cycle disorder
	Beutler screening test	Suspected galactosaemia
	Very long chain fatty acids	Suspected peroxisomal disorder
	White cell enzymes	Dysmorphism, organomegaly, learning difficulties, developmental regression
	Lactate	Suspected mitochondrial disease, glycogen storage disorders
Urine	Organic acids	Organic acidaemia, fatty acid oxidation disorders
	Amino acids	Tubulopathy, cystinosis
	Glycoaminoglycans & oligosaccharides	Mucopolysaccharidoses or oligosaccharidoses

Management

The key principles of management are

1. *Medications*
   - symptomatic therapies, e.g. anticonvulsants, analgesia
   - specific therapies, e.g. ammonia scavengers
   - enzyme replacement therapy – for a limited number of storage disorders (bone marrow transplantation is occasionally an option, see mucopolysaccharidoses (MPS) type I below).

2. *Dietary manipulation*
   There are four key strategies:
   - supplying a deficient product, e.g. regular supply of glucose in hepatic glycogen storage disease type I by regular daytime feeds and continuous overnight feed
   - preventing accumulation of a toxic substrate. In many disorders there is protein restriction, e.g. phenylalanine restriction in phenylketonuria to reduce harmful metabolites. To prevent malnutrition, protein substitutes and vitamin and mineral supplementation is required, guided by a specialist dietician
   - prevention of catabolism. Metabolic demands are increased when ill; if not met, catabolism occurs and certain groups are at risk of metabolic decompensation, e.g. hyperammonaemia in urea cycle disorders. To prevent this, patients have an emergency regimen, i.e. they stop normal diet and are provided with glucose to increase insulin secretion and reduce catabolism. Oral glucose in the form of a glucose polymer, e.g. Polycal, is preferred during minor illnesses as it can be given at home. The drinks are continued regularly during the day and overnight. Vomiting or refusal to achieve their emergency regimen or deterioration despite taking it requires hospital admission for intravenous glucose
   - ketogenic diet. Ketones can be used by the brain as an alternative fuel. Patients with GLUT1 (glucose transporter 1) deficiency are unable to transport glucose in to the central nervous system and thus rely on ketones as an alternative energy source for the brain and so require a ketogenic diet.

Newborn screening

Newborn screening aims to detect treatable conditions prior to their clinical presentation and allow early treatment to improve outcome. It was first introduced in the 1960s for the detection of phenylketonuria and has been extended to include other conditions. It is offered to all newborn babies on day 5–7 of life with drops of blood from a heelprick collected onto filter paper. The conditions tested for are cystic fibrosis, congenital hypothyroidism, haemoglobinopathies, and six inborn errors of metabolism (Table 27.4 and Case History 27.1) In some countries a wider range of disorders are tested for, as they can be diagnosed by tandem mass spectroscopy.

Table 27.4 IEM detectable by newborn screening in the UK

IEM	Incidence	Presentation if not detected/treated	Management
Phenylketonuria (PKU)	1 in 10 000 Carrier frequency 1 in 50	Learning difficulties, seizures, microcephaly	Phenylalanine restricted diet
MCAD (Medium chain acyl-CoA dehydrogenase deficiency)	1 in 10 000	Encephalopathy, often rapidly progressive, collapse after prolonged fast resulting in non-ketotic hypoglycemia and death if untreated	Avoidance of fasting and provision with an emergency regimen
Glutaric aciduria type 1 (GA1)	1 in 30 000 – 1 in 40 000	Macrocephaly with encephalopathic crisis aged 6–18 months resulting in dystonic-dyskinetic movement disorder	Specialist diet, avoidance of fasting and daily carnitine
Isovaleric acidaemia	1 in 250 000	Metabolic acidosis ± hyperammonaemia	Low protein diet, carnitine and glycine
Homocystinuria	1 in 200 000 to 1 in 335 000, but more common in those with Irish ancestry at 1 in 65 000	Marfanoid appearance, learning difficulties, lens dislocation, osteoporosis, thromboembolism	Low protein diet, pyridoxine and folic acid
Maple syrup urine disease (MSUD)	1 in 185 000	Progressive encephalopathy in first week of life	Low protein diet

(Incidence data from Genetics Home Reference page (NIH) https://ghr.nlm.nih.gov/, accessed November 2015)

Case history 27.1

Identification of MCAD (medium chain acyl-CoA dehydrogenase) deficiency on newborn screening

Jack was born at term, birthweight 3.2 kg. On day 5 he had the routine heelprick test for newborn screening. On day 7 it showed he had MCAD deficiency. This was phoned through to the newborn screening nurse who visited the family and checked that Jack was well. She provided them with a 'MCAD deficiency is suspected' leaflet. Jack was seen within 24 hours by the specialist metabolic team, where blood for repeat testing and genetic mutations was taken and urine collected for organic acid analysis. The consultant explained about the condition and that Jack must not go for more than 6 hours without a feed. The specialist dietician provided an emergency regimen for use at times of illness. The family was advised that any future children would have a 1 in 4 risk of also having MCAD deficiency.

Regarding MCAD deficiency:

- although screening is performed, it can present in the first few days of life (i.e. before screening) with sudden onset of encephalopathy. A few babies die every year prior to screening
- any older siblings should be offered testing if they were born prior to newborn screening or in a country where screening does not occur
- families require genetic counselling and future pregnancies should be managed prospectively, ensuring at risk babies receive regular feeds and early biochemical testing.

Table 27.5 Acid-base disturbance

Abnormality	Primary disturbance	pH	pCO$_2$	Base excess	Compensatory response
Respiratory acidosis	↑pCO$_2$	↓	↑	Negative	↑ [HCO$_3^-$]
Metabolic acidosis	↓ [HCO$_3^-$]	↓	N or ↓	Negative	↓pCO$_2$
Respiratory alkalosis	↓pCO$_2$	↑	N or ↓	Positive	↓[HCO$_3^-$]
Metabolic alkalosis	↑ [HCO$_3^-$]	↑	N or ↑	Positive	↑pCO$_2$

Metabolic disease and acid-base disturbance

Acid-base balance is essential for correct cellular functioning. Blood gas measurement can help to identify the primary disturbance (Table 27.5). In general:

- metabolic disturbances are compensated acutely by changes in ventilation and chronically by renal responses
- respiratory disturbances are compensated by renal responses.

Metabolic acidosis is common in severely ill children, but may also be the presenting feature of an IEM. A raised respiratory rate reflects the compensatory hyperventilation that occurs to promote removal of carbon dioxide (Kussmaul respiration). An IEM is more likely if:

- the acidosis is out of keeping with the clinical picture
- abnormalities persist despite standard management
- there is a raised anion gap.

The anion gap

The anion gap is the difference that exists between the commonly measured cations (positively charged ions) and anions (negatively charged ions) in the blood. The anion gap is calculated by:

Anion gap = [Na$^+$ + K$^+$] − [Cl$^-$ + HCO$_3^-$]

Using this equation a normal value is 10–16 mmol/L. This represents the 'unmeasured anions' in the blood. An elevated anion gap most commonly occurs when there is a lactic or ketotic acidosis; but it can occur in the presence of any unmeasured anion such as an organic acid, e.g. methylmalonic or propionic acid (Table 27.6 and Case History 27.2).

Management involves treatment of the underlying aetiology and if acidosis is severe, administration of sodium bicarbonate (see Case History 27.2).

Infection is a common trigger for the presentation of an IEM. Both may require concurrent investigation and treatment

Table 27.6 Metabolic acidosis and the anion gap

With normal anion gap	With raised anion gap
Intestinal loss of base e.g. diarrhoea	Diabetic ketoacidosis
	Renal failure
Renal loss of base e.g. renal tubular acidosis type 1 & type 2	Poisoning with: salicylate, ethanol, methanol, or paraldehyde
	Inborn errors of metabolism

Case history 27.2

An organic acidaemia

Aysha, a 6-day-old girl born at term with a birthweight of 3 kg following an uneventful pregnancy and delivery, presents with reduced feeding and rapid breathing. On examination her respiratory rate is 90 breaths/min and she is unresponsive to stimulation. Blood gas: pH 7.29, pCO_2 2.0 kPa, base excess − 18 mmol/L, HCO_3^- 10 mmol/L, Na^+ 140 mmol/L, K^+ 3.6 mmol/L, Cl^- 110 mmol/L, lactate 8 mmol/L. The anion gap = (140 + 3.6) − (110 + 10) = 23.6 mmol/L. Such a large anion gap would not be generated by this level of lactate. The gas normalises with intravenous 10% dextrose and two half corrections of sodium bicarbonate and she becomes alert and has a normal respiratory rate. In view of the encephalopathy and raised anion gap a urine organic acid analysis is performed and shows increased methylmalonic acid. The diagnosis is later genetically confirmed as methylmalonic acidaemia.

> Always consider an inborn error of metabolism if:
> - unexplained encephalopathy and/or markedly raised anion gap
> - sudden unexplained death of infancy

Hyperammonaemia

Ammonia is a highly toxic chemical derived from bodily nitrogen. It is detoxified to urea by the urea cycle, which principally occurs in the liver. It should be measured when there is:

- unexplained encephalopathy
- respiratory alkalosis as it is a respiratory stimulant
- recurrent vomiting
- unexplained severe illness in a baby or child
- unexplained seizures as it causes cerebral oedema.

Ammonia can also be transiently elevated in severe illness, liver disease, by certain medications and

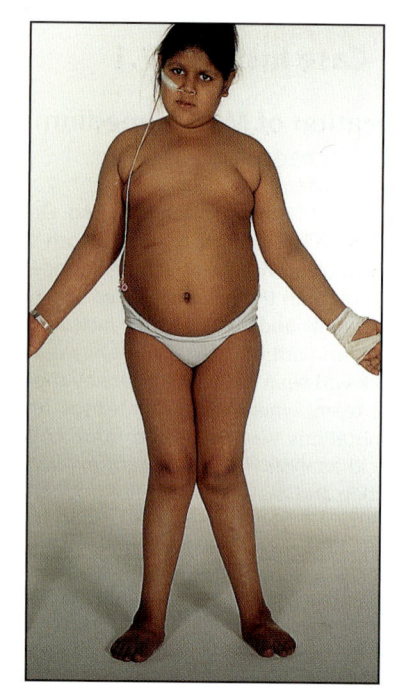

Figure 27.1 Type I glycogen storage disease in a 12-year-old girl. There is truncal obesity with a distended abdomen from an enlarged liver; short stature and hypotrophic muscles; 'doll' faces; nasogastric feeding to maintain blood glucose levels overnight.

transiently in the newborn. Principles of management are to stop feeds, start 10% dextrose, give intravenous ammonia scavenging medications and arginine to support the urea cycle, and arrange urgent transfer to paediatric intensive care for haemofiltration.

Hypoglycaemia

Hypoglycaemia is common in the first day of life in infants who are preterm, growth restricted or ill, and blood glucose measurements are checked routinely in these circumstances. Thereafter, blood glucose should be checked in any child who appears seriously ill, has a prolonged seizure or develops an altered state of consciousness. It is defined as a blood glucose of less than 2.6 mmol/L. Investigation with a hypoglycaemia screen at the time of hypoglycaemia is required to identify an IEM or endocrine cause (Box 26.5, Ch. 26 Diabetes and Endocrinology). The presence or absence of ketones should be specifically sought as their absence is an abnormal response. On physical examination, the presence of hepatomegaly should be sought to identify glycogen storage disorders.

Glycogen storage disorders

The glycogen storage disorders (GSD) are a diverse group and can be divided into hepatic, muscular and cardiac subgroups. The hepatic forms are associated with hypoglycaemia. GSD type 1a exemplifies the hepatic form (Fig. 27.1 and Case History 27.3). It is due to deficiency of glucose-6-phosphatase and leads

Case history 27.3

A glycogen storage disorder

A 4 month old boy with a normal neonatal and past medical history presents with a 1-day history of cough and fever. He has not fed for 12 hours and has reduced wet nappies. On examination he has a cherubic face, the clinical features of moderately severe bronchiolitis and has a 10-cm soft, enlarged liver. His blood glucose is 1.8 mmol/L. On investigation of his hypoglycaemia, he is found to have a lactic acidosis, his serum is milky and triglycerides are raised, The nurses note he becomes sweaty and irritable prior to feeds. Glucose monitoring demonstrates prefeed hypoglycaemia if feeds are more than 2.5 hours apart. GSD type 1a is diagnosed and confirmed on mutation analysis. He is commenced on 2-hourly daytime feeds and a continuous overnight nasogastric feed.

Features of glycogen storage disorders are:

- GSD type 1 often presents when illness prevents feeding or when an infant's feed frequency is reduced
- the hepatomegaly can be easily missed as it has a soft consistency
- lactate is raised because it acts as an alternative fuel
- type 1b is differentiated from type a by the presence of neutropenia.

---

to severe hypoglycaemia because of the inability to mobilise glucose from glycogen or utilise glucose from gluconeogenesis. The most common muscle glycogenosis is GSD V, also called McArdle disease. It is due to deficiency of **myophosphorylase**. Patients characteristically have exercise intolerance relieved by rest, the 'second wind' phenomena. This reflects the ability to utilise free glucose mobilised in the blood stream. They are at risk of the breakdown of muscle tissue (rhabdomyolysis) and its complications, particularly acute kidney injury.

Lysosomal storage disorders

The lysosome is the recycling centre of the cell and contains a number of enzymes. Deficiency of one of these enzymes results in the inability to breakdown a specific chemical leading to its accumulation within the cell. This accumulation typically leads to signs of visceral storage (hepatosplenomegaly) and/or central nervous system involvement with developmental regression or seizures or both. There are a number of groups of lysosomal storage disorders, e.g. mucopolysaccharidoses, oligosaccharidoses (mannasidosis), mucolipidoses (I-cell disease), sphingolipidoses (Fabry disease). Diagnosis is initially based on urinary glycosaminoglycan and oligosaccharide screen and blood testing of the white cell enzymes. These results can then lead to specific enzymology testing.

Mucopolysaccharidoses (MPS)

The mucopolysaccharidoses are the more commonly seen lysosomal disorders. There is defective breakdown of glycosaminoglycans (GAGs). They are progressive multisystem disorders which may affect the neurological, ocular, cardiac, and skeletal systems (Table 27.7). Hepatosplenomegaly is usually present. Most children present with developmental delay following a period of essentially normal growth and development up to 6–12-months of age. Developmental attainment then slows and children may show some loss of skills. It is only in the second 6 months of life that the characteristic facies begin to emerge, with coarsening of the facial features and prominent forehead due to frontal bossing (Fig. 27.2).

The different forms of MPS have highly variable clinical features. The characteristics of five of the varieties are shown in Table 27.8. The diagnosis is made by identifying the enzyme defect and the excretion in the urine of the major storage substances, the glycosaminoglycans (GAGs). Treatment is supportive according to the child's needs and a number of the conditions have enzyme replacement therapies available. Successful enzyme replacement by bone marrow transplantation has been performed for MPS type I but it cannot reverse any established neurological abnormality and has a minimal effect on the skeletal component.

Mitochondrial disease

The Krebs cycle, (also known as the tricarboxylic acid cycle), is found in all cells except red blood cells, which lack mitochondria. It links the pathways of intermediary metabolism with the mitochondrial respiratory chain and is regulated by the pyruvate dehydrogenase (PDH) complex. The primary function of this system is the production of ATP (adenosine triphosphate) from the process of oxidative phosphorylation. Strictly speaking, mitochondrial disorders are those directly resulting from deficits in energy production by oxidative phosphorylation. Mitochondrial disease thus affects those organs with the greatest energy demands, i.e. brain, heart, kidney, retina, skeletal muscle, and clinical presentation is very varied (Case History 27.4). Some clinical syndromes are recognised (Table 27.9). Investigation is difficult and often only symptomatic treatment is possible. Mitochondrial disease should be considered when there is:

- multisystem disease
- elevated lactate; though differential diagnosis is wide, and it is not always present
- MRI brain scans showing characteristic features e.g. in Leigh syndrome.

Lipid storage disorders

Lipid storage diseases are a group of IEM in which enzyme deficiency causes lipid accumulation in cells and tissues (see Table 27.10). This excessive storage of fats can causes permanent cellular and tissue damage,

Mucopolysacharidoses

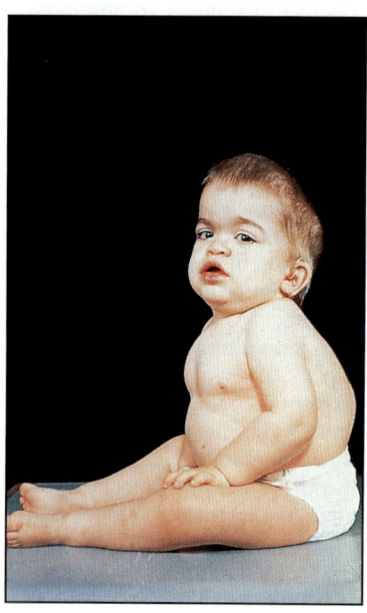

Figure 27.2 Untreated Hurler syndrome showing the characteristic facies and skeletal dysplasia. The prominence of the lower spine is called a 'gibbus'.

Table 27.7 Clinical features of mucopolysaccharidoses

Eyes	Corneal clouding
Skin	Thickened skin
	Coarse facies
Heart	Valvular lesions
	Cardiomyopathy
Neurology	Developmental regression
Skeletal	Thickened skull
	Broad ribs
	Claw hand
	Thoracic kyphosis
	Lumbar lordosis
Other	Hepatosplenomegaly
	Carpal tunnel syndrome
	Conductive deafness
	Umbilical and inguinal hernias

Table 27.8 Types of mucopolysaccharidoses

Type	Inheritance	Cornea	Heart	Brain	Skeletal
MPS I (Hurler)	AR	+++	++	+++	++
MPS II (Hunter)	X-linked	–	+	++	+
MPS III (Sanfilippo)	AR	±	–	+	+
MPS IV (Morquio)	AR	+	+	–	+++
MPS VI (Maroteaux–Lamy)	AR	+++	++	–	++

AR, autosomal recessive.

Table 27.9 Some mitochondrial disorders

Syndrome	Clinical features	Onset (age years)	Common mutations
MERRF	Myoclonic epilepsy with ragged red fibres.	5–15	m.8344G>A
MELAS	Mitochondrial encephalopathy, lactic acidosis, stroke-like episodes. Myopathy, migraine, vomiting, seizures, visual and hearing disturbance.	5–15	80% m.3243A>G
Alpers	Intractable seizures and liver involvement.	Early childhood	POLG

Case history 27.4

Mitochondrial disease

Amy is 8-years-old and presents with a 3-day history of an upper respiratory tract infection and the sudden onset of seizures and encephalopathy. She was admitted to a paediatric intensive care unit and investigations demonstrated rhinovirus in a nasal pharyngeal aspirate and a raised lactate of 9 mmol/L which failed to normalize once seizure control was obtained. An MRI head scan showed basal ganglia calcification and areas of infarction not confined to vascular territories. On history taking there was a significant family history (Fig. 27.3). Amy's presentation and family history suggested a mitochondrial disease, specifically MELAS. Genetic mutation analysis confirmed MELAS. Amy recovered from this episode but died 2 years later from recurrent stroke-like episodes and lactic acidosis.

Features of mitochondrial disease are:
- there may be marked intra-familial variation
- the family history and drawing a family tree are helpful
- infection is often a trigger for acute decompensation.

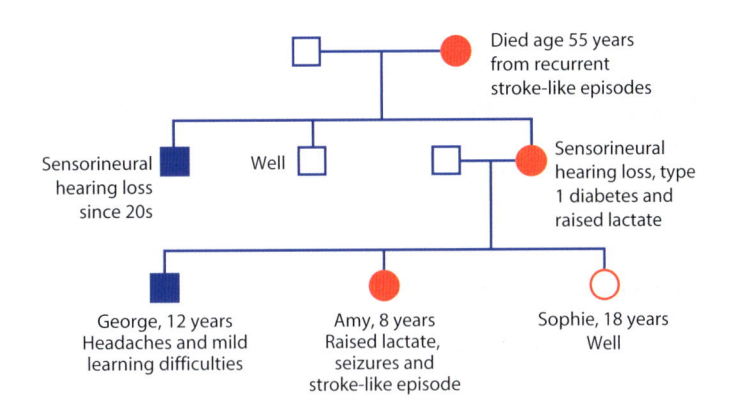

Figure 27.3 Family tree consistent with mitochondrial disease (see Ch. 9. Genetics). Mitochondria are the product of a nuclear and a mitochondrial genome (mtDNA). The mtDNA is inherited exclusively from the mother because after fertilisation of the ova, the sperm derived mitochondria disappear in early embryogenesis. In any one cell there are hundreds of copies of mtDNA. The proportion of copies affected by the mtDNA mutation and the severity of the mutation and the tissue response determine the severity of the clinical phenotype. Here, Amy has MELAS as she has a high proportion of mtDNA, whereas others in the family with lower levels only suffer from type 1 diabetes mellitus and sensorineural hearing loss.

---

affecting the brain, nervous system, liver, spleen and bone marrow. The most common lipid storage disorder is Gaucher disease.

Disorders of lipid metabolism

The most common reason for raised cholesterol in childhood is obesity. However, familial hypercholesterolaemia is the most common inherited disorder of lipid metabolism. The majority of children with the familial disease form are detected on cascade screening because a parent has presented with an acute myocardial infarction. A few children with homozygous familial hypercholesterolaemia may be the index case. They typically present before 5 years of age to dermatologists with lipid deposits (Fig. 27.4). These deposits classically occur in the natal cleft and the extensor surfaces of the elbows.

Treatment of heterozygotes is with the use of a low fat diet and from the age of 8-years, a statin. In homozygous patients the risk of myocardial infarction and stroke in the early teenage years is extremely high. Treatment is started with a low fat diet, a statin and ezetimibe, which lowers cholesterol. If there is a poor response to treatment in homozygous patients, other treatment options include lipid apheresis or liver transplantation.

Abnormally low lipid levels can also be an indicator of metabolic disease, e.g. abetalipoproteinaemia.

Inborn errors of metabolism

Table 27.10 Summary of the features of lipid storage disorders

Disorder	Enzyme defect	Clinical features
Fabry disease	Alpha-galactosidase A	Only X-linked lipid storage disorder
		Males: present in childhood with recurrent acute pain/paraesthesiae in limbs, diminished sweating, angiokeratomas, normal intelligence
		Females: 70% asymptomatic. Presentation tends to be from age 15 years onwards
		Enzyme replacement therapy
Gaucher disease	Beta-glucosidase	Occurs in 1 in 500 Ashkenazi Jews
		Chronic childhood form – splenomegaly, bone marrow suppression, bone involvement, normal IQ
		Splenectomy may alleviate hypersplenism
		Enzyme replacement therapy
		Acute infantile form – splenomegaly, neurological degeneration with seizures
		Carrier detection and prenatal diagnosis are possible
Niemann–Pick disease type C	Cholesterol trafficking disorder	Infantile: neonatal liver disease with hepatosplenomegaly. Usually improves but may be fatal
		Juvenile: age 3–15-years with progressive ataxia, language delay, hepatosplenomegaly, vertical supranuclear gaze palsy, cherry red spot (50%). Death 7 years to adulthood
		Adult: ataxia, dementia, psychiatric illness
		Treatment with substrate reduction therapy
Wolman disease	Lysosomal acid lipase	Neonatal presentation with severe growth faltering, steatorrhoea, massive hepatosplenomegaly and X-ray shows adrenal calcification
		Fatal within first year
		Newly developed enzyme replacement therapy

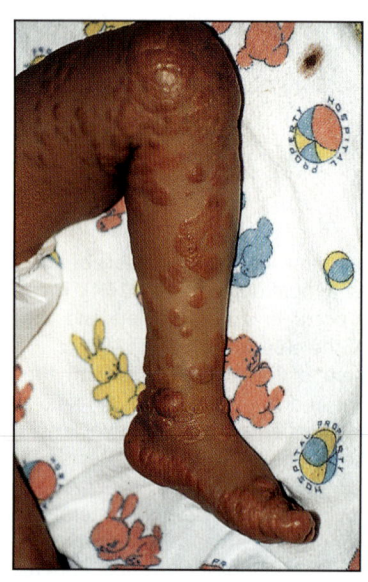

Figure 27.4 Severe skin xanthomata. In this child, it was secondary to liver failure and resolved within weeks of liver transplantation.

> **Summary**
>
> **Inborn errors of metabolism**
> - Are individually rare but collectively not uncommon.
> - Neonatal biochemical screening allows the diagnoses of six inborn errors of metabolism.
> - Present at any age with serious unexplained illness, hepatomegaly/splenomegaly, cardiac failure, drowsiness, seizures, dysmorphic features, developmental regression or sudden unexpected death of infancy.
> - Should also be considered if there is hypoglycaemia, marked metabolic acidosis and anion gap, or respiratory alkalosis of unknown cause.
> - Hyperammonaemia is a time critical medical emergency: rapid diagnosis is essential to allow early treatment to reduce morbidity and mortality.
> - Investigations and management are complex and specialized – consult the specialist metabolic centre.

Acknowledgements

We would like to acknowledge contributors to the section on Inborn Errors of Metabolism in the chapter on Endocrine and Metabolic disorders in previous editions, whose work we have drawn on: Tony Hulse (1st Edition), Jerry Wales (2nd Edition), Ed Wraith (3rd Edition).

Further reading

Clarke JTR: *A Clinical Guide to Inherited Metabolic Disease*, ed 3, 2010, Cambridge University Press.

Websites (Accessed December 2016)

British Inherited Metabolic Disease Group (BIMDG): Available at: www.bimdg.org.uk

NHS newborn blood spot screening programme: Available at: https://www.gov.uk/topic/population-screening-programmes/newborn-blood-spot

Orphanet: Available at: www.orphanet.net
A portal for rare diseases and orphan drugs.

Online Mendelian Inheritance in Man (OMIM): Available at: http://www.ncbi.nlm.nih.gov/omim.
A compendium of human genes and genetic phenotypes.

28

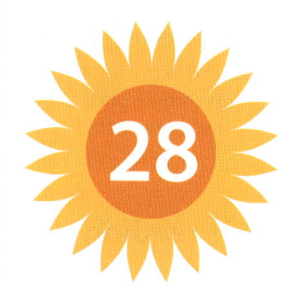

Musculoskeletal disorders

Assessment of the musculoskeletal system	482	The painful limb, knee, and back	486
Variations of normal posture	482	Limp	489
Abnormal posture	484	Arthritis	491
		Genetic skeletal conditions	497

Key features of musculoskeletal disorders in children are:

- physical assessment is with pGALS (Paediatric Gait, Arms. Legs and Spine) and pREMS (paediatric Regional Examination of the Musculoskeletal System)
- many, but not all, concerns of parents about their children's posture are variations of normal alignment in the growing skeleton
- early treatment of talipes equinovarus usually avoids the need for surgery
- limp has a wide differential diagnosis
- juvenile idiopathic arthritis (JIA) is the most common cause of chronic arthritis in children.

Assessment of the musculoskeletal system

This should, as a minimum, include the pGALS assessment (see Chater 2. History and Examination) to identify and localize musculoskeletal problems; any suggestion of a musculoskeletal problem should be followed by more detailed regional musculoskeletal examination (pREMS, see Chapter 2).

Variations of normal posture

Variations are common and may be noticed by parents or on routine developmental surveillance. Most resolve without any treatment but if severe, progressive, painful, functionally limiting or asymmetrical, they should be referred for a specialist opinion.

Bow legs (genu varum)

The normal toddler has a broad base gait. Many children evolve leg alignment with initially a degree of bowing of the tibiae, causing the knees to be wide apart – best observed while the child is standing with the feet together (Fig. 28.1). A pathological cause of bow legs is rickets; check for the presence of other clinical features (see Ch. 13). Severe progressive and often unilateral bow legs is a feature of Blount disease (infantile tibia vara), an uncommon condition predominantly seen in Black children; radiographs are characteristic with beaking of the proximal medial tibial epiphysis.

Knock-knees (genu valgum)

The feet are wide apart when standing with the knees held together (Fig. 28.2). The intermalleolar distance should be less than 8 cm. It is seen in many young children and usually resolves spontaneously.

Flat feet (pes planus)

Toddlers learning to walk usually have flat feet due to flatness of the medial longitudinal arch and the presence of a fat pad which disappears as the child gets older (Fig. 28.3). An arch can usually be demonstrated on standing on tiptoe or by passively extending the big toe. Marked flat feet are common in hypermobility. A fixed flat foot, often painful, presenting in older children with absence of an arch on tip-toeing, may indicate an associated tendo-Achilles contracture (ankle), or tarsal coalition or inflammatory arthropathy (JIA) and referral to paediatric rheumatology or a paediatric orthopaedic surgeon is indicated. Symptomatic flat feet are often helped by footwear advice and, occasionally, an arch support may be required.

In-toeing

There are three main causes of in-toeing

- *Metatarsus varus* (Fig. 28.4a) – an adduction deformity of a highly mobile forefoot.

Variants of normal

Figure 28.1 Bow legs.

Figure 28.2 Knock-knees.

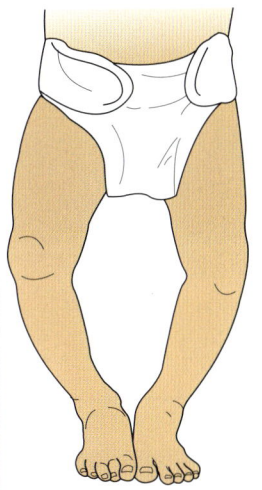

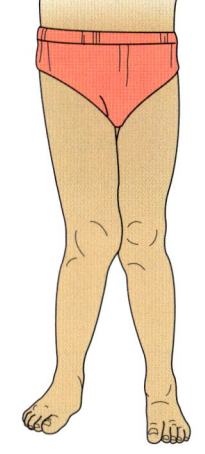

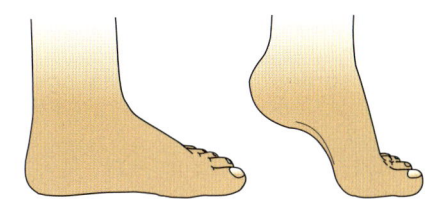

Figure 28.3 Pes planus showing the flat feet of toddlers. The medial longitudinal arch appears on standing on tiptoe.

In-toeing

(a) Metatarsus adductus
(b) Medial tibial torsion
(c) Femoral anteversion

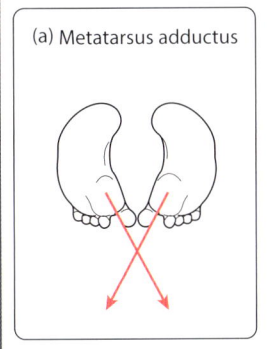

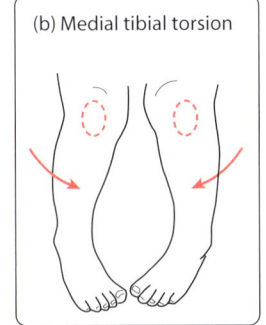

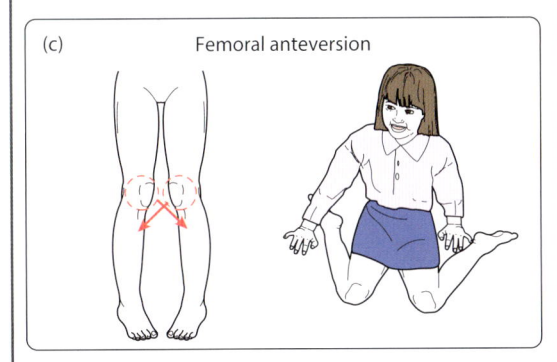

Figure 28.4 In-toeing (a) at the feet; (b) lower leg; and (c) hip, with 'W' sitting.

Box 28.1 Clinical features of in-toeing in children

Metatarsus varus
- Occurs in infants
- Passively correctable
- Heel is held in the normal position
- No treatment required unless it persists beyond 5 years of age and is symptomatic

Medial tibial torsion
- Occurs in toddlers
- May be associated with bowing of the tibiae
- Self-corrects within about 5 years

Persistent anteversion of the femoral neck
- Presents in childhood
- Usually self-corrects by 8 years of age
- May be associated with hypermobility of the joints
- Children sit between their feet with the hips fully internally rotated ('W' sitting)
- Most do not require treatment but femoral osteotomy may be required for persistent anteversion

- *Medial tibial torsion* (Fig. 28.4b) – at the lower leg, when the tibia is laterally rotated less than normal in relation to the femur.
- *Persistent anteversion of the femoral neck* (Fig. 28.4c) – at the hip, when the femoral neck is twisted forward more than normal.

The clinical features are described in Box 28.1.

Toe walking

Common in young children and may become persistent, usually from habit. The child can walk normally on request. Habitual toe walking needs to be distinguished from mild cerebral palsy or tightness of the Achilles tendons or inflammatory arthritis in the foot or ankle. In older boys, Duchenne muscular dystrophy should be excluded.

Summary

Variations of musculoskeletal normality and differential diagnosis

Perceived disorder	Normal age range	Differential diagnoses to consider
Bow legs	1–3 years	Rickets, osteogenesis imperfecta, Blount disease
Knock-knees	2–7 years	Juvenile idiopathic arthritis (JIA)
Flat feet	1–2 years	Hypermobility, congenital tarsal fusion
In-toeing	1–2 years	Tibial torsion, femoral anteversion
Toe walking	1–3 years	Spastic diplegia, muscular dystrophy, JIA, mucopolysaccaridosis

Abnormal posture

Talipes equinovarus (clubfoot)

Positional talipes from intrauterine compression is common. The foot is of normal size, the deformity is mild and can be corrected to the neutral position with passive manipulation (Fig. 10.14). Often the baby's intrauterine posture can be recreated. If the positional deformity is marked, parents can be shown passive exercises by the physiotherapist.

Talipes equinovarus is a complex abnormality (Figs 28.5, 28.6). The entire foot is inverted and supinated, the forefoot adducted and the heel is rotated inwards and in plantar flexion. The affected foot is shorter and the calf muscles thinner than normal. The position of the foot is fixed, cannot be corrected completely and is often bilateral. The birth prevalence is 1 per 1000 live births, affects predominantly males (2:1), can be familial but is usually idiopathic. However, it may also be secondary to oligohydramnios during pregnancy, a feature of a malformation syndrome or of a neuromuscular disorder such as spina bifida. There is an association with developmental dysplasia of the hip (DDH).

Treatment is started promptly with plaster casting and bracing ('Ponsetti method'), which may be required for many months. It is usually successful unless the condition is very severe, when corrective surgery is required.

Summary

Regarding talipes equinovarus:
- Needs to be differentiated from positional talipes.
- Check for neuromuscular disorder or spinal lesion and for developmental dysplasia of the hip (DDH).
- Early plaster casting and bracing usually avoids the need for surgery, and is being adopted world-wide.

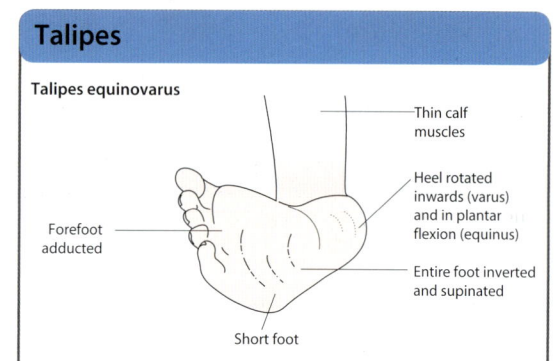

Talipes

Figure 28.5 Abnormalities in talipes equinovarus.

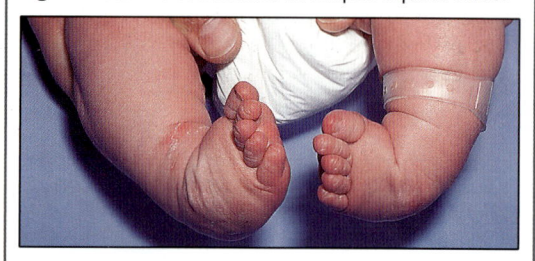

Figure 28.6 Talipes equinovarus.

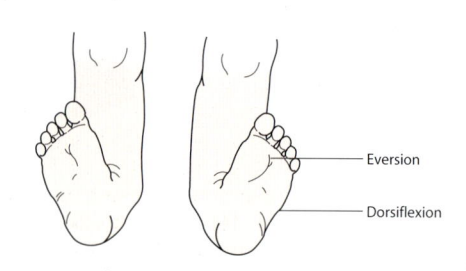

Figure 28.7 Talipes calcaneovalgus.

Vertical talus

Talipes equinovarus needs to be differentiated from the rare congenital vertical talus, where the foot is stiff and rocker-bottom in shape. Many of these infants have other malformations. The diagnosis can be confirmed on X-ray. Surgery is usually required.

Talipes calcaneovalgus

The foot is dorsiflexed and everted (Fig. 28.7). It usually results from intrauterine moulding and self-corrects. Passive foot exercises are sometimes advised. There is an association with DDH (developmental dysplasia of the hip).

Tarsal coalition

This results from lack of segmentation between one or more bones of the foot and coalitions (fibrous or cartilaginous abnormal connections) become symptomatic as they begin to ossify. The foot becomes progressively more rigid with limited foot motion. The feet often become more symptomatic during the preadolescent years. Radiographs may be normal if the coalitions have not yet ossified. Corrective surgery may be required.

Pes cavus

In pes cavus, there is a high arched foot. When it presents in older children, it is often associated with neuromuscular disorders, e.g. Friedreich ataxia and type I hereditary motor sensory neuropathy (peroneal muscular atrophy). Treatment is required if the foot becomes stiff or painful.

Developmental dysplasia of the hip (DDH)

This is a spectrum of disorders ranging from dysplasia to subluxation through to frank dislocation of the hip. Early detection is important as it usually responds to conservative treatment; late diagnosis is usually associated with hip dysplasia, which requires complex treatment often including surgery. Neonatal screening is performed as part of the routine examination of the newborn (see Fig. 10.18), checking if the hip can be dislocated posteriorly out of the acetabulum (Barlow manoeuvre) or can be relocated back into the acetabulum on abduction (Ortolani manoeuvre). These tests are repeated at routine surveillance at 8 weeks of age. Thereafter, presentation of the condition is usually with a limp or abnormal gait. It may be identified from asymmetry of skinfolds around the hip, limited abduction of the hip or shortening of the affected leg.

On neonatal screening, an abnormality of the hip is detected in about 6–10 per 1000 live births. Most will resolve spontaneously. The true birth prevalence of DDH is about 1.3 per 1000 live births. Clinical neonatal screening misses some cases. This may be because of inexperience of the examiner, but in some it is not possible to clinically detect dislocation at this stage, e.g. where there is only a mildly shallow acetabulum. To overcome these problems, some centres perform ultrasound screening on all newborn infants. It is highly specific in detecting DDH but is expensive and has a high rate of false positives, and is not recommended in the UK. It is performed in some centres if infants are at increased risk (family history, breech presentation).

If developmental dysplasia of the hip is suspected, a specialist orthopaedic opinion should be obtained. An ultrasound examination following an abnormal clinical examination allows detailed assessment of the hip, quantifying the degree of dysplasia and whether there is subluxation or dislocation. If indicated, the infant may be placed in a splint or harness to keep the hip flexed and abducted for several months. Progress is monitored by repeat ultrasound or X-ray. The splinting must be done expertly as necrosis of the femoral head is a potential complication. In most instances, a satisfactory response is obtained. Surgery is required if conservative measures fail.

Scoliosis

Scoliosis is a lateral curvature in the frontal plane of the spine.

In structural scoliosis, there is rotation of the vertebral bodies which causes a prominence in the back from rib asymmetry. In most cases, the changes are mild, pain-free and primarily a cosmetic problem; however, in severe cases, the spinal curvature can lead to cardiorespiratory failure from distortion of the chest.

Causes of scoliosis are:

- Idiopathic: the most common, either early onset (<5 years old) or, most often, late onset, mainly girls 10–14-years of age during their pubertal growth spurt.
- Congenital: from a congenital structural defect of the spine, e.g. hemivertebra, spina bifida, syndromes, e.g. Vertebral, Anorectal, Cardiac, Tracheo-oEsophageal, Renal and Limb anomalies (VACTERL) association.
- Secondary: related to other disorders such as neuromuscular imbalance (e.g. cerebral palsy, muscular dystrophy); disorders of bone such as neurofibromatosis or of connective tissues such as Marfan syndrome, or leg length discrepancy, e.g. due to arthritis of one knee in juvenile idiopathic arthritis. Examination should start with inspection of the child's back while standing up straight. In mild scoliosis, there may be irregular skin creases and difference in shoulder height. The scoliosis can be identified on examining the child's back when bent forward (Fig. 28.8). If the scoliosis disappears on forward bending, it is postural although leg lengths should be checked.

Mild scoliosis will resolve spontaneously, or progresses minimally. If more severe, the severity and progression of the curvature of the spine is determined by X-ray. Severe cases are managed in specialist spinal centres where the place of non-medical treatment such as bracing will be considered, with surgery indicated only if severe or there is coexisting pathology such as neuromuscular or respiratory disease.

Torticollis

The most common cause of torticollis (wry neck) in infants is a sternomastoid tumour (congenital muscular torticollis). They occur in the first few weeks of life and present with a mobile, non-tender nodule, which can be felt within the body of the sternocleidomastoid muscle. There may be restriction of head turning and

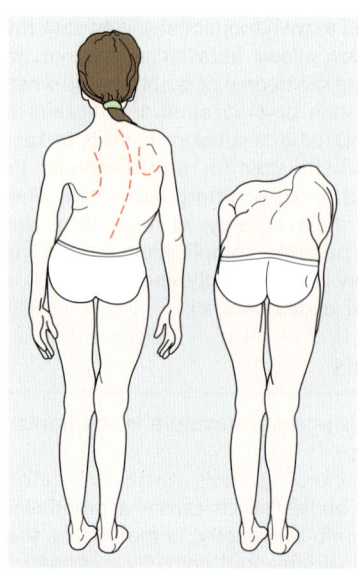

Figure 28.8 Structural scoliosis with vertebral rotation shown by rib rotation on bending forward.

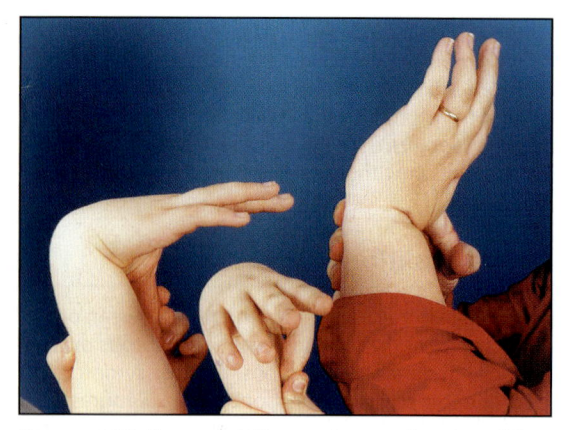

Figure 28.9 Hypermobility syndrome, showing ability of a mother and two of her children to hyperextend the thumb onto the forearm.

tilting of the head. The condition usually resolves in 2–6 months. Passive stretching is advised, but its efficacy is unproven.

Torticollis presenting later in childhood may be due to muscular spasm or secondary to ear, nose or throat infection, spinal tumour (such as osteoid osteoma), cervical spine arthritis or malformation or posterior fossa tumour.

The painful limb, knee, and back

Growing pains

Episodes of generalized pain in the lower limbs, referred to as 'growing pains' or nocturnal idiopathic pain, are common in preschool and school-aged children. The pain often wakes the child from sleep and settles with massage or comforting. The condition is poorly understood. Features to be fulfilled for this diagnosis are often referred to as the 'Rules of Growing Pains', which are:

- age range 3–12 years
- pains symmetrical in lower limbs and not limited to joints
- pains *never* present at the start of the day after waking
- physical activities not limited; no limp
- physical examination normal (including pGALS), with the exception of joint hypermobility in some, and otherwise well.

If the presentation 'does not fit the rules', further assessment is necessary.

Hypermobility

Older children or adolescents with hypermobility may complain of musculoskeletal pain mainly confined to the lower limbs, often worse after exercise. Joint swelling is usually absent or is transient. Hypermobility may be generalized or limited to peripheral joints (such as hands and feet). There is symmetrical hyperextension of the thumbs and fingers that can be hyperextended onto the forearms (Fig. 28.9), elbows and knees can be hyperextended beyond 10°, and palms can be placed flat on the floor with knees straight. Lower limb findings associated with hypermobility are hyperextensibility of the knee joint and flat feet with normal arches on tiptoe, which are over-pronated secondary to ankle hypermobility.

While mild degrees of hypermobility are a normal finding in younger female children, and many children with hypermobility are asymptomatic and find being very flexible an advantage in dancing and gymnastics, some experience recurrent mechanical joint and muscle pain, which is often activity related. These children require specialist assessment and may benefit from advice about footwear, exercises and occasionally orthotics. Hypermobility is also a feature of some chromosomal syndromes, e.g. Down syndrome, and some inherited collagen disorders (e.g. Marfan and Ehlers–Danlos syndrome).

Complex regional pain syndromes

The most dramatic musculoskeletal pain is that encountered in complex regional pain syndromes (CRPS), formerly known as idiopathic pain syndromes, which may be localized or generalized. They usually present in adolescent females.

Localized forms often present with foot and ankle involvement (typically unilateral); the pain can be extreme and incapacitating, often triggered by minor trauma or without a clear precipitant. Presentation to the clinic may be in a wheelchair. In addition to severe pain, there may be hyperaesthesia (increased sensitivity to stimuli), allodynia (pain from a stimulus that does not normally produce pain), and the affected part (often a foot or hand) may be cool to touch, be swollen and mottled, held in flexion with minimal if any active movement, and bizarre posturing is not uncommon. Typically, with distraction, the normal range of passive movements is possible.

Diffuse forms are characterized by severe widespread pain with disturbed sleep patterns, feeling exhausted during the day, with extreme tenderness over soft tissues. The characteristic tender points that are found in adults with fibromyalgia may be absent or fewer in number in children.

The child or adolescent with complex regional pain is otherwise well and physical examination is otherwise normal.

Organic pathology needs to be excluded. The aetiology is unknown, but affected children often have significant associated stresses in their lives.

A multidisciplinary rehabilitation regimen is required, predominantly physical therapy-based, either community or inpatient.

Acute-onset limb pain

Limb pain of acute onset has a number of causes. Trauma is the most common, usually accidental from sports injuries or falls, but occasionally non-accidental. Osteomyelitis, bone tumours and septic arthritis are uncommon but need urgent treatment.

Osteomyelitis

In osteomyelitis, there is infection of the metaphysis of long bones. The most common sites are the distal femur and proximal tibia, but any bone may be affected (Fig. 28.10). It is usually due to haematogenous spread of the pathogen, but may arise by direct spread from an infected wound. The skin is swollen directly over the affected site. Where the joint capsule is inserted distal to the epiphyseal plate, as in the hip, osteomyelitis may spread to cause septic arthritis. Most infections are caused by *Staphylococcus aureus*, but other pathogens include *Streptococcus* and *Haemophilus influenzae* if not immunized. In sickle cell anaemia, there is an increased risk of staphylococcal and salmonella osteomyelitis. Infection may be from tuberculosis; although rare in the UK, it needs to be considered, especially in the immunodeficient child.

Presentation

This is usually with a markedly painful, immobile limb (pseudoparesis) in a child with an acute febrile illness. Directly over the infected site there is swelling and exquisite tenderness, and it may be erythematous and warm. Moving the limb causes severe pain. There may be a sterile effusion of an adjacent joint. Presentation may be more insidious in infants, in whom swelling or reduced limb movement is the initial sign. Beyond infancy, presentation may be with back pain in a vertebral infection or with a limp or groin pain in infection of the pelvis. Occasionally, there are multiple foci (e.g. disseminated staphylococcal or *H. influenzae* infection).

Investigation

Blood cultures are usually positive and the white blood count and acute-phase reactants are raised. X-rays are initially normal, other than showing soft tissue swelling; it takes 7–10 days for subperiosteal new bone formation and localized bone rarefaction to become visible. Ultrasound may show periosteal elevation at presentation. Magnetic resonance imaging (MRI) allows identification of infection in the bone (subperiosteal pus and purulent debris in the bone) and differentiation of bone from soft tissue infection. Radionuclide bone scan (Fig. 28.11) may be helpful if the site of infection is unclear. The X-ray changes of chronic osteomyelitis are shown in Fig. 28.12.

Treatment

Prompt treatment with parenteral antibiotics is required for several weeks to prevent bone necrosis, chronic infection with a discharging sinus, limb deformity and amyloidosis. Antibiotics are given intravenously until there is clinical recovery and the acute-phase reactants have returned to normal, followed by oral therapy for several weeks. Aspiration or surgical decompression of the subperiosteal space may be performed if the presentation is atypical or in immunodeficient children. Surgical drainage is performed if the condition does not respond rapidly to antibiotic therapy. The affected limb is initially rested in a splint and subsequently mobilized.

Summary

Osteomyelitis
- Presents with fever, a painful, immobile limb, swelling and extreme tenderness, especially on moving the limb.
- Blood cultures are usually positive.
- Parenteral antibiotics must be given immediately.
- Surgical drainage if unresponsive to antibiotic therapy.

Malignant disease

Acute lymphoblastic leukaemia may present with bone pain in children (sometimes primarily at night) and even frank arthritis. Neuroblastoma, usually in young children, may present with systemic arthritis or bone pain from metastases which may be difficult to localize.

Bone tumours

Malignant bone tumours – osteogenic sarcoma and Ewing tumour – are rare. They present with pain or swelling, or occasionally with a pathological fracture. Radiographs of a joint should include the long bone above and below, especially with knee pain, as distal femur and proximal tibia are the most common sites for malignant bone tumours. Further features are considered in Chapter 22 Malignant disease.

Osteoid osteoma is a benign tumour affecting adolescents, especially boys, usually involving the femur, tibia, or spine. The pain is more severe at night and improves with nonsteroidal anti-inflammatory drug (NSAID) therapy. There may be some localized tenderness, soft tissue swelling, joint effusion if sited near a joint and scoliosis if in the spine. The X-ray is

Osteomyelitis

Figure 28.10 Possible spread of osteomyelitis. In children, the epiphyseal growth plate limits the spread of metaphyseal infection. In infants, before there has been maturation of the growth plate, infection can spread directly to cause joint destruction and arrested growth.

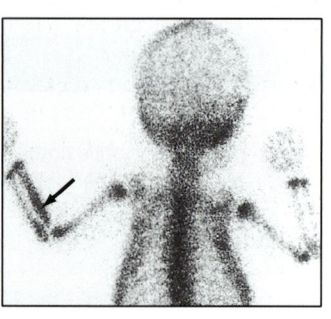

Figure 28.11 Bone scan of osteomyelitis with increased radionuclide uptake of the left radius. (Courtesy of H. Carty.)

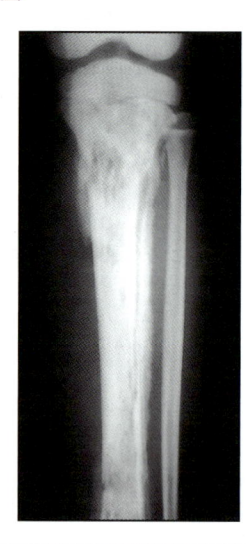

Figure 28.12 Chronic osteomyelitis, showing periosteal reaction along the lateral shaft of the tibia and multiple hypodense areas within the metaphyseal regions.

usually diagnostic, with a sharply demarcated radiolucent nidus of osteoid tissue surrounded by sclerotic bone. MRI or CT scan may be required to confirm the diagnosis, and may be indicated even if the X-ray is normal. Treatment is by surgical removal and carries a good prognosis.

The painful knee

When assessing a painful knee, the hip must always be examined, as hip pain is often referred to the knee.

Osgood–Schlatter disease

This is osteochondritis of the patellar tendon insertion at the knee, often affecting adolescent males who are physically active (particularly football or basketball). Usually presents with knee pain after exercise, localized tenderness and sometimes swelling over the tibial tuberosity. There is often hamstring tightness. It is bilateral in 25–50% of cases. Most resolve with reduced activity and physiotherapy for quadriceps muscle strengthening, hamstring stretches and occasionally orthotics. A knee immobilizer splint may be helpful.

Chondromalacia patellae

There is softening of the articular cartilage of the patella. It most often affects adolescent females, causing pain when the patella is tightly apposed to the femoral condyles, as in standing up from sitting or on walking up stairs. It is often associated with hypermobility and flat feet, suggesting a biomechanical component to the aetiology.

Treatment is with physiotherapy for quadriceps muscle strengthening.

Osteochondritis dissecans (segmental avascular necrosis of the subchondral bone)

This presents as persistent knee pain in the physically very active adolescent, with localized tenderness over the femoral condyles. Pain is caused by separation of bone and cartilage from the medial femoral condyle following avascular necrosis. Complete separation of articular fragments may result in loose body formation and symptoms of knee locking or giving way. Treatment is initially with rest and quadriceps exercises; sometimes arthroscopic surgery is required.

Subluxation and dislocation of the patella

Subluxation of the patella produces the feeling of instability or giving way of the knee. It is often associated with generalized hypermobility. Rarely, dislocation of the patella can occur, usually laterally, suddenly and with severe pain – reduction occurs spontaneously or on gentle extension of the knee. Treatment is with quadriceps exercises. Sometimes surgery is required to realign the pull of the quadriceps on the patellar tendon.

Injuries

Contact sports characteristically result in acute injuries to the knee, while non-contact sports with sustained activity tend to result in chronic injury and overuse syndromes. Sporting injuries to the menisci and ligaments are common in adolescents. MRI scans are helpful to determine the extent of damage. Management is usually conservative. In infants and young children, similar injuries are more likely to result in fractures, as their ligaments are relatively stronger than their bones.

Back pain

Back pain is a symptom of concern in the very young and preadolescent ages as, in contrast to adults, a cause can often be identified. The younger the child, the more likely there will be significant pathology. Red flag clinical features are listed in Box 28.2.

Mechanical causes – there may be muscle spasm or soft tissue pain from injury, often sport-related or from poor posture or abnormal loading (such as carrying heavy school bags on one shoulder).

Tumours: benign or malignant – The spine is a common site for osteoid osteoma. It may also be the site of primary tumours or metastases.

Vertebral osteomyelitis or discitis – there is localized tenderness; in infants there is reluctance to walk or bear weight or pain on spine flexion along with fever and systemic upset. While plain X-rays may show abnormalities suggesting the diagnosis, further imaging (MRI) is often required. Treatment is with intravenous antibiotics.

Spinal cord or nerve root entrapment – from tumour or prolapsed intervertebral disc – often associated with trauma or heavy lifting.

Scheuermann disease – an osteochondrosis of the vertebral body; may present with a fixed thoracic kyphosis with or without back pain. The diagnosis is usually made on X-ray. In many cases, the radiographic changes are a coincidental finding and the patient is asymptomatic.

Spondylolysis/spondylolisthesis – stress fracture of the pars interarticularis of the vertebra. Increased risk with certain sporting activities, e.g. bowling in cricket or gymnastics. If bilateral it can result in spondylolisthesis, forward slip of the vertebral body, and potential cord or nerve root compression. There is pain on spine extension and localized tenderness. Change may be apparent on X-ray but often further imaging (CT scan) is required.

Complex regional pain syndrome (CRPS) – diagnosed when no physical cause is found; may be exacerbated by psychological stress.

> **Box 28.2** Red flag clinical features of back pain
> - Young age – pathology more likely
> - High fever – infection
> - Night waking, persistent pain – osteoid osteoma or tumours
> - Painful scoliosis – infection or malignancy
> - Focal neurological signs including nerve root irritation, loss of bowel/bladder control – nerve root/spinal cord compression
> - Associated weight loss, systemic malaise – malignancy.

Limp

Limp can be divided into acute painful limp and chronic or intermittent limp, where pain may or may not be the presenting feature, and by age (Table 28.1).

Transient synovitis ('irritable hip')

This is the most common cause of acute hip pain in children. It occurs in children aged 2–12 years old. It often follows or is accompanied by a viral infection. Presentation is with sudden onset of pain in the hip or a limp. There is no pain at rest, but there is decreased range of movement, particularly internal rotation. The pain may be referred to the knee. The child is afebrile or has a mild fever and does not appear ill.

It can be difficult to differentiate transient synovitis from early septic arthritis of the hip joint (Table 28.2), and if there is any suspicion of septic arthritis, joint aspiration and blood cultures are mandatory.

In a small proportion of children, transient synovitis precedes the development of Perthes disease. Management of transient synovitis is with bed rest and, rarely, skin traction. It usually improves within a few days.

Perthes disease

This is an avascular necrosis of the capital femoral epiphysis of the femoral head due to interruption of

Table 28.1 Causes of limp

Age	Acute painful limp	Chronic and intermittent limp
1–3 years	Infection – septic arthritis, osteomyelitis of hip or spine Transient synovitis Trauma – accidental/non-accidental Malignant disease – leukaemia, neuroblastoma	Developmental dysplasia of the hip (DDH), talipes Neuromuscular, e.g. cerebral palsy Juvenile idiopathic arthritis (JIA)
3–10 years	Transient synovitis Septic arthritis/osteomyelitis Trauma and overuse injuries Perthes disease (acute) Juvenile idiopathic arthritis (JIA) Malignant disease, e.g. leukaemia Complex regional pain syndrome	Perthes disease (chronic) Neuromuscular disorders, e.g. Duchenne muscular dystrophy Juvenile idiopathic arthritis (JIA) Tarsal coalition
11–16 years	Mechanical – trauma, overuse injuries, sport injuries Slipped capital femoral epiphysis (acute) Avascular necrosis of the femoral head Reactive arthritis Juvenile idiopathic arthritis (JIA) Septic arthritis/osteomyelitis Osteochondritis dissecans of the knee Bone tumours and malignancy Complex regional pain syndrome	Slipped capital femoral epiphysis (chronic) Juvenile idiopathic arthritis (JIA) Tarsal coalition

Table 28.2 Contrast in clinical features of transient synovitis and septic arthritis of the hip

	Transient synovitis	Septic arthritis
Onset	Acute limp, non-weight bearing	Acute onset, non-weight bearing
Fever	Mild/absent	Moderate/high
Child's appearance	Child often looks well	Child looks ill
Hip movement	Comfortable at rest, limited internal rotation and pain on movement	Hip held flexed; severe pain at rest and worse on any attempt to move joint
White cell count	Normal	Normal/high
Acute-phase reactant/ESR	Slight increase/normal	Raised
Ultrasound	Fluid in joint	Fluid in joint
Radiograph	Normal	Normal/widened joint space
Management	Rest, analgesia	Joint aspiration, usually under ultrasound guidance Prolonged antibiotics, rest and analgesia
Course	Resolves <1 week, approx. 3% develop Perthes disease	Progressive and severe joint damage if not treated

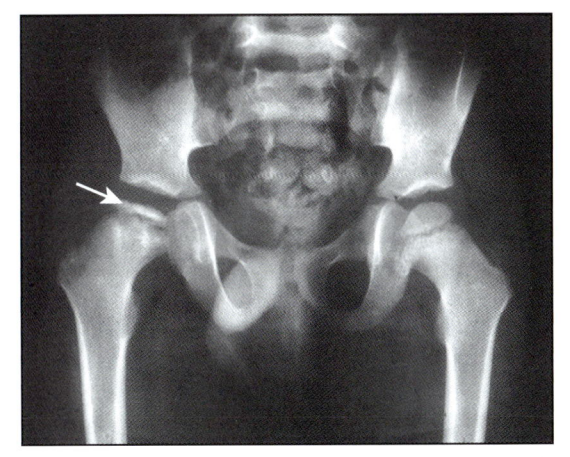

Figure 28.13 Perthes disease, showing flattening with sclerosis and fragmentation of the right femoral capital epiphysis; the left hip is normal.

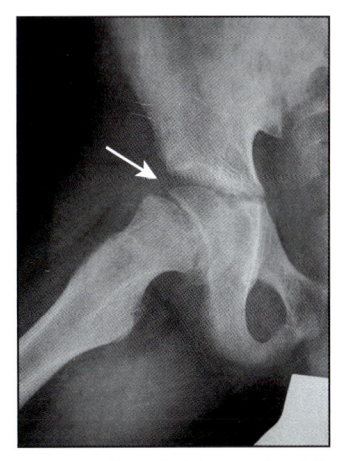

Figure 28.14 Slipped capital femoral epiphysis of the right hip.

the blood supply, followed by revascularization and reossification over 18–36 months. It mainly affects boys (male:female ratio of 5:1) of 5–10 years of age. Presentation is insidious, with the onset of a limp, or hip or knee pain. The condition may initially be mistaken for transient synovitis. It is bilateral in 10–20%. If suspected, X-ray of both hips (including frog views) should be requested; early signs of Perthes include increased density in the femoral head, which subsequently becomes fragmented and irregular (Fig. 28.13).

Even if the initial X-ray is normal, a repeat may be required if clinical symptoms persist. A bone scan and MRI scan can be helpful in making the diagnosis.

Treatment options include rest, physiotherapy to optimize hip movement, and in some cases traction, plaster casts and surgery.

In most children the prognosis is good, particularly in those below 6 years of age with less than half the epiphysis involved. In older children or with more extensive involvement of the epiphysis, deformity of the femoral head and metaphyseal damage are more likely, with potential for subsequent degenerative arthritis in adult life.

Slipped capital femoral epiphysis

Results in displacement of the epiphysis of the femoral head postero-inferiorly, requiring prompt treatment in order to prevent avascular necrosis. It is most common at 10–15 years of age during the adolescent growth spurt, particularly in obese boys, and is bilateral in 20%. There is an association with metabolic endocrine abnormalities, e.g. hypothyroidism and hypogonadism. Presentation is with a limp or hip pain, which may be referred to the knee. The onset may be acute, following minor trauma, or insidious. Examination shows restricted abduction and internal rotation of the hip. Diagnosis is confirmed on X-ray (Fig. 28.14), and a frog lateral view should also be requested. Management is surgical, usually with pin fixation in situ.

> **Summary**
>
> Regarding hip disorders:
> - Developmental dysplasia of the hip (DDH) – identified on screening at birth or 8 weeks, detection of asymmetry of skinfolds around the hip, limited abduction of the hip, shortening of the affected leg, or a limp or abnormal gait.
> - Transient synovitis – most common cause of acute hip pain or a limp; must be differentiated from septic arthritis.
> - Perthes disease – usually school-aged children with hip pain or limp.
> - Slipped capital femoral epiphysis – adolescent with a limp or hip pain.

Arthritis

Acute arthritis presents with pain, swelling, heat, redness and restricted movement in a joint. In a monoarthritis of acute onset, the child is also likely to be systemically unwell with fever; if septic arthritis or osteomyelitis is the cause, urgent diagnosis and treatment is required. With infection, more than one joint can be affected, although a single joint is more common.

The causes of polyarthritis are listed in Table 28.3.

Reactive arthritis

Reactive arthritis is the most common form of arthritis in childhood. It is characterized by transient joint swelling (usually <6 weeks) often of the ankles or knees. It usually follows (or rarely accompanies) evidence of extra-articular infection. The enteric bacteria (*Salmonella, Shigella, Campylobacter* and *Yersinia*) are often the cause in children, but viral infections, sexually transmitted infections in adolescents (chlamydia, gonococcus), Mycoplasma and *Borrelia burgdorferi* (Lyme disease) are other causes. Rheumatic fever and post-streptococcal reactive arthritis are rare in high-income countries but

Table 28.3 Causes of polyarthritis

Infection	Bacterial – septicaemia/septic arthritis, TB
	Viral – rubella, mumps, adenovirus, coxsackie B, herpes, hepatitis, parvovirus
	Other – *Mycoplasma*, Lyme disease, rickettsia
	Reactive – gastrointestinal infection, streptococcal infection
	Rheumatic fever
Inflammatory bowel disease	Crohn's disease, ulcerative colitis
Vasculitis	Henoch–Schönlein purpura, Kawasaki disease
Haematological disorders	Haemophilia, sickle cell disease
Malignant disorders	Leukaemia, neuroblastoma
Connective tissue disorders	Juvenile idiopathic arthritis (JIA), systemic lupus erythematosus (SLE), dermatomyositis, mixed connective tissue disease (MCTD), polyarteritis nodosa (PAN)
Other	Cystic fibrosis

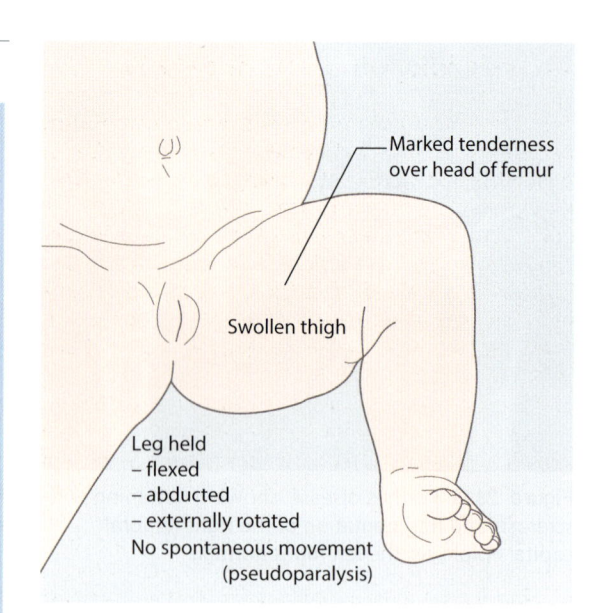

Figure 28.15 Septic arthritis of the hip in infants, showing the characteristic posture to reduce intracapsular pressure. Any leg movement is painful and is resisted.

- Marked tenderness over head of femur
- Swollen thigh
- Leg held
  - flexed
  - abducted
  - externally rotated
- No spontaneous movement (pseudoparalysis)

are frequent in many low and middle-income countries. Fever is low grade. Acute-phase reactants are normal or mildly elevated and X-rays are normal. No treatment or only NSAIDs are required and complete recovery can be anticipated.

Septic arthritis

This is a serious infection of the joint space, as it can lead to bone destruction. It is most common in children less than 2 years old. It usually results from haematogenous spread but may also occur following a puncture wound or infected skin lesions, e.g. chickenpox. In young children, it may result from spread from adjacent osteomyelitis into joints where the capsule inserts below the epiphyseal growth plate. Usually only one joint is affected, with the hip being a particular concern in infants and young children. Beyond the neonatal period, the most common organism is *Staphylococcus aureus*. *H. influenzae* was an important cause in young children prior to Hib immunization and often affected multiple sites. Underlying and predisposing illnesses such as immunodeficiency and sickle cell disease should be considered.

Presentation

This is usually with an erythematous, warm, acutely tender joint, with a reduced range of movement, in an acutely unwell, febrile child. Infants often hold the limb still (pseudoparesis, pseudoparalysis) and cry if it is moved. A joint effusion may be detectable in peripheral joints. Although a sympathetic joint effusion may be present in osteomyelitis, it is accompanied by marked tenderness over the bone. However, in up to 15% of cases of osteomyelitis, there is coexistent septic arthritis. The diagnosis of septic arthritis of the hip can be particularly difficult in toddlers, as the joint is well covered by subcutaneous fat (Fig. 28.15). Initial presentation may be with a limp or pain referred to the knee.

Investigation

There is an increased white cell count and acute-phase reactants. Blood cultures must be taken. Ultrasound of deep joints, such as the hip, is helpful to identify an effusion. X-rays are used to exclude trauma and other bony lesions. However, in septic arthritis, the X-rays are initially normal, apart from widening of the joint space and soft tissue swelling. Further imaging options include MRI scanning or a radioisotope bone scan may be indicated if the site of infection is unclear. Aspiration of the joint space under ultrasound guidance for organisms and culture is the definitive investigation. Ideally, this is performed immediately, unless this would cause a significant delay in giving antibiotics. A prolonged course of antibiotics is required, initially intravenously. Washing out of the joint or surgical drainage may be required if resolution does not occur rapidly or if the joint is deep-seated, such as the hip. The joint is initially immobilizsed in a functional position, but subsequently must be mobilized to prevent permanent deformity.

> **Early treatment of septic arthritis is essential to prevent destruction of the articular cartilage and bone**

Juvenile idiopathic arthritis (JIA)

This is the most common chronic inflammatory joint disease in children and adolescents in the UK. It is defined as persistent joint swelling (of >6 weeks duration) presenting before 16 years of age in the absence of infection or any other defined cause. Ninety-five per cent of children have a disease that is clinically and immunogenetically distinct from rheumatoid arthritis in adults. It has a prevalence of approximately 1 in 1000 children, (i.e. similar to epilepsy), with over 12 000 affected children in the UK.

There are at least seven different subtypes of JIA. The subtypes and their clinical features are shown in Table 28.4. Classification is clinical and based on the number of joints affected in the first 6 months: as polyarthritis (more than four joints) (Fig. 28.16); oligoarthritis (up to and including four joints); or systemic (with fever and rash) (see Case history 28.1). Psoriatic arthritis and enthesitis are further subtypes. Subtyping is further classified according to the presence of rheumatoid factor and HLA B27 tissue type.

Features in the history are gelling (stiffness after periods of rest, such as long car rides), morning joint stiffness, and pain. In the young child, it may present with intermittent limp or deterioration in behaviour or mood or avoidance of previously enjoyed activities, rather than complaining of pain.

Initially, there may be only minimal evidence of joint swelling, but subsequently there may be swelling of the joint due to fluid within it, inflammation, chronic arthritis, proliferation (thickening) of the synovium and swelling of the periarticular soft tissues.

As the presentation can be indolent, especially in young children, and in the most common forms the baseline investigations are often initially normal (i.e. normal full blood count and inflammatory markers, negative rheumatoid factor and radiographs), diagnosis can be difficult (see Case History 28.2). Antinuclear factor may be present in children with JIA, but may be observed in healthy children or transient illness. However, in any child with widespread joint pain, fatigue or multisystem involvement, the possibility of a connective tissue disorder needs to be considered. Long term, with uncontrolled disease activity there may be bone expansion from overgrowth, which in the knee may cause leg lengthening or valgus deformity, in the hands, discrepancy in digit length, and in the wrist, advancement of bone age.

If systemic features are present, sepsis and malignancy must always be considered.

> If JIA is suspected, even if joint abnormality is not clear, referral to paediatric rheumatology is indicated as early treatment radically improves outcome

Complications

Chronic anterior uveitis

This is common but usually asymptomatic in the early stages and if not detected and treated, can lead to severe visual impairment due to cataract and glaucoma. Regular ophthalmological screening using a slit lamp is indicated, especially for children with oligoarticular disease and those who are antinuclear antibody positive.

Flexion contractures of the joints

These occur when the joint is held in the most comfortable position, thereby minimizing intra-articular pressure. Chronic untreated disease can lead to joint destruction and the need for joint replacement. Joint contracture is preventable with early diagnosis and treatment.

Growth failure

This may be generalised from anorexia, chronic disease, and systemic corticosteroid therapy (Fig. 28.17). May also be localized overgrowth such as leg length discrepancy due to prolonged active knee synovitis and

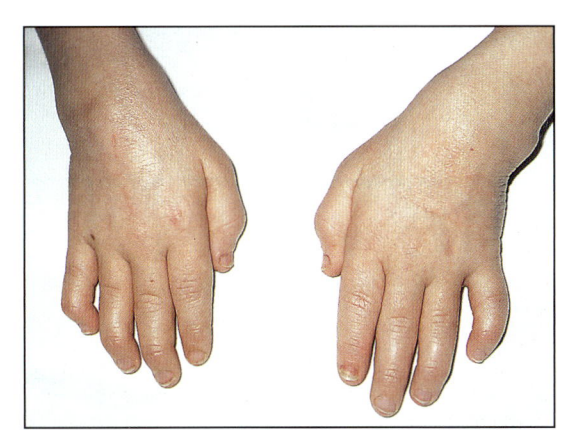

Figure 28.16 Polyarticular juvenile idiopathic arthritis, showing swelling of the wrists, metacarpal, and interphalangeal joints and early swan-neck deformities of the fingers.

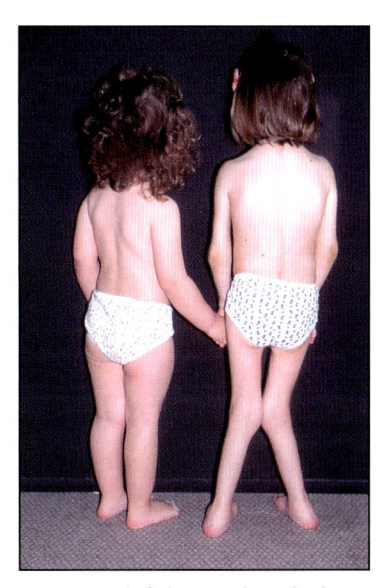

Figure 28.17 Growth failure and marked genu valgum (knock-knees) in an 8-year-old girl with juvenile idiopathic arthritis. For comparison, her sister on the left is 4 years old.

Table 28.4 Classification and clinical features of juvenile idiopathic arthritis (JIA)

JIA subtype (approximate %)	Onset age	Sex ratio (F:M)	Articular pattern	Extra-articular features	Laboratory abnormalities
Oligoarthritis (persistent) (49%)	1–6 years	5:1	1–4 (max) joints involved; knee, ankle or wrist most common	Chronic anterior uveitis in 20%, leg length discrepancy Prognosis excellent	ANA+/–
Oligoarthritis (extended) (8%)	1–6 years	5:1	>4 joints involved after first 6 months. Asymmetrical distribution of large and small joints	Chronic anterior uveitis 20%, asymmetrical growth Prognosis moderate	ANA+/–
Polyarthritis (RF negative) (16%)	1–6 years	5:1	Symmetrical large and small joint arthritis, often with marked finger involvement. Cervical spine and temporomandibular joint may be involved	Low-grade fever, chronic anterior uveitis 5%, late reduction of growth rate Prognosis moderate	
Polyarthritis (RF positive) (3%)	10–16 years	5:1	Symmetrical large and small joint arthritis, often with marked finger involvement	Rheumatoid nodules 10% Similar to adult rheumatoid arthritis Prognosis poor	RF+ (long term)
Systemic arthritis (9%)	1–10 years	1:1	Oligoarthritis or polyarthritis. May have aches and pains in joints and muscles (arthralgia/myalgia) but initially no arthritis	Acute illness, malaise, high daily fever initially, with salmon-pink, macular rash, lymphadenopathy, hepatosplenomegaly, serositis Prognosis variable to poor	Anaemia, raised neutrophils and platelets, high acute-phase reactants
Psoriatic arthritis (7%)	1–16 years	1:1	Usually asymmetrical distribution of large and small joints, dactylitis	Psoriasis, nail pitting or dystrophy, chronic anterior uveitis 20% Prognosis moderate	
Enthesitis-related arthritis (7%)	6–16 years	1:4	Lower limb, large joint arthritis initially, mild lumbar spine or sacroiliac involvement later on	Enthesitis – localized inflammation at insertion of tendons or ligaments into bone, often in feet, Achilles insertion Occasional acute uveitis Prognosis moderate	HLAB27+
Undifferentiated arthritis (1%)	1–16 years	2:1 (variable)	Overlapping articular and extra-articular patterns between ≥2 subtypes or insufficient criteria for subclassification	Prognosis variable	

ANF: Anti-Nuclear Factor; RF: Rheumatoid Factor.

Case history 28.1

Systemic-onset juvenile idiopathic arthritis

A 2-year-old boy presented with a high fever (Fig. 28.18a) and malaise. A salmon-coloured rash was present at times of fever (Fig. 28.18b). Investigation showed markedly raised acute-phase reactants. Shortly afterwards, he developed severe polyarticular joint disease. A diagnosis of systemic-onset juvenile idiopathic arthritis was made on the basis of the clinical presentation and exclusion of other disorders (Table 28.3).

He was treated with high-dose intravenous corticosteroids with rapid improvement, started on low dose oral corticosteroids and weekly methotrexate given by subcutaneous injection. The family were supported by the nursing team, who taught them about his injections and treatments, and physiotherapy, who advised exercises and stretches to improve his joint range and muscle strength. He had further flares of his disease and was started on biological therapy given by monthly intravenous infusion at the paediatric day unit. Within 4 months from diagnosis he had excellent disease control and a year later he was well but still on weekly methotrexate with monthly biological treatment. He will require long term follow-up including regular blood tests and review by the paediatric rheumatology team.

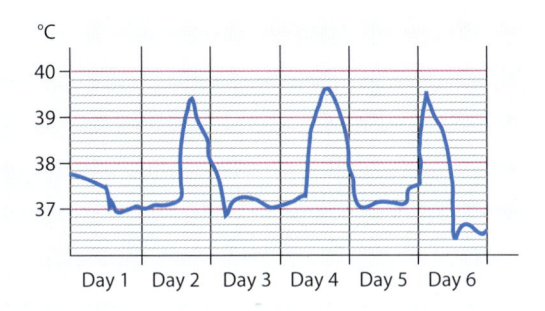

Figure 28.18a Temperature chart showing spikes, often in the evenings, but normal in between times.

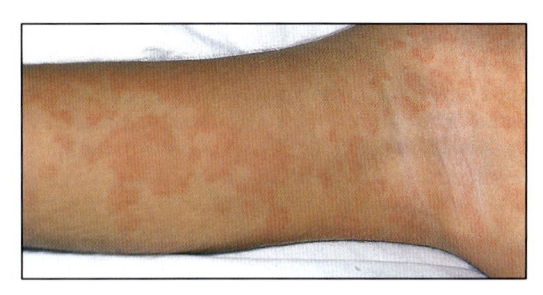

Figure 28.18b Salmon-pink rash.

---

undergrowth, such as micrognathia, usually seen in long-standing or suboptimally treated arthritis due to premature fusion of epiphyses. Growth problems are largely preventable with early diagnosis and treatment.

Constitutional problems

Anaemia of chronic disease, delayed puberty.

Osteoporosis

Multifactorial aetiology, including diet, reduced weight bearing, systemic corticosteroids and delayed menarche. Reduce risk by dietary supplements of calcium and vitamin D; regular weight-bearing exercise; and minimise oral corticosteroid use and sometimes bisphosphonates.

Amyloidosis

Very rare now, causes proteinuria and subsequent renal failure and has a high mortality.

Management

The management of JIA has radically changed in the last decade and improvement in outcome is evident as long as children access appropriate care. Deformity and disability are much less common with current treatment approaches and early diagnosis. The overall management aim is to induce remission as soon as possible.

All children suspected of having JIA should be managed by specialist paediatric rheumatology multidisciplinary teams, often working in shared care with local hospitals; such teams have specific paediatric expertise in the use and monitoring of immunosuppressive treatments (e.g. methotrexate and biological therapies) and intra-articular corticosteroid injections that are now routinely used. There is need for education and support for the child and family, physical therapy to maintain joint function, and links to other specialities including ophthalmology, dentistry and orthopaedics. The team works closely with schools, social services, and primary healthcare providers. The child is encouraged to take part in all activities except contact sports during active flares. With optimal care, most children are managed as outpatients.

Medical management includes:

- *NSAIDs and analgesics* – do not modify disease but help relieve symptoms during flares.
- *Joint injections, increasingly under ultrasound guidance* – effective, first-line treatment for oligoarticular JIA; in polyarticular disease multiple joint injections are used as bridging agent when starting methotrexate. Often requires sedation or inhaled anaesthesia (Entonox).

Case history 28.2

Oligoarticular onset juvenile idiopathic arthritis

A 4 year old girl was noted by her parents to be limping intermittently for several weeks. Her teacher at school commented that she was quieter, less keen to play, and was not able to sit on the floor in story time. Her general practitioner performed a pGALS assessment and observed she had a limp and her right knee was swollen and restricted (Fig. 28.19). She was referred to the paediatric department and then paediatric rheumatology.

Investigations showed that her basic blood tests (full blood count, acute phase reactants) were normal but her ANA (antinuclear antibody) test was positive. She had evidence of chronic anterior uveitis on slit lamp examination, although she had no visual symptoms. Her uveitis was treated with topical corticosteroids. Her knee was injected with corticosteroids under general anaesthesia. She had physiotherapy to improve her joint movement and function. The family received information and support from the paediatric rheumatology multidisciplinary team. Her mobility, mood and energy improved and she returned to normal activities at home and school. Her prognosis is excellent, although further flares of her arthritis and/or uveitis are possible and she needs regular review. This case history demonstrates how prompt diagnosis and early specialist management reduces long-term morbidity.

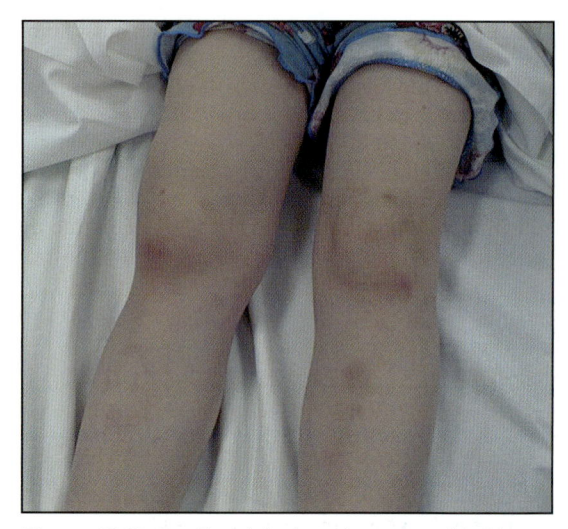

Figure 28.19 Swollen right knee in 4 year old girl with oligoarticular onset juvenile idiopathic arthritis.

- *Methotrexate* – early use reduces joint damage. Effective in approximately 70% with polyarthritis, less effective in systemic features of JIA. It is given as weekly dose (tablet, liquid, or injection) and regular blood monitoring is required (for abnormal liver function and bone-marrow suppression). Nausea is common.
- *Systemic corticosteroids* – avoided if possible, to minimise risk of growth suppression and osteoporosis. Pulsed intravenous methylprednisolone often used for severe polyarthritis as an induction agent. May be life-saving for severe systemic arthritis or macrophage activation syndrome.
- *Cytokine modulators ('biologics') and other immunotherapies* – Many agents (e.g. anti-TNF alpha, IL-1, CTLA-4, or IL-6) now available and useful in severe disease refractory to methotrexate. Costly and given under strict national guidance with registries for long-term surveillance. T-cell depletion coupled with autologous haematopoietic stem cell rescue (bone marrow transplant) is an option for refractory disease.

Prognosis

The prognosis has markedly improved and most children and families can expect good disease control and quality of life. If good disease control is not achieved, there can be significant morbidity from previous inflammation, such as joint damage requiring joint replacement surgery, visual impairment from uveitis, or fractures from osteoporosis. Joint replacements are now rarely needed in childhood, but are still needed in some adults with JIA. Long-term outcome studies have shown that at least one in three children will need ongoing treatment into adult years to maintain remission. There is also significant psychosocial morbidity with impact on schooling and employment outcomes.

Transitional care programmes are increasingly provided to facilitate the changes through adolescence and young adulthood and to help young people learn how to self-manage their chronic disease, live independently, and engage in shared decision making.

Henoch–Schönlein purpura

This is the most common vasculitis of childhood and presents with a purpuric rash over the lower legs and buttocks, usually associated with arthritis of the ankles or knees. Other features are abdominal pain, haematuria and proteinuria (see Ch. 19).

Systemic lupus erythematosus (SLE)

Systemic lupus erythematosus is rare in children, but may present in adolescent females typically with malaise, arthralgia and malar rash (often photosensitive). Organ involvement (kidneys, lung, or central nervous system) are serious complications.

Juvenile dermatomyositis

Juvenile dermatomyositis (JDMS) is rare. It usually begins insidiously with malaise, progressive weakness

Summary

Diagnostic clues regarding musculoskeletal disorders

'Typical' symptom combinations	Pivotal clinical features	Possible diagnoses
Nocturnal wakening with leg pain	Normal child	'Growing pains' Osteoid osteoma
	Anaemia, bruising, irritability, infections	Leukaemia, lymphoma, neuroblastoma (young child)
'Clunk' on hip movement on neonatal and early infant screening, limp in an older infant	Older infant: asymmetrical upper leg skin folds, limited hip abduction	Developmental dysplasia of the hip (DDH)
Febrile, toxic-looking infant, irritability with nappy changing	Restricted joint range (especially hip) or limb movement	Septic arthritis Osteomyelitis
Sudden limp in an otherwise well young child	Unilateral restricted hip movement	Transient synovitis of the hip Perthes disease
Fever, erythematous rash, red eyes, irritability in infant or young child	Erythema/oedema of hands and feet, oral mucositis, cervical lymphadenopathy	Kawasaki disease
Irritability, fever, reluctance to move in an infant or young child	Stiff back, 'tripod' sitting	Discitis Vertebral osteomyelitis
Joint pain, stiffness, and restriction Loss of joint function	Persistent joint swelling Loss of joint range	Juvenile idiopathic arthritis
Hip pain in an obese adolescent boy	Unilateral hip restriction	Slipped capital femoral epiphysis
Lethargy, unwilling to do physical activities, irritability, rash	Eyelid erythema Proximal muscle weakness	Juvenile dermatomyositis
Constitutional symptoms, lethargy, arthralgia in an adolescent female	Multisystem abnormalities, haematuria, facial erythema	Systemic lupus erythematosus

(often difficulty climbing stairs), and facial rash with erythema over the bridge of the nose and malar areas and a violaceous (heliotropic) discoloration of the eyelids (see Fig. 29.10). The skin over the metacarpal and proximal interphalangeal joints may be hypertrophic and pink, and the nailfold capillaries may be dilated and tortuous. Muscle pain is a common, if non-specific, symptom and arthritis is present in 30% of cases. Respiratory failure and aspiration pneumonia may be life-threatening. The condition is described further in Chapter 29.

Genetic skeletal conditions

These are inherited abnormalities resulting in generalized developmental disorders of the bone, of which there are several hundred types. They usually result in reduced growth and abnormality of bone shape rather than impaired strength, except for osteogenesis imperfecta. The bones of the limbs and spine are often affected, resulting in short stature. Intelligence is usually normal. Improved knowledge of the molecular basis of collagen and its disorders is allowing better understanding and delineation of some of these disorders.

Achondroplasia

Inheritance is autosomal dominant, but about 50% are new mutations. Clinical features are short stature from marked shortening of the limbs, a large head, frontal bossing, and depression of the nasal bridge (see Fig. 12.10b). The hands are short and broad. A marked lumbar lordosis develops. Hydrocephalus sometimes occurs.

Thanatophoric dysplasia

This results in stillbirth. The infants have a large head, extremely short limbs and a small chest. The appearance of the bones on X-ray is characteristic. The importance of the correct diagnosis of this disorder is that, in contrast to achondroplasia, its inheritance is sporadic. It may be identified on antenatal ultrasound.

Cleidocranial dysostosis

In this autosomal dominant disorder, there is absence of part or all of the clavicles and delay in closure of the anterior fontanelle and of ossification of the skull. The child is often able to bring the shoulders together in front of the chest to touch each other as a 'party trick'. Short stature is usually present. Intelligence is normal.

Arthrogryposis

This is a heterogeneous group of congenital disorders in which there is stiffness and contracture of joints. The cause is usually unknown, but there may be an association with oligohydramnios, widespread congenital anomalies, or chromosomal disorders. It is usually sporadic. Marked flexion contractures of the knees, elbows and wrists, dislocation of the hips and other joints, talipes equinovarus, and scoliosis are common, but the disorder may be localized to the upper or lower limbs. The skin is thin, subcutaneous tissue is reduced, and there is marked muscle atrophy around the affected joints. Intelligence is usually unaffected. Management is with physiotherapy and correction of deformities, where possible, by splints, plaster casts, or surgery. Walking is impaired in the more severe forms of the disorder.

Osteogenesis imperfecta (brittle bone disease)

This is a group of disorders of collagen metabolism causing bone fragility, with bowing and frequent fractures.

In the most common form (type I), which is autosomal dominant, there are fractures during childhood (Fig. 28.20a) and a blue appearance to the sclerae (Fig. 28.20b) and some develop hearing loss. Treatment with bisphosphonates reduces fracture rates. The prognosis is variable. Fractures require splinting to minimise joint deformity.

There is a severe, lethal form (type II) with multiple fractures already present before birth (Fig. 28.21). Many affected infants are stillborn. Inheritance is variable but mostly autosomal dominant or due to new mutations. In other types, scleral discoloration may be minimal.

Osteopetrosis (marble bone disease)

In this rare disorder, the bones are dense but brittle. The severe autosomal recessive disorder presents with faltering growth, recurrent infection, hypocalcaemia, anaemia and thrombocytopenia. Prognosis is poor, but bone marrow transplantation can be curative. A less severe autosomal dominant form may present during childhood with fractures.

Osteogenesis imperfecta

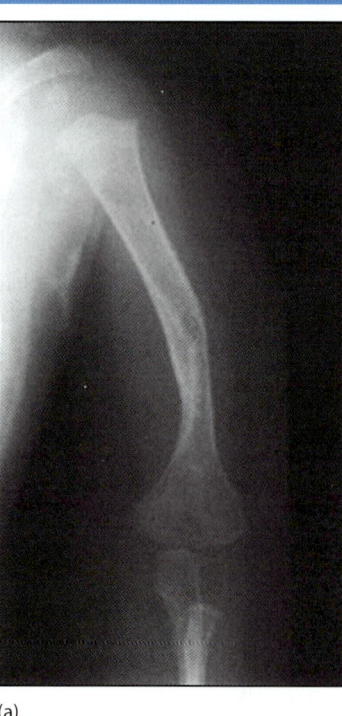

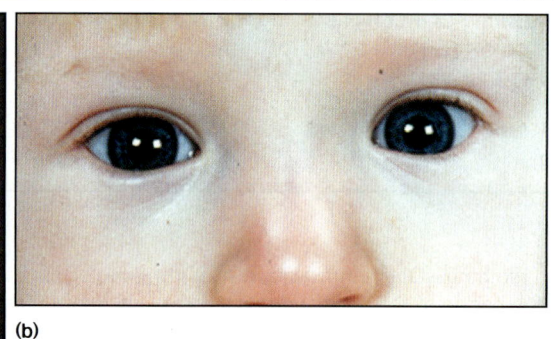

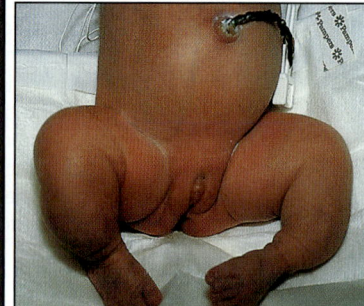

Figure 28.21 Osteogenesis imperfecta (type II) showing shortened, deformed lower limbs from gross deformity of the bones with multiple fractures.

Figure 28.20 Osteogenesis imperfecta type I, showing **(a)** fracture of the humerus and osteoporotic bones; and **(b)** blue sclerae.

> Osteogenesis imperfecta is often considered in the evaluation of unexplained fractures in suspected child abuse.

Marfan syndrome

This is an autosomal dominant disorder of connective tissue associated with tall stature, long thin digits (arachnodactyly), hyperextensible joints, a high arched palate, dislocation (usually upwards) of the lenses of the eyes, and severe myopia. The body proportions are altered, with long, thin limbs resulting in a greater distance between the pubis and soles (lower segment) than from the crown to the pubis (upper segment). The arm span, measured from the extended fingers, is greater than the height. There may be chest deformity and scoliosis. The major problems are cardiovascular, due to degeneration of the media of vessel walls resulting in a dilated, incompetent aortic root with valvular incompetence and mitral valve prolapse and regurgitation. Aneurysms of the aorta may dissect or rupture. Monitoring by echocardiography is required.

Acknowledgements

We would like to acknowledge contributors to this chapter in previous editions, whose work we have drawn on: John Sills (1st, 2nd Editions), Tauny Southwood (3rd Edition), Helen Foster (4th Edition), Sharmila Jandial (4th Edition).

Further reading

Cassidy J, Laxer RM, Petty RE, Lindsley CB: *Textbook of Pediatric Rheumatology*, ed 6, Edinburgh, 2016, Elsevier Saunders.

Foster HE, Brogan P: *Oxford Handbook of Paediatric Rheumatology*, Oxford, 2016, Oxford University Press.

Szer IS, Kimura Y, Malleson PN, Southwood T, editors: *Arthritis in Children and Adolescents: Juvenile Idiopathic Arthritis*, Oxford, 2006, Oxford University Press.

Woo P, Laxer RM, Sherry DD: *Pediatric Rheumatology in Clinical Practice*, New York, 2007, Springer.

Websites (Accessed December 2016)

Arthritis Research UK: Available at: http://www.arthritisresearchuk.org/arthritis_information/information_for_medical_profes/medical_student_handbook.aspx
Free educational materials for medical students including pGALS.

Arthritis Research UK: Available at: http://www.arthritisresearchuk.org/.
Information about arthritis for health professionals.

British Society for Paediatric and Adolescent Rheumatology: Available at: http://www.bspar.org.uk/pages/bspar_home.asp.
Information about clinical guidelines and protocols.

Paediatric Musculoskeletal Matters: Available at: http://www.pmmonline.org
Free educational materials including pGALS, pREMS, interactive cases, and notes on common and significant musculoskeletal conditions. A pGALS app is available.

29

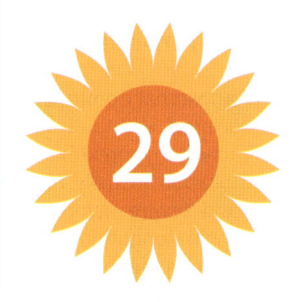

Neurological disorders

Headache	500	Ataxia	517
Seizures	503	Cerebrovascular disease	517
Epilepsies of childhood	506	Microcephaly and macrocephaly	518
Motor disorders	510	Neural tube defects and	
Central motor disorders	511	hydrocephalus	518
Peripheral motor disorders:		The neurocutaneous syndromes	521
the neuromuscular disorders	511	Neurodegenerative disorders	522

Features of neurological disorders in children are:
- recurrent headaches are most often caused by migraine and tension-type headache
- febrile seizures are common and usually have a good prognosis, but any cause of the febrile illness that needs treatment needs to be identified
- the diagnosis of an epilepsy is primarily based on a detailed history and often substantiated by a video
- epilepsy syndromes present at different ages e.g. infantile spasms at 4–6 months, childhood absence epilepsy at 4–12 years
- motor disorders may be central, (involving the corticospinal (pyramidal) tract, basal ganglia or cerebellum), or peripheral (neuromuscular disorders)
- the number of babies born with neural tube defects has declined markedly over the last 50 years.

The central nervous system comprises 100 000 million neurones and when it malfunctions it has the potential to generate a wide spectrum of clinical problems. The site of the dysfunctional neurones determines the nature of the problem, which may involve impaired movement, vision, hearing, sensory perception, learning, memory, consciousness or sleep. They generate "neurological", as well as "emotional" (affective) disorders, e.g. anxiety and depression, and other "mental health" disorders, and some "functional" or "medically unexplained" illnesses. The division of brain disorders into "neurological" and "mental health" is artificial, and although based historically on morbid pathology, is nowadays more based on the therapies offered than on biology. Classifying this wide range of symptom complexes can be problematic.

Headache

Headache is a frequent reason for older children and adolescents to consult a doctor. The International Headache Society has devised a classification, as shown in Box 29.1, which defines

- *Primary headaches*: four main groups, comprising migraine, tension-type headache, cluster headache (and other trigeminal autonomic cephalalgias), and other primary headaches (such as primary stabbing headache). They are thought to be due to a primary malfunction of neurons and their networks.
- *Secondary headaches*: symptomatic of some underlying pathology, e.g. from raised intracranial pressure or space-occupying lesions.
- *Trigeminal and other cranial neuralgias and other headaches* including root pain from herpes zoster.

Primary headaches

Tension-type headache

This is a symmetrical headache of gradual onset, often described as tightness, a band or pressure. There are usually no other symptoms.

Migraine

Migraine without aura

This accounts for 90% of migraine. In children, episodes may last 1–72 hours; the headache is commonly bilateral but may be unilateral. Characteristically pulsatile, over the temporal or frontal area, it is often accompanied by unpleasant gastrointestinal disturbance such

Box 29.1 The classification of headache disorders

Primary headaches
- Migraine
- Tension-type headache
- Cluster headache and other trigeminal autonomic cephalalgias
- Other primary headaches

Secondary headaches
Headache attributed to:
- Medication overuse headache
- Head and/or neck trauma
- Cranial or cervical vascular disorder – vascular malformation or intracranial haemorrhage
- Non-vascular intracranial disorder – raised intracranial pressure, idiopathic intracranial hypertension
- A substance or its withdrawal – alcohol, solvent or drug abuse
- Infection – meningitis, encephalitis, abcess
- Disorder of homeostasis – hypercapnia or hypertension
- Disorder of facial or cranial structures – acute sinusitis
- Associated with emotional disorders

Cranial neuralgias, central and primary facial pain, and other headaches
- Trigeminal and other cranial neuralgias and central causes of facial pain
- Other headaches

---

as nausea, vomiting, abdominal pain, photophobia and phonophobia (sensitivity to sounds). It is typically aggravated by physical activity and relieved by sleep.

Migraine with aura
Accounts for 10% of migraine. The headache is preceded by an aura (visual, sensory, or motor), although the aura may occur without a headache. Features are the absence of problems between episodes and the frequent presence of premonitory symptoms (tiredness, difficulty concentrating, autonomic features, etc.).

The most common aura comprises visual disturbance, which may include:

- negative phenomena, such as hemianopia (loss of half the visual field) or scotoma (small areas of visual loss)
- positive phenomena such as fortification spectra (seeing zigzag lines).

Rarely, there are unilateral sensory or motor symptoms (e.g. hemiplegic migraine).

Migraine attacks usually last for a few hours, during which time children often prefer to lie down in a quiet, dark place.

Symptoms of *tension-type headache* or a *migraine* often overlap. They are probably part of the same pathophysiological continuum, with evidence that both result from primary neuronal dysfunction, including channelopathies, with vascular phenomena as secondary events. There is a genetic predisposition, with first-degree and second-degree relatives often also affected. Bouts are often triggered by a disturbance of inherent biorhythms, such as late nights or early rises, stress, or winding down after stress at home or school. Certain foods, e.g. cheese, chocolate, and caffeine, are only rarely a reliable trigger. In girls, headaches can be related to menstruation and the oral contraceptive pill.

Uncommon forms of migraine
These include

- *Familial hemiplegic migraine* – caused by a calcium channel defect, dominantly inherited.
- *Sporadic hemiplegic migraine*.
- *Basilar-type migraine* – vomiting with nystagmus and/or cerebellar signs.
- *Periodic syndromes* – often precursors of migraine and include:
  - *cyclical vomiting* – recurrent stereotyped episodes of vomiting and intense nausea associated with pallor and lethargy. The child is well in between episodes
  - *abdominal migraine* – an idiopathic recurrent disorder characterised by episodic midline abdominal pain in bouts lasting 1–72 hours. Pain is moderate to severe in intensity and associated with vasomotor symptoms, nausea, and vomiting. The child is well in between episodes
  - *benign paroxysmal vertigo of childhood* – is characterized by recurrent brief episodes of vertigo occurring without warning and resolving spontaneously in otherwise healthy children. Between episodes, neurological examination, audiometric and vestibular function tests are normal.

Secondary headaches

Raised intracranial pressure and space-occupying lesions

Headaches often raise the fear of brain tumours; this may well be the reason for parents to consult a doctor. Headaches due to a space-occupying lesion are worse when lying down and morning vomiting is characteristic. The headaches may also cause night-time waking. There is often a change in mood, personality, or educational performance. Other features suggestive of a space-occupying lesion are:

- visual field defects – from lesions pressing on the optic pathways, e.g. craniopharyngioma (a pituitary tumour)
- cranial nerve abnormalities causing diplopia, new-onset squint or facial nerve palsy. The VIth (abducens) cranial nerve has a long intracranial course and is often affected when there is raised pressure, resulting in a squint with diplopia and inability to abduct the eye beyond the midline. It is a false localising sign. Other nerves are affected depending on the site of lesion, e.g. pontine lesions may affect the VIIth (facial) cranial nerve and cause a facial nerve palsy
- abnormal gait
- torticollis (tilting of the head)
- growth failure, e.g. craniopharyngioma or hypothalamic lesion
- papilloedema – a late feature
- cranial bruits – may be heard in arteriovenous malformations but these lesions are rare
- early or late puberty.

Summary

Headaches

Headaches history

Premonitory symptoms, aura, character, position, radiation, frequency, duration, triggers, relieving and exacerbating factors?
Special consideration:
Triggers – stress, relaxation, food, menstruation?
Emotional or behavioural problems at home or school?
Vision checked – refractive error?
Head trauma?
Alcohol, solvent, or drug abuse?
Analgesia over-use?

Headache type

Tension-type headache – constriction band.
Migraine without aura – bilateral or unilateral, pulsatile, gastrointestinal disturbance, e.g. nausea, vomiting, abdominal pain, photophobia. Lies in quiet, dark place. Relieved by sleep
Migraine with aura – preceded by aura (visual, sensory or motor), premonitory symptoms
Mixed-type headaches – common

Red flag symptoms – space-occupying lesion

Headache – worse lying down or with coughing and straining
Headache – wakes up child (different from headache on awakening, not uncommon in migraine)
Associated confusion, and/or morning or persistent nausea or vomiting
Recent change in personality, behaviour or educational performance

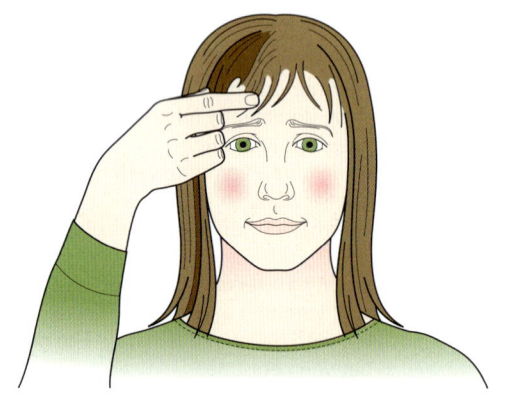

Red flag physical signs – space-occupying lesion

- Growth failure
- Visual field defects – craniopharyngioma
- Squint
- Cranial nerve abnormality
- Torticollis
- Abnormal coordination – for cerebellar lesions
- Gait – upper motor neurone or cerebellar signs
- Fundi – papilloedema
- Bradycardia
- Cranial bruits – arteriovenous malformation

Other physical signs

Visual acuity – for refractive errors
Sinus tenderness – for sinusitis
Pain on chewing – temporomandibular joint malocclusion
Blood pressure – for hypertension

Investigations

Only consider these if Red Flag features

Medication overuse headache

Patients with primary headaches, especially migraine, are at risk of developing a rebound "chronic daily headache" (technically, headache on 15 or more days a month) if they have a bad patch and use acute analgesics or triptans on more than 2 days a week. Withdrawing the offending medication will resolve this in about 2 weeks.

Other causes

These are listed in Box 29.1.

Management

The mainstay of management is a thorough history and examination with detailed explanation and advice. Imaging is unnecessary in the absence of any 'Red flag' features.

Efforts should be made to make a specific headache diagnosis and children and parents informed that recurrent headaches are common. For most there are good and bad spells, with periods of months or even years in between the bad spells, and that they cause no long-term harm. Written child-friendly information for the family to take home is helpful. Children should be advised on how to live with and control the headaches, rather than allowing the headaches to dominate their lives. There is nothing medicine can do to cure this problem but there is much it can offer to make the bad spells more bearable.

Rescue treatments

- Analgesia – paracetamol and nonsteroidal anti-inflammatory drugs (NSAIDs), taken as early as possible in an individual troublesome episode.
- Antiemetics – prochlorperazine or cyclizine, for nausea.
- Triptans (serotonin (5-HT$_1$) agonists), e.g. sumatriptan. A nasal preparation of this is particularly useful in children, early in a migraine attack, together with a NSAID or paracetamol.
- Physical treatments such as cold compresses, warm pads, topical forehead balms.

Prophylactic treatments

Where headaches are frequent and intrusive:

- sodium channel blockers – topiramate or valproate
- beta-blockers – propranolol; contraindicated in asthma
- tricyclics: pizotifen (5-HT$_2$ antagonist) – can cause weight gain and sleepiness, or amitriptyline – can cause dangerous arrhythmias in overdose
- acupuncture.

Psychosocial support

- Psychological support – is it required to ameliorate a particular stressor, e.g. bullying, anxiety over exams, or illness in friends or family?
- Relaxation and other self-regulating techniques, addressing life-style issues: ensuring adequate and regular rest, play, sleep, water, and food.

Seizures

A seizure is a paroxysmal abnormality of motor, sensory, autonomic, and/or cognitive function, due to transient brain dysfunction. The term includes epileptic, syncopal (anoxic), brainstem (hydrocephalic, coning), emotional or functional (psychogenic pseudo-seizures), and as yet undetermined. Regarding seizures as epileptic or non-epileptic will guard against the misdiagnosis of epilepsy, which is common.

Epileptic seizures

What makes a seizure epileptic is the nature of the underlying electrical activity in the brain, especially in the cerebral cortex, so it can sometimes be difficult to tell from a non-epileptic (especially a syncopal seizure) clinically. Epileptic seizures are due to excessive and hypersynchronous electrical activity, typically in neural networks in all or part of the cerebral cortex.

Convulsions

A convulsion is a seizure (epileptic or non-epileptic) with motor components, particularly stiff (tonic), a massive jerk (myoclonic), jerking (clonic), trembling (vibratory), thrashing about (hypermotor); as opposed to a non-convulsive seizure with motor arrest, e.g. an unresponsive stare (as in generalized epileptic absence seizures and some focal epileptic seizures), or drop attack (as in an epileptic atonic seizure).

Epilepsies

An epilepsy is a brain disorder that predisposes the patient to have unprovoked epileptic seizures. Generally, an epilepsy can be recognized after two or more unprovoked epileptic seizures have occurred.

Acute symptomatic epileptic seizures

When epileptic seizures are provoked by an acute brain injury, e.g. from acute cortical ischaemia during arterial ischaemic stroke, or from a cerebral contusion during a traumatic brain injury, or cortical inflammation during meningitis. They do not constitute an epilepsy, even if there were recurrent injuries. These are called acute symptomatic epileptic seizures. The causes of seizures are listed in Box 29.2.

Febrile seizures

A "febrile seizure" or "febrile convulsion" is an epileptic seizure accompanied by a fever in the absence of intracranial infection. These occur in 3% of children, between the ages of 6 months and 6 years. There is a genetic predisposition, with a 10% risk if the child has a first-degree relative with febrile seizures. The seizure usually occurs early in a viral infection when the temperature is rising rapidly. They are usually brief generalized tonic-clonic seizures. About 30–40% will have further febrile seizures. This is more likely

Box 29.2 Causes of seizures

Epilepsies
- **Genetic** (70–80%) – also called "idiopathic", caused by alleles at several loci together rather than a single gene, so inheritance is "complex"
- **Structural, metabolic**
  - Cerebral dysgenesis/malformation
  - Cerebral vascular occlusion
  - Cerebral damage, e.g. congenital infection, hypoxic-ischaemic encephalopathy, intraventricular haemorrhage/ischaemia
  - Cerebral tumour
  - Neurodegenerative disorders
  - Neurocutaneous syndromes e.g. Tuberous Sclerosis

Acute symptomatic seizures
- Due to any cortical brain injury or insult, at the time of the trauma or illness
  - Stroke, traumatic brain injury, intracranial infection
  - Hypoglycaemia, hypocalcaemia, hypomagnesaemia, hyponatraemia/hypernatraemia,
  - Poisons/toxins

Febrile seizures

Non-epileptic seizures
- **Convulsive syncope**
  - Cardiac syncope e.g. prolonged Q-T syndrome
  - Neurally mediated syncope: cardio-inhibitory e.g. reflex asystolic syncope (reflex anoxic seizures); vasodepressor or mixed (vasovagal syncope)
  - Expiratory apnoea syncope ("blue breath-holding spells")
  - Hypovolaemic syncope e.g. with haemorrhage, dehydration or anaphylaxis
- **Sudden rise in intracranial pressure** e.g. hydrocephalic attack, haemorrhage
- **Sleep disorders** e.g. benign neonatal sleep myoclonus, hypnic jerks
- **Functional/medically unexplained** e.g. dissociative states

---

the younger the child, the shorter the duration of illness before the seizure, the lower the temperature at the time of seizure and if there is a positive family history.

Simple febrile seizures do not cause brain damage; the child's subsequent intellectual performance is the same as in children who did not experience a febrile seizure. There is a 1–2% chance of subsequentally developing an epilepsy, similar to the risk for all children.

However, complex febrile seizures; i.e. those which are focal, prolonged, or repeated in the same illness, have an increased risk of 4–12% of subsequent epilepsy.

The acute management of seizures is described in Chapter 6. Examination should focus on the cause of the fever, which is usually a viral illness, but a bacterial infection including meningitis should always be considered. The classical features of meningitis such as neck stiffness and photophobia may not be as apparent in children less than 18 months of age, so an infection screen (including blood cultures, urine culture, and lumbar puncture for cerebrospinal fluid) may be necessary. If the child is unconscious or has cardiovascular instability, lumbar puncture is contraindicated and antibiotics should be started immediately.

Parents need reassurance and information. Advice sheets are usually given to parents. Antipyretics may be given but have not been shown to prevent febrile seizures. The family should be taught the first aid management of seizures. If there is a history of prolonged seizures (>5 min), rescue therapy with buccal midazolam can be supplied. Oral prophylactic antiepileptic drugs are not used as they do not reduce the recurrence rate of seizures, and have a relatively high risk of adverse effects. An EEG is not indicated as it does not predict seizure recurrence.

Summary

Febrile seizures
- Affect 3% of children; have a genetic predisposition.
- Occur between 6 months and 6 years of age.
- Are usually brief, generalised tonic-clonic seizures occurring with a rapid rise in fever.
- If a bacterial infection, especially meningitis, is present, it needs to be identified and treated.
- Advise family about management of seizures, consider rescue therapy.
- If simple – does not affect intellectual performance or risk of developing epilepsy.
- If complex, 4–12% risk of subsequent epilepsy.

Paroxysmal disorders

There is a broad differential diagnosis for children with paroxysmal disorders ('funny turns'). Epilepsy is a clinical diagnosis based on the history from eyewitnesses and the child's own account. If available, videos of the seizures can be of great help. The diagnostic questions are: was it an epileptic seizure, and if so does the child have an epilepsy? Epilepsies can be further delineated as outlined below. If non-epileptic or uncertain, further delineation of the nature of the seizure or paroxysmal event is required (Fig. 29.1). The most common pitfall is that of syncope leading to an anoxic (non-epileptic) tonic-clonic convulsive seizure.

The key to the diagnosis lies in a detailed history, review of video if available, which, together with the

Causes of paroxysmal disorders ('funny turns')

'Blue breath-holding' spells — Temper

Occur in some toddlers when they are upset. The child cries, holds his breath in expiration and goes blue. Sometimes children will briefly lose consciousness but rapidly recover fully. Drug therapy is unhelpful. Attacks resolve spontaneously, but behaviour modification therapy with distraction, may help.

Reflex asystolic syncope — Head trauma, Cold food, Fright, Fever

Also called reflex anoxic seizures. Occur in infants or toddlers. Many have a first-degree relative with a history of faints. Commonest triggers are pain or discomfort, particularly from minor head trauma, cold food (such as ice-cream or cold drinks), fright or fever. Some children with febrile seizures may have experienced this phenomenon. After the triggering event, the child becomes very pale and falls to the floor. The hypoxia may induce a generalised tonic–clonic seizure. The episodes are due to cardiac asystole from vagal inhibition. The seizure is brief and the child rapidly recovers. Ocular compression under controlled conditions often leads to asystole and paroxysmal slow-wave discharge on the EEG.

Syncope (transient loss of consciousness)

Children may faint if in a hot and stuffy environment, on standing for long periods, or from fear. Clonic movements lasting a few seconds are common.

Migraine

May sometimes lead to paroxysmal headache involving unsteadiness or light-headedness as well as the more common visual or gastrointestinal disturbance. In some young people these episodes occur without headache.

Benign paroxysmal vertigo

This is characterised by recurrent episodes of vertigo, lasting from one to several minutes, associated with nystagmus, unsteadiness or even falling. It is a primary headache disorder of childhood occasionally due to a viral labyrinthitis.

Other causes — Prolonged QT interval

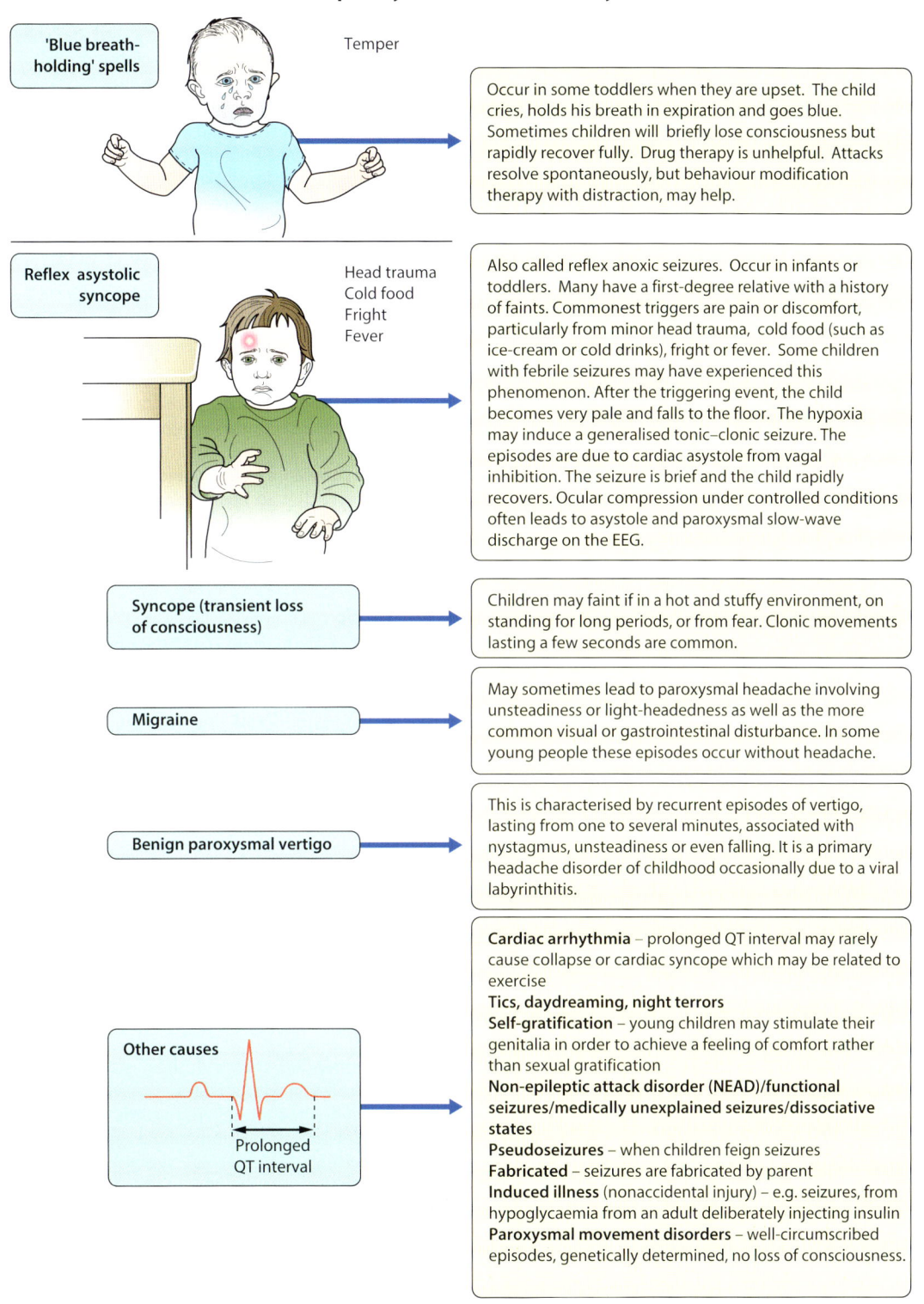

Cardiac arrhythmia – prolonged QT interval may rarely cause collapse or cardiac syncope which may be related to exercise
Tics, daydreaming, night terrors
Self-gratification – young children may stimulate their genitalia in order to achieve a feeling of comfort rather than sexual gratification
Non-epileptic attack disorder (NEAD)/functional seizures/medically unexplained seizures/dissociative states
Pseudoseizures – when children feign seizures
Fabricated – seizures are fabricated by parent
Induced illness (nonaccidental injury) – e.g. seizures, from hypoglycaemia from an adult deliberately injecting insulin
Paroxysmal movement disorders – well-circumscribed episodes, genetically determined, no loss of consciousness.

Figure 29.1 Causes of 'funny turns'.

past history and clinical examination, will lead to a diagnosis of "epilepsy", acute symptomatic or febrile seizure, or non-epileptic seizure. Interictal EEG is useful in categorizing an epilepsy once diagnosed. Ictal EEG can be helpful in difficult to diagnose cases when seizures are frequent enough to capture or can be triggered.

Transient loss of consciousness is most commonly due to syncope, which is caused by a transient impairment of brain oxygen delivery, generally due to impaired cerebral perfusion (see Chapter 18).

Summary

Blue breath-holding spells (expiratory apnoea syncope) and reflex asystolic syncope (reflex anoxic seizures)
In toddlers:
- "blue breath-holding" spells – precipitated by anger or crying and cannot catch his breath which is stuck in expiration, goes blue, stiff then limp, with rapid recovery
- reflex asystolic syncope – precipitated by sudden surprising pain, stops breathing, goes pale, stiff with brief convulsion sometimes, rapid recovery, or if severe sleeps for an hour or more
- other non-epileptic paroxysmal disorders: see Fig. 29.1.

Epilepsies of childhood

Epilepsy has an incidence of about 0.05% (less common during first year of life) and a prevalence of 0.5%. This means that most large secondary schools will have about six children with an epilepsy. Most epilepsy is "genetic" (i.e. "idiopathic") with complex inheritance, but other causes of seizures are listed in Box 29.2.

An international classification of epileptic seizures and epilepsies is used, (International League Against Epilepsy (ILAE) 2011–2013 Classifications). This broadly classifies seizures as either:

- *generalized* – discharge arises from both hemispheres, includes absence, myoclonic, tonic, tonic-clonic, atonic; may be in combination or in sequence
- *focal* – where seizures arise from one or part of one hemisphere.

Focal seizure manifestations will depend on the part of the brain where the discharge originates and moves to:

- *frontal* seizures – involve the motor or pre-motor cortex. May lead to clonic movements, which may travel proximally (Jacksonian march), or a tonic seizure with both upper limbs raised high for several seconds. Asymmetrical tonic seizures can be seen, which may be bizarre and hypermotor and can be mistaken for non-epileptic seizures
- *temporal lobe* seizures– may result in strange warning feelings or aura with smell and taste abnormalities and distortions of sound and shape. Lip-smacking, plucking at one's clothing, and walking in a non-purposeful manner (automatisms) may be seen, following spread to the pre-motor cortex. Déjà-vu feelings are described (intense feelings of having been in the same situation before). Consciousness can be impaired and the seizures are usually longer than absence seizures
- *occipital* seizures – cause stereotyped visual hallucinations
- *parietal lobe* seizures – cause contralateral dysaesthesias (altered sensation), or distorted body image.

In focal seizures, the level of consciousness may be retained, consciousness may be lost, or the seizure may evolve to a secondarily generalised tonic-clonic seizure.

In many children, especially under 5 years old, it may be unclear whether an epileptic seizure is generalised or focal.

The main seizure types are summarised in Fig. 29.2 and the epilepsies in Table 29.1.

Diagnosis

The diagnosis of an epilepsy is primarily based on a detailed history from the child and eyewitnesses, substantiated by a video if available. This is increasingly provided on mobile phones. Particular attention is focussed on any specific triggers and if the child has any impairments, as there may be educational, psychological, or social problems. Clinical examination should include checking for skin markers for a neurocutaneous syndrome or neurological abnormalities. Although epilepsy is usually genetic (idiopathic), it may be the presentation or a complication of an underlying neurological disorder.

Investigation

Remember not all seizures are epileptic!

ECG

It is recommended that a 12-lead standard ECG is done in all children with seizures, especially convulsive seizures, even when an epilepsy seems most likely, as the consequences of missing convulsive syncope due to an arrhythmia, e.g. long-QT syndrome, can be an avoidable fatality (See Ch. 18).

EEG (electroencephalogram)

An inter-ictal EEG is indicated whenever an epilepsy is diagnosed. It can help categorize the epilepsy type and severity. If seizures are frequent then an ictal EEG can make the diagnosis, e.g. in suspected childhood absence epilepsy and suspected infantile spasms (West syndrome). If the standard interictal EEG is normal, a sleep or sleep-deprived record can be helpful. Additional techniques are 24 hour ambulatory EEG or a 5-day video-telemetry EEG. For assessment prior to surgery, more invasive techniques such as subdural electrodes can be used.

Epileptic seizure types

Generalised seizures

Onset in both hemisphere

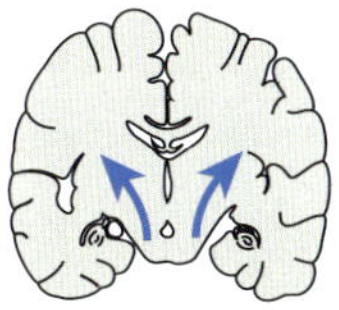

In generalised seizures, there is:
- loss of consciousness if > 3 seconds duration
- no warning
- symmetrical seizure
- bilaterally synchronous seizure discharge on EEG

Absence seizures → Transient loss of consciousness, with an abrupt onset and termination, unaccompanied by motor phenomena except for some flickering of the eyelids and minor alteration in muscle tone. Absences can often be precipitated by hyperventilation

Myoclonic seizures → Brief, often repetitive, jerking movements of the limbs, neck or trunk. Non-epileptic myoclonic movements are also seen physiologically in hiccoughs (myoclonus of the diaphragm) or on passing through stage II sleep (sleep myoclonus)

Tonic seizures → Generalised increase in tone

Tonic–clonic seizures → Rhythmical contraction of muscle groups following the tonic phase.
In the rigid tonic phase, children may fall to the ground, sometimes injuring themselves. They do not breathe and become cyanosed. This is followed by the clonic phase, with jerking of the limbs. Breathing is irregular, cyanosis persists and saliva may accumulate in the mouth. There may be biting of the tongue and incontinence of urine. The seizure usually lasts from a few seconds to minutes, followed by unconsciousness or deep sleep for up to several hours

Atonic seizures → Often combined with a myoclonic jerk, followed by a transient loss of muscle tone causing a sudden fall to the floor or drop of the head

Focal seizures

Onset in neural network limited to one cerebral hemisphere

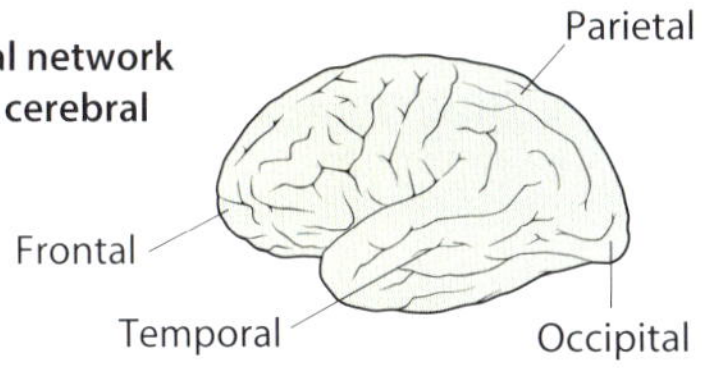

Parietal, Frontal, Temporal, Occipital

Focal seizures:
- originate in a relatively small group of dysfunctional neurones in one of the cerebral hemispheres
- may be heralded by an aura (the sensory symptoms) which reflects the site of origin
- may or may not be associated with change in consciousness or evolve to generalised tonic-clonic seizure

Focal seizures → Frontal seizures – motor phenomena
Temporal lobe seizures – auditory or sensory (smell or taste) phenomena
Occipital – positive or negative visual phenomena
Parietal lobe seizures – contralateral altered sensation (dysaesthesia)

Figure 29.2 Epileptic seizure types.

Brain imaging

- *Structural.* MRI and CT brain scans are generally required routinely for childhood epilepsies unless there is a characteristic history of childhood absence epilepsy, juvenile absence epilepsy, juvenile myoclonic epilepsy, and childhood rolandic epilepsy. MRI fluid-attenuated inversion recovery (FLAIR) sequences are better at detecting mesial temporal sclerosis in temporal lobe epilepsy, which can sometimes be surgically cured.
- *Functional.* While it is not always possible to see structural lesions, techniques have advanced to allow functional imaging to detect areas of abnormal metabolism suggestive of epileptogenic zones. These include PET (positron emission tomography) and SPECT (single photon emission computed tomography), which use isotopes and ligands injected and taken up by metabolically active cells. Both can be used between seizures to detect areas of hypometabolism in epileptogenic lesions. Ictal SPECT can locate areas of hypermetabolism during epileptic seizures. They are used in the work up of patients for possible epilepsy surgery.

Other investigations

Metabolic investigations will be indicated if there is developmental arrest or regression, or seizures are related to feeds or fasting, and should be considered in epilepsies (i.e. not including febrile seizures) starting in the first 2 years of life. Genetic tests are becoming

Table 29.1 Some epilepsy syndromes – arranged by age of onset

Name	Age of onset	Seizure pattern	Comments
Infantile spasms (West syndrome)	3–12 months	Violent flexor spasms of the head, trunk, and limbs followed by extension of the arms, last 1–2 s, often multiple bursts of 20–30, often on waking or many times a day. May be misinterpreted as colic. Social interaction often deteriorates – a useful marker in the history	Most have underlying neurological cause. EEG – hypsarrhythmia (Fig. 29.3). Treatment is vigabatrin and/or corticosteroids; good initial response in 60–70%, but unwanted side effects of therapy, and relapses common. Most will lose skills and develop learning disability and continuing epilepsy.
Lennox–Gastaut syndrome	1–3 years	Multiple seizure types, but mostly atonic, atypical (subtle) absences, and tonic seizures in sleep. Also neurodevelopmental arrest or regression and behaviour disorder.	Many causes, and often other complex neurological problems or history of infantile spasms. EEG shows slow generalized spike and wave (1–3 Hz). Prognosis is poor.
Childhood absence epilepsy	4–12 years	Momentary unresponsive stare with motor arrest, may twitch their eyelids or a hand or mouth minimally. Sudden onset, lasts only a few seconds (<30 s). Child has no recall except realises they have missed something and may look puzzled or say 'pardon' on regaining consciousness. Developmentally normal but can interfere with schooling. Accounts for only 2% of childhood epilepsy.	Two-thirds are female. Episodes can be induced by hyperventilation blowing on a piece of paper or windmill for 2–3 min; useful during EEG. The EEG shows fast generalised spike and wave (3–4 Hz) discharges, bilaterally synchronous during and sometimes between absences (Fig. 29.4). Prognosis good with 80% remission in adolescence; a few evolve into juvenile absence or juvenile myoclonic epilepsy.
Benign rolandic epilepsy (Benign epilepsy with centro-temporal spikes)	4–10 years	Tonic-clonic seizures in sleep, or simple focal seizures with awareness of abnormal feelings in the tongue and distortion of the face (supplied by the rolandic (centro-temporal) area of the brain).	15% of all childhood epilepsies. EEG shows focal sharp waves from the rolandic area. Important to recognise as relatively benign and may not require AEDs. Remits in adolescence.
Panayiotopoulos syndrome (Early-onset benign occipital epilepsy)	1–5 years	Autonomic features with vomiting and unresponsive staring in sleep, with head and eye deviation, progressing sometimes to a convulsive seizure.	Comprises 5% of childhood epilepsies. EEG shows posterior focal sharp waves and occipital discharges when eyes are shut. Remits in childhood. Some have specific learning difficulties.
Juvenile absence epilepsy	10–20 years	Absences, and generalised tonic-clonic seizures, often with photosensitivity. Learning is unimpaired.	Characteristic EEG. Response to treatment is usually good but lifelong. Remission unlikely.
Juvenile myoclonic epilepsy	10–20 years	Myoclonic seizures, generalized tonic-clonic seizures, and absences may occur, mostly shortly after waking. A typical history is throwing drinks or cereal about in the morning as myoclonus occurs at this time. Learning is unimpaired.	Characteristic EEG. Response to treatment is usually good but lifelong. Remission unlikely

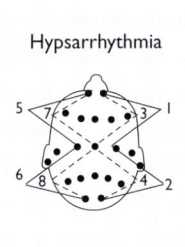

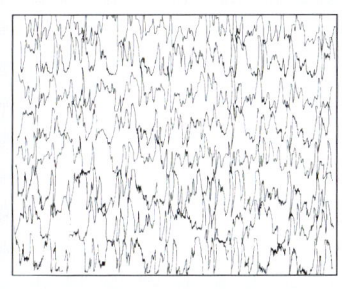

Figure 29.3 EEG of hypsarrhythmia in infantile spasms (West syndrome). There is a chaotic background of slow-wave activity with sharp multifocal components.

Figure 29.4 EEG in a typical absence seizure in childhood absence epilepsy. There is a three per second spike and wave discharge which is bilaterally synchronous during, and sometimes between, attacks.

increasingly useful, especially in intractable epilepsies with developmental arrest or delay ("epileptic encephalopathies").

Management

Management begins with diagnosis, but this is often uncertain initially. So the uncertainty needs explaining and a plan put in place to ensure the child's safety until more information, e.g. from investigations or parental video clips is available. Once diagnosed, a clear explanation of the diagnosis and advice to help adjustment to the condition is needed. A specialist epilepsy nurse may assist families by providing education and continuing advice on lifestyle issues. The decision whether to treat or not is related to the risk of recurrence, how dangerous or impairing, and how upsetting further seizures would be, in the context of the child or young person's life. It is common practice not to institute treatment for typical childhood rolandic epilepsy, and treatment of childhood absence epilepsy is aimed at maximizing their educational potential and supporting their social development.

Antiepileptic drug therapy

Principles governing use are:

- not all children with epileptic seizures require antiepileptic drug (AED) therapy. The decision should be based on the seizure type, epilepsy type, frequency, and the social and educational consequences of the seizures set against the possibility of unwanted effects of the AED
- choose an appropriate AED for the seizure and epilepsy. Inappropriate AEDs may be detrimental, e.g. carbamazepine can make absence and myoclonic seizures worse
- monotherapy at the minimum dosage to prevent the seizures without adverse effects is the desired goal, although in practice more than one AED may be required
- all AEDs have potential unwanted effects and these should be discussed with the child and parent
- AED levels are not measured routinely, but may be useful to check for concordance (adherence) or to see if a dose increase could be considered if a high dose is not working
- children with prolonged epileptic seizures (convulsive epileptic seizures with loss of consciousness >5 min) are given rescue therapy to keep with them. This is usually buccal midazolam
- AED therapy may be discontinued after 2 years free of seizures, but should usually be continued indefinitely in young people with juvenile absence epilepsy or juvenile myoclonic epilepsy.

Guidance regarding treatment options for different seizure types and epilepsies are shown in Table 29.2. Common unwanted effects of AEDs are shown in Table 29.3.

Table 29.2 Choice of antiepileptic drugs (NICE guidelines 2014)

Seizure type	First-line	Second-line
Generalised		
Tonic-clonic	Valproate, carbamazepine*, lamotrigine	Clobazam, levetiracetam, topiramate
Absence	Valproate, ethosuximide, lamotrigine	Clobazam, levetiracetam, topiramate
Myoclonic	Valproate, levetiracitam, topiramate	Clobazam, piracitam
Focal seizures	Carbamazepine, valproate, levetiracetam, lamotrigine	Clobazam, topiramate, gabapentin*, tiagabine*

*Avoid with absence seizures, myoclonic seizures or juvenile myoclonic epilepsy.

Table 29.3 Common or important unwanted effects of antiepileptic drugs

Drug	Adverse-effects
Valproate	Weight gain, hair loss, teratogenic, rare idiosyncratic liver failure
Carbamazepine	Rash, hyponatraemia, ataxia, liver enzyme induction, can interfere with other medication including oral contraception
Lamotrigine	Rash, insomnia, ataxia
Ethosuximide	Nausea and vomiting
Levetiracetam	Irritability
Gabapentin	Insomnia
Topiramate	Weight loss, depression, parasthesia
Vigabatrin	Irritability, restriction of visual fields, which has limited its use to infantile spasms and tuberous sclerosis

All the above drugs may cause drowsiness.

Other treatment options

In children with intractable epilepsies, there are a number of other treatment options.

- *Ketogenic (low-carb, fat-based) diets* may be helpful in some children.
- *Vagal nerve stimulation*, delivered using externally programmable stimulation of a wire implanted around the afferent (left) vagal nerve, may be helpful in some children.
- Epilepsy *surgery*. Cessation of seizures and AED therapy may be achieved in some children whose epilepsy has a well-localised structural cause or epileptogenic zone, as demonstrated by good concordance between ictal EEG, MRI, and functional imaging findings. The main procedure is temporal lobectomy for mesial temporal sclerosis, but other procedures include hemispherotomy (disconnection of the hemisphere) and other focal resections.

Advice and prognosis

The aim is to promote independence and confidence. Some children with epilepsy and their families need psychological help to adjust to the condition. The school needs to be aware of the child's problem and teachers advised on the management of seizures. Unrecognized absences may interfere with learning, which is an indication for being vigilant about 'odd episodes' which may be epileptic seizures. Relatively few restrictions are required, but situations where having a seizure could lead to injury or death should be avoided. This includes avoiding deep baths (showers are preferable) and not swimming unsupervised.

For adolescents, there will be issues to discuss around driving (only after 1 year free of seizures), contraception and pregnancy. There may also be issues with concordance (adherence) and the precipitation of seizures by alcohol and poor sleep routines.

Sudden unexpected death in epilepsy, (SUDEP), is very rare in childhood, but may be discussed and its rarity emphasised. Information is available from self-help groups and organisations such as Epilepsy Action.

Children with epilepsy do less well educationally, with social outcomes and with future employment than those with other chronic illnesses such as diabetes.

Two-thirds of children with epilepsy go to a mainstream school, but some require educational help for associated learning difficulties. One-third attend a special school, but they often have multiple disabilities and their epilepsy is part of a severe brain disorder. A few children require residential schooling where there are facilities and expertise in monitoring and treating intractable epilepsies.

Status epilepticus

Status epilepticus, an epileptic seizure lasting 30 minutes or repeated epileptic seizures for 30 minutes without recovery of consciousness. It is described in Chapter 6 Paediatric emergencies.

> **Summary**
>
> **Epilepsy**
> - Affects 1 in 200 children.
> - Classified according to seizure type, epilepsy type, and underlying aetiology.
> - An inter-ictal EEG is performed whenever an epilepsy is diagnosed to help categorize the epilepsy type. An ictal EEG may make the diagnosis.
> - Antiepileptic drug therapy should be considered where the seizures are intrusive, and selected according to seizure and epilepsy type. Monotherapy is given if possible and chosen for the least potential adverse effects.
> - Requires liaison with the school about how to manage a seizure and avoiding situations which could lead to injury.

Motor disorders

Movement is governed by three main cerebral control centres. Patterns of information, modulated by afferent sensory information (joint position, crude touch, visual, auditory and vestibular), pass down the brainstem and spinal cord, through synapses in the anterior horns and along peripheral nerves to the target muscles. In clinical practice the first question to ask when seeing a child with a motor disorder is whether this is a central

Table 29.4 Causes of movement disorders

Corticospinal (pyramidal) tract disorders	Basal ganglia disorders	Cerebellar disorders
Cerebral dysgenesis, e.g. neuronal migration disorder	Acquired brain injury: – Acute and profound hypoxia-ischaemia – Carbon monoxide poisoning – Post-cardiopulmonary bypass chorea	Acute – medication and drugs, including alcohol and solvent abuse
Global hypoxia–ischaemia		Postviral – particularly varicella infection
Arterial ischaemic stroke		
Cerebral tumour		Posterior fossa lesions or tumours, e.g. medulloblastoma
Acute disseminated encephalomyelitis	Post-streptococcal chorea (rheumatic fever)	Genetic and degenerative disorders, e.g. Friedreich ataxia and ataxia telangiectasia
Postictal paresis	Mitochondrial cytopathies	
Hemiplegic migraine	Wilson disease	
	Huntington disease	
	Vitamin E deficiency	
	Pontocerebellar hypoplasia	

or a peripheral nervous system disorder. The pattern of movement usually gives the answer.

Central motor disorders

The three central movement control centres are:
- *Motor cortex*, lying along the precentral gyrus (the homunculus reflects the body upside down, legs superiorly and face inferiorly, just above the Sylvian fissure, with large areas to govern fine movements of the tongue, fingers and thumb). Information from here passes down the corticospinal (pyramidal) tracts to link with the basal ganglia.
- *Basal ganglia*, deep grey matter structures, store patterns of movement so that we need not put conscious effort into every movement we make.
- *Cerebellum*, controls posture, balance, coordination and speech.

Disorders of these central movement control centres are:
- *Corticospinal (pyramidal) tract disorders* – there is weakness with a pattern of adduction at the shoulder, flexion at the elbow and pronation of the forearm; adduction and internal rotation at the hip, flexion at hip and knee, and plantar flexion at the ankle with brisk hyper-reflexia and extensor plantar reflexes. Fine finger movement will be lost.
- *Basal ganglia disorders* – will lead either to difficulty initiating movement, with fluctuating (largely increased) tone – a 'dystonia' or a 'dyskinesia' where packets of movement information are released to give jerky movement (chorea) or writhing movement (athetosis).
- *Cerebellar disorders* – will lead to difficulty holding a posture; past-pointing (dysmetria); poor alternating movements (dysdiadochokinesis). The gait is wide-based and ataxic. Posterior-column sensory pathway problems may give a similar clinical picture (but with even worse ataxia when the eyes are closed), but are much rarer in childhood. Associated nystagmus and a characteristic scanning dysarthria may be seen. Causes of these disorders are listed in Table 29.4.

Cerebral palsy

This is described in Chapter 4. Developmental problems and the child with special needs.

Peripheral motor disorders: the neuromuscular disorders

Any part of the lower motor neurone pathway can be affected in a neuromuscular disorder, so that anterior horn cell disorders, peripheral neuropathies, disorders of neuromuscular transmission and primary muscle diseases can all occur. The causes of neuromuscular disorders are shown in Fig. 29.5. The key clinical feature of a neuromuscular disorder is weakness, which may be progressive or static. Affected children may present with:

- hypotonia (floppiness)
- delayed motor milestones
- muscle weakness
- unsteady/abnormal gait
- fatiguability
- muscle cramps (suggesting a metabolic myopathy).

History and examination may provide useful clues. Children with myopathy often show a waddling gait

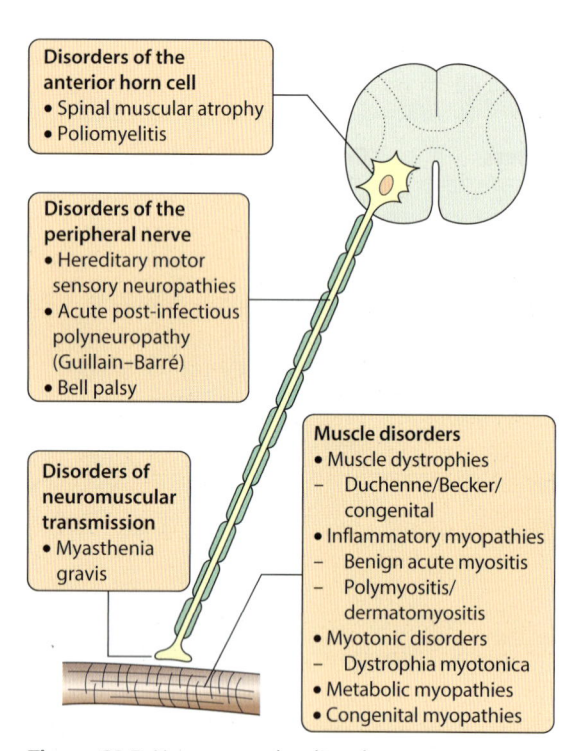

Figure 29.5 Neuromuscular disorders.

Disorders of the anterior horn cell
- Spinal muscular atrophy
- Poliomyelitis

Disorders of the peripheral nerve
- Hereditary motor sensory neuropathies
- Acute post-infectious polyneuropathy (Guillain–Barré)
- Bell palsy

Disorders of neuromuscular transmission
- Myasthenia gravis

Muscle disorders
- Muscle dystrophies
  - Duchenne/Becker/congenital
- Inflammatory myopathies
  - Benign acute myositis
  - Polymyositis/dermatomyositis
- Myotonic disorders
  - Dystrophia myotonica
- Metabolic myopathies
- Congenital myopathies

be more consistent with a disorder of the motor end-plate/neuromuscular junction e.g. myasthenia gravis.

It is usually difficult to differentiate a myopathy from a neuropathy on clinical grounds but there are some broad points to look for:

- anterior horn cell – there are signs of denervation: weakness, loss of reflexes, fasciculation and wasting as the nerve supply to the muscle fails
- neuropathy – often longer nerves affected. Motor neuropathy will give weakness, sensory neuropathy will give impaired perception of pain and temperature or touch, with a loss of reflexes in either
- myopathy – there is weakness (often proximal), wasting, gait disturbance
- neuromuscular junction – as end-plate acetylcholine stores become depleted, there is diurnal worsening through the day, leading to fatiguability.

Investigations

Myopathy:

- Plasma creatine kinase – markedly elevated in Duchenne and Becker muscular dystrophy, congenital muscular dystrophy, many limb girdle muscular dystrophies and inflammatory myopathies.
- Muscle biopsy, usually taken with an open technique – modern histochemical techniques often enable a definitive diagnosis.
- DNA testing – to identify abnormal genes.
- Ultrasound and MRI of muscles – used to diagnose and monitor progress.

Neuropathy:

- Nerve conduction studies – to identify delayed motor and sensory nerve conduction velocities seen in neuropathy.
- DNA testing – for abnormal genes.
- Nerve biopsy – occasionally performed by removing a segment of sural nerve in the leg.
- EMG (electromyography) helps in differentiating myopathic from neuropathic disorders, e.g. fatiguability on repetitive nerve stimulation in myasthenia.

Diagnosis of neuromuscular disorders has been made easier by advances in genetic (DNA) testing, e.g. for spinal muscular atrophy (SMA), Duchenne muscular dystrophy, myotonic dystrophy, the congenital muscular dystrophies, limb girdle muscular dystrophies and hereditary neuropathies.

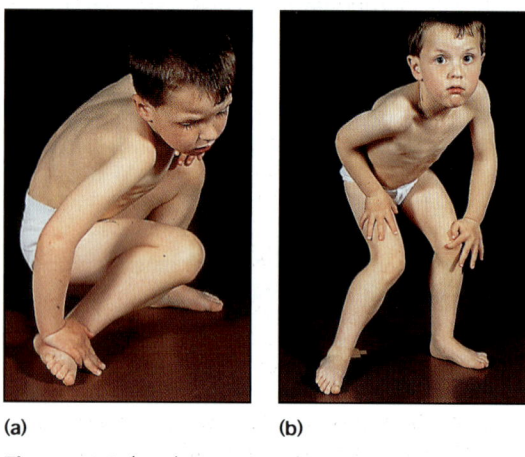

(a) (b)

Figure 29.6 (a, b) Gowers' sign. The child needs to turn prone to rise (the key, early feature of Gowers' sign), then uses his hands to climb up on his knees before standing (late feature), because of poor hip girdle fixation and/or proximal muscle weakness. Any child continuing to turn prone to rise after 3 years of age is likely to have a neuromuscular condition.

or positive Gowers' sign suggestive of proximal muscle weakness. Gowers' sign is the need to turn prone to rise to a standing from a supine position. This is normal until the age of 3 years. It is only when children have become very weak that they 'climb up the legs with the hands' to gain the standing position (Fig. 29.6). A pattern of more distal wasting and weakness, particularly in the presence of pes cavus, suggests a hereditary motor sensory neuropathy. Increasing fatiguability through the day, often with ophthalmoplegia and ptosis, would

Disorders of the anterior horn cell

Presentation is with weakness, wasting and absent reflexes. Poliomyelitis has almost been eradicated globally by immunization.

Spinal muscular atrophy

This is an autosomal recessive degeneration of the anterior horn cells, leading to progressive weakness and wasting of skeletal muscles due to mutations in the

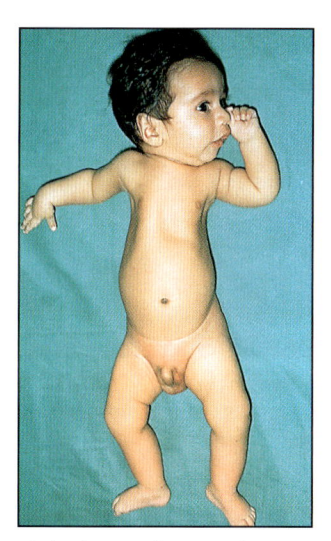

Figure 29.7 Spinal muscular atrophy type 1 (Werdnig–Hoffmann disease) showing proximal muscle wasting, chest deformity from weakness of the intercostal muscles and thighs held abducted because of hypotonia.

survival motor neurone (SMN1) gene. This is the second most common cause of neuromuscular disease in the UK after Duchenne muscular dystrophy. A number of phenotypes are recognised.

Spinal muscular atrophy type 1 (Werdnig–Hoffmann disease)

A very severe progressive disorder presenting from birth to 3 months of age (Fig. 29.7). Diminished fetal movements are often noticed during pregnancy and there may be arthrogryposis (positional deformities of the limbs with contractures of at least two joints) at birth. Typical signs include:

- alert expression
- fasciculation of the tongue
- symmetrical flaccid paralysis
- absent deep tendon reflexes
- intercostal recession
- weakness of bulbar muscles causing weak cry and poor suck with pooling of secretions.

These children never sit unaided. Death is from respiratory failure within about 12 months of age.

There are milder forms of the disorder with a later onset. Children with type 2 spinal muscular atrophy present at age 3 months to 15 months, can sit but never walk independently. Those with the milder type 3 (Kugelberg–Welander) present after 1 year of age and do learn to walk. The most severe form is SMA type 0 and is diagnosed in newborn infants that are born so weak that their survival is limited to only a few weeks.

Peripheral neuropathies

Charcot–Marie–Tooth disease (the hereditary motor sensory neuropathies)

There are many forms of Charcot–Marie–Tooth (CMT) disease, which typically lead to symmetrical, slowly progressive distal muscular wasting. They are caused by mutations in myelin genes. CMT1A accounts for 70–80% and is inherited in an autosomal dominant manner in two thirds, one third developing the mutation de novo. The other types of CMT disease can be inherited by autosomal dominant, recessive or X-linked modes.

Children may present preschool with tripping from bilateral foot drop. Examination shows loss of ankle reflexes progressing to loss of knee reflexes. Pes cavus may be present, the lower limbs being affected more than the upper. Nerve conduction studies show a motor and sensory neuropathy. Affected nerves may be hypertrophic due to demyelination followed by attempts at remyelination. Nerve biopsy typically shows 'onion bulb formation' due to these two processes. The disease is chronic but only rarely do those affected lose the ability to walk. The initial presentation of Friedreich ataxia can be similar.

Guillain–Barré syndrome (acute post-infectious polyneuropathy)

Can occur at any age, and typically presents 2–3 weeks after an upper respiratory tract infection or campylobacter gastroenteritis, with an ascending, progressive, symmetrical weakness over a few days to 2 weeks. There is loss of tendon reflexes and autonomic involvement. Sensory symptoms, usually in the distal limbs or trunk, are less striking than the weakness but can be unpleasant. When present, a bilateral facial weakness is easily missed in young children. Involvement of bulbar muscles leads to difficulty with chewing and swallowing and the risk of aspiration.

Dysautonomia occurs in 70% and manifests as tachycardia, bradycardia and other arrhythmias, hypertension and orthostatic hypotension, urinary retention, ileus and loss of sweating. Hypoventilation can require artificial ventilation, best started before established respiratory failure. The maximum muscle weakness may occur only 2–4 weeks after the onset of illness. Although full recovery can be expected in 90% of cases, this may take up to 2 years.

MRI of the spinal cord (or brain and spinal cord) is the most useful acute investigation, to identify or exclude a spinal cord lesion e.g. a bleed, tumour, or inflammatory transverse myelitis. The CSF white count is not raised, but CSF protein is characteristically markedly raised, but this may not be seen until the second week of illness. Nerve conduction studies typically show reduced velocities but this may not be evident until after the second week.

Management is supportive, particularly of respiration. The disorder is probably due to the formation of antibody attaching itself to protein components of myelin. Corticosteroids have no beneficial effect and may delay recovery. Controlled trials indicate the ventilator-dependent period can be significantly reduced by intravenous immunoglobulin infusion or plasma exchange.

Bell palsy and facial nerve palsies

Bell palsy is an isolated lower motor neurone paresis of the VIIth cranial nerve leading to facial weakness

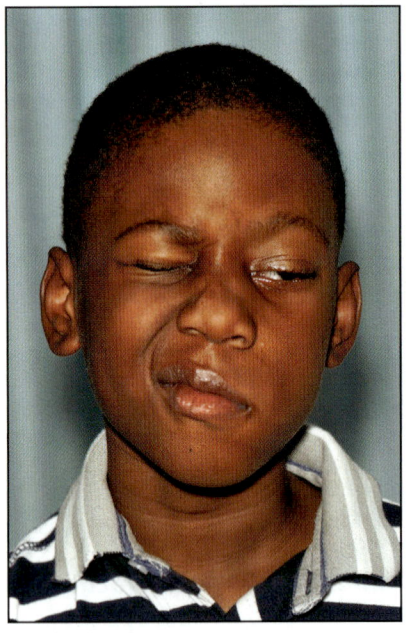

Figure 29.8 Bell palsy. There is left facial weakness of both the upper and lower face.

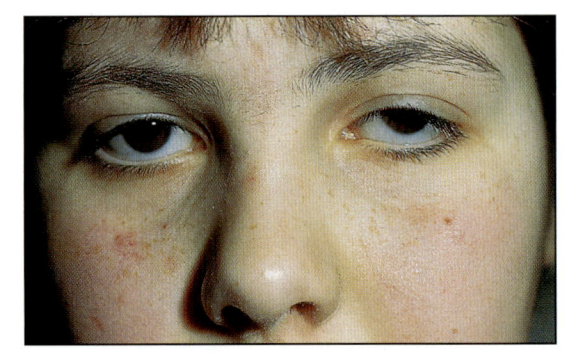

Figure 29.9 Myasthenia gravis showing ptosis from ocular muscle fatigue which improved with edrophonium.

(Fig. 29.8). Although the aetiology is unclear, it may be post-infectious with an association with herpes simplex virus or Lyme disease. The herpes virus may invade the geniculate ganglion and give painful vesicles on the tonsillar fauces and external ear, along with a facial nerve paresis. If herpes is the suspected cause, treatment is with aciclovir.

Corticosteroids can reduce oedema in the facial canal if given during the first week and speed full recovery. Recovery is complete in the majority of cases but may take several months. The main complication is conjunctival infection due to incomplete eye closure on blinking. This may require the eye to be protected with lubricating drops or ointment, a patch or even tarsorrhaphy.

There are important differential diagnoses. If there is also a recent VIth nerve paresis, or ipsilateral cerebellar signs, or contralateral upper motor neurone signs, suspect a brain stem lesion. If there are symptoms of a recent VIIIth nerve paresis, the most likely diagnosis is a compressive lesion in the cerebellopontine angle. Hypertension should be excluded, as there is an association between Bell palsy and coarctation of the aorta and renal failure.

Disorders of neuromuscular transmission

Myasthenia gravis

This presents as abnormal muscle fatiguability which improves with rest or anticholinesterase drugs.

Juvenile myasthenia

This is similar to adult autoimmune myasthenia gravis and is due to binding of antibody to acetylcholine receptors on the postsynaptic membrane of the neuromuscular junction. This reduces the number of functional receptors. Presentation is usually after 10 years of age with ophthalmoplegia and ptosis, loss of facial expression and difficulty chewing (Fig. 29.9). Generalised, especially proximal, weakness may be seen.

Diagnosis is made by observing improvement following the administration of intravenous edrophonium over a few minutes or oral pyridostigmine or neostigmine over days. Identifying acetylcholine receptor antibodies (seen in 60–80%) or, more rarely, anti-MuSK (antimuscle-specific kinase) antibodies will confirm the diagnosis and direct treatment decisions. Treatment is with the choline esterase inhibitors pyridostigmine or neostigmine and immunosuppressive therapy. Immune-modulating drugs such as prednisolone, azathioprine or mycophenolate mofetilis, or even monoclonal antibodies ("biologicals") e.g. rituximab are of value. Thymectomy is indicated if a thymoma is present or in young antibody positive patients with a very acute, severe presentation affecting more than just ocular muscles. Plasma exchange is used for crises.

Congenital myasthenic syndromes

These are rare genetic syndromes which cause neuromuscular junction failure in newborn infants. Features may include ptosis, ophthalmoplegia and bulbar and respiratory muscle weakness and arthrogryposis. These disorders do not always respond to anticholinesterase inhibitors.

Muscle disorders

The muscular dystrophies

This is a group of inherited disorders with progressive muscle degeneration.

Duchenne muscular dystrophy

Duchenne muscular dystrophy is the most common phenotype, affecting 1 in 3000–6000 male infants. It is inherited as an X-linked recessive disorder, although about a third have de novo mutations. It results from a deletion of the gene for dystrophin, which connects the cytoskeleton of a muscle fibre to the surrounding extracellular matrix through the cell membrane.

Where it is deficient, there is an influx of calcium ions, a breakdown of the calcium calmodulin complex and an excess of free radicals, ultimately leading to myofibre necrosis. The plasma creatine kinase (CK) is markedly elevated. Some countries have neonatal screening; affected children are detected by an elevated creatine kinase.

Children present with a waddling gait and/or language delay; they have to mount stairs one by one and run slowly compared with their peers. Although the average age of diagnosis remains 5 years, children often become symptomatic much earlier. They will show Gowers sign (the need to turn prone to rise). There is pseudohypertrophy of the calves because of replacement of muscle fibres by fat and fibrous tissue.

In the early school years, affected boys tend to be slower and clumsier than their peers. The progressive muscle atrophy and weakness means that they are no longer ambulant by the age of about 10–14 years. Life expectancy is reduced to the late twenties from respiratory failure or the associated cardiomyopathy. About one-third of affected children have learning difficulties. Scoliosis is a common complication.

Management
Physiotherapy will help to prevent contractures with the aid of splints. Tendoachilles lengthening and scoliosis surgery may be required. Weakness of intercostal muscles may lead to nocturnal hypoxia. This will present with daytime headache, irritability and loss of appetite. Overnight CPAP (continuous positive airway pressure) or non-invasive positive pressure ventilation, may be provided to improve the quality of life.

Affected children should be reviewed periodically at a specialist regional centre. Ambulant children with Duchenne muscular dystrophy are increasingly treated with corticosteroids to preserve mobility and prevent scoliosis. The precise mechanism by which glucocorticoids help is not known. There is considerable research into exon skipping drugs which may correct the open reading frame of the dystrophin gene. Ataluren is now available for Duchenne boys with a nonsense (stop) mutation (10–15%). This drug allows bypass of the nonsense mutation and production of a small amount of dystrophin.

It is possible to identify female carriers, if they have a mildly raised creatine kinase or if the gene deletion is detected on DNA analysis. Antenatal diagnosis is then possible.

Becker muscular dystrophy
Becker dystrophy is allelic with Duchenne muscular dystrophy (i.e. caused by different mutations in the same gene), but some functional dystrophin is produced. The features are similar to those of Duchenne muscular dystrophy but clinically the disease is milder and progresses more slowly. The average age of onset is 11 years, loss of independent ambulation is in the late twenties, with life expectancy well into middle or old age.

Limb girdle muscular dystrophies
These conditions present with proximal upper and lower limb weakness. Cardiomyopathy and difficulty with breathing may be associated with some. These conditions can have different modes of inheritance. Plasma creatine kinase is usually raised.

Congenital muscular dystrophies
These have autosomal recessive inheritance, and most present at birth or in early infancy with weakness, hypotonia or contractures. Typically the proximal weakness is slowly progressive with a tendency to contracture when the ability to walk is lost. Feeding difficulties and breathing difficulties may occur in some cases. Some may run a more static course. Muscle biopsy shows dystrophic features with a reduction of one of the extracellular matrix proteins such as laminin (most common); or one of several glycosyltransferases. These dystrophies may be linked with central nervous abnormalities, which may result in learning difficulties.

Congenital myopathies
These conditions present at birth or in infancy with defects primarily affecting skeletal muscle fibres, causing muscle weakness and/or hypotonia. They are static or slowly progressive. They are named according to the changes seen on muscle biopsy or electron microscopy. Plasma creatine kinase is normal or only mildly elevated.

Metabolic myopathies
Metabolic conditions can affect muscles, due either to the deposition of storage material or to energy-depleting enzyme deficiencies. Presentation is as a floppy infant or, in older children, with muscle weakness or cramps on exercise. The main causes are:

- glycogen storage disorders (see Ch. 27)
- disorders of lipid metabolism. Fatty acids are important muscle fuel. Fatty acid oxidation occurs in the mitochondria and defects in this pathway can result in weakness. Carnitine palmitoyltransferase II (CPT II) deficiency is the most frequent disorder of lipid metabolism. Defects of fatty acid oxidation can cause a secondary deficiency in carnitine
- mitochondrial cytopathies (see Ch. 9 Genetics and Ch. 27 Inborn errors of metabolism). Rare disorders caused by mutations in the genes for mitochondrial proteins involved in respiratory chain function can be caused by mitochondrial DNA mutations (which are maternally inherited), or nuclear DNA mutations (mostly recessive or X-linked). Myopathy may be the major manifestation or the disorder may be multisystem, with lactic acidosis and encephalopathy. The mutation responsible and mode of inheritance should be determined.

The inflammatory myopathies
Benign acute myositis
This is assumed to be a postviral phenomenon, as it often follows an upper respiratory tract infection and runs a self-limiting course. Pain and weakness occur in affected muscles. Plasma creatine kinase is usually raised.

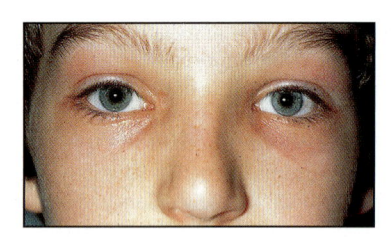

Figure 29.10 Pink-purple rash in dermatomyositis.

Dermatomyositis

This is a systemic illness, probably due to an angiopathy. Onset is usually between 5–10 years of age. This can be acute, but more typically is insidious with fever, misery, and eventually symmetrical muscle weakness, which is mainly proximal. Sometimes pharyngeal muscle involvement affects swallowing. There is also a characteristic violaceous (pink-purple) rash on the eyelids, and periorbital oedema (Fig. 29.10). The rash may also affect the extensor surfaces of joints, e.g. elbow, and with time subcutaneous calcification (calcinosis) can appear. Inflammatory markers (CRP (C-reactive protein), ESR) are sometimes raised, although the creatine kinase is usually raised. Muscle biopsy shows an inflammatory cell infiltrate and atrophy. Physiotherapy is needed to prevent contractures. Corticosteroids are the standard treatment, continued at a tailored dose for 2 years. Other immunosuppressants, e.g. methotrexate, ciclosporin (cyclosporine), may be needed. Mortality is 5–10%. There is a greater risk of cancer in patients with this condition.

Myotonic disorders

Myotonia is delayed relaxation after sustained muscle contraction. It can be identified clinically and by EMG.

Dystrophia myotonica type I

This relatively common illness is dominantly inherited and caused by a nucleotide triplet repeat expansion, CTG in the *DMPK* gene, so this means there can be anticipation through generations, especially when maternally transmitted (see Ch. 9). Newborns with congenital myotonic dystrophy can present with hypotonia and feeding and respiratory difficulties due to muscle weakness. They can have thin ribs, talipes at birth, together with oligohydramnios and reduced fetal movements during pregnancy. It is then useful to examine the mother for myotonia. This manifests as slow release of handshake or difficulty releasing the tightly clasped fist. This may be mild and not previously noticed. Sensitivity is required as diagnosis in a neonate may have repercussions for the family. However, making the diagnosis in family members can help to reduce the risk of potential complications, such as cardiac dysrhythmia and anaesthetic complications. Older children can present with a myopathic facial appearance (Fig. 29.11), learning difficulties and myotonia. Adults develop cataracts and males develop baldness, testicular atrophy and type 2 diabetes. Death is usually due to cardiac conduction defects.

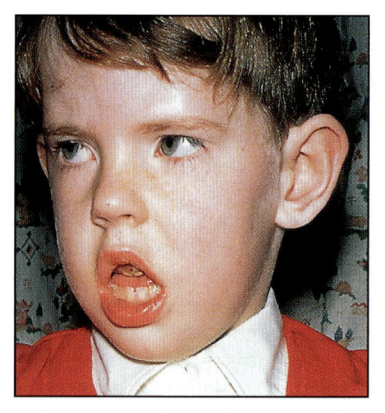

Figure 29.11 Myotonic dystrophy in an 8-year-old who has marked facial weakness and moderately severe learning difficulties.

Box 29.3 Causes of a hypotonic ("floppy") infant

Central	Hypoxic-ischaemic encephalopathy
	Intracranial haemorrhage
	Cerebral malformations
	Chromosome/genetic (e.g. Down syndrome, Prader–Willi syndrome)
	Congenital infections: toxoplamsma, rubella, cytomegalovirus, herpes
	Acquired infections
	Peroxisomal disorders
	Drug effects (e.g. benzodiazepines)
Spinal cord	Birth trauma (especially breech delivery)
	Syringomyelia
Anterior horn cell	Spinal muscular atrophy
Neuromuscular junction	Myasthenia gravis (transient / congenital)
	Infantile botulism
Muscle	Muscular dystrophies (e.g. congenital myotonic dystrophy)
	Congenital myopathies (e.g. central core disease)
Peripheral nerve	Hereditary motor and sensory neuropathies
	Inborn errors of metabolism
Metabolic myopathies	Carnitine deficiency

The hypotonic or 'floppy" infant

Persisting hypotonia can be readily felt on picking up the infant, who tends to slip through the fingers or hang like a rag doll when suspended prone. There will be marked head lag when the head is lifted by the arms from supine. The causes are listed in Box 29.3.

Box 29.4 Causes of ataxia

- Friedreich ataxia
- Ataxia telangiectasia
- Cerebellar agenesis/dysgenesis
- Postinfectious cerebellitis – varicella
- Posterior fossa tumours
- Other hereditary cerebellar ataxias
- Miller Fisher syndrome (a varient of Guillain-Barré syndrome)
- Mitochondrial disease
- Drugs e.g. carbamazepine, lamotrigine
- Toxins e.g. ethanol

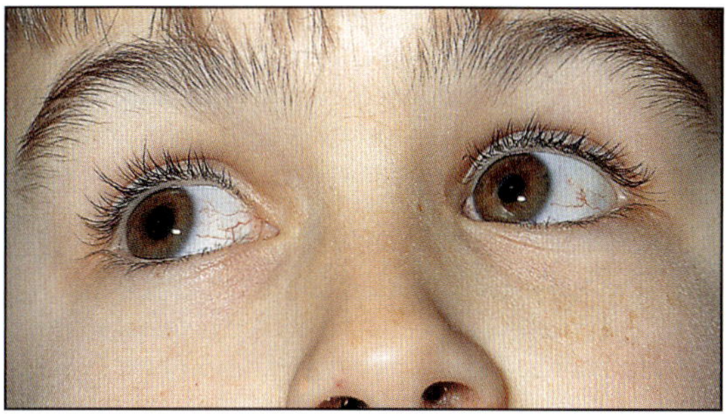

Figure 29.12 Telangiectasia of the conjunctiva are present from about 4 years of age in ataxia telangiectasia.

The clinical examination may help determine the site of the lesion, whether cerebral or neuromuscular. Central hypotonia is associated with poor truncal tone but preserved limb tone. Dysmorphic features suggest a genetic cause. Lower motor neurone lesions are suggested by a frog-like posture (Fig. 29.7), poor antigravity movements and absent tendon reflexes.

Ataxia

The causes of ataxia are listed in Box 29.4.

Friedreich ataxia

This is an autosomal recessive condition. It is due to a triplet repeat in the *FXN* gene causing a lack of the frataxin protein. It presents with worsening ataxia and dysarthria, distal wasting in the lower limbs with absent reflexes and pes cavus. It is similar to Charcot-Marie-Tooth disease, but in Friedreich ataxia there is impairment of joint position and vibration sense (posterior-columns affected), extensor plantars (indicating pyramidal involvement) and typically optic atrophy. The cerebellar component becomes more apparent with age. Evolving kyphoscoliosis, diabetes mellitus and cardiomyopathy can cause cardiorespiratory compromise and death at age 40–50 years.

Ataxia telangiectasia

This disorder of DNA repair is autosomal recessive. The gene codes for a protein kinase mutation which, among other things, is involved in repairing double stranded DNA breaks. There is mild delay in motor development in infancy and oculomotor problems with incoordination and delay in ocular pursuits and saccades (moving eyes to a target); difficulty with balance and coordination becoming evident at school age. There is subsequent deterioration, with a combination of a complex eye movement disorder including nystagmus, dystonia, spasms, jerks and tremors, cerebellar ataxia and dysarthria. Many children require a wheelchair for mobility in early adolescence. Telangiectasia develop in the conjunctiva (Fig. 29.12), and may occur in the neck and shoulders from about 4 years of age. These children:

- have an increased susceptibility to infection, and deficiencies of IgA and IgE
- develop malignant disorders, such as lymphomas and acute leukemias
- develop progressive pulmonary disease with bronchiectasis
- have a raised serum alpha-fetoprotein
- have sensitivity to ionizing radiation.

Most will die of malignancy or chronic lung disease in their twenties.

Other hereditary cerebellar ataxias

There is a growing number of these, largely dominantly inherited (genotypes identified), with a relatively benign course in childhood.

Cerebrovascular disease

Intracranial haemorrhage

Extradural haemorrhage

This usually follows direct head trauma (see Fig. 7.4), often associated with skull fracture (tearing of middle meningeal artery as it passes through the foramen spinosum of the sphenoid bone). It results from arterial or venous bleeding into the extradural space. There is often a lucid interval until the conscious level deteriorates, with seizures secondary to increasing size of the haematoma. There may be focal neurological signs with dilatation of the ipsilateral pupil, paresis of the contralateral limbs, and a false localising unilateral or bilateral VIth nerve paresis. In young children, initial presentation may be with anaemia and shock. The diagnosis is confirmed with a CT scan. Management is to correct hypovolaemia, urgent evacuation of the haematoma and arrest of the bleeding.

Subdural haematoma

This results from tearing of the bridging veins as they cross the subdural space. It is a characteristic lesion in nonaccidental injury caused by shaking or direct trauma in infants and toddlers. Retinal haemorrhages are typical of shaking injury. Subdural haematomas are occasionally seen following a fall from a considerable height, and rarely, in association with brain shrinkage through atrophy or overdrainage of hydrocephalus.

Subarachnoid haemorrhage

This is much more common in adults. Presentation is usually with a severe headache with rapid onset ("thunderclap headache"), vomiting, confusion or a lowered level of consciousness, and sometimes seizures and coma. A CT scan of the head usually identifies blood in the CSF. Occasionally a lumbar puncture is required. The cause is often an aneurysm or arteriovenous malformation. It can be identified on MR angiography, CT, or conventional angiography. Treatment can be neurosurgical or with interventional radiology.

> **Summary**
>
> **Intracranial haemorrhage**
> - History of significant head injury – remember that an extradural haemorrhage may be present even if lucid afterwards.
> - Subdural haematoma and retinal haemorrhages in an infant – consider non-accidental injury caused by shaking or direct trauma.

Stroke

Perinatal stroke is described in Chapter 11. Childhood stroke may be due to vascular, thromboembolic or haemorrhagic disease. The clinical presentation is determined by the vascular territory involved. Commonly there is compromise of the anterior circulation (internal carotid, anterior cerebral arteries and middle cerebral arteries), which leads to contralateral hemiparesis with or without hemianopia, and speech disturbance. Less common is compromise of the posterior circulation (vertebrobasilar arteries) with associated visual and/or cerebellar signs.

Causes include:

- Cardiac: congenital cyanotic heart disease, e.g. Fallot tetralogy, endocarditis.
- Haematological: sickle cell disease; deficiencies of antithrombotic factors, e.g. protein S.
- Postinfective: following varicella or other viral infections.
- Inflammatory: damage to vessels in autoimmune disease, e.g. SLE (systemic lupus erythematosus).
- Metabolic/genetic: homocystinuria, mitochondrial disorders, e.g. **m**yoclonic **e**pilepsy, **l**actic **a**cidosis, and **s**troke (MELAS); **c**erebral **a**utosomal **d**ominant **a**rteriopathy with **s**ubcortical **i**nfarcts and **l**eukoencephalopathy (CADASIL).
- Vascular malformations: arteriovenous malformation or moyamoya disease, in which there is a progressive involution of cerebral arteries. Moyamoya comes from the Japanese for 'puff of smoke', similar to the blurred appearance seen on angiography.
- Trauma: Dissection of carotid or vertebral arteries.

Investigations should include an assessment of cerebral and external carotid vasculature with MRI, MR angiogram, and when indicated, MR venography; echocardiography to detect a source of embolism, along with a thrombophilia and vasculitis screen, and metabolic tests for homocysteine and mitochondrial cytopathy. Often no cause can be identified. Rehabilitation requires the involvement of the multidisciplinary therapy team. Low dose aspirin prophylaxis is recommended after arterial ischaemic stroke.

> **Summary**
>
> **Strokes**
> - Occur in infants and children.
> - In infants, occur in the perinatal period, and may present in late infancy with a hemiplegia or with seizures.
> - In children, are seen in association with cardiac or sickle cell disease, following varicella infection or neck trauma. However, often no cause is evident.

Microcephaly and macrocephaly

These are described in Chapter 12.

Neural tube defects and hydrocephalus

Neural tube defects

Neural tube defects result from failure of normal fusion of the neural plate to form the neural tube during the first 28 days following conception. Their birth prevalence in the UK has fallen dramatically from 4/1000 live births in the 1970s to 0.2/1000 live births (Fig. 29.13). This is mainly because of a natural decline, as well as antenatal screening.

The reason for the natural decline is uncertain, but may be associated with improved maternal nutrition. Mothers of a fetus with a neural tube defect have a 10-fold increase in risk of having a second affected fetus. Folic acid supplementation reduces this risk. High doses are now recommended periconceptually for women with a previously affected infant planning a further pregnancy. Low-dose periconceptual folic acid supplementation is recommended for all pregnancies. In some countries e.g. United States, folic acid is added to cereal grain products.

Anencephaly

This is failure of development of most of the cranium and brain. Affected infants are stillborn or die shortly after birth. It is detected on antenatal ultrasound screening and termination of pregnancy is usually offered.

Encephalocele
There is extrusion of brain and meninges through a midline skull defect, which can be corrected surgically. However, there are often underlying associated cerebral malformations.

Spina bifida occulta
This failure of fusion of the vertebral arch (Fig. 29.14a) is often an incidental finding on X-ray, but there may be an associated overlying skin lesion such as a tuft of hair, lipoma, birth mark or small dermal sinus, usually in the lumbar region. There may be underlying tethering of the cord (diastematomyelia), which, with growth, may cause neurological deficits of bladder function and lower limbs. The extent of the underlying lesion can be delineated using ultrasound and/or MRI scans. Neurosurgical relief of tethering is usually indicated.

Meningocele and myelomeningocele
Meningoceles (Fig. 29.14b) usually have a good prognosis following surgical repair.

Myelomeningoceles (Figs 29.14c, 29.15) may be associated with:

- variable paresis of the lower limbs with hypotonia
- muscle imbalance, which may cause dislocation of the hip and talipes
- sensory loss
- bladder denervation (neuropathic bladder)
- bowel denervation (neuropathic bowel)
- scoliosis
- hydrocephalus from the associated Chiari type 2 malformation (herniation of the cerebellar tonsils and brainstem tissue through the foramen magnum), leading to disruption of CSF flow.

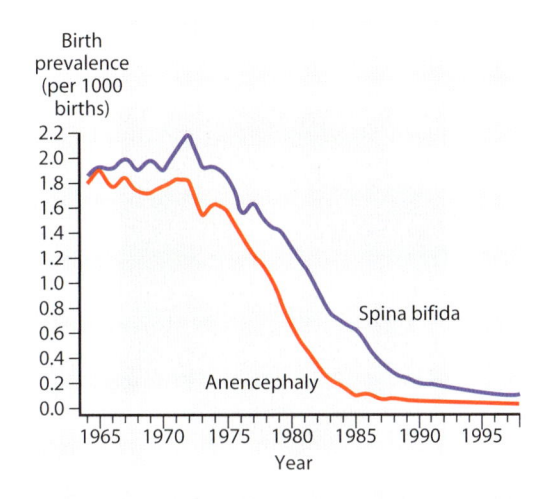

Figure 29.13 The decline in the number of babies born with neural tube defects. This has resulted from a natural decrease together with antenatal diagnosis and termination of pregnancy.

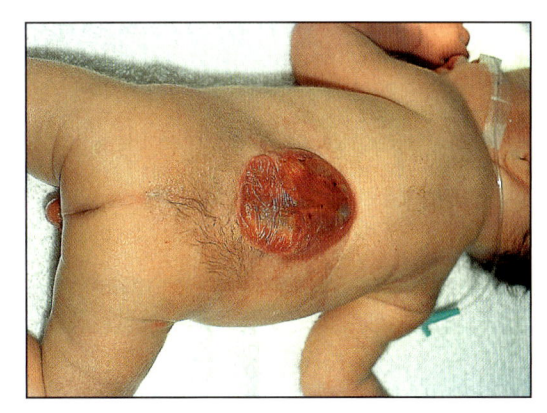

Figure 29.15 Myelomeningocele showing the exposed neural tissue and the patulous anus from neuropathic bowel.

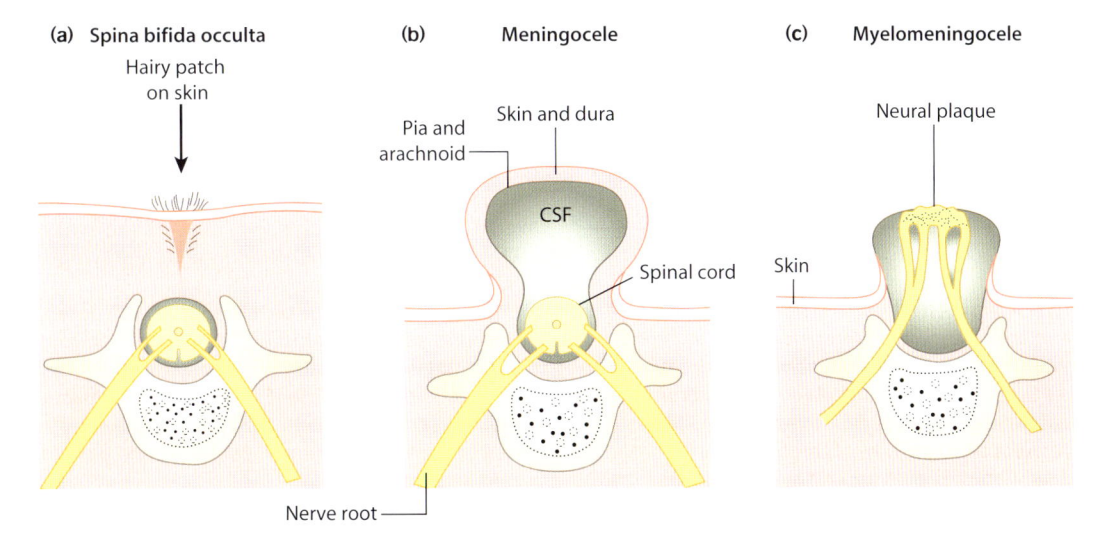

Figure 29.14 Neural tube defects: **(a)** spina bifida occulta; **(b)** meningocele; and **(c)** myelomeningocele.

Management

The back lesion is usually closed soon after birth. Paralysis and muscle imbalance requires physiotherapy to prevent joint contractures. Walking aids or a wheelchair help mobility. Because of the sensory loss, skin care is required to avoid the development of skin damage and ulcers.

The neuropathic bladder is managed with an indwelling catheter or intermittent urinary catheterisation by parents or by older children themselves. There should be regular checks for hypertension, renal function and urinary infection. Prophylactic antibiotics may be necessary. Medication (such as ephedrine or oxybutynin) may improve bladder function and improve urinary dribbling.

Bowel denervation – requires regular toileting, and laxatives and suppositories are likely to be necessary with a low roughage diet for lesions above L3.

Scoliosis – is monitored and may require surgical treatment. Ventricular dilatation associated with a Chiari 2 malformation is often present at birth and 80% of affected infants require a ventriculoperitoneal shunt for progressive hydrocephalus during the first few weeks of life.

The most severely disabled have a spinal lesion above L3 at birth. They are unable to walk, have a scoliosis, neuropathic bladder, hydronephrosis and frequently develop hydrocephalus.

Modern medical care has improved the quality of life for severely affected children. Their care is best managed by a specialist multidisciplinary team.

Summary

Neural tube defects
- Include anencephaly, encephalocele, spina bifida occulta, meningocele, and myelomeningocele.
- The birth prevalence in the UK has fallen dramatically, mainly owing to a natural decline but also to antenatal screening.
- The birth prevalence is reduced by periconceptual folic acid.
- Myelomeningoceles can cause paralysis of the legs, dislocation of the hip and talipes, sensory loss, neuropathic bladder and bowel, scoliosis and hydrocephalus from the Chiari 2 malformation.

Hydrocephalus

In hydrocephalus, there is an accumulation of cerebrospinal fluid in the brain. In babies and children this can be congenital, associated with cerebral malformations, or obstruction to the flow of cerebrospinal fluid leading to dilatation of the ventricular system proximal to the site of obstruction. The obstruction may be within the ventricular system or aqueduct (non-communicating i.e. obstructive hydrocephalus), or at the arachnoid

Box 29.5 Causes of hydrocephalus

Non-communicating (obstruction in the ventricular system)

Congenital malformation:
- Aqueduct stenosis
- Atresia of the outflow foramina of the fourth ventricle
- Chiari malformation (cerebellar tonsils herniation through foramen magnum)

Posterior fossa neoplasm or vascular malformation
Intraventricular haemorrhage in preterm infant

Communicating (failure to reabsorb CSF)

Subarachnoid haemorrhage
Meningitis, e.g. pneumococcal, tuberculous

Some can cause both noncommunicating and communicating hydrocephalus.

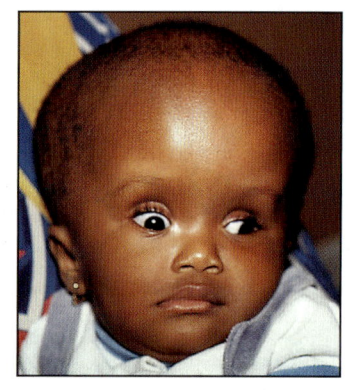

Figure 29.16 Grossly enlarged head and downward deviation of the eyes (setting-sun sign) from untreated hydrocephalus.

villi, the site of absorption of CSF (communicating hydrocephalus) (Box 29.5).

Clinical features

In infants with hydrocephalus, as their skull sutures have not fused, the head circumference will be disproportionately large or show an excessive rate of growth. The skull sutures separate, the anterior fontanelle bulges and the scalp veins become.

Congenital infection distended. An advanced sign is fixed downward gaze or "sun setting" of the eyes (Fig. 29.16). Older children will develop signs and symptoms of raised intracranial pressure.

Hydrocephalus may be diagnosed on antenatal ultrasound screening or in preterm infants on routine cranial ultrasound scanning. For suspected hydrocephalus, initial assessment is with cranial ultrasound (in infants) or CT or MRI head scans. The head circumference should be monitored over time and plotted on a centile chart.

Treatment is required for symptomatic relief of raised intracranial pressure and to minimise the risk of neurological damage. The mainstay is the insertion of a

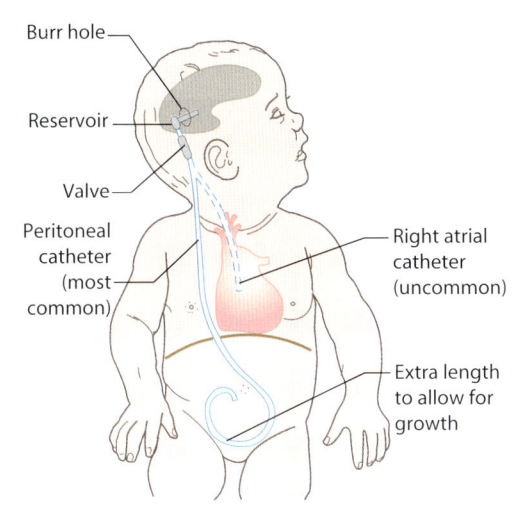

Figure 29.17 Ventriculoperitoneal shunt for drainage of symptomatic hydrocephalus. A sufficient length of shunt tubing is left in the peritoneal cavity to allow for the child's growth. Right atrial catheters require revision with growth.

ventriculoperitoneal shunt (Fig. 29.17), but endoscopic treatment to create a ventriculostomy is sometimes performed. Shunts can malfunction due to blockage or infection (usually with coagulase-negative staphylococci). They then need replacing or revising. Overdrainage of fluid can cause low-pressure headaches but the insertion of programmable valves can help avoid this.

Summary

Hydrocephalus
- In infants, presents with excessive increase in head circumference, separation of skull sutures, bulging of the anterior fontanelle, distension of scalp veins and sun setting of the eyes.
- Older children present with symptoms of raised intracranial pressure.
- Treatment is usually with a ventriculo-peritoneal shunt.

The neurocutaneous syndromes

The nervous system and the skin have a common ectodermal origin. Embryological disruption causes syndromes involving abnormalities to both systems – the neurocutaneous syndromes.

Neurofibromatosis

Neurofibromatosis type 1 (NF-1) affects 1 in 3000 live births. It is an autosomal dominant, highly penetrant condition, with variable expression. It is caused by a mutation in the neurofibromin-1 (*NF1*) gene, which arises in about 50% as a de novo mutation.

In order to make the diagnosis, two or more of these criteria need to be present:

- six or more café-au-lait spots greater than 5 mm in size before puberty, greater than 15 mm after puberty (Fig. 29.18)
- more than one neurofibroma, an unsightly firm nodular overgrowth of any nerve
- axillary freckling (Fig. 29.18)
- optic glioma which may cause visual impairment
- one Lisch nodule: a hamartoma of the iris seen on slit-lamp examination
- bony lesions from sphenoid dysplasia, which can cause eye protrusion
- a first-degree relative with NF-1.

The cutaneous features tend to become more evident after puberty, and there is a wide spectrum of involvement from mild to severe. Neurofibromata appear in the course of any peripheral nerve, including cranial nerves. They may look unsightly or cause neurological signs if they occur at a site where a peripheral nerve passes through a bony foramen. Visual or auditory impairment may result if there is compression of the IInd or VIIIth cranial nerve. Megalencephaly with learning difficulties and epilepsy are sometimes seen.

Neurofibromatosis type 2 (NF-2; multiple inherited schwannomas, meningiomas, and ependymomas) is less common. It is an autosomal dominant syndrome caused by a mutation in the NF2 gene, usually presenting in adolescence. About 50% are due to de novo mutations. Bilateral acoustic neuromata are the predominant feature and present with deafness and sometimes a cerebellopontine angle syndrome with a facial (VIIth) nerve paresis and cerebellar ataxia.

Both NF-1 and NF-2 can be associated with endocrinological disorders, the multiple endocrine neoplasia syndromes.

Other associations are phaeochromocytoma, pulmonary hypertension, renal artery stenosis with hypertension. Rarely, the benign tumours undergo sarcomatous change. However, most people with the disorders carry no features other than the cutaneous stigmata.

Tuberous sclerosis

The prevalence of tuberous sclerosis is 1 in 9000 live births. It is autosomal dominant, with variable penetrance, and up to 70% of mutations arise de novo. The cause is a mutation in the *TSC1* or TSC2 genes.

The cutaneous features consist of:

- depigmented "ash leaf" shaped patches or amelanotic naevi which fluoresce under ultraviolet light (Wood's light)
- roughened patches of skin (shagreen patches) usually over the lumbar spine
- angiofibromata ("adenoma sebaceum") in a butterfly distribution over the bridge of the nose and cheeks, which are unusual before the age of 3 years (Fig. 29.19).

Neurocutaneous syndromes

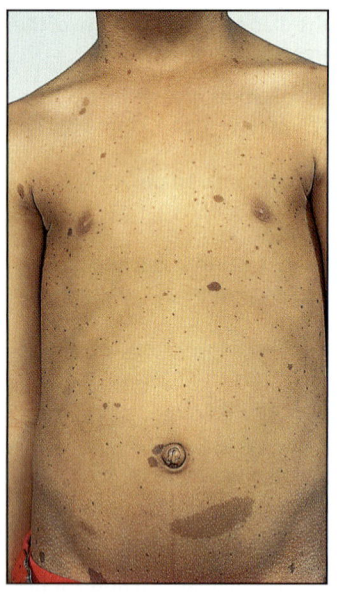

Figure 29.18 Café-au-lait patches and axillary freckling in neurofibromatosis.

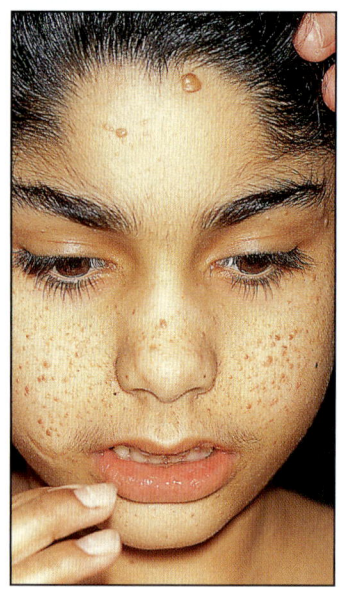

Figure 29.19 Facial angiofibromas in tuberous sclerosis.

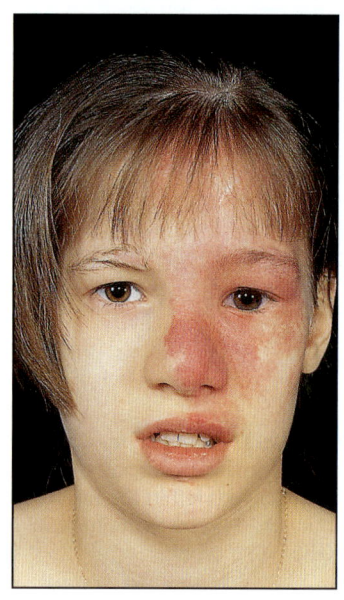

Figure 29.20 Sturge–Weber syndrome. There is a port-wine stain in the distribution of the trigeminal nerve.

Neurological features are seen in 50%, including:
- infantile spasms and developmental delay
- epilepsy – often focal
- intellectual disability, often with autism.

Children with early onset intractable epilepsy have severe learning difficulties and often have autistic features when older.

Other features include:
- fibromata beneath the nails (subungual fibromata)
- dense white areas on the retina (phakomata) from local degeneration
- rhabdomyomata of the heart which are identifiable in the early weeks on echocardiography but usually resolve in infancy
- angiomyolipomas and polycystic kidneys
- cysts in the lungs.

In the brain, even if asymptomatic, there are subependymal nodules and cortical tubers. The subependymal nodules may enlarge over time and form subependymal giant cell astrocytomas which sometimes block the flow of CSF causing headache, vomiting, and hydrocephalus.

Many people who carry the gene have no stigmata other than the cutaneous features and no associated neurological features. CT scans will detect the calcified subependymal nodules and tubers from the second year of life. MRI is more sensitive and more clearly identifies the lesions.

Sturge–Weber syndrome

This is a sporadic disorder with a haemangiomatous facial lesion (a port wine stain) in the distribution of the trigeminal nerve associated with a similar lesion intracranially (ipsilateral leptomeningeal angioma). In the most severe form, it may present with epilepsy, intellectual disability, and a contralateral hemiplegia.

The ophthalmic division of the trigeminal nerve is always involved (Fig. 29.20). Calcification of the gyri used to show characteristic 'rail-road track' calcification on skull X-ray, but MRI is the imaging modality of choice nowadays. Children presenting with intractable epilepsy in early infancy may benefit from hemispherotomy. Laser treatment may be used to lighten or remove the port wine stain. For children who are less severely affected, deterioration is unusual after the age of 5 years, although there may still be seizures and learning difficulties. There is a high risk of ipsilateral glaucoma in 50% of children, which should be assessed in the neonatal period.

Neurodegenerative disorders

These are disorders that cause a deterioration in motor and intellectual function. Abnormal neurological features develop, including seizures, spasticity, abnormal head circumference (macrocephaly or microcephaly), involuntary movement disorders, visual and hearing loss, and behaviour change. While individually rare,

Table 29.5 Some examples of neurodegenerative disorders seen in children

	Presentation	Diagnostic investigations
Age 0–2 years		
Infantile neuronal ceroid lipofuscinosis (NCL)	Developmental arrest by end of first year, seizures and blindness	Skin biopsy, blood enzyme analysis, DNA testing
Krabbe leucodystrophy	Irritability, hypertonia, myoclonus	White cell enzymes
Rett syndrome	Regression by 6–18 months, with characteristic hand wringing	DNA testing
Tay Sachs	Hypotonia, seizures, and blindness.	White cell enzymes.
Age 2–5 years		
Mucopolysaccharidosis type III	Developmental delay, behavioural disturbances, dysmorphism	Urinary glycosaminoglycans and blood white cell enzymes
NCL – late infantile	Myoclonus, motor difficulties, blindness	Skin biopsy, enzymes analysis, DNA testing
Alpers	Seizures, developmental regression, hypotonia and hepatic derangement	Genetic tests
Age 5–12 years		
Juvenile NCL	Cognitive and motor decline. Visual deterioration. Seizures later	Vacuolated lymphocytes on light microscopy, fingerprinting on electron microscopy, DNA testing
Adrenoleucodystrophy	Cognitive development slowed, visual impairment, seizures	VLCFA (Very Long Chain Fatty Acids), DNA testing
Niemann–Pick disease type C	Seizures, vertical gaze palsy	Sea blue histiocytes on bone marrow aspiration, DNA testing
Friedeich ataxia	Ataxia, pyramidal signs, and peripheral neuropathy	DNA testing
Age 12+ years		
Wilson Disease	Psychiatric, extrapyramidal	Plasma copper and caeruloplasmin, penicillamine challenge
Juvenile Huntington	Progressive dystonia, dementia, seizures, corticospinal tract signs	DNA testing

they are numerous and include many inborn errors of metabolism. These are discussed in more detail in Chapter 27 (Inborn errors of metabolism).

Developmental regression or reported loss of previously acquired skills should prompt investigation of the cause. The most commonly encountered neurodegenerative conditions are:

- lysosomal storage disorders, e.g. mucopolysaccharidosis type III, in which absence of an enzyme leads to accumulation of harmful metabolites within the lysosomes. These disorders often have organomegaly associated with them
- peroxisomal enzyme defects, e.g. X-linked adrenoleucodystrophy (see below). Peroxisomes are catalase and oxidase containing organelles involved in long-chain fatty acid oxidation. Enzyme deficiencies can lead to accumulation of very long-chain fatty acids (VLCFAs)
- Wilson disease, from the accumulation of copper, may cause changes in behaviour and additional involuntary movements or a mixture of neurological and hepatic symptoms (see Ch. 21 Liver disease).

Some of the more important examples of neurodegenerative disorders seen in children are summarized in Table 29.5.

Adrenoleukodystrophy

The adrenoleukodystrophies (ALDs) are a group of disorders caused by peroxisomal defects. These organelles are essential for the breakdown of fatty acids in cells. The different forms are:

- neonatal – part of the Zellweger spectrum of disorders, with hypotonia, feeding problems, seizures and may have characteristic facial features
- X-linked ALD (X-ALD) – the most common peroxisomal disorder, with incidence of 1 in 20 000. Caused by mutations in the gene, which is

involved in the import of very long-chain fatty acids (VLCFA) into the peroxisome. This results in damaging effects on the adrenal glands, the brain cells and myelin. There are high levels of very long-chain fatty acids in the blood. There are two forms:
- childhood cerebral form – affects boys aged 4–12 years. Presents with school failure, behaviour changes, regression, ataxia, and adrenal insufficiency. Option for haematopoietic stem cell transplantation if diagnosed early
- adrenomyeloneuropathy – presents in males and less commonly females with slowly progressive spastic paraparesis and dorsal column sensory disturbance
- Addison disease – may be only manifestation.

Acknowledgements

We would like to acknowledge the contributor to this chapter in previous editions, whose work we have drawn on extensively: Richard Newton (1st, 2nd, 3rd, 4th Editions).

Further reading

Bushby K, Finkel R, Birnkrant DJ, Case LE, Clemens PR, Cripe L, et al. The diagnosis and management of Duchenne muscular dystrophy. Part 1: *Lancet Neurology* 2010;9:77–93.

Bushby K, Finkel R, Birnkrant DJ, Case LE, Clemens PR, Cripe L, et al. The diagnosis and management of Duchenne muscular dystrophy. Part 2: *Lancet Neurology* 2010;9:177–189.

Forsyth R, Newton R: *Paediatric Neurology. Oxford Specialist Handbook in Paediatrics,* Oxford, 2012, Oxford University Press.

Newton RW: *Colour Atlas of Pediatric Neurology,* London, 1995, Mosby-Wolfe.
A well-illustrated textbook.

Websites (Accessed November 2016)

British Paediatric Neurology Association: Available at: http://www.bpna.org.uk.

Systematic reviews

Systematic reviews of migraine treatment in children, epilepsy, steroids for facial palsy and treatment of Guillain–Barré syndrome can be found in the Cochrane Library.
Available via: http://www.thecochranelibrary.com.

International Headache Society classification:
Available at: http://www.ihs-headache.org/ichd-guidelines

International League Against Epilepsy (ILAE):
Available at: http://www.ilae.org.

Neuromuscular Disease Center: *(Washington University School of Medicine, St Louis, MO).* Available at: http://neuromuscular.wustl.edu.

NICE Epilepsies: Diagnosis and Management 2016:
Available at: https://www.nice.org.uk/guidance/cg137

30

Adolescent medicine

Communicating with adolescents	525		Mental health problems	531
Consent and confidentiality	527		Health-risk behaviour	531
Range of health problems	528		Sexual health	531
Mortality	528		Health promotion	532
Impact of chronic conditions	529		Transition to adult services	533
Fatigue, headache, and other somatic symptoms	530			

Features of adolescent medicine are:

- the adolescent consultation differs from the paediatric consultation
- the HEADS acronym assists in taking a psychosocial history
- mortality of adolescents aged 15–19 years is now greater than that of young children aged 1–4 years in the UK
- chronic illness may impact on adolescent development, which in turn may impact on the chronic illness, e.g. adherence
- prominent mental health problems are eating disorders and self-harm.

Adolescence is the transition from childhood to adulthood. There is no clearly defined age range, but it is usually considered to be from puberty to 18 years of age. There are 7.4 million adolescents in the UK, 12% of the population, with increased proportions observed in ethnic minority groups.

The transition from being a child to an adult involves many biological, psychological, and social changes (Table 30.1), with adolescent brain development continuing into the third decade. Pubertal development is considered in Chapter 12. Difficulties may arise if the pubertal changes are early or delayed. While general practitioners will see all adolescent medical problems, difficulties may arise when obtaining specialist medical care. Those less than 16 years old are generally looked after by paediatricians; over 16 years old, by either paediatricians or more often by adult physicians and surgeons. However, paediatric facilities, e.g. children's wards, are often geared to the needs of young children rather than adolescents, whilst older adolescents may be overwhelmed by the medical conditions encountered on adult wards and the independence expected of them. Adolescent females with gynaecological problems are often cared for by gynaecologists, usually in adult facilities. Some paediatricians in the UK are now specializing in adolescent medicine in a similar way to North America and Australia, and the number of facilities focusing on the special needs of adolescents is increasing.

Communicating with adolescents

The adolescent consultation differs from the paediatric consultation for young children, in that the adolescent has a greater active role in the consultation.

As well as seeing adolescents with their parents, an integral component of adolescent healthcare is offering young people the opportunity to be seen independently of their parents for at least part of the visit. They, however, still have the right to a chaperone but it should not be assumed the latter can be a parent. Another principle is that the parents should ideally not be seen alone after the adolescent has spent time with the doctor, so that the adolescent can trust that whatever confidences have been disclosed to the doctor have been kept.

Some practical points about communicating and working with adolescents are:

- make the adolescent the central person in the consultation
- be yourself. When establishing rapport, it may be appropriate to engage the adolescent by talking about his/her interests, e.g. football, clothes, or music, but do not try to be cool, false, or patronizing; your relationship should be as his/her doctor, not his/her friend
- consider the family dynamics. Is the mother or father answering for the adolescent? Does the adolescent seem to want this or resent being interrupted?

Table 30.1 Developmental changes of adolescence

	Biological	**Psychological**	**Social**
Early adolescence	Early puberty: Females – breast bud, pubic hair development, start of growth spurt Males – testicular enlargement, start of genital growth	Concrete thinking (Fig. 30.1a), but begin to develop moral concepts and awareness of their sexual identity	The early emotional separation from parents, start of a strong peer identification, early exploratory behaviours, e.g. may start smoking
Mid-adolescence	Females – end of growth spurt, menarche, change in body shape Males – sperm production, voice breaks, start of growth spurt Acne Blushing Need for more sleep	Abstract thinking, but still seen as 'bulletproof', increasing verbal dexterity, may develop a fervent ideology (religious, political)	Continuing emotional separation from parents, strong peer group identification, development of sexual identity and orientation, early vocational plans
Late adolescence	Males – end of puberty, continued growth in height, strength, and body hair	Complex abstract thinking (Fig. 30.1b), identification of difference between law and morality, increased impulse control, further development of personal identity, further development or rejection of ideologies	Social autonomy, may develop intimate relationships, further education or employment, may begin or develop financial independence

From Christie D, Viner R. Adolescent Development. *BMJ* 2005; 330: 301-304 with permission.

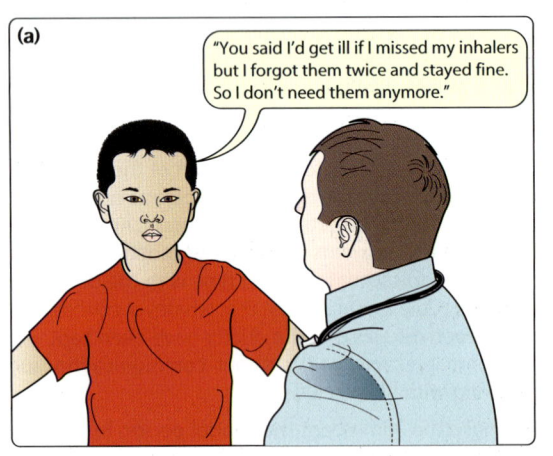

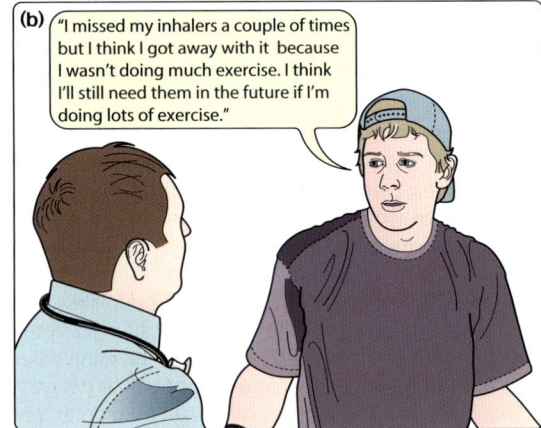

(a) "You said I'd get ill if I missed my inhalers but I forgot them twice and stayed fine. So I don't need them anymore."

(b) "I missed my inhalers a couple of times but I think I got away with it because I wasn't doing much exercise. I think I'll still need them in the future if I'm doing lots of exercise."

Figure 30.1 Example showing the difference between (a) concrete and (b) abstract thinking in the management of asthma in an older child and an adolescent.

- avoid being judgemental or lecturing. Avoid 'You …' statements and use 'I …' statements in preference, e.g. 'I am concerned that you …'. A frank and direct approach works best. Your role should be that of a knowledgeable, trusted adult from whom they can get advice if they so choose

- an authoritarian approach is likely to result in a rebellious stance. Working things out together in a practical way has the best chance of success
- frame difficult questions so they are less threatening and judgemental, e.g. 'some teenagers drink alcohol, do any of your friends drink? How

Table 30.2 HEADS acronym for psychosocial history taking in adolescents

H	**Home life**	Relationships, social support, household chores
E	**Education**	School, exams, work experience, career, university, financial issues
A	**Activities**	Exercise, sport, other leisure activities
		Social relationships, friends, peers, who can they rely on? Bullying?
D	**Driving**	Aged 16 years if has high rate mobility component of the Disability Living Allowance or Enhanced Rate of the Mobility Component of the Personal Independence Payment
	Drugs	Drug use, cigarettes, alcohol. How much? How often?
	Diet	Weight, caffeine (diet drinks), binges/vomits
S	**Sexual health**	Concerns, periods, contraception (and in relation to medication)
	Sleep	How much? Hard to get to sleep? Wake often?
	Suicide/affect	Early waking? Depression, self-harm, body image
	Safety	Safety issues around substance use, sexual activity, Internet use, etc.

much do they drink in a week? Do you drink alcohol – how much do you drink compared with them?' Likewise, when asking sensitive questions on, e.g. sexual health, always give young people warning and explain the rationale of why such questions need to be asked
- do not perpetuate myths in your questions to the young people, e.g. 'Lots of young people smoke – do you?' Only one in ten 15 year olds in the UK currently smoke although this doubles to one in five in the 16-year-old to 24-year-old age group
- confidentiality is particularly important to this age group and must be respected. Explain that you will keep everything you are told confidential, unless they or somebody else is at risk of serious harm. Always assess the adolescent's understanding of confidentiality and correct any misunderstanding
- bear in mind proxy presentations, e.g. abdominal pain, when the real reason is anxiety about the possibility of pregnancy, or sexually transmitted infection (STI) or the result of recreational drug use
- a full adolescent psychosocial history is useful to engage the young person, to assess the level of risk as well as identifying protective or resilient factors and provide information that will aid the formulation of effective interventions. The HEADS acronym may be helpful in this regard (Table 30.2), although questions must always be tailored to stage of development and the right of the young person to not answer should be respected
- communicate and explain concepts appropriate to their cognitive development. For young adolescents, use concrete examples (here and now) rather than abstract concepts (if … then)
- history taking should avoid making the assumption of heterosexuality with questions about romantic and sexual partners asked in a gender neutral way
- if they need to have a physical examination, consider their privacy and personal integrity
  – Who do they want present? As with any age, young people have the right to a chaperone but it should not be assumed the young person will want this to be their parent. Also, find out if they would prefer a doctor of the same sex, if this is an option.

> **Summary**
>
> **Talking and listening with young people**
> - Always give them the opportunity to be seen independently of their parents.
> - Explain and assure confidentiality.
> - Psychosocial screening is useful to:
>   – engage young people
>   – assess risk
> - Identify protective/resilient factors:
>   – they assist formulation of interventions.

Consent and confidentiality

Consent

In the UK, young people can give consent if they are sufficiently informed and either over 16 years old or under 16 years of age and competent to make decisions for themselves. Conflict rarely arises about a treatment, as usually the adolescent, his/her parents and doctors agree that it is necessary. Handling of disagreement over consent is considered in Chapter 5.

Confidentiality

Confidentiality is regarded by adolescents as of crucial importance in their medical care. They want to know that information they have disclosed to their doctor is not revealed to others, whether parents, school, or police, without their permission. In most circumstances, their confidentiality should be kept unless there is a risk of serious harm, either to themselves from physical or sexual abuse, from suicidal thoughts or to others from homicidal intent. Difficulties relating to confidentiality for adolescents are usually about contraception, abortion, STIs, substance abuse, or mental health. It is usually desirable for the parents to be informed and involved in the management of these situations and the adolescent should be encouraged to tell them or allow the doctor to do so. However, if the young person is competent to make these decisions for himself/herself, the courts have supported medical management of these situations without parental knowledge or consent.

Range of health problems

Adolescence is considered a healthy stage of life compared with early childhood or old age. In spite of this, the majority of young people will consult their general practitioner more than once in a year and 15% of adolescents report a chronic illness. The range of health problems affecting adolescents include:

- common acute illnesses: respiratory disorders, skin conditions, musculoskeletal problems including sports injuries, and somatic complaints. Acute serious illness has become rare, with mortality predominantly from trauma
- chronic illness and disability: e.g. asthma, epilepsy, diabetes, cerebral palsy, juvenile idiopathic arthritis, sickle cell disease. The prevalence of some of the common chronic disorders in adolescence is shown in Table 30.3. There is also a range of uncommon disorders with serious chronic morbidity such as malignant disease and connective tissue disorders. In addition, children with many congenital disorders which often used to be fatal in childhood now survive into adolescence or adult life, e.g. cystic fibrosis, Duchenne muscular dystrophy, complex congenital heart disease, metabolic disorders
- high prevalence of somatic symptoms: e.g. fatigue, headaches, backache
- mental health problems including suicide and deliberate self-harm

Table 30.3 Prevalence of some chronic illnesses per 1000 adolescents (12–18 years old)

Disease	Prevalence per 1000 adolescents
Musculoskeletal conditions	41
Skin conditions	32
Significant mental health problems	120
Diabetes	
Type 1	2
Type 2	1–2
Respiratory conditions	150
Asthma	100
Cystic fibrosis	0.1
Epilepsy	4
Hearing problems	18
Cerebral palsy	1.5
Juvenile idiopathic arthritis (JIA)	1

- eating disorders and weight problems
- those associated with health-risk behaviours, such as smoking, drinking, drug abuse and sexual health, contraception, and teenage pregnancy.

Mortality

The dramatic improvement in the mortality of young children seen since the 1960s has not been matched in adolescents, who now have a higher mortality rate than that of 1-year-old to 4-year-old age group (Fig. 30.2). Although deaths in adolescents from communicable diseases have declined markedly, this has not been matched by mortality from road traffic accidents, other injuries and suicide, and these now predominate (Fig. 30.3). Alcohol is thought to be a contributing factor in one-third of these deaths.

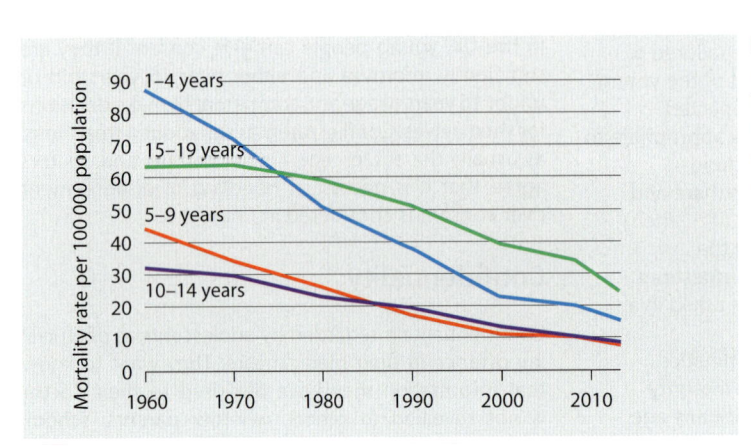

Figure 30.2 Mortality by age group in England and Wales 1960–2013. The graph shows that the mortality rate is now greater at age 15-years to 19-years than at 1-year to 4-years of age. (Data from ONS, 2015.)

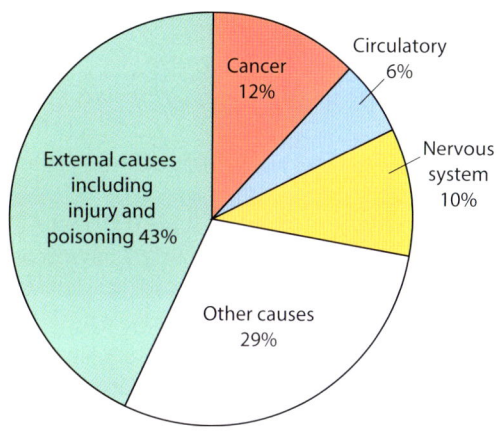

Figure 30.3 Causes of death, 15-years to 19-years of age, in England and Wales, 2013. (Data from ONS, 2015.)

- Cancer 12%
- Circulatory 6%
- Nervous system 10%
- Other causes 29%
- External causes including injury and poisoning 43%

☀ Mortality rate in UK for 15–19 year olds is now greater than for 1–4 year olds

Impact of chronic conditions

Chronic illness may disrupt biological, psychological, and social development. In addition, these developmental changes may affect the control and management of the disorder (Table 30.4). The impact of chronic illness on children, young people and their families is considered in Chapter 24.

Adherence

Poor adherence is a problem for many people, including adolescents as they are beginning to take over management of their health, wish to avoid parental supervision, and may give the management of their illness a lower priority than social and recreational activities. They may not believe that taking the medication really matters, especially if it is preventative or of long-term rather than short-term benefit.

Peer relationships and self-image are very important when considering adherence. For example, it may be more important for an adolescent with diabetes to lunch promptly, so he/she can sit with his/her friends

Adolescent medicine

Table 30.4 Some of the ways in which chronic illness and development interact with each other

	Effect of chronic illness on development	**Effect of development on chronic illness**
Biological	Delayed puberty Short stature Reduced bone mass accretion Malnutrition secondary to inadequate intake due to increased caloric requirement of disease or anorexia Localized growth abnormalities in inflammatory joint disease, e.g. premature fusion of epiphyses	Pubertal hormones may impact on disease, e.g. growth hormone worsens diabetes and increases insulin requirements; females with cystic fibrosis may have deterioration in lung function; corticosteroid toxicity worse in the peripubertal phase Increased caloric requirement may worsen disease control or result in undernutrition – may need dietary supplements or overnight feeding with nasogastric tube or gastrostomy Growth may cause scoliosis
Psychological	Regression to less mature behaviour Adopt sick role Impaired development of sense of attractive/sexual self Parental stress, depression, financial problems in providing care; siblings may suffer	Deny that their health may suffer from their actions Poor adherence and disease control Reject medics like parents
Social	Reduced independence when should be separating Failure of peer relationships Social isolation – unable to participate in sports or social events School absence and decline in school performance, may lower self-esteem Vocational failure	Risk behaviour may adversely affect disease, e.g. smoking and asthma or cystic fibrosis, alcohol and diabetic control, sleep deprivation and epilepsy Chaotic eating habits lead to malnutrition or obesity

Table 30.5 Ways to maximize adherence

Assess the size of the problem and be nonjudgemental	Ask: 'Some people have trouble taking their medication. When was the last time you forgot?'
Take time to explore practicalities	Try to put yourself in the adolescent's shoes and think through the detail of their regimen with them. 'Which is the most difficult dose to remember?' 'How do you fit in taking your tablets into your daily routine?' Make regimen as simple as possible. Do not forget practical issues – poor adherence may be as simple as not having any private space at school to take the treatment
Explore beliefs	May harbour strange or incorrect beliefs about medications, e.g. falsely attribute a side-effect, and therefore refuse to take the medication
Use daily routines to 'anchor' adherence	Find daily activities to anchor taking the medication, e.g. brushing teeth, or 'with breakfast and dinner' instead of 'twice a day'. Find the least chaotic time of day: may be morning or evening! Let the suggestions come from the adolescent
Motivation	Negotiate short-term treatment goals. Search for factors that motivate the young person
Involve and contract	Plan the regimen with the adolescent. Some may respond to a written contract that both sides agree to stick to
Written instructions	Most of what is said has been shown to be forgotten once they leave the room!
Take time to explain	Check level of knowledge on each occasion
Solution-focused approach	Find out what has been going well and why. Use this information, e.g. 'How have you managed to remain out of hospital for 3 weeks this month?'

rather than go to the school nurse first for his insulin injection. Side-effects are also important, particularly those that affect well-being or appearance. They may assess risk differently from adults, so that the risk of not being one of their crowd because of having to adhere to a certain treatment may appear to be more important than the risks attached to not taking any medication.

Adherence may be influenced by lack of knowledge and/or poor recall of previous disease education. The disorder may have presented when the child was much younger, so that the original consultation will have taken place primarily between the doctor and parents. If this communication has not been updated with increasing age, the adolescent's knowledge may be poor, with little understanding about his/her illness, what medications he/she is taking and why. As the responsibility for management moves to the young person, information needs to be provided about medications and treatment appropriate for his/her development. Other ways to maximize adherence are summarized in Table 30.5.

The implications of their condition on the rest of their health and their life needs to be considered. This may include sexual health, future vocational development, including the need for disclosure and their rights under the Equality Act (2010). Similarly, the implications of other health-risk behaviours such as substance use, tattoos, and piercing may need to be discussed.

> **Summary**
>
> **Chronic conditions during adolescence**
> - Chronic illness and/or disability may disrupt adolescent development.
> - Consideration should be made of the impact of the chronic condition on the rest of health (including sexual and reproductive health) as well as education and leisure.

Fatigue, headache, and other somatic symptoms

Fatigue, headache, abdominal pain, backache, and dizziness are common in adolescence. International surveys of adolescents in Europe reveal that two-thirds report morning fatigue more than once a week, 25% have a headache, and 15% stomach ache, backache, or sleep problems more than once a week. In many, these symptoms appear to be a feature of adolescence, although organic disease must be excluded by history, examination, and occasionally, investigation. For a minority, they may be a physical manifestation of psychological problems, and are precipitated by or maintained by factors such as bullying or parental discord.

Occasionally, the symptoms are so severe and persistent that they considerably affect quality of life, with impairment of school attendance, academic results, and peer relationships. This may be from chronic fatigue syndrome or chronic idiopathic pain syndromes. Further investigation and assessment will be required and multidisciplinary rehabilitation and cognitive behavioural therapy within the family may be beneficial. The management of somatic symptoms and chronic fatigue syndrome are considered further in Chapter 24.

Mental health problems

The prevalence of mental health problems in adolescents is estimated to be about 11%. The main problems are listed in Table 30.6.

Deliberate self-harm varies from little actual harm, where there is a wish to communicate distress or escape from an interpersonal crisis, to suicide. About 7% to 14% of adolescents will self-harm, depending on its definition.

Abnormal eating behaviour including eating disorders are common during adolescence. About 40% of females and 25% of males begin dieting in adolescence because of dissatisfaction with their body. In anorexia nervosa and bulimia, there is a morbid preoccupation with weight and body shape. This is discussed in more detail in Chapter 24.

Health-risk behaviour

During adolescence, young people begin to explore 'adult' behaviours, including smoking, drinking, drug use, and sex. These behaviours, often referred to as 'risk-taking' behaviours, may reflect the adolescent's search for pleasure and excitement by participating in new and enjoyable experiences, as well as exerting independence from parents or rebelling against parents' wishes and lifestyle. There is also considerable pressure to fit in with peers.

Adolescents do not always understand the risks involved and may behave as if they are immune from harm. Participating in these activities may also deflect attention away from themselves to mask shyness or anxiety. Unfortunately, health-risk behaviours started in adolescence tend to continue into adult life.

Sexual health

The average age for first sexual intercourse in the UK is 16 years, with one-fifth of 14-year-olds having had intercourse. Having sexual intercourse at an early age is often associated with unsafe sex. This may be because of a lack of knowledge, lack of access to contraception, inability to negotiate obtaining contraception, being drunk or high on drugs, or unable to resist being pressurized by his/her partner.

Risk-taking behaviour in adolescents can result in STIs or unplanned pregnancy. STIs may present with urethral or vaginal discharge, urinary symptoms, pain on micturition, abdominal or loin pain, or postcoital vaginal bleeding. Chlamydia is asymptomatic in 50% of cases and can lead to later infertility. In young teenagers, it is more likely to present with a vaginal discharge. Studies have shown that up to one-third of sexually active teenage girls have an STI. They are also at risk of human immunodeficiency virus (HIV) infection.

Management of sexually transmitted infections

Taking a sexual history from an adolescent should be approached sensitively, in a developmentally appropriate manner, giving the young person warning of the topic, as well as why the questions are being asked. Relevant questions include those related to the risk of STIs: number of partners; any partners during travel abroad; contraception used; whether vaginal, oral, or anal sex; any discharge, lower abdominal pain, urinary symptoms; and last menstrual period. However, many STIs are asymptomatic, especially in younger teenagers, male and female.

If indicated, swabs should be taken for virology and microbiology (to look for human papillomavirus, herpes simplex virus, chlamydia, and gonorrhoea). HIV testing may be indicated. In England, in response to the high rates of chlamydia in the under-25-year-old age group, there is a national chlamydia screening programme enabling them to test themselves with easy-to-use kits.

Treatment regimens vary, depending on prevalent antibiotic resistance. Chlamydia can be treated with azithromycin or doxycycline, gonorrhoea with a cephalosporin. Metronidazole can be added for pelvic inflammatory disease. It is advisable to inform and treat partners.

Table 30.6 Main mental health problems and disorders in adolescents

Problem or disorder	Prevalence (%)
Depression	3–5
Anxiety	4–6
Attention deficit hyperactivity disorder	2–4
Eating disorders	1–2
Conduct disorder	4–6
Substance misuse disorder	2–3

From Michaud P-A, Fombonne E: Common mental health problems. In: Viner R, editor, *ABC of Adolescence*, Oxford, 2005, Blackwell with permission.

Contraception

Most adolescents who are sexually active *are* using contraception, albeit sometimes haphazardly. In the UK, contraception is used by only half at first intercourse. Condoms, followed by the oral contraceptive pill, are the most common forms of contraception used. As teenagers have a relatively high failure rate in their ability to use condoms correctly and with the oral contraceptive pill having irregular use, the 'double Dutch' method of condom and oral contraception is advocated to protect against both STIs and pregnancy.

Adolescents with chronic disease, e.g. diabetes, even without microvascular complications, are generally started on lower doses of the contraceptive pill. Some medications prescribed in adolescents are potentially teratogenic (e.g. retinoids for acne, methotrexate for juvenile idiopathic arthritis or other disorders) and may therefore need to be combined with an oral contraceptive pill or depot hormonal implant. Discussions, however, must also reinforce condom use to prevent STIs. Finally, young people's accessibility to youth friendly contraception services needs to be checked as over half have been reported to be unaware of such services in their local area.

Emergency contraception

Emergency contraception (in the past misleadingly known as the 'morning after pill') can provide significant protection from pregnancy for up to 72 hours after unprotected intercourse. Emergency contraception is available from a pharmacist without prescription for those 16 years and over, and on prescription for those under 16 years. If taken within 72 hours, it has a 2% failure rate. Side-effects include nausea and lethargy. However, knowledge of emergency contraception is poor among many young people.

Teenage parenthood

The UK has the highest rate of teenage pregnancy in Western Europe, though encouragingly with a downward time trend. Teenage girls may present with complaints such as abdominal pain, fatigue, breast tenderness, or appetite changes rather than late or missed menstrual period.

Becoming a teenage parent can be a positive life choice and is influenced by culture. There may be considerable support from the extended family, and this may work well. However, in those where the pregnancy was unintended or who are emotionally deprived themselves or unsupported and live in poverty, there may be many adverse consequences for the mother and child. Children of teenage mothers have a higher infant mortality, a higher rate of childhood accidents, illness, and admission to hospital, being taken into care, low educational achievement, sexual abuse, and mental health problems. Deprivation, from the mother's lack of financial and emotional support and the paucity of her own education and life experiences, is the strongest risk factor. Protective factors are having a supportive family, religious belief, and a stable, long-term relationship with the partner.

Health promotion

The reasons to undertake health promotion in adolescents are:

- it is the period for starting health-risk behaviours (smoking, alcohol, drug misuse, unsafe sexual activity) as well as health-promoting behaviours (regular physical exercise, nutrition)
- health-risk behaviours started in adolescence often continue into adult life
- health behaviours may have a direct effect on their lives, e.g. teenage pregnancy, road traffic accidents
- increasing morbidity, e.g. obesity and diabetes.

The main areas for health promotion are:

- health-risk behaviours
- mental health
- violent behaviour
- physical activity, nutrition, and obesity
- parent–adolescent communication.

There are a number of approaches to health promotion for adolescents:

- provide suitable information in a user-friendly way for young people. There are several websites that provide this
- health promotion by society as a whole, e.g. banning cigarette advertising, making emergency contraception available in pharmacies. These can be very effective. However, there is increasing evidence that improving the socioeconomic circumstances of young people would be the most effective intervention for health promotion. Also, as adolescents often embark on more than one risk behaviour, tackling the underlying problem may reduce other risk-taking behaviours: e.g. a programme to reduce bullying in a whole school may also reduce other behaviour such as drug misuse
- training programmes to improve adolescents' ability to accept or reject certain courses of behaviour can be effective for the individual, but is time consuming and expensive
- health promotion by professionals. Exhorting adolescents not to smoke, to eat a balanced diet, use contraception, etc., has not been found to be effective, and may be counterproductive. Health professionals do have a role in health promotion at an individual level. It is likely to be most effective if targeted at those who are receptive or contemplating change in their health-risk behaviour. However, motivational interviewing techniques (which do not assume that they are ready to change their behaviour, but aim to increase their intrinsic motivation to change) have also been shown to be useful with this age group.

Transition to adult services

The young person with a chronic condition must eventually leave paediatric and adolescent services for adult services. This often involves changing from a treatment model based around close contact between the adolescent and healthcare professionals (e.g. unlimited telephone advice from clinical nurse specialists, possibly home visits, frequent appointments) and involvement with parents and other family members, to one where they are likely to be seen infrequently in a busy adult clinic where parental involvement may be minimal or discouraged.

Young people and their parents need both information about the transfer process and time to prepare including the necessary skills to negotiate the adult healthcare system. Transitional care encompasses this preparation which, by definition, addresses the medical, psychosocial, and educational/vocational needs as a young person moves from child- to adult-centred services. Parents are often concerned that the adult team will not address their teenager's healthcare needs. It is helpful if an identified healthcare professional, often a nurse specialist, is responsible for coordinating transition arrangements.

Whereas transitional care starts in early adolescence, some flexibility in age of transfer is desirable, so that it can occur when the young person is developmentally ready and has the necessary maturity to cope with adult services.

Transfer may be via an adolescent or young adult service with clinics run by both adolescent and adult teams together. Such bridging arrangements have many advantages, but require a sufficient number of patients and medical staff able and willing to provide this service. These clinics are usually for specialist conditions, e.g. diabetes, juvenile idiopathic arthritis, cystic fibrosis, or congenital heart disease. Alternatively, transfer may be successfully accomplished if there is good communication between teams, although it usually involves a radical change in ethos for the adolescent and family. The general practitioner may be a source of continuity between changing specialty practitioners.

> **Summary**
>
> **Transition to adult services**
> - Transitional care aims to address medical, psychosocial, and educational/vocational issues as young people move from child- to adult-centred services.

Acknowledgements

We would like to acknowledge contributors to this chapter in previous editions, whose work we have drawn on: Terry Segal (3rd Edition), Russell Viner (3rd Edition), Janet McDonagh (4th Edition).

> **Summary**
>
> **The main health problems of adolescents**
>
> **Common acute illness:**
> - respiratory disorders, skin conditions, musculoskeletal problems
>
> **Chronic illness and disability,** including previously fatal congenital disorders
>
> **Somatic symptoms:**
> - Fatigue, headache, backache and abdominal pain (see Ch. 24)
>
> **Mental health problems** (see Ch. 24)
>
> **Health-risk behaviours:**
> - Smoking, drinking, drug abuse, road traffic accidents (see Chs 1, 7 and 24)
>
> **Sexual health:**
> - Sexually transmitted infections, contraception, teenage pregnancy
>
> **Eating disorders** (see Ch. 24) **and obesity** (see Ch. 13)

Further reading

Colver A, Longwell S: New understanding of adolescent brain development: relevance to transitional healthcare for young people with long term conditions. *Archives of Disease in Childhood* 98:902–907, 2013.

Viner R: *ABC of Adolescence*, London, 2005, BMJ Books.

White B, Viner RM: Improving communication with adolescents. *Archives of Disease in Childhood Education & Practice* 97:93–97, 2012.

Websites (Accessed November 2016)

Key Data on Adolescence 2015: http://www.youngpeopleshealth.org.uk/key-data-on-adolescence

Lancet commission on adolescent health and wellbeing: *Lancet* 387(10036):2423-2478, 2016. http://www.thelancet.com/commissions/adolescent-health-and-wellbeing

National Health Service England: Available at: http://talklab.nhs.uk/programme

Better Conversations: To improve communication during medical consultations with young people.

National Health Service England: Available at: http://www.nhs.uk/Livewell/teenboys/Pages/teenboyshome.aspx.
Information for young people (boys).

National Health Service England: Available at: http://www.nhs.uk/Livewell/TeenGirls/Pages/teengirlshome.aspx.
Information for young people (girls).

Youth Health Talk: Available at: http://www.healthtalk.org/young-peoples-experiences.

Young people's experiences: Information from young people for young people.

31

Global child health

Child mortality	535
Improving neonatal survival	538
Maternal health and obstetric care	539
Improving the survival of children	540
Mental health	540
Coexisting multiple pathologies: a major threat to child survival	540
Children affected by conflict	542
Future developments	542

Features of global child health are:
- the number of deaths of children <5 years of age per year has halved in the last 25 years, but there is huge intercountry and intracountry variation in mortality rates
- poverty; poor maternal education; conflict; and inadequate access to safe water, sanitation and healthcare are the main determinants of child mortality
- the number of children dying from infectious diseases has declined markedly
- neonatal mortality accounts for an increasing proportion of child deaths, but could be significantly reduced by implementing basic neonatal care.

Child mortality

Worldwide, 5.9 million children under 5 years of age died in 2015 (Fig. 31.1). Neonatal mortality (first 4 weeks of life) accounts for 45% of all under-5-year-old deaths. Infectious diseases, with undernutrition as a major contributing factor, continue to account for about half of the deaths in children beyond the neonatal period (4 weeks to 5 years) (see Fig. 15.1).

- 5.9 million children <5 years of age die each year
- 45% of all deaths in children <5 years of age occur in the neonatal period (first 4 weeks of life)
- After the neonatal period, about half of all child deaths are due to just five preventable and treatable conditions: pneumonia, diarrhoea, malaria, measles and HIV (human immunodeficiency virus)

Where deaths occur

Although only about 48% of the world's estimated 629 million under-5-year-olds live in sub-Saharan Africa and South Asia, 93% of child deaths occur in these two regions (Fig. 31.2). Over half of all child deaths occur in just five countries: India, Nigeria, Democratic Republic of Congo, Pakistan, and China. Mortality rates are useful for comparing the quality of child health outcomes between countries (Table 31.1). The under-5-year-old mortality rate in Sierra Leone (pre-Ebola) was 161/1000 compared with Switzerland's 4/1000. The major discrepancy between mortality between different regions of the world is shown in Fig. 31.2.

Determining child mortality rates and health outcomes in different countries

In order to determine child mortality and health outcomes and monitor change, accurate data need to be collected. There has been considerable effort to

Table 31.1 Mortality rates are useful for comparing the quality of child health outcomes between countries

Mortality rate (per 1000 live births)	Sub-Saharan Africa	UK
Under 5 years old	92	5
Infant (<1 year old)	64	4
Neonatal (< 28 days old)	31	3

Data from: http://www.unicef.org/media/files/Levels_and_Trends_in_Child_Mortality_2014.pdf (Accessed October 4, 2015).

31 Global child health

Deaths in children <5 years old

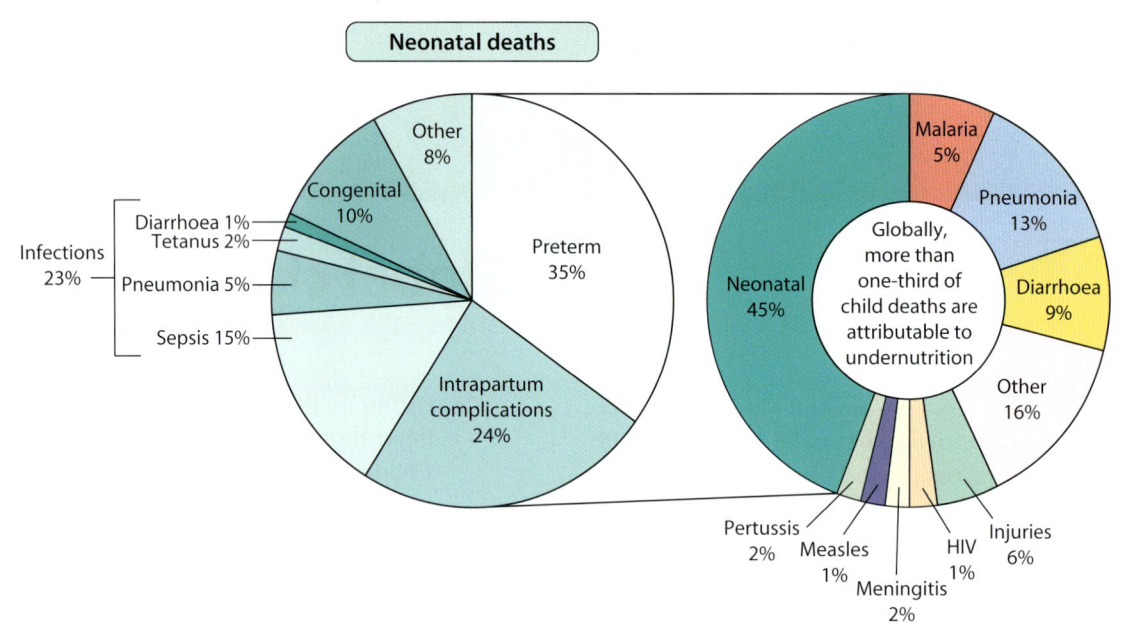

Neonatal deaths

- Other 8%
- Congenital 10%
- Diarrhoea 1%
- Tetanus 2%
- Infections 23%
  - Pneumonia 5%
  - Sepsis 15%
- Preterm 35%
- Intrapartum complications 24%

- Neonatal 45%
- Malaria 5%
- Pneumonia 13%
- Diarrhoea 9%
- Other 16%
- Injuries 6%
- HIV 1%
- Meningitis 2%
- Measles 1%
- Pertussis 2%

Globally, more than one-third of child deaths are attributable to undernutrition

Figure 31.1 Causes of the 5.9 million deaths among children under 5 years of age in 2015. (Data from WHO fact sheet: Available at: www.who.int/mediacentre/factsheets/fs178/en/ and Liu L, Oza S, Hogan D, Perin J, Rudan I, et al: Global, regional, and national causes of child mortality in 2000–13, with projections to inform post-2015 priorities: an updated systematic analysis. *Lancet* 385:430–440, 2015 – Erratum in: *Lancet* 385:420, 2015.)

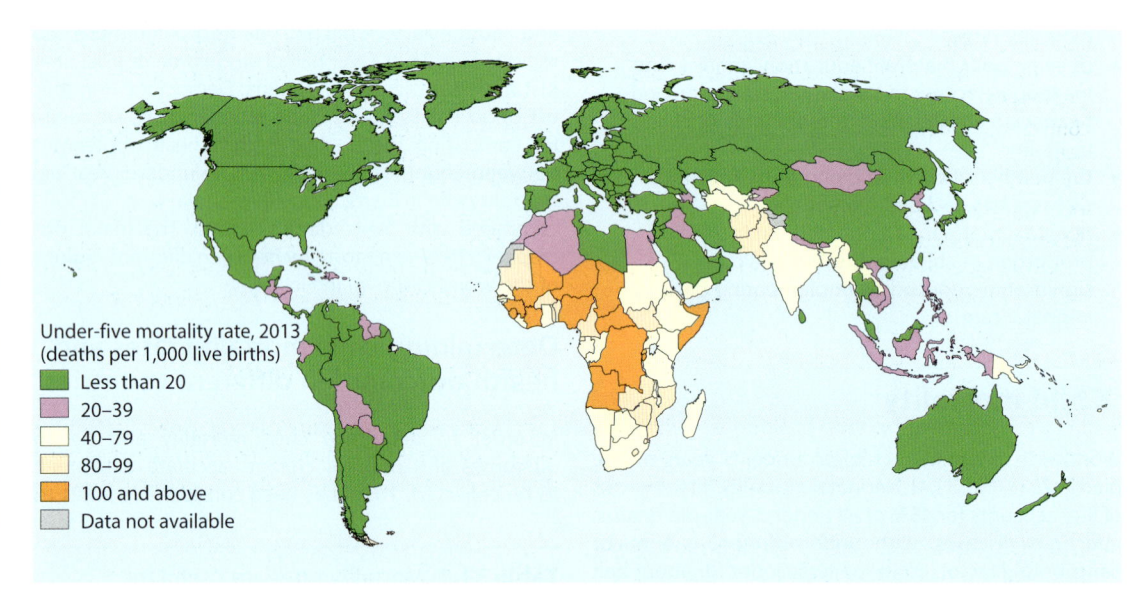

Under-five mortality rate, 2013 (deaths per 1,000 live births)
- Less than 20
- 20–39
- 40–79
- 80–99
- 100 and above
- Data not available

Figure 31.2 Global distribution of under-5-year-old deaths. (Data from Committing to Child Survival: a promise renewed. Progress report 2014, UNICEF.)

improve data collection, but many obstacles remain; even deaths, particularly of newborn infants, are often unreported in countries with poor vital registration systems.

Why is child mortality so high?

Children depend on their environment as well as the provision of healthcare for their survival, as described in Chapter 1 (The child in society). The environment can have major detrimental effects on their chances of survival:

- poverty and social determinants – pervade almost all aspects of health and healthcare. In almost all low-resource countries, there is a marked difference in health outcomes between high-income and low-income groups (Fig. 31.3)
- maternal education – the higher the level of maternal education, the higher the chance of her child's survival (Fig. 31.3)

536

Neonatal mortality rate by household wealth quintile, mother's education, and residence, 2005–2013

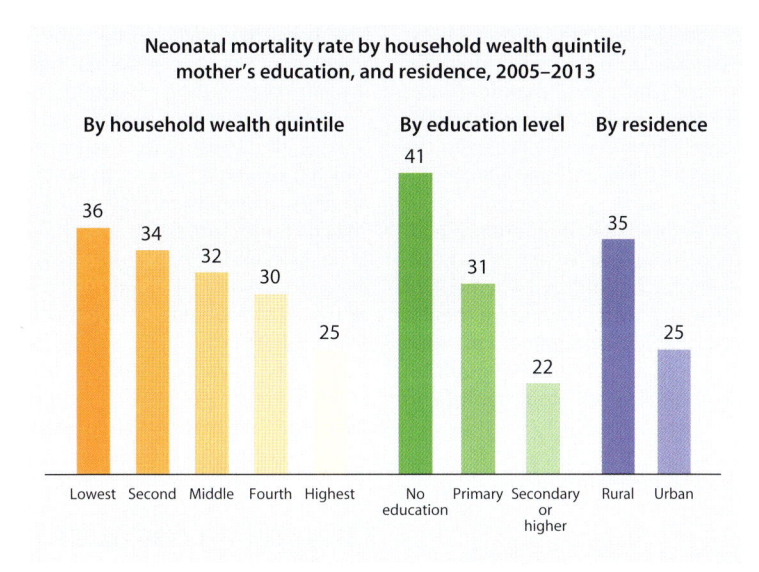

By household wealth quintile: Lowest 36, Second 34, Middle 32, Fourth 30, Highest 25

By education level: No education 41, Primary 31, Secondary or higher 22

By residence: Rural 35, Urban 25

Figure 31.3 Children born to poorer households, to mothers with no formal education, and living in rural areas face a higher risk of dying in the first 28 days of life. (Data from Committing to Child Survival: a promise renewed. Progress report 2014, UNICEF.)

- poor sanitation and unclean water – increase in diarrhoea and infection
- poor food security – malnutrition increases vulnerability and severity of illness, especially infection [see Ch. 13 (Nutrition)]. Chronic malnutrition is reflected in stunting of children
- inadequate housing, air pollution, and overcrowding – promotes the spread of respiratory pathogens (Fig. 31.3)
- conflict – see the 'Children affected by conflict' section
- geographical variation in diseases – large intercountry and inter-regional differences, e.g. malaria is responsible for 15% of deaths in children under-5-years-old in Sub-Saharan Africa compared with 1% in Southeast Asia.

The provision of healthcare in many low and middle-income countries is poor and adversely affects survival:

- limited finance available for healthcare – whereas Sweden spends US$4244/person per year on health (10% of gross domestic product), in 34 low-resource countries it is less than US$50/person per year (WHO 2013)
- disease prevention, e.g. vaccination, insecticide-treated net distribution for protection from malaria – lower coverage in poor areas
- access – difficult to get to health facilities; cost and affordability may be major limiting factors
- community care is limited by lack of trained community health workers
- health centres and hospitals – care compromised by lack of trained staff, equipment, drugs, suitable buildings, etc.
- medical care – lack of trained doctors is a serious problem in almost all these countries. The contrast between the proportion of doctors compared with deaths in children is shown in Figs 31.4 and 31.5.

Reducing child mortality

There has been a major effort by many low and middle-income countries to improve child health. This has been done in conjunction with the international community,

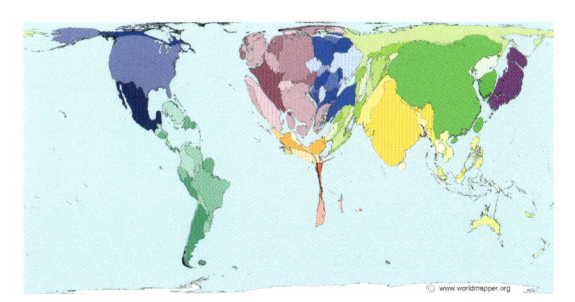

Figure 31.4 Territory size shows the proportion of doctors who work in that territory. (© Benjamin D. Hennig (Worldmapper Project) http://www.worldmapper.org, 2002 data; accessed November 2015.)

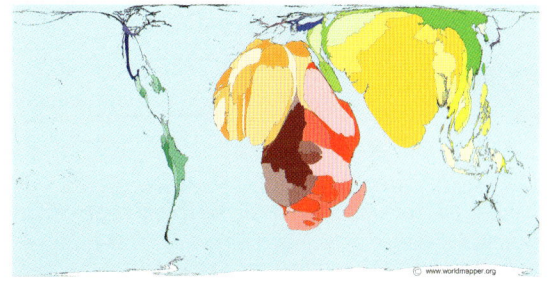

Figure 31.5 Territory size shows the proportion of all deaths of children aged 1 year to 5 years. (© Benjamin D. Hennig (Worldmapper Project) http://www.worldmapper.org, 2002 data; accessed November 2015.)

with programmes of aid (United States Agency for International Development (USAID), Department for International Development (DfID), etc.), charities (Gates Foundation, etc.), and non-governmental organizations (United Nations Children's Emergency Fund, Save the Children, etc.). Some of the major international initiatives are listed in Box 31.1.

The launch of the Integrated Management of Childhood Illness in 1992 was an important step in promoting the comprehensive and holistic management of children attending primary and secondary health facilities. It recognized that an integrated approach to childhood illness is required, including nutrition and preventative care in families and communities. In health facilities, sick children are triaged according to the presence of specific danger signs and management is planned according to algorithms.

A major advance in global child health was the adoption of the Millennium Development Goals (MDGs), which have served as a focus for the international community's commitment to reduce child mortality. The specific target for MDG 4 was to reduce child mortality in children under 5 years of age by two-thirds between the years 1990 and 2015. In 1990 there were 12.7 million deaths of children under 5 years of age compared with the 5.9 million in 2015, a 54% reduction (Fig. 31.6). Contributions were also made by other MDGs, which included reducing maternal mortality (MDG 5) and reducing the burden of HIV (human immunodeficiency virus), malaria, and tuberculosis (MDG 6).

> **Box 31.1** Key international developments in maternal and child health
>
> - 1946: United Nations Children's Emergency Fund (UNICEF) established
> - 1948: World Health Organization (WHO) formed
> - 1974: Extended Programme of Immunisation (EPI) included diphtheria, pertussis, tetanus, polio, tuberculosis, and measles
> - 1980s: GOBI-FFF. Key primary care strategies: growth monitoring, oral rehydration therapy, breastfeeding, immunization, family spacing, female education, and food supplementation
> - 1989: UN Convention on the Rights of the Child
> - 1992: World Summit for Children – Child-to-Child strategy, Baby Friendly Initiative, Integrated Management of Childhood Illness
> - 2000: United Nations endorses Millennium Development Goals
> - 2013 Global Action Plan for Pneumonia and Diarrhoea
> - 2015 United Nations endorses Sustainable Development Goals

Improving neonatal survival

There are 135 million births a year worldwide, and 3 million neonatal deaths. Progress in reducing neonatal mortality has been strikingly slower than in reducing under-5-year-old mortality (Fig. 31.6). Whereas the birth of a baby should be a joyous occasion, globally, every year, 1 million newborns and 125 000 mothers (half of maternal deaths) die during or in the first day after childbirth. There are also 1.2 million stillbirths.

The main causes of neonatal death (Fig. 31.1) are:

- preterm birth
- intrapartum complications, i.e. perinatal asphyxia
- infections such as sepsis and pneumonia.

Neonatal tetanus is an important cause of death in many countries, though this has been markedly reduced by maternal immunization and hygiene at delivery, especially clean cord-care practices. Intrauterine growth restriction is a significant comorbidity in many neonatal deaths. Whereas only 14% of babies in low-resource countries are low birthweight (<2.5 kg), they account for 60% to 80% of deaths.

Millenium Development Goal 4

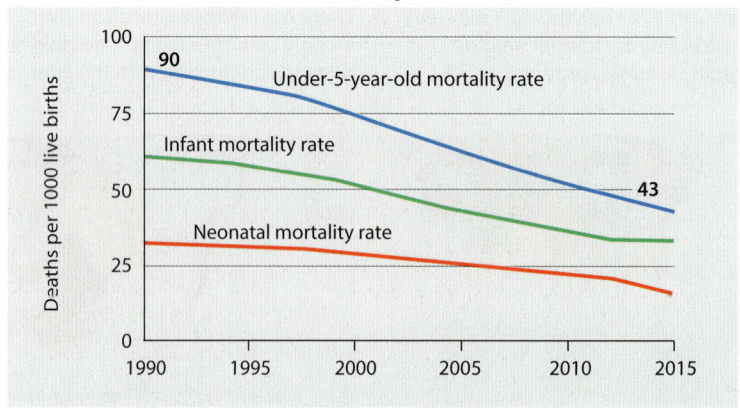

Figure 31.6 Reduction in under-5-year-old and neonatal mortality rates during the Millennium Development Goal period 1990–2015. Under-5-year-old mortality rate estimated to be 43 per 1000 live births and neonatal mortality rate 19 per 1000 live births in 2015. (Data from UN Interagency Group for Child Mortality Estimation (IGME) 2013, Available at: http://www.unicef.org/media/files/Levels_and_Trends_in_Child_Mortality_2014.pdf and Millennium Development Goals Report 2015, UN; accessed August 2016.)

Maternal health and obstetric care

Maternal health and obstetric care are major determinants of neonatal morbidity and mortality. Factors are listed in Table 31.2. About 70% of deliveries worldwide are now by a skilled birth attendant, but their obstetric skills are variable and rapid referral to health facilities able to deal with obstetric emergencies remains problematic. Participatory women's groups, where mothers meet for peer counselling to deal with their local issues, have been shown to markedly reduce both maternal and neonatal mortalities.

Saving newborn lives

It has been estimated that over 1 million newborns could be saved by the provision of essential newborn care (Fig. 31.7).

While, in some settings, provision of more advanced neonatal care or even neonatal intensive care including

Table 31.2 Maternal health and obstetric care that improve neonatal morbidity and mortality

Before conception	Pregnancy	Labour and delivery
• Family planning (encourage delay of first pregnancy to age 18 years and 3 yearly birth interval) • Maternal nutrition optimized, including folic acid to prevent neural tube defects • Chronic conditions stabilized – hypertension, diabetes • Infection prevention and treatment (malaria, tetanus, sexually transmitted infections, HIV (human immunodeficiency virus)	• Complications of pregnancy managed – pre-eclampsia, etc.	• Antenatal steroids for preterm labour • Skilled birth attendant at all births, with newborn resuscitation training • Timely and skilled management of complications, e.g. caesarean section to prevent perinatal asphyxia • Clean delivery practices

Key interventions in the neonatal period

	Essential newborn care	Hospital-level interventions
Neonatal resuscitation	Skilled birth attendants can provide basic neonatal resuscitation (Helping Babies Breathe programme) and identify infants needing additional care	Appropriately trained healthcare professionals (Helping Babies Breathe programme)
Infection prevention	Hand hygiene, clean cord cutting/ligature, chlorhexidine to cord	Hand hygiene, clean equipment
Hypothermia prevention	Drying of baby, skin to skin contact of mother and baby, covering the baby including head, delay bathing the baby	If significantly preterm, place in plastic bag/wrap immediately after birth, then radiant heater or incubator or warming mattress
Feeding	Early and exclusive breastfeeding within 1 h of birth	Supplemental feeding if required (expressed breast milk via cup or nasogastric tube)
Sick, preterm, or low birth weight babies		Antibiotic treatment if at increased risk or signs of infection
		Intravenous fluids and supplemental oxygen if required

Figure 31.7 Key interventions in the neonatal period.

mechanical ventilation may be appropriate, the lives of the largest number of babies could be saved if the essential neonatal care outlined earlier was available.

Case history 31.1

Preterm birth

A baby boy was born at 32 weeks' gestation in Malawi. The mother was transferred to a district hospital to deliver her baby after the spontaneous onset of preterm labour. Following delivery, the infant received oxygen, intravenous antibiotics, and expressed breast milk via a nasogastric tube. After the baby was stabilized, he was nursed by Kangaroo Mother Care, where the mother provides continuous care for her baby on her chest (Fig. 31.8). This provides better thermal care and lower infection rates than incubator care, promotes breastfeeding and maternal bonding to her baby. Breastfeeding was successfully established over a period of 3 weeks.

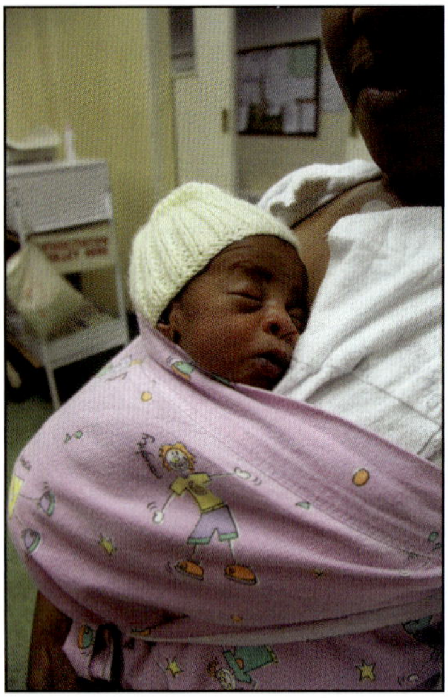

Figure 31.8 Kangaroo Mother Care of preterm infants. This is widely promoted and practiced in many low and middle-income countries, and gaining popularity in high-income countries.

Improving the survival of children

Infection

A major component of the reduction in child mortality has been reduced mortality from infectious diseases. Increasing immunization coverage has been hugely successful. The goal of the World Health Organization Expanded Programme of Immunisation is to provide universal access to vaccines to all at risk. However significant inequity remains in the vaccines offered to children living in different countries as well as in the coverage of vaccination schedules within countries. The strategies adopted to reduce infection are shown in Fig. 31.9.

Nutrition

Exclusive breastfeeding for the first 6 months of life is strongly advocated as it is the ideal milk for babies and there is less risk of gastroenteritis and other infections. To promote successful breastfeeding, the World Health Organization has developed the Baby-Friendly Hospital Initiative, which comprises 10 steps for maternity departments to follow.

Malnutrition remains a major problem in many countries, both acute and chronic [Ch. 13 (Nutrition)]. It is estimated that 1 in 4 children under 5 years of age experiences chronic malnutrition and is stunted; over 90% are in Africa and Asia, the majority in South Asia.

As well as malnutrition, obesity is becoming an increasing problem in low and middle-income countries. Globally, of the 42 million children under the age of 5 years who are overweight, about 31 million live in low-income countries. This is predominantly seen in middle-class families, where energy-dense food and drinks are popular and children do much less exercise than those in poorer communities.

Trauma and road traffic injuries

Sub-Saharan Africa has the highest death rates due to unintentional injury in the world, with 53/100 000 children compared with 39/100 000 globally. The five major causes of injury are road traffic incidents, burns, drowning, poisoning, and falls. Poor living conditions and socioeconomic circumstances place children at increased risk from exposure to dangerous environments. Critically, unintentional injury, mainly through road traffic incidents, is one of the few causes of child mortality that is predicted to increase by 2030. There is also a problem in providing good surgical care following injuries.

Mental health

Globally, 10–20% of children and adolescents have mental health disorders that impact negatively on their health and well-being. The epidemiology of child mental health is poorly described and access to services is scarce, even in middle-income countries. Suicide is a major cause of death in young male adolescents.

Coexisting multiple pathologies: a major threat to child survival

In low and middle-income countries children often have multiple coexisting pathologies as well as multiple adversities relating to the background in which they live. This combination contributes to poor outcomes. Examples are shown in Case Histories 31.2 and 31.3.

Strategies to reduce infection and malnutrition

	Prevention	Community management	Hospital management
Pneumonia	Expanded programme for immunisation (EPI) (Hib, PCV, measles, rotavirus, etc.) Water, Sanitation, and Hygiene (WASH) Vitamin A and zinc supplementation Household food security School-feeding programmes Deworming Breast feeding promotion	Antibiotic therapy Detection of severe pneumonia and hospital referral	Antibiotic and oxygen therapy
Diarrhoea		Oral rehydration therapy (ORS) and continued feeding	ORS or IV fluids if shock
Malnutrition		Ambulatory management of mild or moderate malnutrition with ready-to-use therapeutic food (RTUF)	WHO Ten Steps to Recovery for inpatient management of severe acute malnutrition
Malaria	Insecticide-treated bed nets Vector control, indoor residual spraying	Near-patient Rapid Diagnostic Testing (RDT) for malaria Artemisinin Combination Therapy (ACT)	
TB	Effective adult TB control programme BCG immunization Contact tracing and isoniazid preventative treatment	Effective childhood TB case detection and access to suitable laboratory services Child-friendly TB treatment programmes	
HIV	Prevention of Mother-To-Child Transmission (PMTCT)	Access to HIV serological (antibody) and virological (antigen) testing Child-friendly antiretroviral therapy (ART) treatment programmes	
Guidelines	Integrated management of childhood illness (IMCI)	Training courses e.g. Emergency Triage, Assessment and Treatment (ETAT)	

Figure 31.9 Strategies to reduce infection and malnutrition showing prevention and community and hospital management. HiB, *Haemophilus influenzae* type b vaccination; PCV, pneumococcal conjugate vaccine; IV, intravenous; WHO, World Health Organization.

Case history 31.2

Burns to the face

This girl in rural Niger sustained facial burns (Fig. 31.10). She fell into the open kitchen fire when she had a seizure. Although her epilepsy had initially responded well to phenobarbital, regular supplies were unavailable. Difficulty in finding affordable transport from the village to the health clinic delayed presentation by 4 days, by which time there was secondary infection and increased risk of cataract from conjunctival injury. This simple example highlights the influence of environment on children's health. Although her illness was readily treatable and her injuries were preventable with a fireguard, delayed treatment resulted in complications and only basic medical care was available at the clinic.

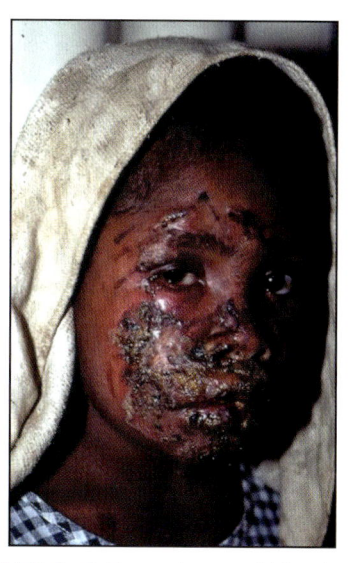

Figure 31.10 Facial burns in a rural Nigerian girl.

Case history 31.3

Malnutrition

This 10-month-old girl in Kenya presented to an urban health clinic with cough and diarrhoea, and was found to be severely malnourished, with a mid-upper-arm circumference less than 115 mm and weight for length more than −3 standard deviations below the median (Fig. 31.11). She was referred to hospital for inpatient therapeutic feeding. In the weeks after her birth, she had moved from a rural area to the city as her 17-year-old mother needed to find work. After exclusively breastfeeding for 3 months, the child had been fed predominantly on *ugali* (maize flour cooked to thick porridge consistency). Her mother had struggled to maintain breastfeeding as she had two manual jobs and could not afford artificial milk. This example shows how poverty can affect infant health. The combination of her mother's conflicting demands between home and work, coupled with the isolation of moving to a new urban environment and her poverty resulted in her daughter develop severe acute malnutrition before seeking help.

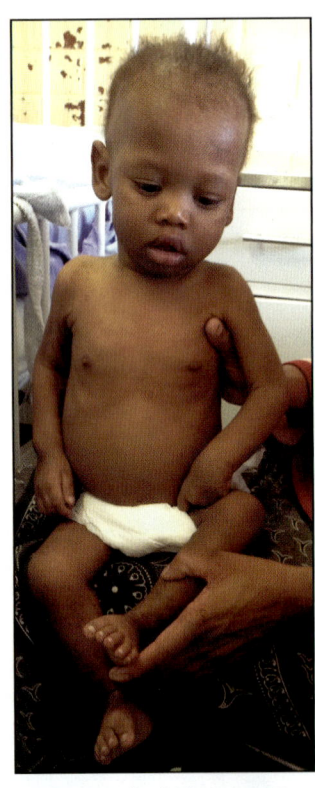

Figure 31.11 A 10-month old in urban Kenya with malnutrition because of poor socioeconomic circumstances. She has oedema of the feet and lower limbs and redness of the hair from kwashiorkor.

Children affected by conflict

The increasing number of conflicts in the Middle East and Africa, many of which are protracted and target civilian populations, means that there are huge numbers of refugees (16.7 million) and internally displaced people (33.3 million). Children and women are disproportionately affected physically and psychologically by conflict.

As well as the threat to life, children living in conflict may suffer in a wide variety of ways. They may lack shelter and endure exposure to harsh weather such as freezing winters. There may be lack of clean water and sanitation and fragile food security and hunger. They may not be able to access education as no schooling is available. There may be a lack of safe birthing facilities and neonatal care. Healthcare is likely to be compromised by poor uptake of vaccinations, limited access to poorly staffed and equipped health facilities, and also low supplies of essential medicines. The direct threat posed to health facilities and healthcare workers combines to undermine the health of children in conflict. The mental health of children may be severely affected by deep-rooted fear and unrelenting anxiety and exposure to violence that undermines normal social development and psychological growth. Family members may have been injured or killed. Feelings of hopelessness and lack of a future as well as witnessed trauma and the direct psychological impact of conflict or civil unrest may lead to post-traumatic stress disorder. There may be a continual fear of physical or sexual violence. Providing even basic healthcare under these conditions is often extremely difficult; it requires innovative strategies adapted to particular circumstances.

Future developments

Sustainable development goals

These were approved by the United Nations in September 2015. The eight MDGs (Millenium Development Goals) have been replaced by 17 Sustainable Development Goals (SDGs), which have broad aspirations, such as ending poverty and hunger, inclusive and equitable quality education for all. Whereas six of the eight MDGs focussed on health, there is only one SDG specifically for health, to 'ensure healthy lives and promote well-being for all at all ages'. This includes ending preventable deaths of newborns and children under 5 years of age, and sets a target of 12 per 1000 live births for neonatal mortality and 25 for children aged under 5 years by 2030. In addition, the focus of other SDGs on ending poverty and hunger, combating climate change, and improving education will have a welcome impact on health. An example is multiple areas of intervention in school-based programmes, such as school feeding; micronutrient supplementation; treatment of soil-transmitted helminths; protection from malaria; and improved water, sanitation, and hygiene. They will all benefit child health in a more holistic way than the current, narrow vertical focus on HIV virus or malaria programmes alone.

Summary

Global child health
- The number of child deaths globally has decreased to 5.9 million under-5-year-old deaths per year, but the proportion of neonatal deaths has risen to 44%.
- Over half of all child deaths occur in just five countries: India, Nigeria, Democratic Republic of Congo, Pakistan, and China.
- The main causes of neonatal mortality are preterm birth, infection, and intrapartum-related conditions.
- The main causes of postneonatal child mortality are pneumonia, diarrhoea, malaria, and injuries.
- Malnutrition contributes to one-third of child deaths.
- Trauma, conflict, being refugees, mental health, and the coexistence of multiple pathologies pose significant and ongoing threats to the wellbeing of children in low and middle-income countries.
- The Sustainable Development Goals, approved by the United Nations in 2015, are setting the agenda for improving global child health until 2030.

Acknowledgements

We would like to acknowledge contributors to the section on global child health in the chapter The Child in Society in previous editions, whose work we have drawn on: Tom Lissuaer (3rd Edition), Mitch Blair (3rd Edition), Stephen Allen (4th Edition), Ike Lagunju (4th Edition), Raúl Pardíñaz-Solís (4th Edition).

Further reading

Websites (Accessed November 2016)

Ending Preventable Child and Maternal Deaths: Available at: http://www.apromiserenewed.org.
A promise renewed.

The Lancet: Available at: http://www.thelancet.com/series/everynewborn.
Every newborn series, 2014.

United Nations: Available at: https://sustainabledevelopment.un.org/?menu=1300.
Sustainable Development Goals, UN.

Appendix

Growth charts	544
Gestational age assessment of newborn infants	555
Management action plan for asthma	556
Blood pressure chart	557
Peak flow chart	557
Imaging in children	557
Blood tests	558

Growth charts

Examples of growth charts used in the UK for:
- preterm infants: males (Fig. A.1a) and females (Fig. A.1b)
- 0–1-year-old, boys (Fig. A.1c) and girls (Fig. A.1d)
- 1–4-year-old, boys (Fig. A.1e) and girls (Fig. A.1f)
- 2–9 year-old boys (Fig. A.1g) and 2–8 year-old girls (Fig. A.1h)
- 9–18 year-old boys (Fig. A1.i) and 8–18 year-old girls (Fig. A.1j).

In the nine-centile UK charts, the interval between each pair of centile lines is the same (two-thirds standard deviation). They show the 0.4 and 99.6 centile lines, which are two and two-thirds standard deviations below and above the median, respectively. The charts for older children also show the timing of the stages of puberty.

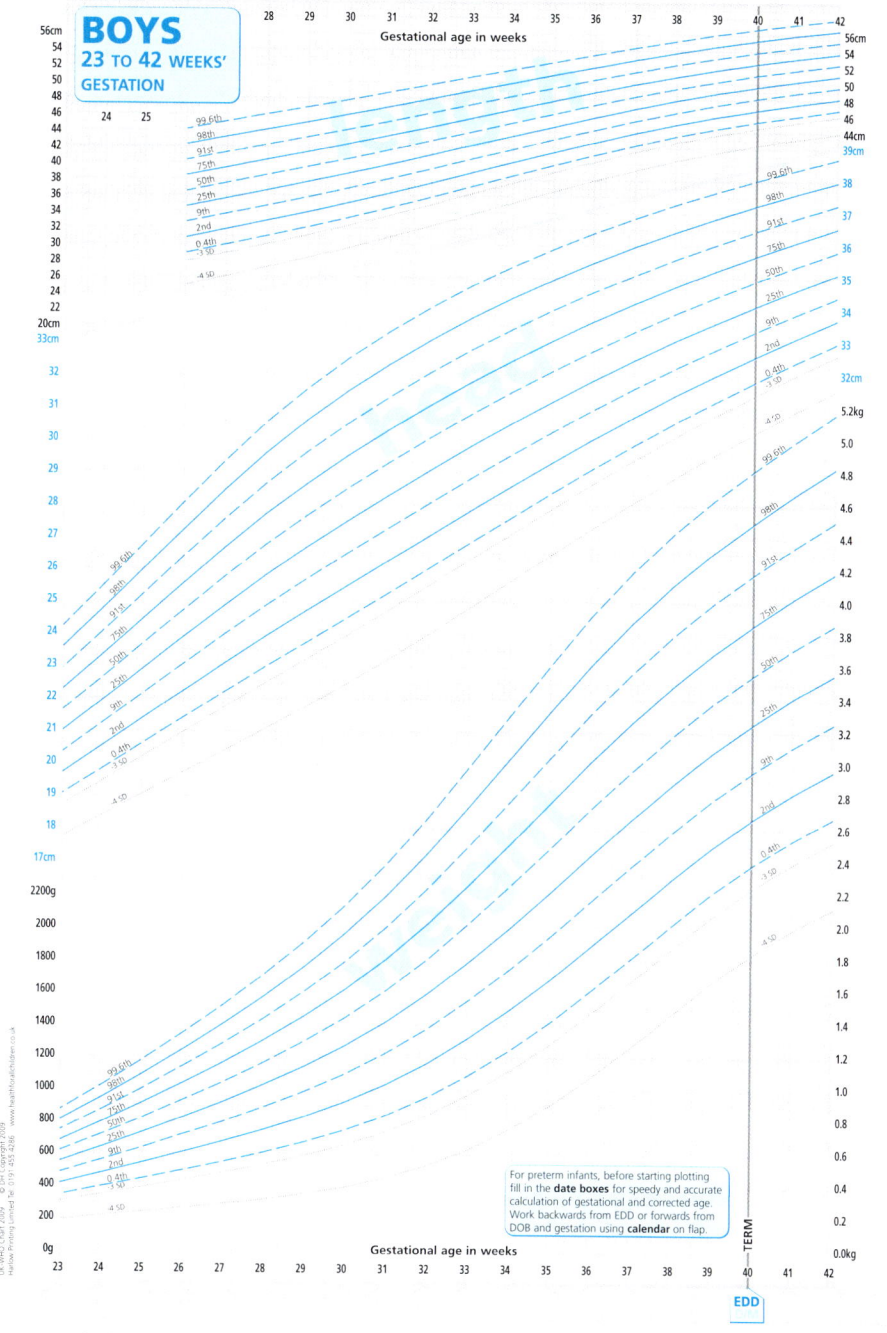

Figure A.1 Growth chart for preterm infants: (**a**) males. (Chart © Child Growth Foundation. Further supplies and information from www.healthforallchildren.co.uk. Reproduced with permission.)

Continued

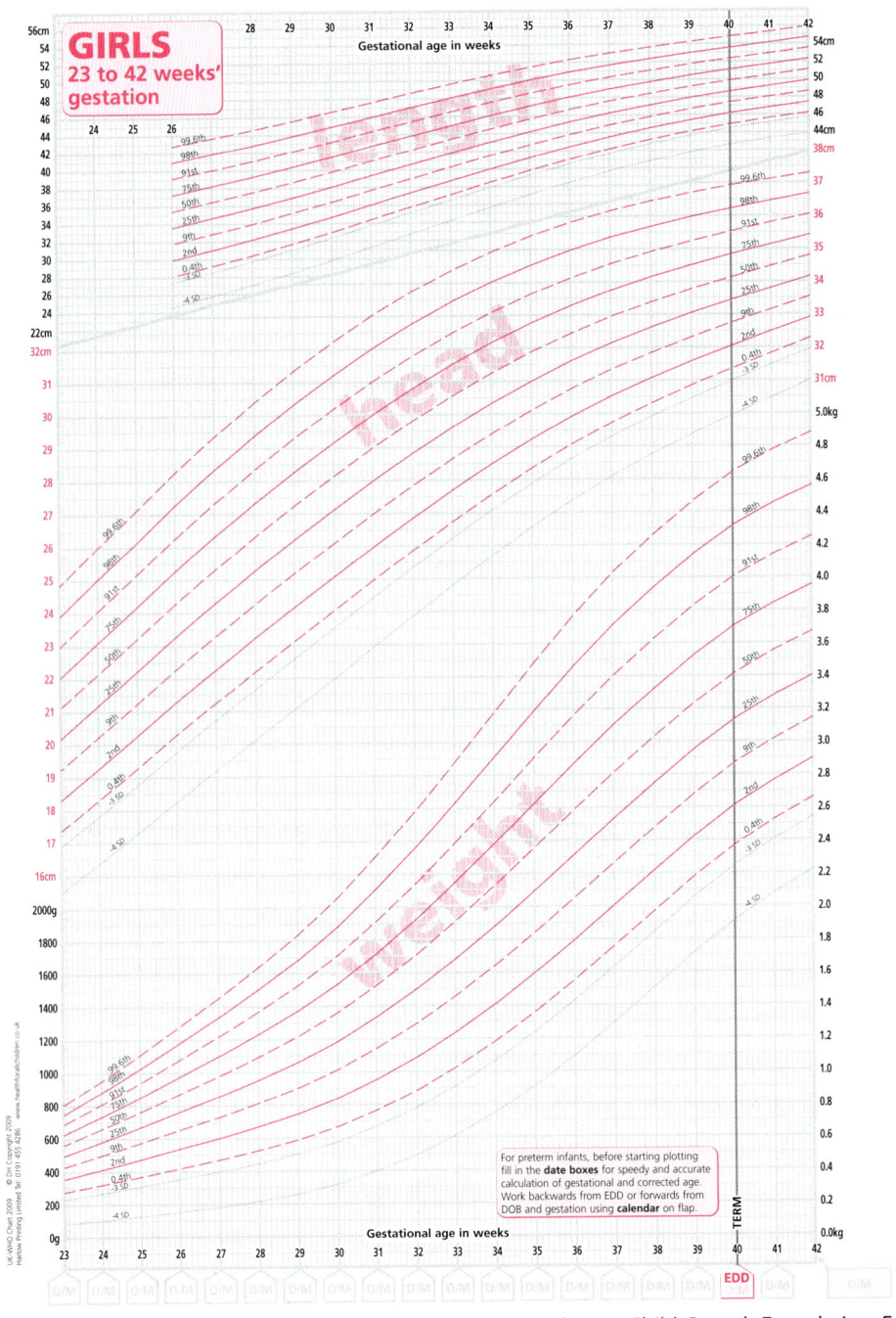

Figure A.1, cont'd Growth chart for preterm infants: (**b**) females. (Chart © Child Growth Foundation. Further supplies and information from www.healthforallchildren.co.uk. Reproduced with permission.)

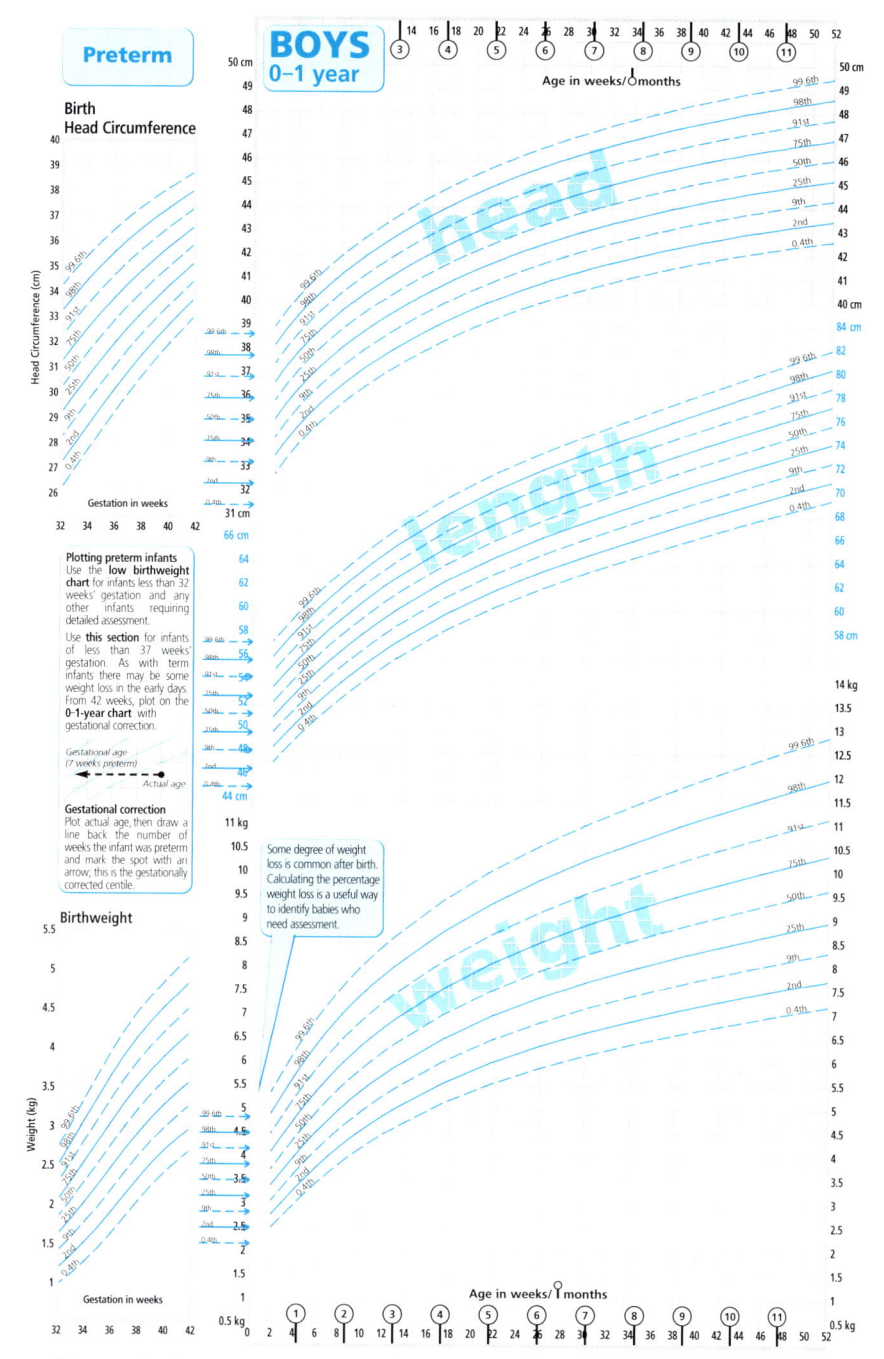

Figure A.1, cont'd Growth chart age 0–1-year: (**c**) Boys. (Chart © Child Growth Foundation. Further supplies and information from www.healthforallchildren.co.uk. Reproduced with permission.)

Continued

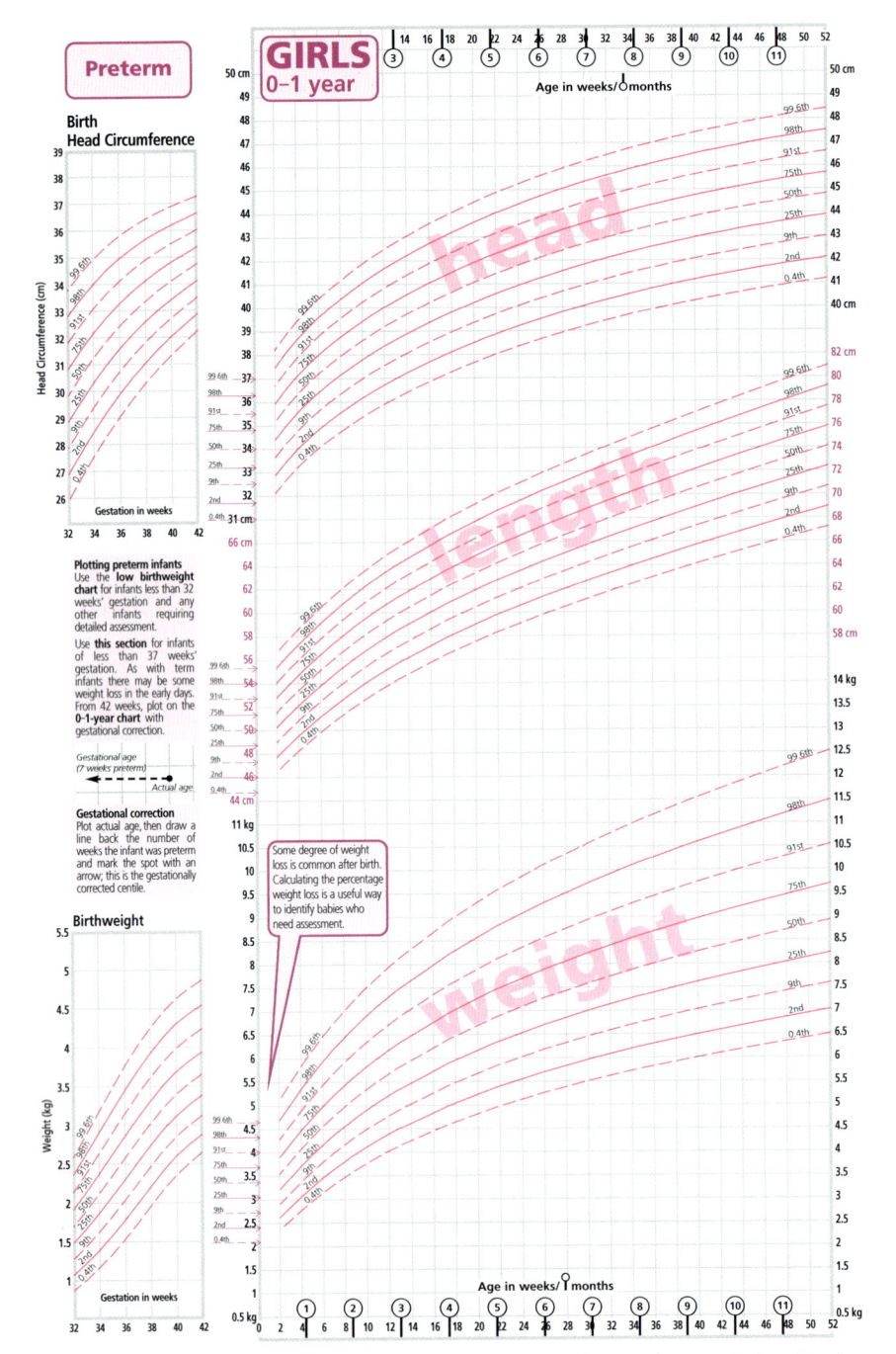

Figure A.1, cont'd Growth chart age 0–1-year: (**d**) girls. (Chart © Child Growth Foundation. Further supplies and information from www.healthforallchildren.co.uk. Reproduced with permission.)

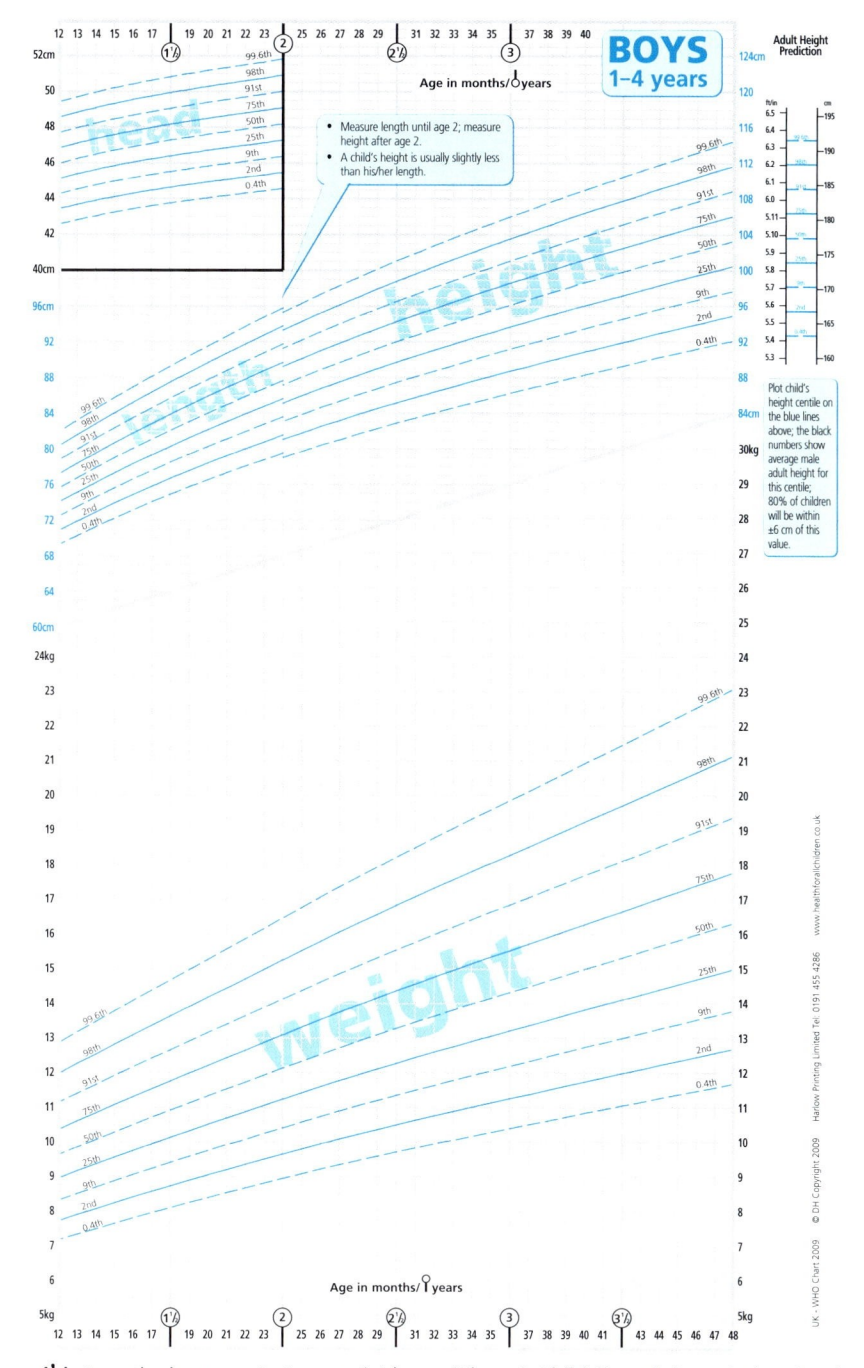

Figure A.1, cont'd Growth chart age 1–4-years: (**e**) boys. (Chart © Child Growth Foundation. Further supplies and information from www.healthforallchildren.co.uk. Reproduced with permission.)

Continued

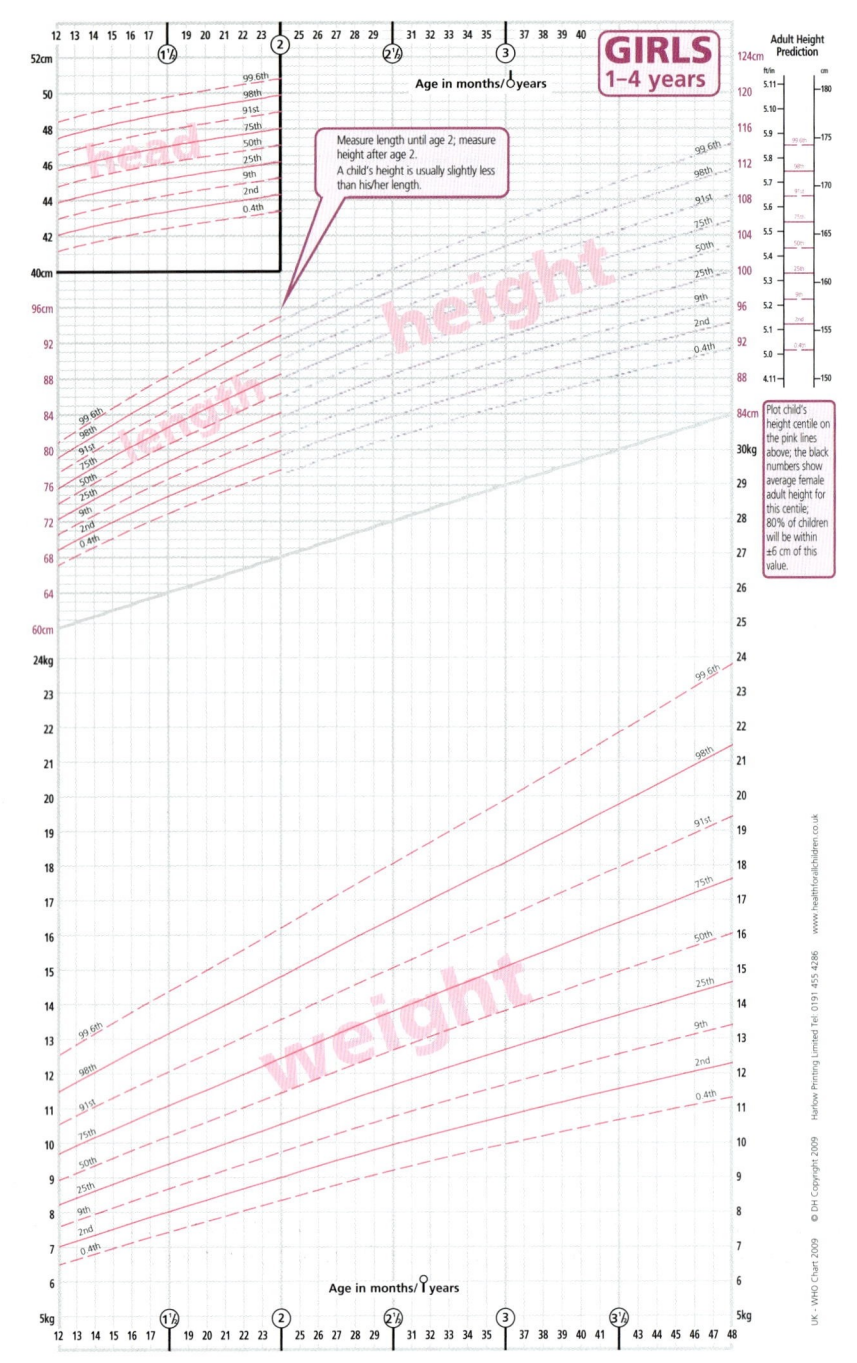

Figure A.1, cont'd Growth chart age 1–4-years: (**f**) girls. (Chart © Child Growth Foundation. Further supplies and information from www.healthforallchildren.co.uk. Reproduced with permission.)

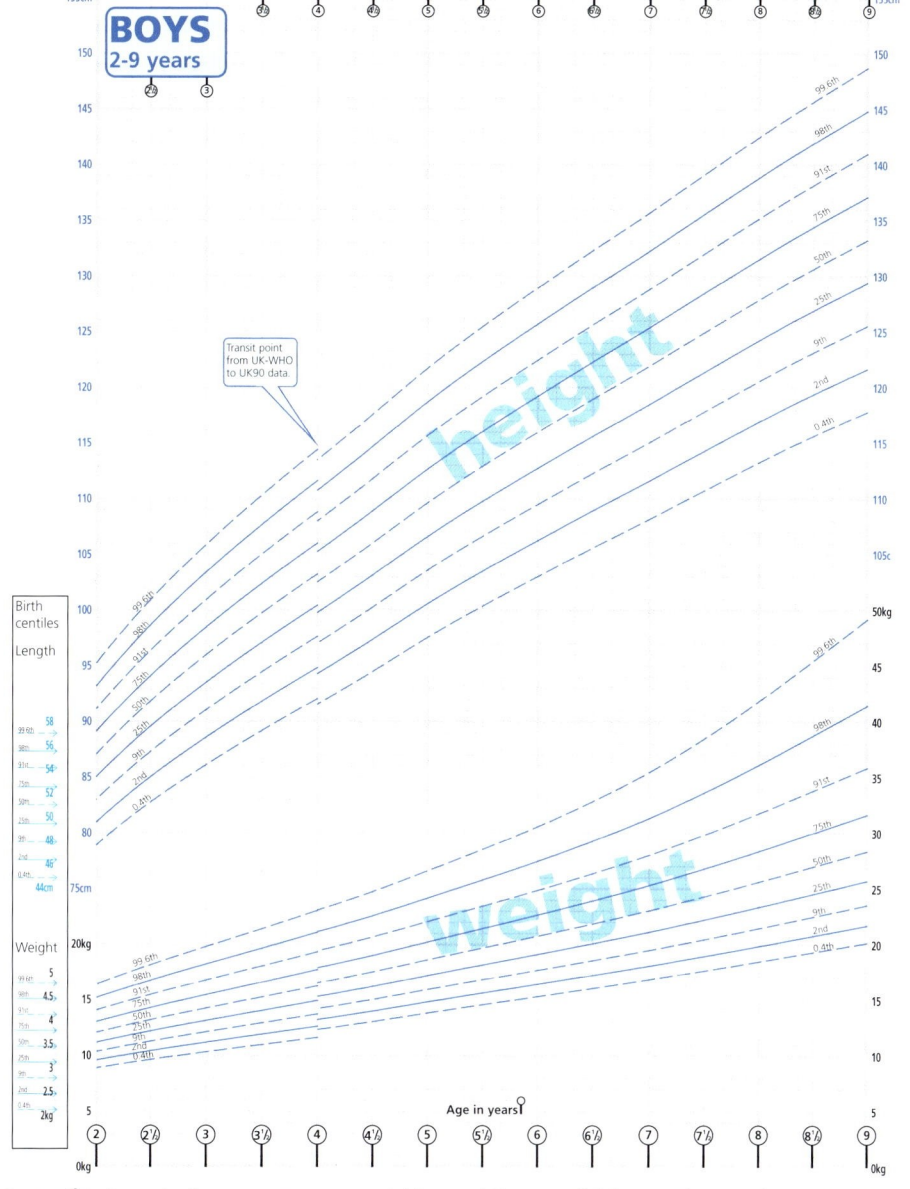

Figure A.1, cont'd Growth chart age 2–9-years: (**g**) boys. (Chart © Child Growth Foundation. Further supplies and information from www.healthforallchildren.co.uk. Reproduced with permission.)

Continued

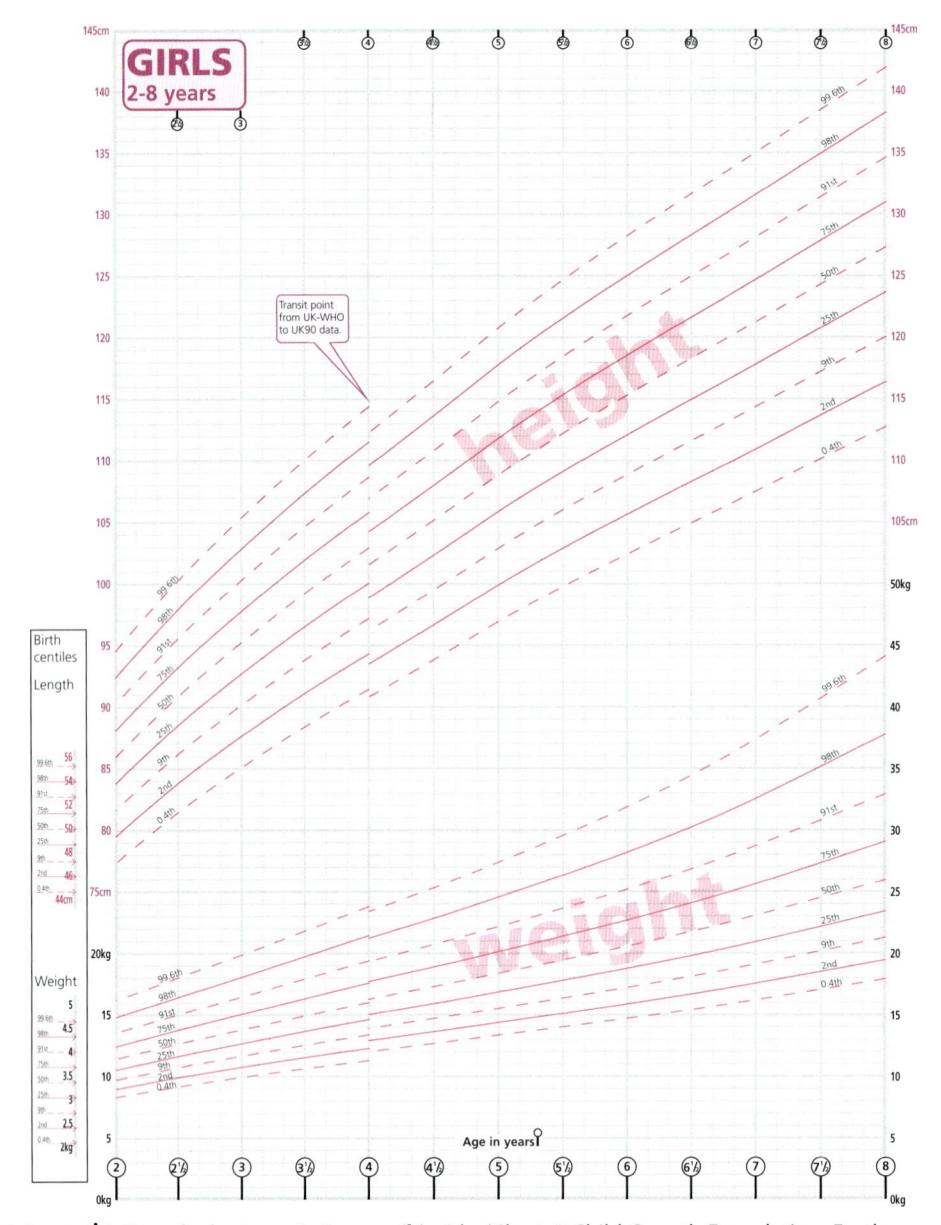

Figure A.1, cont'd Growth chart age 2–8-years: (**h**) girls. (Chart © Child Growth Foundation. Further supplies and information from www.healthforallchildren.co.uk. Reproduced with permission.)

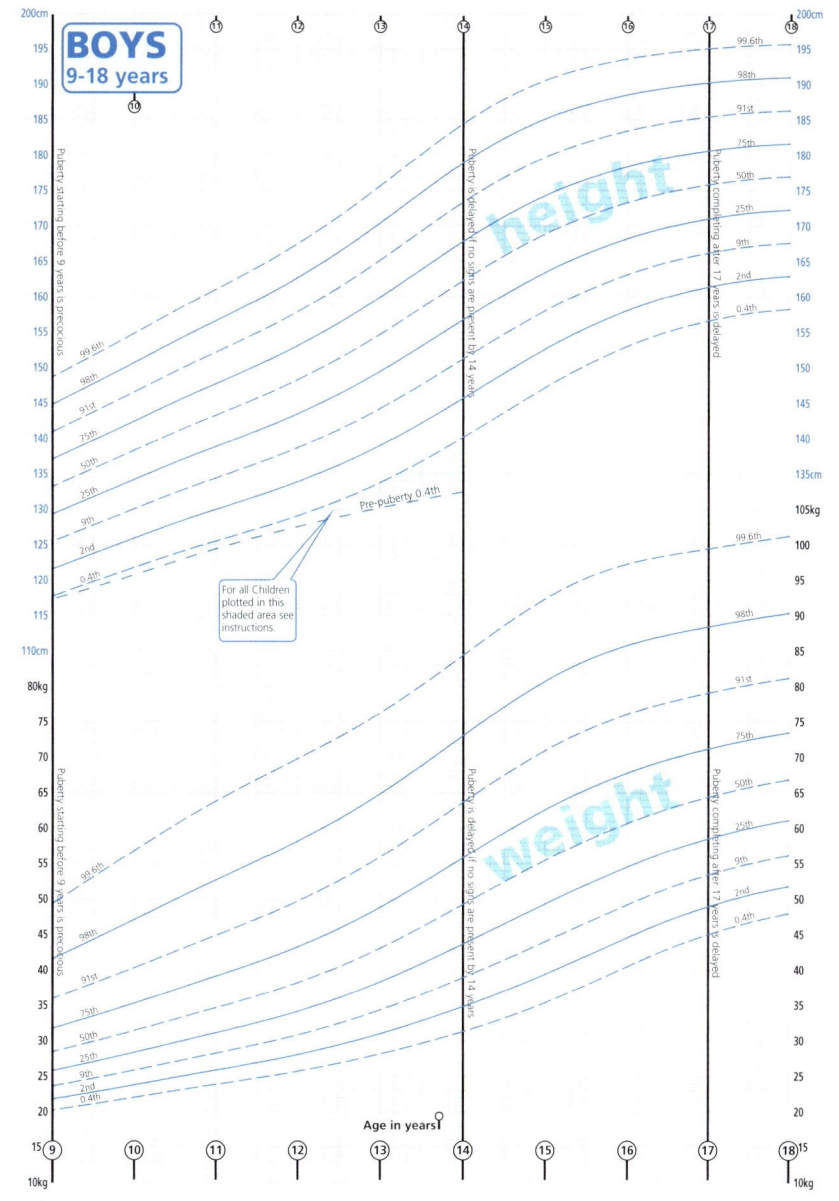

Figure A.1, cont'd Growth chart age 9–18-years: (**i**) boys. (Chart © Child Growth Foundation. Further supplies and information from www.healthforallchildren.co.uk. Reproduced with permission.)

Continued

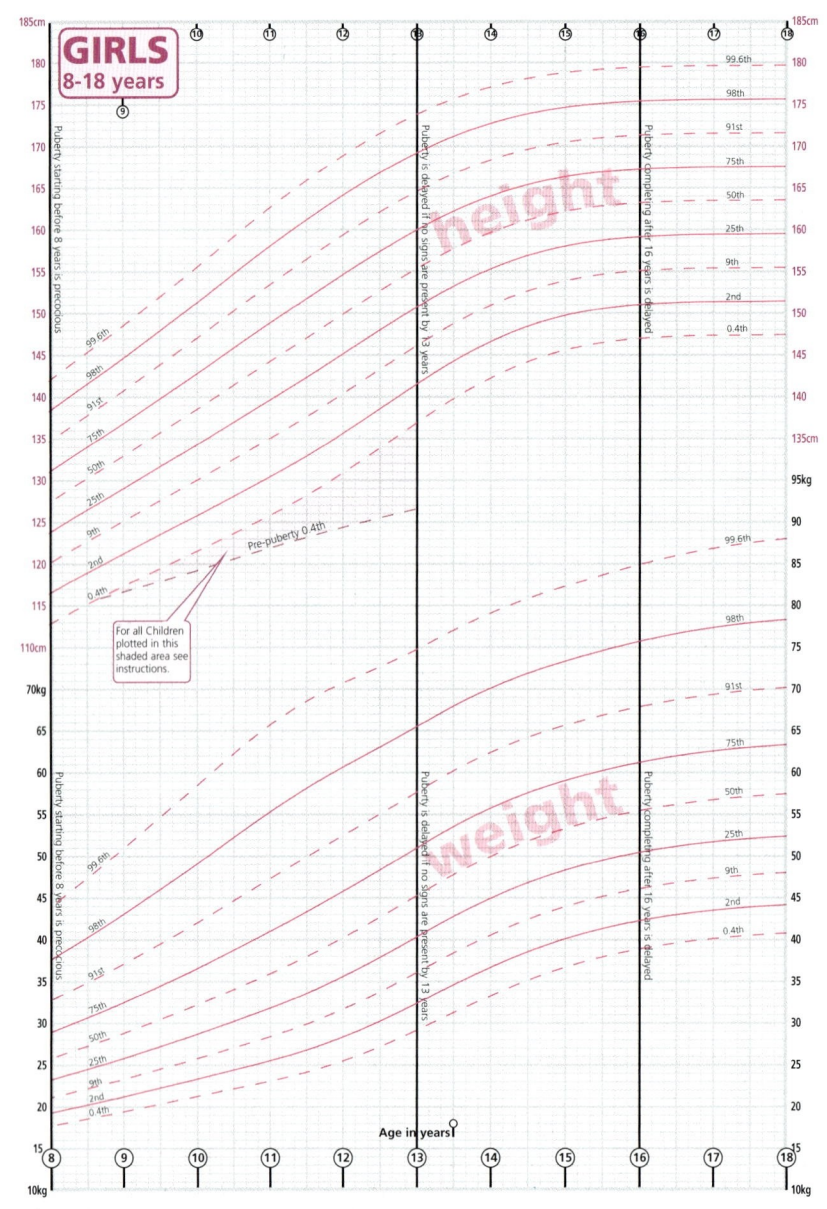

Figure A.1, cont'd Growth chart age 8–18-years: (**j**) girls. (Chart © Child Growth Foundation. Further supplies and information from www.healthforallchildren.co.uk. Reproduced with permission.)

Gestational age assessment of newborn infants (Fig. A.2)

a) Neuromuscular maturity

	−1	0	1	2	3	4	5
Posture							
Square window (wrist)	>90°	90°	60°	45°	35°	0°	
Arm recoil		180°	140°–180°	110°–140°	90°–110°	<90°	
Popliteal angle	180°	160°	140°	120°	100°	90°	<90°
Scarf sign							
Heel to ear							

b) Physical maturity

Skin	Sticky, friable, transparent	Gelatinous, red, translucent	Smooth pink, visible veins	Superficial peeling and/or rash, few veins	Cracking pale areas rare veins	Parchment, deep cracking, no vessels	Leathery, cracked, wrinkled
Lanugo	None	Sparse	Abundant	Thinning	Bald areas	Mostly bald	
Plantar surface	Heel-toe 40–50 mm: −1 <40 mm: −2	>50 mm no crease	Faint red marks	Anterior transverse crease only	Creases ant. 2/3	Creases over entire sole	
Breast	Imperceptible	Barely perceptible	Flat areola, no bud	Stippled areola 1–2-mm bud	Raised areola 3–4-mm bud	Full areola 5–10-mm bud	
Eye/ear	Lids fused loosely: −1 tightly −2	Lids open Pinna flat, stays folded	Sl. curved pinna; soft; slow recoil	Well-curved pinna; soft but ready recoil	Formed and firm, instant recoil	Thick cartilage, ear stiff	
Genitalia male	Scrotum flat, smooth	Scrotum empty, faint rugae	Testes in upper canal, rare rugae	Testes decending, few rugae	Testes down, good rugae	Testes pendulous, deep rugae	
Genitalia female	Clitoris prominent, labia flat	Prominent clitoris, small labia minora	Prominent clitoris, enlarging minora	Majora and minora equally prominent	Majora large, minora small	Majora cover clitoris and minora	

c) Maturity rating

Score	Weeks
−10	20
−5	22
0	24
5	26
10	28
15	30
20	32
25	34
30	36
35	38
40	40
45	42
50	44

Figure A.2 Scoring system for assessment of gestational age in newborn infants (Ballard score). This is a method of assessing gestational age according to neuromuscular (**a**) and physical maturity (**b**). The infant's gestation or age (±2 weeks) is determined from the total score using the conversion chart (**c**). (Adapted from Ballard JL, Khoury JC, Wedig K, et al: New Ballard score, expanded to include extremely premature infants. *Journal of Pediatrics* 119:417–423, 1991.)

Management action plan for asthma (Fig. A.3)

Green zone – GO

Your asthma is under control if:
- your breathing feels good
- you do not have a cough or wheeze
- you can take part in normal activities and play games / sport.
- your are sleeping through the night
- you are not missing school because of your asthma

Peak flows are between:

....

....

Green zone action –
Your normal medicines are:
Preventer

....

....

Other medicines

....

....

Reliever

....
as required.
Remember: If necessary take this before exercise or if you have cold-like symptoms. Take 2–4 puffs every 4 hours if you need it. If there is no improvement, move to the Amber zone.

Amber zone – WARNING

Your asthma is getting worse if you:
- wake at night with asthma symptoms
- have a cough, wheeze, or 'tight' chest
- need to use the reliever inhaler once a day, more than usual or, it is not lasting for 4 h.

Peak flows are between:

....

....

Amber zone action –
Take all medicines as normal.

Take 4–10 puffs of reliever – one puff at a time as taught. Use a spacer if you have one and shake the MDI in between puffs. Take every 4 hours if needed.

- If no improvement – make an appointment to see your doctor for that day.
- If you have a Symptom/Peak flow Diary – start filling it in and take it with you to the doctor.

Or
Start your home prednisolone
…….mg daily, if you have it. See your doctor if you are not better after 12 hours.

Remember: If no better after 10 puffs of reliever, move to Red zone.

Red zone – DANGER

Your asthma is severe if after taking 10 puffs of reliever you:
- are still breathing hard and fast
- can't talk or feed easily
- are exhausted
- are frightened and look anxious
- are very pale/grey/blue in colour

Peak flow reading (if able) below:

....

....

Red zone action –
   Call an ambulance now

- Keep taking one puff of reliever every 20–30 s or four slow breaths or, if you have one, nebulized reliever with oxygen until the ambulance arrives.
- Take a dose of oral steroids if not already taken.
- Don't move about
- Keep calm

Figure A.3 Example of patient management action plan for asthma.

Blood pressure chart (Fig. A.4)

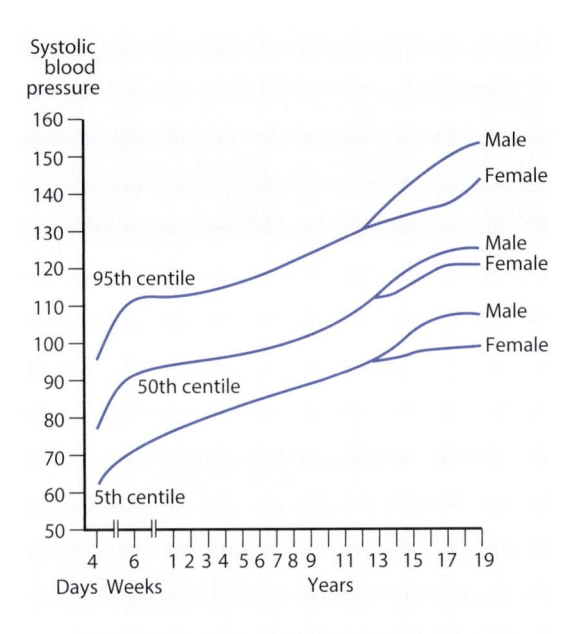

Figure A.4 Systolic blood pressure according to age. Blood pressure charts are also available according to height. (Data from de Swiet M, Fayers P, Shinebourne EA: Blood pressure in a population of infants in the first year of life: the Brompton Study. *Pediatrics* 65:1028–1035, 1980 and de Man SA, André JL, Bachmann H, Grobbee DE, Ibsen KK et al: Blood pressure in childhood: pooled findings of six European studies. *Journal of Hypertension* 9:109–114, 1991.)

Peak flow chart (Fig. A.5)

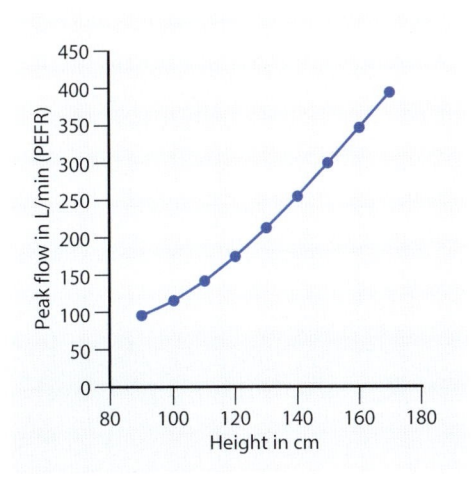

Figure A.5 The normal range of peak flow measurements according to height.

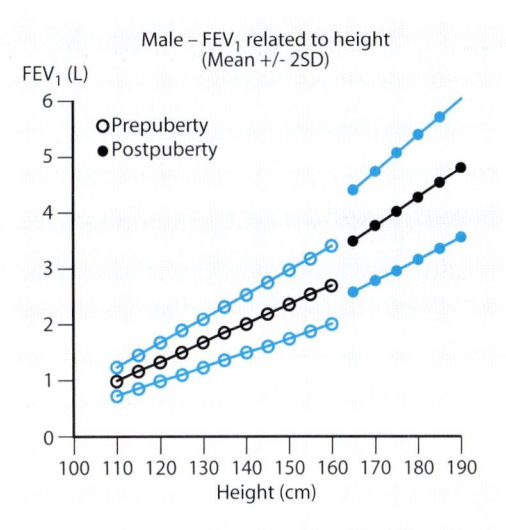

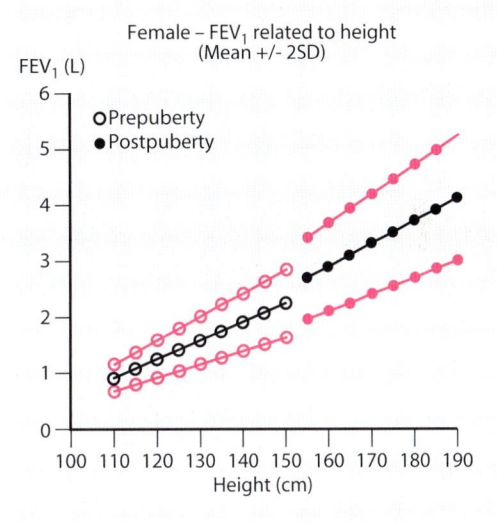

Figure A.6 The normal range of forced expiratory volume in 1 second (FEV_1). It varies with height, gender, and before and after puberty. It is the change over time that is most important in determining the effectiveness of a treatment.

Imaging in children

Principles relating to the use of imaging are:
- X-rays – use is minimized to avoid the risk of ionizing radiation. If used, the minimum number of exposures with the lowest radiation dose is used
- ultrasound – is good at identifying structures where there is a fluid/solid interface, but images are not obtained through bone. It is highly operator dependent, and paediatric expertise is required
- MRI (magnetic resonance imaging) scans – provide detailed images but the child has to lie still. This may require sedation or co-operation, or even a general anaesthetic

- CT (computerised tomography) scans – can usually be obtained quickly and are less distorted by movement artefact, but involve ionizing radiation. They are useful for acute head injury (where time is crucial) and for chest imaging.

Blood tests

All children dislike needles. It is also time consuming. Before requesting a blood test, consider 'Can I get this information in another way?' and 'Is this essential – will it alter management and benefit the child?' Some investigations are required when a child is seriously ill.

Taking blood from children

If a blood test is necessary, consider the kindest and safest way to do it. Be patient whenever possible. Local anaesthetic cream reduces the pain of venepuncture, but requires at least 30 minutes to be effective; cold spray/ice can also be effective if time is limited. Distraction can be very helpful for some children, but needs to be tailored to the child's age and the procedure. Experience in performing the procedure helps reduce pain and upset. The most common blood tests undertaken in paediatric clinical practice are summarized in Tables A.1, A.2, and A.3.

Table A.1 Common blood tests and their interpretation

Blood test		Normal value	Interpretation
Urea and electrolytes	Sodium	130–150 mmol/L	Low in relative water excess (or sodium loss). High in water loss (i.e. dehydration)
	Potassium	3.5–4.7 mmol/L	Elevated in renal failure/dysfunction. Low in recurrent vomiting
	Urea		Elevated in dehydration but also in gastrointestinal bleeding
	Creatinine		Elevated in renal disease (and dehydration)
Full blood count	Haemoglobin	110–140 g/L	See Table A.3 for variation with age
	Mean cell volume		If low, suggests either iron deficiency or haemoglobinopathy
	White cell count		High in infection, low in severe infection. Very high or low in malignancy
	Platelet count	$150–450 \times 10^9$/L	High in infection. Low if consumed, i.e. DIC (disseminated intravascular coagulation), ITP (immune thrombocytopenic purpura)
Blood gas (capillary)	pH	pH 7.31–7.41	Low is acidosis, high is alkalosis
	Partial pressure of carbon dioxide	4.5–6 kPa	High values suggest respiratory cause for any acidosis [see Tables A.2 and 27.5 for further details]
Blood glucose	Glucose	2.6–6.0 mmol/L	High in diabetes, elevated by stress. Low in children with metabolic diseases
Inflammatory markers	C-reactive protein (CRP)	<5 mg/L (laboratory values vary)	Elevated in infection or proinflammatory state. Rises and falls more quickly than ESR
	Erythrocyte sedimentation rate (ESR)	<10 mm/h (laboratory values vary)	
Blood culture	Bacteraemia		Will identify bacteria in the blood if sufficient volume. Typically takes 48 h to achieve growth in culture
Thyroid function tests	Thyroid stimulating hormone (TSH)	0.3–5.5 mIU/L	Elevated in hypothyroidism (unless due to hypopituitarism, when thyroid-stimulating hormone will remain low and free T3/T4 is required)
	Free T3/T4		

Table A.2 Capillary blood gas interpretation. Sometimes used to measure blood pH and blood carbon dioxide (CO_2) on very small volumes of blood. Digit must be warm and free flowing blood sample. Bicarbonate (HCO_3) and base excess values are calculated. Abnormal results should always be repeated.

a) **General guide**

	Parameters	Normal	Acidosis	Alkalosis
Acidotic or alkalotic?	pH	7.31–7.41	<7.31	>7.41
Respiratory cause?	CO_2	4.6–6 kPa	↑	↓
Metabolic cause?	HCO_3	22–26 mmol/L	↓	↑
	Base excess	−2 to +2		

b) **More detailed analysis**

pH	CO_2	HCO_3	Interpretation
Normal	Normal	Normal	Normal
<7.31	↑	Normal	Respiratory acidosis
<7.31	Normal	↓	Metabolic acidosis
<7.31	↑	↓	Mixed respiratory and metabolic acidosis
Normal	↑	↑	Compensated respiratory acidosis
Normal	↓	↓	Compensated metabolic acidosis
>7.41	↓	Normal	Respiratory alkalosis
>7.41	Normal	↑	Metabolic alkalosis
>7.41	↓	↑	Mixed respiratory and metabolic alkalosis

Table A.3 Normal ranges: haematology

Age	Haemoglobin (g/L)	Mean corpuscular volume (fl)	White blood cells (×10⁹/L)	Platelets (×10⁹/L)
Birth	145–215	100–135	10–26	150–450 at all ages
2 weeks	134–198	88–120	6–21	
2 months	94–130	84–105	6–18	
1 year	113–141	71–85	6–17.5	
2–6 years	115–135	75–87	5–17	
6–12 years	115–135	77–95	4.5–14.5	
12–18 years:				
Male	130–160	78–95	4.5–13	
Female	120–160	78–95	4.5–13	

Index

Page numbers followed by "*f*" indicate figures, "*t*" indicate tables, and "*b*" indicate boxes.

A

Abdomen
  associated signs, 16
  colicky pain, 359
  distension, 16, 234*b*, 235, 240, 244, 249, 253–255, 255*f*
  injuries to, 100
  recurrent pain, 243–244, 244*b*, 244*f*
  X-ray, 172
Abdominal examination, 16, 17*b*
Abdominal migraine, 243, 501
ABO incompatibility, 181, 184
Abscess, cerebral, 261
Absence seizures, 507, 508*t*, 509*t*
Absent reflexes, 20
Abstract thought, 36
Abuse *see* Child abuse
Acanthosis nigricans, 455*f*
Accident and Emergency department, 65, 65*b*
Accidents, 97–102, 97*f*
  burns and scalds, 102, 541
  choking, suffocation and strangulation, 101, 101*b*, 101*f*
  drowning, 101–102
  poisoning, 103
  prevention, 98, 98*f*
  road traffic, 98, 540
  types affecting children, 98
Achondroplasia, 128, 201*f*, 497
Aciclovir, 189
Acid-base disturbance, 475*t*, 559*t*
Acidosis, 364
Acne vulgaris, 451
Acrodermatitis enteropathica, 251*f*
Acute abdomen/abdominal pain, 238–242
  adolescents, 240*b*
  appendicitis, 17, 239–240, 239*f*
  auscultation, 18
  causes, 239*f*
  intussusception, 18, 240–241, 241*b*, 241*f*
  malrotation, 242, 242*b*, 242*f*
  Meckel diverticulum, 242, 242*b*, 242*f*
  mesenteric adenitis, 240
  non-specific, 240
  older children, 240*b*
  rectal examination, 18
Acute asthma, 305–309, 306*f*
Acute epiglottitis, 298–299, 298*t*, 299*b*, 299*f*
Acute kidney injury, 361–363, 362*b*–363*b*

Acute liver failure (fulminant hepatitis), 380, 380*t*
Acute lymphatic leukaemia, case history, 74*b*
Acute lymphoblastic leukaemia (ALL), 390
  case history in, 391*b*, 391*f*
  management of, 390–391
  prognostic factors in, 391*t*
Acute myeloid leukaemia/acute nonlymphocytic leukaemia (AML/ANLL), 390
Acute nephritis, 358–359, 358*b*, 360*b*
Acute otitis media, 296–297, 296*f*, 297*b*
Acute post-infectious polyneuropathy (Guillain-Barré syndrome), 513
Acute renal failure, 93*t*
Acute scrotum, 371, 373*b*
Acute symptomatic epileptic seizures, 503
Addison disease, 468–469, 468*b*, 468*f*
Adenocarcinoma of colon, 253
Adenoidectomy, 297
Adenosine deaminase deficiency, 137–138
Adherence, 529–530, 530*t*
Adolescents
  acute abdominal pain in, 240*b*
  anaphylaxis in, 89–90, 90*b*
  chronic conditions in, 529–530, 529*t*, 530*b*
  communication with, 525–527, 526*f*, 527*b*
  confidentiality in, 527–528
  consent in, 527
  developmental changes, 526*t*
  diabetes management, 461–462
  emotional abuse, 116
  fatigue, headache, and other somatic symptoms, 530–531
  health problems, 528, 528*t*, 533*b*, 533*f*
  health promotion, 532
  health-risk behaviour, 531
  heart failure in, 322*b*
  lymphomas, 393
  malignant disease in, 385
  medicine in, 525–534
  mental health of, 424–441
  mental health problems, 531, 531*t*
  mortality, 528–529, 528*f*–529*f*
  pregnancy, 532
  problems of, 435–439
    anorexia nervosa In, 435–436, 437*b*
    chronic fatigue syndrome in, 437, 437*b*
    cognitive style in, 435, 435*b*
    deliberate self-harm in, 438
    depression in, 437–438, 437*b*
    drug misuse in, 438–439
    psychosis in, 439
    self-harm in, how to ask about, 438, 438*b*
  psychosocial history in, 527*t*
  self-harm, 104, 438

sexual health, 531–532
teenage parenthood and, 532
transition to adult services, 533, 533b
Adrenal crisis, 469
Adrenal disorders, 466–469
Adrenal hyperplasia, congenital, 466–468, 467b–468b, 467f
Adrenal insufficiency, primary, 468–469, 468b–469b
Adrenal steroid biosynthesis, 467f
Adrenaline, nebulized, 298
Adrenarche (premature pubarche), 208–209
Adrenoleukodystrophy, 523–524
Adult Learning Disability Teams, 62–63
Advanced life support, paediatric, 83, 85f
Adversities, in family, 427–428, 427b
Age of child
abnormal development and, 47, 47f
adapting, 12–13
developmental questioning, 36–37
emotional abuse, 116
with fever, 256
haemoglobin concentration, 402f
history-taking/examination, 9
neurodevelopmental problems, 44–45, 45t
pneumonia and, 311
respiratory infections, 294f
vision testing, 43t
see also Adolescents; Infants; Neonates
Aggressive behaviour, 431, 431f
Alagille syndrome, 376–378, 377f
Alarm, enuresis, 431–432
Albinism, 444, 444f
Alcohol, 7
effect on fetus, 143, 149–150, 149f
Allergen avoidance, in asthma, 304–305
Allergic facies, 290f
Allergic rhinitis, 292, 292b
Allergy, 288–293
allergic march, 289
asthma and, 292
defined, 288b
food, 290–292, 291f, 292b
IgE-mediated and non-IgE mediated, 290–291
management of, 290, 292
mechanisms of allergic disease, 288–289
paediatric, 290b
prevention of allergic diseases, 289–290
Allopurinol, 390
Alopecia areata, 450, 451f
Alport syndrome, 359
Amblyopia, 59
Aminophylline, 306–308
Aminosalicylates, 253
Ammonia, 476
Amniocentesis, 122–123, 144f
Amoxicillin, 244, 296, 311
Amphetamine abuse, 150
Amyloidosis, 495
Anaemia, 402–413, 414b
aplastic, inherited, 413
bone marrow suppression, 388
causes in infants & children, 403f
defined, 402
diagnostic approach to, 404f
due to impaired red cell production, 403
haemolytic, 406–412
ineffective erythropoiesis in, diagnosis of, 403–406
iron deficiency, 403–405
kidney disorder, 364
in newborn, 412–413
of prematurity, 413

Anaesthesia, epidural, during labour, 150
Analgesia, 503
Anaphylaxis, 89–90, 90b, 90f, 288b, 293
ANCA (antineutrophil cytoplasm antibodies), 359
Anencephaly, 518–519
Angelman syndrome, 133, 134f
Angioedema, 293, 293b
Anion gap, 475, 476b, 476t, 559t
Anorexia nervosa, 221, 435–436, 437b
Antenatal diagnosis, 143–146, 144f–145f, 145b
cardiac disorders, 322
case history, 145b, 145f
fetal medicine, 143–146
fetal surgery, 146
kidney and urinary tract disorders, 344–348, 346f, 348f
screening tests, 144b
Anterior horn cell, disorders of, 512–513
Anthropometry, 222
Antibiotic therapy
bacterial meningitis, 261
epiglottitis, acute, 299
gastroenteritis, 248, 278
impetigo, 264–265
intravenous, 256, 299
macrolide antibiotics, 310
otitis media, 296–297
parenteral, 259
pneumonia, 186, 311
for preterm or sick infants, 172
tonsillitis, 296
Antidiarrhoeal drugs, 248
Antiemetics, 248
Antiepileptic drug therapy, 509, 509t–510t
Antihistamines, 447
Anti-IgE therapy, 304
Antiphospholipid syndrome, with SLE, 149
Anti-Ro or anti-La antibodies, 340
Antisocial behaviour, 433–434, 434b
α_1-Antitrypsin deficiency, 378
Antitumour necrosis factor agents, 252–253
Antiviral agents, 447
Anxiety, 434
Aorta
coarctation of *see* Coarctation of aorta
interruption of the aortic arch, 338, 338f
Aortic stenosis, 335, 335b, 335f
Apgar score, 153, 153t
Aplastic anaemia, inherited, 413
Aplastic crisis, 407
Apnoea
in bronchiolitis, 301
in preterm infants, 174
in whooping cough, 310
Apparent life-threatening events, 94
Appearance, general, examining, 14
Appendicectomy, 240
Appendicitis, 17, 239–240, 239f
Applied behavioural analysis, 54
Arnold-Chiari malformation, 145b
Array comparative genomic hybridization (microarray), 126–127, 127f
Arrhythmias, 340
cardiac, 339–340
Arterial lines, 172
Arthritis, 491–497
juvenile idiopathic, 493–496, 493f
reactive, 491–492
septic, 490t, 492, 492f
Arthrogryposis, 498
Ascites, 18, 383, 384f

Asperger syndrome, 53–54
Asphyxia, 152–153
    perinatal, 167
Aspirin, 341–342
Association, in birth defects classification, 136
Asthma, 301–305
    acute, 305–309, 306f
    add-on therapy, 304
    allergen avoidance in, 304–305
    atopic, 302
    clinical features, 303
    examination, 15t
    exercise-induced, 304
    hospital admission criteria, 305–306
    investigations, 303
    management of, 303, 304t, 306–308, 307f
    management action plan, 556
    pathophysiology, 302, 302f
    patient education, 308–309, 309f
    peak flow, 303, 557
    treatment, stepwise approach, 305f
Astigmatism, 59
Astrocytoma, 391
Asylum seekers, 3
Asymmetric heads, 205, 207f
Ataxia, 517
Ataxia telangiectasia, 285, 517, 517f
Ataxic (hypotonic) cerebral palsy, 51
Athetosis, 51
Atlantoaxial instability, 122
Atopic asthma, 302
Atopic dermatitis, 445–447, 446b–447b, 446f–447f
Atopic eczema, 292, 445–447, 446b–447b, 446f–447f
Atopy, 288b
Atresia
    biliary, 375–376, 383f
        case history, 377b, 377f
    duodenum, jejunum or ileum, 191–192, 192f
    mitral, 333–334
    oesophageal, 191, 191f
    rectal, 192
    tricuspid, 334, 334f
Atrial septal defect, 325–326, 326b, 326f
Atrioventricular septal defect, complete, 333, 334f
Attention deficit hyperactivity disorder (ADHD), 55–56, 56b, 425b
Audiogram, 56, 57f
Audiometry, 42
    auditory brainstem response, 39, 40f
    impedance tests, 57
    threshold, 42
    visual reinforcement, 39, 41f
Auditory brainstem response audiometry, 39, 40f
Auscultation
    cardiovascular system examination, 16
    masses, abnormal, 18
    respiratory system examination, 13f, 14
Autism spectrum disorders, 53–54, 53b, 425b
Autoimmune thrombocytopenic purpura (AITP), 149
Autonomy, 72–73
Autosomal dominant inheritance, 128, 129b, 129f
Autosomal dominant polycystic kidney disease (ADPKD), 345–348, 346f
Autosomal recessive inheritance, 129–130, 130b, 130f
Autosomal recessive polycystic kidney disease (ARPKD), 345–348, 346f
AVPU, 81

B

Back pain, 489, 489b
'Back to Sleep' campaign, 94–95, 95f
Bacterial infections, 263–265
    meningitis see Bacterial meningitis
    secondary, 267
        see also Respiratory infections
Bacterial meningitis, 259–261
    organisms causing, 259, 259t
    partially treated, 261
Bacterial peritonitis, spontaneous, 383–384
Bacterial tracheitis (pseudomembranous croup), 299
Ballard score, 555
Bariatric surgery, 231
Basal metabolic rate (BMR), 212, 212f
Basal-bolus insulin, 456f
Basic life support, paediatric, 83, 84f
Basilar-type migraine, 501
BCG immunization, against TB infection, 275, 282, 284
Becker muscular dystrophy, 515
Beckwith-Wiedemann syndrome, 160
Bedtime, sleep at, difficulty in, 429, 429b
Behavioural difficulties, 7
Bell palsy, 513–514, 514f
Beneficence, 72–73
Benign acute myositis, 515
Benign paroxysmal vertigo of childhood, 501
Benign rolandic epilepsy, 508t
Benzathine penicillin, 342
Bernard-Soulier syndrome, 419
Best interests, 73
Bicycle handlebar injuries, 100
Bilateral hydronephrosis, 347f
    antenatal diagnosis, 348f
Bilevel positive airway pressure (BiPAP), 318
Biliary atresia, 375–376, 383f
    case history, 377b, 377f
Bilirubin, 182f–183f,
    acute liver failure and, 380
    conjugated, 376
    unconjugated, 181
Biochemical screening (Guthrie test), 165, 185, 314, 474
Biopsychosocial formulation, 427–428, 428b, 428t
Birth asphyxia see Hypoxic-ischaemic encephalopathy
Birth defects, clinical classification, 135–136
Birth injuries, 169–170, 170b
Birth size see Size at birth
Bite, human, 115f
Bladder
    exstrophy, 348
    incomplete emptying, 351
    neuropathic, 353–354
Blalock-Taussig shunt insertion, 334
Bleeding disorders, 413–421, 418b, 418f
    evaluating, clinical features in, 416b
        see also Disseminated intravascular coagulation; Immune thrombocytopenic purpura (ITP)
Blepharitis, 267
Blindness, 75
Blood tests, 558, 559
Blood gas analysis, 559
Blood glucose monitoring, 457–458, 457b–458b, 457f–458f
Blood loss, 413
Blood pressure
    examining, 24
    measurement, 24f, 80, 360, 360b, 557
Blood vessels, 414–415
Blue breath-holding spells, 506b
Body composition, 211f

Body mass index (BMI), 227–228
    centile chart, 230f
Boils, 265
Bone age, 198, 198f, 199–203
Bone lesions, in Langerhans cell histiocytosis, 398, 399f
Bone marrow failure syndromes, 413
Bone marrow suppression, in malignant disease, 388
Bone mineralization, poor in preterm infants, 175–176
Bone tumours, 396–397, 397f, 487–488
Bones and joints, examining, 20
Borderline IQ, 54
Bordetella pertussis, 310
Bottom-shuffling, 29, 48
Bow legs (genu varum), 482, 483f
Bowel obstruction, 191–192, 192f
Brachial nerve palsy, 169
Bradycardia, 153
    in preterm infants, 174
Brain
    haemorrhages, 176
    injury, 116–118, 176–178, 176f–177f
    magnetic resonance imaging (MRI), 167–169, 169f
    rapid growth and development of, 212
Brain tumours, 385, 385f, 387, 391–393, 392b, 392f
    clinical features of, 392
    investigations in, 392–393
    late effects of, 393
    management of, 393
Brainstem glioma, 391
Breast enlargement, in newborn, 162b, 162f
Breast milk jaundice, 183
Breastfeeding, 213–215
    advantages of, 214, 215b
    constipation and, 253
    establishing, 214–215
    physiology of, 216f
    potential complications, 214, 216b
    prevalence of, 214f
Breasts, premature development, 208, 209b, 209f
Breath holding spells, 505f
Breathing disorders, examination of child, 13
Breech delivery, 169
Brittle bone disease, 118
Bronchiectasis, 313, 313f
Bronchiolitis, 87b, 87f, 180f, 300–301, 301f
    acute wheezing in, 309
    examination, 15t
Bronchitis, 313
Bronchodilator therapy, asthma, 303–304
Bronchopulmonary dysplasia, 178, 178f
Bronchoscopy, 309b
Bruising, 115f, 116–118, 169, 420t
Buccal pigmentation, 468f
Bullous impetigo, 442, 442f
Bullying, 110–111, 116
Burkholderia species, 314
Burkitt lymphoma, 393–394, 394f
Burns, 102, 103b, 541
    assessment, 102, 103f
    case history, 541b, 541f
    cigarette, 118
    depth, 103b
    management, 102
    surface area, 102, 102f

C

^{13}C breath test, 243–244
Café-au-lait spots, 209f
Campylobacter jejuni infection, 245

Cancer *see* Malignant disease
Candida infection, 445, 445f
Capillary leak, 89
Capillary refill time, 81f
Captopril, 328
Caput succedaneum, 169
Cardiac disorders, 320–343
    aetiology, 321
    antenatal diagnosis, 322
    cardiomyopathy, 342
    care following cardiac surgery, 339
    circulatory changes at birth, 321, 321f
    common mixing (blue and breathless), 333–334, 334b
    congenital heart disease *see* Congenital heart disease
    cyanosis *see* Cyanosis
    diagnosis, 323, 325b
    epidemiology, 320, 320b
    heart failure, 16, 322–323, 322b, 324b, 324f
    heart murmurs, 322
    infective endocarditis, 342
    Kawasaki disease, 343
    left-to-right shunts, 325–329, 329b
    myocarditis, 342
    nomenclature, 325
    outflow obstruction in sick infant, 337–339, 339b
    outflow obstruction in well child, 335–337, 337b
    presentation, 322–323, 325b
    pulmonary hypertension, 186, 343
    rheumatic fever, 340–342
    right-to-left shunts, 329–333
Cardiomyopathy, 342
Cardiopulmonary resuscitation, 83, 85f
Cardiovascular disorders, systems review, 11
Cardiovascular system, 14–16, 16b
Care plan, 71
Catheter shunts, 146
Cefotaxime, 259
Ceftriaxone, 259, 261
Cefuroxime, 299
Centile charts, 13–14, 194–196, 544–554
Central nervous system (CNS), acute lymphoblastic leukaemia and, 391
Cephalhaematoma, 169, 170f
Cephalosporin, 259, 261
    resistance to, 261
Cerebral abscess, 261
Cerebral calcification, 151
Cerebral infarction, 261
Cerebral palsy, 48–51, 51b, 51f, 511
    ataxic (hypotonic), 51
    causes, 49
    clinical presentation, 49–51
    defined, 48
    dyskinetic, 51
    example, 51b, 51f
    late walking and, 29f
    management, 51
    patterns, 52b
    spastic, 49–51, 62f
    types, 52f
Cerebrospinal fluid (CSF), 177, 259
Cerebrovascular disease, 517–518
Charcot-Marie-tooth disease, 513
Chemotherapy
    acute lymphoblastic leukaemia, 391
    bone tumours, 397
    malignant disease, 387
        short-term side-effects of, 388f
    soft tissue sarcomas, 396
    Wilms' tumour, 396

Index

Chest
- common disorders, 15t
- compressions, 84–85, 157
- injuries to, 100
- pains in, 340
- shape of, 14, 15f
- syndrome, acute sickle, case history, 410

Chest X-ray
- acute sickle chest syndrome, 410b, 410f
- aortic stenosis, 335
- asthma, 305–306
- atrial septal defect, 325
- coarctation of the aorta, 338
  - adult-type, 336–337
- cystic fibrosis, 315f
- leukaemia, 390
- preterm infants, 172
- pulmonary stenosis, 336
- tetralogy of Fallot, 330f, 331
- transposition of the great arteries, 331, 332f
- ventricular septal defect, 328

Chickenpox, 267–268, 268b–269b
Chikungunya, 278
Chignon, 169, 170f
Child
- mental health, 424–441, 540
- mortality, 5–6, 6f, 535–538
  - causes, 536f
  - global distribution, 536f
  - poverty, 536, 537f
  - rates, 535–536, 535t
  - reducing, 537–538, 538b
- nutritional vulnerability, 211–213, 213b
- reasons for talking, 25t

Child abuse, 110b, 120b
- case history, 110b, 119b, 119f
- emotional abuse, 110–111, 116, 117b, 117t
- fabricated or induced illness as, 111
- investigation, 116–118
- management of, 118–120
- neglect, 110–111, 116, 117b
- physical abuse, 110, 114b, 114f
- presentation, 113–116
- prevalence, 111–113, 112t
- risk factors, 113, 113b
- severe, 114b, 114f
- sexual abuse, 111, 116, 118f
- types, 110–111

Child development *see* Development
Child development service, 60, 61f, 122
Child protection, 109–120, 120b
- *see also* Child abuse

Child Protection Plan, 119
Childhood absence epilepsy, 508t, 509f
Child-rearing, cultural attitudes to, 3–4
Children's coma scale, 92t
Child's world, 1–5, 2f
Chlamydia trachomatis eye infection, 188, 189f
Choking, 101, 101b, 101f
Cholangitis, sclerosing, 380
Choledochal cysts, 376
Chondromalacia patellae, 488
Chordee, 372, 373f
Chorea, 51
Chorionic villus sampling, 144f
Chromosomal abnormalities, 121–122
- deletions, 126, 139
  - Down syndrome, 122–124
- duplications, 126–127
  - Edwards syndrome, 125, 125b, 125f
  - Klinefelter syndrome, 126, 126b, 202, 210b
- numerical or structural, 121–122
  - Patau syndrome, 125, 125b
  - reciprocal translocations, 126
  - short stature and, 199
  - Turner syndrome *see* Turner syndrome (45, X)

Chromosome 13, 386
Chromosome 14, 378
Chronic anterior uveitis, 493
Chronic fatigue syndrome, 437, 437b
Chronic granulomatous disease, 285
Chronic illness, on mental health, 425b
Chronic kidney disease, 363–365, 365b
- causes, 364t
- grading of severity, 364t

Chronic lung infection, 313
Cigarette smoking *see* Smoking
Ciliary dyskinesia, primary, 317
Ciliopathies, 381
Circulatory changes, at birth, 321, 321f
Circulatory support, sepsis, 89
Circumcision, 372
Cirrhosis, 382–383, 382f–383f
Cisplatin, 388
Clarithromycin, 244
Clavicle, fracture at birth, 170
Cleft lip and palate, 190, 190f
Cleidocranial dysostosis, 498
Climbié, Victoria, 109
Clinical examination *see* Examination
Clubbing of fingers or toes, 14, 15f
Coagulation, acquired disorders of, 419
Coagulation cascade, 363
Coagulation factors, 413
Coagulation inhibitors, 413
Coagulation pathway, 415f
Co-amoxiclav, 311
Coarctation of aorta, 324f, 338
- adult-type, 336–337, 337b, 337f
- examination, 16

Cocaine abuse, 150
Cochlear implants, 56, 57f
Coeliac disease, 199, 249, 250b, 250f
Cognitive development, 30–36
Cognitive skills, slow acquisition *see* Learning difficulties
Cognitive style, 426, 426b, 435, 435b
Colectomy, 253
'Colic,' infant, 238
Collodion baby, 444, 444f
Coloboma, 164
Colostrum, 214
Coma
- assessment and management of, 92f, 93
- pupillary signs in, 92f

Commando crawling (creeping), 29, 48
Common arterial trunk, 333–334
Common Assessment Framework, 60
Common cold (coryza), 296
Common mixing (blue and breathless), 333–334, 334b
Communicating serious problems, 71, 72b
Communication aids, 61, 62f
Compensated/uncompensated shock, 87
Complete atrioventricular septal defect, 333, 334f
Complex regional pain syndromes, 486–487, 489
Concomitant squints, 59
Conductive hearing loss, 56–57, 58t
Confidentiality, 72–73, 527–528
Congenital adrenal hyperplasia (CAH), 208–209
Congenital cataract, 164b, 164f
Congenital central hypoventilation syndrome, 318

Congenital complete heart block, 340, 340f
Congenital dislocation of the hip (CDH), 160
Congenital heart disease, 122
    causes, 321t
    complex, 333–334
    cyanotic, 330f, 333b
    diagnosis, 323
    genetic causes, 321
    lesions, 320b
    oxygen saturation screening, 165
    presentation, 323t
        see also Cardiac disorders
Congenital hypothyroidism, 185
Congenital infections, 150–151, 150b, 183
Congenital malformations, 135, 135b
    in diabetic mothers, 148, 148b
    multiple births, 147
Congenital muscular dystrophies, 515
Congenital myasthenic syndromes, 514
Congenital myopathies, 515
Congenital nephrotic syndrome, 357
Conjunctivitis, 188, 189f, 267, 292, 292b
Connelly, Peter (Baby P), 109
Consanguinity, autosomal recessive inheritance, 129–130
Consent, 73, 527
Constipation, 253–255
    management, 254f
    'red flag' symptoms, 253b
Constitutional delay in growth and puberty (CDGP), 199, 200f, 210b
Contact tracing, tuberculosis, 277
Continuing therapy, acute lymphoblastic leukaemia, 391
Continuous positive airways pressure (CPAP), 171, 318
Contraception, 532
Coordination, neurological examination, 20
Corneal light reflex test, 59, 59f
Coronary heart disease, 213f
Corticosteroids
    excess, 202
    inhaled, for asthma, 304
    systemic, 496
    topical, 374, 446
Coryza (common cold), 296
Cotrimoxazole, 391
Cough, 310–311
    in bronchitis, 313
    persistent or recurrent, 310–311, 311b
        see also Whooping cough (pertussis)
Cover test, 59, 59f
Cow's milk, 216–217
    compared with human milk, 217t
    formula, 215, 217
Cranial irradiation, 202
Cranial nerves, neurological examination, 19
Cranial ultrasound, preterm infants, 177b, 177f
Craniofacial disorders, 190–191
Craniopharyngioma, 202, 391
Craniosynostosis, 205–206, 207b, 207f
Craniotabes, 226
Crawling, 29
Cri du-chat syndrome, 126
Crohn's disease, 201, 252–253, 252f
Croup, 298, 298t
Crouzon syndrome, 207f
Crying, 237–238
Cryptorchidism, 348
Cultural attitudes to child-rearing, 3–4
Cushing syndrome, 202, 469, 469b, 469f
Cyanosis, 14, 323
    respiratory system examination, 14
Cyanotic congenital heart disease, 330f, 333b

Cyclical vomiting, 501
Cyclophosphamide, 388
Cystic fibrosis, 313–317, 381
    asthma and, 303
    clinical features, 314–315, 314b, 315f
    diagnosis, 315
    epidemiology, genetics and basic defect, 313, 314f
    examination, 14
    gene-based therapies, 137–138
    management of, 315–317, 316f
    nutritional management, 316
    pathophysiology, 314
    respiratory management, 315–316
    screening for, 165
    in teenagers and adults, 316–317
Cysts, choledochal, 376
Cytogenetic analysis techniques, 127t
Cytogenetics, Down syndrome, 122–124
Cytokine modulators, 5, 496
Cytomegalovirus (CMV), 150f, 151, 269–270
Cytoplasmic inheritance, 132–133

D

Databases, genetic, 121
Day-case surgery, 66
Daytime enuresis, 353–354, 355b
De novo mutation, autosomal dominant inheritance, 128
Deafness, in otosclerosis, 128
Defiance, 430–431
Deformation, 135
Dehydration, 215–216, 245–247
    clinical assessment, 246t
    management, 247f
    shock from, clinical features, 246f
Delayed puberty, 209–210, 210b
    causes, 210b
    constitutional delay, 199, 210b
Deletions, chromosomal abnormalities, 126
    de novo, 133
    mutation analysis, 139
ΔF508 mutation, in cystic fibrosis, 313
Dengue fever, 278
Dental caries, 232, 232f
Denver Developmental Screening Test, 37
Depression, 437–438, 437b
Dermatological disorders, 442–452
Dermatomyositis, 516, 516f
Desaturation, preterm infants, 174
Desmopressin (DDAVP), 417, 432
Developed countries
    breastfeeding advantages, 214
    gastroenteritis, 248
Development
    abnormal see Developmental problems
    assessing, 30b
    child health surveillance, 38–39, 39b
    cognitive, 30–36
    fields of, 28, 35b–36b
    functional areas, 28f
    goals, global, 538f, 542
    hearing, 29, 33f, 39–42, 42b
        impairment, 56–57, 58b
    heredity, influence of, 27–28, 28f
    history-taking, 12, 12f
    motor skills see Fine motor skills; Gross motor development
    normal child, 27–43

pattern of, 29
    child, 30
    variation in, 29
prematurity, adjusting for, 29
screening and assessment, 37–38, 38b
skills in serial way, 36f
social, emotional and behavioural, 28, 34f
speech and language, 33f
    disorders, 53
vision, 42, 42b
    abnormalities, 58–60, 60b
Developmental coordination disorder, 54–55
Developmental delay, 44–45, 47
    conditions causing, 46t
    investigations, 48t
    terminology, 46
Developmental dysplasia of the hip (DDH), 160, 164b, 164f, 485
Developmental milestones, 28–36
    abnormal development patterns and, 50f
    by median age, 36
Developmental problems, 44–63, 47b, 62b
    abnormal motor development, 47–51, 50f
    clinical signs, 45
    with concentration and attention, 55–56
    concepts, 46–47
    features, 44–45
    gap between normal and abnormal development, 47, 47f
    hearing impairment, 56–57, 58b
    learning difficulties see Learning difficulties
    patterns of abnormal development, 46–47, 47f
    severity, 46–47
    social/communication skills, 53–54
    speech and language, 53
    visual impairment, 58–60, 60b
Developmental progress, analysing, 29–30, 36–37, 37b
    detailed assessment, 36–37
    equipment, developmental testing, 37
    observation during questioning, 37
    short-cut approach, 36–37
    whether normal, 29–30
Developmental skills, examining, 13
Dexamethasone, 261, 277, 298
Diabetes, 453–471
Diabetes mellitus, 93t, 453–462, 455b, 462b
    affecting fetus, 148, 148b
    assessment of child with, 461b, 461f
    blood glucose monitoring, 457–458, 457b, 457f
    case history, 74b
    classification, 453b
    clinical features, 454, 455f
    cystic fibrosis and, 316
    hypoglycaemia in, 458–459
    impact of, 462t
    long-term management, 459–462
    reduced, in breastfeeding, 214
    stages, 454f
    symptoms and signs, 454b
    type 1, 454
Diabetic ketoacidosis, 239, 459, 460b, 460f
Dialysis, 363–365
Diamond-Blackfan anaemia (DBA), 405–406
Diaphragmatic hernia, 186–187, 187f
Diarrhoea
    antidiarrhoeal drugs, 248
    chronic, 251, 251b
    in toddlers, 251
    zinc deficiency, 248
        see also Gastroenteritis; Inflammatory bowel disease

Diet, 456–457
Digoxin, 143, 339–340
Diphtheria, 282–284
Diplegia, 51
Dipstick testing, 350t
Disabilities, children with, 62b
    education, 62
    rights of, 63
    terminology, 46
    transition of care to adult services, 62–63
        see also Learning difficulties
Disability, 7
Discrimination testing, performance and speech, 39–42, 41f
Disease, in adult life, nutritional deficiency, 213, 213f
Disobedience, 430–431, 430b
Disruption, 135
Disseminated intravascular coagulation (DIC), 89, 415, 420–421
Distal intestinal obstruction syndrome, 317
Distraction testing, 39, 41f
DMSA scan, 345t, 353f
Donor breast milk, 175
'DOPE,' and neonatal resuscitation, 157b
Double inlet left ventricle, 333–334
Down syndrome (trisomy 21), 122–124, 123b–124b, 123f
    clinical features, 122
    cytogenetics, 122–124
    inheritance, 124b
    maternal age, 124t
    mosaicism, 124
    non-disjunction, meiotic, 122–123, 124f
    pre-pregnancy care, 143
    short stature, 199
    translocation, 124, 124f
Doxorubicin, 388
Doxycycline, 531
Drawing, 32
Drowning, 101–102
Drug abuse, 5, 143, 150
    in adolescence, 438–439
Drug allergy, 293
Drugs, 7
Dry powder inhaler, 308b, 308f
Duchenne muscular dystrophy, 138, 514–515
Duodenal ulcers, 243
Duodenum, atresia or stenosis of, 191
Duplex kidney, 346f, 348
Duty, 72
Dyscalculia, 55
Dysgraphia, 55
Dyskinetic cerebral palsy, 51
Dyslexia, 55
Dysmorphology, 135–136, 137b
    birth defects, clinical classification of, 135–136
    pathogenic mechanisms, 135
Dysplasia, 135
Dysplastic kidney, 348
Dyspnoea, 14
Dyspraxia, 54–55
Dystonia, 51
Dystrophia myotonica type I, 516, 516f

E

Eardrum, 296–297, 296f
Early relationships, mental health problems, 426–427, 426f, 427b
Ears, examining, 23
Eating disorders, 221, 435–436, 440

ECG *see* Electrocardiography/electrocardiogram (ECG)
Echocardiography
    atrial septal defect, 325
    tetralogy of Fallot, 331
    transposition of the great arteries, 331
    ventricular septal defect, 328
Economic wealth, 5
Eczema, 303
    allergy, 292
    atopic, 445–447, 446b–447b, 446f–448f
Eczema herpeticum, 267, 267f
Educational underachievement, 435, 435b
Edwards syndrome (trisomy 18), 125, 125b, 125f
Effusion
    otitis media with *see* Otitis media with effusion
    subdural, 261
Eisenmenger syndrome, 333, 333f
Electrocardiography/electrocardiogram (ECG)
    aortic stenosis, 335
    atrial septal defect, 325
    coarctation of the aorta, 338
        adult-type, 337
    epilepsies, 506
    pulmonary stenosis, 336
    tetralogy of Fallot, 330f, 331
    transposition of the great arteries, 331, 332f
    ventricular septal defect, 328
Electroencephalogram (EEG), epilepsies, 506
Emergencies, 65, 65b
    paediatric, 80–96
Emergency contraception, 532
Emollients, 446
Emotional abuse, 110–111, 116, 117b, 117t
Emotional and behavioural problems, 424–427
    management, 439–441, 440b, 440t
        cultural considerations, 439
        treatment, 439–441, 440b, 441f
Emotional difficulties, 7
Encephalitis, 261–262, 262b, 262f, 267
    chickenpox and, 267
    enteroviruses and, 270–271
    measles and, 271
    mumps and, 272
Encephalocele, 519
Encephalopathic illness, 90
Encephalopathy, 93t, 261–262
    liver disease, 382
Endocarditis, infective, 342, 342f
Endocrine and metabolic disorders
    Cushing syndrome, 202, 469
    diabetes mellitus *see* Diabetes mellitus
    hyperthyroidism, 148–149, 465, 465b, 465f
    hypothyroidism *see* Hypothyroidism
    parathyroid disorders, 466
Endocrinology, 453–471
Endoscopy, 243, 252–253
Ensembl genome browser, 122f
Enteral feeding, 175
Enterococcus faecalis, 187–188
Enteroviral neonatal sepsis syndrome, 271
Enteroviruses, 270–271, 271b
Enucleation of eye, 397–398
Enuresis, 353–355, 355b
    daytime, 353–354
    nocturnal, 353, 431–432, 432b
Environment of child
    child abuse, 113
    influence of heredity, 27–28, 28f
Ependymoma, 391
Epicanthic folds, 23
EPICure study, 181

Epidermolysis bullosa, 444, 444f
Epididymitis, 370f
Epidural anaesthesia, 150
Epiglottitis, acute, 298–299, 298t, 299b, 299f
Epilepsies of childhood, 506–510, 510b
    advice and prognosis, 510
    brain imaging, 507
    diagnosis, 506
    investigation, 506–509
    management of, 509–510
    surgery, 510
    syndromes, 508t
    see also Seizures
Epinephrine, nebulized, 298
Epstein-Barr virus (EBV), 269, 296, 380
Erb palsy, 169, 170f
Erythema multiforme, 452b
Erythema nodosum, 451b
Erythema toxicum (neonatal urticaria), 162b, 162f
Erythromycin, 311
Escherichia coli, 187–188, 350–351
Essential newborn care, 539f
Ethics, 72–75, 75b
    application, 72–73
    terminology, 72
European countries, comparison with other, 6
Evidence-based paediatrics, 75–78, 76f–77f, 79b
    practice based on, 78
    range of evidence, 78b
Ewing sarcoma, 387, 396–397, 397f
Examination, 13–23
    abdomen, 16–18
    age of child, 9
    approach to, 14
    blood pressure, 24
    bones and joints, 20
    cardiovascular system, 14–16
    cerebral palsy, 49
    child's cooperation, 13
    communicating with children, 24
    developmental problems, 44–45
    developmental skills, 13
    ears, 23, 23f
    eyes, 23
    general appearance, 14
    initial observations, 13–14
    masses, abnormal, 18
    neck, 23
    neurology/neurodevelopment, 18–20
    of newborn infant, 160–165, 161b–162b, 161f
    respiratory system, 14
    short stature, 202, 203t
    summary and management plan, 24–26
    throat, 23, 23f
    undescended testes, 368
    undressing children, 13
    see also History-taking; Investigations
Exchange transfusion, jaundice, 184–185
Executive functions, disorder of, 55
Exercise-induced asthma, 304
Exomphalos, 192, 192f
Extended family, 3
Extra digits, infant, 163b, 163f
Extracellular fluid depletion, 245–246
Extracorporeal membrane oxygenation (ECMO), 186
Extradural haemorrhage, 99, 517
Extrauterine life, adaptation to, 152–153, 152f–153f, 153t
Eyes
    examining, 23
    retinoblastoma, 397–398

F

Fabricated or induced illness, 111
Facial nerve palsies, 169, 513–514
Factor V Leiden mutation, 422
Faecal masses, 18
Faecal soiling, 432, 432b
Failure to thrive, 217 see weight faltering
Family history, 11, 12f
Family nurse partnership, 7–8
Family tree, 128
Family structure, 1–3, 2f
Fanconi anaemia, 413
Fanconi syndrome (generalized proximal tubular dysfunction), 361, 361b
Fasting, 463
Fat-soluble vitamins, 382, 382t
Febrile child, 256–259, 258f, 259b
    causes of fever, 266t
    clinical features, 256–259
    identification of fever, 256
    management of, 259
    prolonged fever, 273–275, 273b
    tropics, returning from, 277, 278b
Febrile seizures, 503–504, 504b
Female genital mutilation, 111, 112f
Female puberty, 196–197, 198f, 199b
    precocious, 206–207
Females, genital examination, 18
Femoral pulses, examining, 16
Femur, fracture at birth, 170
Fertility preservation, in cancer treatment, 389
Fetal alcohol syndrome, 149–150, 149f
Fetal blood sampling, 144f
Fetal circulation, 152
Fetal growth, 194
Fetal medicine, 143–146
Fetal surgery, 146
α-Fetoprotein (αFP), 387, 398
Fetoscopy, 144f
Fetus
    drug abuse affecting, 150
    growth-restricted, monitoring, 146, 159
    hearing in, 39
    labour drugs affecting, 150
    maternal conditions affecting, 148–149, 148b, 148f
    maternal drugs affecting, 149–150, 149t
    obstetric conditions affecting, 146–147
    serum immunoglobulin (antibody) levels in, 257f
    smoking affecting, 142, 149–150
        see also Infants; Neonates; Perinatal medicine; Pregnancy
Fibrinolysis, 413
Fibropolycystic liver disease, 381
Fields of development, 28
Fine motor skills, development, 28, 32f
Fingers, clubbing of, 14, 15f
    respiratory system examination, 14
Flat feet (pes planus), 482, 483f
Flecainide, 143
Flexion contractures of joints, 493
Fluids
    balance, preterm infants, 175
    intravenous, 237
        during labour, 150
    resuscitation, 88, 88b, 88f
    sepsis, 89
Fluorescence in situ hybridization (FISH), 122, 126, 127f, 137
Fluoride, 232
Folic acid deficiency, 229t

Folic acid supplements, 143
Follicle-stimulating hormone (FSH), 206
Fontan operation, 334
Food allergy/intolerance, 290–292, 291f, 292b, 447
Forceps marks, 169
Foreign body inhalation, 101f, 309, 309b, 309f
Foreskin, 371–372
    hooded, 372
    infancy, 371, 371f
    non-retractile, 371–372, 373b
        see also Circumcision
Formoterol, 304
Formula feeding, 215–216
Fractures, 119b, 119f
    at birth, 170, 170b
Fragile X syndrome, 132, 133b, 133f
Friedreich ataxia, 517
Frontal seizures, 506
Functional dyspepsia, 243–244
Fundoscopy, 23
Fungal infections, 187–188, 448–449
Funny turns, 505
FVIII concentrate, recombinant, 417

G

G6PD deficiency, 183, 407
Gait, examining, 20
Galactosaemia, 378, 463b
Galactose, 378
Gall stones, 243
Gastric banding, 231
Gastritis, 243–244
Gastroenteritis, 244–248, 249b
    assessment, 245–246
    case history, 248b, 248f
    conditions mimicking, 245b
    investigation, 246–247
    management of, 247–248
    nutrition, 248
    postgastroenteritis syndrome, 248
Gastroenterology, 234–255
    acute abdominal pain see Acute abdomen/abdominal pain
    constipation, 253–255
    gastroenteritis, 244–248
    Hirschsprung disease, 254–255, 255b
    inflammatory bowel disease, 252–253
    malabsorption, 249–251
    recurrent abdominal pain, 243–244
    vomiting, 234–237, 234b, 235f
Gastrointestinal disorders
    from cancer treatment, 388
    in newborn, 191–192
    systems review, 11
Gastrointestinal infection, reduction of, in breastfeeding, 214
Gastro-oesophageal reflux, 235–237
    case history, 236b, 236f
    complications, 236b
    investigation, 236–237
    management, 237, 237b
Gastroschisis, 192
Gastrostomies, 222–223, 222f
Gaucher disease, 5, 480t
Gaussian distribution, 134
Gene therapy, 317
Genetic counselling, 134, 139–140, 140b
    couples at risk, 143
    syndrome diagnosis and, 137b, 137f

Genetic services, 138–140
Genetics/genetic disorders, 121–141
    chromosomal abnormalities, 121–122
    chromosomal disorder/syndromes, 199
    cystic fibrosis, 313
    dysmorphology, 135–136, 137b
    fragile X syndrome, 132, 133b, 133f
    gene-based therapies, 137–138
    genetic counselling, 134, 139–140, 140b, 143
    genetic services, 138–140
    heart disease and, 16
    imprinting, 133, 134b, 134f
    investigations, 138–139, 138t
    Mendelian inheritance, 127–132, 128f
    polygenic, multifactorial or complex inheritance, 134–135, 135b, 135f
    presymptomatic (predictive) testing, 140
    short stature, 199
    trinucleotide repeat expansion mutations, 132, 139
    uniparental disomy, 133, 134f
    unusual genetic mechanisms, 132–133
Genital area, examination, 18
Genital disorders, 367–374
    in girls, 374, 374b
    inguinoscrotal conditions, 367–371
Genitourinary disorders, systems review, 11
Germ cell tumours (GCTs), 387, 398
German measles, 143, 150–151, 150f, 151b, 272–273, 273b
Gestational age assessment, 555
Gestational diabetes, 148
Gingivostomatitis, 266–267, 266f
Girls
    genital disorders, 374, 374b
    puberty see Female puberty
Glandular fever (infectious mononucleosis), 269
Glasgow Coma Scale, 90, 92t
Glenn or hemi-Fontan operation, 334, 339
Global child health, 535–543
    future development, 542
    maternal health and obstetric care, 539–540, 539f, 539t
    mental health, 540
    neonatal survival, 538
    survival of children, 540
Glomerular filtration rate (GFR), 344, 344f, 345
Glucocorticoid therapy, 143, 171
Glucose-6-phosphate dehydrogenase (G6PD) deficiency, 407, 407b
Glycogen storage disorders (GSD), 463b, 476–477, 476f, 477b
Gonadoblastoma, 126
Gonococcal infection, 188
Gowers' sign, 20, 512f
Gram-negative infections, 188, 388
Granuloma annulare, 450, 451f
Graves disease, 148–149, 465, 465f
Griffiths Infant Developmental Scale, 37–38
Grommets, 57
Gross motor development, 30, 31f
Gross Motor Function Classification System, 49t
Gross Motor Function Measure (GMFM), 38
Growing pains, 486
Growth, 194–210
    abnormal
        in fetus, monitoring of, 146, 159
        of head, 204–206
        in infant, 159
        large-for-gestational-age infants, 160
        monitoring growth-restricted fetus, 159
        patterns, 158–159, 159f
    chart, 196, 545–554
    childhood phase, 194
    constitutional delay of, 199, 210b
    failure, in juvenile idiopathic arthritis (JIA), 493–495, 493f
    faltering see weight faltering
    features, 194
    fetal, 158, 194
    high nutritional demands for, 211–212
    infantile, 194
    measurements, 194–196, 195f–196f, 196b
    pubertal spurt, 194
    puberty, 196–199, 199b
        see also Short stature; Tall stature
Growth hormone deficiency, 202
Growth hormone treatment, 203, 203b, 203f
Guarding, abdominal examination, 17
Guillain-Barré syndrome, 513
Guthrie test (biochemical screening), 165, 185, 465

H

Haematological disorders, 401–423
    anaemia see Anaemia
    bleeding disorders, 413–421
    bone marrow failure syndromes, 413
    haematological values, at birth and the first few weeks of life, 402, 402f
    haemoglobin production, in fetus and newborn, 401, 401t, 402b, 402f
    thrombosis, 421–422, 422b
Haematuria, 357–359, 358b
Haemodialysis, 363
Haemoglobin (Hb), 182f, 401, 401t, 402b, 402f
Haemoglobin SC disease, 410
Haemoglobinopathies, 408, 408f, 408t
Haemolytic anaemia, 406–412, 406f
Haemolytic disease of the newborn, 413
Haemolytic disorders, 181–183, 406–412
Haemolytic uraemic syndrome (HUS), 363
Haemophilia, 416–418, 416t, 417b, 417f
Haemophilus influenzae
    cystic fibrosis, 314
    epiglottitis, acute, 298
    immunization, 282f, 283f
    in meningitis, 259, 261
    otitis media, 296–297
    pneumonia, 311
Haemophilus influenzae infection, 264
Haemopoiesis, 401
Haemorrhages
    brain, 176
    extradural, 517
    intracranial, 93t, 517–518, 518b
    intraventricular, 176–178
    subaponeurotic, 169, 170f
    subarachnoid, 518
    subconjunctival, 310
Haemorrhagic disease of the newborn, 161–165, 378, 419
Haemostasis, normal, 413–415
Hand, foot and mouth disease, 270
Hand dominance, 48
Handicap, defined, 46
Hands, X-rays, 198, 198f
Harrison's sulcus
    asthma and, 303, 303f
    examination, 14
    rickets and, 226, 227f
HbH disease, 412

Head
- abnormal growth of, 204–206, 206b–207b
- asymmetric heads, 205, 207f
- circumference, 195
- injuries to, 98–100, 99b–100b, 99f
  - case history, 100b, 100f
- lag, 19
- soft tissue sarcomas, 396
  - see also Brain; Neck

Head lice, 450f
Headache, 392f, 500–503, 502b
- in adolescent, 530–531
- classification, 501b
- management of, 503
- medication overuse, 503
- primary, 500–501
- prophylactic treatments, 503
- psychosocial support, 503
- rescue treatment, 503
- secondary, 502–503
  - see also Migraine

HEADS acronym, psychosocial history taking, 527t
Health, child, inequalities in, 7
Health promotion, 532
Health service delivery, 4
Health surveillance, 38–39, 39b
Healthy child programme, 7–8, 38, 38t
Hearing, 29, 33f, 39–42, 42b
- checklist for parents, 42b
- development, 28
- in fetus, 39
- impairment, 56–57, 58b, 122, 261
  - see also Deafness
- in newborn, 39
- normal compared to impaired, 57f
- parental concern, 42
- screening, in newborn, 165
- tests, 39–42, 40b

Hearing aids, 57
Heart failure, 322–323, 322b
- case history, 324b, 324f
- drug therapy, 328
- in infants, 16
- symptomatic, 341–342

Heart murmurs, 322
- examining, 16

Heart rate, 16, 80
Heart sounds, examining, 16, 16f
Height
- measuring, 195
- normal human growth, 194, 195f
- socioeconomic status, 212
- standard deviation, 196, 196f
- velocity charts, 195f, 199
  - see also Growth; Short stature; Tall stature

Heimlich manoeuvre, 101f
Helicobacter pylori, 243–244
Hemiplegia, 49–51
Henoch-Schönlein purpura, 358–359, 359f, 496
Hepatic dysfunction, 375f
Hepatic failure, 93t
Hepatitis, 18, 150
- autoimmune, 380
- fulminant, 380
- hepatitis A virus (HAV), 378
- hepatitis B virus (HBV), 189, 284, 378, 379b
  - chronic B, 378–379
- hepatitis C virus (HCV), 379
- hepatitis D virus (HDV), 379
- hepatitis E virus (HEV), 379–380
- neonatal syndrome, 376–378
- viral, 378–380
- worldwide prevalence, 379f
  - see also Epstein-Barr virus (EBV)

Hepatocellular carcinoma, 398
Hepatomegaly, 16
- causes of, 17f, 17t

Hereditary cerebellar ataxias, 517
Hereditary motor sensory neuropathies, 513
Hereditary spherocytosis (HS), 186, 406–407
Hernia
- diaphragmatic, 186–187, 187f
- inguinal, 180f, 367, 368f–369f

Herpangina, 270
Herpes simplex virus (HSV), 261–262, 266–267, 267b, 446
- encephalitis, 267
- in newborn, 189

Herpetic whitlows, 267
Hib, 264, 264b, 282
High throughput sequencing, 121
Hirschsprung disease, 192, 254–255, 255b, 255f
History-taking, 10–12, 26b
- case history, 12b

HIV (human immunodeficiency virus) infection, 279–281, 279f–280f, 281b
Hodgkin lymphoma, 393, 393f–394f, 394b
Homocystinuria, 474t
Homozygosity, autosomal dominant inheritance, 128
Hormonal abnormalities, 364
Horseshoe kidney, 346f, 348
Hospital care, 64
- admission rates, 65–66, 65f–66f, 66t
- child-orientated environment, 67
- children, 67–68, 68b
- discharge from, 68, 68f
- family-centred care, 67
- multidisciplinary, 67
- psychosocial support, 67
- skilled staff, 67
- tertiary, 67–68
  - see also Medications; Pain

Human genome project, 121
Human herpesvirus 6 (HHV-6) and 7, 270
Human papillomavirus (HPV) vaccine, 283
Human parvovirus B19, 270, 270b
Humerus, fracture at birth, 170
Huntington disease, 132, 140
Hyaline membrane disease *see* Respiratory distress syndrome (RDS)
Hydatid of Morgagni, 370
Hydrocele, 367–368, 368f–369f, 373b
Hydrocephalus, 145b, 151, 393, 520–521, 521b
- causes, 520b
- clinical features, 520–521, 520f–521f
- infections, 261

Hydrocortisone, 447
Hygiene hypothesis, 289, 289f
Hyperammonaemia, 476
Hyperbilirubinaemia, conjugated, 185
Hypercholesterolaemia, 356
Hyperexpanded chest, 15f
Hypergonadotropic hypogonadism, 210b
Hypermetropia, 59
Hypermobility, 486, 486f
Hypernatraemic dehydration, 215–216, 245–246
- management, 247–248

Hyperoxia (nitrogen washout) test, 329
Hyperparathyroidism, 466
Hypersensitivity, 288b
Hypertension, 93t, 214, 360, 360b, 557f
Hyperthyroidism, 23, 148–149, 465, 465b, 465f
Hypertrophic cardiomyopathy, 148

Hypocalcaemia, 159, 225–226, 466
    clinical features of, 227b
Hypoglycaemia, 93t
    in diabetes, 458–459, 464b
    in fetus, 148
    in glycogen storage disorders, 476–477
    in newborn, 159, 189
    seizures and, 189–190
Hyponatraemic dehydration, 245
Hypoparathyroidism, 466
Hypoplastic left heart syndrome, 338–339, 338f
Hypospadias, 372, 373b, 373f
Hypothermia, 158, 167–169, 174–175, 223
Hypothyroidism, 23, 122
    acquired, 465
    congenital, 185, 464–465, 464b–465b, 464f
    short stature, 202
Hypotonic ("floppy") infant, 20f, 516–517, 516b
Hypovolaemia, 356
Hypoxic-ischaemic encephalopathy (HIE), neonates, 78, 167–169, 168b–169b, 168f–169f

I

Idiopathic short stature, 202
IgA nephropathy, 359
IgE-mediated food allergy, 290–291, 291f
Ileostomy, 253
Ileum, atresia or stenosis of, 191
Illness
    in adult life, poor appetite associated with, 199–202
    chronic, present with short stature, 199–202
    effects of, and nutrition, 212
    fabricated or induced, 111
    severity, 13
Imaging
    Crohn's disease, 252
    internal injuries, 100
    kidneys and urinary tract, 345t
    principles for use, 559
    see also Ultrasound screening
Immune thrombocytopenic purpura (ITP), 118f, 419–420, 421b, 421f
Immunity, 256–286
Immunization, 281–284, 282f–283f
    against pneumonia, 311
    rationale behind, 282–284
Immunocompromised host, infection in, 267
Immunodeficiency, 284–286, 284b
    from chest infections, 317
Immunoglobulin, 214, 257f
Immunohistochemistry, 387
Immunomodulators, 446
Immunoreactive trypsinogen (IRT), 314
Immunosuppression, infection from, 388
Impairment
    hearing see Hearing, impairment
    terminology, 46
    visual see Vision, severe impairment
Impetigo, 264–265, 264f, 442
Imprinting, 133, 134b, 134f
Inborn errors of metabolism, 93t, 463b, 472–481, 473t, 480b
    examples, 472t
    frequency, 473t
    hypoglycaemia, 476–477
    lipid metabolism disorders, 479, 480f
    lysosomal storage disorders, 477
    metabolic disease, and acid-base disturbance, 475, 475t
    mitochondrial disease, 477, 478t, 479b
    newborn screening, 474, 474t, 475b
Increased work of breathing, 14
Incubators, 174–175
Inequalities, causes, 7
Infant feeding, 213–217
    breastfeeding, 213–215
    formula feeding, 215–216
    weaning, 217
Infant formula, specialized, 217
Infantile seborrhoeic dermatitis, 445, 445f
Infantile spasms (West syndrome), 508t, 509f
Infants
    colic, 238
    general appearance, 14
    growth-restricted, 159
    head injuries, 100
    heart failure, 16, 322–323, 322b
    infections see under Infections
    large-for-gestational-age, 160
    nutritional vulnerability of, 211–213, 213b
    post-resuscitation care, 158
    preterm see Preterm infants
    serum immunoglobulin (antibody) levels in, 257f
        see also Neonates; Sudden infant death syndrome (SIDS)
Infarct, intracranial, 93t
Infection meningitis, 93t
Infections, 187–189, 256–286, 257f, 536f, 541f
    bacterial, 263–265
    congenital, 150–151, 150b, 183
    early-onset, 187
    with fever see Febrile child
    focus for, 258
    gram-negative, 188, 388
    group A streptococcal, 264–265, 265b
    HIV, 279–281
    immunization, 281–284
    immunodeficiency, 284–286
    from immunosuppression, 388
    in infants/newborns, 176
    jaundice and, 183
    Kawasaki disease, 273–275, 274b–275b, 274f
    L. monocytogenes infection, 188
    late-onset, 187–188, 187b
    life-threatening, 259–263
    Listeria, 143
    Lyme disease, 281
    nephrotic syndrome, 356
    pneumococcal, 264, 264b
    pneumonia in, 311
    prolonged fever, 273–275, 273b
    respiratory see Respiratory infections
    risk factors, 258
    skin see Skin disorders
    staphylococcal, 264–265, 265b
    streptococcal see Streptococcal infections
    survival of children, 540, 541f
    tropical, 256, 277
    tuberculosis, 275–277
    umbilical, 188
    urinary tract see Urinary tract infection (UTI)
    viral, 265–273
Infectious mononucleosis (glandular fever), 269, 296
Inflammatory bowel disease, 252–253
Inflammatory myopathies, 515–516
Inguinal hernia, 180f, 367, 368f–369f, 373b
Inguinoscrotal conditions, 367–371
Inhaler, 308b
Inherited aplastic anaemia, 413
Initial interview, 71

Injuries
    at birth, 169–170, 170b
    brain, 116–118, 176–178, 176f–177f
    child abuse, 115t
    head, 98–100, 99b–100b, 99f, 202
    internal, 100
    seriously injured child, 83, 86f
    sport, 489
    unintentional *see* Accidents
Insect sting hypersensitivity, 293, 293b
Inspection
    of abdomen, 16–17
    cardiovascular system examination, 15
Insulin, 455–456, 456f
Insulin infusion pump, 458b
Insulin-like growth factor (IGF-1), 194, 202–203
Integrated Management of Childhood Illness (IMCI), 538
Intensification, in acute lymphoblastic leukaemia, 391
Intensive care unit, paediatric, neonatal intensive care, 147
Intestinal malabsorption, rickets, 226b
Intestinal obstruction, 191–192
Intimate partner violence, 111
In-toeing, 482–483, 483b
Intracranial haemorrhage, 517–518, 518b
Intracranial pressure, raised, 391–393, 392f, 502
Intracranial tumour, 93t
Intracytoplasmic sperm injection, 317
Intraosseous infusion, 85
Intrarenal reflux, 351
Intrauterine growth restriction (IUGR), 146–148, 158–159
    short stature and, 203
Intrauterine shunting, 146
Intravenous immunoglobulin (IVIG), 263
Intraventricular haemorrhage, 176–178
Intubation, 85, 156–157
Intussusception, 18, 240–241, 241b, 241f
Investigations
    developmental delay, 48t
    gastroenteritis, 246–247
    genetic, 138–139, 138t
    malnutrition, 222
    in preterm or sick infants, 172
    short stature, 202, 203t
    see also Examination
Ipratropium bromide, 304
    nebulized, 306
IQ tests, 37–38
Iron
    deficiency, 403–405
        case history, 405b
        clinical features, 404–405
        diagnosis, 405
        management, 405
        treatment of, with normal Hb, 405
    dietary sources, 405b
    requirements, during childhood, 404f
Irritable bowel syndrome, 243
Isonatraemic dehydration, 245
Isovaleric acidaemia, 474t
Itchy rashes, 446b

J

Jaundice, 181–185, 182f, 185b, 375
    within 24 hours of birth, 181–183
    age at onset, 181, 182t
    breast milk, 183
    clinical condition, 183
    clinical evaluation, 181–183
    dehydration, 183
    gestation, 183
    infection, 183
    kernicterus, 181, 183f
    management of, 183–185
    prolonged, 182–185, 376b
    physiological, 183
    rate of change, 183
    severity of, 183
    at two days to three weeks of age, 183
Jejunum, atresia or stenosis of, 191
Joint pain, nephritis, 359
Justice, 72–73
Juvenile absence epilepsy, 508t
Juvenile dermatomyositis (JDMS), 496–497
Juvenile idiopathic arthritis (JIA), 493–496, 493f
    classification, 494t
    complications, 493–495
    management, 495–496
    oligoarticular onset, 496b, 496f
    prognosis, 496
    systemic-onset, 495b, 495f
Juvenile myasthenia, 514
Juvenile myoclonic epilepsy, 508t

K

Kangaroo mother care, 540f
    case history, 540
Kaposi sarcoma, 398
Kartagener syndrome, 317
Kasai procedure, 377f
Kawasaki disease, 273–275, 274b–275b, 274f, 343, 343f
Kernicterus, 181, 183f
Ketoacidosis, 148
Ketogenic diet, 510
Kidney and urinary tract disorders, 344–366
    absence of both kidneys, 344–345
    acidosis, 364
    acute kidney injury, 361–363
    antenatal treatment, 348
    antenatal ultrasound screening, 344–348
    assessment of kidneys and urinary tract, 344
    chronic disease, 363–365, 364t, 365b
    congenital abnormalities, 344–348, 346b
    dialysis, 363–365
    duplex, 346f, 348
    enuresis, 353–355
    examining, 18
    haematuria, 357–359, 358b
    haemolytic uraemic syndrome, 363
    hypertension, 360
    normal, ultrasound, 347f
    palpable kidneys, 360b
    posterior urethral valves, 347, 348
        case history, 349b, 349f
    postnatal management, 348
    proteinuria, 355–357
    radiological investigation, 345t
    renal calculi (stones), 360–361
    renal failure *see* Renal failure
    renal masses, 360
    renal scarring, 352–353
    renal tubular disorders, 361
    salt and water balance, controlling, 364
    transplantation, 364–365, 365b, 365f
    transport defects, 362f
    urinary tract infection *see* Urinary tract infection (UTI)
    urinary tract obstruction, 347b, 348
Klebsiella, 187–188, 350–351

Klinefelter syndrome (47, XXY), 126, 126b
Knee, painful, 488–489
Knock-knees (genu valgum), 482, 483f
Knudson two-hit hypothesis, autosomal dominant inheritance, 128
Kwashiorkor, 223, 224f, 541f, 542f

L

L. monocytogenes infection, 188
La (SS-B) antigen, 149
Labial adhesions, 374
Labour
    drugs given during, affecting fetus, 150
    preterm, 147
        see also Preterm infants
Lactose intolerance, 217
Langerhans cell histiocytosis (LCH), 398
Language impairment, 425b
Laparoscopy, undescended testes, 370
Large bowel obstruction, 192
Laron syndrome, 202
Laryngotracheal infections, 298
Laryngotracheobronchitis ('croup'), 298
Laser therapy, in fetus, 146
Lead poisoning, 104
Learning difficulties
    causes, 46t
    comorbidities, 55
    concentration problems, 55
    general, 54
    management of, 55
    severe, 54
    specific, 54–56
    terminology, 46
Left-to-right shunts, 325–329, 329b
'Lemon-shaped' skull, 145, 145f
Lennox-Gastaut syndrome, 508t
Leukaemia, 385, 385f
    clinical presentation, 390
    investigations, 390
    signs and symptoms, 390f
Leukotriene receptor antagonist, 304
Levator palati, 19
Lice, 450f
Limb girdle muscular dystrophies, 515
Limb tone, 19
    in cerebral palsy, 49–51
Limbs, inspection, 19–20
Limit ages, 28–29
Limp, 489–491, 490t, 491b
Lipid storage disorders, 477–479, 480t
Listeria infection, 143
Liver
    biopsy, 376
    percussion, 18
    tenderness in, 18
Liver disorders, 375–384
    acute liver failure, 380, 380t
    cirrhosis, 382–383, 382f–383f
    fibropolycystic, 381
    hepatitis see Hepatitis
    hypertension, portal, 382–383, 382f–383f
    neonatal cholestasis, 375–378, 376b
    non-alcoholic fatty liver disease, 381
    in older children, 380–381, 380b
    tumours, 398
Liver transplantation, 384
    in cystic fibrosis, 316
Locomotor patterns, early, 29f

Lomotil, 248
Long sight, 59
Long-acting β_2-agonists (LABAs), 304
Long-term blood transfusion, complications of, in children, 412b
Looked after children, 2–3
Loperamide, 248
Lumbar puncture, 177, 260
Lund and Browder chart, 102f
Lung function tests, 24
Lyme disease, 261, 281
Lymph nodes, examining, 23
Lymphadenopathy, in rubella, 272–273
Lymphomas, 393–394
    Burkitt, 393–394, 394f
    Hodgkin, 393, 393f–394f, 394b
    non-Hodgkin, 393
Lysosomal storage disorders, 477

M

Macrocephaly, 205
Macrolide antibiotics, 310
Macrosomia, 148, 148f
MAG3 renogram, 345t
Magnetic resonance imaging (MRI), brain, 167–169, 169f
Magnetic resonance spectroscopy, 392–393
Malabsorption, 249–251
    causes, 251, 251f
    diagnosis, 249
    management, 249
        see also Coeliac disease
Malaria, 278
Male puberty, 197, 197f–198f
    precocious, 207, 209b, 209f
Males, genital examination, 18
Malformation see Congenital malformations
Malignant disease, 385–400, 385f–386f, 389b
    aetiology, 386, 386f
    bone tumours, 396–397, 487–488
    brain tumours, 385, 385f, 387, 391–393
    chemotherapy, 387, 388f
    clinical presentation, 386
    drug-specific side-effects, 388
    end-of-life care, 399
    fertility preservation, 389
    gastrointestinal damage, 388
    germ cell tumours, 387, 398
    high-dose therapy with stem cell rescue, 387
    investigations, 386–387
    Langerhans cell histiocytosis, 398
    leukaemia see Leukaemia
    liver tumours, 386, 398
    long-term survivors, 398–399, 399t
    lymphomas, 393–394
    management of, 387
    melanoma, 137–138
    musculoskeletal disorder, 487–488
    nausea and vomiting, 388
    neuroblastoma, 387, 394–395, 394b–395b, 395f
    nutritional compromise, 388
    palliative care, 399
    pathology, 387
    presentation in children, 400b
    psychosocial support, 389
    radiology, 386–387
    radiotherapy, 387–388
    rare tumours, 398
    soft tissue sarcomas, 396

staging, 387
supportive care, 388–389
surgery, 388
targeted therapies, 387
in teenagers and young adults, 387
treatment, 387–388
  side-effects, 388–389
tumour marker studies, 387
venous access, 389, 389f
Wilms' tumour, 18, 395–396, 396b, 396f
Malnutrition, 211, 221–224, 224b–225b, 540, 541f
case history, 542b, 542f
consequences, 222
Malrotation, 242, 242b, 242f
with volvulus, 191
Maple syrup urine disease (MSUD), 474t
Marasmus, 223, 224f, 541f, 542
Marble bone disease, 498
Marfan syndrome, 499
Mask ventilation, 153, 154f–157f
Masses, abnormal
examination, 18
renal, 360
MCAD (medium chain acyl-CoA dehydrogenase deficiency), 474t
Meal refusal, in preschool years, 428, 429b
Measles, 271, 271b–272b, 272f, 282–283
Measles, mumps and rubella vaccine (MMR), 282
Measurements, growth, 194–196, 195f–196f, 196b
Meckel diverticulum, 242, 242b, 242f
Meconium aspiration, 158, 186
Meconium ileus, 192
Meconium plug, 192
Media and technology, 5
Medial tibial torsion, 483, 483f
Median ages, 29
developmental milestones, 28–29, 36
gross motor development, 31f
vision and fine motor skills, 32f
Medical care, child mortality, 537, 537f
Medical history, 11
Medications
absorption, 70
accidental poisoning by, 103, 104t
antibiotics *see* Antibiotic therapy
asthma, 303, 304t
biology, 70
clearance, 70
distribution, 70–71
fetus, maternal drugs affecting, 149–150, 149t
induced illness and, 111
during labour, affecting fetus, 150
past and present, 11
prescribing for children, 70–71, 71b
see also Drug abuse
Medium chain acyl-CoA dehydrogenase deficiency (MCAD), 474t
Medulloblastoma, 391
Melanocytic naevi (moles), 442–443, 443f
Mendelian inheritance, 127–132, 128f
autosomal dominant inheritance, 128, 129b, 129f
autosomal recessive inheritance, 129–130, 130b, 130f
X-linked inheritance, 130–131
Y-linked inheritance, 132
Meningitis, 202, 259–261, 262b
assessment and investigation, 260f
bacterial, 259–261
cerebral complications, 261
enteroviruses, 270–271
group C meningococcal, 261
seizures and, 189–190
tuberculous, 259, 277
uncommon pathogens, 261
viral, 261, 272
Meningocele, 519–520, 519f
Meningococcal infection, 263–264, 264f, 282–283
Meningococcal septicaemia, 89b, 89f
case histories, 263b, 263f
Meningoencephalitis, 93t
Menstruation, 198–199
Mental health
child and adolescent, 424–441, 540
chronic illness on, effect, 425b
disorders of, diagnosable, prevalence, 424t
problems
in adolescence, 435–439
biological/developmental factors in, 425
in childhood, 425
in middle childhood, 431–435
in preschool years, 428–431
prevalence of, 424t
psychological factors in, 425–426
social factors in, 426–427
specific paediatric, 428–439
Mental health problems, adolescents, 531, 531t
Mesenteric adenitis, 240
Metabolic acidosis, 475, 476t, 559t
Metabolic myopathies, 515
Metastatic disease, 396
Metatarsus varus, 482, 483f
Methicillin-resistant *S. aureus*, 263
Methicillin-sensitive *S. aureus*, 263
Methotrexate, 496
Metronidazole, 244
Microarray techniques, 121
Microcephaly, 205, 205f–206f, 206b
Micturating cystourethrogram (MCUG), 345t, 349f, 353f
Middle childhood, problems, 431–435
antisocial behaviour, 433–434, 434b
educational underachievement, 435
faecal soiling, 432, 432b
nocturnal enuresis, 431–432, 432b
school refusal, 434, 434b
tics, 433
Midstream sample of urine, 350
Migraine, 500–501
with aura, 501
uncommon forms, 501
without aura, 500–501
Milestones, developmental, 28–38
Milia, in newborn, 162b, 162f
Milk aspiration, in newborn, 186
Millennium Development Goals (MDGs), 538, 538f, 542
Mitochondrial disease, 132–133, 477, 478t, 479b, 479f
Mitral atresia, 333–334
MMR (measles, mumps and rubella) vaccine, 282
Moles, 442–443, 443f
Molluscum contagiosum, 448, 448f
Mongolian spots, 116
in newborn, 162f
Moraxella catarrhalis, 296–297
Mortality, child, 97, 535–538
adolescent, 528–529, 528f–529f
causes, 97, 536f
global distribution, 536f
neonatal/perinatal, 142b, 537f, 538–540
poverty, 536, 537f
rates, 97, 535–536, 535t
reduction in, 5–6, 537–538, 538b
Mosaicism, Down syndrome, 124

Motor development, 29
    abnormal, 47–51, 50f
    normal see Fine motor skills, development; Gross motor development
Motor disorders, 510–511, 511t
    central, 511
    cerebral palsy see Cerebral palsy
    investigations, 512
    muscle disorders, 514–516
    neuromuscular transmission, 514
    peripheral, 511–517
Movement patterns, neurological examination, 20
Mucopolysaccharidoses (MPS), 477, 478b, 478f, 478t
Multicystic dysplastic kidney (MCDK), 345–348, 346f
Multidisciplinary child development services, 60–62, 61f
Multiple births, 147, 147b
Mumps, 272
Murmurs, heart see Heart murmurs
Muscle bulk, 19
Muscle tone, 19
Muscular dystrophies, 514–515
Musculoskeletal assessment, regional, 22f
Musculoskeletal disorders, 482–499
    abnormal posture, 484–486
    arthritis, 491–497
    diagnostic clues regarding, 497b
    genetic skeletal conditions, 497–499
    limp, 489–491, 490t, 491b
    musculoskeletal system, assessment, 21–22, 482
    painful limb, knee and back, 486–489
    systems review, 11
    variations of normal posture, 482–483, 483b–484b
Mutation analysis, 138–139
Myasthenia gravis, 514, 514f
Mycobacterium tuberculosis, 275, 311
Mycoplasma pneumoniae, 311
Myelomeningocele, 519–520, 519f
Myocardial dysfunction, 89
Myocarditis, 271, 342
Myopathy, 20
Myopia (short sight), 59
Myotonic disorders, 516

N

Napkin rash, 445b, 445f
Narcotics, maternal drug abuse with, 150
Nasogastric tube feeding, 173f
National and international environment, 5
National Institute of Clinical Excellence (NICE)
    on diabetes, 148
    on fever, 259
National Service Framework, 7
Natural disasters, 5
Nebulizer, 308b, 308f
Neck
    examining, 23
    injuries to, 98–100
    soft tissue sarcomas in, 396
    stiffness in, 259–260
    see also Head
Necrotizing enterocolitis, 176, 176b, 176f
Necrotizing fasciitis/cellulitis, 263
Neglect, 110–111, 116, 117b
Neighbourhood, 4
Neonatal cholestasis, 375–378, 376b
Neonatal hepatitis syndrome, 376–378
Neonatal metabolic liver disease, 378
Neonatal resuscitation, 153–158, 154f–157f, 157b

Neonates
    anaemia in, 412–413
    birth injuries, 169–170, 170b
    child protection, 192
    craniofacial disorders, 190–191
    features, 166, 166f
    gastrointestinal disorders, 191–192
    hearing in, 165
    heart failure, 322b
    heat loss prevention in, 175
    hypoxic-ischaemic encephalopathy, 167–169, 168b–169b
    infections see under Infections
    medicine, 166–193
    mortality, 142b, 536–540
    perinatal stroke, 190, 190f
    preterm see Preterm infants
    respiratory distress, 185–187, 186t
    routine examination, 160–165, 161b–162b, 161f, 165t
    screening, 474, 474t, 475b
    seizures, 189–190, 190b
    significant abnormalities detected, 163b
    transient tachypnoea of newborn, 185–186
    see also Infants
Nephritis
    acute, 358–359, 358b, 360b
    familial, 359
    post-streptococcal and post-infectious, 358
Nephroblastoma (Wilms' tumour), 395–396, 396b, 396f
Nephrotic syndrome, 355–357, 355f, 357b
    case history, 356b
    congenital, 357
    facial oedema, 356f
    investigations, 356b
    steroid-resistant, 357, 357t
    steroid-sensitive, 355–357, 356f, 357b
Nerve palsies, at birth, 169, 170b, 170f
Neural tube defects, 518–520, 519f, 520b
Neuroblastoma, 18, 387, 394–395
    case history, 395, 395f
    clinical features, 394
    investigations, 394–395
    management, 395
    presentation, 394b
Neurocutaneous syndromes, 521–522, 522b
Neurodegenerative disorders, 522–524, 523t
Neurodevelopmental problems see Developmental problems
Neurofibromatosis, 521, 522f
Neurological disorders, 500–524
    ataxia, 517, 517b
    cerebral palsy see Cerebral palsy
    cerebrovascular disease, 517–518
    epilepsies of childhood, 506–510, 510b
    headache see Headache; Migraine
    hydrocephalus see Hydrocephalus
    macrocephaly in, 518
    microcephaly in, 518
    motor disorders see Motor disorders
    neural tube defects, 518–521, 519f, 520b
    neurocutaneous syndromes, 521–522, 522b
    neurodegenerative disorders, 522–524, 523t
    seizures see Seizures
    systems review, 11
Neurological emergencies, 90
Neurology/neurodevelopment examination, 18–20
Neuromuscular disorders, 511–517, 512f
Newborn see Neonates
Next-generation sequencing, 139
Niemann-Pick disease type C, 480t
Niferex, 405

Night terrors, 429–430
Nightmares, 429
Nissen fundoplication, 237
Nitrogen losses, 212
Nocturnal enuresis, 431–432, 432b
　explanation, 431
Non-alcoholic fatty liver disease, 381
Non-disjunction, meiotic, (Down syndrome), 122–124, 124f
Non-Hodgkin lymphoma (NHL), 393
Non-maleficence, 72
Non-penetrance, autosomal dominant inheritance, 128, 129f
Non-specific abdominal pain, 240
Nontuberculous mycobacterial infections, 277
Noonan syndrome, 136b, 136f
Norwood procedure, 339
Nutrition, 211–233
　brain growth and development and, 212
　compromise, from cancer treatment, 388
　Crohn's disease, 252
　in cystic fibrosis, 316
　deficiency in, long-term outcome of, 212–213
　early childhood caries and, 232
　enteral, 222–223
　failure to thrive *see* Failure to thrive
　gastroenteritis, 248
　high demands, for growth, 211–212
　infantile growth, 194
　intensive support, role, 222–224
　kidney disease and, 364
　liver disease and, 382
　low stores, in infants and children, 211
　malnutrition, 211, 221–224, 224b–225b, 541f, 542
　obesity and, 202, 227–231
　parenteral, 172, 223, 223f
　during pregnancy, 142
　in preterm infants, 175–176
　short stature and, 199–202
　status of, assessment, 221–222, 222b, 222f
　survival of children, 540
　vitamin deficiency *see* Vitamin deficiency, vitamin A; Vitamin deficiency, vitamin D
　vulnerability of infants and children, 211–213, 213b
Nystagmus, 19, 58

O

Obesity, 7, 227–231, 231b
　aetiology, 213, 228–229
　complications, 228b
　definitions, 227–228
　drug treatment, 231
　endogenous causes, 231
　low birthweight and, 194
　management of, 231
　prevalence, 230f
　prevention, 229–231
　reduced, in breastfeeding, 214
　surgery, 231
Obstructive sleep apnoea, 317, 318f
Occipital plagiocephaly, 205
Occipital seizures, 506
Occlusive bandages, 447
Oesophageal atresia, 191, 191f
Oesophageal varices, 383
Oesophagitis
　acid-related, 237
　eosinophilic, 244
Omalizumab, 304

Omeprazole, 237
Omphalocele, 192
Ophthalmoscopy, 23
Opiates, maternal drug abuse with, 150
Orchidopexy, 369
Orchitis, 272
Organophosphorus pesticides, 104, 106t–107t
Orlistat, 231
Osgood-Schlatter disease, 488
Osteochondritis dissecans, 489
Osteogenesis imperfecta, 118, 128, 498, 498b, 498f
Osteoid osteoma, 487–488
Osteomalacia, 225
Osteomyelitis, 487, 487b–488b, 488f
Osteopenia of prematurity, 175–176
Osteopetrosis, 498
Osteoporosis, 495
Osteosarcoma, 396–397
Otitis media, acute, 77, 296–297, 296f, 297b
Otitis media with effusion, 296f, 297
Otoacoustic emmision hearing test, 40
Otosclerosis, 128
Outflow obstruction
　in sick infant, 337–339, 339b
　in well child, 335–337, 337b
Oxygen dissociation curve, 402f
Oxygen therapy, preterm infants, 174b
Oxytocin, 150

P

Paediatric allergy, 290b
Paediatrics, governed by age, 10b, 10f
Pain
　back, 489, 489b
　chest, 340
　children, 69–70
　　acute, 69
　　chronic, 69
　　management of, 69–70, 69b
　　postoperative, 70
　　reassessing, 70
　　recognising, 69, 69f
　　responding, 69–70
　limb, 487–488
Palliative care
　children, 66, 66f, 71
　malignant disease, 399
Palpation
　abdominal examination, 17
　cardiovascular system examination, 15
　respiratory system examination, 14
Panayiotopoulos syndrome, 508t
Pancreatic exocrine insufficiency, in cystic fibrosis, 314–315
Parainfluenza viruses, 298
Paralytic squints, 59
Paraphimosis, 372
Parasitic infestations, 449–450
Parathyroid disorders, 466
Parathyroid hormone, 225
Paravertebral tumours, 394
Parental chromosomal analysis, 124
Parental employment, 3
Parenteral nutrition, 172, 223, 223f
Parenting styles, 3
Parietal lobe seizures, 506
Paroxysmal disorders, 504–506, 505f
Parvovirus B19 infection, 270, 405
Patau syndrome (trisomy 13), 125, 125b

Patella, subluxation and dislocation of, 489
Patent ductus arteriosus, 152, 174–175, 328–329, 328b, 328f
PATHOS instrument, 438, 438b
Peak expiratory flow rate (PEFR), 303, 557f
Peak flow meter, 24f
Peak flow tests, 24
Pectus carinatum (pigeon chest), 14
Pectus excavatum (hollow chest), 14
Pedestrian road traffic accidents, 98
Pediculosis capitis, 449–450
Peer group, 4
Pelvic kidney, 346f, 348
Pelviureteric junction (PUJ) obstruction, 243, 347f
Penicillin resistance, 261
Penis
    abnormalities, 371–372
    circumcision, 372
    hypospadias, 372, 373f
    paraphimosis, 372
Peptic ulceration, 243–244
Percussion
    cardiovascular system examination, 16
    masses, abnormal, 18
    respiratory system examination, 14
Percutaneous endoscopic gastrostomy, 222f
Performance IQ (PIQ), 37–38
Periarticular oedema, 359
Pericarditis, 271
Perinatal isoimmune thrombocytopenia, 146
Perinatal medicine, 142–165
    antenatal diagnosis, 143–146, 144f–145f, 145b
    congenital infections, 150–151, 150b
    defined, 142, 142b
    features, 142
    neonatal resuscitation, 153–158, 154f–157f, 157b
    pre-pregnancy care, 142–143
    routine examination of newborn, 160–165, 161b–162b, 161f, 165t
    size at birth, 158–160, 159b
    see also Fetus
Periorbital cellulitis, 265, 265f
Peripheral intravenous line, 172
Peripheral neuropathies, 513–514
Peristalsis, gastric, 237, 238f
Peritonitis, 239
Periventricular leucomalacia (PVL), 177–178
Periventricular white matter brain injury, 177–178
Persistent ductus arteriosus (PDA), 152, 174–175, 328–329, 328b, 328f
Persistent pulmonary hypertension of newborn, 186
Perthes disease, 489–491, 491f
Pertussis, 178, 282, 283f, 310, 310b
Pes cavus, 485
PGALS (paediatric Gait, Arms, Legs, Spine) screen, 20, 21f–22f
Pharyngitis, 296
Phenylketonuria (PKU), 474t
Phimosis, 371–372, 372f
Phototherapy, jaundice, 184, 184b, 184f
Physical abuse, 110, 114b, 114f
Physiological jaundice, 183
PIC lines (peripherally inserted central line), 172
Pierre Robin sequence, 191, 191f
Pituitary disorders, 466, 466b
Pituitary-derived gonadotropins, 206
Pityriasis rosea, 450
Placental insufficiency, 146
Plantar responses, neurological examination, 20
Platelets, 413–414
Pleurodynia (Bornholm disease), 271

Pluripotent haematopoietic stem cells, 401
Pneumococcal infections, 264
Pneumococcal vaccination, 282, 283
Pneumonia, 311–312
    antibiotic for, 186
    clinical features, 311, 312f–313f
    examination, 15t
    management of, 311–312
    prognosis and follow-up for, 312
    see also Streptococcal infections
Pneumothorax
    in preterm infants, 171–174, 174f
    in term infants, 186
Point mutations, 139
Poisoning, 93t, 97f, 103–104
    accidental, 103, 108b
    case history, 108b
    chronic, 104
    drug overdose and, 107t
    lead, 104
    management of, 104, 105b, 105f
    poisons, 106t–107t
Poliovirus infection, 282–283
Polyarthritis, 492t
Polycystic kidney disease, 345, 346
Polycystic ovarian syndrome (PCOS), 208–209
Polycythaemia, 148
Polyhydramnios, 144b, 148
Polymerase chain reaction (PCR), DNA analysis, 138
Populations, linear growth, 212
Portal hypertension, 382–383, 382f–383f
Port-wine stain, 163b, 163f, 522, 522f
Positional talipes, in newborn, 162b, 162f
Positron emission tomography (PET) scanning, 393
Posseting, 234
Posterior urethral valves, 347f, 348, 349b
Postoperative pain, 70
Post-term infants, defined, 142b
Postural reflexes, 30t
Potter syndrome, 135, 345–348, 346f
Poverty, children living in, 4
Power, neurological examination, 19–20
Prader-Willi syndrome (PWS), 133, 134f, 136b, 136f, 203, 231
Precocious puberty (PP), 206–207, 208f
Prednisolone, 298, 304, 306
Pre-eclampsia, 146
Pregnancy
    antenatal diagnosis, 143–146, 144f–145f, 145b
    pre-pregnancy care, 142–143
    teenage, 532
Preimplantation genetic diagnosis (PGD), 143, 144f
Prematurity
    adjusting, 29
    anaemia of, 402, 413
    extreme, 199
    sexual development, 206–209
        see also Preterm infants; Retinopathy of prematurity
Preoperational thought, 30–36
Preschool years
    problems, 428–431
        aggressive behaviour, 431, 431f
        attention deficit hyperactivity disorder, 431
        autism spectrum disorder, 431
        defiance, 430–431
        disobedience, 430–431
        meal refusal, 428, 429b
        sleep-related, 429–430
        tantrums, 430–431, 430b, 431f
    thought, quality, 426b

Prescribing medicines, 70–71
Presenting symptoms, 10–11, 11f
Pressurized metered dose inhaler and spacer, 308b, 308f
Presymptomatic (predictive) testing, 140
Preterm birth, 540b, 540f
Preterm delivery, 146–147, 147f
Preterm infants, 171–178, 173f
    apnoea, 174
    bradycardia, 174
    brain injury, 176–178, 176f–177f
    breastfeeding, 214, 214f
    bronchopulmonary dysplasia, 178, 178f
    compared with term, 173t
    crying in, 238
    defined, 142b
    desaturation, 174
    fluid balance, 175
    infections see under Infections
    jaundice, 181–185, 182f, 185b
        see also Jaundice
    maturational changes, 173b
    medical problems, 171b
    necrotizing enterocolitis, 176, 176b, 176f
    nutritional issues, 175–176
    patent ductus arteriosus, 174–175
    pneumothorax, 171–174, 174f
    pre-eclampsia in mother and, 146
    problems following discharge, 178, 179b, 179f, 181f
    respiratory distress syndrome, 171, 174b, 174f
    resuscitation, 158
    retinopathy of prematurity, 178
    stabilizing, 171, 172b, 172f
    surfactant therapy in, 171
    temperature control, 174, 175b, 175f
    very low birthweight, 178, 180b, 180f
        see also Infants; Jaundice; Neonates
Prevenar 13, 311
Preventer therapy, 304
Primary care, 64–65, 64f
Primary immunodeficiencies, 284, 285f, 286t
Primary nocturnal enuresis, 353
Primitive reflexes, 30t, 49
Prolonged fever, 273–275, 273b
Prolonged jaundice, 182–185
Prostaglandin F2, 150
Protection, child, 7
Protein, requirements, reference values, 212t
Proteinuria, 355–357
    causes of, 355b
Proteus infection, 350–351
Proton-pump inhibitors, 237
Prune-belly syndrome, 346f
Pruritus, liver disease, 382
Pseudohypoparathyroidism, 466
Pseudomembranous croup (bacterial tracheitis), 299
Pseudomonas, 187–188
Pseudomonas aeruginosa, 314
Pseudopseudohypoparathyroidism, 466
Psoriasis, 450, 450f
Psychosis, 439
Psychosocial deprivation, short stature and, 202
Psychosocial support
    atopic eczema, 447
    hospital care, 67
    malignant disease, 389
Puberty, 196–199, 199b
    in both sexes, 198, 198f
    delayed, 209–210, 210b
        constitutional delay, 199, 210b
    diabetes management, 461–462
    in females, 196, 197f
    growth spurt, 194
    in males, 197, 197f–198f
    precocious, 206–207, 208f
    Tanner stages, 197f–198f
    timing of, 198f
        see also Adolescents
Public child health, major, initiatives, 7–8
Public health issues, 5–7
Pulmonary hypertension, 343, 343b
    in newborn, 186
Pulmonary hypoplasia, 186–187
Pulmonary interstitial emphysema (PIE), 171–174
Pulmonary stenosis, 336, 336b, 336f
Pulse oximetry, 301
Pulses
    cardiovascular system examination, 14–15
    femoral, 16, 161
    normal resting, in children, 16t
Pupillary signs, in coma, 92f
Purpura fulminans, 267
P wave, 339
Pyelonephritis, 349, 351
Pyloric stenosis, 237, 237b–238b, 238f
Pyloromyotomy, 237

Q

QRS complex, 339
Quadriplegia, 51, 51f

R

Radiological investigation
    kidney and urinary tract disorders, 345t
    malignant disease, 386–387
Radiotherapy
    brain tumours, 393
    malignant disease, 387–388
Rapid assessment of level of consciousness, 81b
Rashes, 444–447
    in febrile child, 258, 266t
    nephritis, 359
    systemic disease and, 451–452, 451b–452b, 451f–452f
    systemic Langerhans cell histiocytosis, 398, 399f
    systems review, 11
        see also Meningitis
RB gene, 386
Reactive arthritis, 491–492
Reconstituted families, 2
Rectal atresia, 192
Rectal examination, 18
Recurrent abdominal pain, 243–244
    management of, 243
Red blood cells
    abnormally shaped, 406f
    destruction of, increased, 406–412
    production of, reduced, 412
Red cell aplasia, 405–406
Reflex asystolic syncope, 506b
Reflexes
    absent, 20
    neurological examination, 20
    postural, 30t
    primitive, 30t, 49
    red, for eye abnormalities, 160, 164b
Refractive errors, 59
Refugees, 3
Regurgitation, 234

Relapse, treatment, 391
Relievers (short-acting β₂-agonists), 303
Remission induction, in acute lymphoblastic leukaemia, 390
Renal agenesis, 344–345
Renal calculi, 360–361, 360f
Renal failure, 361–363
　acute, 363t
　liver disease and, 384
　postrenal, 361–363
　prerenal, 361
　　see also Kidney and urinary tract disorders; Urinary tract infection (UTI)
Renal function, assessment in children, 345t
Renal masses, 360
Renal osteodystrophy, prevention, 364
Renal scarring, 352–353
Renal stones, 360–361, 360f
Renal transplantation, 363–365
　case history, 365
Renal tubular disorders, 361
Research in paediatrics, ethics of, 73–75
Resilience, 427
Respiratory disorders, 294–319
　asthma see Asthma
　chronic lung infection, 313
　cough, persistent or recurrent, 310–311
　cystic fibrosis see Cystic fibrosis
　sleep-disordered breathing, 317–318
　systems review, 11
　　see also Respiratory distress; Respiratory distress syndrome (RDS); Respiratory infections
Respiratory distress
　in infancy, 83b
　in term infants, 185–187, 186t
Respiratory distress syndrome (RDS), 148
　in preterm infants, 171, 174b, 174f
　very low birthweight, 178, 180b, 180f
Respiratory failure, 83–87, 93t
　assessment, 83, 83b
　invasive ventilatory support, 87, 87b
　noninvasive ventilation, 83–87
　oxygen, 83
　supportive therapy, 83
Respiratory infections
　age distribution, 294f
　bronchiolitis, 180f, 300–301
　bronchitis, 313
　pneumonia see Pneumonia
　upper respiratory tract, 295–297
　whooping cough (pertussis), 310
　　see also Specific infection
Respiratory rate, 15, 80
Respiratory syncytial virus (RSV), 178, 296
Respiratory system, examination, 14, 15b, 15t
Resuscitation
　cardiopulmonary, paediatric, 83–85
　diaphragmatic hernia, 186–187
　drowning, 101–102
　failure to respond, in neonate, 158
　fluid, 88, 88b, 88f
　neonatal, 153–158, 154f–157f, 157b
Retina, development, 42
Retinoblastoma, 397–398, 398f
Retinoids, 143
Retinopathy, toxoplasmosis and, 151
Retinopathy of prematurity, 178
Reynell language scale, 38
Rhabdomyosarcoma, 396, 397f
Rhesus haemolytic disease, 181
Rhesus isoimmunization, 146

Rheumatic fever, 340–342
　Jones criteria, 341f
Rhinoconjunctivitis, 292, 292b
Riboflavin, deficiency, 229t
Rickets, 225–227, 227b
　aetiology, 226
　causes, 226b
　clinical features, 227b
　clinical manifestations, 226
　diagnosis, 226
　management, 226–227
　nutritional, 226
　seizures and, 228b
　severe, 227f
Rifampicin, 261, 277, 299
Rights, 72, 110
Right-to-left shunts, 329–333
Ringworm, 448–449, 449f
Ro (SS-A) antigen, 149
Road traffic injuries, 97f, 97–98, 540
Robertsonian translocation, 124, 124f
Rotavirus infection, 244–245
Rotavirus vaccine, 282
Rubella, 143, 150–151, 150f, 151b, 272–273, 273b
Russell-Silver syndrome, 200f–201f

S

Safeguarding, 113–120
Salbutamol, 303
　intravenous, 306–308
Salmeterol, 304
Scabies, 449, 449b, 449f
Scalds, 102
　child abuse, 115f, 118
Schedule of Growing Skills, 37
Scheuermann disease, 489
School refusal, 434, 434b
Schools, 4
Scoliosis, 485, 486f
Screening, neonatal biochemical, 474, 474t
Secondary (onset) enuresis, 354–355, 355b
Sedatives, during labour, 150
Seizures, 503–506
　absence, 507, 509f
　acute symptomatic epileptic, 503
　causes, 504b
　convulsion, 503
　epilepsies of childhood see Epilepsies of childhood
　epileptic, 503, 507f
　febrile, 503–504, 504b
　focal, 506
　frontal, 506
　generalized, 506
　infantile spasms, 508t, 509f
　neonatal, 189–190, 190b
　occipital, 506
　parietal lobe, 506
　paroxysmal disorders, 504–506, 505f
　rickets and, 228b
　temporal lobe, 506
Self-esteem, 425–426
Self-harm, 438
Self-help groups, 432
Sensation, neurological examination, 20
Sensorineural hearing loss, 56, 58t
Sepsis, 88–89, 89b, 89f, 187
Septic arthritis, 490t, 492, 492f
Septic screen, 257b
Septicaemia, meningococcal, case histories, 263b

Sequence birth defects, 135
Seriously ill child, 80–81, 81f–82f, 83b
    with fever *see* Febrile child
    severity of, 258
    stabilizing, 171, 172b
Seriously injured child, 83, 86f
Seronegative hepatitis, 380
Serratia species, 187–188
Sex development, disorders of, 469–470, 470f
Sexual abuse, 111, 116, 118f, 349
Sexual development, premature, 206–209
Sexual exploitation, 111
Sexual health, 531–532
Sexually transmitted infections, management of, in adolescents, 531
Shigella, 245, 363
Shingles (herpes zoster), 268, 269f
Shock, 87–88, 93t, 244–248, 324b
    case history, 87b, 87f, 324b, 324f
    clinical features, 87–88, 88b, 245, 246f, 246t, 247, 247f, 248
    compensated, 87
    fluid loss, 87
    fluid resuscitation, 88, 88b, 88f
    intravenous fluid requirement, 88t
    management, 88, 245, 246f, 246t, 247, 247f, 248
    uncompensated, 88
Short-bowel syndrome, 251
Short stature, 199–203
    assessment of child with, 204b, 204f
    causes, 200f–201f
    disproportionate, 202
    endocrine factors, 202
    examination and investigation, 202, 203t
    extreme, 202
    familial, 199
    growth hormone treatment, 203
    psychosocial, 202
    in Turner syndrome, 125–126, 125f, 203b, 203f
    see also Growth; Tall stature
Short-acting β_2-agonists (relievers), 303
SHOX (short stature homeobox) gene, 202
Shunts *see* Left-to-right shunts; Right-to-left shunts
Shwachman-Diamond syndrome, 413
Siblings, 3
Sick children, care of, 64–79
    after death, 71
    care plan, 71
    caring for staff, 71
    communicating serious problems, 71, 72b
    end-of-life, 71
    ethics, 72–75, 75b
    hospital care *see* Hospital care
    medications *see* Medications
    pain *see* Pain
    palliative, 71
    place, 71
    primary, 64–65, 64f
    secondary, 65–66, 67b
Sickle cell disease, 130, 408–410
    acute crises, 410
    brain, 410f
    case history, 410b, 410f
    chronic problems, treatment, 410
    clinical manifestations, 409f
    dactylitis in, 409f
    families with, ethnic origin, 411f
    management, 408–410
    pathogenesis, 408
    prenatal diagnosis, 410
    prognosis, 410
    screening, 410
Sickle cell trait, 410–411
Side-effects, drug-specific, 388
Single-parent households, 2, 3t
Single-system birth defects, 135
Sinus arrhythmia, 14
Sinusitis, 297
Size at birth, 158–160, 159b, 194
    see also Growth; Short stature
Skin disorders, 448b
    boils, 265
    fungal infections, 448–449
    impetigo, 264–265, 264f
    in newborn, 442–444
    parasitic infestations, 449–450
    rashes *see* Rashes
    viral infections, 448
Skin lesions, primary, 443t
Skin prick test, 291
Skin-to-skin contact, 173f, 540f
Sleep terrors, 429–430
Sleep-disordered breathing, 317–318, 318b
Sleep-related problems
    preschool years, 429–430
    see also Nocturnal enuresis
Slipped capital femoral epiphysis, 491, 491f
Small bowel obstruction, 191–192, 192f
Small for gestational age or small-for-dates, 158, 159f, 199
Smegma, 371f
Smoke inhalation, 102
Smoking, 7
    affecting fetus, 142, 149–150
    asthma and, 304–305
    persistent or recurrent cough, 310
Snoring, 317–318
Social environment, immediate, 1–4
Social history, 11
Social/communication skills, abnormal *see* Autism spectrum disorders
Society, child in, 1–8
    well-being, 5
Socioeconomic status, 4, 4f, 212
Sodium valproate, 143
Soft tissue injuries, at birth, 169, 170b, 170f
Soft tissue sarcomas, 396, 397f
Somatic symptoms, 432–433, 433b, 530–531
Sore throat (pharyngitis), 296
Soya milk, 217
Space-occupying lesions, 502
Spastic cerebral palsy, 49–51, 62f
Special needs, child with, 44–63
Speech and language
    delay, 53
    development, 28
        abnormal, 53
    discrimination hearing test, 39–42
    disorders, 53
Speech therapy, 53
Spherocytosis, 183, 406–407
Sphygmomanometer, blood pressure measurement, 24
Spina bifida, 144b–145b, 145f, 165t, 519
Spina bifida occulta, 519, 519f
Spinal muscular atrophy, 512–513
Spleen, percussion, 18
Splenomegaly, 18
    causes, 17t
Sporadic hemiplegic migraine, 501
Sputum, 15b
Squint, 42, 58–59, 59b
Staghorn calculus, 360f

Standing, observing, 20
Staphylococcal infections, 264–265
    scalded skin syndrome, 265, 265f
    Staphylococcus aureus see *Staphylococcus aureus*
Staphylococcus aureus
    bacterial tracheitis, 299
    boils, 265
    cystic fibrosis, 314
    eczema, 442
    late-onset infection, 187–188
    methicillin-resistant or sensitive, 263
    necrotizing fasciitis/cellulitis, 263
    toxic shock syndrome, 262–263
Staphylococcus pneumoniae, 264, 264b
Star chart, nocturnal enuresis, 431
Status epilepticus, 510
    convulsive, 90, 91f, 93t
Stem cell transplantation, 401
Stenosis
    aortic, 335, 335b, 335f
    of duodenum, 191
    of ileum, 191
    of jejunum, 191
    pulmonary, 336, 336b, 336f
    pyloric, 237, 237b–238b, 238f
Stevens-Johnson syndrome, 451–452, 452f
Stillbirth, 142b
Strabismus (squint), 58–59, 59b
Strangulation, accidental, 101
Strawberry naevus, infant, 163b, 163f
Streptococcal infections, 264–265
    Group B, 188–189
    Streptococcus pneumoniae, 311
    Streptococcus viridans, 342
Stridor, 295, 295f, 297–300, 298b, 298f, 300b, 300f
    examination, 11
    physiology, 295, 295f
Stroke, 190, 518, 518b
Sturge-Weber syndrome, 163, 522, 522f
Subaponeurotic haemorrhage, 169
Subarachnoid haemorrhage, 518
Subchondral bone, segmental avascular necrosis of, 489
Subdural effusion, 261
Subdural haematoma, 517–518
Sudden infant death syndrome (SIDS), 75, 94–95, 96b
    age distribution, 94f
    'Back to Sleep' campaign, 94–95, 95f
    case history in, 95b
    risk factors associated with, 95f
Sudden unexpected death in infancy (SUDI), 94
Suffocation, 101
Suprapubic aspiration (SPA), 350
Supraventricular tachycardia, 339–340, 339f
Surfactant therapy, in preterm infants, 171
Surgical treatment
    cardiac, care following, 339
    circumcision, 372
    fetal, 146
    gastro-oesophageal reflux, 237
    hypospadias, 372
    inguinal hernia, 367, 368f
    malignant disease, 388
    obesity, 231
    tonsillectomy and adenoidectomy, 297
    undescended testes, 370
Sustainable development goals, 542
Symbolic Toy test, 53
Syncope, 340, 505
Syndrome, 136, 136b
    genetic counselling and, 137b, 137f

Syphilis, 150f, 151
Systemic lupus erythematosus (SLE), 149, 359, 419, 496
Systems review, 11
Sytron, 405

T

T cell, 390
Tachypnoea, 14
    transient, of newborn, 185–186
Talipes calcaneovalgus, 484f, 485
Talipes equinovarus (clubfoot), 145, 160–162, 484, 484b, 484f
Tall stature, 204, 205t
    see also Short stature
Tanner stages of puberty, 196–199, 197f, 198f
Tantrums, 430–431
    analyzing, 430b
    management strategies for, 430b
    1-2-3 principle for, 431f
Tarsal coalition, 485
Tay-Sachs disease, 130
Teething, 238
Temperature control, preterm infants, 172
Temporal lobe seizures, 506
Tenderness, abdominal, 17–18
Tension-type headache, 500
Terbutaline, 303
Testes
    detection, undescended, 160
    impalpable, 369
    normal, 368f
    palpable, 368–369
    retractile, 369
    torsion of, 370, 370f
    undescended see Undescended testes
Testicular appendage, torsion of, 370
Testicular torsion, 370, 370f
Testicular volume, assessing, 198f
Tetralogy of Fallot, 329–331, 330b, 330f
β-Thalassaemia major, clinical features and complications, 412b, 412f
β-Thalassaemia trait, 411
Thalassaemias, 130, 411–412
α-Thalassaemias, 411–412
β-Thalassaemias, 411
Thanatophoric dysplasia, 497
Thelarche (premature breast development), 208, 209b, 209f
Theophylline, slow-release oral, 304
Thiamine, deficiency, 229t
Threshold audiometry, 42
Throat, examining, 23
Thrombocytopenia, 116, 146, 149, 419–420, 420t, 421, 422b, 422f
Thrombosis, 356, 421–422, 422b
Thyroid, examining, 23
Thyroid disorders, 464–465
Tics, 433
Tinea capitis, 448–449, 449b
Tissue factor (TF), 413
Toddlers, diarrhoea in, 251
Toe walking, 483
Toes, clubbing of, 14
Tonsillectomy, 297
Tonsillitis, 296
    recurrent, 297
Torsion, testicular, 370, 370f
Torticollis, 485–486
Tosers, building, 32

Toxic shock syndrome, 262–263, 263f
Toxoplasmosis, 143, 150f, 151
Trachea, examination of child, 14
Tracheitis, bacterial, 299
Tracheostomy, 318, 318t
Transient erythroblastopenia of childhood (TEC), 406
Transient synovitis, 489, 490t
Translocation
    Down syndrome, 124, 124f
    reciprocal, 126
Transposition of the great arteries, 331–333, 332b, 332f
Trauma, 93t
    birth, 160
    internal injuries, 100
    survival of children, 540
Travel, 5
Tricuspid atresia, 334, 334f
Triglycerides, long-chain, 217
Trinucleotide repeat expansion mutations, 132, 139
Triplet repeat disorder, 132
Trisomy 13 (Patau syndrome), 125, 125b
Trisomy 18 (Edwards syndrome), 125, 125b, 125f
Trisomy 21 (Down syndrome) *see* Down syndrome (trisomy 21)
Tropical infections, 256, 277, 278b, 278f
Truncal tone, 19
Truncus arteriosus, 333–334
Truth telling, 72–73
    case history, 74b
Tuberculosis (TB), 275–277, 276f, 277b, 317
Tuberous sclerosis, 521–522, 522f
Tumour, intracranial, 93t
Tumour marker studies, 387
Turner syndrome (45, X), 125–126, 125b, 125f, 203, 203f
Twin-twin transfusion syndrome (TTTS), 146, 147
Typhoid, 278

U

Ulcerative colitis, 253
Ultrasound screening, 186–187
    antenatal diagnosis, 186–187, 344–348, 348f
    cerebral, 189–190
    cranial, in preterm infants, 177b, 177f
    Wilms' tumour, 396
Umbilical infection, 188
Umbilical venous catheter, 172
Undescended testes, 368–370, 368f, 373b
    bilateral, 369
    examination, 368
    retractile, 369
Undressing children, for examination, 13
Unexpected death, of child, 94–95
Unilateral hydronephrosis, 347f
    antenatal diagnosis, 348f
Uniparental disomy, 133, 134f
United Nations Convention on the Rights of the Child, 63, 109, 110b
Universal neonatal hearing screening, 40f
Upper respiratory tract infection (URTI), 295–297
Urease, 243–244
Urgent care, 65, 65b
Urinalysis, 24
Urinary tract infection (UTI), 349–353
    acute abdominal pain, 239
    acute scrotum, 371
    bacterial and host factors, predisposing to, 350–351
    case history, 353b
    clinical features, 349
    dipstick testing, 350, 350t
    first, 352f, 354b, 354f
    haematuria, 357
    incomplete bladder emptying, 351
    infecting organism, 350–351
    investigation, 351–352, 352f
    management of, 352
    presentation in infancy/childhood, 349b
    prevention, medical measures, 352
    recurrent, follow-up, 352–353
    sample collection, 350
    see also Kidney and urinary tract disorders
Urinary tract obstruction, 347b, 347f, 348
Urticaria, 89–90, 293, 293b, 452
    neonatal, 162b, 162f
Utility, 72

V

VACTERL association, 136, 191
Vagal nerve stimulation, for epilepsies of childhood, 510
Vaginal discharge, 374
Varicella zoster, 151
Varicocele, 368, 369f
Vasculitis, 261
    kidney disorder, 359
Venous lines, 172
Ventilation
    long-term, 318–319, 319f
    neonatal resuscitation, 153
Ventricular fibrillation, 85
Ventricular septal defect (VSD), 326–328, 327b, 327f
Ventricular tap, 177
Verbal IQ (VIQ), 37–38
Vernix caseosa, 442
Vertebral osteomyelitis, 489
Vertical talus, 484
Vesicoureteric reflux (VUR), 351, 351f
Vincristine, 388
Viral episodic wheeze, 302
Viral infections
    hepatitis, 378–380
        see also Hepatitis
    human herpes virus, 266–267
    meningitis, 261
    warts, 448
    see also Respiratory infections
Vision, 42, 42b
    abnormalities, 58–60, 60b
        causes, 60b
    development, 27
    motor skills, development, 32f
    severe impairment, 59–60
Vision testing, 42
Visual reinforcement audiometry, 39
Vital signs, 80, 80f
Vitamin D, metabolism, 225, 225f
Vitamin deficiency
    vitamin A, 229t
    vitamin B_1, 229t
    vitamin B_2, 229t
    vitamin D, 225–227, 229t
    vitamin E, 229t
    vitamin K, 161–165, 229t, 378, 419
Vitamin K therapy, 161–165
VLBW (very low birthweight infants), 178, 180b, 180f
Vomiting, 234–237, 235b
    causes, 235f
    'red flag' clinical features, 234b

von Willebrand disease (VWD), 416t, 417f, 418–419
Vulvovaginitis, 374

W

Waking, at night, 429
Walking, late, 48
War and natural disasters, 5, 542
Warfarin, 143
Warm, clean hands, examining, 13
Warts, viral, 444
Wealth, economic, 5
Weaning, 214, 217
Weight faltering, 217–221, 221b
    case history, 220b, 220f
    causes, 218, 219f
    clinical features, 218–219
    defined, 217
    identifying, 218
    investigations, 218–219, 221b
    management, 219–220
    organic, 218
    outcome, 221
Werdnig-Hoffmann disease, 513, 513f
Wheelchairs, 62, 62f
Wheeze, 300–309, 302b, 302f
    multiple trigger, 302
    physiology of, 295, 295f
    viral episodic, 302

Whooping cough (pertussis), 310, 310b
Williams syndrome, 126, 136b, 136f
Wilms' tumour, 18, 395–396, 396b, 396f
Wilson disease, 381, 381f
Wiskott-Aldrich syndrome, 285, 419
Wolff-Parkinson-White syndrome, 339
Wolman disease, 480t
World Health Organization (WHO)
    on breastfeeding, 213
        Child Growth Standards, 194–196, 544–554
Wound management, burns and scalds, 102
Wrist, expansion of, rickets, 228f
Wrist, X-rays, 198f, 228

X

X-linked dominant disorders, 131
X-linked recessive inheritance, 131b–132b, 131f

Y

Y-linked inheritance, 132

Z

Zika virus, 278
Zinc deficiency, 248